W9-DFA-279

Sonography

Principles and Instruments

Ninth Edition

Sonography

Principles and Instruments

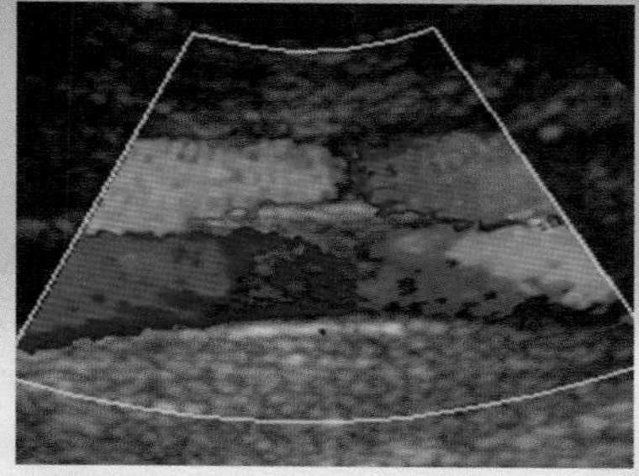

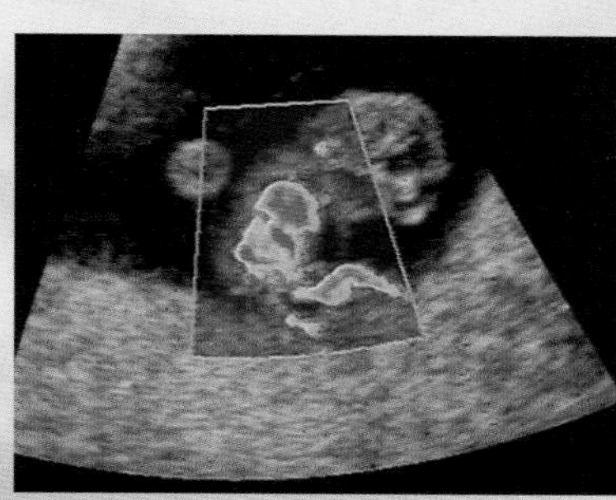

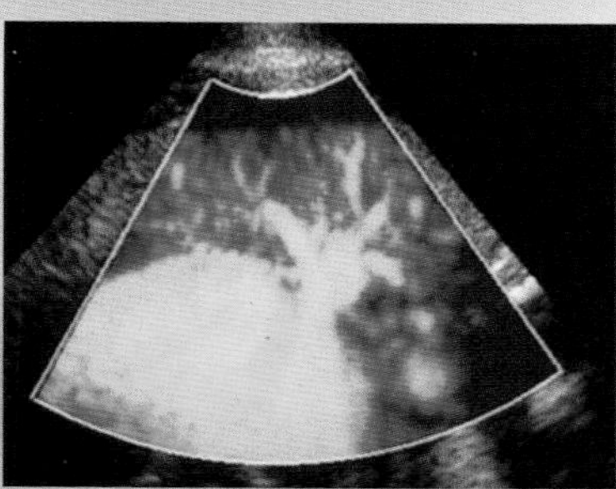

Frederick W. Kremkau, PhD
Professor of Radiologic Sciences
Director, Program for Medical Ultrasound
Center for Applied Learning
Wake Forest University School of Medicine
Winston-Salem, North Carolina

with contributions by:
Flemming Forsberg, PhD
Professor of Radiology
Jefferson Medical College
Thomas Jefferson University
Philadelphia, Pennsylvania

ELSEVIER

ELSEVIER

3251 Riverport Lane
St. Louis, Missouri 63043

SONOGRAPHY: PRINCIPLES AND INSTRUMENTS, Ninth Edition ISBN: 978-0-323-32271-3

Notices

Knowledge and best practice in this field are constantly changing. As new research and experience broaden our understanding, changes in research methods, professional practices, or medical treatment may become necessary.

Practitioners and researchers must always rely on their own experience and knowledge in evaluating and using any information, methods, compounds, or experiments described herein. In using such information or methods they should be mindful of their own safety and the safety of others, including parties for whom they have a professional responsibility.

With respect to any drug or pharmaceutical products identified, readers are advised to check the most current information provided (i) on procedures featured or (ii) by the manufacturer of each product to be administered, to verify the recommended dose or formula, the method and duration of administration, and contraindications. It is the responsibility of practitioners, relying on their own experience and knowledge of their patients, to make diagnoses, to determine dosages and the best treatment for each individual patient, and to take all appropriate safety precautions.

To the fullest extent of the law, neither the Publisher nor the authors, contributors, or editors assume any liability for any injury and/or damage to persons or property as a matter of products liability, negligence or otherwise, or from any use or operation of any methods, products, instructions, or ideas contained in the material herein.

Library of Congress Cataloging-in-Publication Data

Kremkau, Frederick W., author.
Sonography : principles and instruments / Frederick W. Kremkau ; with contributions by Flemming Forsberg. -- Ninth edition.
p. ; cm.
Includes bibliographical references and index.
ISBN 978-0-323-32271-3 (hardcover : alk. paper)
I. Forsberg, Flemming, author. II. Title.
[DNLM: 1. Ultrasonography--methods. 2. Ultrasonography--instrumentation. WN 208]
RC78.7.U4
616.07'543--dc23

2015024189

Publisher: Loren Wilson
Executive Content Strategist: Sonya Seigafuse
Content Development Manager: Billie Sharp
Associate Content Development Specialist: Sarah Vora
Publishing Services Manager: Catherine Jackson
Senior Project Manager: Clay S. Broeker
Design Direction: Julia Dummitt

Printed in China

Last digit is the print number: 9 8 7 6 5 4 3 2

To the next generation of professionals—Myra, Donna, Shelley, Cara, and Olivia.

REVIEWERS

Debra Krukowski, BS, RT(R), RDMS
Program Coordinator/Faculty
Triton College
River Grove, Illinois

Cherie Pohlmann, MS, RT(R), RDMS
Senior Instructor
Department of Radiologic Science
University of South Alabama
Mobile, Alabama

David Sloan, BA, RDMS, RVT
Program Director
Diagnostic Medical Sonography Degree Program
School of Health and Patient Simulation
Springfield Technical Community College
Springfield, Massachusetts

PREFACE

This book is intended for sonography students, allied-health personnel, and physicians who seek understanding of the principles and instrumentation of diagnostic sonography. Applying these underlying principles in practice improves the quality of medical care involving sonography. The best sonographers and image interpreters understand these principles and apply them in their practice.

The purpose of this book is to explain how contemporary diagnostic sonography works. It serves as a principles textbook in sonography educational programs and helps readers handle artifacts properly, scan safely, and prepare for registry and board examinations. The content of the book is driven by the author's assessment of contemporary technology in the field and his experience in teaching this material in the medical-school classroom and at conferences and seminars. The book does not describe how to perform diagnostic examinations or how to interpret the results. Other Elsevier books cover these topics.

Although this latest edition includes newer developments in the field, the emphasis is on the fundamentals. For the sake of beginners, the text is simplified, yet at the same time it maintains its integrity and usefulness for more experienced users. Although the book is designed for *non*-physicist and *non*-engineering readers, digestion of the material will require some effort. Admittedly, for such readers, the material can be difficult. It cannot be made easy for everyone and still maintain the necessary level for appropriate application in practice. However, 40 years of lecturing and publication experience have convinced the author that the material *can* be understood with reasonable preparation and effort on the part of the student. It is assumed that the student has completed courses in basic physics (including mechanics, waves, and electricity) and mathematics (including algebra, trigonometry, and statistics), which are normal prerequisites in sonography programs. The following topics are *not* covered in this textbook: the history of the development of sonography, therapy applications, and investigational techniques. They are covered in other books and journal articles.

DIFFERENCES WITH EARLIER EDITIONS AND NATIONAL EXAMINATIONS

There are several differences between each new edition compared with earlier editions and compared with the content of registry and specialty-board examinations. This is because this text is up to date with current technology, whereas examinations change more slowly because of the necessarily thorough and time-consuming process, which requires practice surveys; committee decisions; and item generation, review, and approval. Outmoded descriptions of technology and instrument features that are no longer largely present in the field are eliminated with each new edition. Thus the book tends to change more rapidly than the examinations. The philosophy of the book is to be, with each new edition, as consistent as possible with contemporary sonographic technology and usage.

FEATURES

- Comprehensive coverage of the principles of sonography
- Preparation for the ARDMS SPI examination
- Latest developments in commercially available sonographic technology
- Hundreds of color illustrations and images
- Hundreds of exercises with answers
- Comprehensive multiple-choice examination with annotated answers
- Consistent pedagogy, including learning objectives, chapter outlines, and key terms
- Key points set off by icons
- Descriptive subheadings
- Boxes and tables
- Math review
- Glossary

NEW TO THIS EDITION

- New illustrations and images demonstrating the latest and best images from the newest equipment
- Expanded content on volume imaging, shear-wave and acoustic-radiation-force elastography, and sophisticated echo acquisition techniques, keeping students up to date on the latest technology
- The latest instrument output data and official safety statements
- Alignment with the ARDMS examination specifications, making this a useful text for preparing for the SPI examination

FOR THE STUDENT

This book should be read in sequential chapter order, as each chapter builds on material previously presented. Key terms are listed at the beginning of each chapter, are highlighted in blue in the chapter, and are defined in the Glossary at the back of the book.

After studying this text, the student should be able to:

- Describe what ultrasound is
- Explain how ultrasound is sent into the body
- Explain how ultrasound detects and locates anatomic structures
- Discuss how echoes are received from the body and processed in the instrument
- Describe how anatomic information is presented on the display

- Explain how ultrasound detects and measures tissue motion and blood flow
- List the ways motion and flow information are presented
- Explain how flow detection is localized to a specific site in tissue
- List the common artifacts that can occur in diagnostic sonography
- Discuss how performance of sonographic instruments is tested
- Describe the risk and safety issues associated with diagnostic sonography

FOR THE INSTRUCTOR

The material in Chapter 4 has been rearranged to enable treatment of more fundamental aspects first, followed by more advanced features.

The following resources are available at *http://evolve.elsevier.com/Kremkau/ultrasound.*

- *Instructor's Electronic Resource* containing an instructor's manual, PowerPoint slides, a test bank, and an image collection
  - The instructor's manual includes outlines and summaries of textbook chapters, visual learning exercises, lab and learning assignments, and review questions.
  - The PowerPoint presentation includes notes for instructors.
  - The test bank, available in Examview or Word, includes over 400 questions.
  - The image collection can be downloaded in PowerPoint or as jpeg files.
- Real-time videos of the following:
  - Use of a sonographic phantom as a patient surrogate
  - Effect of frequency on attenuation and penetration
  - Image formats of various transducer types
  - Impact of output and gain controls on the image
  - Color-Doppler displays and control effects
  - Spectral-Doppler displays and control effects
  - Aliasing artifact and ways to correct it

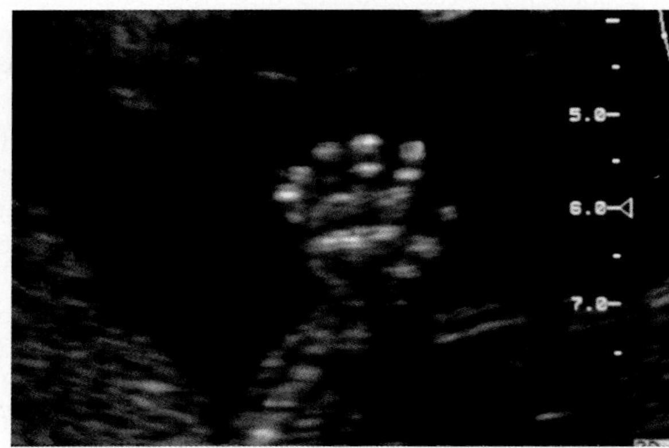

Any questions?

ACKNOWLEDGMENTS

For assistance with illustrations, the author thanks:

Amy Lex
Heather Mareth and Neeta Mhatra
Sherri Pyron
Jake Zeimantz
Philips Healthcare
Siemens Healthcare
GE Healthcare
Spencer Technologies

For their cooperation and assistance, he thanks:

The American Institute of Ultrasound in Medicine (AIUM)
The American Registry for Diagnostic Medical Sonography (ARDMS)
Sonya Seigafuse, Sarah Vora, and Billie Sharp at Elsevier Inc.

CONTENTS

1

Introduction

LEARNING OBJECTIVES

After reading this chapter, the student should be able to do the following:

- Explain the pulse-echo principle used in sonographic imaging.
- Describe the image formats used in sonography.
- Explain how the Doppler effect is applied in sonography.
- List the ways in which Doppler information is presented.

OUTLINE

KEY TERMS

Color-Doppler display
Doppler effect
Gray-scale image
Image
Linear image
Pulse-echo technique
Scan line
Sector image
Sonography
Spectral-Doppler display
Transducer
Ultrasound
Volume imaging

Bats, dolphins, and other animals used **ultrasound** long before humans adopted it for their needs. These animals use ultrasound to detect, locate, determine the motion of, and capture prey; to avoid obstacles; to detect and avoid predators; and to court their mates. One way humans have applied ultrasound techniques is by using **sonography** in diagnostic medicine. Sonography is the use of ultrasound in medical anatomic and flow imaging. Diagnostic ultrasound encompasses sonography and Doppler ultrasound. Doppler ultrasound includes the detection, quantization, and evaluation of tissue motion and blood flow by using the **Doppler effect** with ultrasound. This chapter presents an overview of the principles of sonography and Doppler ultrasound. Here, we are water skiing over the principles. In subsequent chapters we will scuba dive into the details.

SONOGRAPHY

The word *sonography* comes from the Latin *sonus* (sound) and the Greek *graphein* (to write). Diagnostic sonography is medical two-dimensional (2D) and three-dimensional (3D) anatomic and flow imaging with the use of ultrasound. Ultrasound is sound that is higher in pitch than the range of human hearing. Ultrasound imaging is not a passive push-button activity; rather, it is an interactive process that involves a sonographer (an allied health professional who acquires the images), a patient, an ultrasound **transducer**, an instrument, and a sonologist (a physician who interprets the images). Understanding and application of the underlying physical and electronic principles presented in this book will strengthen the expertise of the sonographer and the sonologist, and thus improve the quality of medical care that involves diagnostic sonography.

Medical imaging with ultrasound is called *sonography.*

An **image** (from the Latin term for *imitate*) is a reproduction, representation, or imitation of the physical form of a person or object. An ultrasound image is the visible counterpart of an invisible object, produced in an electronic instrument by the interaction of ultrasound with the object. Ultrasound provides a noninvasive way of looking inside the human body (Figure 1-1) to image otherwise hidden anatomy. Anatomic imaging with ultrasound is accomplished with a **pulse-echo technique**. Pulses of ultrasound generated by a transducer are sent into the patient (Figure 1-2), where they produce echoes at organ boundaries and within tissues. These echoes return to the transducer, where they are detected and presented on the display of a sonographic instrument. The transducer (Figure 1-3) generates the ultrasound pulses and receives the returning echoes. Sonography requires knowledge of the location of origin of each echo and its strength as it returns from the patient. The ultrasound instrument (Figure 1-4) processes the echoes and presents them as visible dots, which form the anatomic image on the display. The brightness

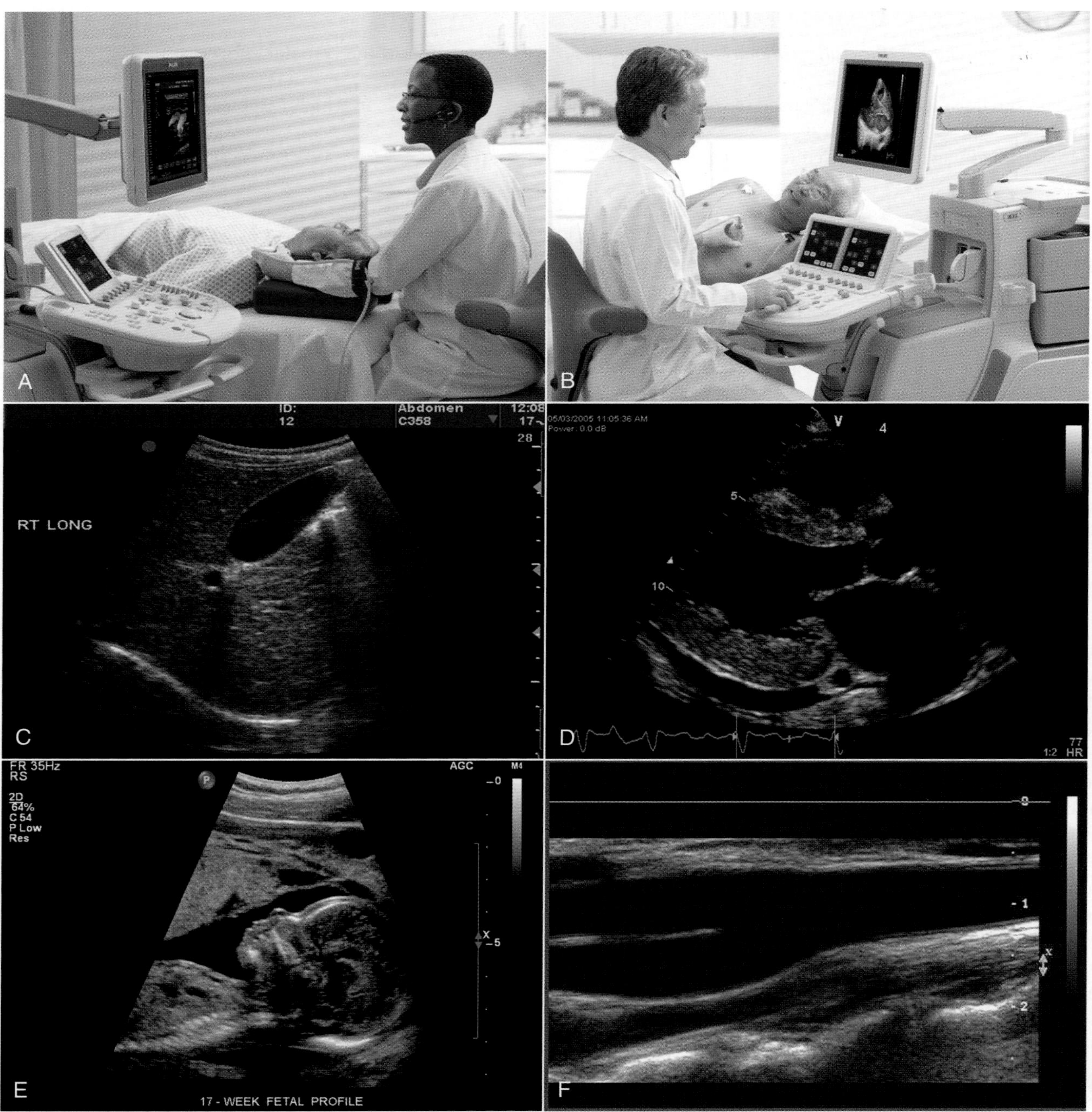

FIGURE 1-1 Ultrasound provides a window into the human body, allowing us to see what would otherwise be hidden from view (**A-B**). Images shown are as follows: **C**, abdominal; **D**, cardiac; **E**, obstetric, and **F**, vascular.

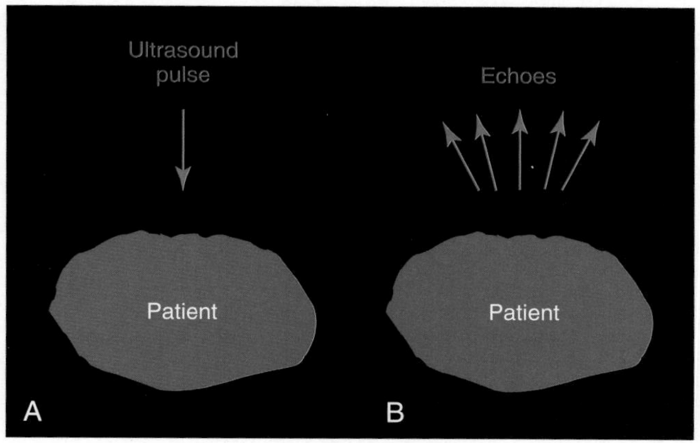

FIGURE 1-2 **Pulse-echo technique.** **A**, In diagnostic ultrasound, ultrasound pulses are sent into the tissues to interact with them and to obtain information about them. **B**, Echoes return from the tissues, providing information that enables anatomic imaging and observation of motion and flow, thus contributing to diagnosis.

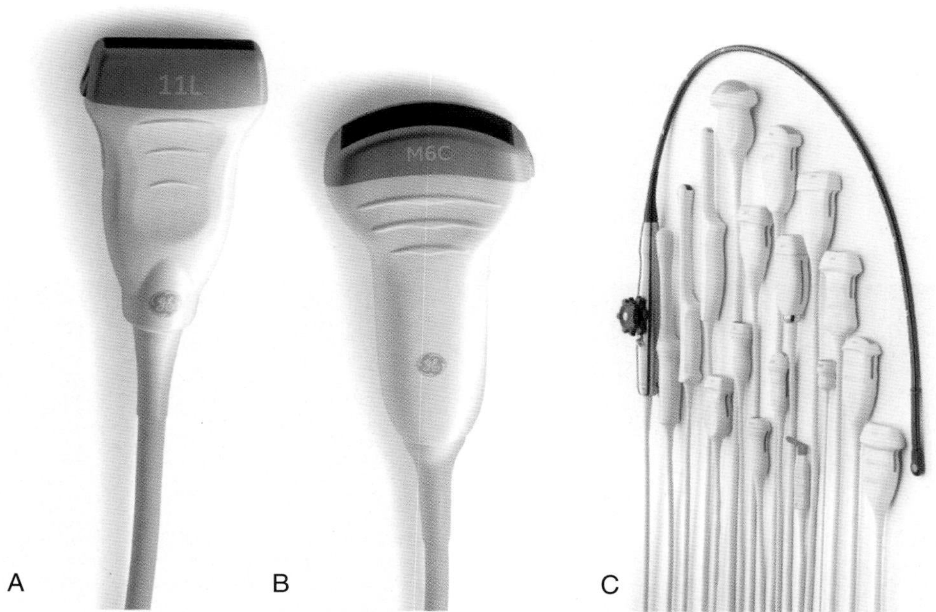

FIGURE 1-3 **A-C**, Transducers.

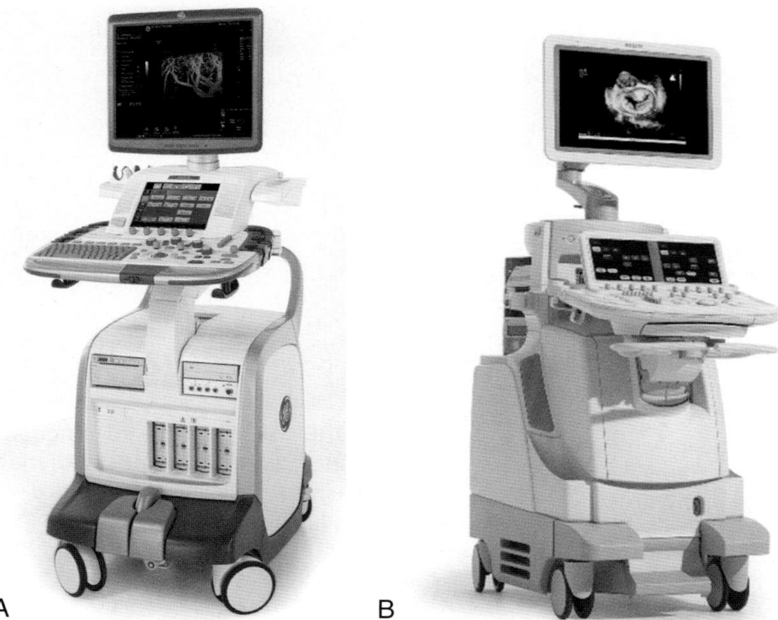

FIGURE 1-4 Sonographic instruments by: **A** and **D**, GE Healthcare, **B**, Philips Healthcare, and **C**, Sonosite, Inc.

Continued

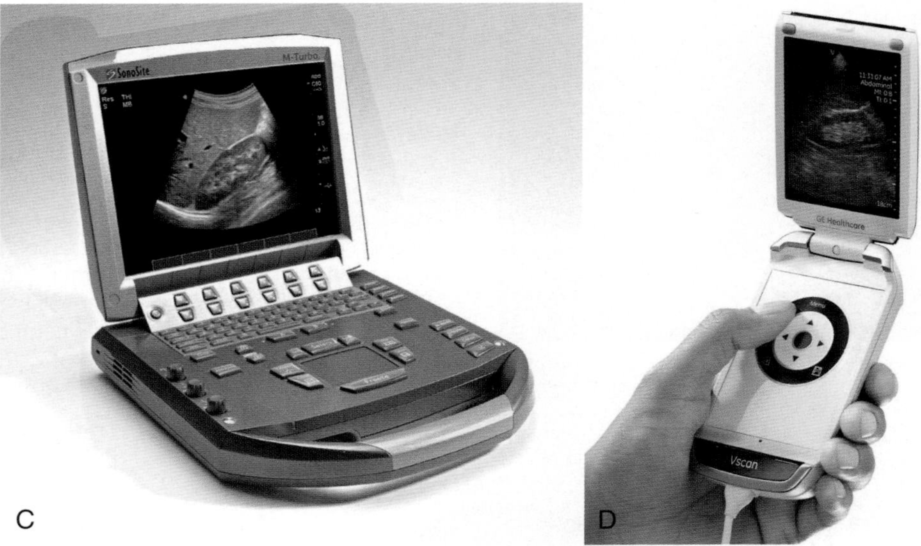

FIGURE 1-4, cont'd

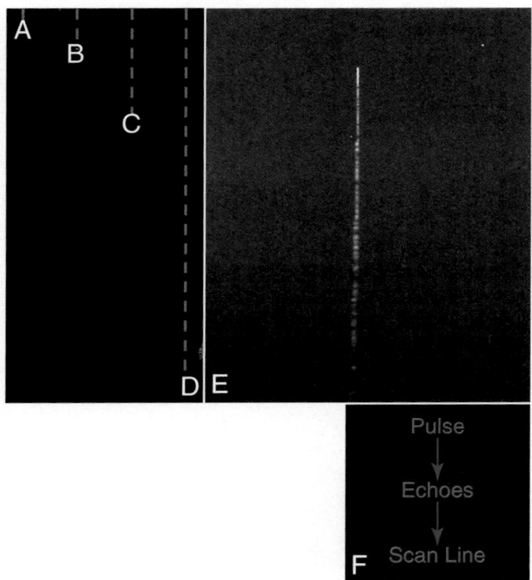

FIGURE 1-5 One pulse of ultrasound generates a single scan line (series of echoes) as it travels through tissue. Echoes are presented in sequence on a scan line while they return from tissue during pulse travel. **A**, The first echo is displayed.**B**, The second echo is added. **C**, Three more echoes are added. **D**, All the echoes from a single pulse have been received and displayed as a completed scan line. **E**, A complete scan line results from one emitted pulse. In practice, this is accomplished in less than one-thousandth of a second. **F**, According to the pulse-echo imaging principle, one pulse traveling through tissues produces a stream of echoes that become one scan line on the display.

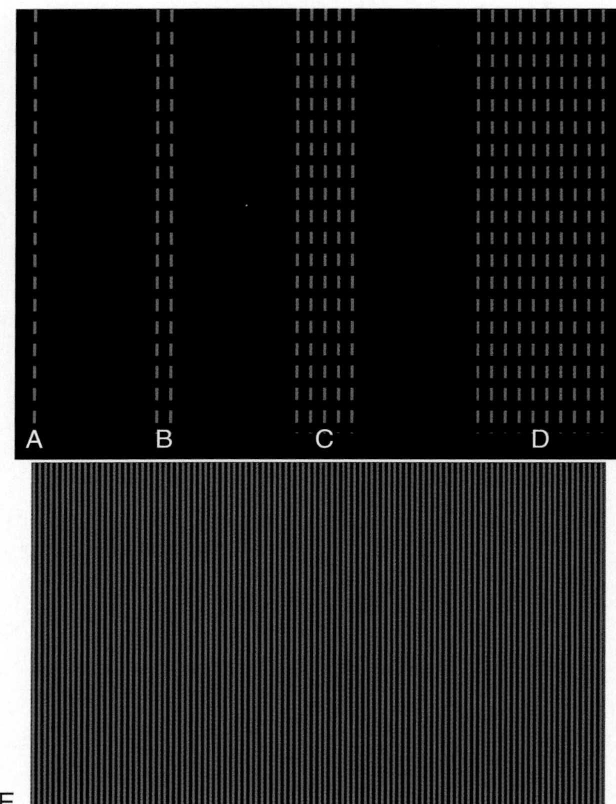

FIGURE 1-6 A single rectangular image or scan (also called a *frame*) is composed of many vertical parallel scan lines. Each scan line represents a series of echoes returning from a pulse traveling through the tissues. **A**, One scan line from one pulse, as generated in Figure 1-5. **B**, A second scan line is added. **C-D**, Five and ten scan lines, respectively. **E**, A complete frame consisting of (in this example) 100 scan lines.

of each dot corresponds to the echo strength, producing what is known as a **gray-scale image**. The location of each dot corresponds to the anatomic location of the echo-generating structure. Positional information is determined by knowledge of the direction of the pulse when it enters the patient and by measurement of the time it takes for each echo to return to the transducer. The proper location to present the echo can then be determined from a starting point on the display (usually at the top). With knowledge of the sound speed, the instrument uses the echo arrival time to determine the depth of the structure that produced the echo.

> Sonography is accomplished with a pulse-echo technique.

> Echoes from anatomic structures represent these structures in a sonographic image.

If one pulse of ultrasound is sent into tissue, a series of dots (one line of echo information, specifically, an echo line, data line, or **scan line**) is displayed (Figure 1-5). Not all of the ultrasound pulse is reflected back from any structure. Rather, most of the original pulse continues on to be reflected back from deeper structures. The echoes from one pulse appear as one scan line (see Figure 1-5, *E-F*). If the process is repeated, but with different starting points for each subsequent pulse, a cross-sectional image of the anatomy is constructed (Figure 1-6). Pulses travel in the same direction from different points and yield vertical parallel scan lines and a rectangular image, as shown in Figure 1-7. These cross-sectional images are produced with vertical parallel scan lines that are so close together they cannot be identified individually. The rectangular display resulting from this procedure often is called *a linear scan,* or **linear image**, referring to the linear-array transducer that is used to produce it. A second approach to sending ultrasound pulses through the anatomy to be imaged is shown in Figure 1-8. With this method, each pulse originates from the same starting point, but subsequent pulses go out in slightly different directions. This approach results in a sector scan, or **sector image**, which has a shape similar to a slice of pie (Figure 1-9). Figure 1-10 shows a format that is a combination of the two just described; that is, pulses (and scan lines) originate from

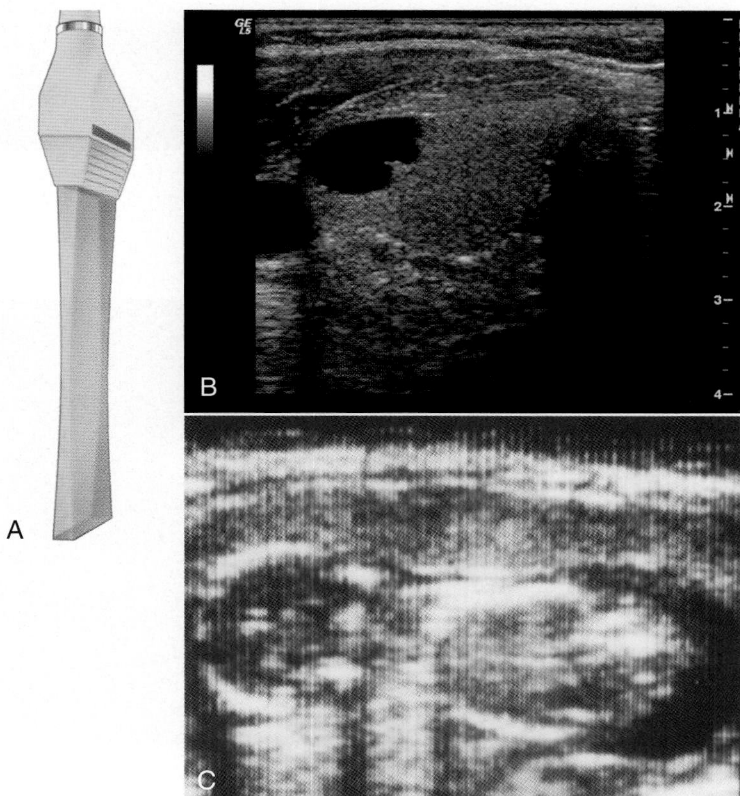

FIGURE 1-7 A, Ultrasound sent through a thin rectangular volume of tissue produces a rectangular image, commonly called a *linear image* or *linear scan.* B, Clinical linear (rectangular) scan. C, Poor-quality (by current standards) fetal image from the late 1970s, revealing the 120 vertical parallel scan lines of which it is composed.

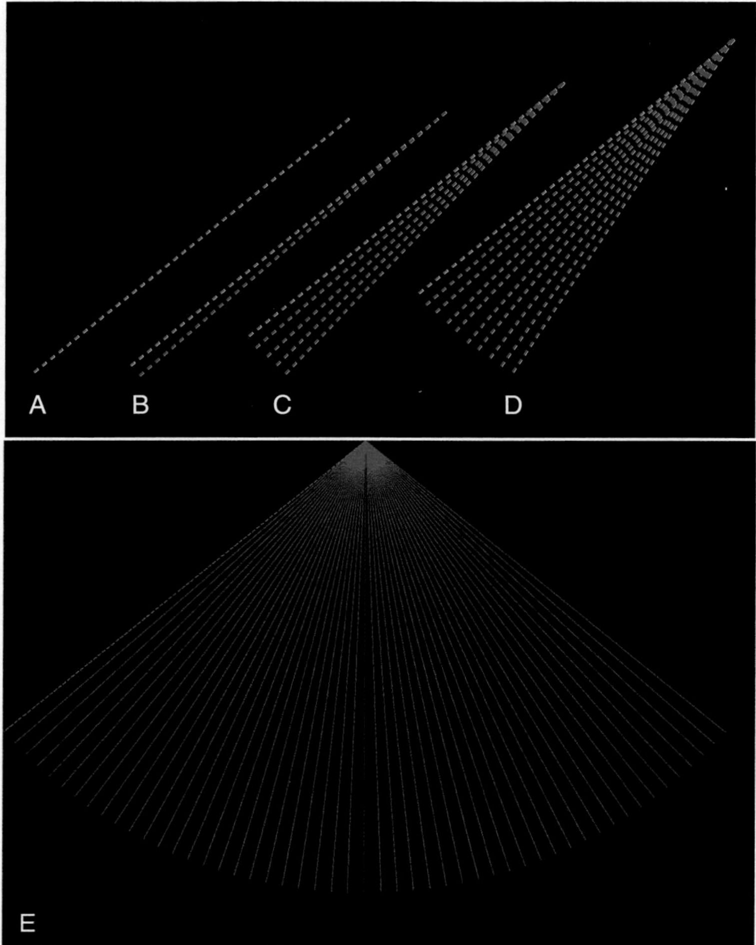

FIGURE 1-8 A single sector frame is progressively built up with 1 (A), 2 (B), 5 (C), 10 (D), and 100 (E) scan lines in sequence. All originate from a common origin and travel out in different directions.

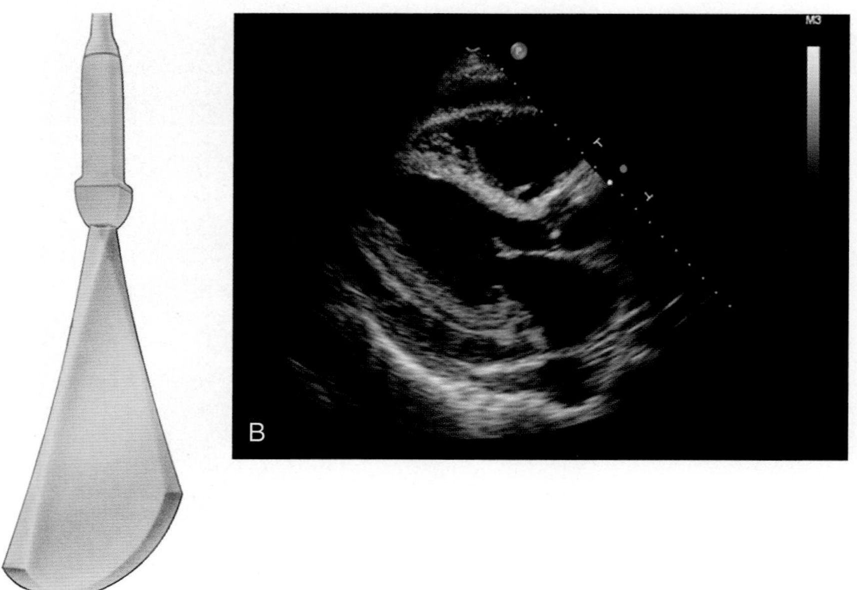

FIGURE 1-9 A, Ultrasound sent through a thin pie-slice–shaped volume of tissue produces an image commonly called a *sector image* or *sector scan.* B, Sector scan of adult heart.

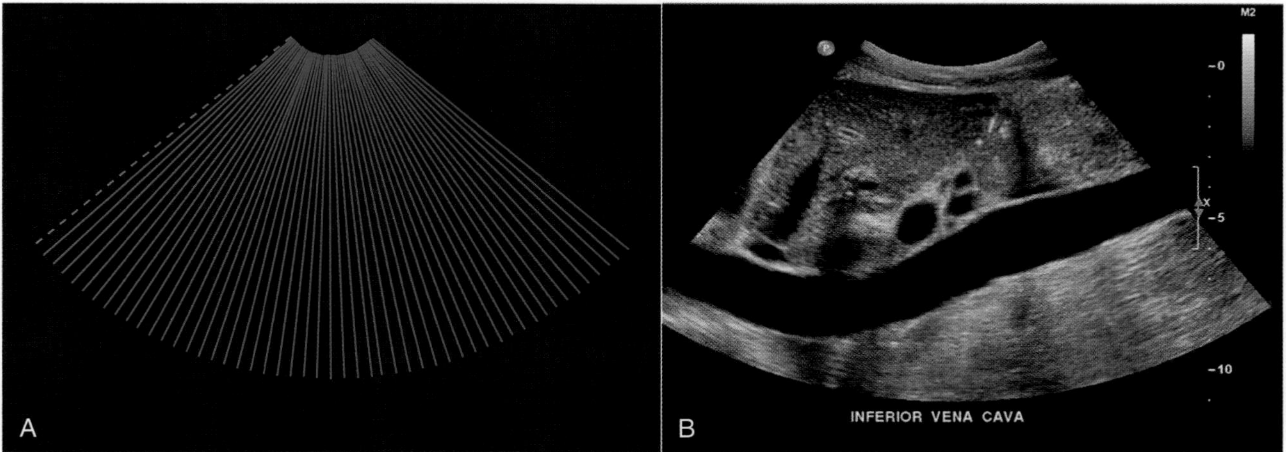

FIGURE 1-10 **A**, A modified form of a sector scan is produced when pulses and scan lines originate from different points across the curved top of a sector display. **B**, Abdominal scan with use of the scan format shown in **A**.

different starting points (as in a linear image), but each pulse (and scan line) travels in a slightly different direction from that of the previous one (as in a sector image). In this example, the starting points form a curved line across the top of the scan, rather than a straight line, as in the linear scans shown in Figure 1-7.

 Sonographic images are composed of many scan lines.

Sonographic scan formats commonly are limited to three types: (1) linear, (2) sector, and (3) a combination of the two. Other formats may be used occasionally, but in any case, what is required is that ultrasound pulses be sent through all portions of the anatomy that are to be imaged. Each pulse generates a series of echoes, resulting in a series of dots (a scan line) on the display. The resulting cross-sectional image is composed of many (typically 96 to 256) of these scan lines. The scan format determines the starting points and paths for individual scan lines, according to the starting point and path for each pulse used to generate each scan line. The clinical cross-sectional gray-scale sonographic images produced are sometimes called *B scans.* This term implies that the images are produced by scanning the ultrasound through the imaged cross-section (i.e., sending pulses through all regions of the cross-section) and converting the echo strength into the brightness of each represented echo on the display (hence, *B* [brightness] scan). The terms *B scan* and *gray-scale scan* have the same meaning.

2D images are presented in linear (rectangular) and sector forms.

For decades, sonography was limited to 2D cross-sectional scans (or "slices") through the anatomy. Today, 2D imaging, while still being used extensively, has been extended to 3D scanning and imaging, also called **volume imaging**. This method requires scanning the ultrasound through many adjacent 2D tissue cross-sections to compose a 3D volume of echo information similar to a loaf of sliced bread (Figure 1-11). This 3D volume of echoes can then be processed and accessed to present 2D or 3D images of the anatomy.

 Sonographic images are of 2D and 3D types.

DOPPLER ULTRASOUND

Echoes produced by moving objects have frequencies that are different from the pulses sent into the body. This phenomenon is called the Doppler effect, which is put to use in detecting and measuring tissue motion and blood flow. The Doppler effect is named after Christian Andreas Doppler, the Austrian physicist who conducted an extensive investigation into its nature.

The use of Doppler radar in weather forecasting, aviation safety, and vehicle speed detection (police radar) has made *the Doppler effect* a household term. In addition to its observation in everyday life (as demonstrated by the changing pitch of a siren or horn heard as the vehicle passes by), the Doppler effect has been applied to automatic door openers in public buildings (Figure 1-12) and to other motion-detecting devices.

The Doppler effect is a change in frequency caused by moving objects.

Doppler ultrasound has been used in diagnostic medicine for decades. Long-standing applications include monitoring the fetal heart rate during labor and delivery and evaluating blood flow in the heart and in the arteries and veins of circulation. Rapid scanning and processing of Doppler data

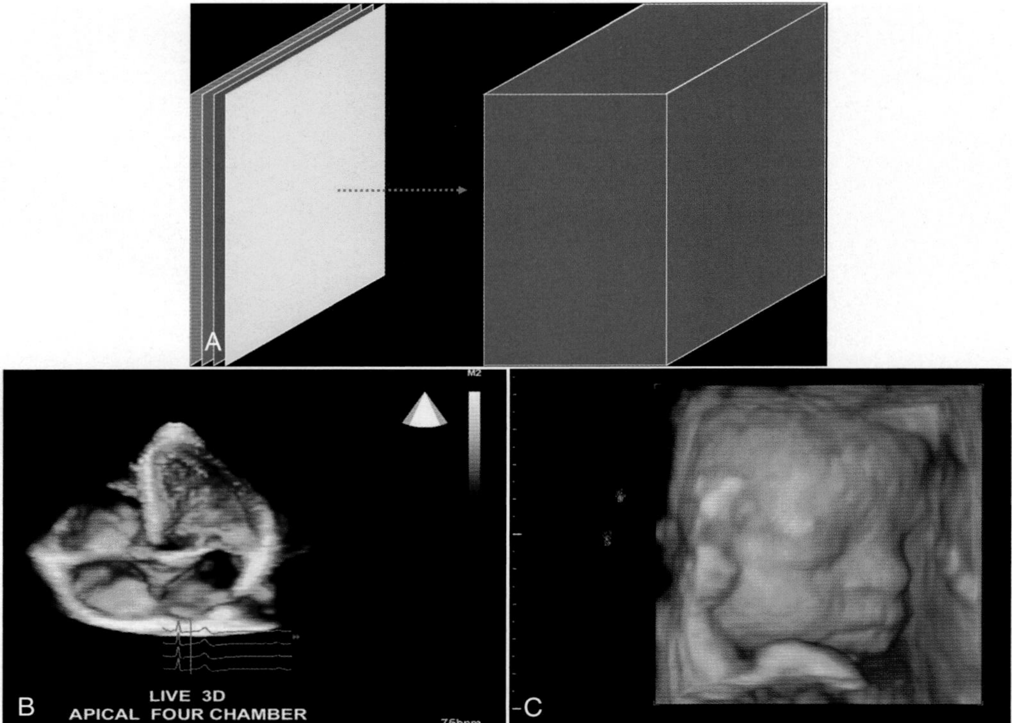

FIGURE 1-11 Three-dimensional (volume) sonographic images. **A**, Three-dimensional echo data acquired by obtaining many two-dimensional sections of echo information *(colored slices)* from the imaged anatomy, forms a three-dimensional volume of stored echo information *(blue box)*. **B**, Cardiac four-chamber view. **C**, Fetal head.

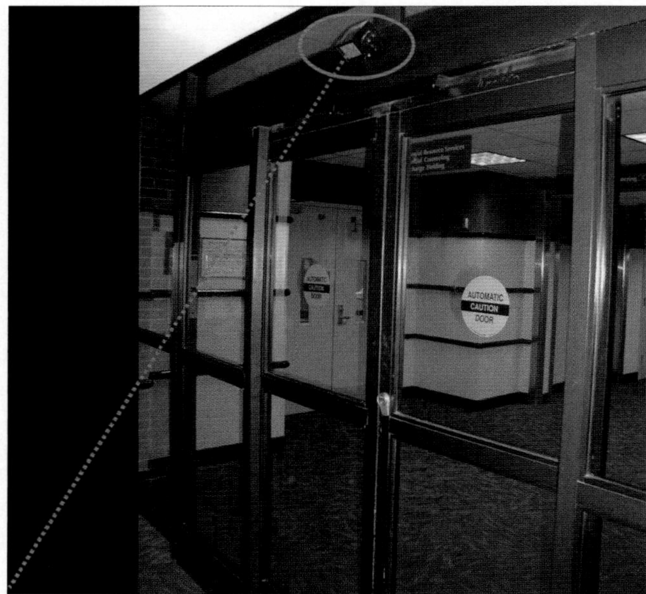

FIGURE 1-12 An ultrasonic automatic door opener *(circle)*.

enable color-coded 2D and 3D presentations of Doppler information (**color-Doppler displays**) to be superimposed on gray-scale anatomic images (Figure 1-13). Doppler information is applied to loudspeakers for audible evaluation and to **spectral-Doppler displays** for quantitative analysis (Figure 1-14). The spectral-Doppler operation includes anatomic imaging to determine the location(s) from which the spectral information is acquired (Figure 1-15).

> Doppler information is presented in audible, color-Doppler, and spectral-Doppler forms.

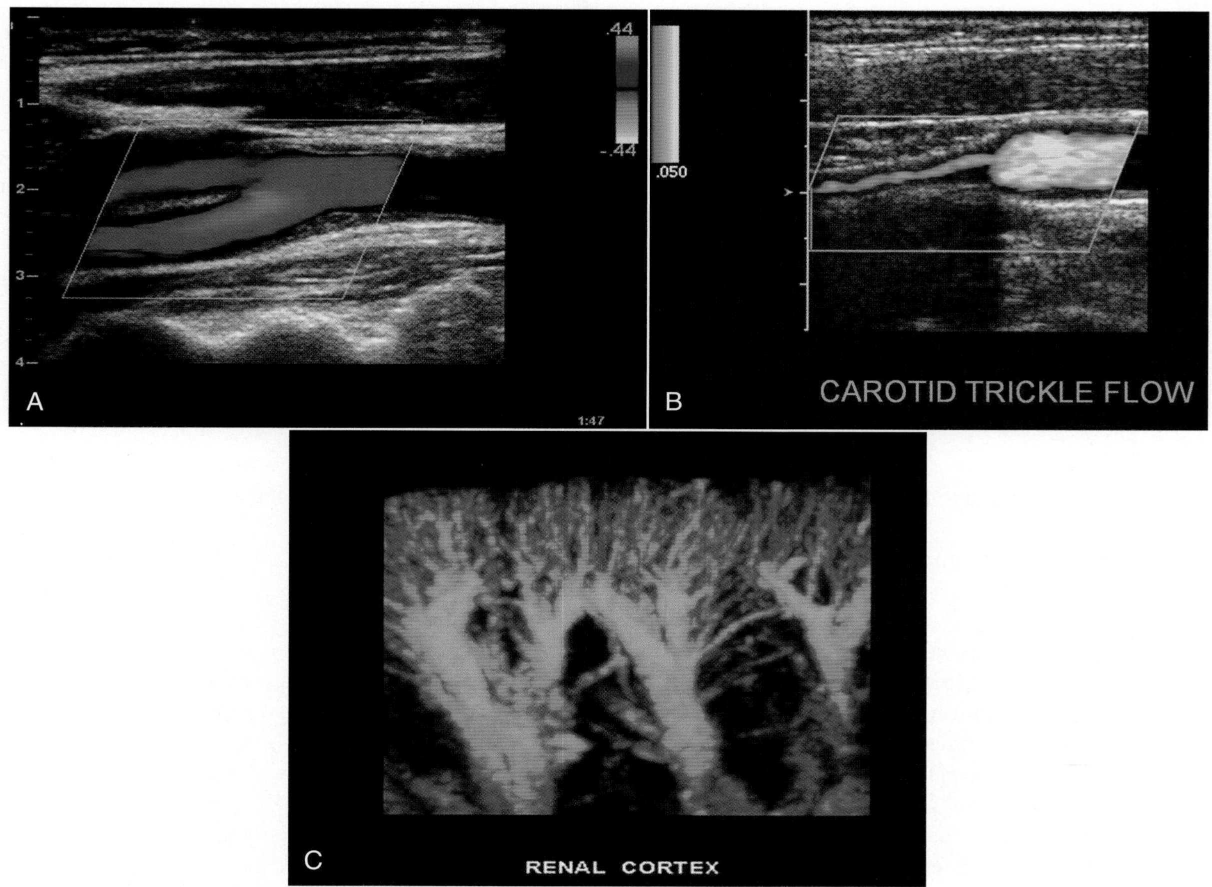

FIGURE 1-13 Color-Doppler displays of blood flow. Presented in forms called **(A)** color-Doppler shift, **(B)** color-Doppler power, and **(C)** three-dimensional color-Doppler power displays.

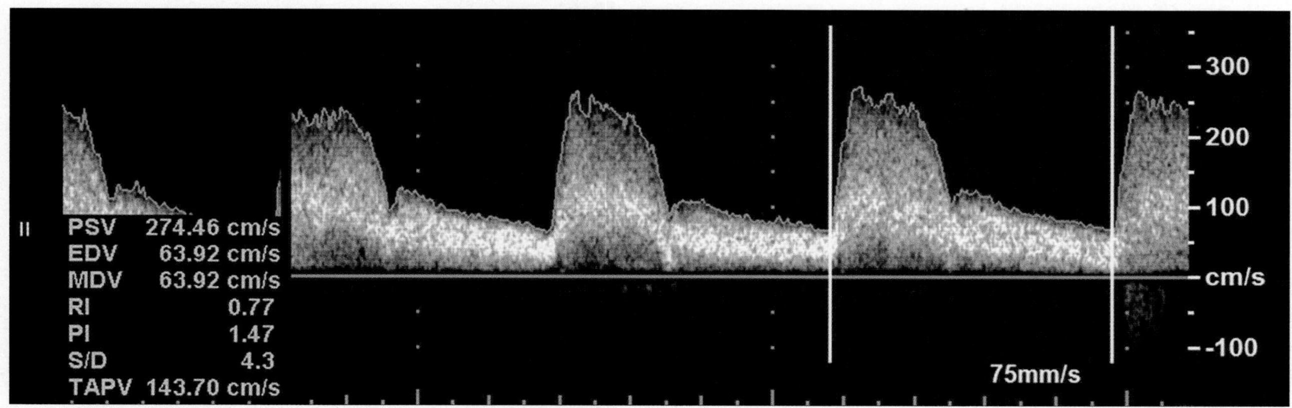

FIGURE 1-14 Spectral-Doppler display of arterial blood flow with presentation of calculated flow velocity data.

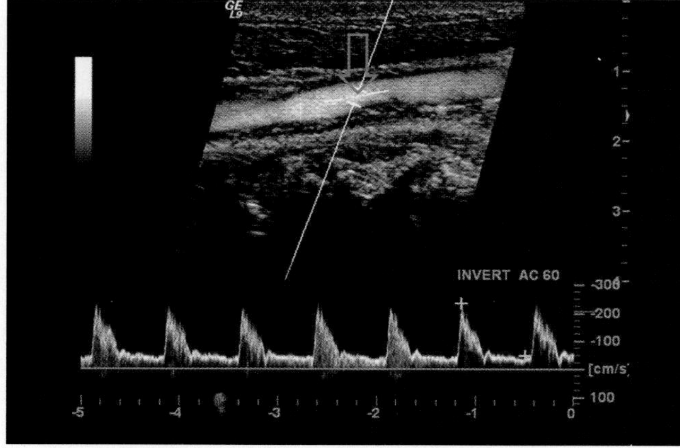

FIGURE 1-15 Spectral-Doppler display of blood flow in the carotid artery. The anatomic image shows the location (*arrow*) from which the spectral-Doppler information was acquired.

REVIEW

The following key points are presented in this chapter:

- Medical imaging with ultrasound is called *sonography.*
- Sonography is accomplished with a pulse-echo technique.
- Echoes from anatomic structures represent these structures in a sonographic image.
- Sonographic images are composed of many scan lines.
- 2D images are presented in linear (rectangular) and sector forms.
- Sonographic images are of 2D and 3D types.
- The Doppler effect is a change in frequency caused by moving objects.
- Doppler information is presented in audible, color-Doppler, and spectral-Doppler forms.

EXERCISES

Answers appear in the Answers to Exercises section at the back of the book.

1. The diagnostic ultrasound imaging (sonography) method has two parts:
Sending ____________ of ____________ into the body and (2) using ____________ received from the anatomy to produce a(n) ____________ of that anatomy.
   a. packs, sound, information, listing
   b. pulses, frequencies, echoes, description
   c. ultrasound, scans, power, image
   d. pulses, ultrasound, echoes, image

2. Ultrasound gray-scale scans are ____________-____________ images of tissue cross-sections and volumes.
   a. pulse-echo
   b. virtual-anatomic
   c. pseudo-gray
   d. artificially presented

3. The brightness of an echo, as presented on the display, represents the ____________ of the echo.
   a. strength
   b. location
   c. origin
   d. frequency

4. A linear scan is composed of many ____________, ____________ scan lines.
   a. horizontal, parallel
   b. horizontal, curved
   c. vertical, parallel
   d. vertical, curved

5. A sector scan is composed of many scan lines with a common ____________.
   a. length
   b. brightness
   c. origin
   d. direction

6. A linear scan has a ____________ shape.
   a. linear
   b. round
   c. square
   d. rectangular

7. The shape of a sector scan is similar to a ____________ of ____________.
   a. slice, pie
   b. slice, bread
   c. scoop, pudding
   d. loaf, bread

8. A sector scan can have a(n) ____________ or a ____________ top.
   a. angled, straight
   b. pointed, curved
   c. normal, inverted
   d. curved, angled

9. Figure 1-16 is an example of an image in which the scan lines do not originate at a common ________.
   a. amplitude
   b. disease
   c. origin
   d. time

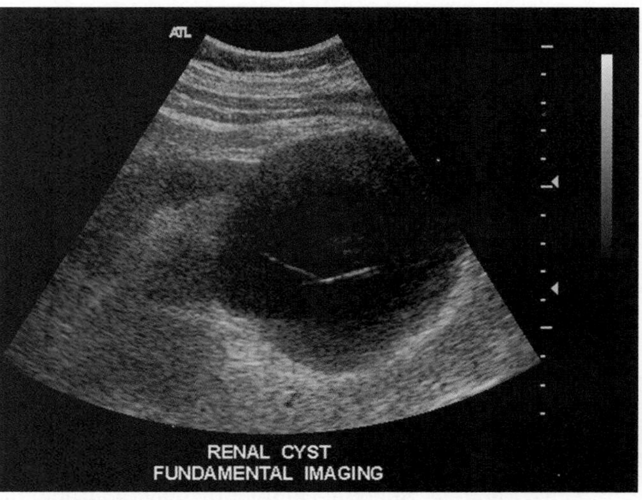

FIGURE 1-16 Illustration to accompany Exercise 9.

10. Sonography is accomplished by using a pulse-echo technique. The important information gained from this technique includes the ___________ from which each echo originated and the __________ of each echo. From this information, the instrument can determine the echo __________ and _________ on the display.
   a. location, strength, location, brightness
   b. location, frequency, frequency, color
   c. anatomy, time, delay, color
   d. anatomy, strength, delay, brightness

11. The ____________ is the interface between the patient and the instrument.
   a. sonographer
   b. Doppler

c. transducer
d. display

12. Transducers generate ultrasound ___________ and receive returning ___________.
a. pulses, echoes
b. waves, images
c. echoes, pulses
d. images, echoes

13. 3D echo information is presented on ___________ displays.
a. TV
b. 2D
c. 3D
d. 4D

14. Acquisition of a 3D echo data volume requires scanning the ultrasound through several tissue ___________.
a. angles
b. orientations
c. types
d. cross-sections

15. The Doppler effect is a change in echo ___________.
a. amplitude
b. intensity
c. impedance
d. frequency
e. arrival time

16. The change referred to in Exercise 15 is a result of ___________.
a. pathology
b. motion
c. pulses
d. echoes

17. The motion that produces the Doppler effect is that of the ___________.
a. transducer
b. sound-beam
c. display
d. reflector

18. In medical applications, the flow of ___________ is commonly the source of the Doppler effect. Doppler information is applied to ___________ for audible evaluation and to ___________ for visual analysis.
a. urine, loudspeakers, computers
b. blood, earphones, computers
c. lymph, earphones, displays
d. blood, loudspeakers, displays

19. The visual display of Doppler information can be in the form of a ___________-Doppler display or a ___________-Doppler display.
a. color, spectral
b. gray-scale, color
c. linear, sector
d. static, temporal

20. Color-Doppler displays can present Doppler-___________ and Doppler-___________ information in color.
a. frequency, shift
b. frequency, power
c. shift, power
d. bandwidth, shift

21. Figure 1-17 shows a ___________.
a. 2D linear image
b. 2D sector image
c. modified sector image
d. 3D gray-scale image
e. spectral display

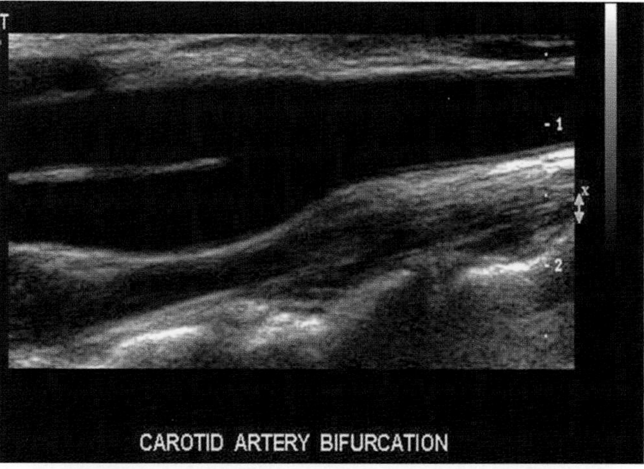

FIGURE 1-17 Illustration to accompany Exercise 21.

22. Figure 1-18 shows a ___________.
a. 2D linear image
b. 2D sector image
c. modified sector image
d. 3D gray-scale image
e. spectral display

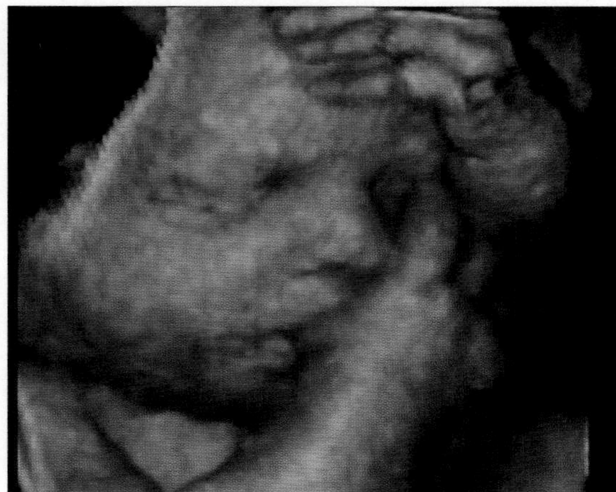

FIGURE 1-18 Illustration to accompany Exercise 22.

23. Figure 1-19 shows a ___________.
a. 2D linear image
b. 2D sector image
c. modified sector image
d. 3D gray-scale image
e. spectral display

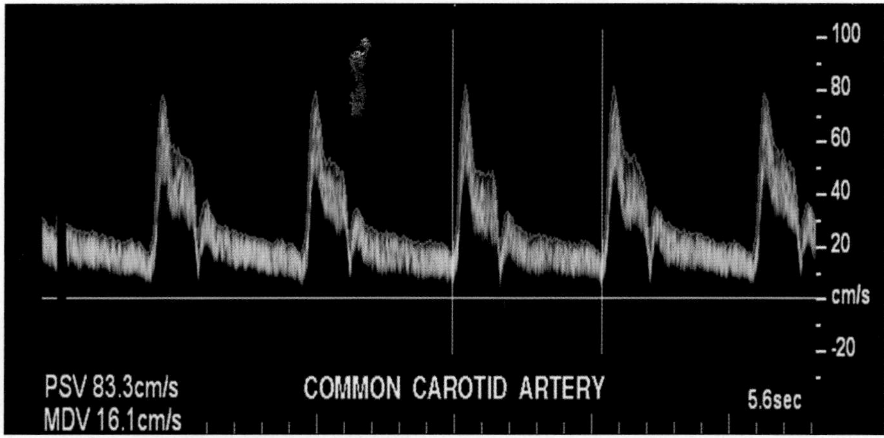

FIGURE 1-19 Illustration to accompany Exercise 23.

24. Figure 1-20 shows a ___________.
  a. 2D linear image
  b. 2D sector image
  c. modified sector image
  d. 3D gray-scale image
  e. spectral display

25. Figure 1-21 shows a ___________.
  a. 2D linear image
  b. 2D sector image
  c. modified sector image
  d. 3D gray-scale image
  e. spectral display

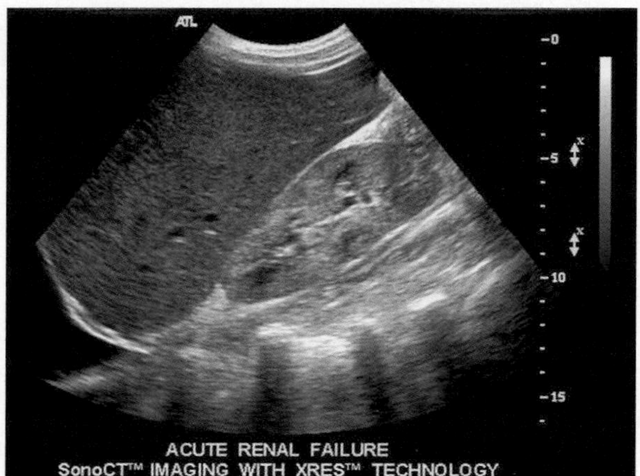

FIGURE 1-20 Illustration to accompany Exercise 24.

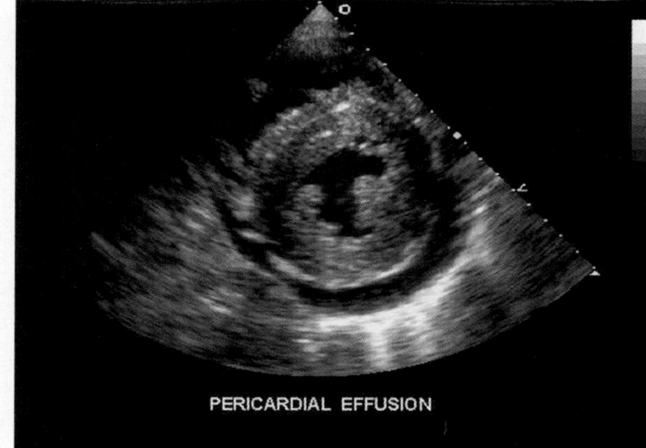

FIGURE 1-21 Illustration to accompany Exercise 25.

2

Ultrasound

LEARNING OBJECTIVES

After reading this chapter, the student should be able to do the following:

- Explain the concept of frequency and its importance in sonography.
- Define *ultrasound* and describe its behavior.
- Discuss how harmonics are generated.
- Compare continuous with pulsed ultrasound.
- Describe the weakening of ultrasound while it travels through tissue.
- Discuss the generation of echoes in tissue.

OUTLINE

KEY TERMS

Absorption
Acoustic
Acoustic variables
Amplitude
Attenuation
Attenuation coefficient
Backscatter
Bandwidth
Compression
Constructive interference
Continuous wave
Contrast agent
Coupling medium
Cycle
Decibel
Density
Destructive interference
Duty factor
Echo
Energy
Fractional bandwidth
Frequency
Fundamental frequency
Harmonics
Hertz
Impedance
Incidence angle
Intensity
Intensity reflection coefficient
Intensity transmission coefficient
Interference
Kilohertz
Longitudinal wave
Medium
Megahertz
Nonlinear propagation
Oblique incidence
Penetration
Period
Perpendicular
Perpendicular incidence
Power
Pressure
Propagation
Propagation speed
Pulse
Pulse duration
Pulse-repetition frequency
Pulse-repetition period
Pulsed ultrasound
Range equation
Rarefaction
Rayl
Reflection
Reflection angle
Reflector
Refraction
Scatterer
Scattering
Sound
Spatial pulse length
Speckle
Specular reflection
Stiffness
Strength
Transmission angle
Transverse wave
Ultrasound
Wave
Wavelength

Ultrasound is similar to the ordinary **sounds** we hear except that its frequency is higher than the range of human hearing. While ultrasound travels through the human body, it interacts with the anatomy in ways that allow us to use it for diagnostic imaging. In this chapter, we consider what ultrasound is, how it is described, and how it travels through and interacts with human anatomy. After exploring this material, you will be prepared to learn in subsequent chapters how ultrasound is generated, received, and processed to produce anatomic, sonographic images.

SOUND

Waves

Diagnostic sonography uses ultrasound to produce images of anatomy and of flow. Ultrasound is a form of sound. Through our sense of hearing we experience sound daily. But what is sound? In spoken communication, sound is produced by a speaker and is heard by a listener. Sound travels from the speaker to the listener, so it is something that travels (i.e., propagates) through a **medium** such as air. But what is this sound that is traveling through air? Sound is a traveling variation in **pressure** (Figure 2-1, *A*). When the speaker speaks, variations in pressure are produced in the throat and mouth. These pressure variations travel through air to the listener, where they stimulate the auditory response in the ear and brain.

In more general terms, we can say that sound is a wave. A **wave** is a traveling variation in one or more quantities, such as pressure. For example, a water wave is a traveling variation in water surface height. Dropping a pebble into a pond disturbs the surface of the water, causing it to move up and down. These up-and-down movements then travel across the surface of the pond so that motion, similar to that generated where the pebble entered the water, eventually occurs at the far shore. Similar to water waves, sound involves mechanical motion in the medium through which it travels. The pressure variations in the sound wave cause the particles of the medium to vibrate back and forth.

 A wave is a traveling variation of a quantity or quantities.

Associated with pressure variations in a sound wave, density variations also exist. **Density** is the concentration of matter (mass per unit volume). Pressure, density, and particle vibration are called **acoustic variables** because they are quantities that vary in a sound wave (the term **acoustic** is derived from the Greek word for hearing). While sound travels through a medium, pressure and density go through **cycles** of increase and decrease, and particles of the medium oscillate. At any point in the medium, pressure and density increase and decrease in repetitive cycles while the sound wave travels past that point. Regions of low pressure and density are called **rarefactions**, and regions of high pressure and density are called **compressions**. Compressions and rarefactions travel through a medium with a sound wave (see Figure 2-1, *B*). Sound requires a medium to travel through; that is, it cannot pass through a vacuum. Sound is a mechanical compressional wave in which back-and-forth particle motion is parallel to

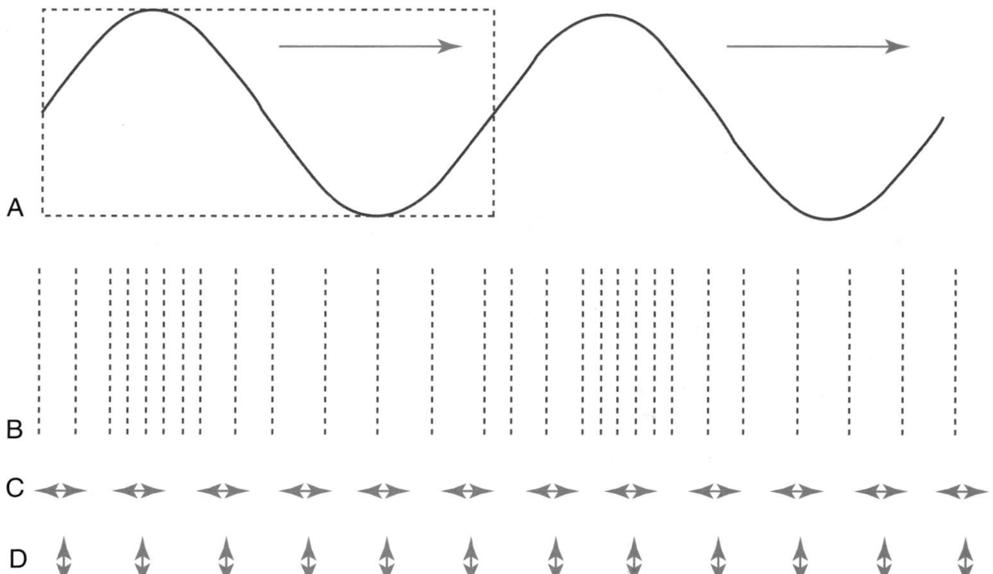

FIGURE 2-1 A, Sound is a traveling pressure variation. The box encloses one cycle of pressure variation. The pressure wave in this example is traveling to the right as indicated by the arrows. B, Sound is also a traveling density variation. Regions of compression (high density) and rarefaction (low density) travel along with the high- and low-pressure regions of the wave. C, Particles vibrate back and forth in a sound wave. This vibratory motion is parallel to the direction of travel of the wave. Such a wave is called a longitudinal wave. Thus sound is a longitudinal, compressional pressure wave. D, A transverse wave involves motion perpendicular to the direction of wave travel.

the direction of wave travel (see Figure 2-1, *C*). Such a wave is called a **longitudinal wave**.

The up-and-down motion of a water surface is **perpendicular** to the direction of wave travel. This type of wave is called a **transverse wave** (see Figure 2-1, *D*). Electromagnetic waves such as light, radio, and microwaves are transverse waves of electric and magnetic fields that involve no particle motion. The particle motion of sound waves is commonly parallel to the direction of wave travel, although, in some cases that are discussed later, the motion may be transverse.

Sound is a traveling variation of acoustic variables.

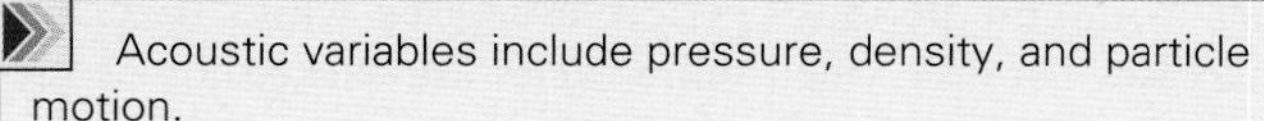

Acoustic variables include pressure, density, and particle motion.

Sound is described by terms that are used to describe all waves. These terms include *frequency, period, wavelength,* **propagation speed**, **amplitude**, and **intensity**. Amplitude and intensity are covered in the later section on **attenuation**.

Frequency

Frequency (f) is a measurement of how often something happens. For example, there are 365 days in a year and 24 hours in a day. Frequency as it relates to sound is a count of how many complete variations (cycles) of pressure (or any other acoustic variable) occur in 1 second. As shown in Figure 2-1, *A*, pressure starts at its normal (undisturbed) value. This would be the pressure in the medium if no sound were propagating through it. While a sound wave travels through a medium, the pressure at any point in the medium increases to a maximum value, returns to normal, decreases to a minimum value, and returns to normal. This is a description of a complete cycle of variation in pressure as an acoustic variable.

A cycle is one complete variation in pressure or other acoustic variable.

The positive and negative halves of a pressure cycle correspond to compression and rarefaction, respectively. In other words, when the pressure is higher, the medium is more dense (more tightly packed), and when the pressure is lower, the medium is less dense. While a sound wave travels past a point in the medium, this cycle of increasing and decreasing pressure and density is repeated over and over. The number of times it is repeated in 1 second is called *frequency* (Figure 2-2). Thus frequency is the number of cycles that occur per second. Frequency units include **hertz** (Hz), **kilohertz** (kHz), and **megahertz** (MHz). One hertz is one cycle per second. One kilohertz equals 1000 Hz. One megahertz equals 1,000,000 Hz.

Frequency is the number of cycles in a wave that occur in 1 second.

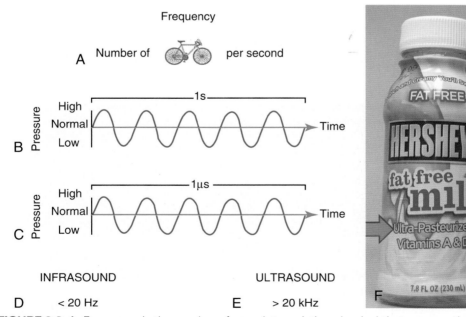

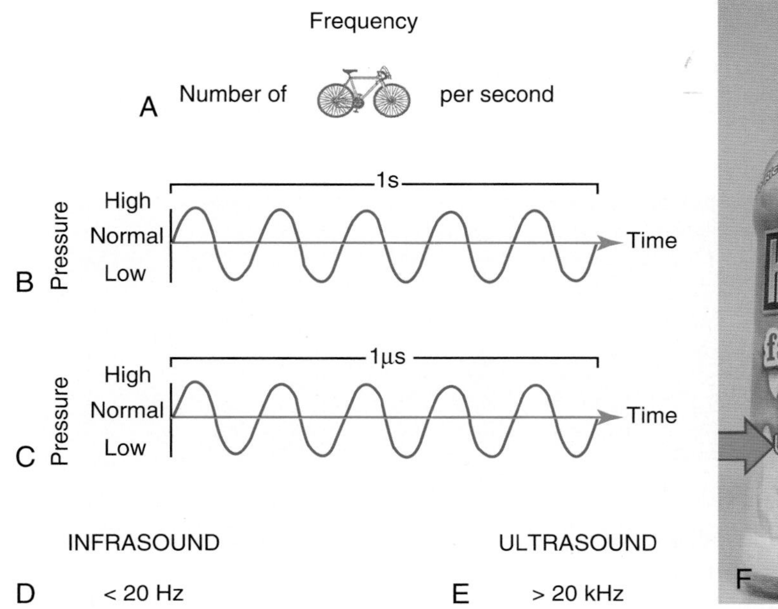

FIGURE 2-2 **A**, Frequency is the number of complete variations (cycles) that an acoustic variable (pressure, in this case) goes through in 1 second. **B**, Five cycles occur in 1 second; thus the frequency is five cycles per second, or 5 Hz. **C**, If five cycles occur within one millionth of a second, also known as a microsecond (1 μs) (i.e., five million cycles occurring in 1 second), the frequency is 5 MHz. **D**, Infrasound is sound that human beings cannot hear because the frequencies are too low (less than 20 Hz). **E**, Ultrasound is sound that human beings cannot hear because the frequencies are too high (greater than 20 kHz). **F**, Ultra (*arrow*) is a prefix meaning "beyond."

> One hertz equals one cycle per second. The abbreviation for hertz is *Hz*.

> One kilohertz equals 1000 cycles per second. The abbreviation for kilohertz is *kHz*.

> One megahertz equals one million cycles per second. The abbreviation for megahertz is *MHz*.

Human hearing operates in a frequency range of approximately 20 to 20,000 Hz, although great variation exists on the upper frequency limit in individuals. Sound with a frequency of less than 20 Hz is called *infrasound* because its frequency is too low for human hearing (*infra* derives from the Latin word for *below*). Sound with a frequency of 20,000 Hz or higher is called *ultrasound* (*ultra* derives from the Latin word for *beyond*) because its frequency is too high for human hearing. Frequency is important in diagnostic ultrasound because of its impact on the resolution and **penetration** of sonographic images. Frequency is controlled by the choice of transducer and by the sonographic instrument.

> Infrasound is sound of a frequency too low for human hearing.

> Ultrasound is sound of a frequency too high for human hearing.

Period

Period (T) is the time that it takes for one cycle to occur (Figure 2-3). In ultrasound, the common unit for period is the microsecond (μs). One microsecond equals one millionth of a second (0.000001 second). For example, the period for 5 MHz ultrasound equals 0.2 μs. Because 5 MHz ultrasound contains five million cycles in a second, each cycle has only one fifth of a millionth of a second (0.2 μs) to occur. The importance of period will become apparent when **pulsed ultrasound** is considered in the next section. Table 2-1 lists common periods. Period decreases while frequency increases because, when more cycles are packed into 1 second, there is less time for each one. Indeed, period equals 1 divided by frequency.

$$T(\mu s) = \frac{1}{f(MHz)}$$

> Period is the time that it takes for one cycle to occur.

> If frequency increases, period decreases.

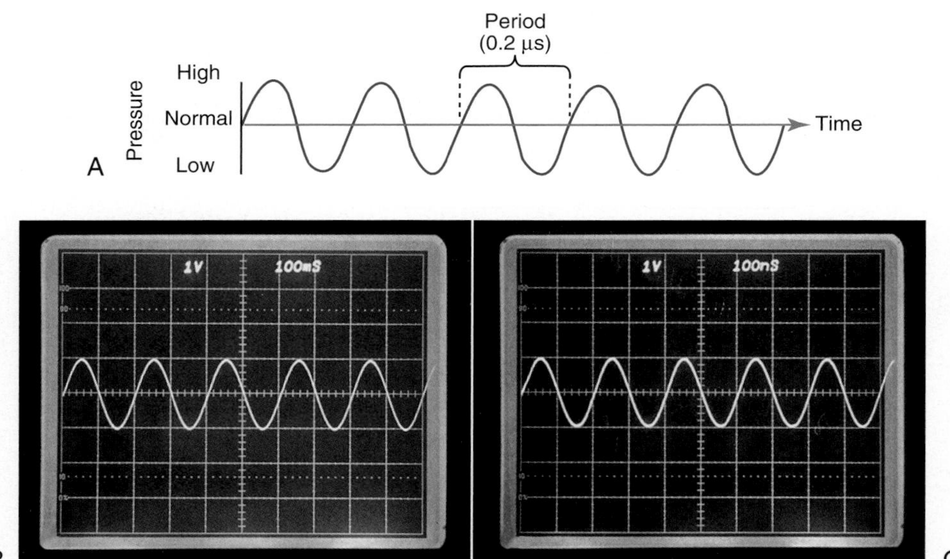

FIGURE 2-3 Period is the time it takes for one cycle to occur. A, Each cycle occurs in 0.2 μs, so the period is 0.2 μs. If one cycle takes 0.2 (or ⅕) millionths of a second to occur, it means that five million cycles occur in 1 second, so the frequency is 5 MHz. **B**, Photograph of a tracing of a 5-Hz wave. The total screen width represents 1 second. One can see that five cycles occur in 1 second and that each cycle takes one fifth (0.2) of a second to occur (period). If this were a pressure wave, it would be an example of infrasound (frequency is 5 Hz, i.e., less than 20 Hz). **C**, In this tracing, the total screen width is 1 μs. If five cycles occur in 1 μs, the period is 0.2 μs and the frequency is 5 MHz, as in **A**. If this were a pressure wave, it would be an example of ultrasound (frequency greater than 20 kHz).

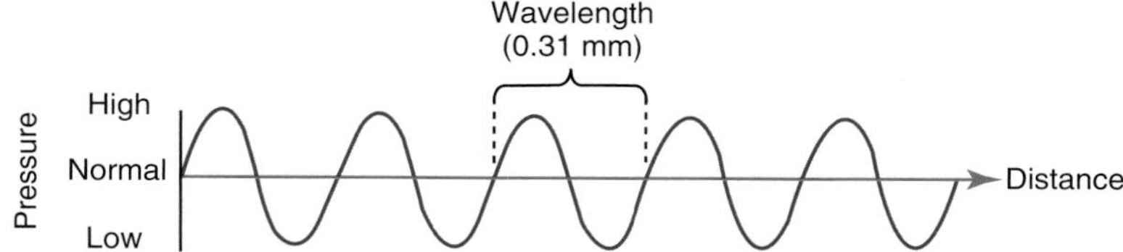

FIGURE 2-4 Wavelength is the length of space over which one cycle occurs. In this figure, each cycle covers 0.31 mm. Thus the wavelength is 0.31 mm. This figure differs from Figures 2-2 and 2-3 in that the horizontal axis represents distance rather than time. For a propagation speed of 1.54 mm/µs and a frequency of 5 MHz, the wavelength is 0.31 mm.

TABLE 2-1 Common Ultrasound Periods and Wavelengths in Tissue

Frequency (MHz)	Period (µs)	Wavelength (mm)*
2.0	0.50	0.77
3.5	0.29	0.44
5.0	0.20	0.31
7.5	0.13	0.21
10.0	0.10	0.15
15.0	0.07	0.10

*Assuming a (soft tissue) propagation speed of 1.54 mm/µs (1540 m/s).

Wavelength

Wavelength (λ) is the length of space that one cycle takes up (Figure 2-4). If we could stop a sound wave, visualize it, and measure the distance from the beginning to the end of one cycle, the measured distance would be the wavelength of the sound wave. Wavelength is the length of a cycle from "front" to "back." More precisely, it could be called *cycle length,* but traditionally it has been called *wavelength.* For ultrasound, wavelength is commonly expressed in millimeters. One millimeter (1 mm) is one thousandth of a meter (0.001 m). The importance of wavelength will be evident when detail resolution of images is considered. Table 2-1 lists common wavelengths in sonography.

 Wavelength is the length of a cycle in space.

Propagation Speed

Propagation speed (c) is the speed with which a wave moves through a medium. For sound, **propagation** speed is the speed at which a particular value of an acoustic variable moves (Figure 2-5), at which a cycle moves, and at which the entire wave moves. All of these are the same speed. Relevant propagation speed units include meters per second (m/s) and millimeters per microsecond (mm/µs).

Propagation speed is the speed at which a wave moves through a medium.

Wavelength depends on frequency and propagation speed. The relationship between the three is that wavelength is equal to propagation speed divided by frequency.

$$\lambda(\text{mm}) = \frac{c(\text{mm}/\mu\text{s})}{f(\text{MHz})}$$

This equation predicts that wavelength will decrease when frequency increases. This prediction is confirmed in Table 2-1.

 If frequency increases, wavelength decreases.

An example of the relationship among frequency, wavelength, and propagation speed is seen by comparing Figures 2-3, *C*; 2-4; and 2-5. In these figures, frequency is 5 MHz, wavelength is 0.31 mm, and propagation speed is 1.54 mm/µs. These values apply to the same wave because they are a compatible set according to the following equation:

$$\lambda(\text{mm}) = \frac{c(\text{mm}/\mu\text{s})}{f(\text{MHz})} = \frac{1.54\text{mm}/\mu\text{s}}{5\text{MHz}} = 0.31\text{mm}$$

Propagation speed is determined by the medium, primarily its stiffness (hardness). **Stiffness** is the resistance of a material to compression. Stiffness is the inverse of compressibility; that is, a compressible material such as a sponge has low stiffness, and a stiff (hard) material such as a rock has low compressibility. Stiffer media have higher sound speeds. Thus propagation speeds are lower in gases (which are highly compressible), higher in liquids, and highest in solids (which are nearly incompressible). The average propagation speed in soft tissues is 1540 m/s, or (in more relevant units for our purposes) 1.54 mm/µs. Values for soft tissues range from 1.44 to 1.64 mm/µs. Not surprisingly, because soft tissue is mostly water, these values are similar to those for liquids such as water.

Propagation speeds are highest in solids and lowest in gases.

The average propagation speed of sound in tissues is 1.54 mm/µs.

In lung tissue, because it contains gas, the propagation speed of sound is much lower than in other soft tissues. However, this

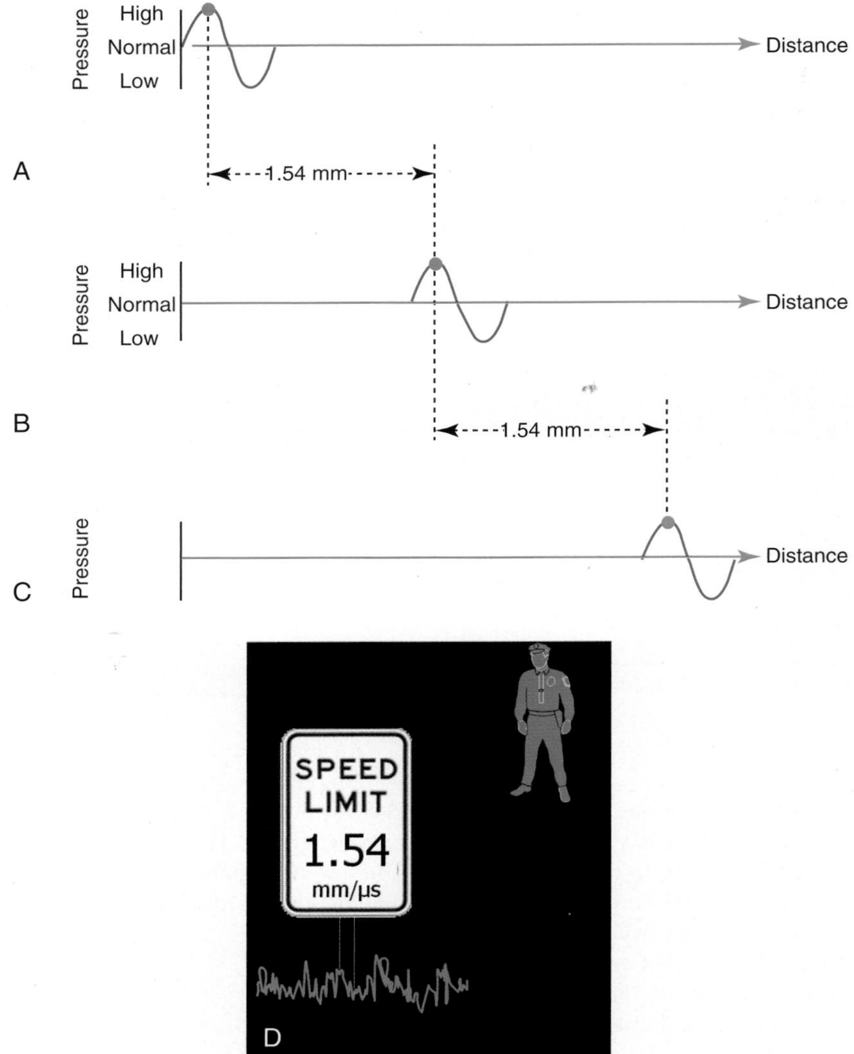

FIGURE 2-5 **Propagation speed is the speed with which a particular value of an acoustic variable (also the rest of the cycle and, indeed, the entire wave) travels through a medium.** **A**, The movement of a maximum (identified by the *red dot*) is shown in this figure. **B**, 1 μs after A. **C**, 1 μs after B and 2 μs after **A**. The maximum (dot) moves 1.54 mm in 1 μs and 3.08 mm in 2 μs. The propagation speed is 1.54 mm/μs. The propagation speed in this figure (1.54 mm/μs), when divided by the frequency in Figure 2-3, *C* (5 MHz), equals the wavelength in Figure 2-4 (0.31 mm). **D**, Propagation speeds in soft tissue average 1540 m/s, or 1.54 mm/μs.

difference is not important because ultrasound does not penetrate air-filled lung tissue well enough for imaging. In bone, because it is a solid, propagation speeds are higher (3 to 5 mm/μs) than in soft tissues. Soft-tissue propagation speeds are within a few percent of the average, so the average can be assumed for all soft tissues with little error. Fat is farthest from the average, about 6% lower. Propagation speed is important because sonographic instruments use it to accurately locate echoes on the display.

Harmonics

The dependence of propagation speed on pressure causes strong sound (pressure) waves to change shape while they travel (Figure 2-6), because the higher-pressure portions of the wave travel faster than the lower-pressure portions.

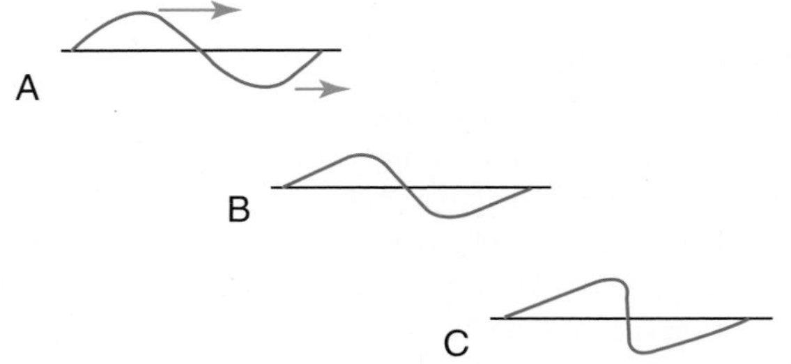

FIGURE 2-6 **In nonlinear propagation, propagation speed depends on pressure.** **A**, Higher-pressure portions of the wave travel faster than the lower-pressure portions. **B-C**, Thus the wave changes shape while it travels. This change from the initial sinusoidal shape introduces harmonics that are even and odd multiples of the fundamental frequency.

This movement produces a wave that originally has a smooth curve shape (called *sinusoidal;* illustrated in Figure 2-6, *A*) that progresses toward a nonsinusoidal shape (see Figure 2-6, *C*). Propagation in which speed depends on pressure and the shape of the wave changes is called **nonlinear propagation**. A continuous (not pulsed) sinusoidal waveform is characterized by a single frequency (equal to the number of cycles per second). Any other wave shape contains additional frequencies that are even and odd multiples of the original frequency. The original frequency is called the **fundamental frequency**. The even and odd multiples are called *even* and *odd* **harmonics**, respectively. A frequency analysis of the wave in Figure 2-6, *A,* would yield a single (fundamental) frequency such as 2 MHz. Analysis of parts *B* and *C* would reveal, in addition to fundamental frequency, harmonics such as 4, 6, and 8 MHz. While the shape becomes less sinusoidal, the harmonics become stronger. Therefore they are stronger in part *C* than in part *B*. The use of harmonic frequency echoes (harmonic imaging is discussed later) improves the quality of sonographic images.

> Harmonics are even and odd multiples of fundamental frequency.

PULSED ULTRASOUND

Thus far we have discussed terms (*frequency, period, wavelength,* and *propagation speed*) that are sufficient to describe **continuous wave** (CW) ultrasound in which cycles repeat indefinitely. For sonography and most of Doppler ultrasound, pulsed ultrasound is used rather than continuous wave. Pulsed ultrasound is not on continuously. An ultrasound pulse is a few cycles of ultrasound. **Pulses** are separated in time with gaps of no ultrasound. Ultrasound pulses are described by some additional parameters that we will now discuss.

> With continuous wave ultrasound, cycles repeat indefinitely. Pulsed ultrasound consists of pulses separated by gaps in time. A pulse is a few cycles of ultrasound.

Pulse-Repetition Frequency and Period

The term *frequency,* when unqualified, is the number of cycles occurring per second for a continuous wave. For a pulsed wave, it is the number of cycles per second that would occur if it were a continuous wave. When qualified with the adjectives *pulse-repetition,* **pulse-repetition frequency** (PRF) is the number of *pulses* that occur in 1 second (Figure 2-7). Diagnostic ultrasound involves a few thousand pulses per second, so PRF is commonly expressed in kilohertz (kHz). One kilohertz equals 1000 Hz. Frequency (the number of cycles per second) and PRF (the number of pulses per second) are independently controlled by the sonographic instrument.

The term *period,* when unqualified, refers to the time for one cycle to occur. When qualified with the adjectives *pulse-repetition,* **pulse-repetition period** (PRP) refers to the time from the beginning of one pulse to the beginning of the next (Figure 2-8). Its common units are milliseconds (ms, or one thousandth of a second). The PRP is the reciprocal of PRF. The pulse-repetition period decreases while PRF

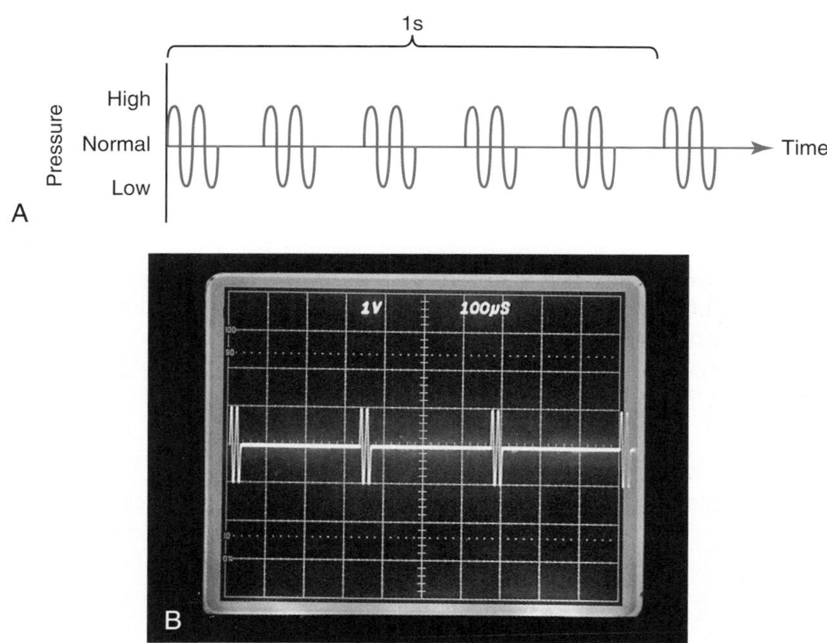

FIGURE 2-7 Pulse-repetition frequency (PRF) is the number of pulses that occur in 1 second. **A**, Five pulses (containing two cycles each) occur in 1 second; thus the PRF is 5 Hz. **B**, In this photograph, three pulses occur in 1 ms (or one thousandth of a second); thus the PRF is 3 kHz. The scaled screen width is 1 ms.

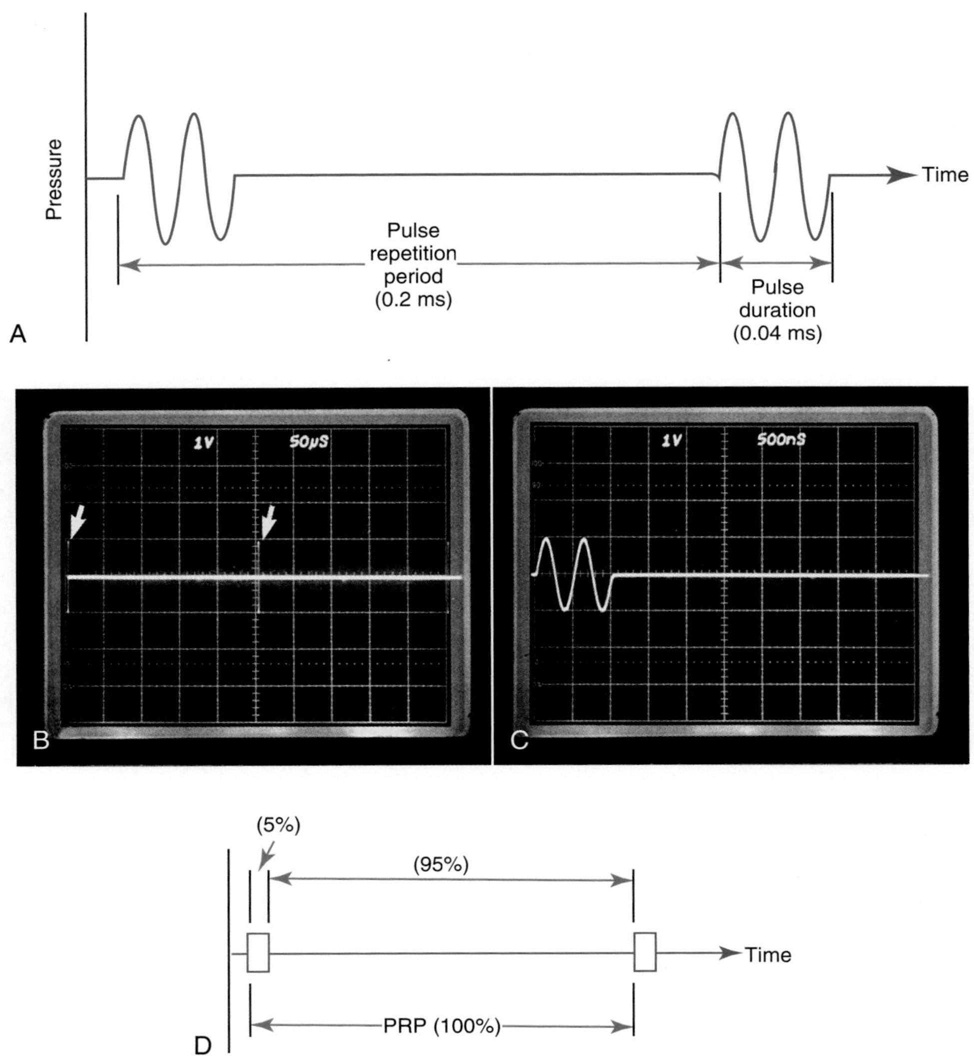

FIGURE 2-8 The pulse-repetition period (PRP) is the time from the beginning of one pulse to the beginning of the next. **A**, The PRP is 0.2 ms (200 μs). Therefore the pulse-repetition frequency is 5 kHz. The pulse duration (PD) is the time that it takes for one pulse to occur. The PD is equal to the period multiplied by the number of cycles in the pulse. The PD is 40 μs. The duty factor (DF) is the fraction of time that the sound is on. The DF is 40/200, which equals 0.2, or 20%. **B**, This photograph shows that the PRP is 0.25 ms (the pulse-repetition frequency is 4 kHz). The period is 0.5 μs, as shown expanded in **C**, and the PD is 1 μs. From one pulse to the next (PRP of 0.25 ms, or 250 μs), the sound is on (PD) for 1 μs. The DF in this example is 0.004, or 0.4%. The screen width is 0.5 ms in **B** and 5 μs in **C**. **D**, The DF is the fraction of time that pulsed ultrasound is actually on. In this example, the PRP represents 100% of the time from the start of one pulse to the start of the next one. Of this time, the sound is on 5% of the time (PD divided by PRP) and off 95% of the time.

increases because, when more pulses occur in a second, the time between them decreases.

$$\text{PRP (ms)} = \frac{1}{\text{PRF (kHz)}}$$

PRF is controlled automatically by sonographic instruments to satisfy requirements that are discussed later. With Doppler techniques, the operator controls PRF, which is also described in later chapters. PRF is important because it determines how quickly images are generated. For example, with a PRF of 5 kHz, 5000 pulses are produced each second, generating 5000 scan lines per second. If, for example, each image has 100 scan lines, 50 images will be produced per second. Later this will be called *frame rate,* and it will determine how well rapidly moving structures can be followed.

 PRF is the number of pulses that occur in 1 second.

 PRP is the time from the beginning of one pulse to the beginning of the next one.

If PRF increases, PRP decreases.

Pulse Duration

Pulse duration (PD) is the time that it takes for one pulse to occur (see Figure 2-8). PD is equal to the period (the time for one cycle) times the number of cycles in the pulse (n) and is expressed in microseconds. Sonographic pulses are typically two or three cycles long. Compared with longer ones, shorter pulses improve the quality of sonographic images. Doppler ultrasound pulses are typically 5 to 30 cycles long.

$$PD(\mu s) = n \times T(\mu s)$$

 Sonographic pulses are typically two or three cycles long. Doppler pulses are typically 5 to 30 cycles long.

PD decreases if the number of cycles in a pulse is decreased or if the frequency is increased (reducing the period). The instrument operator chooses the frequency.

PD is the time for a pulse to occur.

If frequency is increased, period is decreased, reducing PD. If the number of cycles in a pulse is reduced, PD is decreased. Shorter pulses improve the quality of sonographic images.

Duty Factor

Duty factor (DF) is the fraction of time that pulsed ultrasound is on (see Figure 2-8, *D*). Continuous wave ultrasound is on 100% of the time. Pulsed ultrasound, by definition, is not on all of the time. The DF indicates how much of the time the ultrasound is on. Longer pulses increase the DF because the sound is on more of the time.

 DF is the fraction of time that pulsed ultrasound is on.

DF is the fraction of the PRP that the sound is on. The remainder of the time to the next pulse is the listening time for reception of echoes that will form a scan line on the instrument display. Higher pulse-repetition frequencies increase the DF because there is less listening time between pulses. Thus the DF increases with increasing pulse duration or PRF. DF has no units because it is a fraction with time in both the numerator and denominator. Thus the DF is simply expressed as a decimal, such as 0.10 or 0.25, or as a percentage, such as 10% or 25%. The importance of the DF will become evident when intensities and safety issues are discussed later. The DF is equal to PD divided by the PRP, because PD represents the amount of time that the sound is on, and the PRP is the time from one pulse to the next. Thus the ratio of the two represents the fraction of time that pulsed ultrasound is on.

$$DF = \frac{PD(\mu s)}{PRP(\mu s)} = \frac{PD(\mu s) \times PRF(kHz)}{1000(kHz/MHz)}$$

The factor of 1000 converts kilohertz to megahertz to be consistent with microseconds of pulse duration. Multiplying the DF by 100 expresses it as a percentage. For example, if the pulse duration is 2 μs and the PRP is 250 μs, then

$$DF = \frac{2}{250} = 0.008 = \text{or } 0.8\%$$

A range of DFs is encountered in diagnostic ultrasound because of the various conditions chosen by the instrument and the operator. Typical DFs for sonography are in the range of 0.1% to 1.0%. For Doppler ultrasound, because of longer pulse durations, the range of typical DFs is 0.5% to 5.0%.

 If the PD increases, the DF increases.

If PRF increases, PRP decreases and duty factor increases.

Spatial Pulse Length

If we could stop a pulse, visualize it, and measure the distance from its beginning to its end, the measured distance would be spatial pulse length (SPL). **Spatial pulse length** is the length of a pulse from front to back (Figure 2-9, *A*). SPL is equal to the length of each cycle times the number of cycles in the pulse. The length of each cycle is wavelength. Thus SPL increases with wavelength and increases with the number of cycles in the pulse.

$$SPL(mm) = n \times \lambda(mm)$$

 SPL is the length of space occupied by a pulse.

Because wavelength decreases with increasing frequency, SPL decreases with increasing frequency (Figure 2-9, *B-C*). Units for SPL are millimeters. SPL is an important quantity when considering image resolution, because shorter pulse lengths improve resolution.

 If the number of cycles in a pulse increases, SPL increases. If frequency increases, wavelength and SPL decrease.

 Shorter pulses improve sonographic image resolution.

Frequency

Recall that frequency expresses the number of cycles in a wave that occur in 1 second. This is fine for continuous wave ultrasound; however, in pulsed ultrasound, gaps exist between pulses, thus some of the cycles are missing. For example, in 5-MHz frequency continuous wave ultrasound, five million cycles occur in 1 second. But what about 5-MHz pulsed ultrasound? The frequency, 5 MHz, gives the number of cycles per second, as if the wave were a continuous wave, even though it is not. The actual number of cycles that occur in 1 second for pulsed ultrasound depends on the DF. For example, if the DF is 0.01, or 1%, the ultrasound is on only one hundredth of the time, and the actual number of cycles per second is 50,000, or 50 kHz. The quiet time between pulses eliminates 99% of the cycles in this example, even though the frequency implies that there are five million cycles per second. However, the frequency for pulsed ultrasound is still given as 5 MHz because the behavior of the pulses (regarding period, wavelength, propagation speed, and other characteristics such as attenuation) is similar to that of 5-MHz continuous wave ultrasound.

Bandwidth

In contrast to continuous wave ultrasound, which can be described by a single frequency, ultrasound pulses contain a range of frequencies called **bandwidth** (Figure 2-9, *D-E*). The shorter the pulse (the fewer the number of cycles), the higher the number of frequencies it contains (broader bandwidth). **Fractional bandwidth** is bandwidth divided by operating frequency. Fractional bandwidth is unitless. It describes how large the bandwidth is compared with operating frequency. The reciprocal of fractional bandwidth (operating frequency divided by bandwidth) is called *quality factor* (Q).

> Bandwidth is the range of frequencies contained in a pulse.

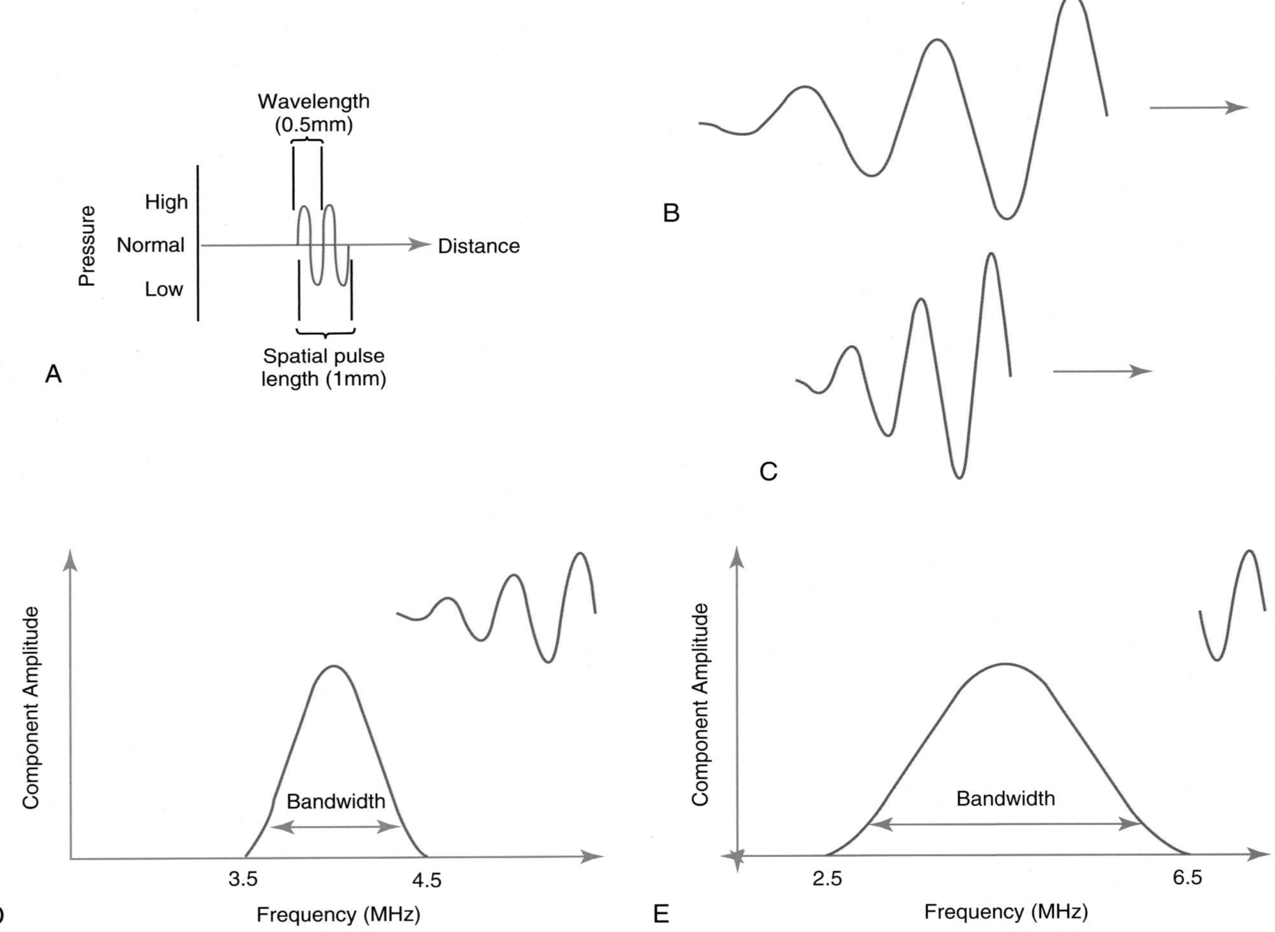

FIGURE 2-9 **A**, Spatial pulse length (SPL) is the length of space over which a pulse occurs. SPL is equal to wavelength multiplied by the number of cycles in the pulse. In this figure, the wavelength is 0.5 mm, there are two cycles in each pulse, and the SPL is 0.5 × 2, or 1 mm. This figure differs from Figures 2-7, A, and 2-8, **A**, in that the horizontal axis represents distance rather than time. **B-C**, Three-cycle damped (decreasing in amplitude) pulses of ultrasound traveling to the right. **B** shows lower-frequency pulse with longer wavelength and SPL. **C** shows higher-frequency pulse with shorter wavelength and SPL. **D-E**, Plots of the frequencies present in two ultrasound pulses. Component amplitude is the amplitude of each frequency component present. Bandwidth is the range of frequencies present. Compare the bandwidth for a narrow band, longer pulse (**D**) with the bandwidth for a broadband, shorter pulse (**E**).

Frequency is the number of cycles per second. Frequency determines the resolution and penetration achieved in sonographic images, as discussed later. PRF is the number of pulses produced per second. It determines the number of scan lines produced per second and the number of images produced per second (the frame rate which is discussed later).

ATTENUATION

We now consider the magnitude of the cyclic variations in a continuous or pulsed ultrasound wave. Amplitude and intensity are indicators of the **strength** of the sound. They are related to how loud the sound would be if it could be heard. Ultrasound, however, cannot be heard, so loudness is irrelevant. Nevertheless, amplitude and intensity are important indicators of how strong or "intense" the ultrasound is.

Amplitude

Amplitude is the maximum variation that occurs in an acoustic variable. Amplitude is a measure of how far a variable gets away from its normal, undisturbed value (its value if there were no sound present). Amplitude is the maximum value minus the normal (undisturbed or no-sound) value (Figure 2-10, *A*). Amplitude is expressed in units that are appropriate

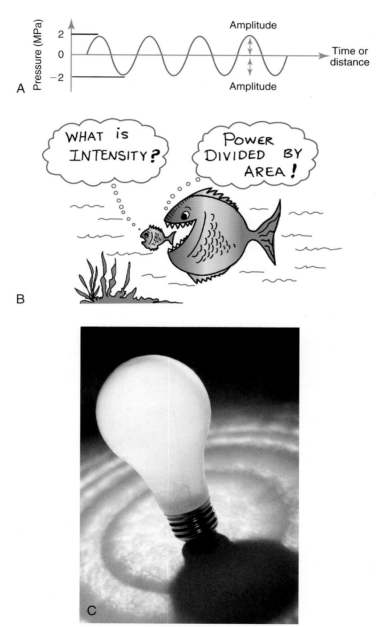

FIGURE 2-10 **A**, Amplitude is the maximum amount of variation that occurs in an acoustic variable (pressure, in this case). In this figure, the amplitude is 2 megapascals (Mpa). **B**, Intensity is the power in a sound wave divided by the area over which the power is spread (the beam area). **C**, A watt is the unit of power for a light bulb.

for the acoustic variable considered. For example, megapascals (MPa) are the units that express pressure amplitude.

Intensity

Energy is the ability to accomplish work. Heat, light, x-rays, microwaves, and mechanical motion are forms of energy. Sound is a form of mechanical energy that can do work. For example, it can vibrate objects in its path or raise the temperature of a medium through which is traveling. **Power** is the rate at which energy is transferred from one part of a system to another (e.g., a lamp plugged into a wall outlet) or from one location to another (e.g., energy that travels down a laser or ultrasound beam). Power is energy transferred divided by the time required to transfer energy, that is, the transfer rate. Power units include watts (W) (see Figure 2-10, *C*) and milliwatts (mW). One milliwatt is one thousandth of a watt.

Intensity (I) is the rate at which energy passes through a unit area. It is equal to the power in a wave divided by the area (A) over which the power is spread (see Figure 2-10, *B*). Ultrasound is generated by transducers in the form of beams, somewhat similar to laser beams, but as sound instead of light. Beam area is expressed in centimeters squared (cm^2). Intensity units include milliwatts per centimeter squared (mW/cm^2) and watts per centimeter squared (W/cm^2). The average intensity of a sound beam is the total power in the beam divided by the cross-sectional area of the beam.

$$I(mW/cm^2) = \frac{P(mW)}{A(cm^2)}$$

An increase in power increases intensity. An increase in area decreases intensity because power is less concentrated. A decrease in area (focusing) increases intensity because power is more concentrated.

> If beam power increases, intensity increases. If beam area decreases (focusing), intensity increases.

Intensity is an important quantity in describing the sound that is sent into the body by a transducer and in discussing bioeffects and safety. An analogy may be made to the effect of sunlight on dry kindling (Figure 2-11). Sunlight normally will not ignite the kindling, but if the same light power from the sun is concentrated into a small area (increased intensity) by focusing it with a magnifying glass, the kindling can be ignited. In this example, increasing intensity produces an effect, even though power remains the same. The beam area is determined by the transducer, in particular, how it focuses the beam. Intensity is proportional to amplitude squared. Thus, if amplitude is doubled, intensity is quadrupled. If amplitude is halved, intensity is quartered.

Attenuation

Attenuation (a) is the weakening of sound while it propagates (Figure 2-12). It is important to understand attenuation because (1) it limits imaging depth and (2) its weakening effect on the image must be compensated by the diagnostic instrument. With an unfocused beam in any medium, such as tissue, amplitude and intensity will decrease while the sound travels through the medium. This reduction in amplitude and intensity as sound travels is called *attenuation* (Figure 2-13). Attenuation encompasses the **absorption** (conversion of sound to heat) of sound while it travels and the **reflection** and **scattering** of the sound (echoes) while it encounters tissue interfaces and heterogeneous tissues. Absorption is the dominant factor that contributes to attenuation of ultrasound in soft tissues. The generation of echoes by the reflection and scattering of sound is crucial to sonographic imaging but contributes little to attenuation in most cases. **Decibels** are the units used to quantify attenuation. The **attenuation coefficient** (a_c) is the attenuation that occurs with each centimeter the sound wave travels: Its units are decibels per centimeter (dB/cm). The farther the sound travels, the greater the attenuation.

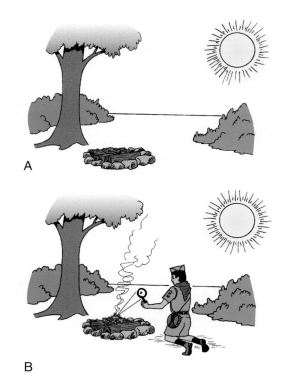

FIGURE 2-11 A, Sunlight does not normally ignite a fire. B, However, when the sunlight is focused, intensity increases, and ignition can occur.

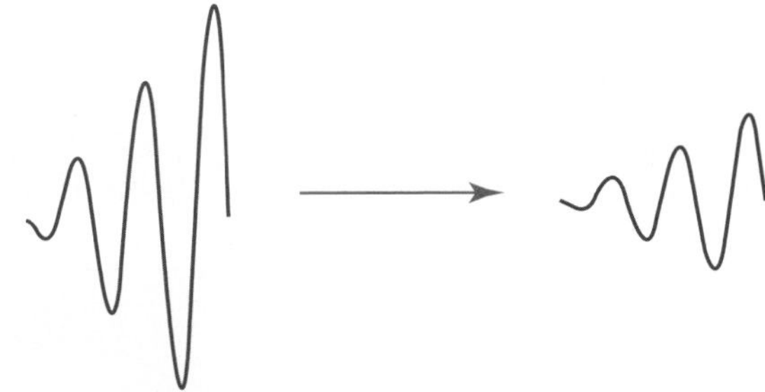

FIGURE 2-12 An ultrasound pulse is weakened (reduction of amplitude) as it travels through a medium (in this case from left to right). This weakening is called *attenuation.*

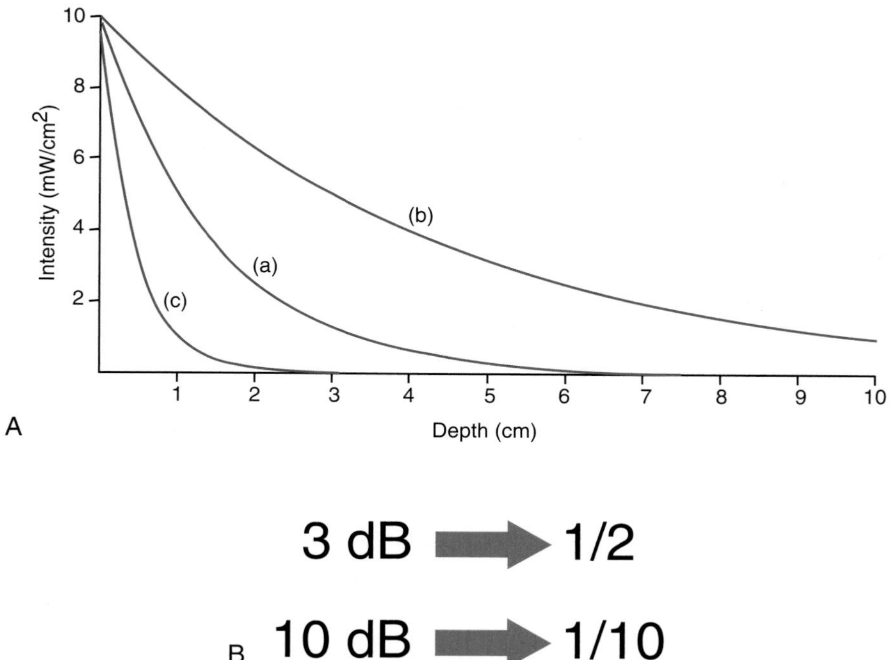

FIGURE 2-13 Attenuation of sound while it travels through a medium. A, *(a)*, The intensity decreases by 50% for each 1 cm of travel. This corresponds to an attenuation coefficient of 3 dB/cm. In *(b)*, the attenuation coefficient is 1 dB/cm, whereas in *(c)*, the attenuation coefficient is 10 dB/cm. **B**, Two easy-to-remember values for decibels and their corresponding intensity reductions are (1) a 3-dB attenuation corresponds to an intensity reduction (50%) to one half the original value, and (2) a 10-dB attenuation corresponds to an intensity reduction (90%) to one tenth the original value.

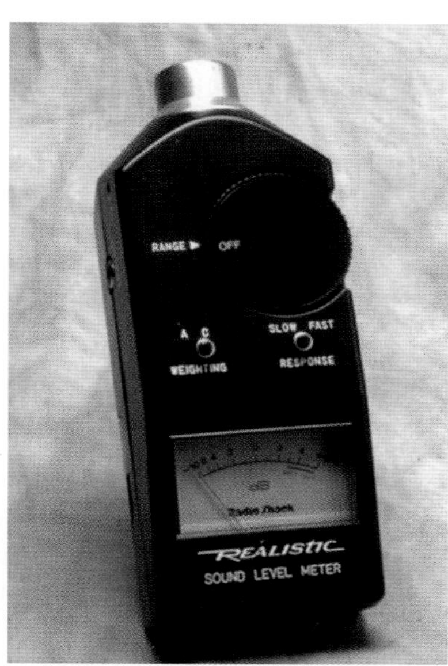

FIGURE 2-14 A sound level meter based on decibels.

TABLE 2-2 Sound Levels

Sound	Level (dB)
Pain threshold	130
Rock concert	115
Chain saw	100
Lawn mower	90
Vacuum cleaner	75
Normal conversation	60
Whisper	30
Hearing threshold	0

Decibels are useful units to make comparisons. For example, they describe the relationships between various measured sound levels (Figure 2-14) and the threshold of human hearing (the weakest sound we can hear). Table 2-2 gives examples of various values. Decibels involve the logarithm of the ratio of two powers or intensities. In the case of attenuation, they are the intensities before and after attenuation has occurred. Two decibel values have particular usefulness: 3 dB corresponds to an intensity ratio of one half, that is, an intensity reduction of 50%; and 10 dB corresponds to an intensity ratio of one tenth, that is, an intensity reduction of 90% (see Figures 2-13 and 2-15).

Example 2-1

Compare the following two intensities in decibels.

$I_1 = 20\,mW/cm^2, I_2 = 10\,mW/cm^2$.

I_2 is one half of I_1. Therefore, I_2 is 3dB less than I_1.

Example 2-2

Compare (in decibels) I_2 with I_1, where $I_1 = 10$ mW/cm² and $I_2 = 0.01$ mW/cm².

Each factor of 10 is equivalent to 10 dB. I_1 is 1000 times I_2, so I_2 is 30 dB less than I_1.

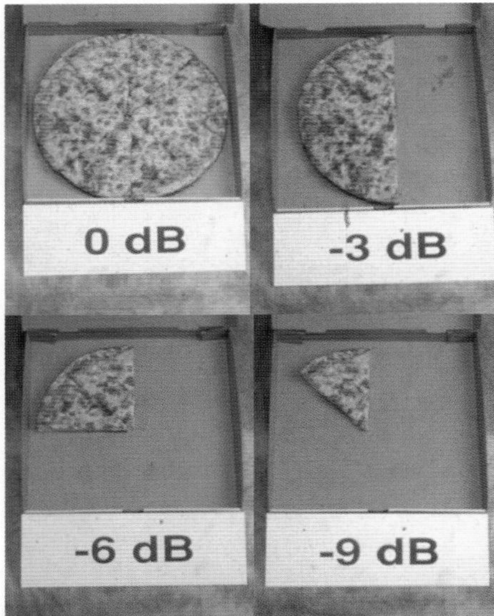

FIGURE 2-15 Each reduction of 3 dB corresponds to removing half of the pizza.

Example 2-3

While sound passes through tissue, its intensity at one point is 1 mW/cm^2. At a point 10 cm farther along, it is 0.1 mW/cm^2. What are the attenuation and attenuation coefficient values?

Because intensity is reduced to one tenth from the first point to the second, attenuation is 10 dB. The attenuation coefficient is attenuation divided by the separation between the two points. In this case,

$$a_c = \frac{10\,\text{dB}}{10\,\text{cm}} = 1\,\text{dB/cm}$$

Table 2-3 lists various values of intensity ratio and percentage values with corresponding decibel values of attenuation. To determine attenuation in decibels, multiply the attenuation coefficient by the sound path length (L) (how far the sound has traveled) in centimeters.

$$a\,(\text{dB}) = a_c\,(\text{dB/cm}) \times L\,(\text{cm})$$

If the attenuation coefficient increases, attenuation increases.

If the path length increases, attenuation increases.

Attenuation increases with increasing frequency. Persons who live in apartments or dormitories experience this fact when they hear mostly the bass notes through the wall from a neighbor's sound system. For soft tissues, there is approximately (values of 0.3 to 0.7 are used by authors for various purposes) 0.5 dB of attenuation per centimeter for each megahertz of frequency (Table 2-4). In other words, the average attenuation coefficient in decibels per centimeter for soft tissues is approximately equal to one half the frequency in megahertz. To calculate the attenuation in decibels, multiply one half of the frequency in megahertz by the path length in centimeters.

TABLE 2-3 Attenuation for Various Intensity Ratios*

Attenuation (dB)	Intensity Ratio	Percent Intensity Ratio
0	1.00	100
1	0.79	79
2	0.63	63
3	0.50	50
4	0.40	40
5	0.32	32
6	0.25	25
7	0.20	20
8	0.16	16
9	0.13	13
10	0.10	10
15	0.032	3.2
20	0.010	1.0
25	0.003	0.3
30	0.001	0.1
35	0.0003	0.03
40	0.0001	0.01
45	0.00003	0.003
50	0.00001	0.001
60	0.000001	0.0001
70	0.0000001	0.00001
80	0.00000001	0.000001
90	0.000000001	0.0000001
100	0.0000000001	0.00000001

*The intensity ratio is the fraction of the original intensity remaining after attenuation.

 If frequency increases, attenuation increases.

$$a\,(\text{dB}) = \frac{1}{2}\,(\text{dB/cm-MHz}) \times f\,(\text{MHz}) \times L\,(\text{cm})$$

The intensity ratio corresponding to the number of decibels may be obtained from Table 2-3. This ratio is equal to the fraction of the intensity (at the beginning of the path) that remains at the end of the path. If the intensity at the beginning is known, the intensity at the end may be found by multiplying the beginning intensity by the intensity ratio. The following is a summary of this four-step process:

1. Multiplying the frequency by one half yields the approximate attenuation coefficient.
2. Multiplying the attenuation coefficient by the path length yields attenuation.
3. The intensity ratio is then determined for the decibel value calculated in step 2 (by using Table 2-3). This is the fraction of the original intensity that remains at the end of the path.
4. Multiplying the intensity ratio by the intensity at the start of the path yields the intensity at the end of the path.

TABLE 2-4 Average Attenuation Coefficients in Tissue

Frequency (MHz)	Average Attenuation Coefficient for Soft Tissue (dB/cm)	Intensity Reduction in 1-cm Path (%)	Intensity Reduction in 10-cm Path (%)
2.0	1.0	21	90
3.5	1.8	34	98
5.0	2.5	44	99.7
7.5	3.8	58	99.98
10.0	5.0	68	99.999

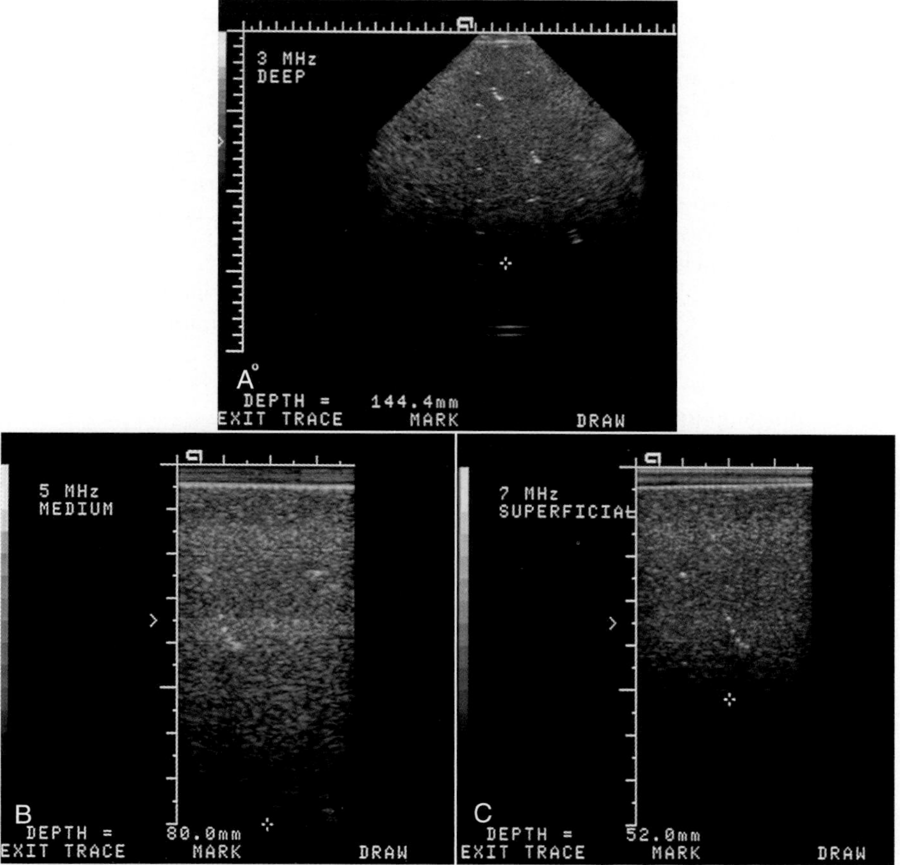

FIGURE 2-16 Examples of penetration in a tissue-equivalent phantom at 3 MHz (**A**), 5 MHz (**B**), and 7 MHz (**C**). Penetration decreases while frequency increases.

Example 2-4

If 4-MHz ultrasound with 10 mW/cm^2 intensity is applied to a soft tissue surface, what is the intensity 1.5 cm into the tissue?

Step 1: Multiply frequency by one half to yield an attenuation coefficient of 2 dB/cm.

Step 2: Multiply the attenuation coefficient (2 dB/cm) by path length (1.5 cm) to yield an attenuation of 3 dB.

Step 3: From Table 2-3 as a reference, an attenuation of 3 dB corresponds to an intensity ratio of 0.5. Thus 50% of intensity remains after the sound travels through this path.

Step 4: Multiply the intensity ratio (0.5) by the intensity at the beginning of the path (10 mW/cm^2) to yield the intensity at the end of the path. The result is 5 mW/cm^2.

Attenuation is higher in the lung than in other soft tissues because of the air present in this organ. Attenuation is higher in bones than in soft tissues.

A practical consequence of attenuation is that it limits the depths of images (penetration) obtained. Penetration decreases while frequency increases (Figure 2-16). Table 2-5 lists attenuation coefficients and typical imaging depths for various frequencies in soft tissue.

 If frequency increases, penetration decreases.

The depths needed to reach various parts of human anatomy determine the frequencies used in diagnostic ultrasound,

TABLE 2-5 Common Values for Attenuation Coefficient and Penetration

Frequency (MHz)	Attenuation Coefficient (dB/cm)	Penetration (cm)
2.0	1.0	30
3.5	1.8	17
5.0	2.5	12
7.5	3.8	8
10.0	5.0	6
15.0	7.5	4

which range from 2 to 20 MHz for most applications. Within this range, lower frequencies are used for deeper penetration and higher frequencies are used for superficial applications and invasive transducers (rectal, vaginal, and esophageal). Even higher frequencies (as high as 50 MHz) are used for some specialized applications, including skin and ophthalmologic imaging and intravascular imaging with catheter-mounted transducers. Frequencies less than 2 MHz are used in large-animal applications.

ECHOES

Ultrasound is useful as an imaging tool because of the reflection and scattering of sound waves at organ and tissue interfaces and scattering within heterogeneous tissues. The reflected and scattered sound waves produce the pattern of echoes that is necessary for diagnostic pulse-echo imaging with ultrasound. These phenomena are considered in this section. We consider two cases, perpendicular and oblique incidence. Perpendicular, considered first, is the simpler case, whereas oblique is in practice the more common case.

Perpendicular Incidence

Perpendicular incidence denotes a direction of travel of the ultrasound wave perpendicular to the boundary between two media (Figure 2-17). The incident sound may be reflected back into the first medium or transmitted into the second medium; most often, both occur. When there is perpendicular incidence, reflected sound travels back through the first medium in a direction opposite to the incident sound (i.e., the reflected sound returns to the sound source along the same path the incident took). In the case of perpendicular incidence, the transmitted sound does not change direction; it continues to move through the second medium in the same direction as the incident sound did in the first. The intensities of the reflected sound (the echo) and the transmitted sound depend on the incident intensity at the boundary and the impedances of the media on either side of the boundary.

Impedance

Impedance (z) determines how much of an incident sound wave is reflected back into the first medium and how much is transmitted into the second medium. Impedance is equal to the density (ρ) of a medium, multiplied by the propagation speed in it. Impedance increases if density increases or if propagation speed increases. Impedance units are rayls. The average soft tissue impedance is 1,630,000 rayls.

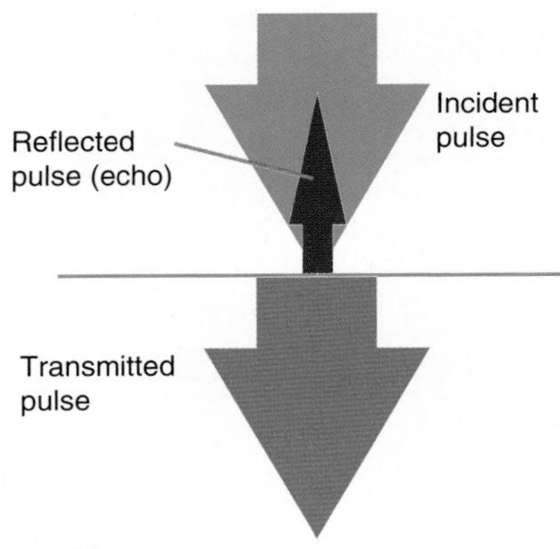

FIGURE 2-17 Reflection and transmission at a boundary with perpendicular incidence. The incident pulse is partially reflected (echo) with the remainder (transmitted pulse) continuing into the second medium. The strengths of the reflected and transmitted pulses are determined by the impedances of the two media at the boundary.

$$z\ (\text{rayls}) = \rho\ (\text{kg/m}^3) \times c\,(\text{m/s})$$

> Impedance increases if density increases or if propagation speed increases.

Dividing the reflected (echo) intensity by the incident intensity yields the fraction of the incident intensity that is reflected. This fraction is called the intensity reflection coefficient (IRC). For example, if the incident intensity (I_i) is 10 mW/cm^2 and echo, or reflected, intensity (I_r) is 1 mW/cm^2, the IRC is one tenth, or 0.1. In this case one tenth (10%) of the incident sound is reflected. Dividing the transmitted intensity (I_t) by the incident intensity yields the fraction of the incident intensity that is transmitted into the second medium. This fraction is called the intensity transmission coefficient (ITC). For example, if the incident intensity is 10 mW/cm^2 and the transmitted intensity is 9 mW/cm^2, the ITC is nine tenths, or 0.9. In this case nine tenths (90%) of the incident sound is transmitted into the second medium. The sum of the reflection and transmission coefficients must equal 1 (i.e., 100%) to account for all the incident sound intensity (what is not reflected at the boundary must be transmitted into the second medium). The two previous examples are really the same example, because if 10% of the sound is reflected back into the first medium, then 90% is transmitted into the second medium; that is, 100% of the incident sound arriving at the boundary is accounted for.

For perpendicular incidence, the reflection coefficient depends on the impedances as follows:

$$\text{IRC} = \frac{I_r(\text{W/cm}^2)}{I_i(\text{W/cm}^2)} = \left[\frac{(z_2 - z_1)}{(z_2 + z_1)}\right]^2$$

From this relationship between the reflection coefficient and the impedances, we see that the coefficient depends on the difference between the impedances. The greater the difference between the impedances, the stronger the echo. The greater the similarity of the impedances, the weaker the echo. If the media impedances are the same, the difference between them is zero, and there is no echo.

> If the difference between the impedances increases, the intensity reflection coefficient (and echo intensity) increases.

The transmission coefficient depends on the reflection coefficient as follows:

$$ITC = \frac{I_t(W/cm^2)}{I_i(W/cm^2)} = 1 - IRC$$

Because the coefficients must add up to 1 (100%), larger reflection coefficients mean smaller transmission coefficients, and vice versa. As you would expect, if more of the incident sound is reflected (stronger echo), less remains to travel into the second medium.

> If intensity reflection coefficient increases, the intensity transmission coefficient decreases.

If the impedances are equal, there is no echo, and the transmitted intensity is equal to incident intensity. This is what we expect: if no sound is reflected at a boundary, then all of it travels into the second medium as if there were no boundary. Conversely, we can conclude that if there is no reflection, the media impedances must be equal. If the impedances are equal, then there is no echo, and the transmitted intensity equals the incident intensity.

For perpendicular incidence and equal impedances, there is no reflection, and transmitted intensity equals the incident intensity. If a large difference exists between the impedances, there will be nearly total reflection (an intensity reflection coefficient close to 1, and an intensity transmission coefficient close to 0). An example of this is an air–soft tissue boundary. For this reason, a gel **coupling medium** is used to provide a good sound path from the transducer to the skin (eliminating the thin layer of air that would reflect the sound, preventing entrance of the sound into the body).

Example 2-5

For impedances of 40 and 60 rayls, determine the intensity reflection and transmission coefficients.

$$IRC = \left[\frac{(60-40)}{(60+40)}\right]^2 = \left(\frac{20}{100}\right)^2 = 0.2^2 = 0.2 \times 0.2 = 0.04$$

$$ITC = 1 - 0.04 = 0.96$$

In Example 2-5, the intensity reflection coefficient can be expressed as 4%, and the intensity transmission coefficient as 96%. The sum of the two coefficients is 100%, emphasizing the fact that all of the incident intensity must be reflected or transmitted.

If the incident intensity is known, the reflected and transmitted intensities can be calculated by multiplying the incident intensity by the intensity reflection coefficient and the intensity transmission coefficient, respectively.

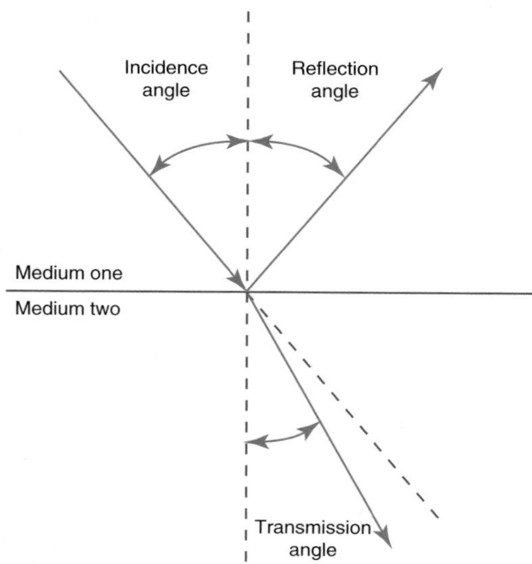

FIGURE 2-18 Reflection and transmission at a boundary with oblique incidence. Incidence and reflection angles are equal. The transmission angle depends on the incidence angle and the media propagation speeds.

Example 2-6

For Example 2-5, if the incident intensity is 10 mW/cm², calculate the reflected and transmitted intensities.

From Example 2-5, the intensity reflection and transmission coefficients are 0.04 and 0.96, respectively, thus

$$I_r = 10 \times 0.04 = 0.4\,mW/cm^2$$
$$I_t = 10 \times 0.96 = 9.6\,mW/cm^2$$

The coefficients give the fractions of the incident intensity that are reflected and transmitted. By multiplying the coefficients by 100, these fractions are expressed in percentages. Their sum must always equal 1 (or 100%). In Example 2-5, all of the incident intensity is accounted for (0.4 mW/cm² reflected, 9.6 mW/cm² transmitted, for a total of 10 mW/cm², or 100% of the incident intensity).

Oblique Incidence

Oblique incidence denotes a direction of travel of the incident ultrasound that is not perpendicular to the boundary between two media (Figure 2-18). This situation is common in diagnostic ultrasound. The direction of travel with respect to the boundary is given by the **incidence angle** (θ_i) as shown in Figure 2-18. In geometry, angles are measured from a line perpendicular to the surface. For perpendicular incidence, the incidence angle is zero. The reflected and transmitted directions are given by the **reflection angle** (θ_r) and

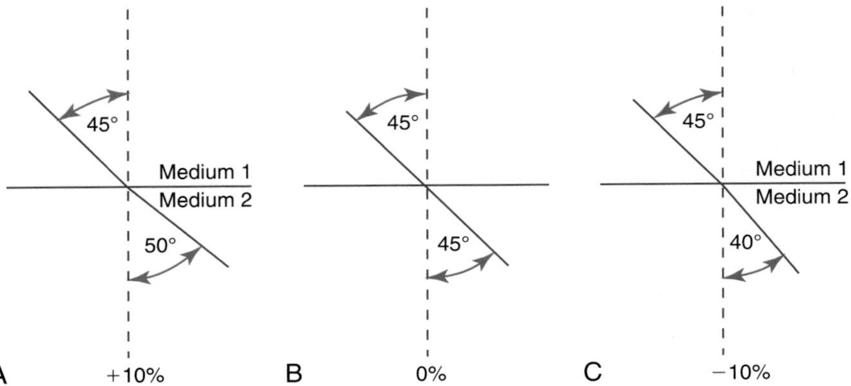

FIGURE 2-19 Transmission angles for an incidence angle of 45 degrees and propagation speeds through medium 2 that are 10% greater than (A), equal to (B), and 10% less than (C) propagation speed through medium 1.

transmission angle (θ_t), respectively. The incidence angle always equals the reflection angle.

$$\theta_i(\text{degrees}) = \theta_r(\text{degrees})$$

This phenomenon is also observed in optics (e.g., a laser beam reflecting off a mirror). The transmission angle depends on the propagation speeds in the media. Note that for oblique incidence, the reflected sound does not return to the transducer but travels off in some other direction.

Refraction

If the direction of sound changes when it crosses a boundary, it means that the transmission angle is different from the incidence angle. A change in the direction of sound when it crosses a boundary is called **refraction** (from the Latin term for *to turn aside*). If the propagation speed through the second medium is greater than through the first medium, then the transmission angle is greater than the incidence angle (Figure 2-19).

$$\text{If } c_1 < c_2, \text{then } \theta_i < \theta_t. \text{ If } c_1 > c_2, \text{then } \theta_i > \theta_t$$

The changes are approximately proportional. For example, if the speed increases by 1% when the sound enters the second medium, the transmission angle will be approximtely1% greater than the incidence angle. Similarly, if the speed in the second medium is less than in the first, the transmission angle is less than the incidence angle. No refraction occurs if the propagation speeds are equal. Also, if the incidence angle is zero (perpendicular incidence), there is no refraction, even though there may be different propagation speeds in the media. Thus the two requirements for refraction to occur are as follows:

1. Oblique incidence
2. Different propagation speed on either side of the boundary

Refraction is important because when it occurs, lateral position errors (refraction artifacts) occur on an image.

Example 2-7

If the incidence angle is 20 degrees, the propagation speed in the first medium is 1.7 mm/μs, and the propagation speed in the second medium is 1.6 mm/μs, what are the reflection and transmission angles? The incidence and reflection angles are always equal, thus the reflection angle is 20 degrees. The ratio of the media speeds is 1.6/1.7, which is equal to 0.94. This result indicates a 6% reduction in speed when the sound crosses the boundary. Because the speed decreases by 6%, the transmission angle is 6% less than the incidence angle, that is, 94% of the incidence angle (0.94 × 20 = 19 degrees).

Refraction occurs with light, sound, and any other type of wave. It is the principle on which lenses operate. Refraction is also the cause of the distorted view of objects seen in a fish bowl or swimming pool. As with sound, when light crosses a boundary obliquely and a change in the speed of the light occurs, the direction of the light changes.

Scattering

The discussion thus far has assumed that a boundary is flat and smooth. The resulting reflections are called *specular* (from the Latin term for *mirror-like*) reflections. If, however, the size of the reflecting object is comparable with that of the wavelength or smaller, or if a larger object does not have a smooth surface, the incident sound will be scattered. Scattering is the redirection of sound in many directions by rough surfaces or by heterogeneous media (Figure 2-20), such as (cellular) tissues, or particle suspensions, such as blood. These cases are analogous to light in which **specular reflections** occur at mirrors. But with rougher surfaces such as a white wall, light is scattered at the surface and mixed up while it travels back to the viewer's eyes. Therefore an observer does not see his or her reflected image when facing a wall. When light passes through fog, which is a suspension of water droplets in air, it is also scattered. This effect limits the viewer's ability to see through fog. Although scattering inhibits vision (we cannot see ourselves reflected in a wall, and we cannot see well through fog), it is of great benefit in sonographic imaging. Scattering benefits the goal of ultrasound, which is to see the "wall" (tissue interface) itself, not the reflection of "oneself" (the transducer in this case). The sonographer also desires to

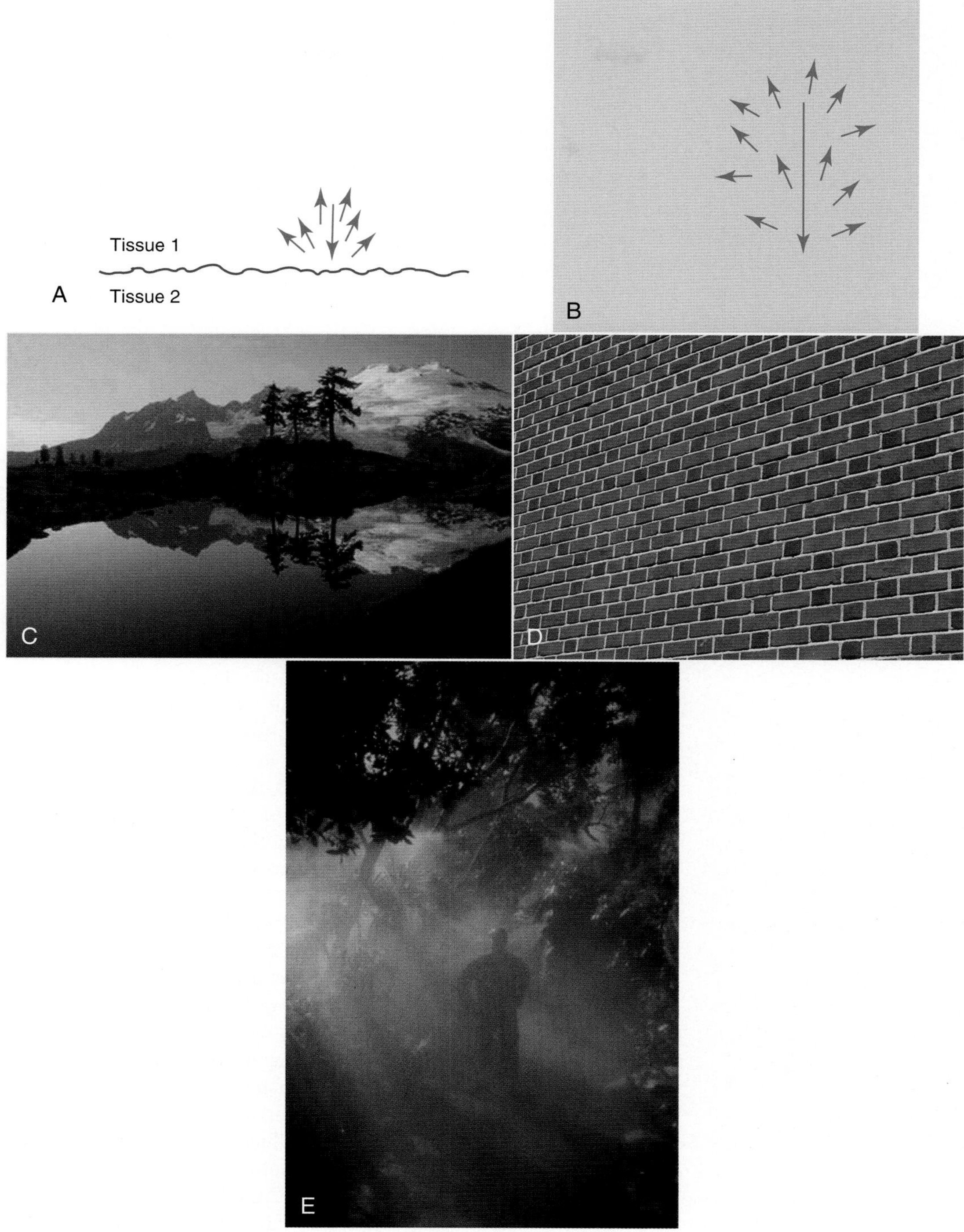

FIGURE 2-20 A sound pulse may be scattered by a rough boundary between tissues (**A**) or within tissues because of their heterogeneous character (**B**). The differences between a specular surface (smooth lake) (**C**), a scattering surface (brick wall) (**D**), and a scattering medium (fog) (**E**) are illustrated.

see the "fog" (tissue parenchyma) itself, not just the objects beyond it.

Backscatter (sound scattered back in the direction from which it originally came) intensities from rough surfaces and heterogeneous media vary with frequency and scatterer size. Normally, scatter intensities are less than boundary specular-reflection intensities, and they increase with increasing frequency. The intensity received by the sound source from specular reflections is highly angle dependent. Scattering from boundaries helps make echo reception less dependent on incidence angle. Unlike the reflection from specular boundaries, scattering permits ultrasound imaging of tissue

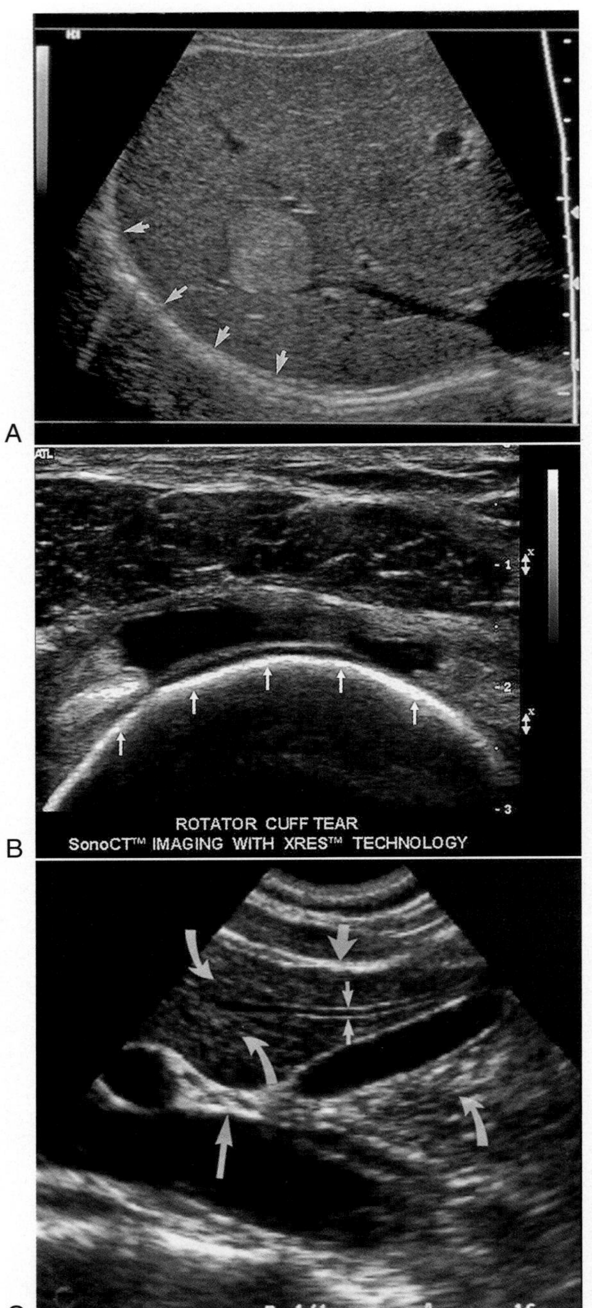

FIGURE 2-21 **A**, Longitudinal abdominal scan in which the diaphragm is imaged, even where it is not (*arrows*) perpendicular to the beam and scan lines. **B**, Strong echoes (*arrows*) from a tissue boundary. **C**, Abdominal scan showing echoes from tissue boundaries (*straight arrows*) and regions of scattering from within tissues (*curved arrows*), allowing parenchymal imaging.

boundaries that are not necessarily perpendicular to the direction of the incident sound (Figure 2-21, *A-B*). Scattering also allows for imaging of tissue parenchyma (Figure 2-21, *C*) in addition to organ boundaries. Scattering is relatively independent of the direction of the incident sound and therefore is more characteristic of the scatterers. Most surfaces in the body are rough for imaging purposes. Reflections from smooth boundaries (e.g., vessel intima) depend not only on the acoustic properties at the boundaries but also on the angles involved.

Speckle

An ultrasound pulse, with its finite length and width, simultaneously encounters many scatterers at any instant in its travel. Thus several echoes are generated simultaneously within the pulse while it interacts with these scatterers. The echoes may arrive at the transducer in such a way that they reinforce (**constructive interference**) or partially or totally cancel (**destructive interference**) each other (Figure 2-22, *A-B*). While the ultrasound beam is scanned through the tissues, with scatterers moving into and out of the beam, the **interference** alternates between being constructive and being destructive, resulting in a displayed dot pattern—a grainy appearance—that does not directly represent scatterers but, rather, represents the interference pattern of the scatterer distribution scanned. This phenomenon is called *acoustic speckle* and is similar to the speckle observed with lasers. **Speckle** is a form of acoustic noise in sonographic imaging (see Figure 2-22, *C*).

Contrast Agents

Liquid suspensions that can be injected into the circulation intravenously to increase echogenicity have been developed. These materials are called ultrasound **contrast agents**.[1,2] Contrast agents must be capable of easy administration, nontoxic, and stable for a sufficient examination time, small enough to pass through capillaries, and large enough and echogenic enough to improve sonography through an alteration in ultrasound–tissue interaction. Almost all agents contain microbubbles of gas that are stabilized by a protein, lipid, or polymer shell (although free gas microbubbles and solid particle suspensions have been used). These agents enhance echogenicity from vessels and perfused tissues in gray-scale sonography and Doppler ultrasound and "opacify" (fill normally anechoic regions with echoes) cardiac chambers (Figure 2-23). Contrast agents produce echoes because of the impedance mismatch between the suspended particles and the suspending medium (i.e., blood). Microbubbles in suspension are especially strong echo producers because the impedance of the gas is so much less than that of the suspending liquid. Bubbles also expand and contract unequally, that is, nonlinearly, under the influence of an ultrasound pulse, thus echoes that contain harmonics of the incident pulse frequency are produced. Because bubbles generate stronger harmonics than tissue, detecting harmonic frequency echoes increases the contrast between the contrast agent and the surrounding tissue. This is called *contrast harmonic imaging* or *harmonic contrast imaging.* Encapsulation of the gas slows its diffusion back into the solution, lengthening the duration of the contrast effect. To further slow diffusion out of an encapsulated bubble, low-solubility gases such as perfluorocarbons are used. Three agents are currently approved for clinical cardiac use (left ventricular opacification and endocardial border detection) in the United States: (1) Definity (octafluoropropane-containing liposomes), (2) Imagent (dimyristoyl lecithin), and (3) Optison (perfluoropropane-filled albumin). In addition to these, other agents—such as Sonazoid, Levovist, and SonoVue—are

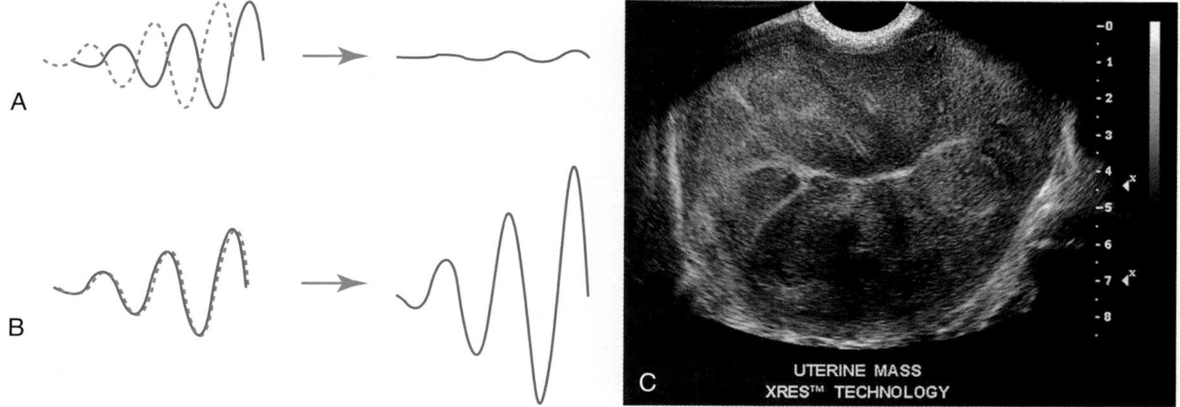

FIGURE 2-22 A, Two similar echoes with slightly different arrival times sum to a nearly zero amplitude (destructive interference). B, Two similar echoes arriving nearly simultaneously sum to nearly double amplitude (constructive interference). C, Speckle, the grainy appearance of the tissues, is seen in this image.

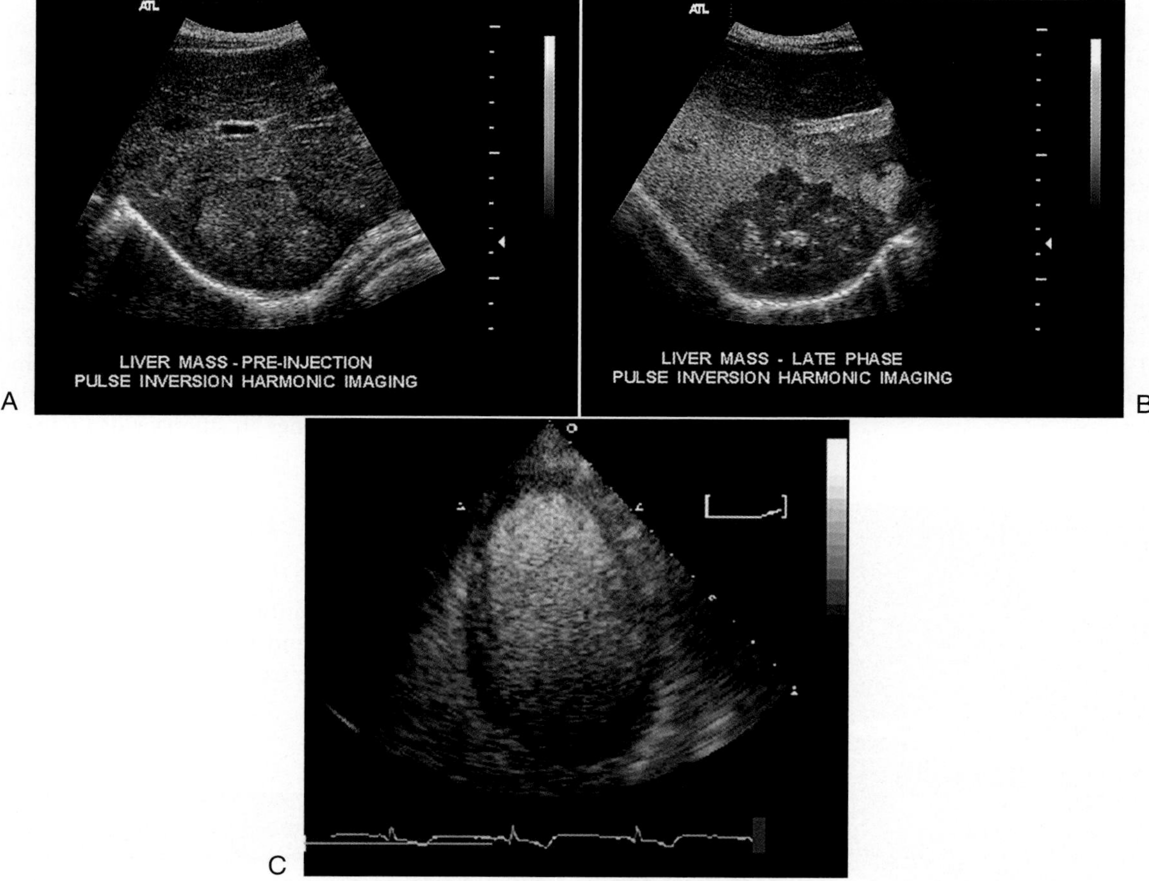

FIGURE 2-23 Contrast agents enhance echogenicity from perfused tissues. Liver mass before (A) and after (B) injection of the contrast agent. The agent has perfused the normal tissue better than the mass, yielding an improved contrast difference between normal and mass. C, Left ventricular "opacification" with a contrast agent.

approved for use in Canada, Europe, and Japan. Contrast agents improve (1) lesion detection when lesion echogenicity is similar to that of the surrounding tissue, (2) lesion characterization by showing both the arterial and portal phases of the agent in real time, and (3) Doppler ultrasound detection when Doppler signals are weak (deep, slow, and small-vessel flows), often rescuing an otherwise failed examination. Ultrasound pulses of sufficiently high pressure amplitude can fragment the bubbles, allowing the gas to dissolve and eliminating the contrast effect. Subsequent lower-amplitude imaging then can show the return of the contrast effect, thus giving an indication of tissue or organ perfusion rate.

Range

Now that sound propagation, reflection, and scattering have been considered, we can discuss an important aspect of sonography: the determination of the distance (range) from the transducer to an echo-generating structure and thus the appropriate location for each echo's placement on its scan line. To position the echoes properly on the display, the following two items of information are required:

1. The direction from which the echo came (which is assumed to be the direction in which the emitted pulse is launched).
2. The distance to the **reflector** or scatterer where the echo was produced.

With regard to point 2, the instrument cannot measure distance directly; rather, it measures travel time and determines the distance from it. Similarly, directly measuring the distance between two cities would be inconvenient (a long measuring tape would be required), but we could determine the distance by asking someone to drive from one city to the other and observe the time required. Of course, we would not know when the person arrived at the other city if we were not a passenger in the car, so we would instruct the driver to return immediately after arriving at the destination (Figure 2-24) to give us that information. Let us say that the round trip took exactly 4 hours. What was the distance traveled? We, of course, cannot determine the answer unless we know the speed traveled. If the driver was traveling at a speed of exactly 50 mph for the entire round trip (a difficult achievement), then we can determine that the distance traveled was 200 miles (50 mph × 4 hours). Therefore the distance to the city is 100 miles. Note that the total distance was halved because round-trip travel time was used to determine the one-way distance.

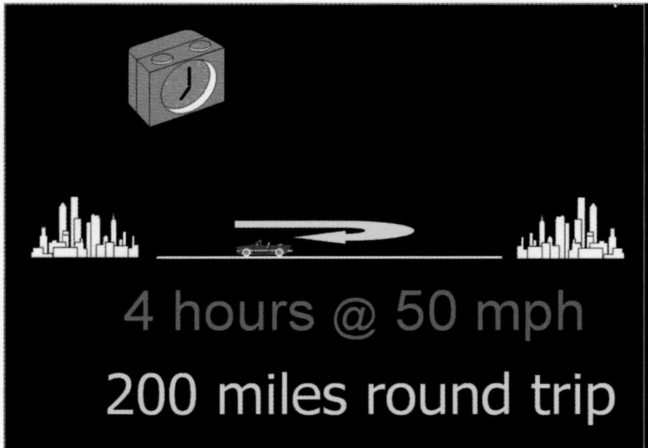

FIGURE 2-24 The distance between two cities can be determined by making a round trip by car. Multiplying the speed of travel by one half of the round-trip travel time yields the distance between the cities. If the speed is 50 mph and the round-trip travel time is 4 hours, the distance between the cities is 100 miles. In this example, the round-trip distance traveled is 200 miles, obtained by multiplying the speed (50 mph) by the elapsed travel time (4 hours).

Thus the distance (d) to a reflector is calculated from the propagation speed and pulse round-trip travel time (t) according to the following **range equation**:

$$d\,(\text{mm}) = \frac{1}{2}[c\,(\text{mm}/\mu\text{s}) \times t\,(\mu\text{s})]$$

> While round-trip time increases, calculated reflector distance increases.

To determine the distance from the source to the reflector, the propagation speed in the intervening medium must be known or assumed, and the pulse round-trip time must be measured. The reason that the factor one half appears is that the round-trip time is the time for the pulse to travel to and return from the reflector. However, only the distance to the reflector is the desired information. The average propagation speed in soft tissue (1.54 mm/μs) is assumed in using the range equation. Because multiplying 1.54 by one half yields 0.77, the distance (millimeters) to the reflector can be calculated by multiplying 0.77 by the round-trip time (microseconds).

In the problem that involves determining the distance between cities, 50 mph is equivalent to 0.83 mile/min or 1.20 min/mile. Thus, at this speed, 2.4 minutes of round-trip travel are required for each mile of distance separating the cities. Similarly, sound speed in tissue is 1.54 mm/μs, so 0.65 μs is required for each millimeter of travel. Thus 6.5 μs are required for 1 cm of travel. Therefore 13 μs of round-trip travel time are required for each centimeter of distance from the transducer to the reflector. To confirm this, substitution of 13 μs for t in the foregoing range equation yields a reflector distance of 10 mm (1 cm).

$$d = \frac{1}{2}(c \times t) = \frac{1}{2}(1.54 \times 13) = \frac{1}{2}(20) = 10\,\text{mm} = 1\,\text{cm}$$

All of this information leads to the important 13 μs/cm rule: the pulse round-trip travel time is 13 μs for each centimeter of distance from source to reflector (Table 2-6;

TABLE 2-6 Pulse Round-Trip Travel Time for Various Reflector Depths

Depth (cm)	Travel Time (μs)
0.5	6.5
1	13
2	26
3	39
4	52
5	65
10	130
15	195
20	260

Figure 2-25). Figure 2-26 illustrates the correspondence between echo arrival time and reflector depth.

Example 2-8

If an echo returns 104 µs after a pulse was emitted by a transducer, at what depth is the echo-producing structure located?

With the range equation:

$$d(mm) = 0.77\,mm/\mu s \times 104\,\mu s = 80\,mm = 8.0\,cm$$

With the 13 µs/cm rule:

$$d(mm) = \frac{104\,\mu s}{13\,\mu s/cm} = 8\,cm$$

Table 2-7 gives common values for several parameters of sonography. Table 2-8 summarizes how various parameters change with frequency.

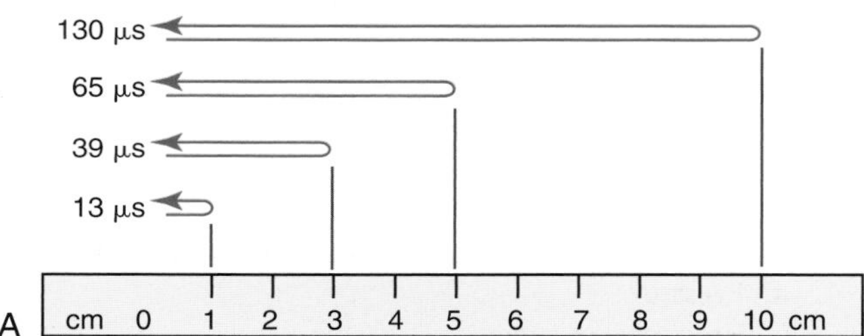

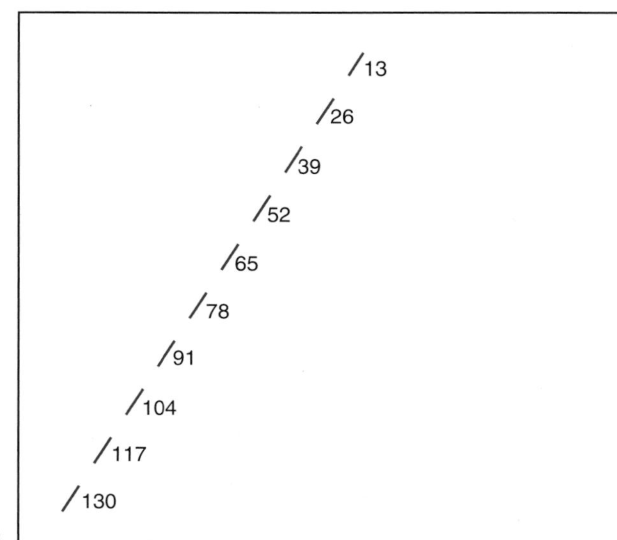

FIGURE 2-25 A, Echo arrival times for 1-, 3-, 5-, and 10-cm reflector distances. B, Echoes from 1-, 2-, 3-, 4-, 5-, 6-, 7-, 8-, 9-, and 10-cm depths arrive at the times (microseconds) indicated.

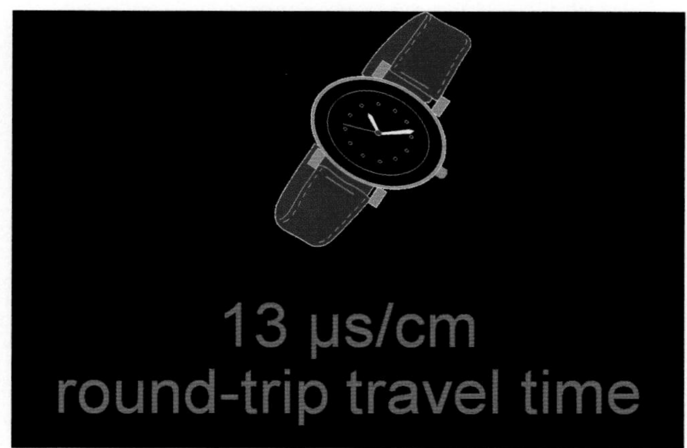

FIGURE 2-26 Substituting the average speed of sound in soft tissues into the range equation yields the 13 µs/cm round-trip travel time rule.

TABLE 2-7 Sonographic Parameters in Tissue

	SYMBOL OR RANGE OF PARAMETER	
	Abbreviation	**Common Values**
Frequency	f	2-20 MHz
Period	T	0.05-0.5 µs
Wavelength	λ	0.08-0.8 mm
Propagation speed	c	1.44-1.64 mm/µs
Impedance	z	1,300,000-1,700,000 rayls
Pulse-repetition frequency	PRF	4-15 kHz
Pulse-repetition period	PRP	0.07-0.25 ms
Cycles per pulse	n	1-3
Pulse duration	PD	0.1-1.5 µs
Spatial pulse length	SPL	0.1-2.5 mm
Duty factor	DF	0.1%– 1%
Pressure amplitude	p	0.1-4 MPa
Intensity*	I_{SPTA}	0.01-100 mW/cm^2
Attenuation coefficient	a_c	1-10 dB/cm

*Spatial-peak, temporal average.

TABLE 2-8 Dependence of Various Factors on Increasing (↑) Frequency

Symbol or Dependence Parameter	Abbreviation	↑ Increase ↓ Decrease
Period	T	↓
Wavelength	λ	↓
Pulse duration	PD	↓
Spatial pulse length	SPL	↓
Attenuation	a	↑
Penetration	pen	↓

REVIEW

The following key points are presented in this chapter:

- Sound is a wave of pressure and density variations and particle vibration.
- Ultrasound is sound that has a frequency greater than 20 kHz.
- Frequency denotes the number of cycles occurring in 1 second.
- Harmonic frequencies are generated while sound travels through tissue.
- Wavelength is the length of a cycle in space.
- Propagation speed is the speed of sound through a medium.
- The medium determines propagation speed.
- The average propagation speed of sound through soft tissue is 1.54 mm/μs.
- Pulsed ultrasound is described by PRF, PRP, PD, DF, and SPL.
- Amplitude and intensity describe the strength of sound.
- Attenuation is the weakening of sound caused by absorption, reflection, and scattering.
- Attenuation increases with frequency and path length.
- The average attenuation coefficient for soft tissues is 0.5 dB/cm for each megahertz of frequency.
- Imaging depth decreases with increasing frequency.
- Impedance is the density of a medium multiplied by propagation speed.
- When sound encounters boundaries between media with different impedances, part of the sound is reflected and part is transmitted.
- With perpendicular incidence, and if the two media have the same impedance, there is no reflection.
- The greater the difference in the impedances of the media at a boundary, the greater is the intensity of the echo that is generated at the boundary.
- With oblique incidence, the sound is refracted at a boundary between media for which propagation speeds are different.
- Incidence and reflection angles at a boundary are always equal.
- Scattering occurs at rough media boundaries and within heterogeneous media.
- Contrast agents are used to enhance echogenicity in sonography and Doppler ultrasound.
- Pulse-echo round-trip travel time (13 μs/cm) is used to determine the distance to a reflector.

EXERCISES

Answers appear in the Answers to Exercises section at the back of the book.

1. A wave is a traveling variation in quantities called *wave* __________
   a. lengths
   b. variables
   c. cycles
   d. periods
2. Sound is a traveling variation in quantities called __________ variables.
   a. wave
   b. pressure
   c. density
   d. acoustic
3. Ultrasound is sound with a frequency greater than __________ Hz.
   a. 2
   b. 15
   c. 20,000
   d. 1540
4. Acoustic variables include __________, __________, and particle motion.
   a. stiffness, density
   b. hardness, impedance
   c. amplitude, intensity
   d. pressure, density
5. Which of the following frequencies is in the ultrasound range?
   a. 15 Hz
   b. 15,000 Hz
   c. 15 kHz
   d. 30,000 Hz
   e. 0.004 MHz
6. Which of the following is *not* an acoustic variable?
   a. Pressure
   b. Propagation speed
   c. Density
   d. Particle motion
7. Frequency is the number of __________ an acoustic variable goes through in a second.
   a. cycles
   b. amplitudes
   c. pulse lengths
   d. DFs
8. The unit of frequency is __________, which is abbreviated __________.
   a. hertz, Hz
   b. megahertz, mHz
   c. kilohurts, khts
   d. cycles, cps
9. Period is the __________ that it takes for one cycle to occur.
   a. length
   b. amplitude
   c. time
   d. height
10. Period decreases while __________ increases.
   a. wavelength
   b. pulse length
   c. frequency
   d. bandwidth

11. Wavelength is the length of __________ over which one cycle occurs.
    a. time
    b. space
    c. propagation
    d. power
12. Propagation speed is the speed with which a(n) __________ moves through a medium.
    a. wave
    b. particle
    c. frequency
    d. attenuation
13. Wavelength is equal to __________ __________ divided by __________.
    a. propagation speed, frequency
    b. media density, stiffness
    c. pulse length, frequency
    d. wave amplitude, period
14. The __________ and __________ of a medium determine propagation speed.
    a. amplitude, intensity
    b. wavelength, period
    c. impedance, attenuation
    d. density, stiffness
15. Propagation speed increases if __________ is increased.
    a. amplitude
    b. frequency
    c. density
    d. stiffness
16. The average propagation speed in soft tissues is __________ m/s or __________ mm/μs.
    a. 10, 3
    b. 1540, 1.54
    c. 3, 10
    d. 1.54, 1540
17. Propagation speed is determined by the ________.
    a. frequency
    b. amplitude
    c. wavelength
    d. medium
18. Place the following classifications of matter in order of increasing sound propagation speed.
    a. gas, solid, liquid
    b. solid, liquid, gas
    c. gas, liquid, solid
    d. liquid, solid, gas
19. The wavelength of 7-MHz ultrasound in soft tissues is __________ mm.
    a. 1.54
    b. 0.54
    c. 0.22
    d. 3.33
20. Wavelength in soft tissues __________ while frequency increases.
    a. is constant
    b. decreases
    c. increases
    d. weakens
21. It takes __________ μs for ultrasound to travel 1.54 cm in soft tissue.
    a. 10
    b. 0.77
    c. 154
    d. 100
22. Propagation speed in bone is __________ that in soft tissues.
    a. lower than
    b. equal to
    c. higher than
    d. 10 m/s greater than
23. Sound travels fastest in __________.
    a. air
    b. helium
    c. water
    d. steel
24. Solids have higher propagation speeds than liquids because they have greater __________.
    a. density
    b. stiffness
    c. attenuation
    d. propagation
25. Sound travels most slowly in __________.
    a. gases
    b. liquids
    c. tissue
    d. bone
26. Sound is a __________ __________ wave.
    a. mechanical expressional
    b. electromagnetic transverse
    c. electromagnetic longitudinal
    d. mechanical longitudinal
27. If propagation speed is doubled (a different medium) and frequency is held constant, the wavelength is __________.
    a. decreased
    b. doubled
    c. halved
    d. unchanged
29. If frequency in soft tissue is doubled, propagation speed is __________.
    a. decreased
    b. doubled
    c. halved
    d. unchanged
30. If wavelength is 2 mm and frequency is doubled, the wavelength becomes __________ mm.
    a. 4
    b. 1
    c. 2.5
    d. unchanged
30. Waves can carry __________ from one place to another.
    a. information
    b. density
    c. impedance
    d. speed

31. From given values for propagation speed and frequency, ____________ can be calculated.
a. amplitude
b. impedance
c. wavelength
d. intensity

32. If two media have different stiffnesses, the one with the higher stiffness will have the higher propagation speed. True or false?

33. The second harmonic of 3 MHz is ____________ MHz.
a. 2
b. 3.2
c. 6
d. 9

34. Odd harmonics of 2 MHz are ____________ MHz.
a. 1, 3, 5
b. 2, 4, 6
c. 6, 9, 12
d. 6, 10, 14
e. 10, 12, 14

35. Even harmonics of 2 MHz are ____________ MHz.
a. 1, 3, 5
b. 2, 4, 6
c. 4, 8, 12
d. 6, 10, 14
e. 10, 12, 14

36. Nonlinear propagation means that ____________.
a. the sound beam does not travel in a straight line
b. propagation speed depends on frequency
c. harmonics are not generated
d. the waveform changes shape while it travels

37. In nonlinear propagation, additional frequencies appear that are ____________ and ____________ multiples of the fundamental frequency. They are called ____________.
a. double, triple, harmonics
b. double, triple, subharmonics
c. odd, even, harmonics
d. odd, even, subharmonics

38. If the density of a medium is 1000 kg/m^3 and the propagation speed is 1540 m/s, the impedance is ____________ rayls.
a. 1540
b. 2540
c. 540
d. 1,540,000

39. If two media have the same propagation speed but different densities, the one with the higher density will have the higher impedance. True or false?

40. If two media have the same density but different propagation speeds, the one with the higher propagation speed will have the higher impedance. True or false?

41. Impedance is ____________ multiplied by ____________.
a. density, propagation speed
b. frequency, oblique incidence
c. wavelength, propagation speed
d. attenuation, PD

42. The abbreviation *CW* stands for ____________.
a. corrected waveform
b. continuous window
c. continuous wave
d. contrast waveform

43. PRF is the number of ____________ occurring in 1 second.
a. cycles
b. pulses
c. periods
d. wavelengths

44. Pulse-repetition ____________ is the time from the beginning of one pulse to the beginning of the next.
a. frequency
b. time
c. duration
d. period

45. The PRP ____________ while PRF increases.
a. increases
b. decreases
c. is unchanged
d. is undetermined

46. PD is the ____________ it takes for a pulse to occur.
a. frequency
b. time
c. duration
d. period

47. SPL is the ____________ of ____________ that a pulse occupies while it travels.
a. length, time
b. length, space
c. amount, amplitude
d. intensity, energy

48. ____________ ____________ is the fraction of time that pulsed ultrasound is actually on.
a. PD
b. Pulse intensity
c. DF
d. Duty frequency

49. PD equals the number of cycles in the pulse multiplied by ____________.
a. frequency
b. period
c. wavelength
d. amplitude

50. SPL equals the number of cycles in the pulse multiplied by ____________.
a. frequency
b. period
c. wavelength
d. amplitude

51. The DF of continuous wave sound is ____________.
a. 1
b. undefined
c. 1540
d. 10

52. If the wavelength is 2 mm, the SPL for a three-cycle pulse is ___________ mm.
a. 6
b. 0.6
c. 0.4
d. 1

53. The SPL in soft tissue for a two-cycle pulse of frequency 5 MHz is ___________ mm.
a. 6
b. 0.6
c. 0.4
d. 1

54. The PD in soft tissue for a two-cycle pulse of frequency 5 MHz is ___________ μs.
a. 6
b. 0.6
c. 0.4
d. 1

55. For a 1-kHz PRF, the PRP is ___________ ms.
a. 6
b. 0.6
c. 0.4
d. 1

56. For Exercises 54 and 55 together, the DF is ___________.
a. 0.0004
b. 0.004
c. 0.04
d. 0.4

57. How many cycles are there in 1 second of continuous wave 5-MHz ultrasound?
a. 5
b. 500
c. 5000
d. 5,000,000
e. None of the above

58. How many cycles are there in 1 second of pulsed 5-MHz ultrasound with a DF of 0.01 (1%)?
a. 5
b. 500
c. 5000
d. 5,000,000
e. None of the above

59. In Exercise 58, how many cycles did pulsing eliminate?
a. 100%
b. 99.9%
c. 99%
d. 50%
e. 1%

60. For pulsed ultrasound, the DF is always ___________ ___________ 1.
a. less than
b. greater than
c. equal to

61. ___________ is a typical DF for sonography.
a. 0.1
b. 0.5
c. 0.7
d. 0.9

62. Amplitude is the maximum ___________ that occurs in an acoustic variable.
a. time
b. variation
c. distance
d. frequency

63. Intensity is the ___________ in a wave divided by ___________.
a. amplitude, power
b. area, power
c. power, amplitude
d. power, area

64. A unit for intensity is ___________.
a. mW/cm^2
b. mHz/cm^2
c. cm/MHz
d. mm/cm^2

65. Intensity is proportional to ___________ squared.
a. mW
b. watts
c. attenuation
d. amplitude

66. If power is doubled and area remains unchanged, intensity is ___________.
a. unchanged
b. halved
c. doubled
d. quadrupled

67. If area is doubled and power remains unchanged, intensity is ___________.
a. unchanged
b. halved
c. doubled
d. quadrupled

68. If both power and area are doubled, intensity is ___________.
a. unchanged
b. halved
c. doubled
d. quadrupled

69. If amplitude is doubled, intensity is ___________.
a. unchanged
b. halved
c. doubled
d. quadrupled

70. If a sound beam has a power of 10 mW and a beam area of 2 cm^2, the spatial average intensity is ___________ mW/cm^2.
a. 10
b. 2
c. 20
d. 5

71. Attenuation is the reduction in ___________ and ___________ as a wave travels through a medium.
a. amplitude, intensity
b. amplitude, wavelength
c. intensity, speed
d. amplitude, speed

72. Attenuation consists of ___________, ___________, and ___________.
 a. amplitude, intensity, power
 b. amplitude, wavelength, power
 c. absorption, reflection, scattering
 d. scattering, amplitude, speed
73. The attenuation coefficient is attenuation per ___________ of sound travel.
 a. second
 b. centimeter
 c. cycle
 d. wavelength
74. Attenuation and the attenuation coefficient are given in units of ___________ and ___________, respectively.
 a. dB, dB/cm
 b. mW/cm^2
 c. dB, dB/cm^2
 d. dB^2, mW
75. For soft tissues, there is approximately ___________ dB of attenuation per centimeter for each megahertz of frequency.
 a. 1.54
 b. 3
 c. 5
 d. 0.5
76. For soft tissues, the attenuation coefficient at 3 MHz is approximately ___________.
 a. 15 dB/cm
 b. 3 dB
 c. 1.5 dB/cm
 d. 15 dB
77. The attenuation coefficient in soft tissue _______ while frequency increases.
 a. increases
 b. decreases
 c. weakens
 d. decelerates
78. For soft tissue, if frequency is doubled, attenuation is ___________. If path length is doubled, attenuation is ___________. If both frequency and path length are doubled, attenuation is ___________.
 a. doubled, doubled, quadrupled
 b. doubled, doubled, doubled
 c. doubled, quadrupled, quadrupled
 d. quadrupled, quadrupled, quadrupled
79. If frequency is doubled and path length is halved, attenuation is ___________.
 a. doubled
 b. halved
 c. quadrupled
 d. unchanged
80. Absorption is the conversion of ___________ to ___________.
 a. energy, amplitude
 b. heat, sound
 c. sound, heat
 d. sound, intensity
81. Absorption can be greater than attenuation in a given medium at a given frequency. True or false?
82. Attenuation is higher in bone than in soft tissue. True or false?
83. The imaging depth (penetration) ___________ while frequency increases.
 a. increases
 b. decreases
 c. is unchanged
 d. is undetermined
84. If the intensity of 4-MHz ultrasound entering soft tissue is 2 W/cm^2, the intensity at a depth of 4 cm is ___________ W/cm^2.
 a. 0.16
 b. 0.32
 c. 0.48
 d. 0.64
85. If the intensity of 40-MHz ultrasound entering soft tissue is 2 W/cm^2, the intensity at a depth of 4 cm is ___________ W/cm^2.
 a. 0.00002
 b. 0.000002
 c. 0.0000002
 d. 0.00000002
86. The depth at which half-intensity occurs in soft tissues at 7.5 MHz is ___________.
 a. 0.6 cm
 b. 0.7 cm
 c. 0.8 cm
 d. 0.9 cm
87. When ultrasound encounters a boundary with perpendicular incidence, the ___________ of the tissues must be different to produce a reflection (echo).
 a. impedances
 b. densities
 c. speeds
 d. hardnesses
88. With perpendicular incidence, two media ___________ and the incident ___________ must be known to calculate the reflected intensity.
 a. impedances, amplitude
 b. amplitudes, impedance
 c. impedances, intensity
 d. amplitudes, intensity
89. With perpendicular incidence, two media ___________ must be known to calculate the intensity reflection coefficient.
 a. densities
 b. speeds
 c. hardnesses
 e. impedances
90. For an incident intensity of 2 mW/cm^2 and impedances of 49 and 51 rayls, the reflected intensity is ___________ mW/cm^2, and the transmitted intensity is ___________ mW/cm^2.
 a. 0.8, 1.2
 b. 0.08, 1.92

c. 0.008, 1.992
d. 0.0008, 1.9992

91. If the impedances of the media are equal, there is no reflection. True or false?

92. With perpendicular incidence, the reflected intensity depends on the ___________.
a. density difference
b. impedance difference
c. impedance sum
d. b and c
e. a and b

93. Refraction is a change in ___________ of sound when it crosses a boundary. Refraction is caused by a change in ___________ ___________ at the boundary.
a. speed, sound direction
b. direction, propagation speed
c. amplitude, media impedance
d. direction, media attenuation

94. Under what two conditions does refraction *not* occur?
a. perpendicular incidence or equal media propagation speeds
b. oblique incidence or equal media propagation speeds
c. perpendicular incidence or unequal media propagation speeds
d. oblique incidence or unequal media propagation speeds

95. The low speed of sound in fat is a source of image degradation because of refraction. If the incidence angle at a boundary between fat (1.45 mm/μs) and kidney (1.56 mm/μs) is 30 degrees, the transmission angle is ___________ degrees.
a. 28
b. 30
c. 32
d. 33

96. Reflection of sound in many directions while it encounters rough media junctions or particle suspensions (heterogeneous media) is called _________.
a. specular
b. refraction
c. propagation
d. scattering

97. Backscatter helps make echo reception less dependent on incident angle. True or false?

98. What must be known to calculate the distance to a reflector?
a. Attenuation, speed, and density
b. Attenuation and impedance
c. Attenuation and absorption
d. Travel time and speed
e. Density and speed

99. No reflection will occur with perpendicular incidence if the media ___________ are equal.
a. impedances
b. speeds
c. densities
d. attenuations

100. Scattering occurs at smooth boundaries and within homogeneous media. True or false?

3

Transducers

LEARNING OBJECTIVES

After reading this chapter, the student should be able to do the following:

- Describe the construction of a transducer and the function of each part.
- Explain how a transducer generates ultrasound pulses.
- Explain how a transducer receives echoes.
- Describe a sound beam and list the factors that affect it.
- Discuss how sound beams are focused and automatically scanned through anatomy.
- Compare linear, convex, phased, and vector arrays.
- Define detail resolution.
- Differentiate among the three aspects of detail resolution.
- List the factors that determine detail resolution.

OUTLINE

KEY TERMS

Aperture
Apodization
Array
Axial
Axial resolution
Beam
Composite
Convex array
Crystal
Curie point
Damping
Detail resolution
Disk
Dynamic aperture
Dynamic focusing
Element
Elevational resolution
Far zone
Focal length
Focal region
Focal zone
Focus
Grating lobes
Lateral
Lateral resolution
Lead zirconate titanate
Lens
Linear
Linear array
Linear phased array
Linear sequenced array
Matching layer
Natural focus
Near zone
Operating frequency
Phased array
Phased linear array
Piezoelectricity
Probe
Resolution
Resonance frequency
Scanhead
Sector
Sensitivity
Side lobes
Sound beam
Source
Transducer
Transducer assembly
Ultrasound transducer
Vector array

This chapter describes transducers, the devices that generate and receive ultrasound. Transducers form the connecting link between the ultrasound–tissue interactions described in Chapter 2 and the instruments described in Chapters 4 and 5. The sound produced by these transducers is confined in beams rather than traveling in all directions away from the source. These beams are focused and are automatically scanned through tissue by the transducers.

CONSTRUCTION AND OPERATION

A transducer converts one form of energy to another. Ultrasound transducers (Figure 3-1) convert electric energy into ultrasound energy, and vice versa. The electric voltages applied to transducers are converted to ultrasound. Ultrasound echoes incident on the transducers produce electric voltages. Loudspeakers (Figure 3-2, *A*), microphones (see Figure 3-2, *B*), and intercoms accomplish similar functions with audible sound.

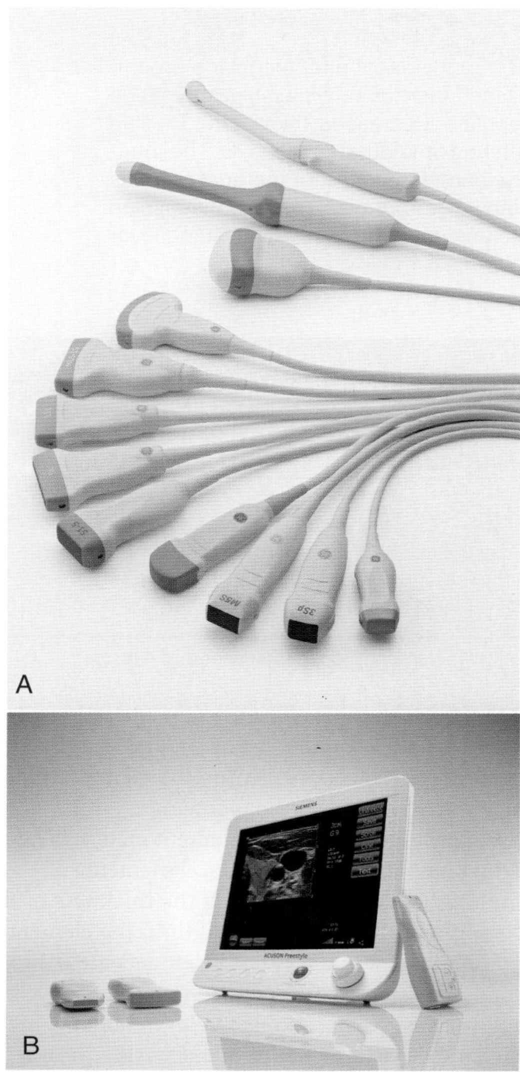

FIGURE 3-1 A, Transducers of various types. B, Cable-free transducers are commercially available. (A, Courtesy of GE Healthcare, B, Courtesy of Siemens Healthcare.)

Some transducers include internally some parts of the electronics that are otherwise located in the instrument.

Piezoelectric Element

Ultrasound transducers operate according to the principle of piezoelectricity. The word piezoelectricity is derived from the Greek word *piezo,* meaning "to press," and *elektron,* meaning "amber," the organic plant resin that was used in early studies of electricity. This principle states that some materials, when deformed by an applied pressure, produce a voltage. Conversely, piezoelectricity also results in the production of a pressure when an applied voltage deforms these materials. Various formulations of lead zirconate titanate are used commonly as materials in the production of modern ultrasound transducer elements. Ceramics such as these are not naturally piezoelectric. They are made piezoelectric during their manufacture by being placed in a strong electric field while they are at a high temperature. If a critical temperature (the Curie point) subsequently is exceeded, the element will lose its piezoelectric properties. These ceramics often are combined with a nonpiezoelectric polymer to create materials called *piezo-composites.* These composites have lower impedance and improved bandwidth, sensitivity, and resolution.

> Piezoelectric elements convert electric voltages into ultrasound pulses and convert returning echoes back into voltages.

Single-element transducers take the form of disks (Figure 3-3, *A*). Linear array transducers contain numerous elements that have a rectangular shape (see Figure 3-3, *B*). When an electric voltage is applied to the faces of either type, the thickness of the element increases or decreases, depending on the polarity of the voltage (see Figure 3-3, *C*). The term *transducer element* (also called *piezoelectric element, active element,* or *crystal*) refers to the piece of piezoelectric material (see Figure 3-3, *D*) that converts electricity to ultrasound, and vice versa. Elements, with their associated case and damping and matching materials (see Figure 3-3, *E*), are called a *transducer assembly,* probe, scanhead, or, simply, *transducer.*

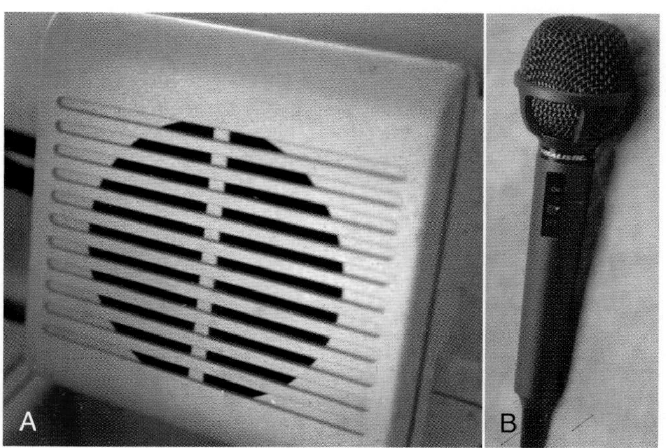

FIGURE 3-2 A, Loudspeaker. B, Microphone.

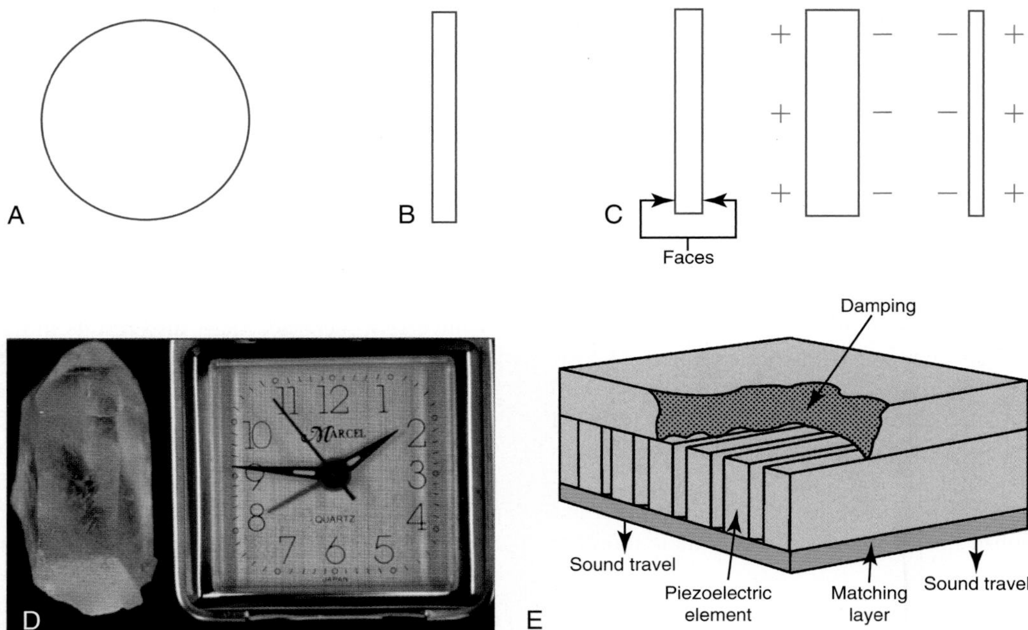

FIGURE 3-3 A, Front view of a disk transducer element. **B**, Front view of a rectangular element. **C**, Side view of either element with no voltage applied to faces (normal thickness), with voltage applied (increased thickness), and with opposite voltage applied (decreased thickness). **D**, Thin slices of quartz crystals (*left*) are used in electric clocks, watches, and other devices. E, The internal parts of a transducer assembly (scanhead or probe). The damping (backing) material reduces pulse duration, thus improving axial resolution. The matching layer improves sound transmission into the tissues. *Note:* Not included in this illustration are a lens and a protective/insulating layer that commonly are attached to the front of the assembly.

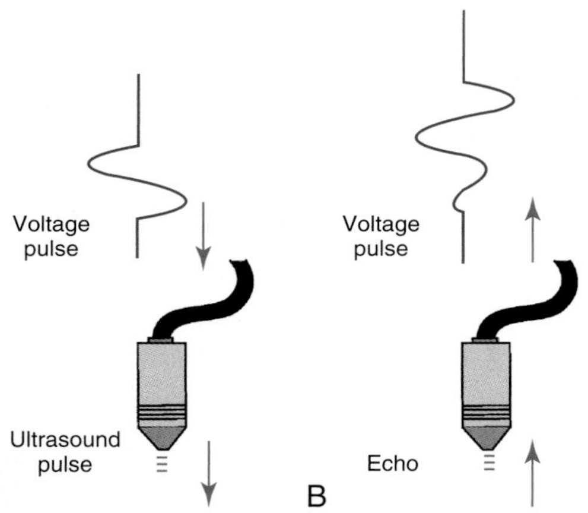

FIGURE 3-4 A transducer converts electric voltage pulses into ultrasound pulses (**A**) and converts received echoes into electric voltage pulses (**B**).

TABLE 3-1 Transducer Element Thickness* for Various Operating Frequencies

Frequency (MHz)	Thickness (mm)
2.0	1.0
3.5	0.6
5.0	0.4
7.5	0.3
10.0	0.2

*Assuming an element propagation speed of 4 mm/μs.

Transducers typically are driven by one cycle of alternating voltage for sonographic imaging. This single-cycle–driving voltage produces a two- or three-cycle ultrasound pulse. Longer-driving voltages, typically 5 to 30 cycles, are used for Doppler techniques. This operation produces an alternating pressure that propagates from the transducer as a sound pulse (Figure 3-4, *A*). The frequency of the sound produced is equal to the frequency of the driving voltage, which must be reasonably near the **operating frequency** (f_o) of the transducer for operation with acceptable efficiency. The operating frequency (sometimes called **resonance frequency**) is the preferred, or natural, frequency of operation for the element. Operating frequency is determined by the following:

- The propagation speed of the element material (c_t).
- The thickness (*th*) of the transducer element.

Operating frequency is such that the thickness of the element corresponds to half a wavelength in the element material. Typical diagnostic ultrasound elements are 0.2 to 1 mm thick (Table 3-1) and have propagation speeds of 4 to 6 mm/μs. Because wavelength decreases while frequency increases, thinner elements yield higher frequencies (Figure 3-5). This is analogous to smaller bells producing higher-pitched sounds (see Figure 3-5, *C*). The transducer converts the returning echo into an alternating voltage pulse (see Figure 3-4, *B*).

$$f_0(\text{MHz}) = \frac{c_t\,(\text{mm}/\mu\text{s})}{2 \times \text{th}(\text{mm})}$$

Thinner elements operate at higher frequencies.

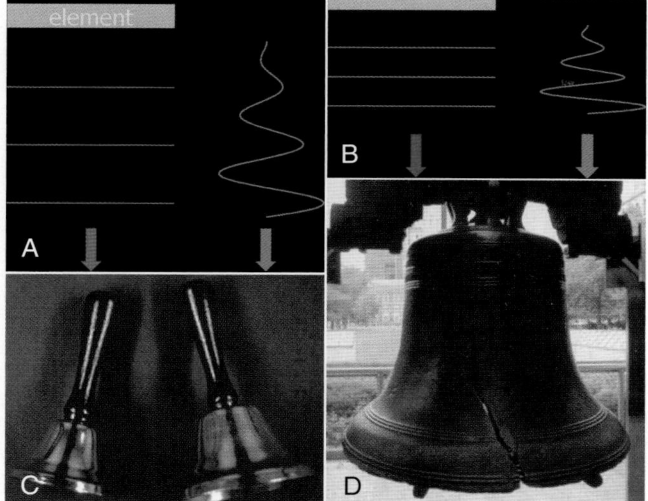

FIGURE 3-5 **A**, Thicker elements operate at lower frequencies. **B**, Thinner elements operate at higher frequencies. **C-D**, Smaller and larger bells ring with higher and lower pitches, respectively.

With wide-bandwidth transducers (e.g., those having a fractional bandwidth of at least 70%), voltage excitation can be used selectively to operate the same transducer at more than one frequency (Figure 3-6). The transducer is driven at one of two or three selectable frequencies by voltage pulses with the selected frequency. The two or three frequencies must fall within the transducer bandwidth. Choosing the higher frequency yields better **detail resolution**. If the resulting penetration is not sufficient for the study at hand, however, a lower frequency can be selected (resulting in some degradation in resolution). Push-button frequency switching is quicker, more convenient, and more cost-effective than changing of transducers. Wide bandwidth also allows harmonic imaging, in which echoes of twice the frequency sent into the body are received to improve the image.

Damping Material

Voltage pulse repetition frequency is equal to the voltage pulse repetition frequency. This is the number of voltage pulses sent to the transducer each second, which is determined by the instrument driving the transducer. Pulse duration is equal to period multiplied by number of cycles in the pulse. Damping (also called *backing*) material, a mixture of metal powder and a plastic or epoxy resin, is attached to the rear face of the transducer elements to reduce the number of cycles in each pulse (see Figures 3-3, *E*, and 3-7). Damping reduces pulse duration and spatial pulse length and improves resolution. This method of damping is analogous to packing foam

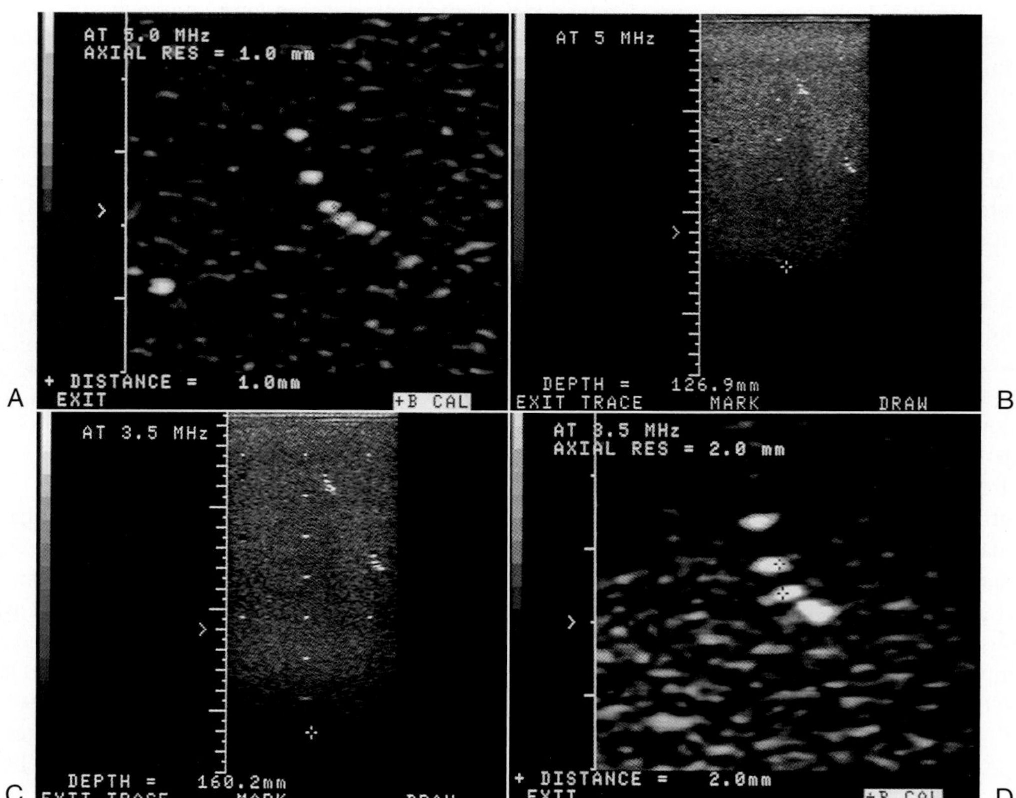

FIGURE 3-6 Multiple-frequency operation allows the transducer to provide (at a higher frequency) selectively better detail resolution (**A**) with reduced penetration (**B**) or (at a lower frequency) deeper penetration (**C**) with some degradation of resolution (**D**).

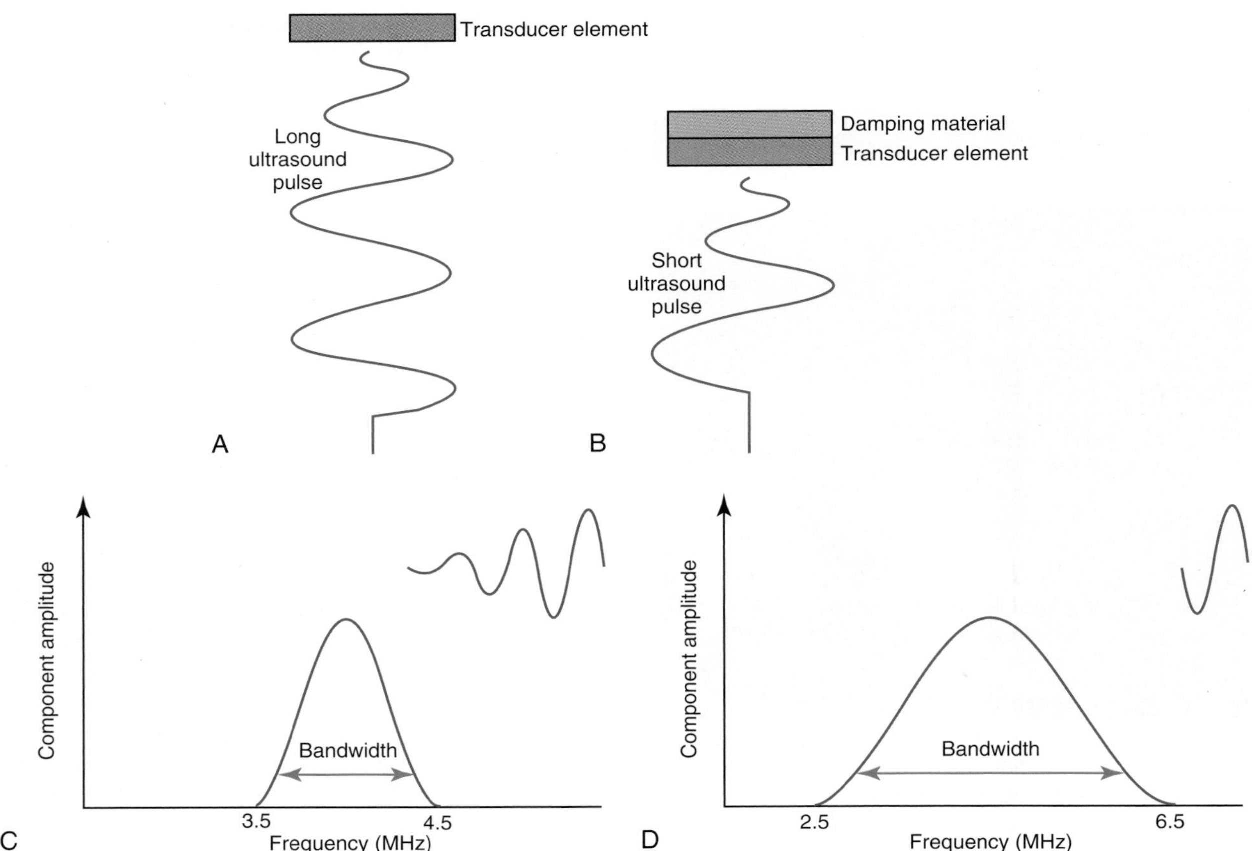

FIGURE 3-7 **A**, Without damping, a transducer element produces a long ultrasound pulse of many cycles. **B**, With damping material on the rear face of the transducer element, a short ultrasound pulse of a few cycles is produced. This figure shows each pulse traveling (*down*) away from the transducer in space so that the bottom end is the beginning or leading edge of the pulse while it travels down. **C-D**, Plots of the frequencies present in the ultrasound pulses (from **A** and **B**, respectively). Component amplitude is the amplitude of each frequency component present. Bandwidth is the frequency range within which the amplitudes exceed a reference value. Compare the frequency spectrum for a narrowband, undamped pulse (**C**) with the frequency spectrum for a broadband, damped pulse (**D**).

rubber around a bell that is rung by a tap with a hammer. The rubber reduces the time that the bell rings after the tap. The rubber also reduces the loudness of the ringing. In the case of ultrasound transducers, the damping material additionally reduces the ultrasound amplitude and thus decreases the efficiency and sensitivity (ability to detect weak echoes) of the system (an undesired effect). This is the price paid for reduced spatial pulse length (a desired effect resulting in improved resolution) with damping. Typically, pulses of two to three cycles are generated with (damped) diagnostic ultrasound transducers. Shortening the pulses broadens their bandwidth. Typical bandwidths for modern transducers range from 50% to 100%. An example of a 100% bandwidth is a 5-MHz operating frequency with a bandwidth of 5 MHz, that is, from 2.5 to 7.5 MHz.

> Composites and damping material shorten pulses and improve resolution.

> Transducers intended for continuous wave Doppler ultrasound use are not damped because pulses are not used in this application. These transducers have higher efficiencies because energy is not lost to damping material.

Matching Layer

Because the transducer element is a solid (having high density and sound speed), it has an impedance that is approximately 20 times that of tissues. Without compensation, this factor would cause approximately 80% of the emitted intensity to be reflected at the skin boundary. Thus most of the sound energy would not enter the body. A returning echo also would have about 80% of its intensity reflected, so only a small portion would enter the transducer. Therefore the received echo intensity for a perfect (100%) reflector would be only 4% ($0.2 \times 1.00 \times 0.2$) because only approximately 20% of the intensity enters and only about 20% of the echo intensity exits the body. To solve this problem, a **matching layer** is usually placed on the transducer face (see Figure 3-3, *E*). This material has an impedance of some

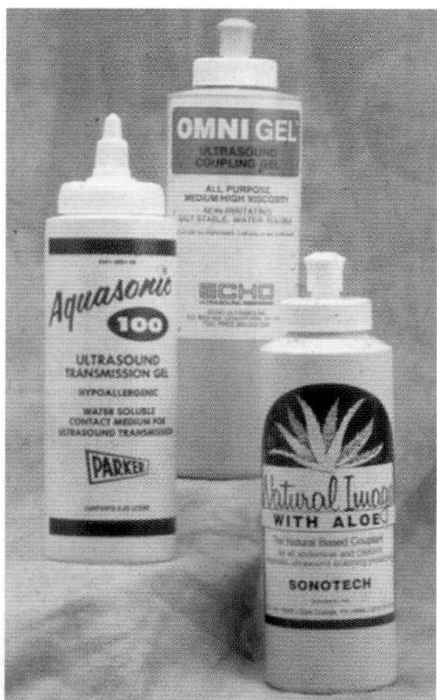

FIGURE 3-8 Coupling gel improves sound transmission into and out of the patient by eliminating air reflection.

intermediate value between those of the transducer element and the tissue. The material reduces the reflection of ultrasound at the transducer element surface, thereby improving sound transmission across it. This is analogous to the coating on eyeglasses or camera lenses that reduces light reflection at the air–glass boundary. Many frequencies (the bandwidth) and wavelengths are present in short ultrasound pulses. Thus multiple matching layers improve sound transmission across the element–tissue boundary better than does a single layer. Typically, two layers are used, although in some cases, one or three layers are used. The lower impedance of piezocomposite elements assists in the impedance-matching process, allowing more of the ultrasound energy to exit the front of the element into the patient rather than being lost as heat in the damping material.

Coupling Medium

Because of its very low impedance, even a very thin layer of air between the transducer and the skin surface reflects virtually all the sound, preventing any penetration into the tissue. For this reason, a coupling medium, usually an aqueous gel (Figure 3-8), is applied to the skin before transducer contact. This eliminates the air layer and facilitates the passage of sound into and out of the tissue. Thus the combination of matching layers with the coupling medium enables the efficient passage of ultrasound into the body and the return of echoes from the body into the transducer.

> Matching layers and coupling media facilitate the passage of ultrasound across the transducer–skin boundary.

Invasive Transducers

Some transducers are designed to enter the body (Figure 3-9) via the vagina, rectum, esophagus, or a blood vessel (catheter-mounted type). These approaches allow the transducer to be placed closer to the anatomy of interest, thus avoiding intervening tissues (e.g., lung or gassy bowel) and reducing the sound transmission path length. This reduction in path length, which yields lower attenuation, allows higher frequencies to be used and improves resolution.

BEAMS AND FOCUSING

A continuous wave ultrasound beam is filled with ultrasound similarly to a flashlight beam being filled with light. A pulsed beam is not. What is meant by "the beam," then, in the case of pulsed ultrasound? The term *beam* refers to the width of a pulse as it travels away from the transducer. Generally, the width in the scan plane is not the same as the width perpendicular to the scan plane. The width in the scan plane determines the **lateral resolution**, whereas the width perpendicular to the scan plane determines the extent of the section thickness artifact.

A single-element **disk** transducer operating in continuous wave mode provides a simple approximation to beams produced by sonographic transducers. The transducer produces a **sound beam** with a width that varies according to the distance from the transducer face, as shown in Figure 3-10. The intensity is not uniform throughout the beam, but the beam shown includes nearly all the power in the beam. Sometimes, significant intensity travels out in some directions not included in this beam. These additional beams are called **side lobes**. They are a source of artifacts.

Near and Far Zones

The region extending from the element to a distance of one near-zone length is called the **near zone**, *near field,* or *Fresnel zone.* The beam width decreases with increasing distance from the transducer in the near zone. Near-zone length (NZL; also called *near-field length*) is determined by the size and operating frequency of the element. Near-zone length increases with increasing frequency or element size, which is also called **aperture** (ap).

> An ultrasound beam consists of near and far zones.

> If aperture increases, near-zone length increases.

> If frequency increases, near-zone length increases.

Table 3-2 lists near-zone lengths for various disk element frequencies and diameters. The region that lies beyond a distance of one near-zone length is called the **far zone**, *far field,* or Fraunhofer zone. The beam width increases with increasing distance from the transducer in the far zone.

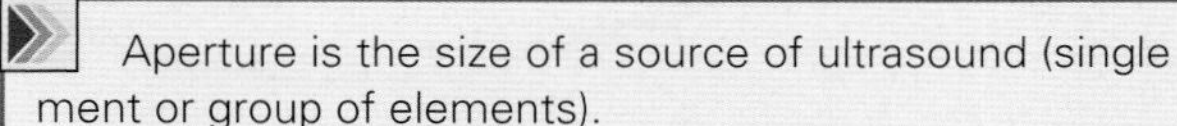

> Aperture is the size of a source of ultrasound (single element or group of elements).

What is somewhat surprising but true is that even in the case of this flat, unfocused transducer element, there is some beam narrowing. This narrowing is sometimes called **natural focus**. Modern diagnostic transducer arrays contain rectangular elements. Beams from rectangular elements are similar but not identical to those from disk elements.

Example 3-1

For a 10-mm, 5-MHz flat (unfocused) disk transducer, what are the beam widths at the near-zone length and at two times the near-zone length?

At the end of the near zone, the beam width is approximately equal to one half the width of the transducer element, or 5 mm. At double the near-zone length, the beam diameter is approximately equal to the diameter of the transducer element, or 10 mm.

The effects of frequency and aperture on near-zone length are shown in Figures 3-11 and 3-12, respectively. An increase in frequency or in aperture increases the near-zone length. At a sufficient distance from the transducer, an increase in frequency or transducer size can decrease the beam diameter, as shown in the figures.

The beam in Figure 3-10, *A*, is for continuous wave mode, but it can be used to describe pulses in the rest of the figure. The beam for pulses is similar, but not identical to, that for continuous sound.

Focusing

To improve resolution, diagnostic transducers are focused. Focusing sound in the same manner as focusing light

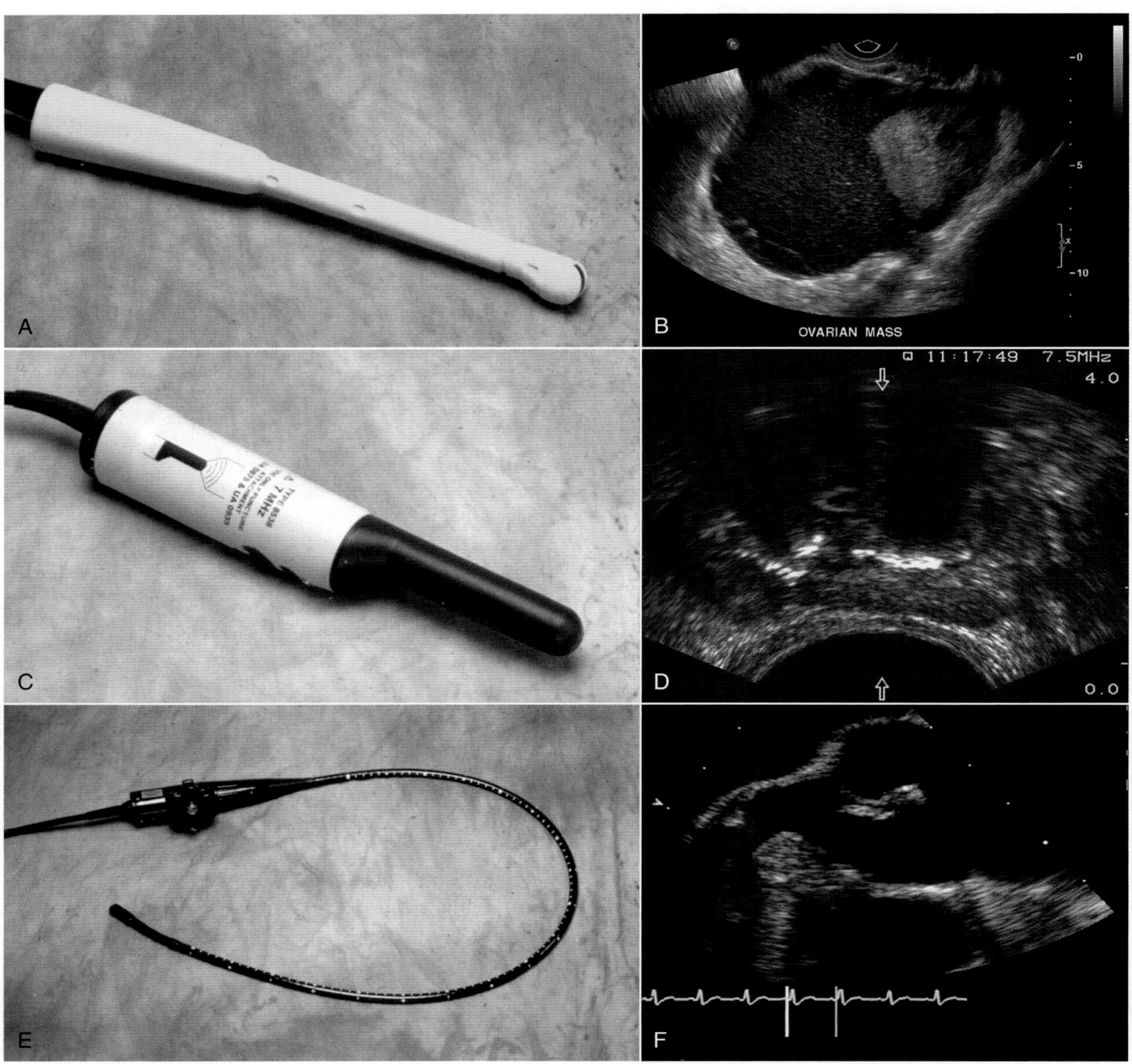

FIGURE 3-9 **A**, Vaginal transducer. **B**, Transvaginal view of an ovarian mass. **C**, Rectal transducer. **D**, Transrectal view of the prostate. **E**, Transesophageal probe for echocardiography. **F**, Transesophageal view of the adult heart.

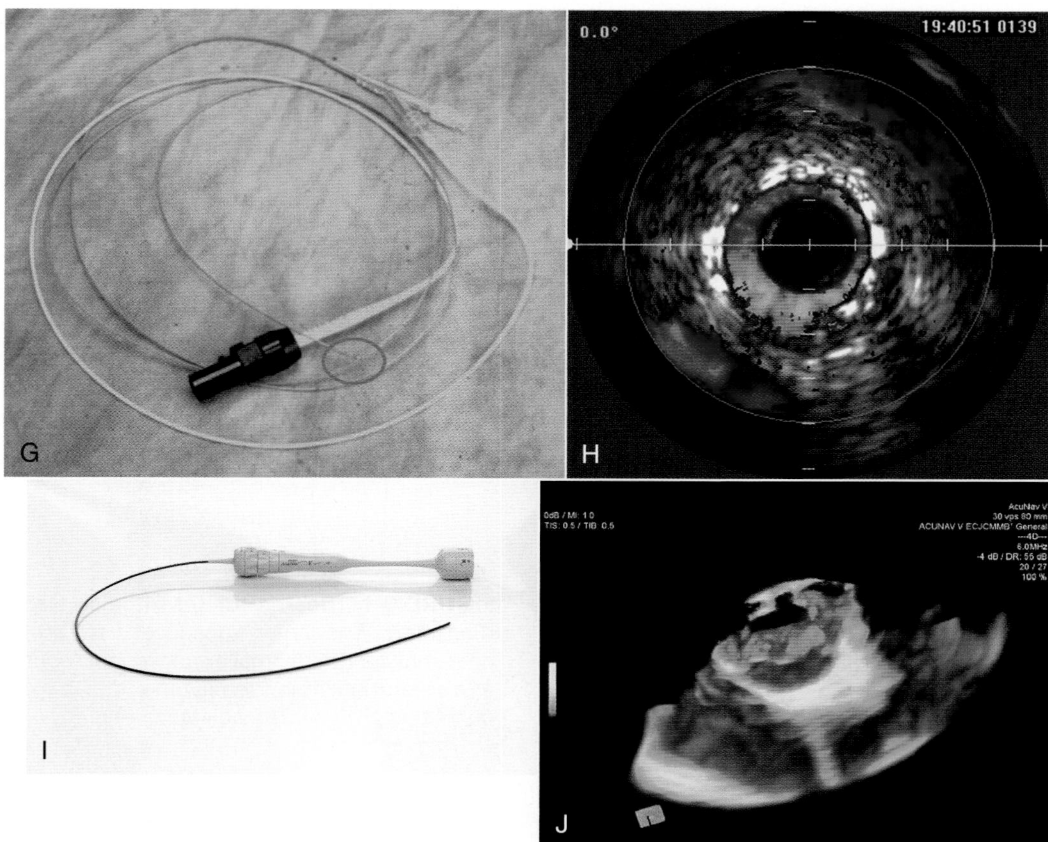

FIGURE 3-9, cont'd **G**, Catheter-mounted transducer (*circle*) for viewing the interior of a blood vessel. **H**, Interior view of a blood vessel. **I**, Intracardiac catheter transducer. **J**, View of aortic valve with the intracardiac catheter transducer. (**I** and **J**, Courtesy of Siemens Healthcare.)

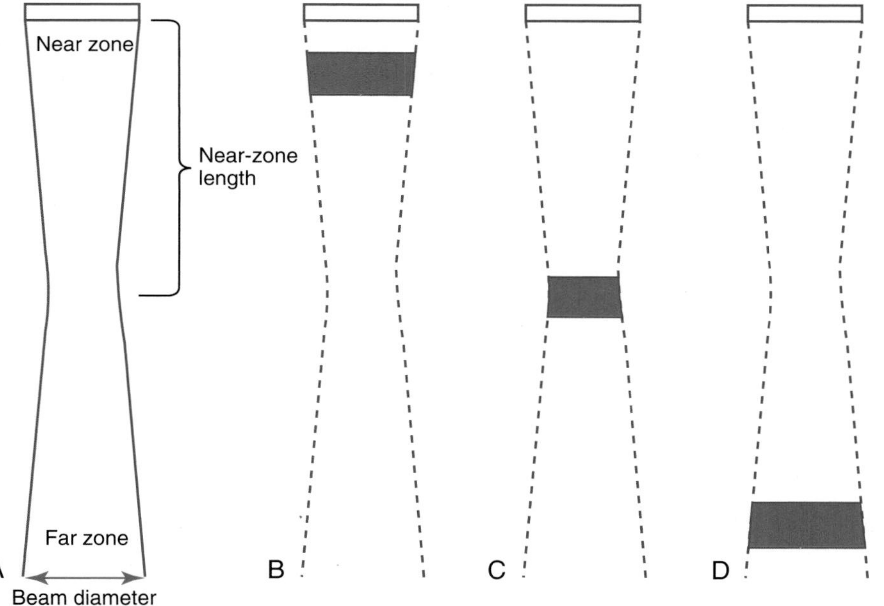

FIGURE 3-10 **A**, Beam width for a single-element unfocused disk transducer operating in continuous wave mode. The near zone is the region between the disk and the minimum beam width. The far zone is the region beyond the minimum beam width. Intensity varies within the beam, with the greatest variations in the near zone. This beam approximates the changing pulse diameter while an ultrasound pulse travels away from a transducer. **B**, An ultrasound pulse shortly after leaving the transducer. **C**, Later, the ultrasound pulse is located at the end of the near-zone length, where its width is at a minimum. **D**, Still later, the pulse is in the far zone, where its width increases while it travels.

TABLE 3-2 Near-Zone Length (NZL) for Unfocused Elements

Frequency (MHz)	Width (mm)	NZL (cm)
2.0	19	12
3.5	13	10
3.5	19	20
5.0	6	3
5.0	10	8
5.0	13	14
7.5	6	4
10.0	6	6

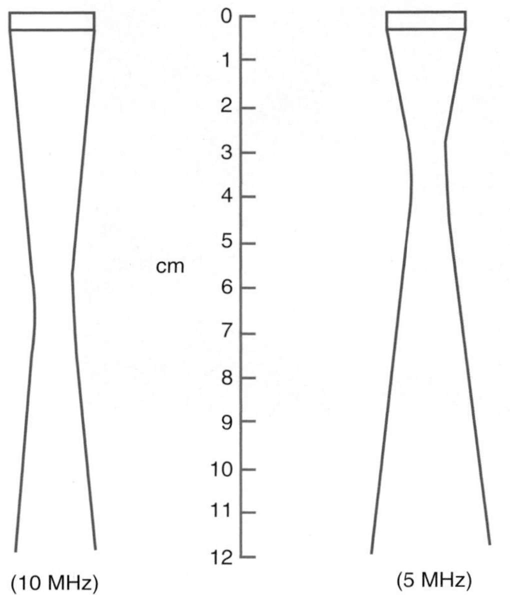

FIGURE 3-11 Beams for disk transducers with a diameter of 6 mm at two frequencies. Higher frequencies produce smaller beam diameters (at a distance greater than 4 cm in this case) and longer near-zone lengths.

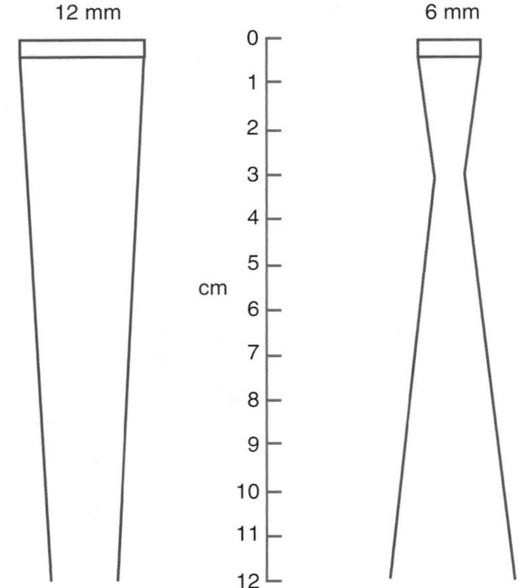

FIGURE 3-12 Beams for 5-MHz disk transducers of two diameters. The larger transducer (*left*) produces the longer near-zone length. A smaller transducer (*right*) produces a larger-diameter beam in the far zone. In this example, the beam diameters are equal at a distance of 8 cm.

reduces beam width. Sound may be focused (Figure 3-13) by using curved (rather than flat) transducer elements, by using a **lens**, or by phasing (discussed later). Focusing moves the end of the near zone toward the transducer and narrows the beam. Beam width is decreased in the **focal region** and in the area between it and the transducer, but it is widened in the region beyond (Figure 3-14). Focal length (fl) is the distance from the transducer to the center of the focal region. Focusing can be accomplished only in the near zone of the comparable unfocused transducer. **Focal zone** length (called *depth of field* in photography) is the distance between equal beam widths that are some multiple (e.g., ×2) of the minimum value (at the **focus**).

> Focusing can be achieved only in the near zone of a beam.

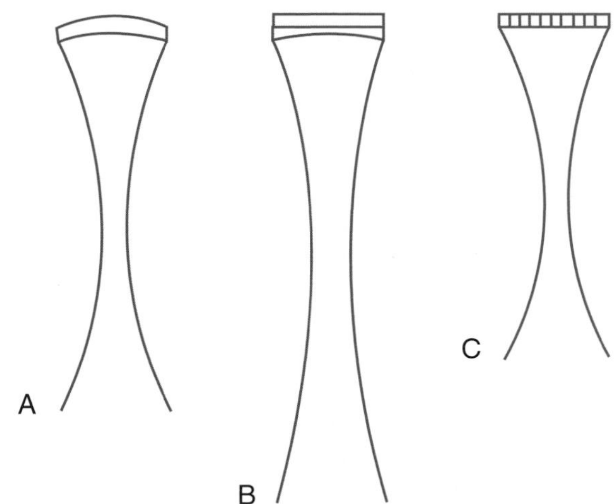

FIGURE 3-13 Sound focusing by a curved transducer element, lens, or phased array. Lenses focus because the propagation speed through them is higher than through tissues. Refraction at the surface of the lens forms the beam so that a focal region occurs. The operation of phased arrays is described later in this chapter. **A**, Curved transducer element. **B**, Lens. **C**, Phased array.

While the element or lens is increasingly curved (or phase-delay curvature in a **phased array** is increased), the focus moves closer to the transducer and becomes "tighter" (i.e., the beam width at the focus decreases). The limit to which a beam can be narrowed depends on wavelength, aperture, and **focal length**.

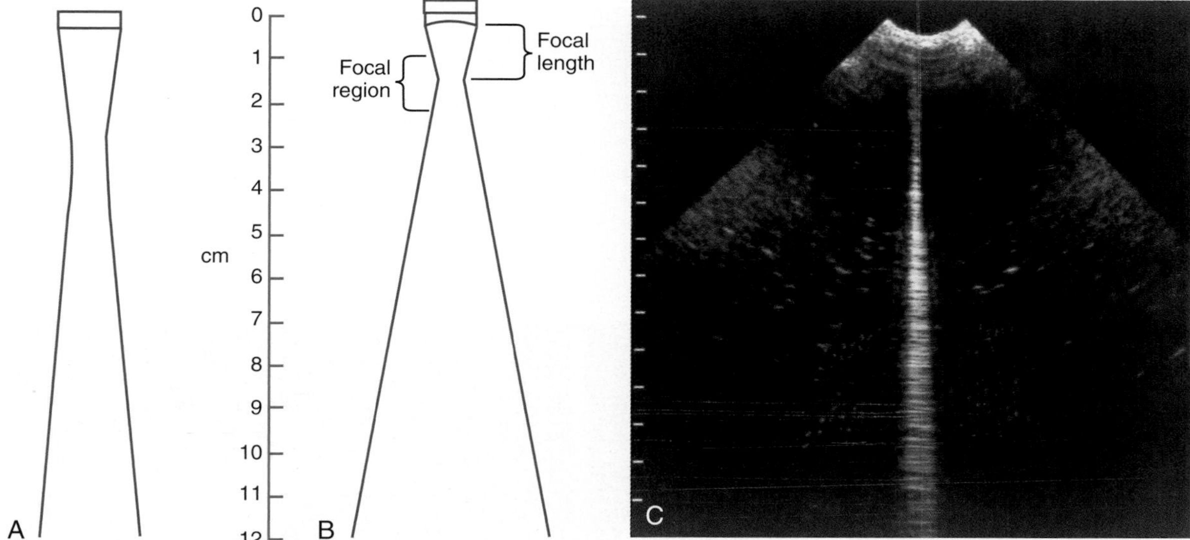

FIGURE 3-14 Beam diameter for a 6-mm, 5-MHz transducer without (**A**) and with (**B**) focusing. Focusing reduces the minimum beam width compared with that produced without focusing. However, well beyond the focal region, the width of the focused beam is greater than that of the unfocused beam. **C**, A focused beam. This is an ultrasound image of a beam profile test object containing a thin vertical scattering layer down the center. Scanning this object generates a picture of the beam (the pulse width at all depths). In this case the focus occurs at a depth of approximately 4 cm (this image has a total depth of 15 cm). Depth markers (in 1-cm increments) are indicated on the left edge of the figure.

ARRAYS

Not only must the transducer emit ultrasound pulses and receive echoes, but it must also send the pulses through the many anatomic paths required to generate an image. This sometimes is called *scanning, sweeping,* or *steering* the beam through the tissue cross-sections to be imaged. Scanning is done rapidly and automatically so that many images, called *frames,* can be acquired and presented in rapid sequence within a second. Presenting images in a rapid sequential format, similar to a movie, is called *real-time sonography.*

Automatic scanning of a sound beam is performed electronically, providing a means for sweeping the sound beam through the tissues rapidly and repeatedly.

Electronic scanning is performed with arrays. Transducer arrays are transducer assemblies with several transducer elements. The elements are rectangular and are arranged in a straight line (linear array; see Figures 3-3, *E,* and 3-15, *A*) or curved line (**convex array**; see Figure 3-15, *B*). **Linear** is the adjectival form of the word "line." Convex means "bowed outward."

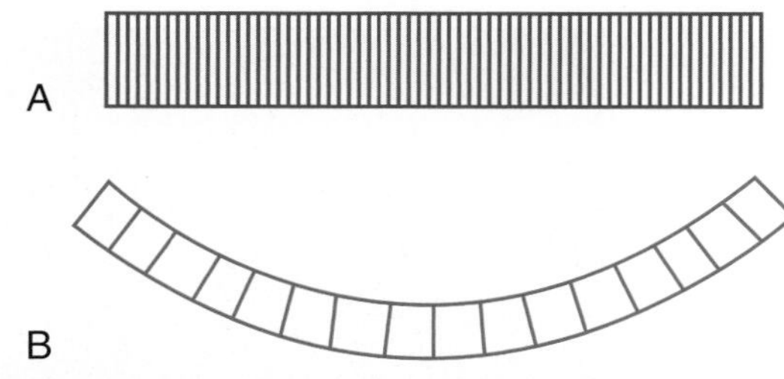

FIGURE 3-15 **A**, Front view of a linear array with 64 rectangular elements. **B**, Side view of a convex array with 16 elements.

Linear Array

Arrays are operated in two ways, called *sequencing* and *phasing.* A more complete name for what is commonly called a *linear array* is **linear sequenced array**. This array contains a straight line of rectangular elements, each approximately one wavelength wide, and is operated by applying voltage pulses to groups of elements in succession (Figure 3-16). Each group of elements acts similarly to a larger transducer element, providing an aperture large enough to confine the ultrasound to a fine enough beam for satisfactory resolution. As different groups are energized, the origin of the sound beam moves across the face of the **transducer assembly** from one end to the other, thus producing the same effect as would manual linear scanning with a single element the size (aperture) of the energized groups. Such electronic scanning, however, can be done rapidly and consistently without involving moving parts or a coupling liquid. If this electronic scanning is repeated rapidly enough, real-time presentation (many images per second) of visual information can result. Real-time presentation requires scanning the beam across the transducer assembly several times per second. The aperture is the size of the group of elements energized to produce each pulse. The width of the entire image is approximately equal to the length of the array (Figure 3-17). The linear image consists of parallel scan lines produced by pulses originating at different points across the surface of the array (and across the top of the image) but that all travel in the same vertical direction (parallel) (see Figure 1-6). This produces a rectangular image, as shown in Figures 3-16, *G,* and 3-17.

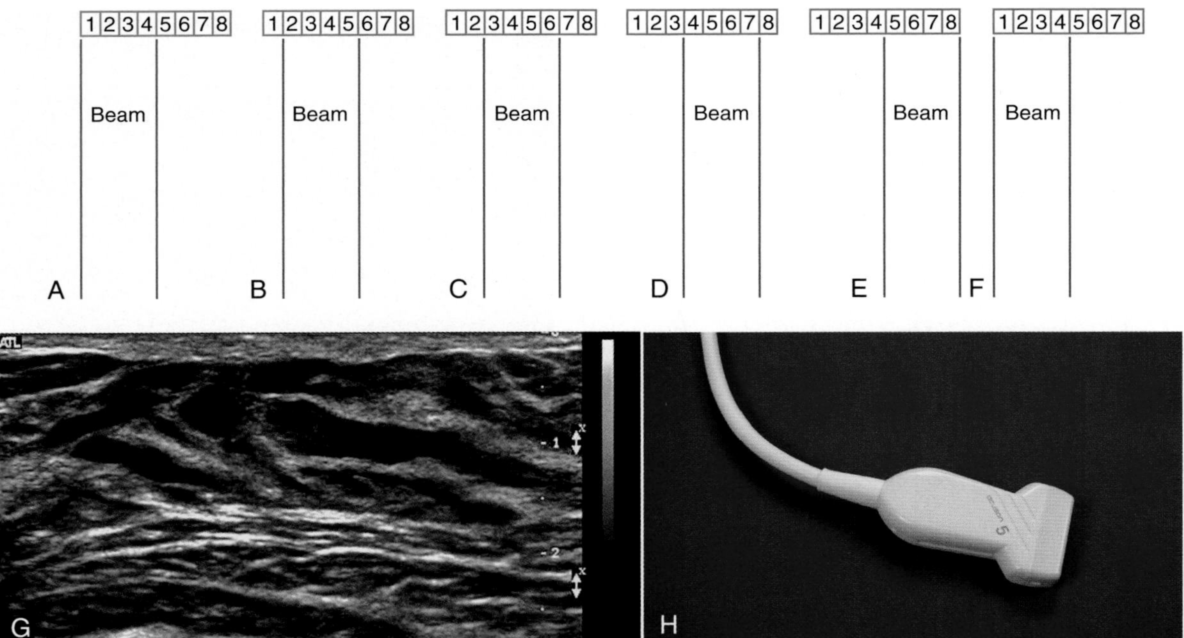

FIGURE 3-16 A linear sequenced array (side view). A voltage pulse is applied simultaneously to all elements in a small group: first to elements 1 to 4 (for example) as a group (**A**), then to elements 2 to 5 (**B**), and so on across the transducer assembly (**C-E**). The process is then repeated (**F**). **G**, An image generated from a linear array. **H**, A linear array transducer.

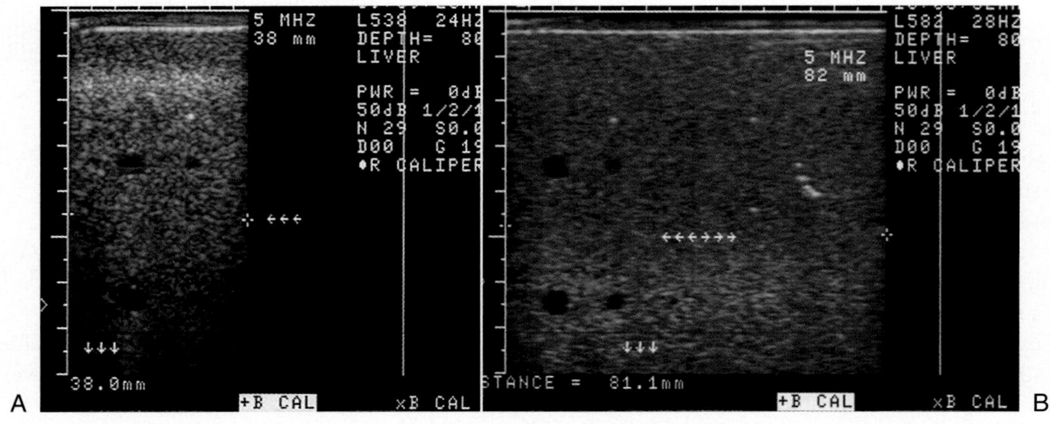

FIGURE 3-17 The linear image width is determined by the length of the linear array used. **A**, In this example, a 5-MHz, 38-mm linear array (L538) produces an image that is 38 mm wide. **B**, A 5-MHz, 82-mm linear array (L582) produces an image that is 81 mm wide.

> A linear array produces rectangular images composed of many parallel, vertical scan lines.

The pulsing sequence described in Figure 3-16 (eight elements, pulsed in groups of four) yields only five scan lines to make up the image. This would certainly be a limited image. A 128-element array pulsed in groups of four would yield a 125-line display. Pulsing these elements individually (rather than in groups of four) would yield a 128-line display, but the small aperture (a single element less than 1 mm in size) would cause excessive beam spreading and poor resolution. If the pulsing sequence alternated groups of three and four elements (e.g., elements 1 to 3, then 1 to 4, 2 to 4, 2 to 5, 3 to 5, 3 to 6, 4 to 6, 4 to 7, and on through the array), the number of scan lines would be doubled, to 250, thereby increasing scan-line density and improving the quality of the image.

Convex Array

A convex array, also called a *curved array,* is constructed as a curved line of elements rather than a straight one. The operation of a convex array is identical to that of the linear sequenced array (sequencing groups of elements from one

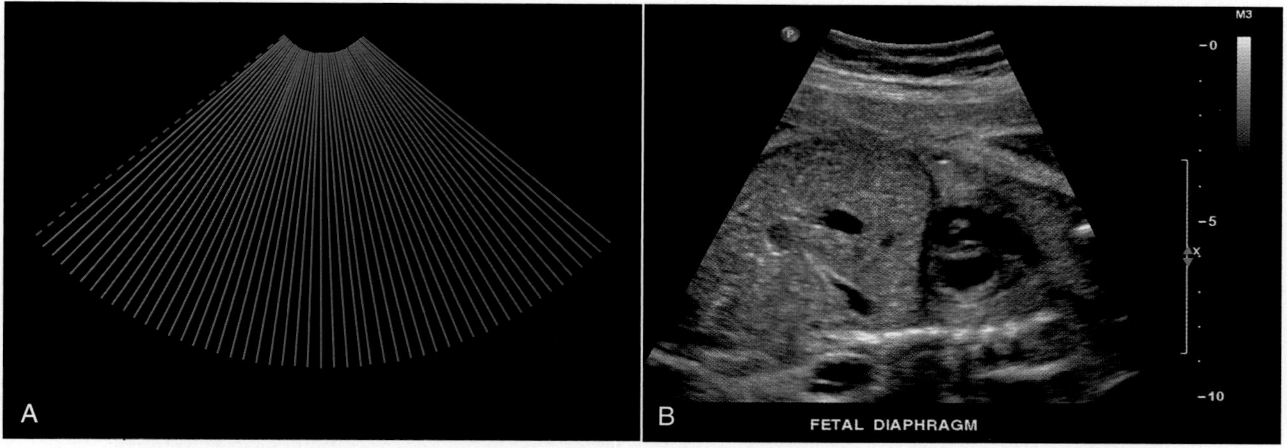

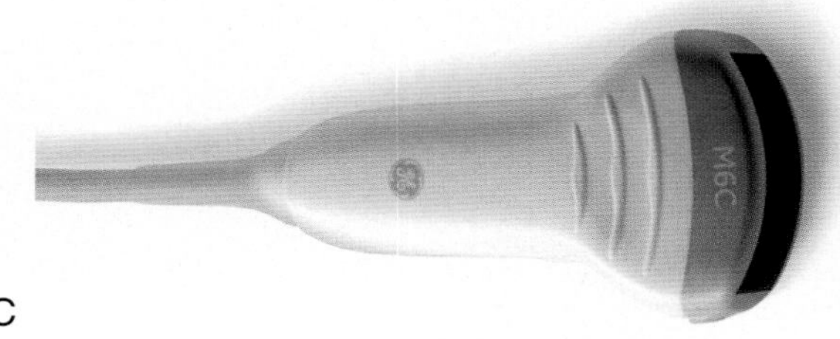

FIGURE 3-18 A, Convex arrays send pulses out in different directions from different points across the curved array surface. B, A sector-type image with a curved top is produced by a convex array. C, A convex array transducer.

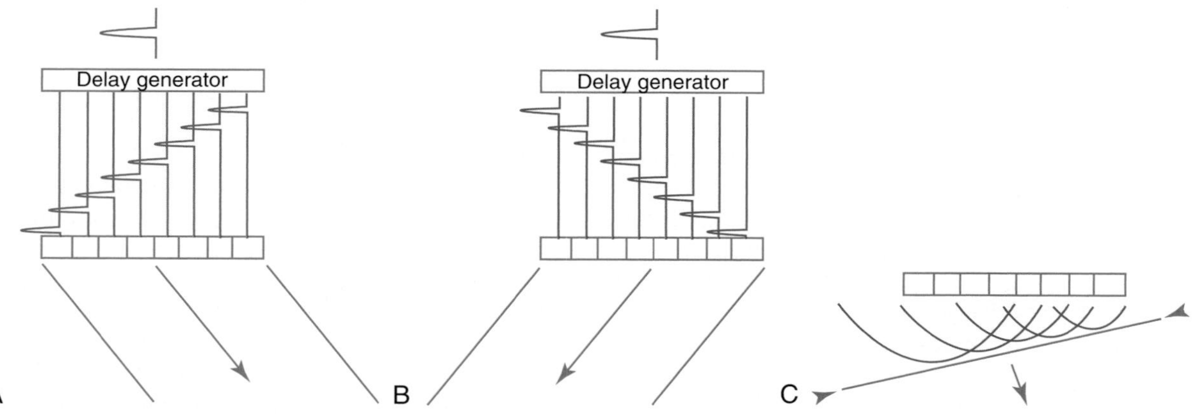

FIGURE 3-19 A linear phased array (side view). A, When voltage pulses are applied in rapid progression from left to right, one ultrasound pulse is produced that is directed to the right. B, Similarly, when voltage pulses are applied in rapid progression from right to left, one ultrasound pulse is produced that is directed to the left. C, The delays in A produce a pulse, the combined pressure wavefront of which (*arrowheads*) is angled from lower left to upper right. A wave always travels perpendicular to its wavefront, as indicated by the *arrow*.

end of the array to the other), but because of the curved construction, the pulses travel out in different directions, producing a sector-type image (Figure 3-18). The complete name for this transducer is *convex sequenced array.*

> The convex array operates similarly to the linear array but produces a sector image.

Phased Array

A linear phased array (commonly called *phased array*) contains a compact straight line of elements, each about one quarter of a wavelength wide. The phased array is operated by applying voltage pulses to most or all elements (not a small group) in the assembly, but with small (less than 1 μs) time differences (called *phasing*) between them, so that the resulting sound pulse is sent out in a specific path direction, as shown in Figure 3-19. If the same time delays were used each time the process was repeated,

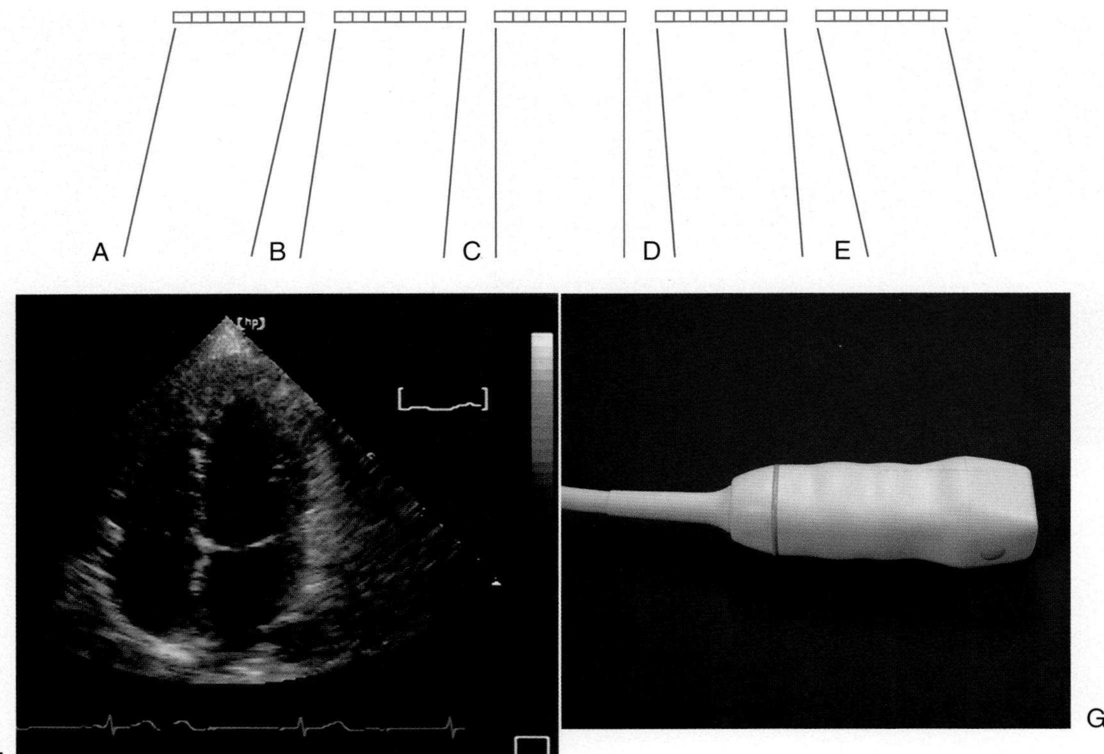

FIGURE 3-20 A five-pulse sequence in which each pulse travels out in a different direction. **A**, The rapid voltage-application progression is from right to left across the array. **B**, A right-to-left progression with slightly shorter time delays. **C**, No delays (all elements energize simultaneously). **D**, A left-to-right progression. **E**, A left-to-right progression with slightly longer delays. **F**, A cardiac sector image produced by a phased array. The image comes to a point at the top. **G**, A phased array transducer.

the subsequent pulses would travel out in the same direction repeatedly. However, the time delays automatically are changed slightly with each successive repetition so that subsequent pulses travel out in slightly different directions, and the beam direction continually changes (Figure 3-20). This process results in the sweeping of the beam, with beam direction changing with each pulse, to produce a sector image (see Figure 3-20, *F*), the same effect as with manual rotation of a single element. Such electronic sector scanning, however, can be done rapidly and consistently without involving moving parts or a coupling liquid. The phased array is sometimes called an *electronic sector transducer.*

> A phased array scans the beam in sector format with short time delays.

Phasing is applied to some linear and convex arrays to steer the beam from each element group in several directions by sending out several pulses from each group with different phasing. Thus echoes can be generated from a specific anatomic location with several viewing angles. The echo information from these multiple views is processed to present an image of improved quality. This is a form of electronic "compounding" of an image. This is discussed in more detail in the next chapter.

Electronic Focus

In addition to steering the beam, the phased array can focus the beam as well (Figure 3-21). An increase in the curved delay pattern (greater time delays between elements) moves the focus closer to the transducer, whereas a decrease (shorter delays) in curvature moves it deeper. Thus phasing provides electronic control of the location of the focus (Figure 3-22). Multiple foci can be used to achieve, in effect, a long focus (Figure 3-23). One pulse can be focused at only one depth. Therefore multiple foci require multiple pulses (per scan line), each focused at a different depth. Echoes from the focal region of each pulse are displayed, and the rest are discarded. The resulting image is a montage of the focal regions of the different pulses, which improves detail resolution. However, the use of multiple pulses per scan line takes more time, and the frame rate is reduced, which degrades temporal resolution (discussed later). Thus temporal resolution is sacrificed in this approach to improving detail resolution.

> Electronic focusing is accomplished with a curved pattern of phased delays. An increase or decrease in the curvature of the delay pattern moves the focus shallower or deeper, respectively.

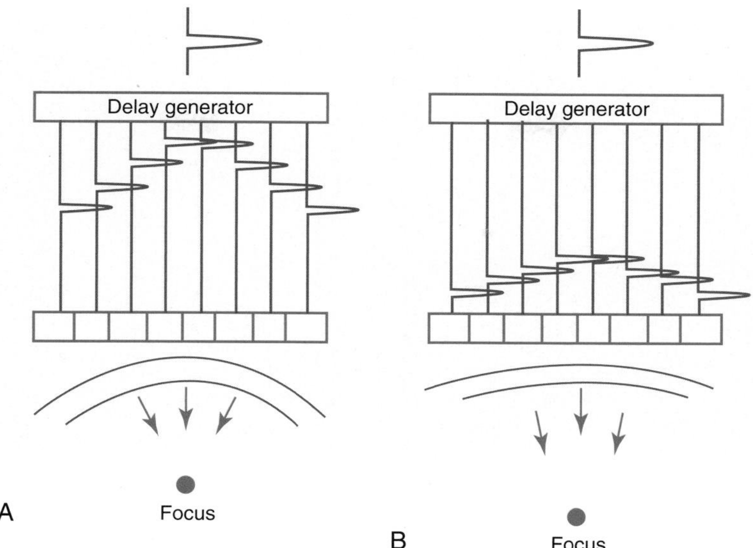

FIGURE 3-21 By adding curvature to the phase delay pattern, a pulse is focused. **A**, Greater curvature places the focus closer to the transducer. **B**, Less curvature moves the focus deeper.

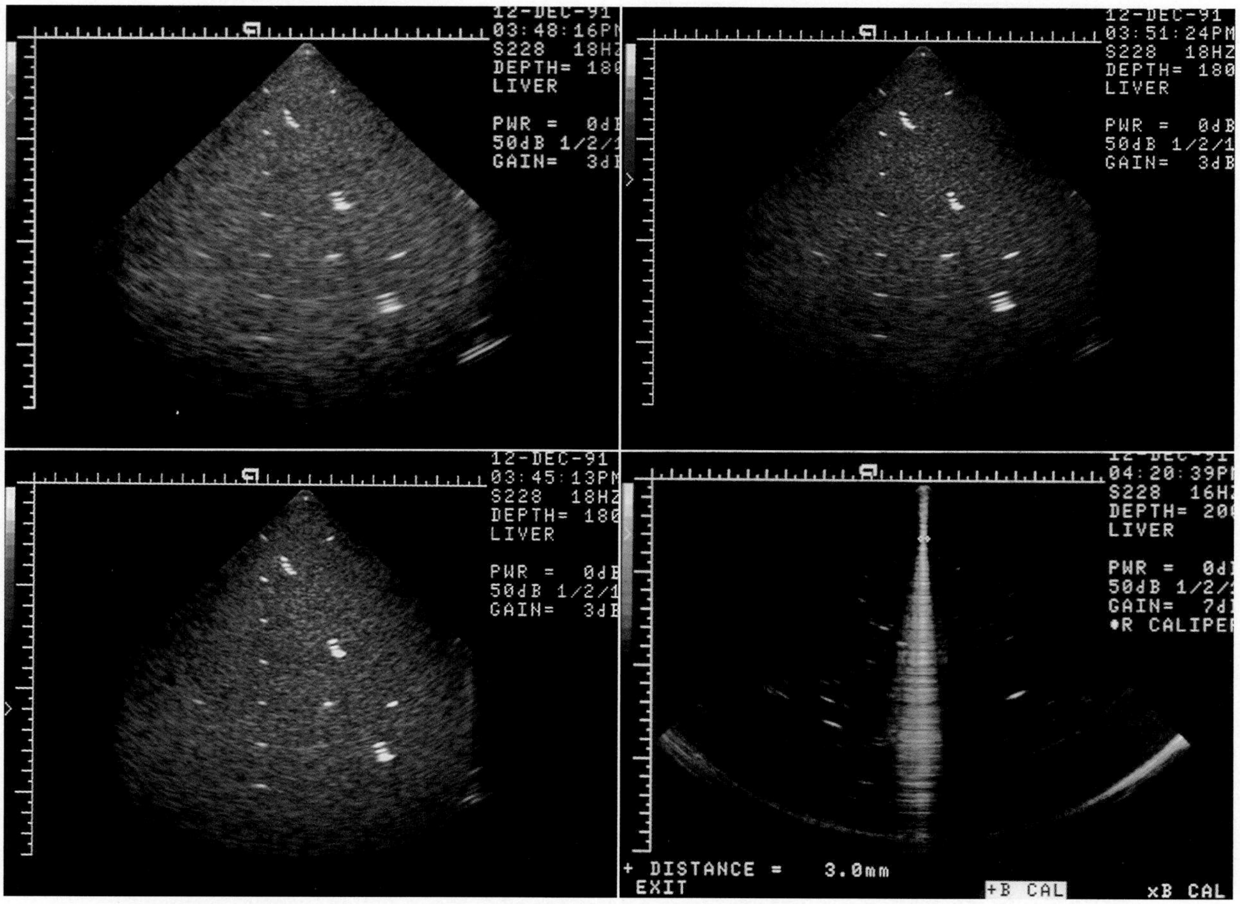

FIGURE 3-22 Phase control of focal length. Focus located at 3 cm (**A**), 7 cm (**B**), and 11 cm (**C**). Beam profiles show foci located at 3 cm (**D**), 7 cm (**E**), and 13 cm (**F**).

Continued

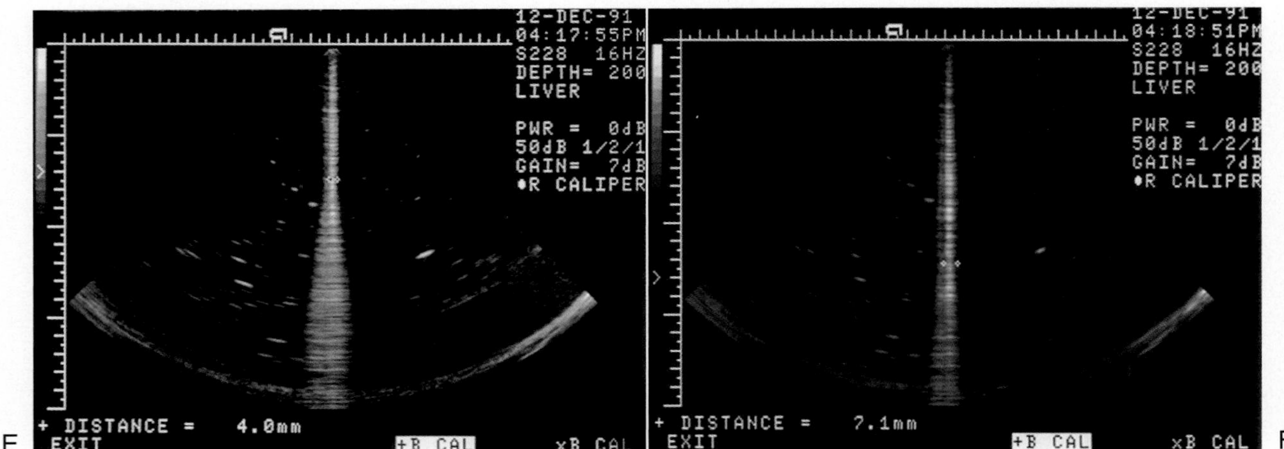

FIGURE 3-22, cont'd

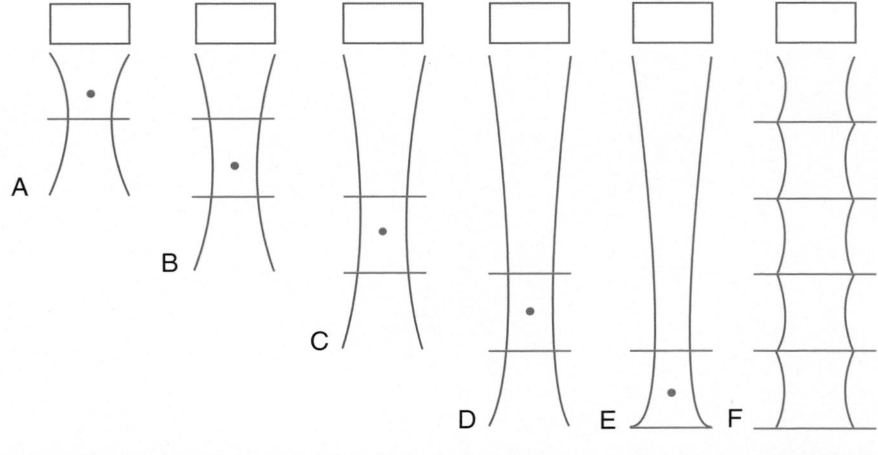

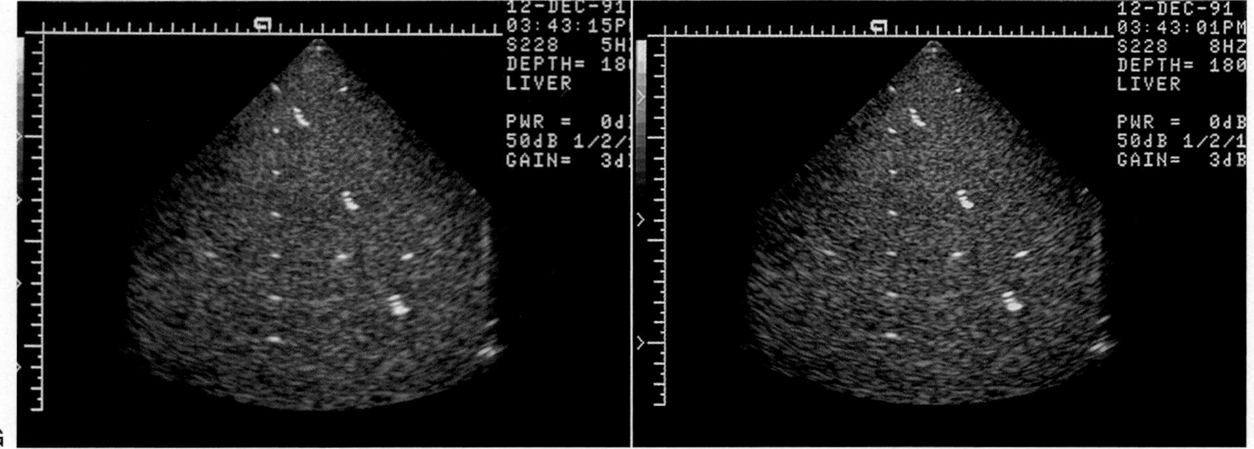

FIGURE 3-23 Multiple-transmit focus uses a pulse for each focus. In this example, five pulses focused at different depths (**A-E**) are needed to produce a montage image (**F**) with an effectively long focus (narrow beam). Only the echoes from the focal region of each pulse are used to produce the image. The rest are discarded. **G**, Five foci at 2, 5, 8, 12, and 16 cm. **H**, Triple foci at 3, 9, and 15 cm. Note the reduced frame rates (5 and 8 Hz, compared with 18 and 16 Hz in Figure 3-22).

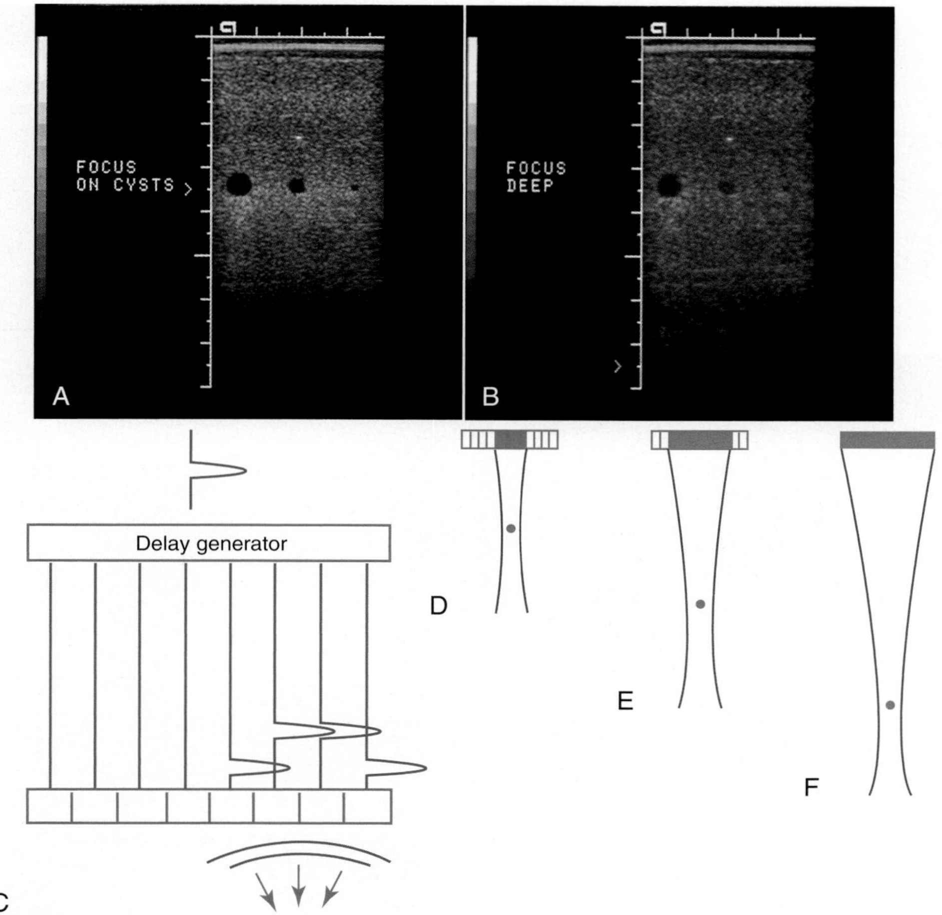

FIGURE 3-24 **A**, A phased linear array with the focus located at 3.5 cm produces a clear image of the small cystic object. **B**, When the focus is located at 7.5 cm (less phase delay curvature), a loss of image quality results for cystic objects. **C**, Phased delays are applied to each element group to focus the pulse. **D-F**, Variable aperture. To maintain comparable focal beam width at different depths, more array elements are used (increasing the aperture) while the focus is moved deeper. **D**, Four elements. **E**, Eight elements. **F**, Twelve elements.

Phasing is also applied to linear arrays to provide electronic focal control (Figure 3-24, *A-B*). The term **phased linear array** indicates that phased focus control is applied to a linear sequenced array. Rather than each group of elements being pulsed simultaneously, as in Figure 3-16, the outer elements are pulsed slightly ahead of the inner ones (see Figure 3-24, *C*). This produces a curved pulse that is focused at a depth determined by the delay between the firing of the outer and inner elements. These pulses are focused, but not steered, by phasing. They still travel straight down to produce parallel vertical scan lines and a rectangular display. In a similar way, phased focusing is applied to convex arrays.

Variable Aperture

Recall that aperture, focal length, and wavelength determine the beam width at the focus. To maintain the same beam width at the focus for increasing focal lengths, the aperture must also be increased. This means that, in fact, not all elements of a phased array are used to generate all pulses. Smaller groups are used for short focal lengths, whereas larger groups are used for foci of increasing depth (see Figure 3-24, *D-F*).

Two-Dimensional Arrays

A single line of elements can electronically focus or steer only in the scan plane. Focus (fixed at one depth) can be achieved in the third dimension with a lens or with curved elements. With at least three rows of elements—that is, a two-dimensional array—phasing can be applied to focus the third dimension electronically. Electronic focusing in the third dimension eliminates the need for a lens or curved elements. This dimension, perpendicular to the scan plane, is called *slice thickness dimension* or *section thickness dimension.* Beam width in this dimension is important with regard to section thickness artifacts, also called *partial-volume artifacts.* This third dimension and its associated section thickness are shown in Figures 1-7, *A*, and 1-9, *A*.

Conventional arrays scan in rectangular or sector format in one dimension (Figure 3-25, *A*). Two-dimensional arrays

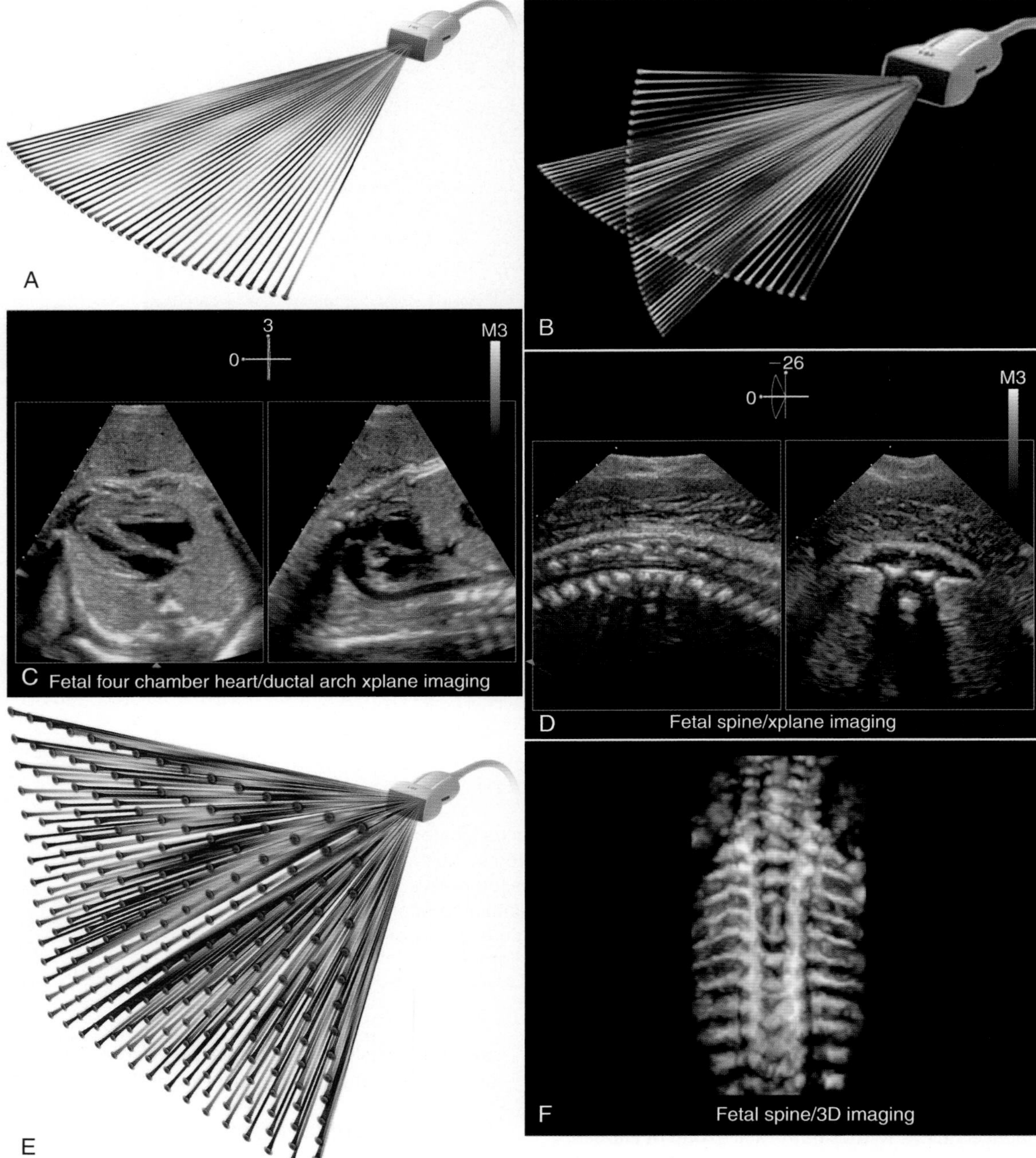

FIGURE 3-25 A, Conventional two-dimensional scan. B-D, Biplane imaging. E-F, Rapid electronic volume (3D) imaging. (Courtesy of Philips Healthcare.)

with hundreds or thousands of elements have the ability to steer and focus in two-dimensions rather than one. Biplane imaging (see Figure 3-25, *B-D*) and rapid electronic volume imaging (see Figure 3-25, *E-F*) are thus facilitated.

Grating Lobes

In addition to side lobes, a characteristic of single-element transducers, arrays have **grating lobes**, which are additional beams resulting from their multielement structure. Grating lobes can be reduced by driving the elements in a group nonuniformly (i.e., with different voltage amplitudes). Outer elements are driven at lower amplitudes than inner elements. Echo reception sensitivity is also less for outer elements. This is called **apodization**. Because optimal apodization changes continually with focusing and steering, it is called *dynamic apodization*. The downside of apodization is that some broadening of the main beam occurs with degradation of resolution. Subdicing of each element into a group of smaller **crystals** is also done to weaken grating lobes and to reduce interelement interaction for improved electronic focusing. The subelements are tied together electrically so that they function as one element.

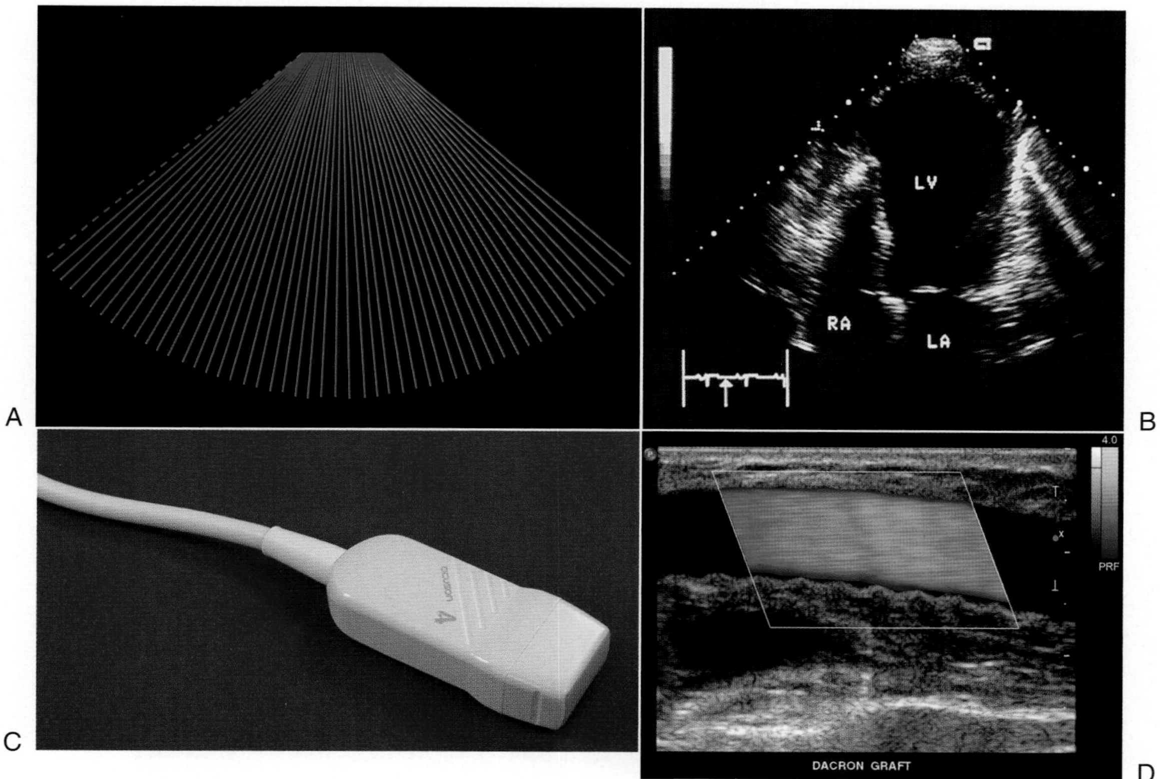

FIGURE 3-26 **A,** A vector array sends pulses out in different directions from different starting points across the flat surface of the array. **B,** A cardiac scan produced by a vector array. **C,** A vector array transducer. **D,** A phased linear array producing a parallelogram-shaped color-Doppler display.

Vector Array

Phasing can be applied to each element group in a linear sequenced array to steer pulses in various directions, in addition to initiating them at various starting points across the array. Vector array is the name applied to this type of transducer (Figure 3-26). This transducer converts the image format of a linear array from rectangular to sector. Scan lines originate from different points across the top of the display and travel out in different directions. The image format is similar to that of a convex array except that the contact surface (footprint) is smaller and the top of the display is flat. More elements can be used at a time, allowing for larger apertures than can be achieved with convex arrays. Phasing can be applied to linear sequenced arrays as well in such a way that each pulse travels in the same direction (but not straight down). This converts a rectangular display to a parallelogram-shaped display useful in color-Doppler imaging (see Figure 3-26, *D*).

> The vector array is a combination of linear and phased array operations. It presents a sector display with a nonzero width at the top.

Reception Steering, Focus, and Aperture

When an array is receiving echoes, the electric outputs of the elements can be timed so that the array is sensitive in a particular direction, with a listening focus at a particular depth (Figure 3-27). This reception focus depth may be increased continually as the transmitted pulse travels through tissues and the echoes arrive from deeper and deeper locations. This continually changing reception focus is called dynamic focusing. Dynamic focusing is similar to the continual change in focusing that occurs with a video camera, for example, when filming a child riding away on a bicycle. The combination of transmission focus (particularly multizone focusing) and dynamic reception focus improves detail resolution over large depth ranges in images. As the focus continually changes during echo reception, the aperture increases to maintain a constant focal width. This is called dynamic aperture. The terms used to describe arrays describe their construction and function as shown in Table 3-3. Boxes 3-1 and 3-2 and Tables 3-4 and 3-5 summarize transducer types, terminology, characteristics, and display formats.

> With phasing, the reception "beam" is steered and dynamically focused.

DETAIL RESOLUTION

Imaging resolution has three aspects:

- Detail
- Contrast
- Temporal

Contrast and temporal resolutions relate more directly to instruments. Detail resolution (Figure 3-28) relates more

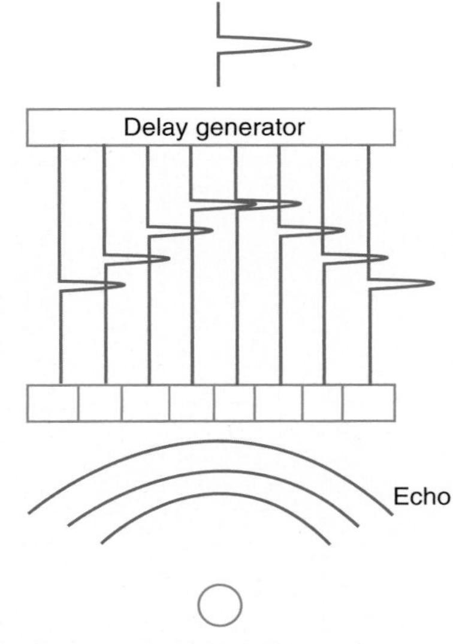

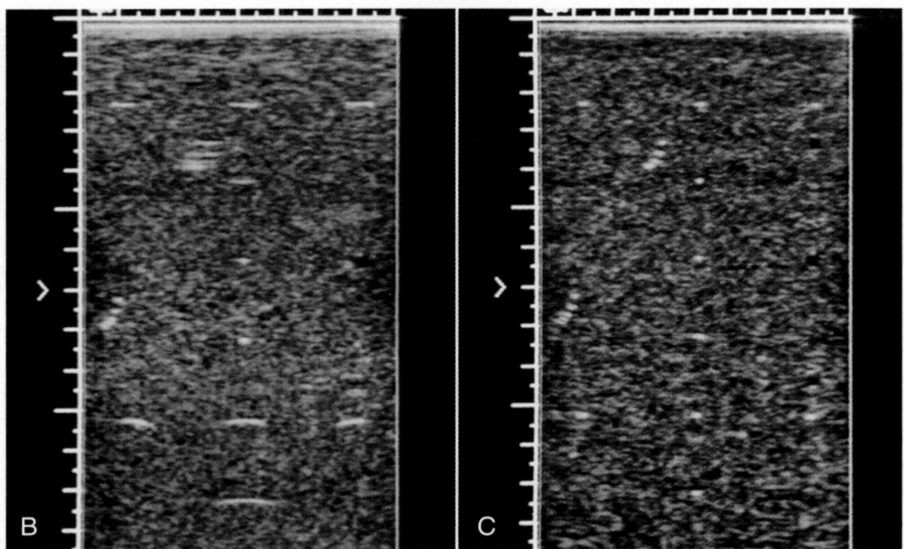

FIGURE 3-27 **A**, A spherically shaped echo arrives at array elements at different times, producing noncoincident voltages in the various channels. If simply combined, a weak, long voltage (with poor resolution and sensitivity) would result. However, with proper delays, the voltages are made to coincide, producing a strong, short (good resolution and sensitivity) voltage. While echoes return from deeper and deeper locations, their curvature is reduced. Thus the delay correction must be reduced while echoes return. This is called **dynamic focusing**. **B**, Dynamic focus is off. **C**, When the dynamic focus is on, resolution improves.

TABLE 3-3 Terms Used to Describe Arrays

Term	Construction	Scanning	Focusing
Array	√		
Linear	√		
Sequenced		√	
Convex	√		
Phased		√	√

BOX 3-2 Array Terminology

- (Phased) linear (sequenced) array
- (Phased) convex (sequenced) array
- (Linear) phased array
- (Phased and sequenced) (linear) vector array

The words in parentheses are implied in the abbreviated common terminology.

BOX 3-1 Common Transducer Types

- Linear array
- Convex array
- Phased array
- Vector array

TABLE 3-4 Transducer Characteristics

Type	Beam Scanned by Sequencing	Beam Scanned by Phasing	Beam Focused by Phasing
Linear array	√		√
Convex array	√		√
Phased array		√	√
Vector array	√	√	√

TABLE 3-5 Display Formats

Type	Rectangle or Parallelogram	Sector	Flat Top	Curved Top	Pointed Top
Linear array	√		√		
Convex array		√		√	
Phased array		√			√
Vector array		√	√		

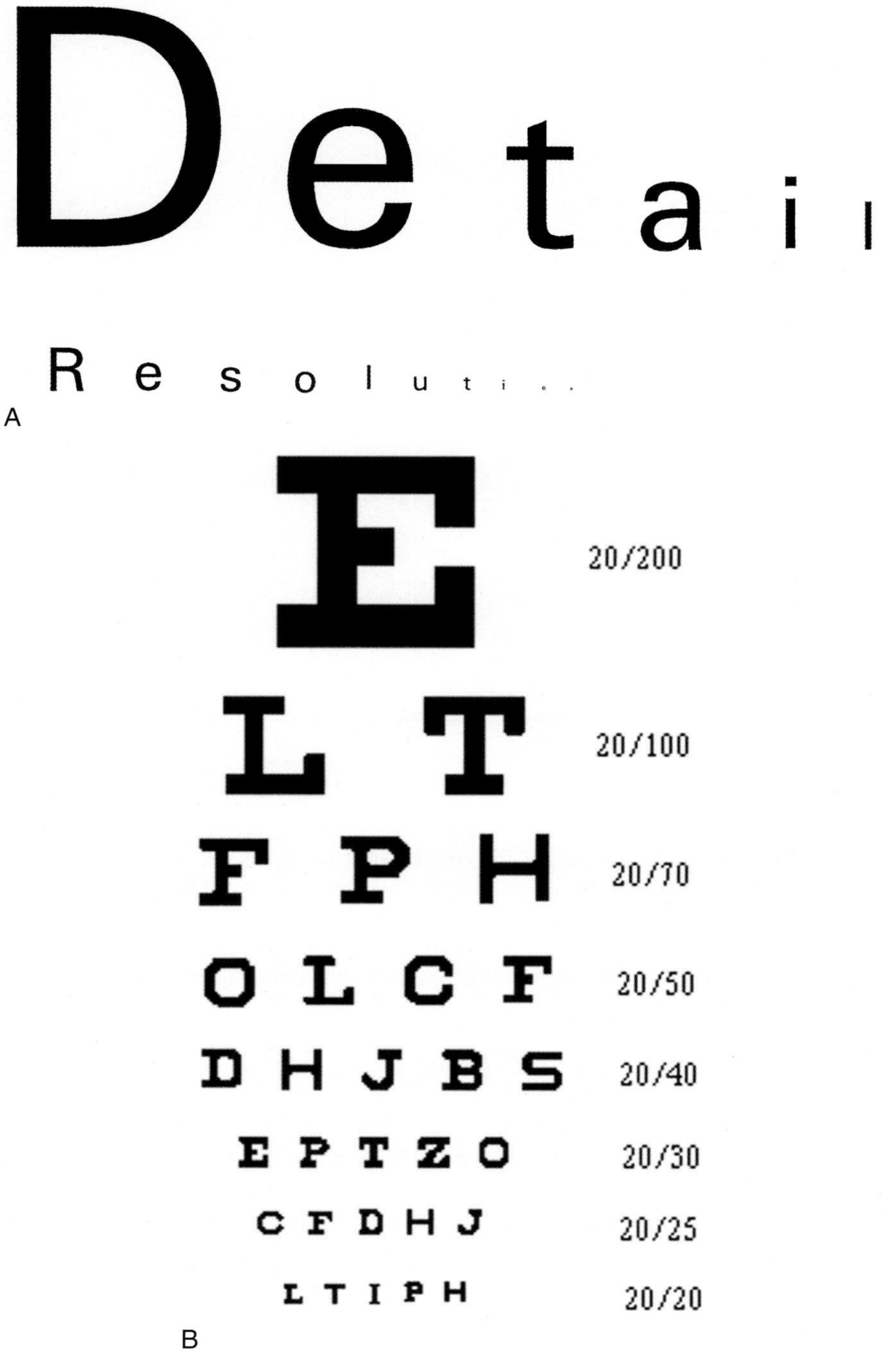

FIGURE 3-28 A, Excellent detail resolution is the ability to image fine detail. Smaller is better, that is, tinier details can be discerned. B, Snellen vision testing chart.

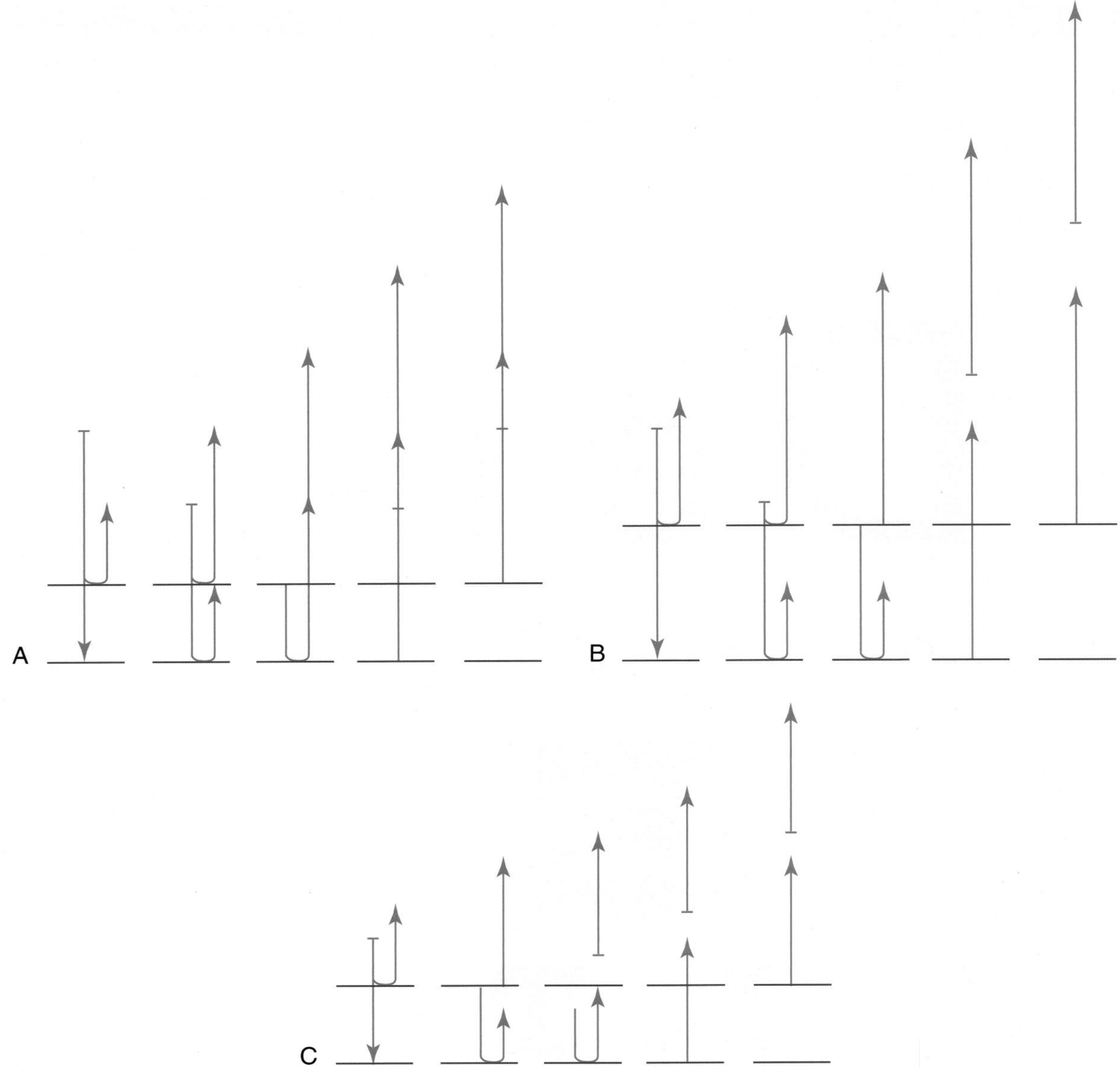

FIGURE 3-29 **Axial resolution.** Action proceeds in time from left to right in each part of the figure. **A,** The separation of the reflectors is less than half of the spatial pulse length and thus echo overlap occurs. Separate echoes are not produced. The reflectors are not resolved on the display. **B,** The reflector separation is increased so that it is greater than half of the spatial pulse length. Echo overlap does not occur. Separate echoes are produced, and the reflectors are resolved on the display. **C,** The reflector separation is the same as in **A,** but resolution is achieved by shortening the pulse to yield separate echoes.

directly to transducers and is therefore discussed in this section. If two reflectors are not separated sufficiently, they produce overlapping (not distinct) echoes that are not separated on the instrument display. Rather, the echoes merge together and appear as one. Thus the echoes are not resolved. If distinct (separated by a gap) echoes are not generated initially in the anatomy, the reflectors will not be separated on the display. In ultrasound imaging, two aspects of detail resolution are **axial** and **lateral**, which depend on the different characteristics of ultrasound pulses as they travel through tissues.

Axial Resolution

Axial resolution (AR) is the minimum reflector separation required along the direction of sound travel (along the scan line) to produce separate echoes (Figure 3-29). The important factor in determining AR is spatial pulse length. AR is equal to one half of the spatial pulse length.

$$\text{AR (mm)} = \frac{\text{SPL (mm)}}{2}$$

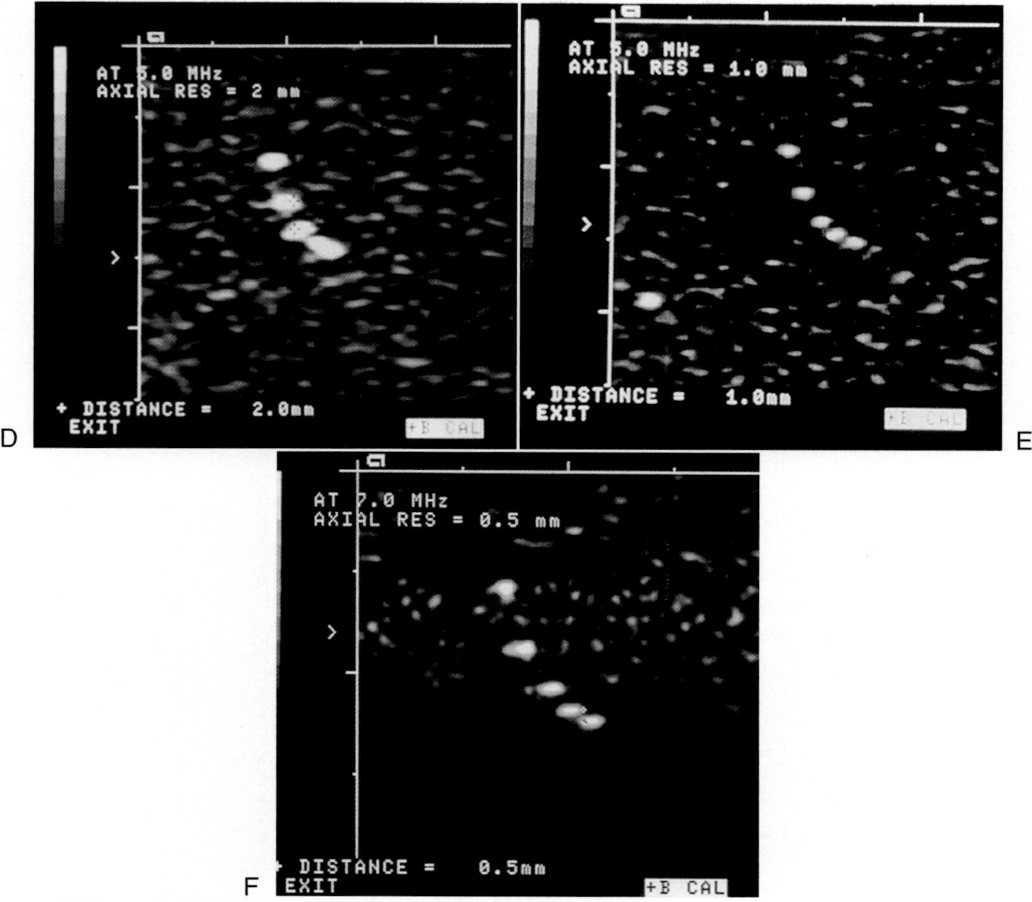

FIGURE 3-29, cont'd D-F, Axial resolution improves while frequency increases: **D**, 5.0 MHz, with a resolution of 2.0 mm; **E**, 5.0 MHz, with a resolution of 1.0 mm; **F**, 7.0 MHz, with a resolution of 0.5 mm.

> AR is the minimum reflector separation necessary to resolve reflectors along scan lines. AR (millimeters) equals spatial pulse length (millimeters) divided by 2.

Note that the numeric value of detail resolution decreases as frequency increases. AR is similar to a shopping-mall sale, a weight-loss program, or a golf score: smaller is better. The smaller the AR, the finer the detail that can be displayed; thus the two reflectors can be closer along the sound path and still be seen distinctly, thereby allowing tinier objects or finer detail to be displayed. To improve AR, spatial pulse length must be reduced. Because spatial pulse length is wavelength multiplied by number of cycles in the pulse, one or both of these factors must be reduced. Wavelength is reduced by increasing frequency. The number of cycles in each pulse is reduced by transducer damping. Because the number of cycles per pulse has been reduced to a minimum (one to three) by transducer design, the only way the instrument operator can improve axial resolution further is to increase frequency. With an increase in frequency, however, comes a reduction in penetration (imaging depth) because attenuation increases while frequency increases. Thus in sonographic imaging, there is a trade-off between resolution and penetration with changing frequency. This is, in fact, an image quality–quantity trade-off.

Lateral Resolution

Lateral resolution (LR) is the minimum reflector separation in the direction perpendicular to the beam direction (that is, across scan lines) that can produce two separate echoes when the beam is scanned across the reflectors (Figure 3-30). LR is equal to the beam width (w_b) in the scan plane.

$$LR(mm) = w_b\ (mm)$$

> Lateral resolution is the minimum reflector separation necessary to resolve reflectors across scan lines. Lateral resolution (millimeters) equals beam width (millimeters).

As with axial resolution, smaller LR is better. A smaller value indicates an improvement (finer detail and the ability to image tinier objects). Just as beam width varies with the distance from the transducer, so, too, does LR. If the lateral

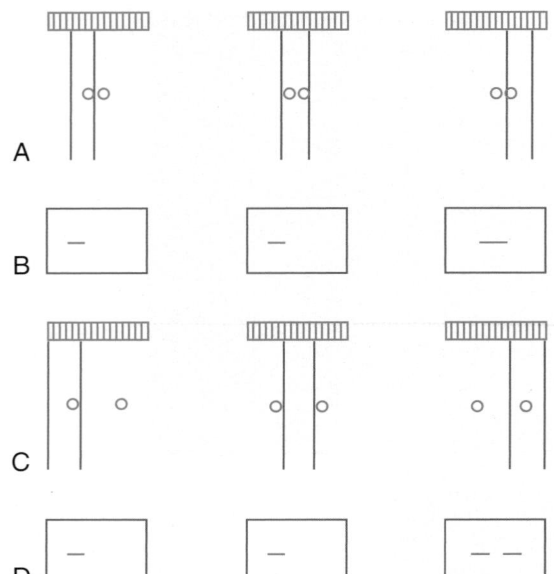

FIGURE 3-30 Lateral resolution. Reflector separation (perpendicular to beam direction) is less than beam diameter in **A** and **B**, whereas in **C** and **D**, reflector separation is greater than the beam diameter. Action proceeds in time from left to right in each part of the figure. **A**, The beam first encounters the left reflector, then is reflected by both reflectors, and finally is reflected by the right reflector. **B**, This scanning sequence results in continual reflection from one or both reflectors. Separate echoes are not produced, and the reflectors are not resolved. **C**, The beam encounters the left reflector, then fits between both reflectors (yielding no echo), and, finally, is reflected by the right reflector. **D**, Separate echoes are produced, and the reflectors are resolved on the display.

separation between two reflectors is greater than the beam diameter, two separate echoes are produced when the beam is scanned across them. Thus the echoes are resolved, or detected, as separate reflectors.

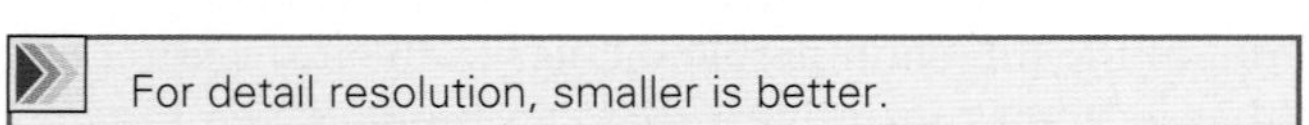

For detail resolution, smaller is better.

If frequency increases, detail resolution improves, but penetration decreases.

LR is improved by reducing the beam diameter, that is, by focusing (Figure 3-31). Figure 3-32 shows a focused beam. The lateral smearing of a thin layer of scatterers indicates the beam width and lateral resolution at various depths. The best resolution is obtained at the focus (Figure 3-33; see also Figure 3-24). Diagnostic ultrasound transducers often have better axial resolution than lateral resolution, although the two may be comparable in the focal region of strongly focused beams. Figure 3-34 shows examples of typical detail resolution.

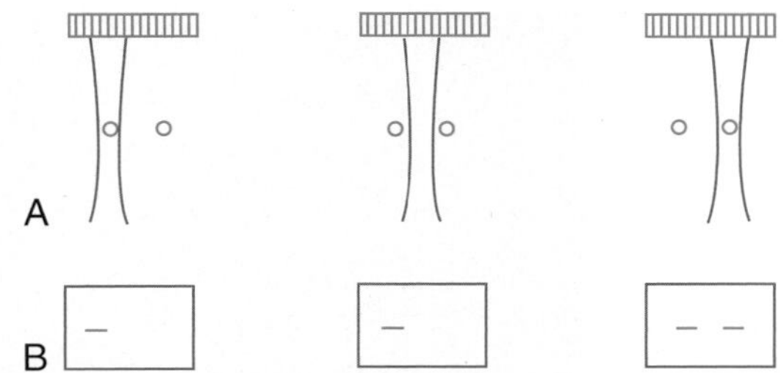

FIGURE 3-31 A, Two separate echoes are generated because the beam is focused and is narrower than the reflector separation. **B**, The two reflectors are resolved on the display. Without focusing, in this case, they would not have been resolved.

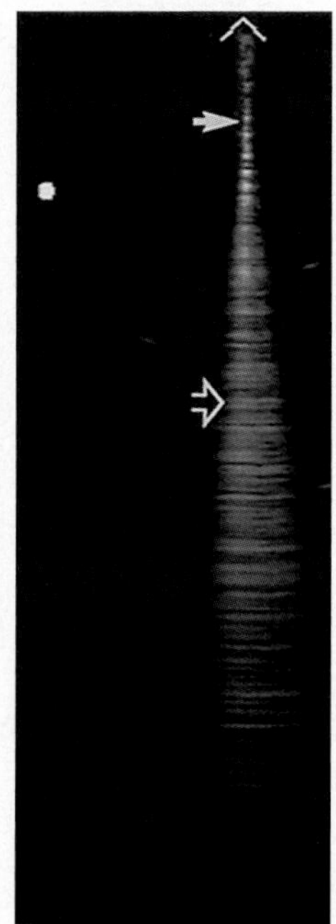

FIGURE 3-32 Beam width is shown as lateral smearing of a thin vertical scattering layer in a test object. The beam indicates the lateral resolution at each depth. In this example, beam width is approximately 2 mm at the focus (*closed arrow*) and approximately 10 mm at a depth of 6 cm (*open arrow*), well beyond the focus.

Elevational Resolution

Section thickness can be considered a third aspect of detail resolution and therefore is sometimes called **elevational resolution**. Elevational resolution contributes to section thickness artifact, also called *partial-volume artifact.* This artifact is a filling in of what should be anechoic structures, such as cysts. This filling in occurs when the section thickness is larger than the size of the structure. Thus echoes from outside the structure are included in the image, and the structure appears to be echoic. The thinner the section, the less its negative effect on sonographic images. Focusing in the section-thickness plane reduces section-thickness artifacts.

The effect of elevational resolution is different from that of axial and lateral resolutions. They cause axial and lateral

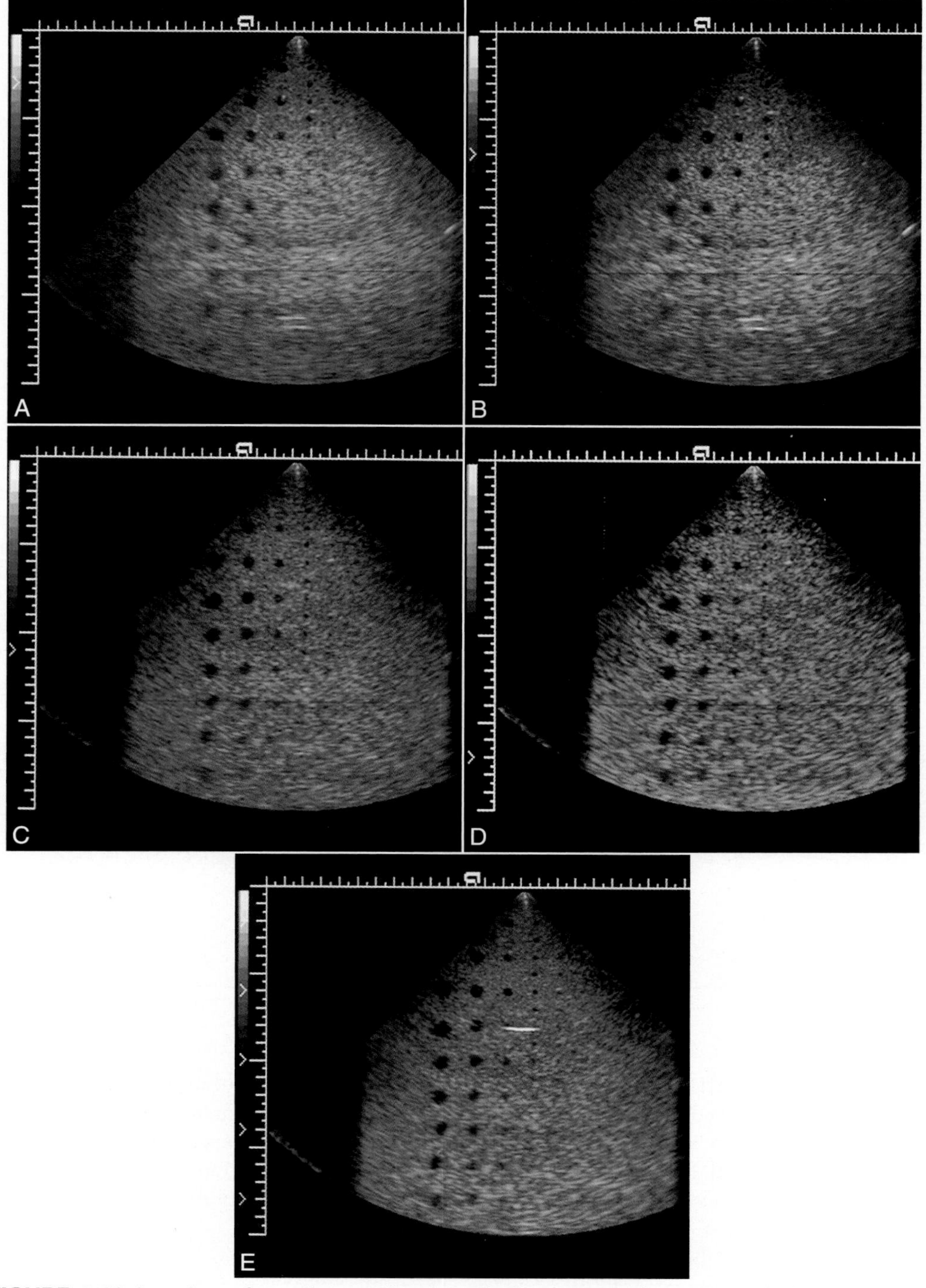

FIGURE 3-33 **Imaging of small cysts involves both aspects of detail resolution: axial and lateral.** Resolution improves at various depths when the focus is located there. Focus at 3 cm (**A**), 7 cm (**B**), 11 cm (**C**), and 17 cm (**D**). With multiple foci (**E**), resolution is improved throughout depth.

smearing of small structures, whereas section thickness brings structures into the image that should be outside. Section-thickness artifact is discussed and illustrated in a later chapter.

Useful Frequency Range

To meet resolution and penetration requirements reasonably, the useful frequency range for most diagnostic applications is 2 to 20 MHz. The lower portion of the range is useful when increased depth (e.g., in an obese subject) or high attenuation (e.g., in transcranial studies) is encountered. The higher portion of the frequency range is useful when little penetration is required (e.g., in imaging breast, thyroid, or superficial vessels or in pediatric imaging). In most large patients, 3 to 5 MHz is a satisfactory frequency; however, in thin

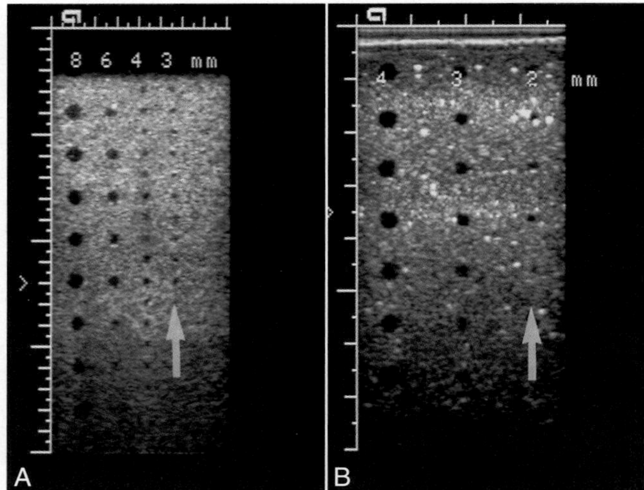

FIGURE 3-34 **A**, An image of a resolution penetration phantom that contains circular anechoic regions ("cysts") in tissue-equivalent material. From left to right, the cysts are 8, 6, 4, 3, and 2 mm in diameter and occur every 1 or 2 cm in depth of the image. Close examination reveals that the 3-mm cysts are the smallest that can be resolved. This image was produced with a 3.5-MHz transducer. **B**, The same phantom is imaged with a 7-MHz transducer. In this instance, the 2-mm cysts can be seen. Note the loss of penetration compared with that shown in **A** (8 cm versus 20 cm). Detail resolution can be improved by increasing the frequency of the ultrasound beam, but at the expense of decreasing the imaging depth.

TABLE 3-6 Typical Imaging Depth and Axial Resolution (Two-Cycle Pulse) in Tissue

Frequency (MHz)	Imaging Depth (cm)	Axial Resolution (mm)
2.0	30	0.77
3.5	17	0.44
5.0	12	0.31
7.5	8	0.20
10.0	6	0.15
15.0	4	0.10

patients and in children, 7.5 and 10 MHz often can be used. If frequencies less than 2 MHz are used, detail resolution is insufficient. If frequencies higher than 20 MHz (less than 20 MHz in deeper applications) are used, the depth is not sufficient in many applications. In the case of ophthalmologic, dermatologic, and intravascular imaging (the latter involving use of catheter-mounted transducers), frequencies as high as 50 MHz are used because penetration of only a few millimeters is sufficient. Table 3-6 lists values for typical imaging depths and axial resolutions for various frequencies.

REVIEW

The following key points are presented in this chapter:

- Transducers convert energy from one form to another.
- Ultrasound transducers convert electric energy to ultrasound energy, and vice versa.
- Transducers operate on the piezoelectric principle.
- Transducers are operated in pulse-echo mode.
- Operating frequency depends on element thickness.
- Axial resolution is equal to one half of the spatial pulse length.
- Pulsed transducers have damping material to shorten spatial pulse length for acceptable resolution.
- Transducers produce sound in the form of beams with near and far zones.
- Lateral resolution is equal to beam width.
- Beam width can be reduced by focusing to improve lateral resolution.
- Detail resolution improves with increasing frequency.
- *Linear* and *convex* are types of array construction.
- *Sequenced, phased,* and *vector* are types of array scanning operations.
- Phasing also enables electronic control of focus.

EXERCISES

Answers appear in the Answers to Exercises section at the back of the book.

1. A transducer converts one form of ____________ to another.
   a. energy
   b. force
   c. image
   d. scan
2. Ultrasound transducers convert ____________ energy into ____________ energy, and vice versa.
   a. electric, light
   b. heat, electric
   c. heat, light
   d. electric, ultrasound
3. Ultrasound transducers operate on the ____________ principle.
   a. piezomagnetic
   b. piezoelectric
   c. electropiezo
   d. electromagnetic
4. Single-element transducers are in the form of ____________.
   a. squares
   b. rectangles
   c. disks
   d. ovals
5. The ____________ of a transducer element changes when voltage is applied to its faces.
   a. width
   b. height
   c. length
   d. thickness
6. The term *transducer* is used to refer to a transducer ____________ or to a transducer ____________.
   a. element, assembly
   b. matching, element
   c. backing, damping
   d. backing, assembly
7. A transducer ____________ is part of a transducer ____________.
   a. assembly, element
   b. element, assembly
   c. cable, matching
   d. backing, damping
8. An electric voltage pulse, when applied to a transducer, produces an ultrasound ____________ of a(n) ____________ that is equal to that of the voltage pulse.
   a. pulse, amplitude
   b. intensity, amplitude
   c. pulse, frequency
   d. pulse, duration
9. The resonance frequency of an element is determined by its ____________.
   a. width
   b. height
   c. length
   d. thickness
10. Operating frequency ____________ when transducer element thickness is increased.
    a. increases
    b. decreases
    c. is unchanged
    d. none of the above
11. The addition of damping material to a transducer reduces the number of ____________ in the pulse, thus improving ____________ ____________. It increases ____________.
    a. amplitudes, detail resolution, frequency
    b. amplitudes, lateral resolution, bandwidth
    c. cycles, lateral resolution, frequency
    d. cycles, axial resolution, bandwidth
12. Damping material reduces the ____________ of the transducer and ____________ of the diagnostic system.
    a. efficiency, sensitivity
    b. frequency, sensitivity
    c. frequency, efficiency
    d. frequency, penetration
13. Ultrasound transducers typically generate pulses of ____________ or ____________ cycles.
    a. five, ten
    b. five, six
    c. one, three
    d. two, three
14. For a particular transducer element material, if a thickness of 0.4 mm yields an operating frequency of 5 MHz, the thickness required for an operating frequency of 10 MHz is ____________ mm.
    a. 0.1
    b. 0.2
    c. 0.3
    d. 0.5
15. Which of the following transducer frequencies would have the thinnest elements?
    a. 2 MHz
    b. 3 MHz
    c. 5 MHz
    d. 7 MHz
    e. 10 MHz
16. The matching layer on the transducer surface reduces ________ caused by impedance differences.
    a. attenuation
    b. amplitude
    c. transmission
    d. reflection
17. A coupling medium on the skin surface eliminates reflection caused by ____________.
    a. air
    b. skin
    c. matching layer
    d. element

18. Damping lengthens the pulse. True or false?
19. Damping increases efficiency. True or false?
20. The damping layer is in front/back of the element.
21. The matching layer is in front/back of the element.
22. The matching layer has ___________ impedance.
 a. high
 b. low
 c. intermediate
 d. zero
23. Elements in linear arrays are in the form of___________.
 a. rectangles
 b. squares
 c. rings
 d. disks
24. Transducer assemblies are also called ___________.
 a. transducers
 b. probes
 c. scanheads
 d. scan converters
 e. skinheads
 f. more than one of the above
25. Operating frequency is also called ___________ ___________.
 a. operating mode
 b. bandwidth mode
 c. operating bandwidth
 d. resonance frequency
26. Mixtures of a piezoelectric ceramic and a nonpiezoelectric polymer are called ___________.
 a. composites
 b. piezopolymers
 c. ceramopolymers
 d. piezocomposites
27. To operate a transducer at more than one frequency requires ___________ ___________.
 a. narrow bandwidth
 b. moderate bandwidth
 c. broad bandwidth
 d. no bandwidth
28. Is it practical to attempt to operate a 5-MHz transducer with a bandwidth of 1 MHz at 6 MHz?
29. Is it practical to attempt to operate a 5-MHz transducer with a bandwidth of 2.5 at 3 and 7 MHz?
30. A beam is divided into two regions, called the ___________ zone and the ___________ zone.
 a. near, far
 b. narrow, wide
 c. forward, reverse
 d. low, high
31. The dividing point between the two regions referred to in Exercise 30 is at a distance from the transducer equal to ___________ ___________ length.
 a. narrow zone
 b. near zone
 c. wide zone
 d. far zone
32. Transducer size is also called ___________.
 a. aperture
 b. zone
 c. bandwidth
 d. width
33. Near-zone length increases with increasing source ___________ and ___________.
 a. amplitude, intensity
 b. amplitude, frequency
 c. aperture, frequency
 d. aperture, amplitude
34. Which transducer element has the longest near zone?
 a. 6 mm, 5 MHz
 b. 6 mm, 7 MHz
 c. 8 mm, 7 MHz
35. A higher-frequency transducer produces a ___________ near-zone length.
 a. longer
 b. shorter
 c. unchanged
 d. none of the above
36. A smaller aperture produces a(n) ___________ near-zone length.
 a. longer
 b. shorter
 c. unchanged
 d. none of the above
37. A transducer with a near-zone length of 10 cm can be focused at 12 cm. True or false?
38. Which of the following transducer(s) can focus at 6 cm?
 a. 5 MHz, near-zone length of 5 cm
 b. 4 MHz, near-zone length of 6 cm
 c. 4 MHz, near-zone length of 10 cm
 d. b and c
 e. None of the above
39. Sound may be focused by using a ___________.
 a. curved element
 b. lens
 c. phased array
 d. more than one of the above
40. Focusing reduces the beam diameter at all distances from the transducer. True or false?
41. The distance from a transducer to the location of the narrowest beam width produced by a focused transducer is called focal ___________.
 a. length
 b. width
 c. depth
 d. height
42. Transducer arrays are transducer assemblies with several transducer ___________.
 a. elements
 b. layers
 c. cables
 d. backings

43. Linear arrays scan beams by ____________ element groups.
a. phasing
b. steering
c. delaying
d. sequencing

44. A phased linear array with a single line of elements can focus in ____________ dimension(s).
a. one
b. two
c. three
d. five

45. Focusing in section thickness can be accomplished with ____________ elements or a ____________.
a. curved, sequencer
b. round, sequencer
c. curved, lens
d. round, lens

46. Electronic focusing in section thickness requires multiple rows of ____________.
a. lenses
b. matchers
c. dampers
d. elements

47. Match the following (answers may be used more than once):
a. Linear array ________.
b. Phased array ________.
c. Convex array ________.
  1. Voltage pulses are applied in succession to groups of elements across the face of a transducer.
  2. Voltage pulses are applied to most or all elements as a group, but with small time differences.

48. If the elements of a phased array are pulsed in rapid succession from right to left, the resulting beam is ____________.
a. steered right
b. steered left
c. focused

49. If the elements of a phased array are pulsed in rapid succession from outside in, the resulting beam is ____________.
a. steered right
b. steered left
c. focused

50. ____________ and ____________ describe how arrays are constructed.
a. linear
b. phased
c. sequenced
d. vector
e. convex

51. ____________, ____________, and ____________ describe how arrays are operated.
a. linear
b. phased
c. sequenced
d. vector
e. convex

52. Shorter time delays between elements fired from outside in result in ____________ curvature in the emitted pulse and a ____________ focus.
a. no, weak
b. less, shallower
c. less, deeper
d. greater, shallower
e. greater, deeper

53. A rectangular image is a result of linear scanning of the beam. This means that pulses travel in ____________ ____________ direction(s) from ____________ starting point(s) across the transducer face.
a. two different, one
b. many different, many
c. the same, one
d. the same, different

54. A sector image is a result of sector steering of the beam. This means that pulses travel in ____________ direction(s) from a common ____________ at the transducer face.
a. two different, end
b. different, origin
c. the same, point
d. the same, end

55. In ____________ and ____________ arrays, pulses travel out in different directions from different starting points on the transducer face.
a. linear, convex
b. convex, phased
c. phased, vector
d. convex, vector

56. Axial resolution is the minimum reflector separation required along the direction of the ____________ ____________ to produce separate ____________.
a. scan lines, echoes
b. sound travel, amplitudes
c. double reflectors, lines
d. scan lines, amplitudes

57. Axial resolution depends directly on ____________ ____________ ____________.
a. the peak amplitude
b. spatial echo distance
c. spatial pulse length
d. spatial pulse width

58. Smaller axial resolution is better. True or false?

59. If there are three cycles of a 1-mm wavelength in a pulse, the axial resolution is ____________ mm.
a. 1.0
b. 1.5
c. 2.5
d. 3.0

60. For pulses traveling through soft tissue in which the frequency is 3 MHz and there are four cycles per pulse, the axial resolution is ____________ mm.
a. 1.0
b. 1.5
c. 2.5
d. 3.0

61. If there are two cycles per pulse, the axial resolution is equal to the ___________. At 5 MHz in soft tissue, this is ___________ mm.
   a. wavelength, 5.0
   b. wavelength, 0.3
   c. duration, 1.54
   d. duration, 0.2
62. Doubling the frequency causes axial resolution to be ___________.
   a. doubled
   b. increased
   c. degraded
   d. halved
63. Doubling the number of cycles per pulse causes axial resolution to be ___________.
   a. doubled
   b. increased
   c. degraded
   d. halved
64. When studying an obese subject, a higher frequency likely will be required. True or false?
65. If better resolution is desired, a lower frequency will help. True or false?
66. If frequencies less than ___________ MHz are used, axial resolution is not sufficient.
   a. 0.1
   b. 2
   c. 5
   d. 20
67. If frequencies higher than ___________ MHz are used, penetration is not sufficient.
   a. 0.1
   b. 2
   c. 5
   d. 20
68. Increasing frequency improves resolution because ___________ is reduced, thus reducing ___________ ___________ ___________.
   a. attenuation, depth of penetration
   b. attenuation, spatial pulse length
   c. wavelength, spatial pulse length
   d. wavelength, depth of penetration
69. Increasing frequency decreases penetration because ___________ is increased.
   a. reflection
   b. heating
   c. speed
   d. attenuation
70. Lateral resolution is the minimum ___________ between two reflectors at the same depth such that when a beam is scanned across them, two separate ___________ are produced.
   a. separation, propagations
   b. amplitude, propagations
   c. separation, echoes
   d. amplitude, echoes
71. Lateral resolution is equal to ___________ ___________ in the scan plane.
   a. beam width
   b. pulse length
   c. beam length
   d. pulse height
72. Lateral resolution does not depend on ___________.
   a. frequency
   b. aperture
   c. phasing
   d. depth
   e. damping
73. For an aperture of a given size, increasing frequency improves lateral resolution. True or false?
74. Lateral resolution varies with distance from the transducer. True or false?
75. For a given frequency, a smaller aperture always yields improved lateral resolution. True or false?
76. Lateral resolution is determined by ___________. (There is more than one correct answer to the question.)
   a. damping
   b. frequency
   c. aperture
   d. number of cycles in the pulse
   e. distance from the transducer
   f. focusing
77. Match the following transducer assembly parts with their functions:
   a. Cable ________
   b. Damping material ______
   c. Piezoelectric element ______
   d. Matching layer ________
      1. Reduces reflection at transducer surface
      2. Converts voltage pulses to sound pulses
      3. Reduces pulse duration
      4. Conducts voltage pulses
78. Which of the following improve sound transmission from the transducer element into the tissue? (more than one correct answer)
   a. Matching layer
   b. Doppler effect
   c. Damping material
   d. Coupling medium
   e. Refraction
79. A 5-MHz unfocused transducer with an element thickness of 0.4 mm, an element width of 13 mm, and a near-zone length of 14 cm produces two-cycle pulses. Determine the following:
   a. Operating frequency if thickness is reduced to 0.2 mm: ___________ MHz
   b. Axial resolution in the case of (a): ___________ mm
   At 5 MHz:
   c. Depth at which lateral resolution is best: ___________ cm
   d. Lateral resolution at 14 cm: ___________ mm
   e. Lateral resolution at 28 cm: ___________ mm
   f. This transducer can be focused at depths less than ___________ cm.

80. Lateral resolution is improved by ___________.
a. damping
b. pulsing
c. focusing
d. matching
e. absorbing

81. For an unfocused transducer, the best lateral resolution (minimum beam width) is ___________ the transducer width. This value of lateral resolution is found at a distance from the transducer face that is equal to the ___________ ___________ length.
a. equal to, near zone
b. half, near zone
c. equal to, far zone
d. half, far zone

82. For a focused transducer, the best lateral resolution (minimum beam width) is found in the ___________ region.
a. near
b. far
c. local
d. focal

83. An unfocused 3.5-MHz, 13-mm transducer will yield a minimum beam width (best lateral resolution) of ___________ mm.
a. 3.5
b. 13
c. 26
d. 6.5

84. An unfocused 3.5-MHz, 13-mm transducer produces three-cycle pulses. The axial resolution in soft tissue is ___________ mm.
a. 0.7
b. 1.4
c. 13
d. 26

85. In Exercises 83 and 84, axial resolution is better than lateral resolution. True or false?

86. Axial resolution is often not as good as lateral resolution in diagnostic ultrasound. True or false?

87. The two resolutions may be comparable in the ___________ region of a strongly focused beam.
a. near
b. far
c. local
d. focal

88. Beam diameter may be reduced in the near zone by focusing. True or false?

89. Beam diameter may be reduced in the far zone by focusing. True or false?

90. Match each transducer characteristic with the sound beam characteristic it determines (answers may be used more than once):
a. Element thickness: ________, ________, and ________
b. Element width: ___________
c. Element shape (flat or curved): ________
d. Damping: ________
1. Axial resolution
2. Lateral resolution
3. Operating frequency

91. The principle on which ultrasound transducers operate is the ___________
a. Doppler effect
b. Acousto-optic effect
c. Acoustoelectric effect
d. Cause and effect
e. Piezoelectric effect

92. Which of the following is not decreased by damping?
a. Refraction
b. Pulse duration
c. Spatial pulse length
d. Efficiency
e. Sensitivity

93. Which three things determine beam diameter for a disk transducer?
a. Pulse duration
b. Frequency
c. Aperture
d. Distance from disk face
e. Efficiency

94. A two-cycle pulse of 5-MHz ultrasound produces separate echoes from reflectors in soft tissue separated by 1 mm. True or false?

95. The lower and upper limits of the frequency range useful in diagnostic ultrasound are determined by ___________ and ___________ requirements, respectively.
a. penetration, attenuation
b. penetration, resolution
c. resolution, penetration
d. attenuation, resolution

96. The range of frequencies useful for most applications of diagnostic ultrasound is ___________ to ___________ MHz.
a. 0.1, 15
b. 2, 20
c. 1, 10
d. 1, 5

97. Because diagnostic ultrasound pulses are usually two or three cycles long, axial resolution is usually equal to ___________ to ___________ wavelengths.
a. 2, 3
b. 4, 6
c. 1, 3.5
d. 1, 1.5

98. What are the axial resolutions in Figure 3-35, *A-B*?
a. 5 mm, 4 mm
b. 4 mm, 3 mm
c. 3 mm, 2 mm
d. 2 mm, 1 mm

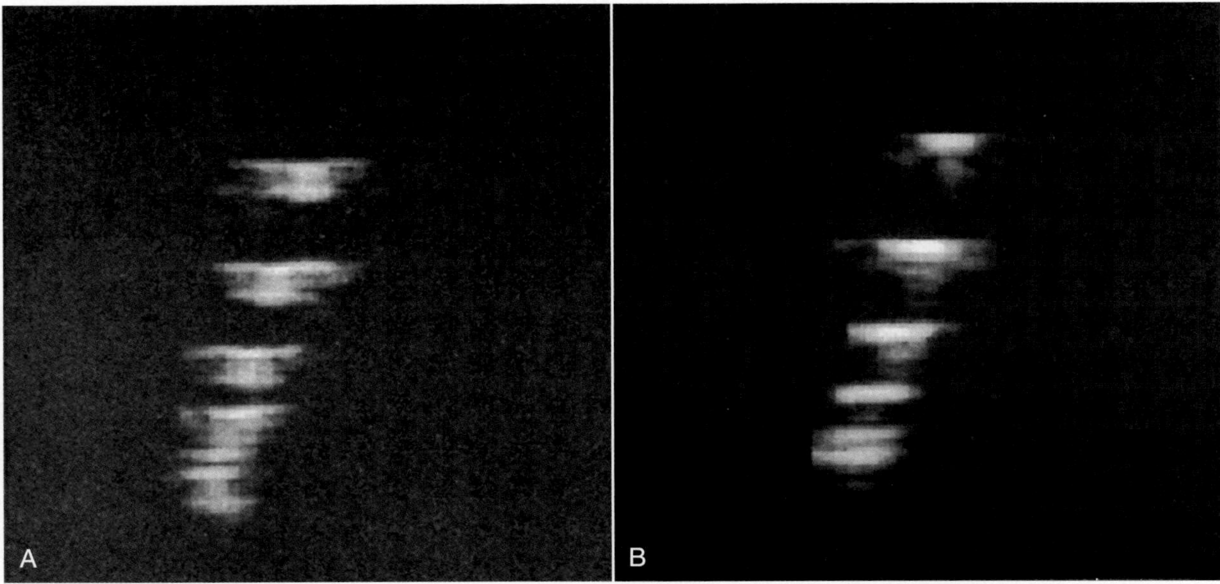

FIGURE 3-35 Illustration to accompany Exercise 98. **A**, An image of a set of six rods in a test object. They are separated by 5, 4, 3, 2, and 1 mm from top to bottom. This scan was made with a transducer that produces 3.5-MHz ultrasound. The first three rods have been separated, whereas the images of the last three rods have merged. This image also shows small reverberation echoes behind each rod. **B**, The same rods imaged with a 5-MHz transducer. Higher-frequency transducers produce shorter pulse lengths and therefore provide improved axial resolution.

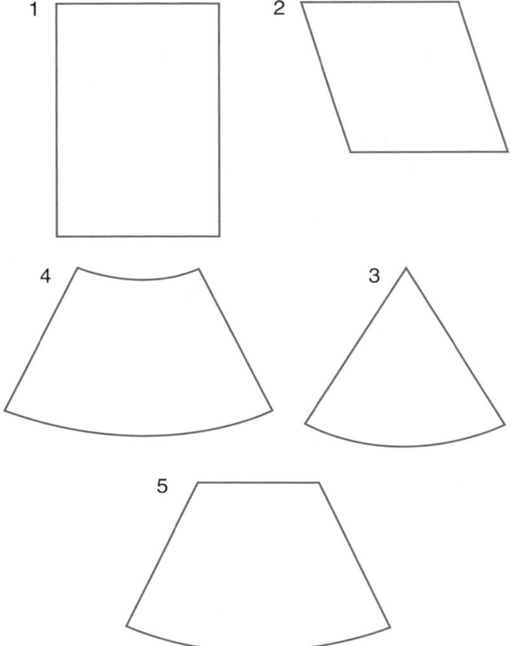

FIGURE 3-36 Display formats. Illustration to accompany Exercise 100.

99. At what depth is the best lateral resolution in Figure 3-14, *C*?

a. 1 cm
b. 2 cm
c. 3 cm
d. 4 cm

100. Match the transducer type with the display formats in Figure 3-36.

a. Linear array ____________
b. Convex array ____________
c. Phased array ____________
d. Vector array ____________
e. Phased linear array ____________

4

Instruments

LEARNING OBJECTIVES

After reading this chapter, the student should be able to do the following:

- Explain how sonographic instruments work.
- List the primary components of sonographic instruments.
- List the functions of each component.
- Describe how images are stored electronically.
- Compare preprocessing with postprocessing.
- Compare signal processing and image processing.
- Explain how displays work.
- List the common display modes.
- Define contrast resolution and list the factors that influence it.
- Define temporal resolution and list the factors that influence it.
- Discuss the purposes of coded excitation, gain, compensation, detection, and compression.
- Describe how elastography differs from conventional gray-scale anatomic imaging

OUTLINE

KEY TERMS

A mode
Amplification
Amplifier
Analog
Analog-to-digital converter
B mode
B scan
Bandpass filter
Beam former
Bistable
Bit
Channel
Cine loop
Coded excitation
Compensation
Compression
Contrast resolution
Demodulation
Depth gain compensation
Detection
Digital
Digital-to-analog converter
Display
Dynamic range
Elastography
Flat-panel display
Frame
Frame rate
Freeze-frame
Gain
Gray scale
Image memory
Image processor
Lateral gain control
M mode
Panoramic imaging
Persistence
Picture archiving and communications systems
Pixel
Postprocessing
Preprocessing
Radio frequency
Real-time
Real-time display
Refresh rate
Scan line
Scanning

KEY TERMS—cont'd

Shear wave
Signal
Signal processor
Spatial compounding
Strain
Stress
Temporal resolution
Time gain compensation
Volume imaging
Young's modulus

In the preceding chapters, we discussed the means by which ultrasound is generated and how it interacts with tissues. We now consider the instruments that receive echo voltages from the transducer and display them in the form of anatomic images. Diagnostic ultrasound systems are pulse-echo instruments. They determine echo strengths and locations of echo-generation sites. The directions and arrival times of echoes returning from tissues determine the locations of echo-generation sites. This chapter describes how the instrument drives the transducer and what it does with the returning echoes.

Sonographic systems (Figure 4-1) produce visual displays from the echo voltages received from the transducer. Figure 4-1, *A*, presents a diagram of the organization of a pulse-echo

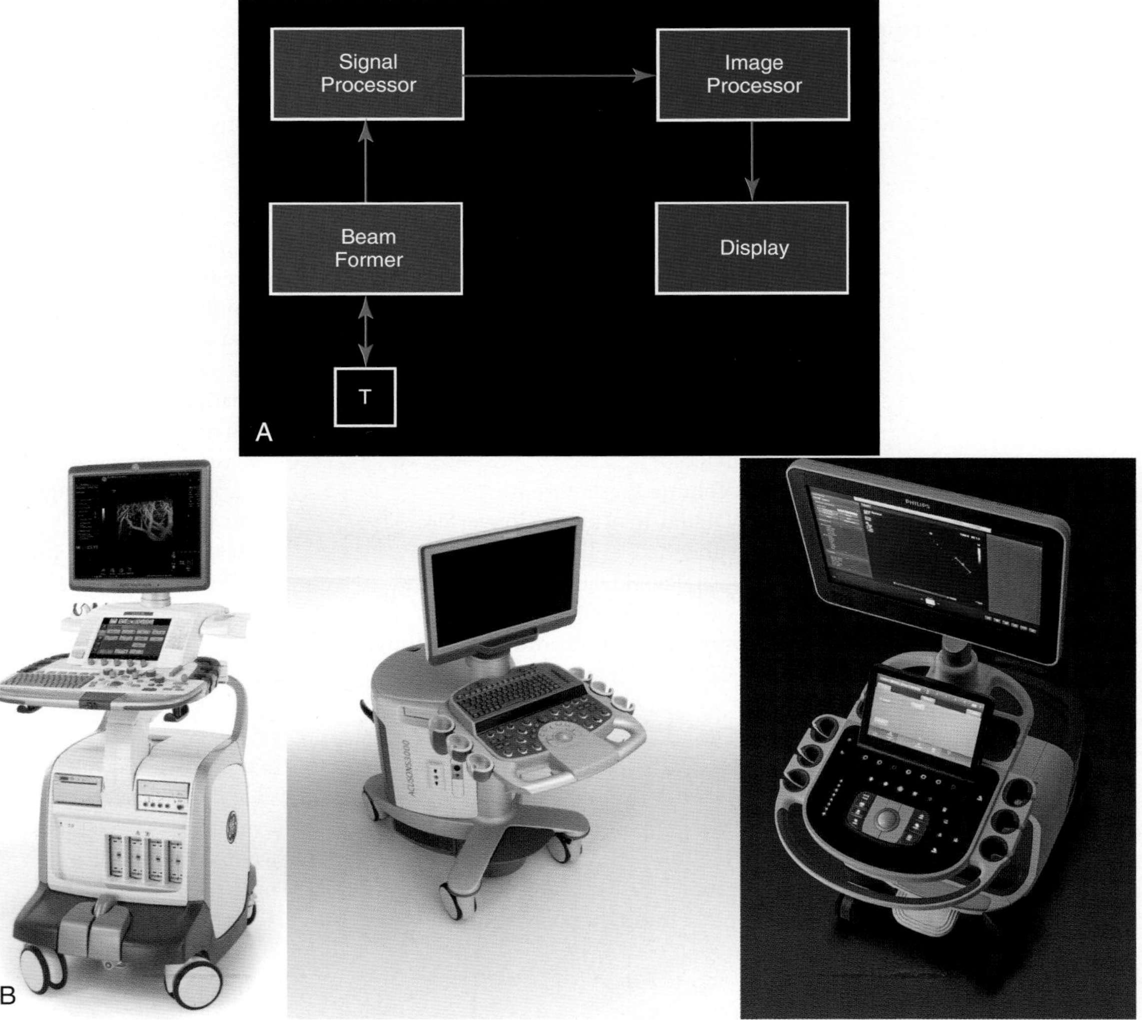

FIGURE 4-1 A, The organization of a pulse-echo imaging system. The beam former produces electric pulses that drive the transducer and performs initial functions on the returning echo voltages from the transducer. The transducer produces an ultrasound pulse for each electric pulse applied to it. For each echo received from the tissues, an electric voltage is produced by the transducer. These voltages go through the beam former to the signal processor, where they are processed to a form suitable for input to the image processor. Electric information from the image processor drives the display, which produces a visual image of the cross-sectional anatomy interrogated by the system. B, Fully featured sonographic instruments.

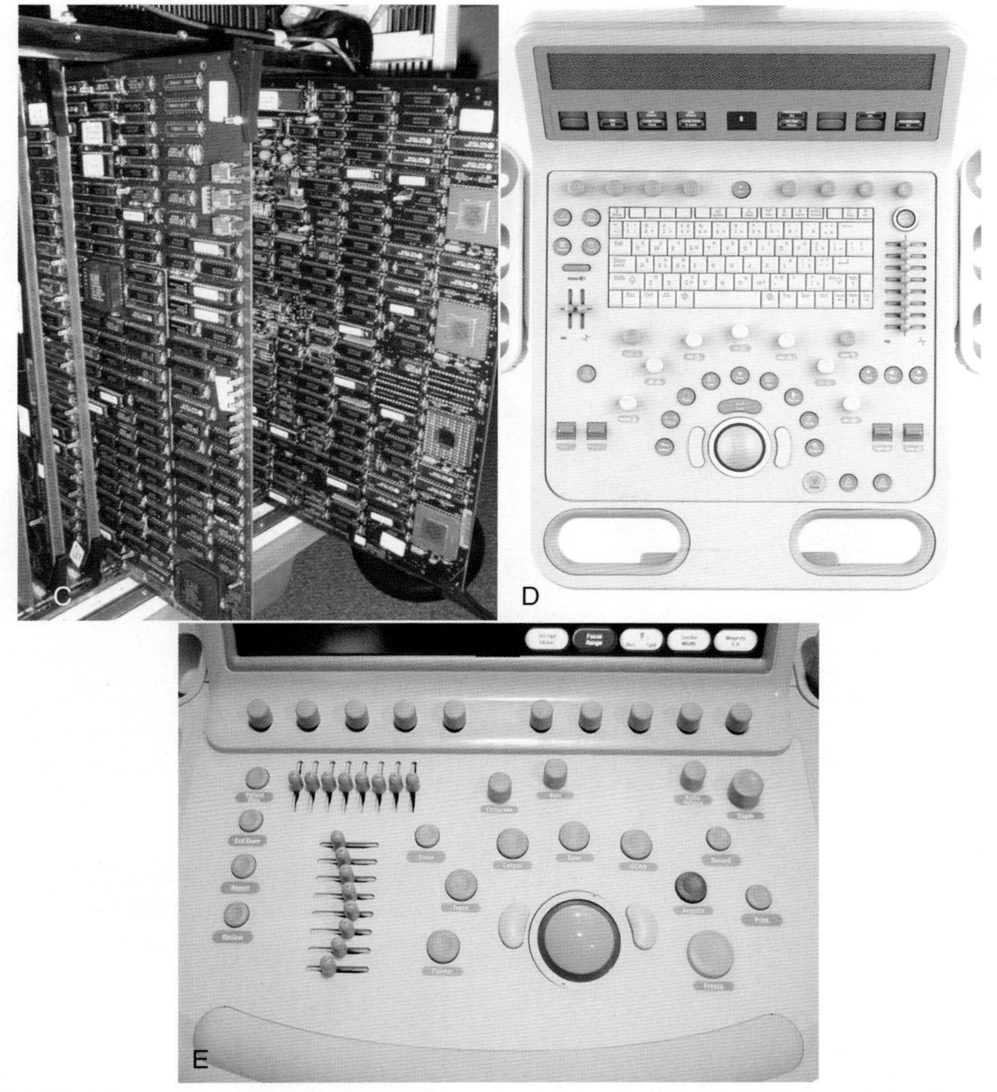

FIGURE 4-1, cont'd C, Sonographic instruments contain circuit boards, integrated circuits, and other electronic components. D-E, Instrument control panels.

Continued

sonographic imaging system. The instrument is composed of a **beam former**, a **signal processor**, an **image processor**, and a **display**.

BEAM FORMER

The beam former is where the action originates. The beam former is diagrammed in Figure 4-2. It consists of a pulser, pulse delays, transmit/receive (T/R) switch, **amplifiers**, analog-to-digital converters, echo delays, and a summer. Box 4-1 lists the functions of a beam former.

Pulser

The pulser produces electric voltages (Figure 4-3) that drive the transducer, forming the beam that sweeps through the tissue to be imaged. The driving voltages are typically in the form of a single cycle of voltage of the desired operating frequency. In response, the transducer produces ultrasound pulses that travel into the patient. The frequency of the voltage pulse determines the frequency of the resulting ultrasound pulse (see Figure 4-3, *B-E*). Frequency ranges from 2 to 20 MHz for most applications.

> The pulser generates the voltages that drive the transducer.

Pulse repetition frequency (PRF) is the number of voltage pulses sent to the transducer each second and thus the number of ultrasound pulses produced per second. PRF ranges from 4 to 15 kHz (5 to 30 kHz for Doppler applications). The ultrasound PRF is equal to the voltage PRF because one

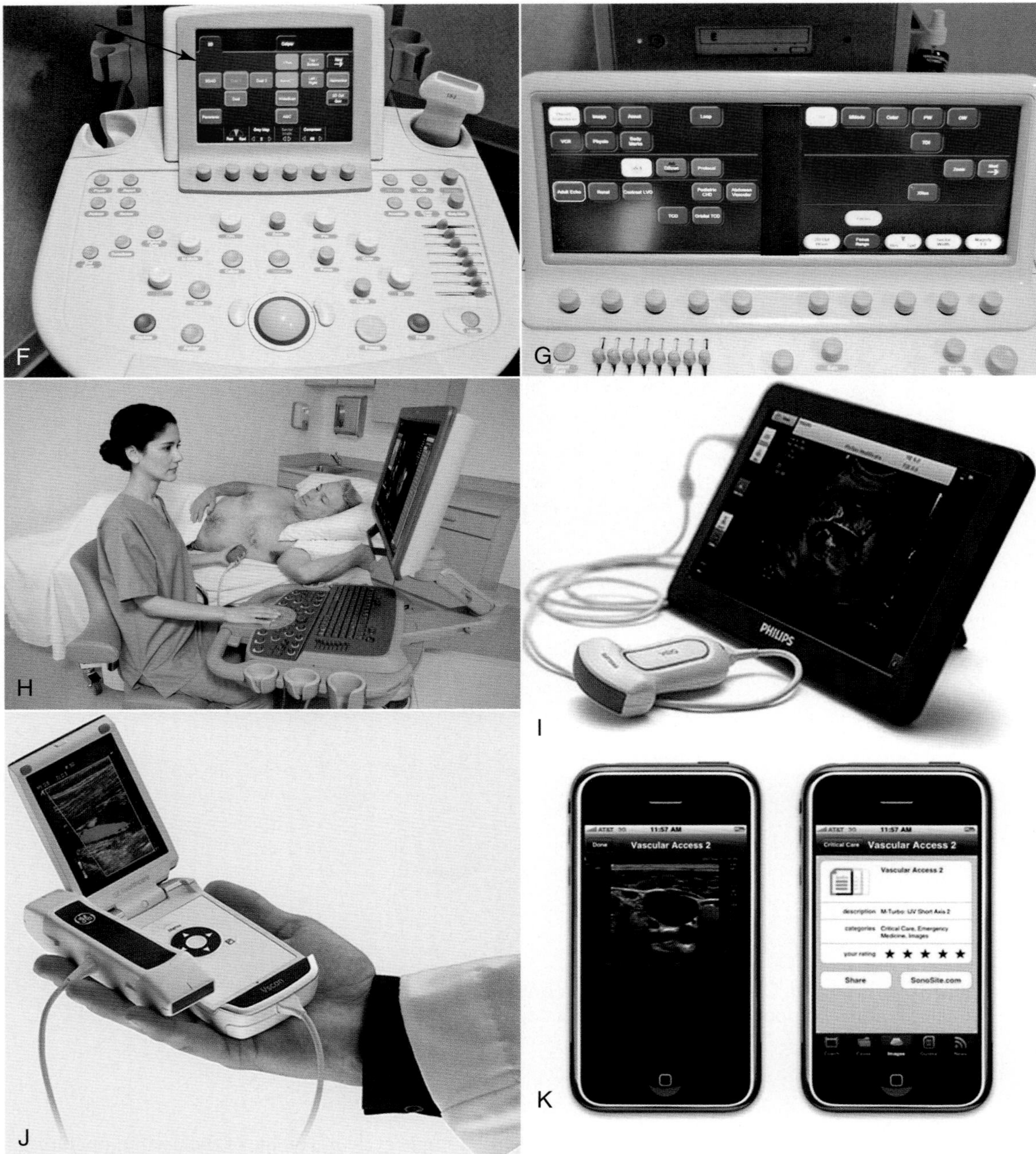

FIGURE 4-1, cont'd F-G, Point-and-click software controls for image control, transducer selection, and other functions. H, Cart system. I-K, Portable systems. (B, Courtesy of GE Healthcare, Siemens Healthcare, and Philips Healthcare. H, Courtesy of Siemens Healthcare. J, Courtesy of GE Healthcare.)

ultrasound pulse is produced for each voltage pulse. Similarly, the ultrasound pulse repetition period is equal to the voltage pulse repetition period. This is the time from the beginning of one pulse to the beginning of the next. The operator does not normally have direct control of PRF. Rather, the pulser adjusts it appropriately for the current imaging depth. To receive information for display at a rapid rate, a high PRF is desirable. PRF, however, must be limited to provide proper display of returning echoes. The timing sequence that is initiated by the pulse is shown in Figure 4-4. To avoid echo misplacement, all echoes from one pulse must be received before the next pulse is emitted. For deeper imaging, echoes take longer to return, thus forcing a reduction in PRF and the number of images that are generated each second, called *frame rate.* Imaging

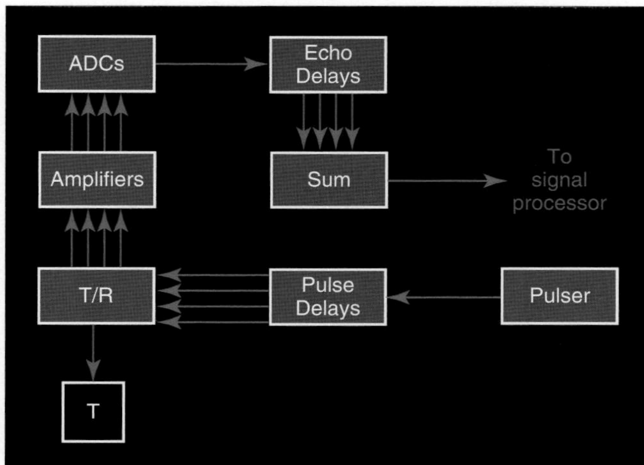

FIGURE 4-2 The beam former consists of a pulser, delays, transmit/receive (T/R) switch, amplifiers, analog-to-digital converters (ADCs), and a summer. The beam former sends digitized echo-voltage streams to the signal processor. *T* is the transducer.

depth—that is, penetration (*pen*) in centimeters—multiplied by PRF (in kilohertz) must not exceed 77 if echo misplacement is to be avoided.

$$\text{pen}\,(\text{cm}) \times \text{PRF}\,(\text{kHz}) \leq 77\,(\text{cm/ms})$$

The symbol ≤ means "less than or equal to."

The instrument automatically achieves the highest PRF while avoiding echo misplacement. While operating frequency is reduced and penetration increases, PRF is reduced to avoid echo misplacement.

BOX 4-1 Functions of the Beam Former

- Generating voltages that drive the transducer.
- Determining PRF, coding, frequency, and intensity.
- Scanning, focusing, and apodizing the transmitted beam.
- Amplifying the returning echo voltages.
- Compensating for attenuation.
- Digitizing the echo voltage stream.
- Directing, focusing, and apodizing the reception beam.

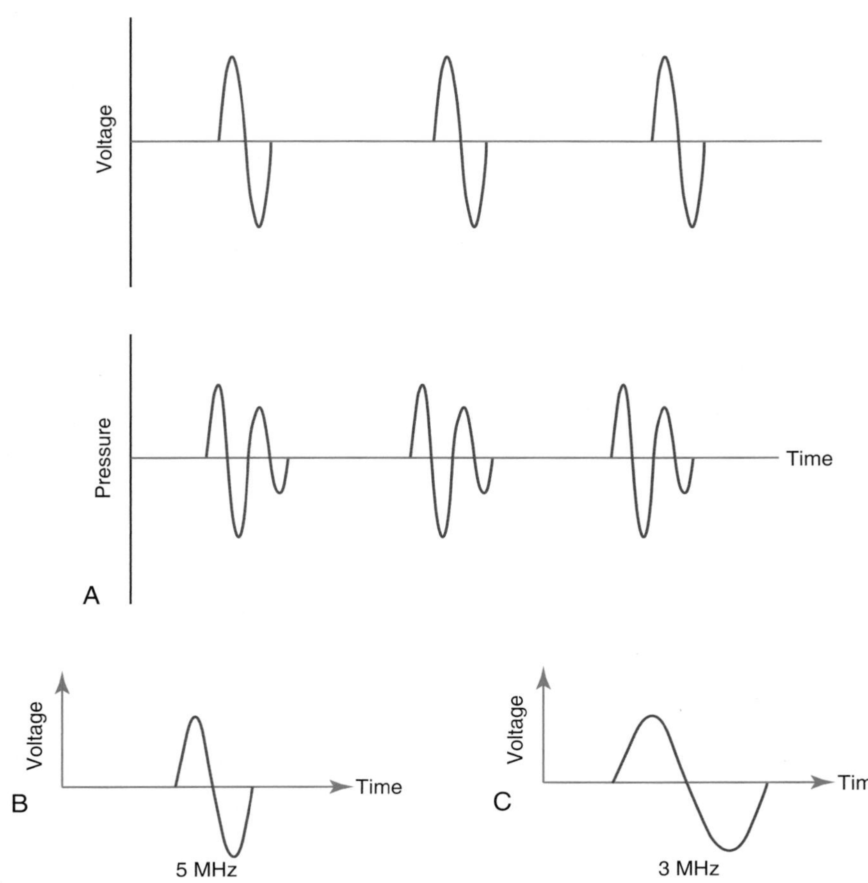

FIGURE 4-3 With every voltage pulse applied (**A**), an ultrasound pulse is produced by the transducer. Voltage pulses of different frequencies (**B** and **C**) produce ultrasound pulses of different frequencies. The operator can change the operating frequency without changing transducers.

Continued

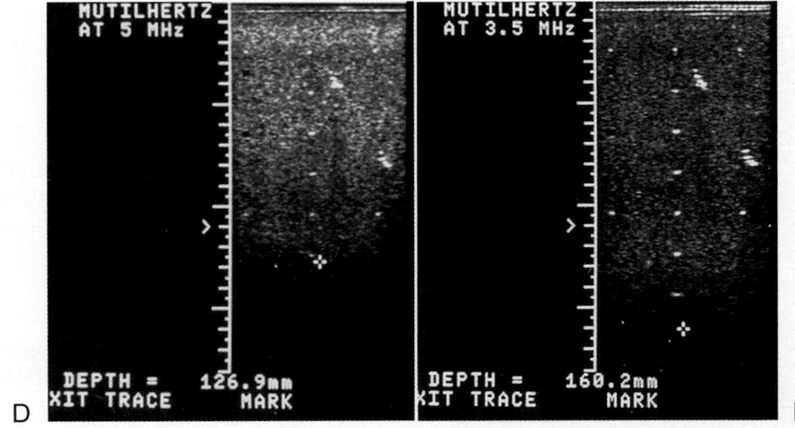

FIGURE 4-3, cont'd D-E, Images with 5- and 3.5-MHz frequencies, respectively, with the same transducer.

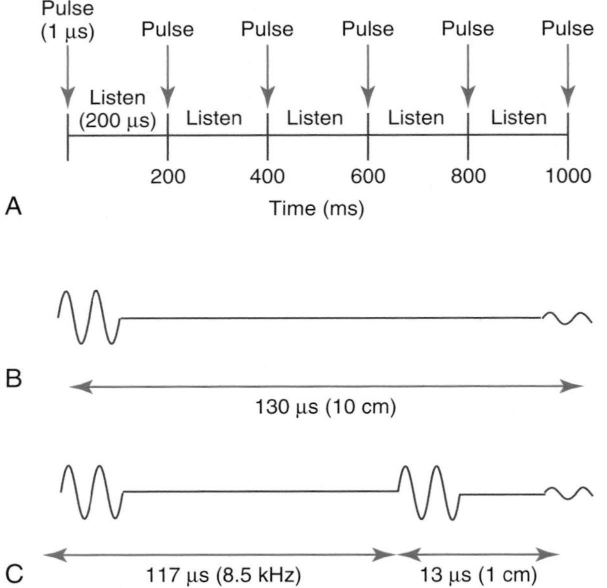

FIGURE 4-4 A, Timing sequence for pulse-echo ultrasound imaging. The sequence is initiated by the production of a 1-μs pulse of ultrasound when the pulser sends a voltage pulse to the transducer. This is followed by a period of as long as 250 μs during which echoes are received from the tissue by the transducer. The length of this time is determined by the maximum depth from which the echoes return. For example, at a frequency of 5 MHz, echoes can return from as deep as 15 cm. The round-trip travel time (13 μs/cm × 15 cm) to this depth is 195 μs. This listening period is followed (5 μs later) by the next pulse. In this illustration, the listening period is 200 μs; that is, the pulse repetition period is 200 μs (the pulse repetition frequency [PRF] is 5 kHz). If PRF were greater, the pulse repetition period would be decreased, resulting in emission of the next pulse before the reception of all the (deeper) echoes from the previous pulse. This would produce range-ambiguity artifact (see Chapter 6) and thus should be avoided. The PRF is automatically adjusted to avoid this problem: higher PRFs are used for superficial imaging, whereas lower PRFs are used for deep imaging (to allow for the longer time required for the arrival of deeper echoes). The latter causes a reduction in frame rate. **B**, An echo (from a 10-cm depth) arrives 130 μs after pulse emission. **C**, If the pulse repetition period were 117 μs (corresponding to a PRF of 8.5 kHz), the echo in B would arrive 13 μs after the next pulse was emitted. The instrument would place this echo at a 1-cm depth rather than the correct value. This is known as *range-ambiguity artifact*.

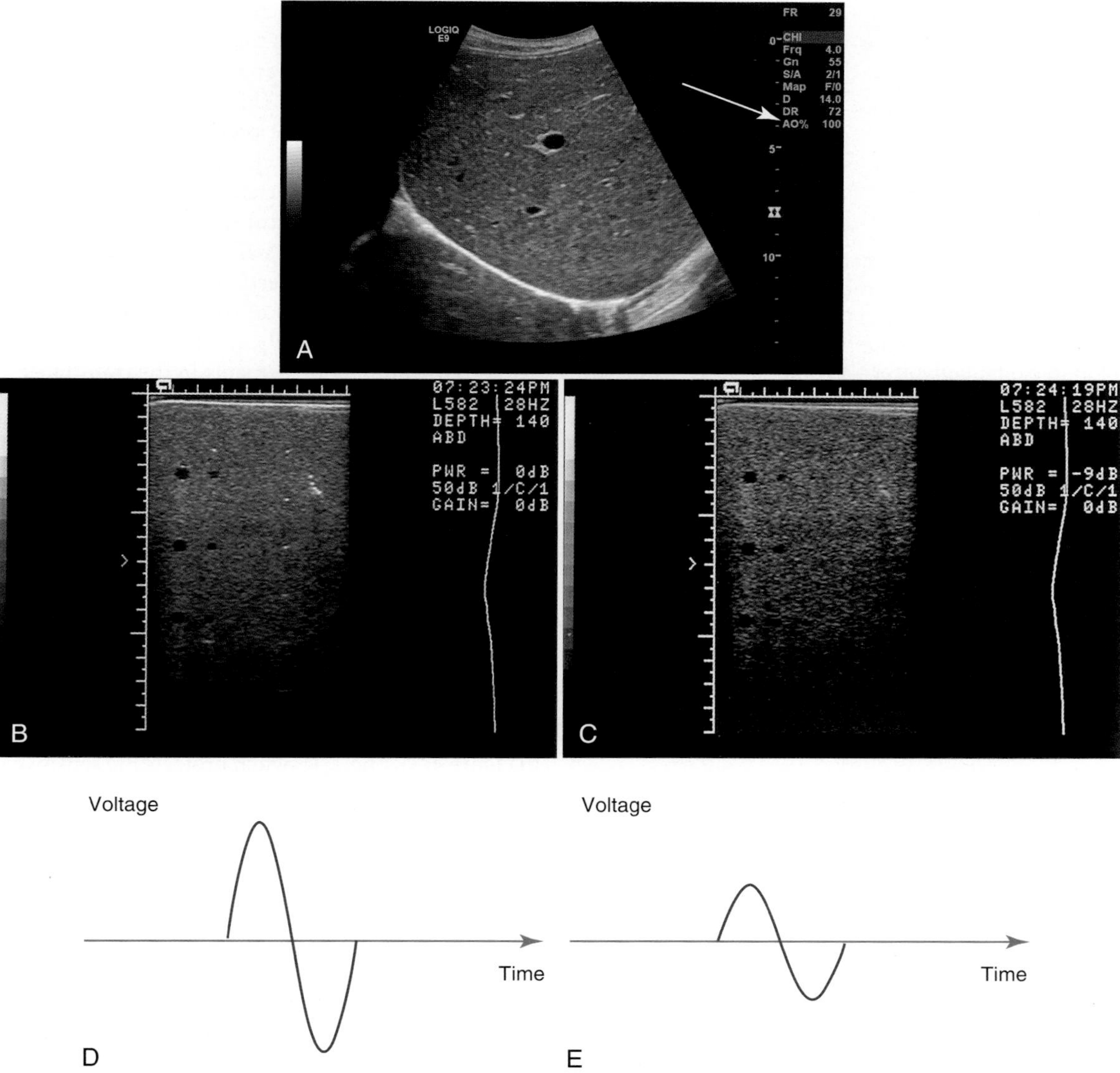

FIGURE 4-5 A, The output indicator (*arrow;* AO = acoustic output) shows a percentage relative to the maximum (100% in this example). B-C, The output indicator here shows decibels relative to the maximum. An output of 0 dB (100%) is compared with one of -9 dB (12.5%), in which the weaker echoes produce a darker image. D-E, Driving voltages from pulser to transducer for 0 and -6 dB, respectively. The voltage amplitude in E is half that in D, yielding one fourth the power and intensity, thus -6 dB output compared with D.

The greater the voltage amplitude produced by the pulser, the greater the amplitude and intensity of the ultrasound pulse produced by the transducer. Transducer driving–voltage amplitudes range to approximately100 V. Output level is sometimes shown on the display in terms of a percentage or decibels relative to maximum (100% or 0 dB) output (Figure 4-5). Other output indicators account for relevant risk mechanisms. Reduction of acoustic output reduces received echo amplitude (see Figure 4-5, *C*). An increase in amplifier gain can compensate for this. A reduction in imaging depth also occurs, but this is surprisingly small. For example, a reduction of 50% in output from a 5-MHz transducer corresponds to only a 5% penetration reduction (from approximately12.0 to 11.4 cm).

Pulse Delays

Thus far, the job of the beam former appears simple, but we must remember that with arrays, complicated sequencing and phasing operations are involved. Sequencing, phase delays, and variations in pulse amplitudes, which are necessary for the electronic control of beam scanning, steering, transmission focusing, aperture, and apodization, must be accomplished. The pulser and pulse delays carry out all of these tasks.

Channels

The pulse delays have a single input from the pulser but multiple outputs to the transducer elements; that is, there are actually many delay paths in the pulse delay circuitry. The

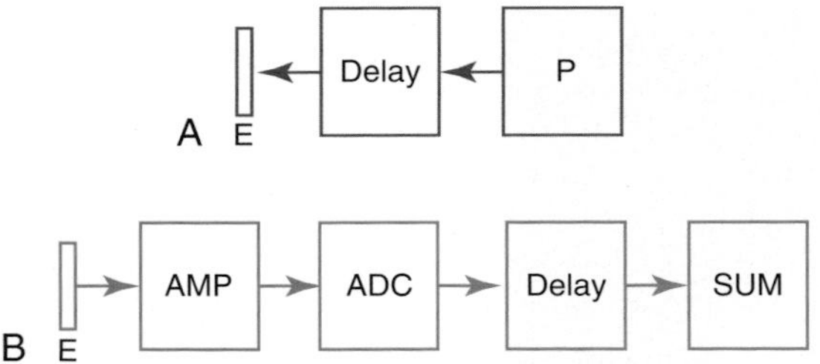

FIGURE 4-6 **A,** A transmission channel consists of an independent delay and transducer element *(E)* combination. Several channels emanate from the pulser *(P)*. **B,** A reception channel consists of an independent element *(E)*, amplifier *(AMP)*, analog-to-digital converter *(ADC)*, and delay. The signals from many channels are combined in the summer *(SUM)*.

reason for this is that each of the many elements in the array needs a different delay to form the ultrasound beam properly. Each independent delay and element combination constitutes a transmission **channel** (Figure 4-6). An increased number of channels allows more precise control of beam characteristics. On reception, each independent element, amplifier, analog-to-digital converter, and delay path constitutes a reception channel. Typical numbers of channels in modern sonographic instruments are 64, 128, and 192. Larger numbers are sometimes advertised, but a looser definition (than the one presented here) of the term *channel* is used in such advertisements. Normally, the number of channels does not exceed the number of elements in the transducer.

> A channel is an independent signal path consisting of a transducer element, delay, and possibly other electronic components.

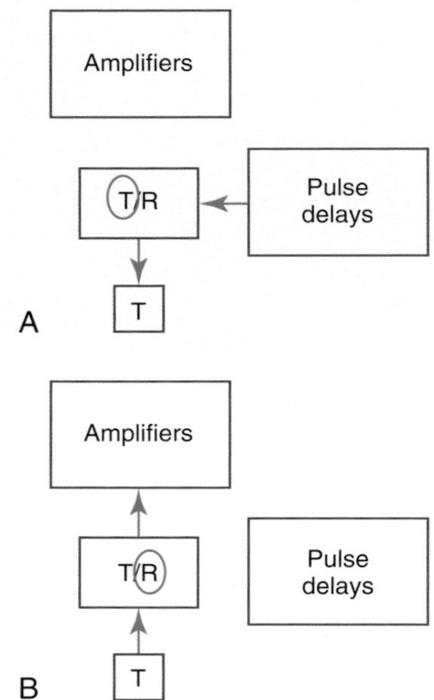

FIGURE 4-7 Transmit/receive (T/R) switch. A, During transmission (energizing the transducer to send a pulse into the body), the T/R switch opens the path from the pulser to the transducer elements. **B,** During echo reception, the T/R switch opens the path from the elements to the reception amplifiers.

Transmit/Receive Switch

The transmit/receive (T/R) switch directs the driving voltages from the pulser and pulse delays to the transducer during transmission and then directs the returning echo voltages from the transducer to the amplifiers during reception (Figure 4-7). The T/R switch protects the sensitive input components of the amplifiers from the large driving voltages from the pulser.

Amplifiers

Amplifiers increase voltage amplitude. The beam former has one amplifier for each channel. **Amplification** is the conversion of the small voltages received from the transducer elements to larger ones suitable for further processing and storage (Figure 4-8). **Gain** is the ratio of amplifier output to electric power input. The power ratio, which is expressed in decibels, is equal to the voltage ratio squared because electric power depends on voltage squared. For example, if the input voltage amplitude to an amplifier is 2 mV and the output voltage amplitude is 200 mV, the voltage ratio is 200/2, or 100. The power ratio is 100^2,

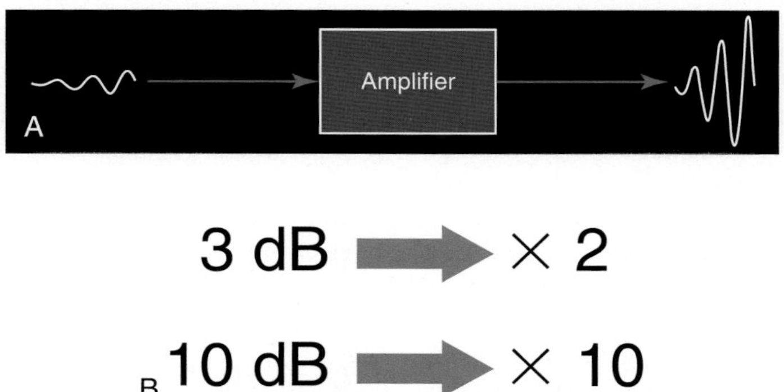

FIGURE 4-8 Gain. A, Amplification (gain) increases voltage amplitude and electric power. **B,** A gain of 3 dB corresponds to an output power equivalent to input power × 2; 10 dB corresponds to an input power × 10.

or 10,000. As shown in Table 4-1, the gain is 40 dB. Beam former amplifiers typically have 60 to 100 dB of gain. Voltages from transducers to these amplifiers range from a few microvolts (μV; for example, from blood) to a few hundred millivolts (mV; for example, from bone or gas). For a 60-dB gain amplifier, the output power is 1,000,000 times the power input, and the output voltage is 1000 times the input. For a 10-μV voltage input, the output voltage is 10 mV. If the gain of this amplifier is increased to 100 dB, the output voltage increases to 1 V.

TABLE 4-1 Gain (Expressed in Decibels) and Corresponding Power and Amplitude Ratios*

Gain (dB)	Power Ratio	Amplitude Ratio
0	1.0	1.0
1	1.3	1.1
2	1.6	1.3
3	2.0	1.4
4	2.5	1.6
5	3.2	1.8
6	4.0	2.0
7	5.0	2.2
8	6.3	2.5
9	7.9	2.8
10	10	3.2
15	32	5.6
20	100	10
25	320	18
30	1,000	32
35	3,200	56
40	10,000	100
45	32,000	180
50	100,000	320
60	1,000,000	1,000
70	10,000,000	3,200
80	100,000,000	10,000
90	1,000,000,000	32,000
100	10,000,000,000	100,000

*The power (amplitude) ratio is output power (amplitude) divided by input power (amplitude).

> Amplifiers increase voltage amplitudes. This increase is called *gain.*

Two useful decibel values to remember are 3 and 10 (see Figure 4-8, *B*). Whereas 3 dB corresponds to a power gain of ×2, 10 dB corresponds to ×10. Values also can be combined; for example, 6 dB corresponds to two doublings (×4); 20 dB corresponds to ×10×10, or ×100; and 13 dB corresponds to ×10×2, or ×20.

Gain control (Figure 4-9) determines how much amplification is accomplished in the amplifier. Gain control is similar in function to the level control on your sound system at home. With too little gain, weak echoes are not imaged. With too much gain, saturation occurs; that is, most echoes appear bright, and differences in echo strength are lost.

> Gain is set subjectively so that echoes appear with appropriate brightnesses.

The amplifiers must also compensate for the effect of attenuation on the image. **Compensation** (also called **time gain compensation** [TGC] and **depth gain compensation**) equalizes differences in received echo amplitudes caused by different reflector depths. Reflectors with equal reflection coefficients will not result in echoes of equal amplitude arriving at the transducer (Figure 4-10) if their travel distances are different (i.e., if the distances between the transducer and the reflectors are different) because sound weakens as it travels (attenuation). Display of echoes from similar reflectors in a similar way is desirable. These echoes may not arrive with the same amplitude because of different path lengths, therefore their amplitudes must be adjusted to compensate

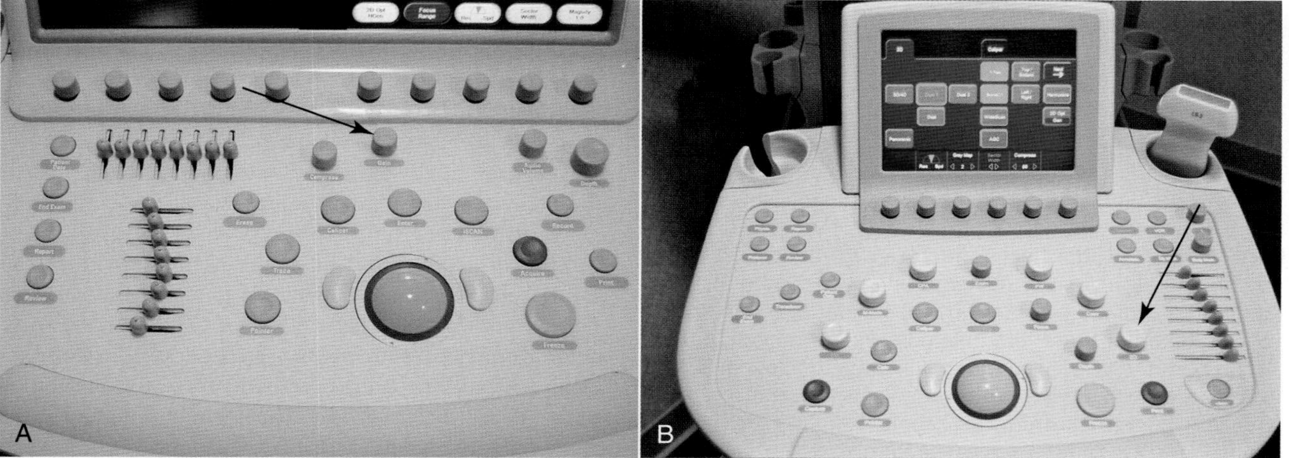

FIGURE 4-9 A-B, Gain controls *(arrows).*

Continued

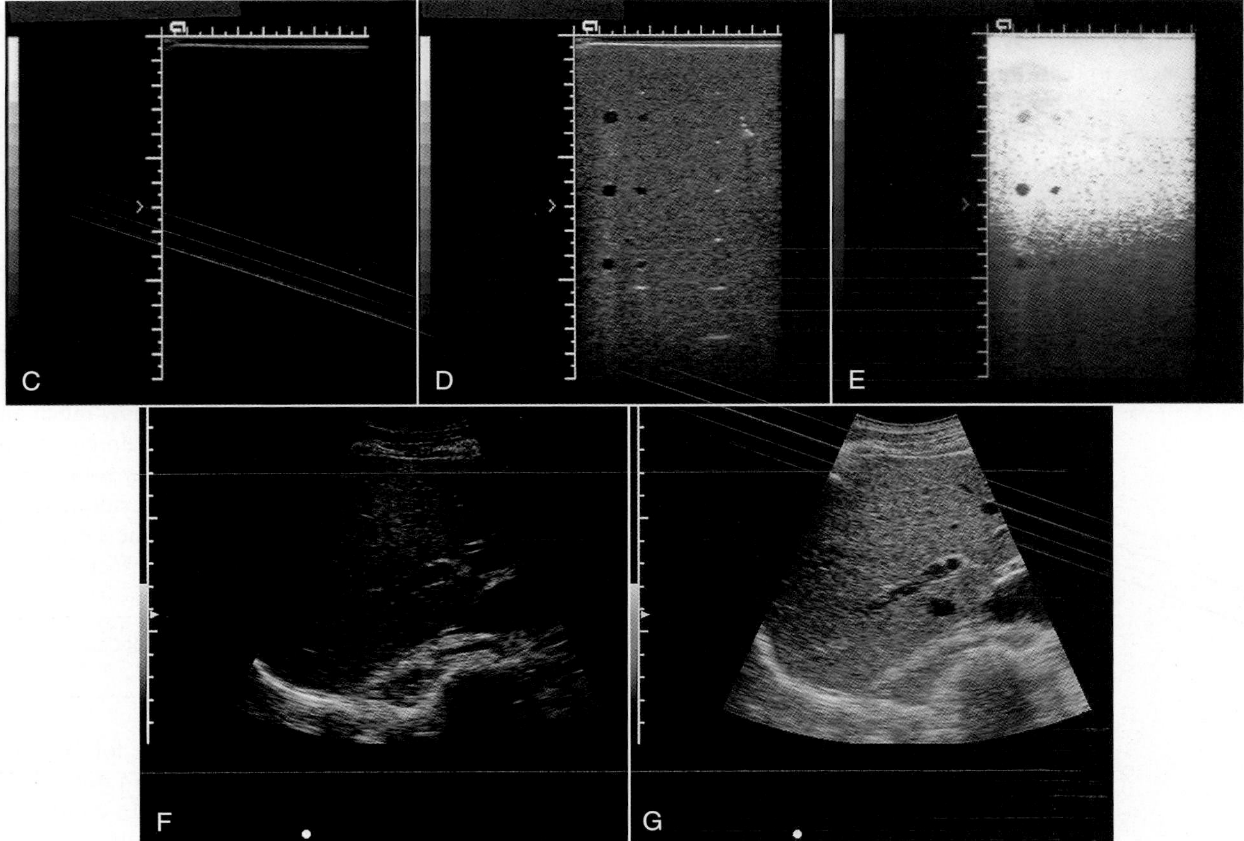

FIGURE 4-9, cont'd C, Gain is too low. D, Proper gain. E, Gain is too high, causing saturation. Abdominal scans with low (F) and proper (G) gain.

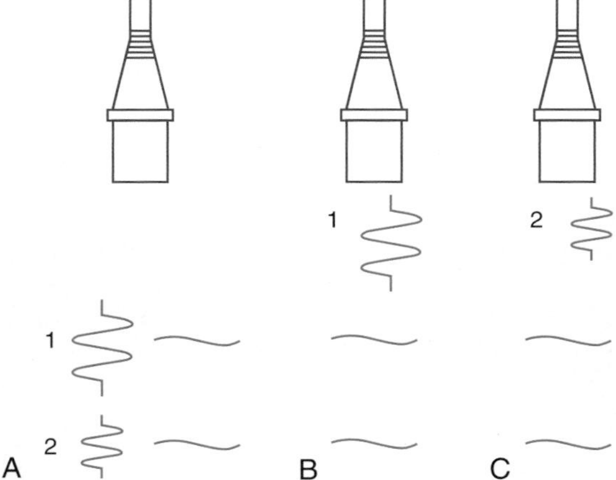

FIGURE 4-10 Two identical reflectors are located at different distances from the transducer. A, The echo at the second reflector is weaker because the incident pulse had to travel farther to get there, thereby increasing attenuation. B, The echo from the first reflector arrives at the transducer. The echo is weaker than it was in A because of attenuation on the return trip. C, The echo from the second reflector arrives at the transducer later and in a weaker form than the first one did because of the longer path to the second reflector.

for differences in attenuation. Longer path lengths result in greater attenuation and later arrival times. Therefore if voltages from echoes arriving later are amplified correctly to a greater degree than are earlier ones, attenuation compensation is accomplished. This is the goal of compensation (Figure 4-11). In other words, the later an echo arrives, the farther it has traveled and the weaker it will be. However, the later it arrives, the more it will be amplified. If this compensation is done properly, the resulting amplitude will be the same as if there had been no attenuation.

The increase of gain with depth is commonly called *time gain compensation slope* because it is sometimes displayed graphically as a line with increasing deflection to the right. This slope can be expressed in decibels of gain per centimeter of depth. When properly adjusted, the slope should correspond to the average attenuation coefficient in the tissue, expressed in decibels per centimeter of depth. Remember that each centimeter of depth corresponds to 2 cm of round-trip sound travel, so the resulting slope should be about 1 dB/cm-MHz because average attenuation in soft tissue is 0.5 dB/cm-MHz. The former refers to centimeters of depth, whereas the latter refers to centimeters of travel. Because attenuation depends on the frequency of

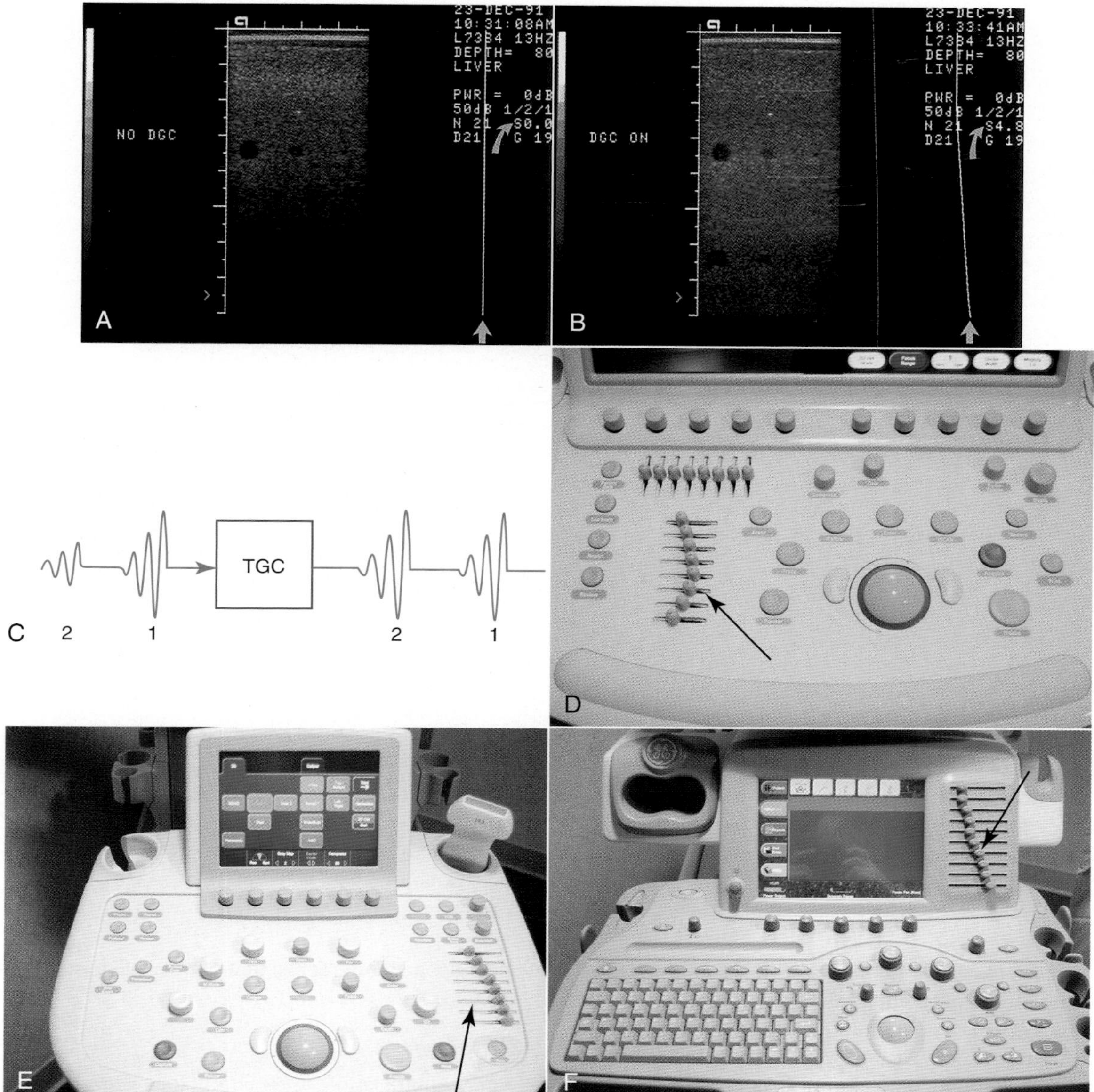

FIGURE 4-11 **Time gain compensation (TGC).** Two scans of a tissue-equivalent phantom imaged at 7 MHz without **(A)** and with **(B)** TGC. Without TGC, the echo brightness (amplitude, intensity, strength) declines with depth (top to bottom). On the display, TGC settings are shown graphically *(straight arrows).* The slopes *(curved arrows)* are 0 dB/cm **(A)** and 4.8 dB/cm **(B)**. Average tissue attenuation is 0.5 dB/cm-MHz. This is calculated per centimeter of sound propagation. Average attenuation then is 1 dB/cm-MHz when the centimeter value is the distance from the transducer to the reflector. The sound must travel twice this distance (round-trip), so the attenuation number doubles. Typical TGC slopes then will be about 1 dB/cm-MHz. **C,** Uncompensated echoes from identical structures at differing depths enter the TGC amplifier. The second *(2)* is weaker than the first *(1)* because it has come from a deeper site and has experienced more attenuation. After TGC, the amplitudes are identical. **D-F,** TGC controls *(arrows).*

the ultrasound beam, the operator subjectively adjusts the time gain compensation to compensate for the frequency used and the attenuation of the tissues being imaged. Time gain compensation is set by the operator to achieve, on average, uniform brightness throughout the image. The average attenuation in the tissue cross-section at the operating frequency has been compensated when this is accomplished.

> Time gain compensates for the effect of attenuation on an image.

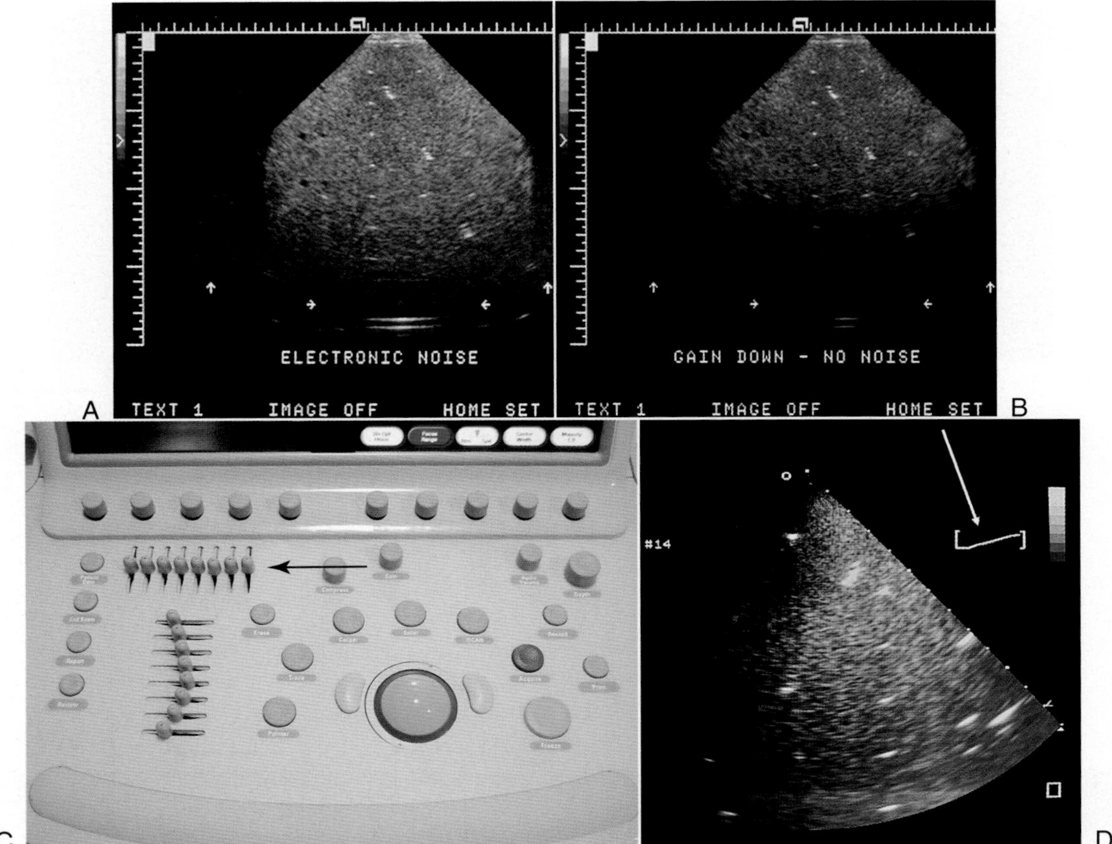

FIGURE 4-12 **A,** Under conditions of high gain, electronic noise (with its fuzzy appearance) can be seen on the display *(arrows)*. **B,** With reduced gain, these weak voltages are not amplified enough to be visualized. **C,** Lateral gain controls *(arrow)*. **D,** Lateral gain adjusted to increase gain from left to right.

Typical time gain compensation amplifiers compensate for approximately 60 dB of attenuation. At the depth at which maximum gain has been achieved, the echo brightness begins to decrease because the time gain compensation can no longer compensate (the amplifier gain cannot be increased further). Thus attenuation and maximum amplifier gain determine the maximum imaging depth. Maximum amplifier gain is determined by noise. Electronic noise (Figure 4-12, *A-B*) exists in all electronic circuits. High-quality input amplifier circuit noise levels are a few microvolts in amplitude. At maximum gain, the amplifier noise and the weak echoes being amplified have comparable amplitude. Any further increase in gain would only increase the noise, with weaker echoes being lost in the noise and thus being unobservable.

Some instruments have **lateral gain control**, which allows adjustment of gain laterally across the image (see Figure 4-12, *C-D*). Regions with different attenuation values located laterally to each other can be compensated to yield similar image brightnesses.

The overall gain control is adjusted first to yield a perceptible image on the display. Then the time gain compensation (and possibly the lateral gain) controls are adjusted to yield on-average uniform brightness over the image. Attenuation variations throughout the image are thus compensated for, yielding a good representation of the tissue cross-section imaged.

Digitizer

After amplification, the echo voltages are digitized; that is, they pass through **analog-to-digital converters** (ADCs). An ADC (also called a *digitizer*) converts the voltage from analog to digital form (Figure 4-13). The term **analog** means "proportional," and the term **digital** means "in the form of discrete numbers." Thus far in the instrument, the echo voltage has been proportional to the echo pressure. After the ADC, echo voltages are replaced by a series of numbers, and further manipulation of the echoes is accomplished as digital signal processing (mathematical manipulation of numbers representing echoes). This is similar to what is done in all digital electronics such as CD and DVD players and digital cellular telephones that handle, store, and process sound and pictures in digital form. The ADC interrogates the incoming voltage at regular intervals and determines its value at each interrogation instant. The interrogation rate must be twice the highest frequency involved in the interrogated voltage to preserve (in the subsequent digital number stream) all the harmonics contained in the interrogated voltage. For example, to digitize a 5-MHz continuous wave voltage properly,

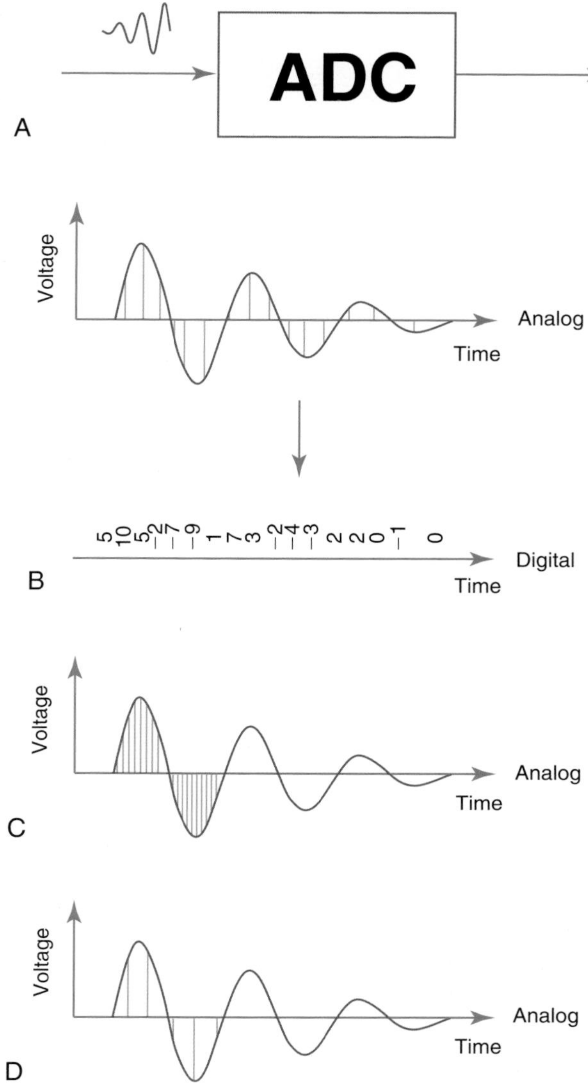

FIGURE 4-13 A, The analog-to-digital converter (*ADC*) converts (**B**) the analog (proportional) echo voltage into a series of numbers representing the sampled voltage. The higher the sampling rate of the analog-to-digital converter, the better the temporal detail of the voltage is preserved. **C,** High sampling rate. **D,** Low sampling rate.

the digitizing rate must be at least 10 MHz; that is, the voltage is interrogated 10 million times per second, yielding a stream of 10 million digitized values per second describing the original analog voltage.

ADCs convert the analog voltages representing echoes to numbers for digital signal processing and storage.

Echo Delays

After amplification and digitizing, the echo voltages pass through digital delay lines to accomplish reception dynamic focus and steering functions.

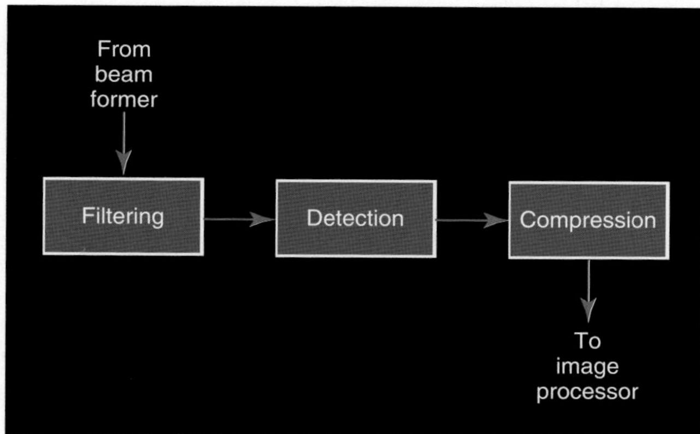

FIGURE 4-14 The signal processor performs filtering, detection, and compression functions. The processor receives digital signals from the beam former and, after processing, sends them on to the image processor.

BOX 4-2 Functions of the Signal Processor

- Bandpass filtering
- Amplitude detection
- Compression (dynamic range reduction)

Summer (Adder)

After all the channel signal components are delayed properly to accomplish the focus and steering functions, they are added together in the adder to produce the resulting scan line, which, along with all the others, will be displayed after signal processing and image processing. Reception apodization and dynamic aperture functions are also accomplished as part of this summing process.

The beam former is responsible for electronic beam scanning, steering, focusing, apodization, and aperture functions with arrays.

SIGNAL PROCESSOR

The reception portion of the beam former amplifies and combines the contributions from the individual elements and channels to form the stream of echoes returning from each transmitted pulse and sends them on to the signal processor. Operations carried out here include filtering, detection, and compression. The signal processor is diagrammed in Figure 4-14. Box 4-2 lists the functions of the signal processor.

Filtering

Tuned amplifiers are used to reduce noise in the electronics. They operate at a specific frequency with a bandwidth that includes the frequencies in the returning echoes and eliminates the electronic noise outside that bandwidth. A tuned amplifier is simply an amplifier with an electronic filter called the *bandpass filter.* A bandpass filter is one that passes a range

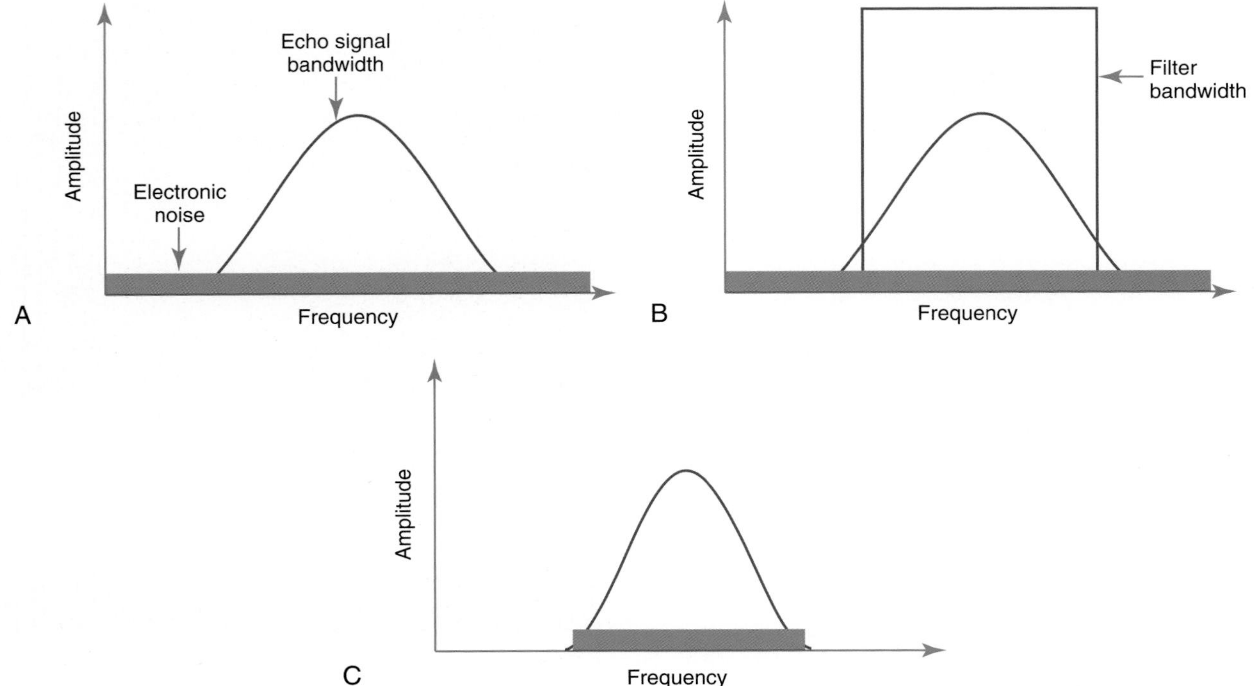

FIGURE 4-15 **A,** Input to filter includes the echo signal bandwidth and the electronic noise with unlimited bandwidth. **B,** The filter bandwidth is designed to accommodate the signal bandwidth. **C,** The output from the filter has the frequencies above and below its bandwidth removed. Only the noise frequencies within the filter bandwidth remain.

of frequencies (its bandwidth) and rejects those above and below the acceptance bandwidth (Figure 4-15). Some tuned amplifiers dynamically move the frequency range of the filter to track the bandwidth of the returning series of echoes from a pulse. The echo bandwidth decreases while the echoes return because the higher frequencies in the bandwidth are attenuated more than the lower ones.

Filtering eliminates frequencies outside the echo bandwidth while retaining those that are most useful in a given type of operation.

Detection

Detection (also called **demodulation**) is the conversion of echo voltages from **radio frequency** form to amplitude form (Figure 4-16). This is done by detecting and connecting the maxima of the cyclic variations. The cyclic voltage form is called *radio frequency* because it is similar to voltages found in a radio receiver, and the frequencies are similar to those in the low end of the shortwave radio band. The detected form retains the amplitudes. Because diagnostic ultrasound pulses do not have constant amplitude, when demodulated, they do not have the simplified blocked appearance shown in Figure 4-16. Detection is not an operator-controllable function.

> Detection is the conversion of echo voltages from radio frequency form to video form. The video form retains amplitudes of the echo voltages.

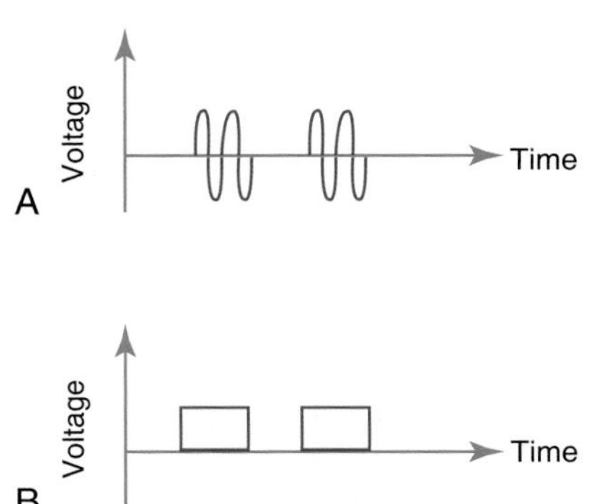

FIGURE 4-16 Echo voltages are produced in a complicated cyclic form **(A)** called *radio frequency* (RF), which would be difficult to store and display. Furthermore, only the amplitude of each echo is needed for a gray-scale display of anatomy. Thus the RF form is converted to the simpler amplitude form **(B)**, which retains the amplitude of each echo voltage.

Compression

The ratio of the largest to the smallest amplitude or power that a system can handle is called **dynamic range** (Figure 4-17). Dynamic range is expressed in decibels. For example, if an amplifier is insensitive to voltage amplitudes of less than 0.01 mV (because they are buried in the electronic noise) and cannot properly handle voltage amplitudes of greater than 1000 mV, the ratio of usable voltage extremes is 1000/0.01, or 100,000. The power ratio is equal to the square of the voltage ratio: $100{,}000^2$, or 10,000,000,000. According to Table 4-1, the

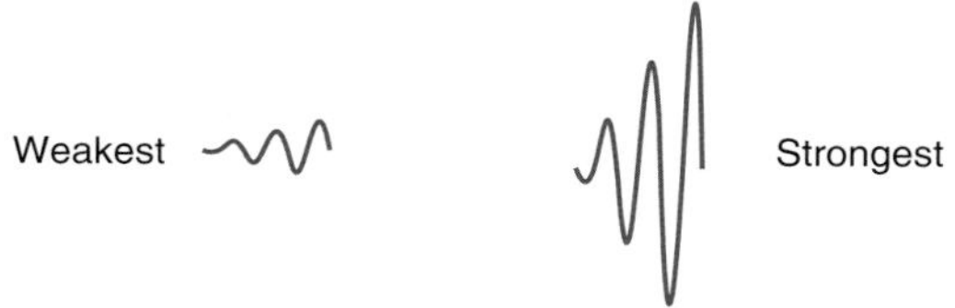

FIGURE 4-17 Dynamic range is the relationship between the weakest and strongest echoes and is expressed in decibels.

dynamic range of the amplifier is 100 dB. Amplifiers have typical dynamic ranges of 100 to 120 dB. System dynamic ranges are claimed to be as high as 170 dB. Greater values indicate the ability to detect weaker echoes, that is, greater sensitivity. The higher dynamic ranges assume some bandwidth reduction (to reduce electronic noise) and improvement yielded by the reception beam–forming process with several reception channels. Other portions of the electronics (especially the display) have much smaller dynamic range capability. Displays have dynamic ranges of as high as 30 dB. Furthermore, human vision is limited to a dynamic range of approximately 20 dB. The largest power (brightness) can be only approximately 100 times the smallest for our viewing of the display. Thus the largest voltage amplitude can be only approximately 10 times the smallest. The echo dynamic range remaining after compensation is typically 50 to 100 dB. Compression is the process of decreasing the differences between the smallest and the largest echo amplitudes to a usable range (Figure 4-18). Amplifiers that amplify weak inputs more than strong ones accomplish this. A compressor would have to compress the intensity ratio (100,000) corresponding to 50 dB to an intensity ratio of 100 (acceptable for the display).

> Compression reduces dynamic range with selective amplification.

Compression is operator adjustable as a dynamic range control (Figure 4-19). This control reduces dynamic range by assigning some weak echo amplitude values to zero or by assigning some of the strongest to maximum. Reassigned echoes may be at either end of the dynamic range or at both ends (see Figure 4-19, *J-L*). A smaller dynamic range setting presents a higher-contrast image. Gain control moves the dynamic range graph to the left or right (down or up the dynamic range) as gain is increased or decreased (see Figure 4-19, *M-N*).

> Signal processing includes digital filtering, detection, and compression of echo data. The order in which these processes occur in the signal processor is usually filtering first, with detection and compression following in either order.

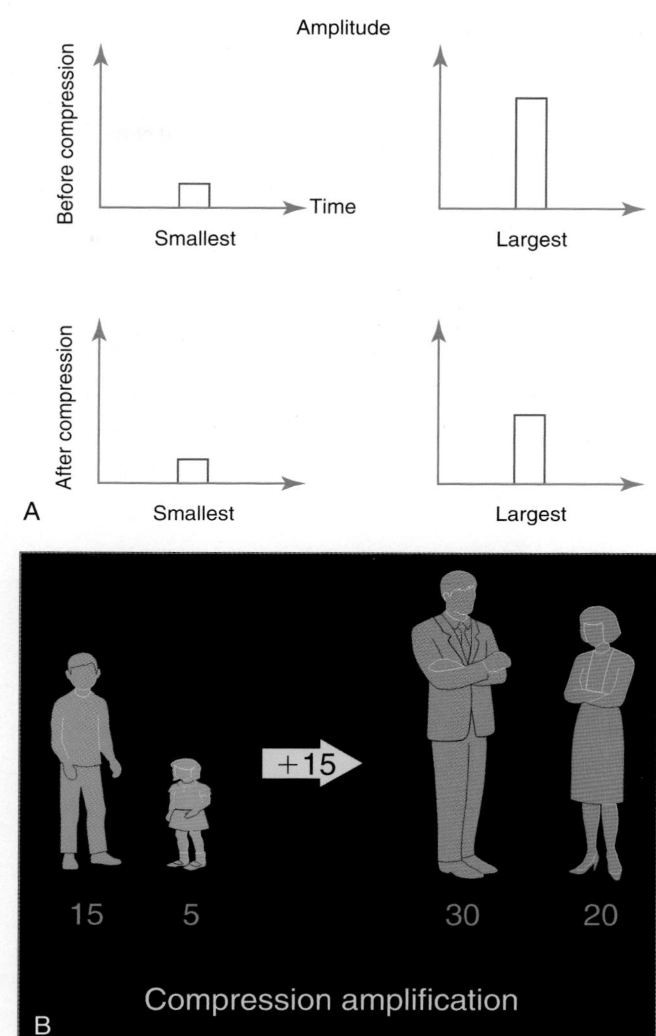

FIGURE 4-18 **Compression decreases the difference between the smallest and largest amplitudes passing through the system. A,** In this example, the ratio of largest to smallest amplitudes before compression is 5. After compression, the ratio is 3. **B,** A family illustration of compression amplification. Big brother (age 15 years) is twice as tall (large dynamic range) as his little sister (age 5 years). Fifteen years later, the brother (age 30 years) is just slightly taller than the sister (age 20 years). Both have grown (amplification), but the shorter child grew more than the taller one, reducing the difference between them (compression).

IMAGE PROCESSOR

Until this point (through the beam former and signal processor), the echo data are traveling in scan-line form serially through the system, that is, one scan line at a time. No image has yet been formed. The image processor converts the digitized, filtered, detected, and compressed serial scan-line data into images that are stored in **image memory**, all in preparation for presentation on the instrument display. After detection of the echo voltage amplitudes in the signal processor, the scan-line data enter the image processor, where they are preprocessed and stored in image form and then are processed in image form (Figure 4-20). Box 4-3 lists the functions of the image processor.

With use of a display scan format, the image processor provides a means for displaying the acquired information that is initially in a linear or sector ultrasound scan-line format.

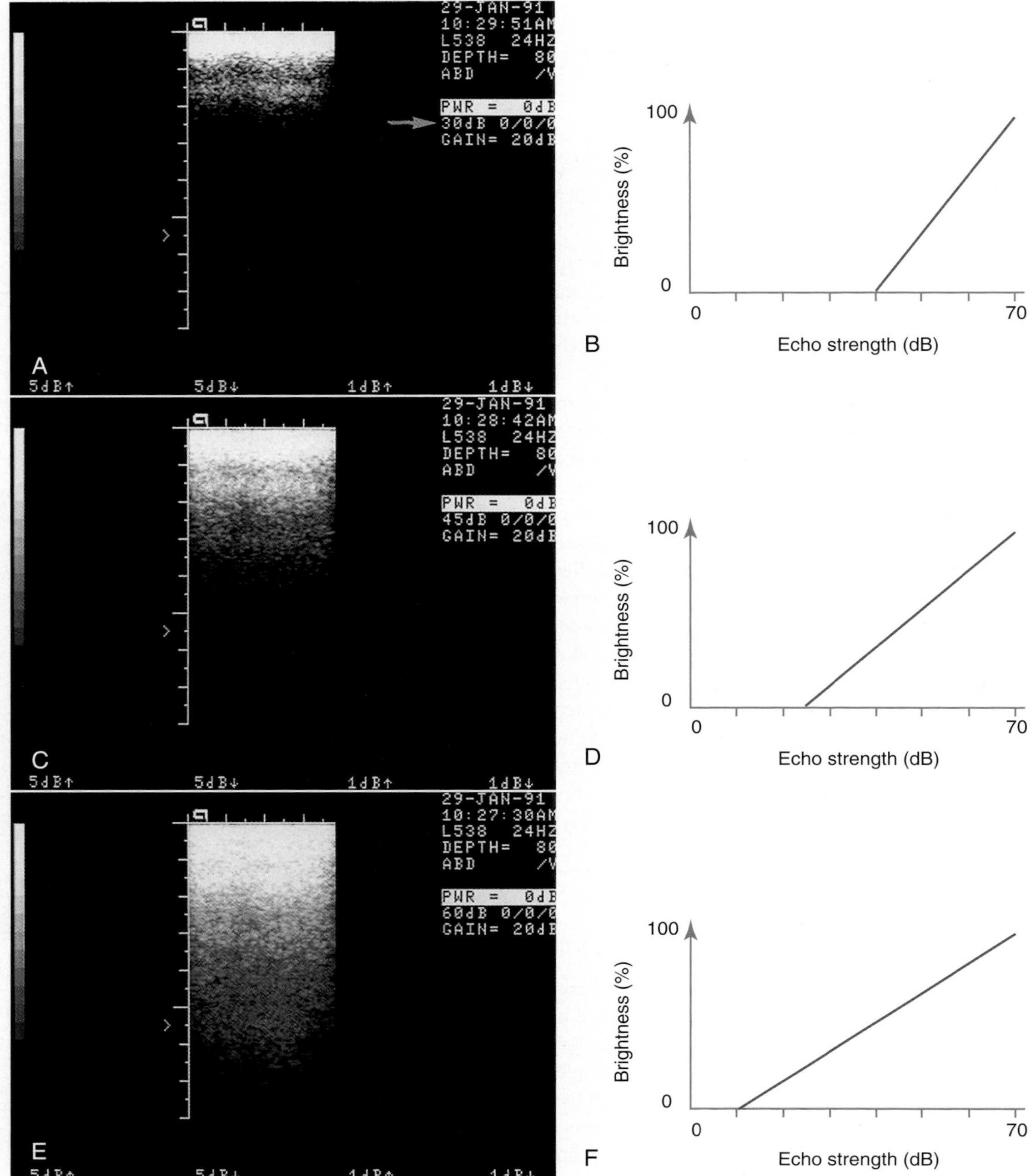

FIGURE 4-19 **A,** The dynamic range setting *(arrow)* is 30 dB. The lower 40 dB of echoes returning from a tissue-equivalent phantom are set to 0 *(black portion).* The remainder show high contrast, with brightness progressing from black for 40-dB echoes to white for 70-dB echoes. **B,** A 30-dB dynamic range setting assigns the weakest 40 dB of echo dynamic range to zero *(black)* and the remaining 30 dB of dynamic range to linearly higher brightnesses. **C,** A display with a dynamic range of 45 dB. **D,** Brightness assignment for a 45-dB dynamic range. **E,** A display with a dynamic range of 60 dB. **F,** Brightness assignment for a 60-dB dynamic range.

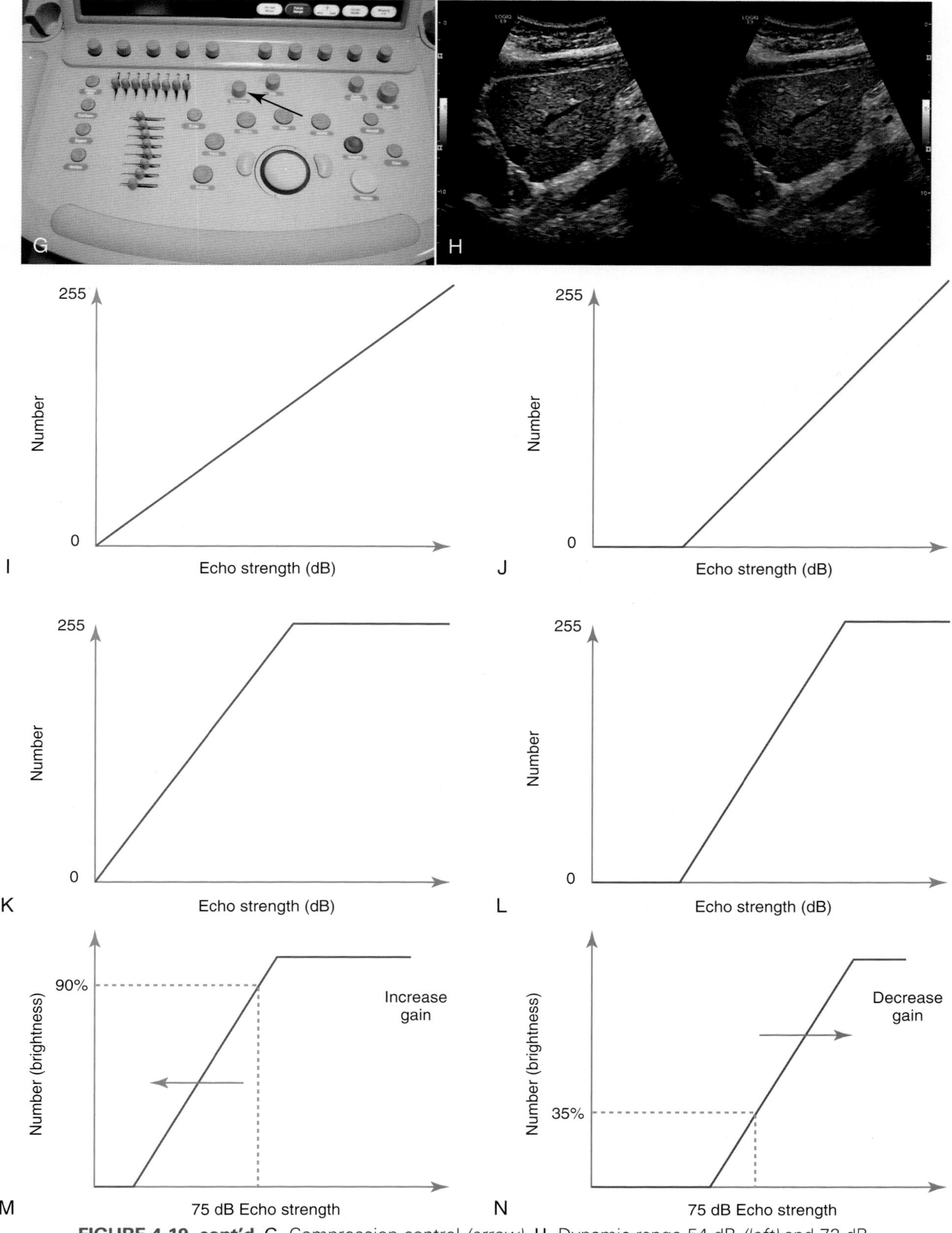

FIGURE 4-19, cont'd G, Compression control *(arrow)*. H, Dynamic range 54 dB *(left)* and 72 dB *(right)*. I, Full system dynamic range displayed. J, Dynamic range reduced by setting a weaker portion to 0 *(black)*. K, Dynamic range reduced by setting a stronger portion to maximum *(white)*. L, Dynamic range reduced by setting weaker and stronger portions to black and white, respectively. M, This graph of brightness versus echo strength moves to the left as gain is increased. A midrange echo appears bright. N, The graph moves to the right for decreasing gain. The midrange echo appears dark.

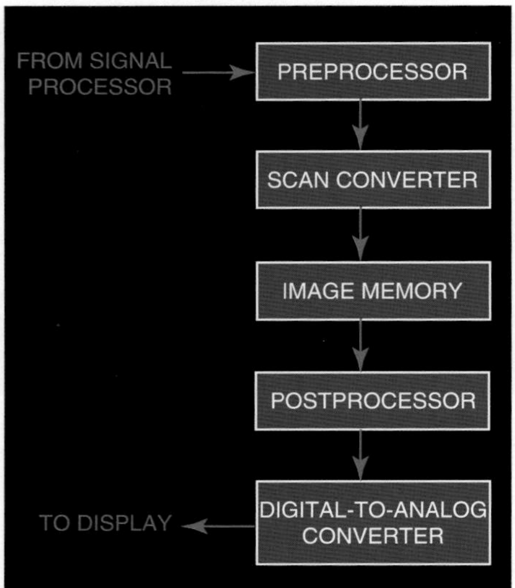

FIGURE 4-20 The image processor converts scan-line data into images, processes the images before storing them in the image memory, processes them as they come out of the memory, converts them from digital form to analog form, and sends them on to the display.

BOX 4-3 Functions of the Image Processor

- Preprocessing
- Persistence
- Three-dimensional acquisition
- Storing image frames
- Cine loop
- Postprocessing
- Gray scale
- Color scale
- Three-dimensional presentation
- Digital-to-analog conversion

The direction of each scan line and the location of echoes in depth down each scan line are used to determine the proper location in the image memory (and thus on the display) for each echo. For example, a pulse emitted from the transducer straight down into the body will result in a series of echoes that are located in appropriate memory locations straight down a column in memory at various depths, that is, various row locations (Figure 4-21, *A*). A pulse emitted in an off-vertical direction will result in a series of echoes that must be located in various rows and columns (see Figure 4-21, *B*). The image processor properly locates each series of echoes corresponding to each scan line for each pulse emitted from the transducer, filling up the memory with echo information. This is accomplished in a fraction of a second, yielding one scan or **frame** of image information. This process is repeated several times per second to produce a rapid sequence of frames stored in the memory and presented on the display. This rapid-sequence presentation is called **real-time display**, and the entire process is called *real-time sonography.* Image depth control (see Figure 4-21, *C*) determines the depth to be displayed and thus the depth range covered by the image memory in the scan conversion process.

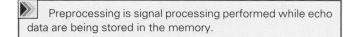

> The image processer formats echo data into image form for image processing, storage, and display.

Preprocessing

As part of the process of scan-line information going into the image memory, various processing functions may be performed on the image. This is called **preprocessing** because it occurs before the echo data are stored in the image memory. Examples of preprocessing include edge enhancement (a function that sharpens boundaries to make them more detectable and measurements more precise), pixel interpolation, persistence, and three-dimensional acquisition.

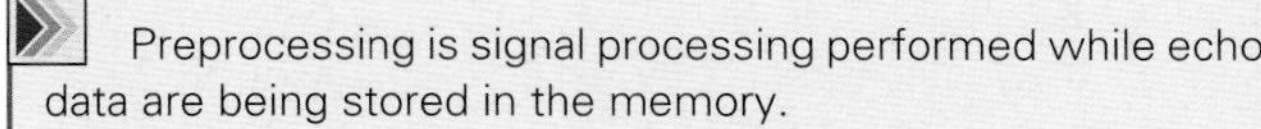

> Preprocessing is signal processing performed while echo data are being stored in the memory.

Pixel Interpolation

Image improvement can be accomplished by filling in missing **pixels**. A common situation in which this occurs is sector scans in which scan lines have increasing separation with distance from the transducer and intervening pixels are left out. Interpolation assigns a brightness value to a missed pixel, based on an average of brightnesses of adjacent pixels (see Figure 4-21, *D*).

Persistence

Persistence is the averaging of sequential frames to provide a smoother image appearance and to reduce noise (Figure 4-22). Noise, primarily speckle, is reduced because it is a random process. When several frames containing random content are averaged, the random content is reduced. Speckle reduction improves dynamic range and **contrast resolution**. But frame averaging, in effect, reduces frame rate because averaged frames are no longer independent. Operator control permits averaging of a selectable number of sequential frames from zero up to some maximum. Lower levels of persistence, or none at all, are appropriate for following rapidly moving structures. Higher levels are appropriate for slower-moving structures.

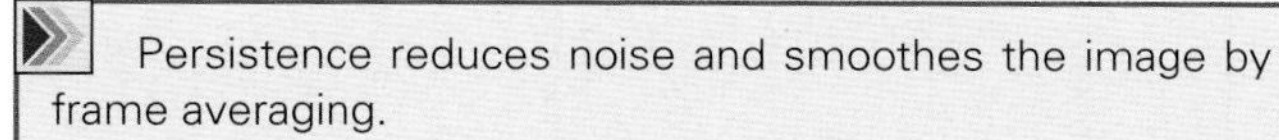

> Persistence reduces noise and smoothes the image by frame averaging.

Volume Imaging

Three-dimensional imaging (3D, **volume imaging**) is accomplished by acquiring many parallel two-dimensional (2D-slice imaging) scans (Figure 4-23, *A*) and then processing this 3D volume of echo information in appropriate ways for presentation on 2D displays. The multiple 2D frames are obtained by (1) manual scanning of the transducer, with position-sensing devices keeping track of scan-plane location and orientation; (2) automated mechanically scanned transducers; or

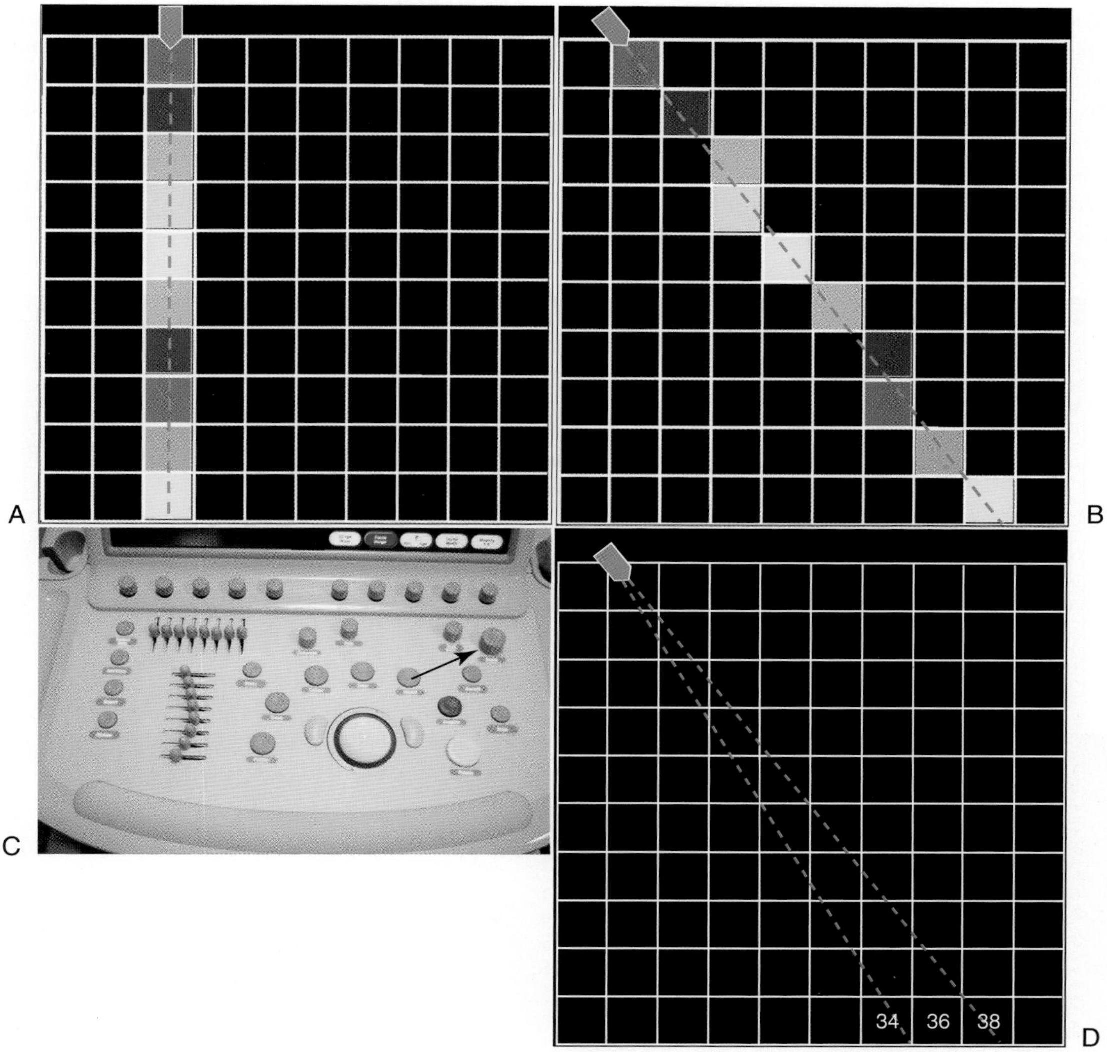

FIGURE 4-21 **A,** A pulse emitted straight down into the body *(arrowhead and dashed line)* results in echoes located in a column of memory locations. **B,** A pulse emitted in another direction results in echoes located in various rows and columns. **C,** Image depth control. **D,** Pixel interpolation. Part of the image memory pixel grid is shown along with the paths of two pulses. At the bottom of the grid, the paths have separated sufficiently so that the pixel between them is missed. The interpolation calculation determines the mean value of the two adjacent pixels (34 and 38), which is 36. That value then is entered in the intervening pixel.

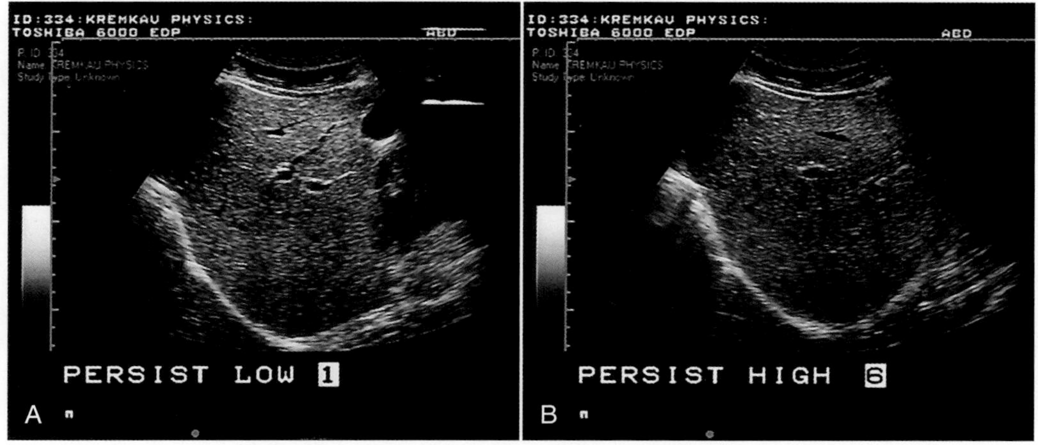

FIGURE 4-22 **A,** Persistence off. **B,** Persistence on.

(3) electronic scanning with 2D element-array transducers. Common ways of presenting the 3D echo data include surface renderings (see Figure 4-23, *B*), 2D slices through the 3D volume, and transparent views. The advantage of 2D slice presentation is that it is possible to present image-plane orientations that are impossible to obtain with conventional 2D scanning. Serial slice presentations similar to those in other imaging modes (magnetic resonance imaging [MRI] and computed tomography [CT]) can be presented (see Figure 4-23, *C-H*). Surface renderings are popular in obstetric imaging and echocardiography. Transparent views allow "see-through" imaging of the anatomy, as with plain-film radiographs.

> 3D images are acquired by assembling several 2D scans into a 3D volume of echo information in the image memory.

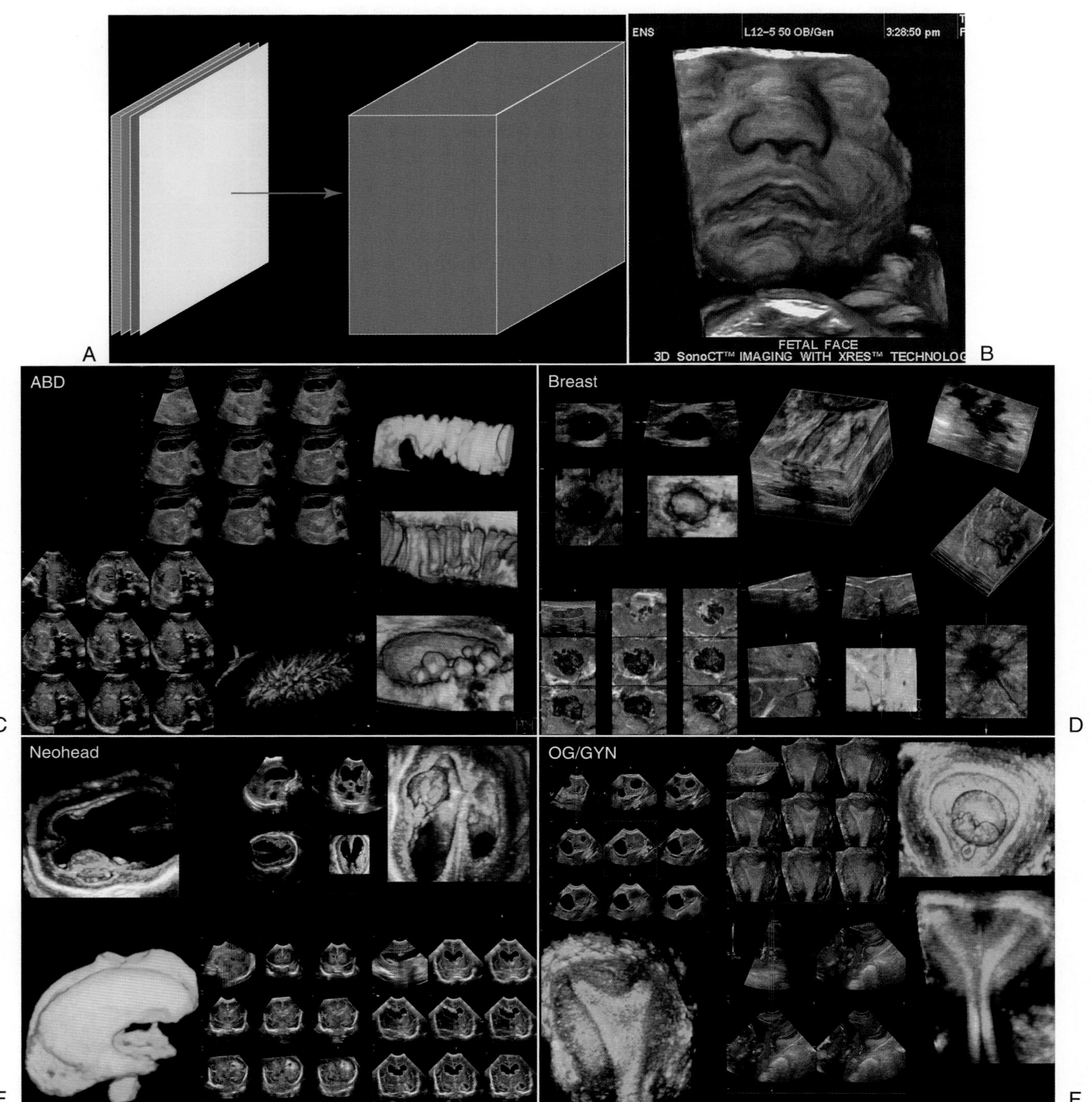

FIGURE 4-23 **Three-dimensional sonographic images. A,** Three-dimensional echo data are acquired by obtaining many parallel two-dimensional sections of echo information from the imaged anatomy yielding **(B)** a three-dimensional fetal surface-rendered image.

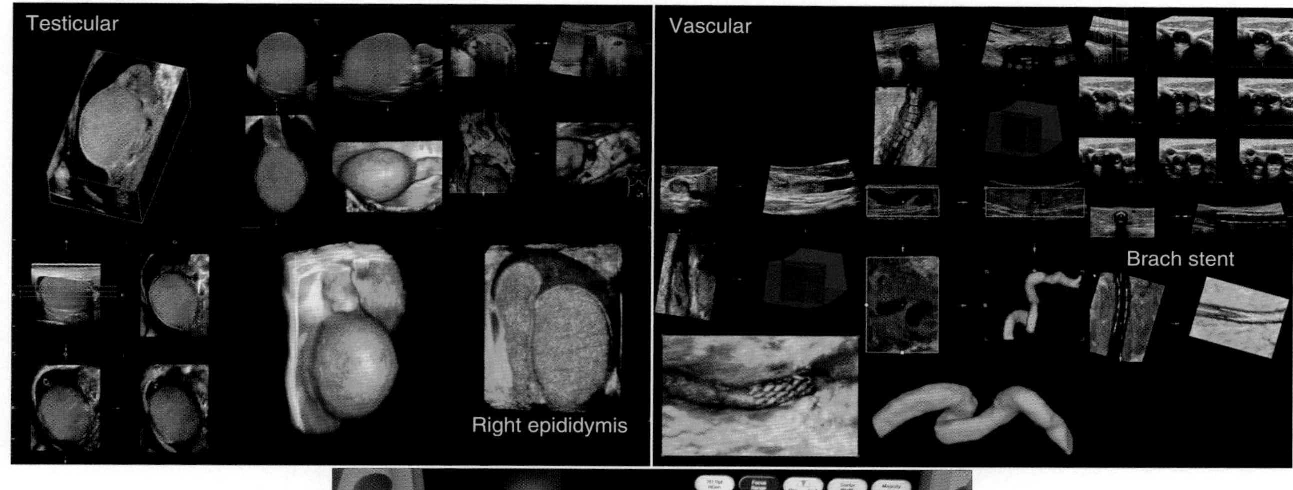

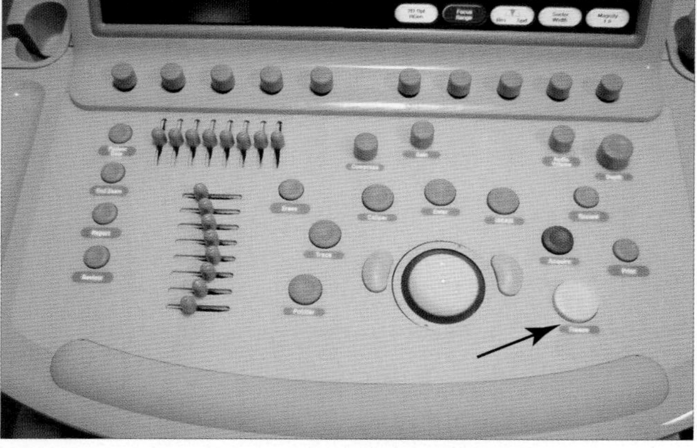

FIGURE 4-23, cont'd C-H, Various presentations of volume imaging of the abdomen, breast, neonatal head, obstetric/gynecologic cases, testicle, and blood vessel. I, The freeze button *(arrow)* stops the scanning and saves the last several image frames in the image memory.

3D images can be acquired at rates sufficient for "live" or **real-time** presentations. The current tendency is to call this *4D imaging,* in which the fourth dimension is time. Although this term sounds fashionable for marketing purposes, it is inconsistent with previous terminology. Real-time 2D imaging is not called *3D*; nevertheless, this moniker has caught on to some extent.

Image Memory

While echo data are preprocessed, the image frames are stored in the image memory. Storing each image in the memory while the sound beam is scanned through the anatomy permits display of a single image (frame) out of the rapid sequence of several frames acquired each second in real-time sonographic instruments. Holding and displaying one frame out of the sequence is known as **freeze-frame** (see Figure 4-23, *I*). Instruments typically store the last several frames acquired before freezing. This is called **cine loop**, cine review, or image review feature.

Pixels and Bits

Image memories used in sonographic instruments are digital; that is, they are computer memories that store numbers (digits) just as digital cameras do (Figure 4-24, *A*). The 2D image plane is divided, similar to a checkerboard (see Figure 4-24, *B*), into squares called *pixels* (picture elements), in a rectangular matrix, for example, 1024 × 768 or 512 × 384. The pixels number several thousands (786,432 and 196,608 in the previous examples), so they are tiny and not normally noticed unless magnified sufficiently. A number that corresponds to the echo strength received from the location within the anatomy corresponding to that memory position (see Figure 4-24, *C*) is stored in each of the pixel locations in the memory. The more pixels there are, the finer the spatial detail in the stored image (see Figure 4-24, *D-G*). If the digital memory were composed of a single-layer matrix checkerboard, each pixel location could store only one of two numbers: a zero or a one. The reason is that the memory element assigned to each pixel is an electronic device that is binary (*bi* meaning "two"), similar to an on–off switch (Figure 4-25, *A*) and thus can operate only in two conditions corresponding to one or zero. This would allow only **bistable** (black-and-white) imaging (see Figure 4-25, *B-C*). To image **gray scale** (several shades of gray or brightness, in addition to black and white), storage of one of several possible numbers in each

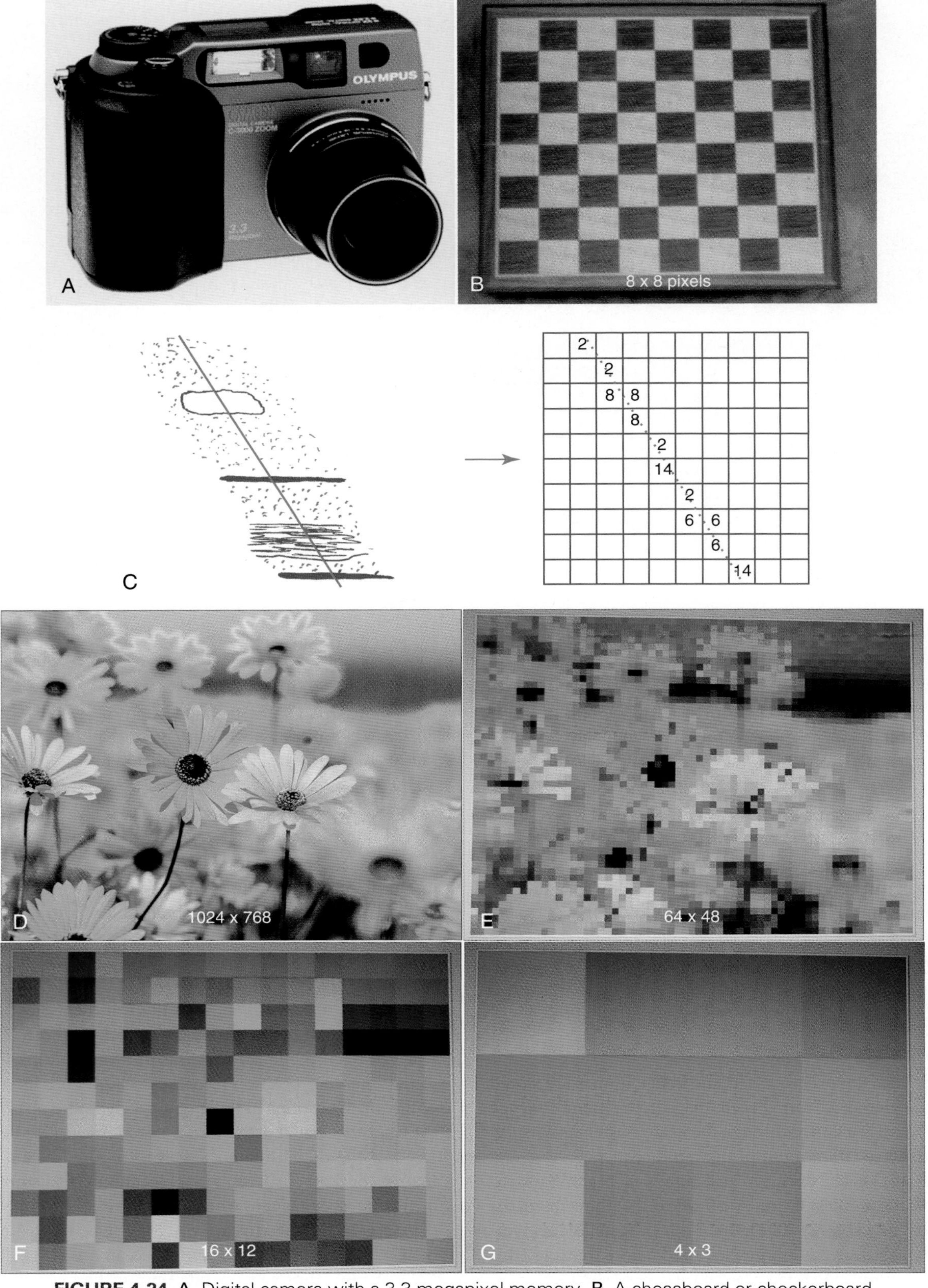

FIGURE 4-24 **A,** Digital camera with a 3.3 megapixel memory. **B,** A chessboard or checkerboard is divided into eight rows and eight columns of squares, for a total of 64 "pixels." **C,** Anatomic cross-section to be scanned, and the front view of a portion of the image memory. Numbers are stored in the memory elements according to the intensity of the echoes received from corresponding anatomic locations as an ultrasound pulse passes through them. **D-G,** Digital photos at pixel resolutions of 1024 × 768, 64 × 48, 16 × 12, 4 × 3, respectively.

memory location is necessary. This requires the memory to have more than one matrix. These "checkerboards" can be thought of as being layered back to back. In a four-binary-digit memory, there are four checkerboards back to back (see Figure 4-25, *D*) so that each pixel has 4 **bits** (binary digits) associated with it. In the binary numbering system, this allows numbers from 0 to 15 to be stored (a 16-shade system). Thus a 4-bit memory is a 16-shade memory. A 4-bit memory has four binary digits assigned to each pixel, that is, four layers of memory.

> The memory divides the image into pixels, such as a matrix of 512 × 384.

Binary Numbers

Because the memory elements are binary, digital memories use the binary numbering system to store echo information in the image memory. Computer memories and processors use binary numbers to carry out their functions because they

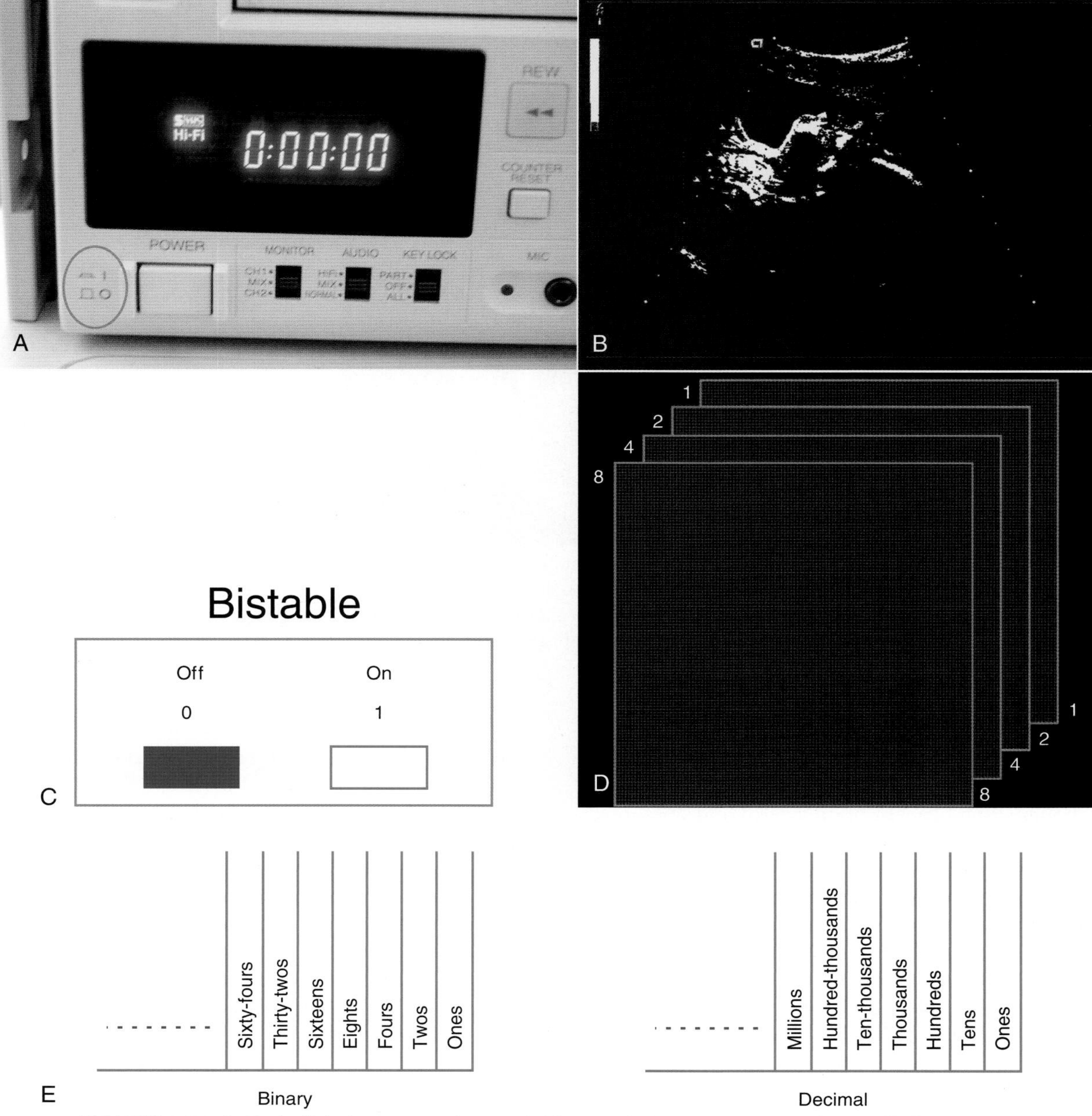

FIGURE 4-25 **A,** Each digital memory element is like a switch, with 1 as on and 0 as off. **B,** Bistable image of fetal head and neck. **C,** In bistable imaging, only two values are used: memory element off represents 0 and is presented as black; memory element on represents 1 and is presented as white. **D,** A 10 × 10-pixel, 4-bit-deep (4 bits per pixel) digital memory. **E,** Columns in decimal numbers represent multiples of 10, whereas those in binary numbers represent multiples of 2.

Continued

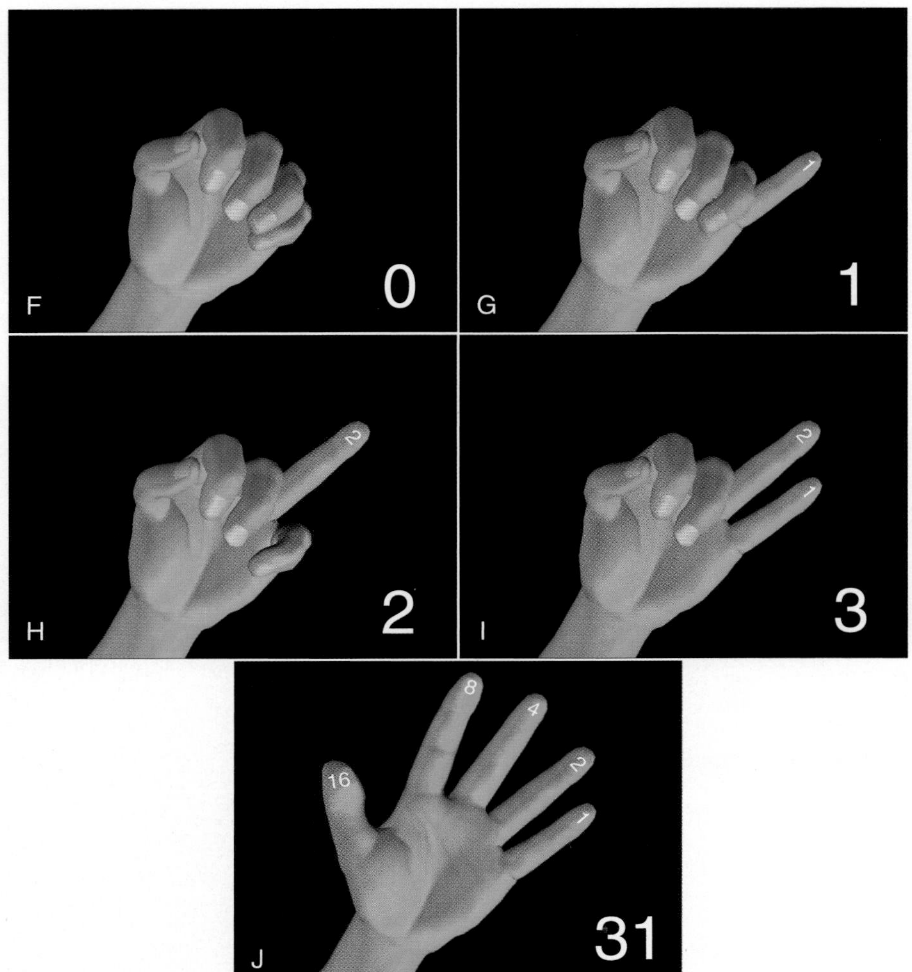

FIGURE 4-25, cont'd F-J, Conventional counting with fingers assigns the value 1 to each finger. Counting is much more efficient if different values are assigned to different fingers. Using the binary assignment procedure, each finger represents double the value of the previous finger. Normally we count only to 5 on one hand, but in this manner we can count to 31 (1 + 2 + 4 + 8 + 16) and to 1023 on two hands.

contain electronic components (switches) that operate in only two states, representing the numbers 0 and 1.

Binary digits (bits) consist of only zeros and ones, represented by their respective numeric symbols, 0 and 1. Other values must be represented by moving these symbols to different positions (columns). In the decimal system, in which there are 10 different symbols, 0 through 9, there is no single symbol for the number 10 (9 is the largest number for which there is a single symbol). To represent 10 in symbolic form then, the symbol for 1 is used, but it is moved to the left, to the second column. A 0 is placed in the right column to clarify this, resulting in the symbol 10. The same symbol used to represent 1 is used, but in such a way (that is, in the second column) that it no longer represents 1, but rather 10.

A similar procedure is used in the binary numbering system. The symbol 1 represents the largest number (1) for which there is a symbol in this system. To represent the next number (2), the same thing is done as in the decimal system; that is, the symbol 1 is placed in the next column to represent the number 2. In this case a 1 in the second column represents a value of 2 rather than 10, as in the decimal system. Columns in the two systems represent values as shown in Figure 4-25, *D-J*. In the decimal system, each column represents 10 times the column to its right. In the binary system, each column represents 2 times the column to its right.

Table 4-2 lists the binary forms of the decimal numbers 0 to 63. Numbers 64 to 127 would have one additional digit (representing the "sixty-fours" column), and so forth with higher multiples of 2.

> Binary numbers use only the digits 0 and 1. Each column of a binary number represents double the column to its right.

Table 4-3 gives several examples of digital memories. Figure 4-25, *D*, shows a 4-bit (per pixel) memory. Table 4-4 gives the total number of memory elements in various digital memories. A group of 8 bits is called a *byte,* and 1024 bytes (8192 bits) are called a *kilobyte.* In today's ultrasound instruments, 6-, 7-, and 8-bit memories are present. Human vision can differentiate approximately 100 gray levels. More than the 256 shades of an 8-bit system are not directly perceived by human vision.

In summary, then, the procedure for entering the echo information required for display of the 2D cross-sectional image into a digital memory is as follows:

- The beam is scanned through the patient in such a way that it "cuts," similar to a knife, through the tissue cross-section.
- Echoes received from all points on this cross-section are converted to numbers that are stored at corresponding pixel locations in the digital memory.
- All the information necessary for displaying this cross-sectional image now is stored in the memory.
- The information then can be taken out of the memory and presented on a 2D display in such a way that the numbers coming out of the memory are displayed with corresponding pixel brightnesses on the face of the display (Figure 4-26).

Figure 4-27 shows examples of such presentations. To enlarge the pixels, read magnification (sometimes called *zoom*) is used. In this presentation, rather than showing all the pixels in the memory, the monitor shows a smaller group of pixels in expanded (magnified) fashion. This increases pixel size, making the pixel composition of the image more obvious. Read zoom is a postprocessing function. Write magnification is also available on some instruments. This allows a smaller anatomic field of view to be written into the entire memory, thereby enlarging the image without enlarging the pixel size (Figure 4-28). Write zoom is a preprocessing function.

Digital (derived from the Latin term *digitus,* meaning "finger" or "toe") memories are discrete rather than continuous, which means that they can store only whole numbers in each pixel location. These numbers range from zero to a maximum that is determined by the number of bits per pixel (see Table 4-3).

For a 256 × 512 matrix in which the represented anatomic width and depth are 10 and 20 cm, respectively, each pixel represents an anatomic dimension of 0.4 mm. This represents the spatial (detail) resolution of the memory matrix. If the width and

TABLE 4-2 Binary and Decimal Number Equivalents

Decimal	Binary	Decimal	Binary
0	000000	32	100000
1	000001	33	100001
2	000010	34	100010
3	000011	35	100011
4	000100	36	100100
5	000101	37	100101
6	000110	38	100110
7	000111	39	100111
8	001000	40	101000
9	001001	41	101001
10	001010	42	101010
11	001011	43	101011
12	001100	44	101100
13	001101	45	101101
14	001110	46	101110
15	001111	47	101111
16	010000	48	110000
17	010001	49	110001
18	010010	50	110010
19	010011	51	110011
20	010100	52	110100
21	010101	53	110101
22	010110	54	110110
23	010111	55	110111
24	011000	56	111000
25	011001	57	111001
26	011010	58	111010
27	011011	59	111011
28	011100	60	111100
29	011101	61	111101
30	011110	62	111110
31	011111	63	111111

TABLE 4-4 Bits (Binary Digits or Memory Elements) in Digital Memories with 512 × 512 (262,144) Pixels

Bits per Pixel	Total Bits	Total Kilobytes*
4	1,048,576	128
5	1,310,720	160
6	1,572,864	192
7	1,835,008	224
8	2,097,152	256

*1 byte = 8 bits; 1 kilobyte = 1024 bytes, or 8192 bits.

TABLE 4-3 Characteristics of Digital Memories

	LOWEST NUMBER STORED		HIGHEST NUMBER STORED		
Bits per Pixel	Decimal	Binary	Decimal	Binary	Number of Shades
4	0	0000	15	1111	16
5	0	00000	31	11111	32
6	0	000000	63	111111	64
7	0	0000000	127	1111111	128
8	0	00000000	255	11111111	256

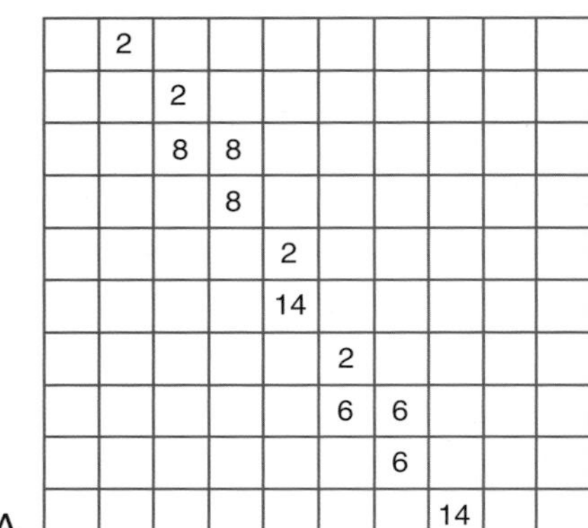

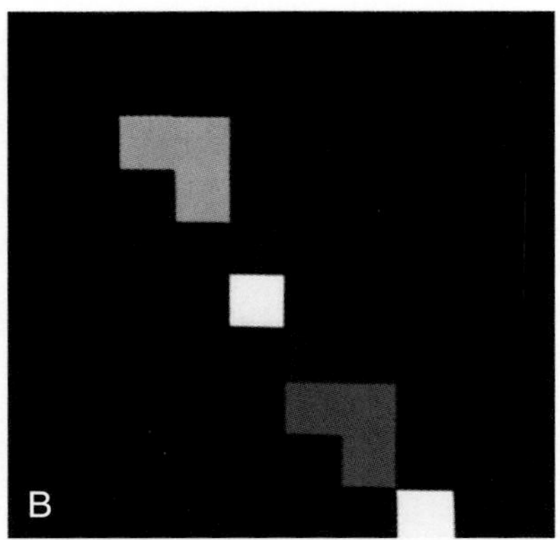

FIGURE 4-26 For display of scanned anatomic structures, numbers are read out of pixel locations in digital memory (**A**) and applied to the display in such a way that pixel brightness corresponds to those stored numbers (**B**). The display for the scan line acquired in Figure 4-24, *C*, is shown.

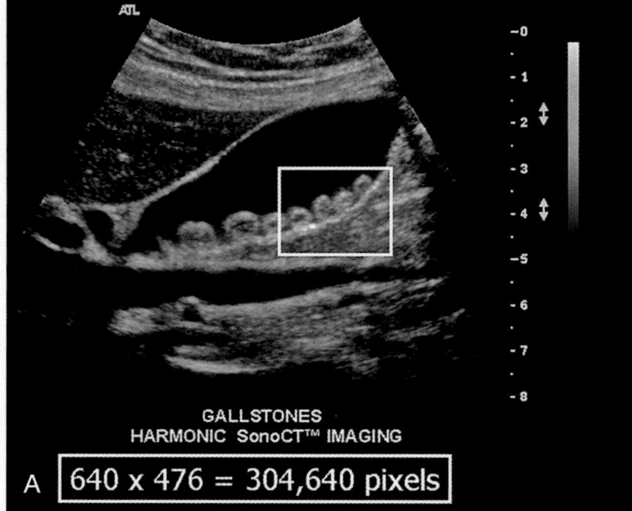

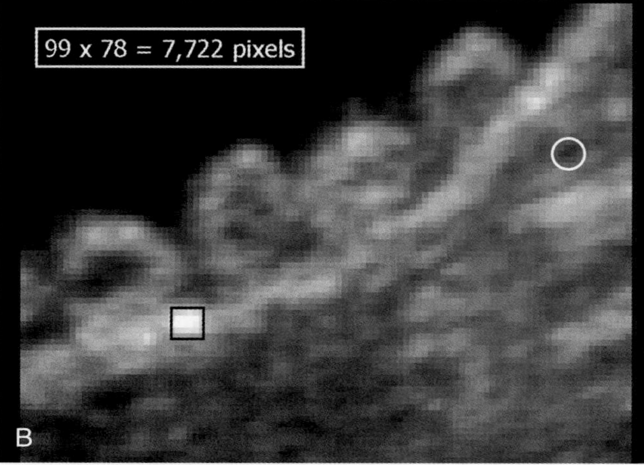

FIGURE 4-27 Displays of pixels of various brightnesses representing various numbers in the corresponding memory locations. The display is magnified *(zoom)* here to make the square pixels more easily discernible. Normally, the pixels are too small and numerous to be noticed individually. **A,** Unmagnified abdominal image containing 304,640 unresolved pixels. The box encloses the region magnified in **B.** Magnification reveals the 7722 pixels included within the box in **A.** The circle and the box enclose regions of small and large numbers (weak and strong echoes, respectively) in the image memory, respectively.

depth are 5 and 10 cm, then the memory spatial resolution is 0.2 mm. Detail resolution is usually limited by spatial pulse length and beam width rather than by pixel density in the memory.

Postprocessing

Signal processing and image processing performed before storage of the echo information in the image memory are called *preprocessing.* In general, preprocessing includes all that is done to echoes before they are stored in the memory (Figure 4-29). Image processing that is accomplished after the echoes are stored in the memory is called *postprocessing.* In general, postprocessing includes all of the procedures performed with echoes while they are brought out of the memory to be displayed. Read magnification is an example. **Postprocessing** is the assignment of specific display brightnesses to numbers retrieved from the memory (Figure 4-30). Some aspects of preprocessing, such as persistence and **spatial compounding**, are operator controllable. Postprocessing is also an operator-controllable operation.

> Postprocessing is image processing performed on image data retrieved from the memory. Postprocessing determines how echo data stored in the memory will appear on the display.

On most instruments, preprogrammed postprocessing brightness assignment schemes are selectable by the operator. A linear assignment (see Figure 4-30) equally divides the display brightness range among the stored gray levels of the system. This can be in white-echo (see Figure 4-30, *D*) or black-echo (see Figure 4-30, *E*) form, although the latter is seldom used. The assignment rules for these two schemes are the inverse of each other (see Figure 4-30, *A-B*). Other schemes (Figure 4-31 and 4-32, *A-B*) that allow assignment of more of the brightness range to certain portions of the stored number range capability of the system may also be used. This can improve the presentation and perception of small echo strength differences stored in the memory (improved contrast resolution, discussed later).

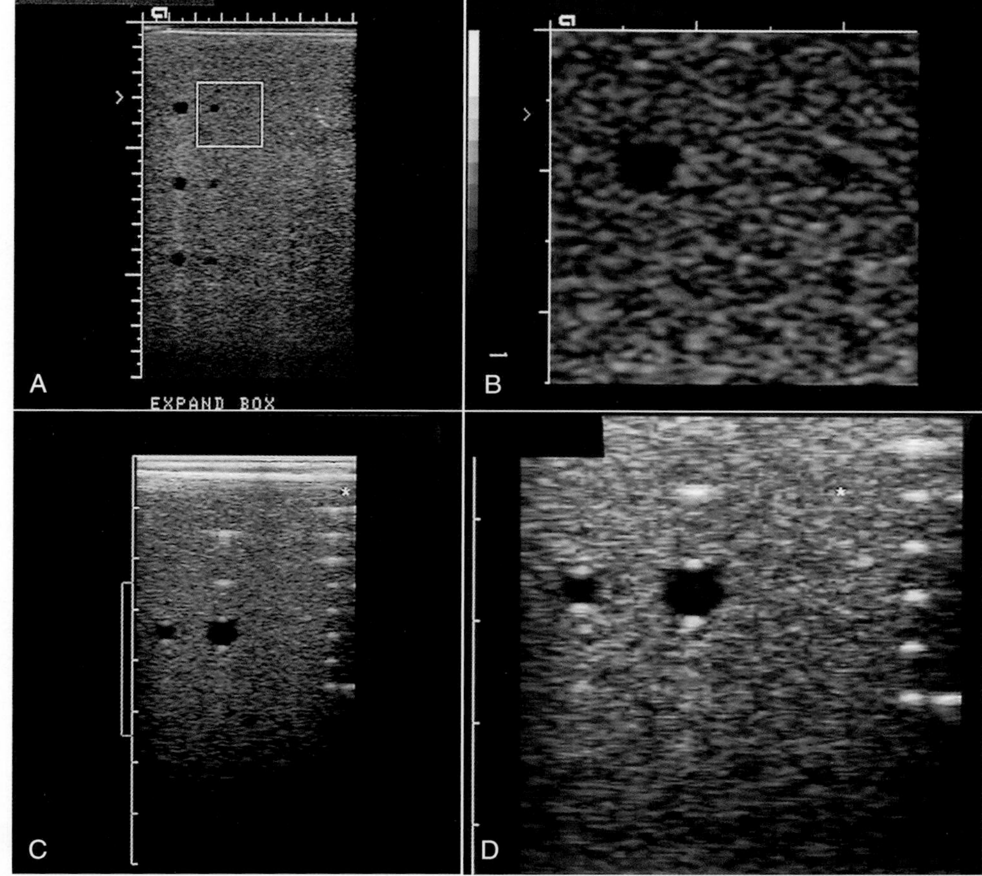

FIGURE 4-28 **Write and read zoom or magnification. A,** A scan of a phantom without write magnification. **B,** A scan using write magnification. Included are 4- and 2-mm simulated cysts. Read magnification, or zoom, when applied to an "unzoomed" image (**C**), magnifies the stored pixels (**D**).

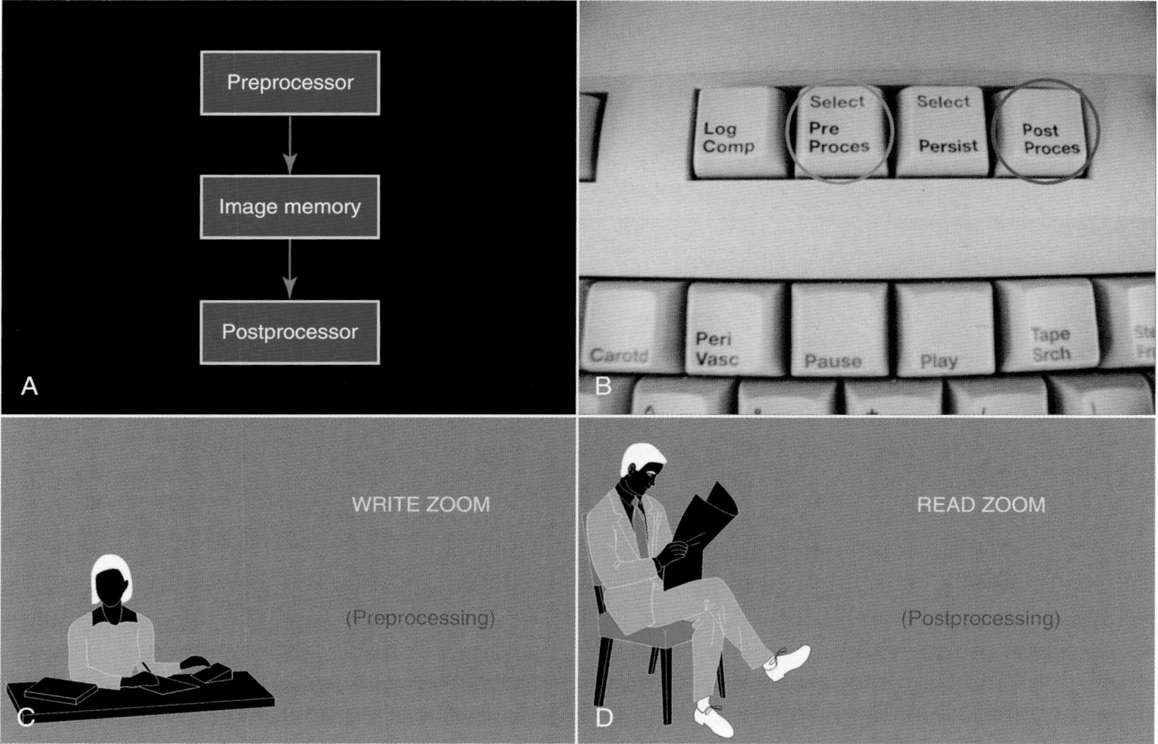

FIGURE 4-29 A, Preprocessing *(red circle in* B*)* includes operations performed on echoes before storage in memory. B, Postprocessing *(blue circle)* includes operations performed after information is stored in memory. Write (**C**; see Figure 4-28, *B*) and read (**D**; see Figure 4-28, *D*) magnification are examples of preprocessing and postprocessing, respectively.

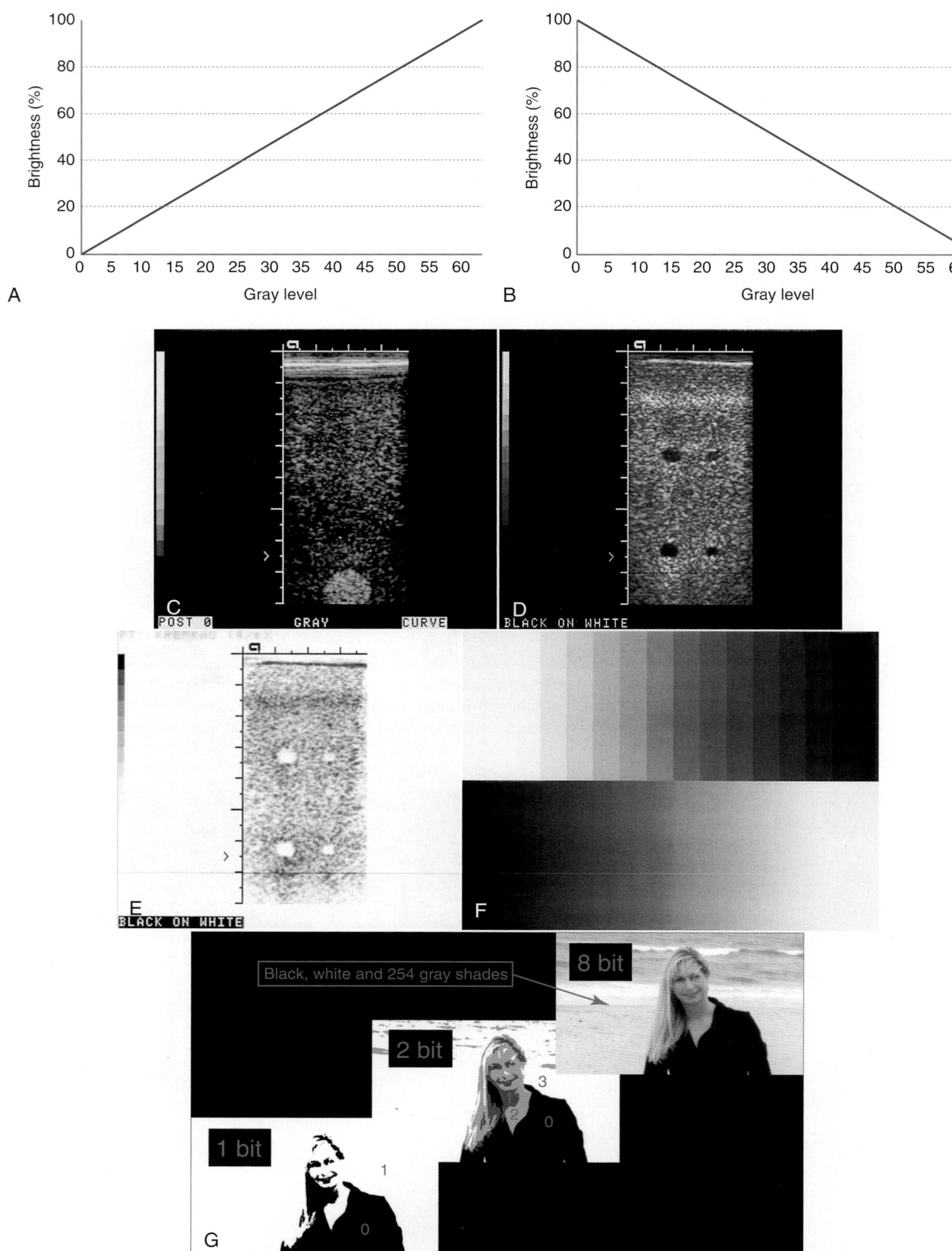

FIGURE 4-30 **Postprocessing is the assignment of specific display brightnesses to numbers derived from specific pixel locations in memory.** **A,** Brightness increases with increasing echo intensity (i.e., gray level stored in the memory). This is called *white-echo display.* **B,** Brightness increases with decreasing echo intensity *(black-echo display).* Both forms of display were common in the early days of gray-scale imaging. The latter is now seldom used because the white-echo display has been shown to be superior. **C-D,** Examples of the numerical assignment shown in **A**. **E,** Example of the numerical assignment shown in **B**. **F,** The upper portion shows 16 shades using a numerical assignment similar to that of **B**. The lower portion shows 256 shades and uses a numerical assignment similar to that of **A**. In both cases, echo strength increases to the right. **G,** Digital photographs with 1-, 2-, and 8-bit gray-scale resolutions. They yield 2 (black and white), 4 (black, white, and two grays), and 256 shades, respectively.

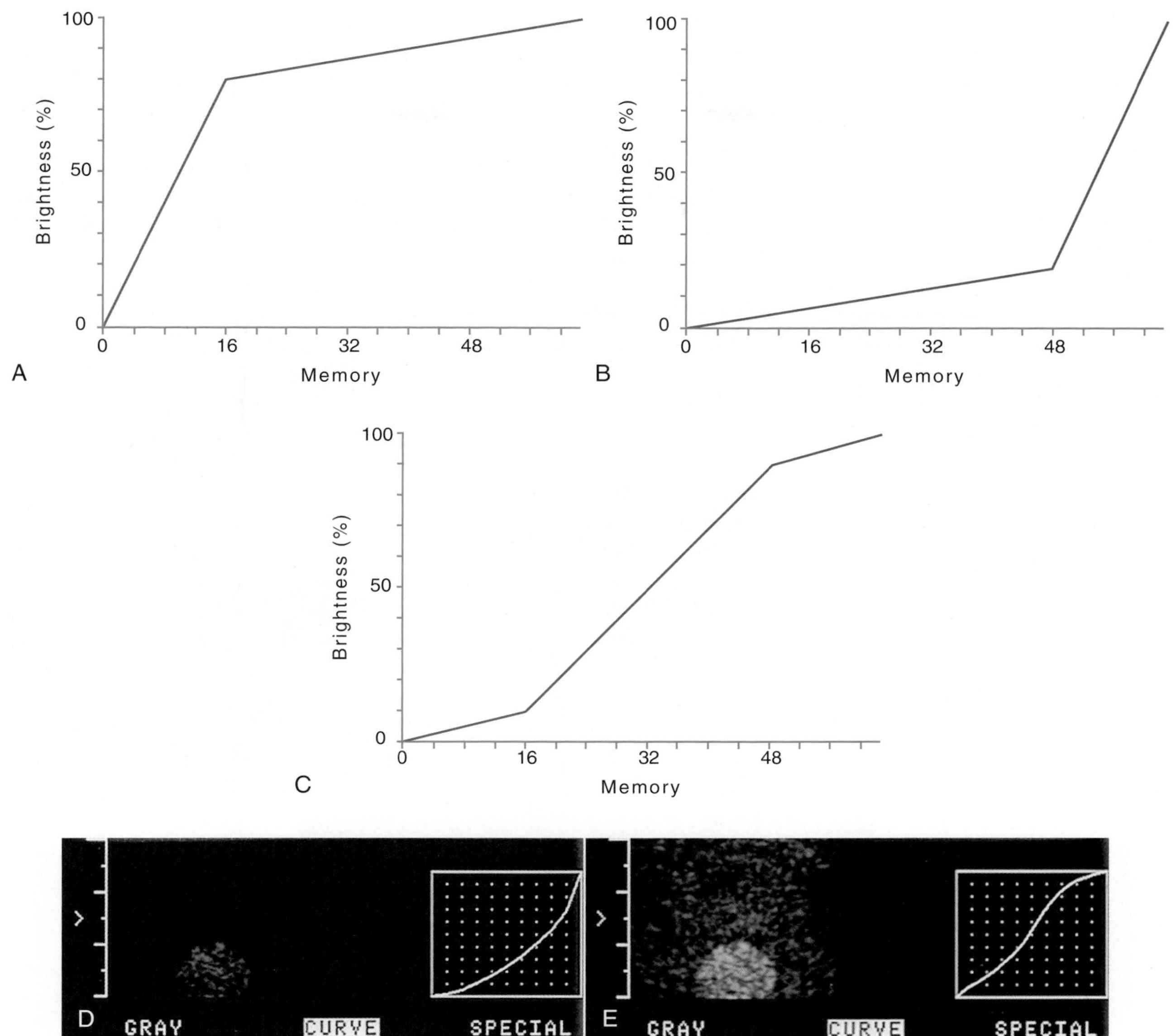

FIGURE 4-31 Nonlinear postprocessing assignment schemes. A large brightness range is reserved for weak (**A**), strong (**B**), and intermediate-strength (**C**) echoes. Each area has improved contrast resolution (discussed later) at the expense of poorer contrast resolution in the remainder of the dynamic range. **D,** A display using a postprocessing curve similar to that in **B**. **E,** A display using a postprocessing curve similar to that in **C**. Compare **D** and **E** with the linear case in Figure 4-30, *A, C*.

B Color

Some instruments have the postprocessing ability to present different echo intensities in various colors rather than in gray shades, that is, the ability to colorize echoes. In this case different colors, rather than gray levels, are assigned to various echo intensities. Because the eye can differentiate more color tints than gray shades, color displays offer improved contrast resolution capability (discussed later). This process is called *B color* or *color scale* (compared with gray scale). A color bar is included in such displays to show how colors are assigned to various echo strengths. Figure 4-32, *C-E* provides some examples.

> B color is a form of postprocessing that assigns colors, rather than gray shades, to different echo strengths.

Volume Presentation

Common ways of presenting 3D echo data (volume imaging) (Figure 4-33) include surface renderings, 2D slices through the 3D volume, and transparent views. The advantage of 2D slice presentation is that it is possible to present image-plane orientations that are difficult or impossible to obtain with conventional 2D scanning. Surface renderings are popular in obstetric and cardiac imaging. Transparent views allow "see-through" imaging

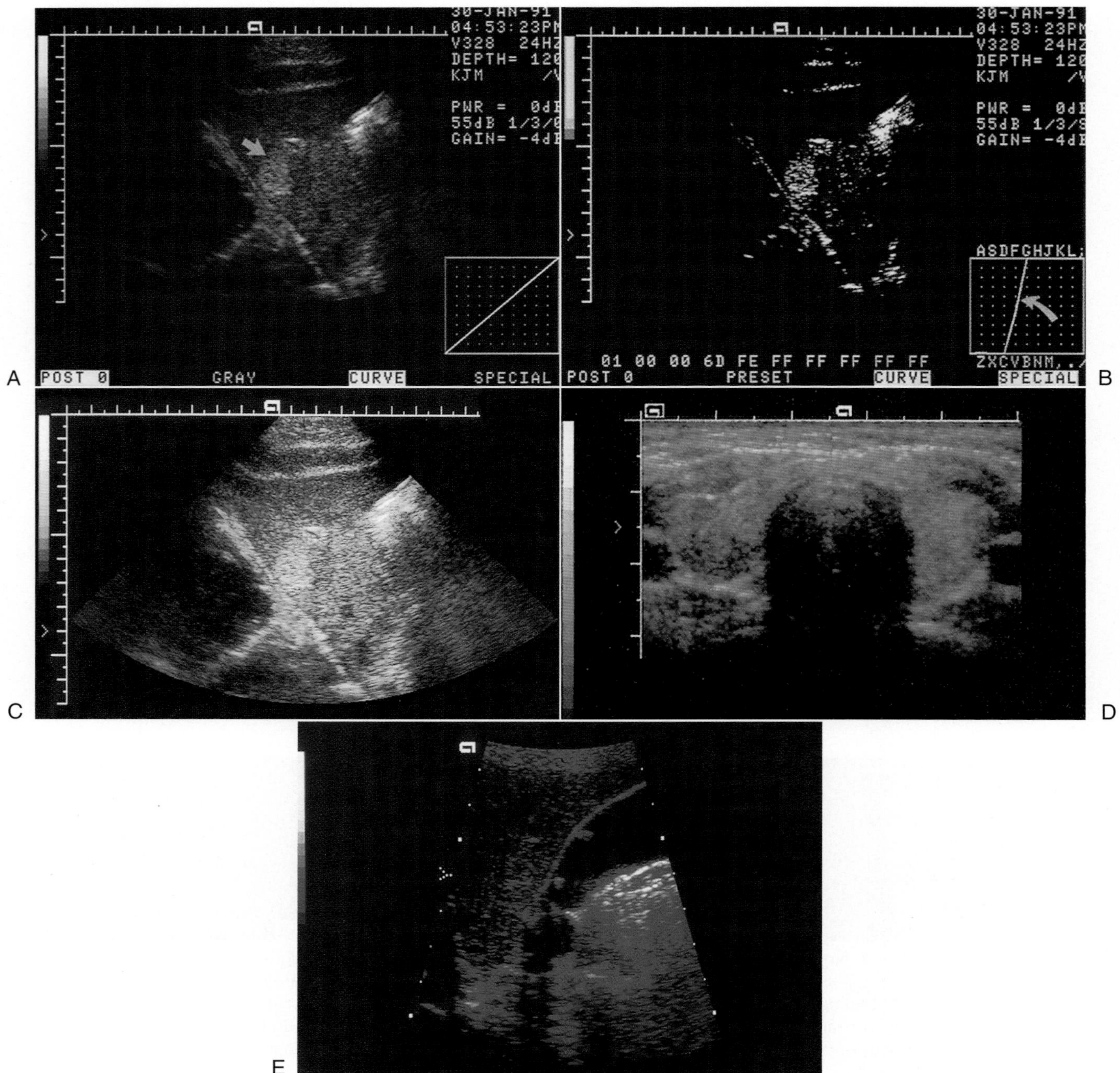

FIGURE 4-32 **A,** An image of a hemangioma *(arrow)* obtained by using linear postprocessing. **B,** An image of a hemangioma with a steep postprocessing assignment *(curved arrow)* designed to produce a great contrast between these normal and abnormal tissue echoes. **C-E,** Color displays of a hemangioma (**C**; compare with **A** and **B**), thyroid (**D**), and gallbladder (**E**). Color assignments, shown in the color bars on the left, are designated as follows: (**C**) temperature (increasing intensity assigned dark orange through yellow to white), (**D**) magenta (dark magenta through light magenta to white), and (**E**) rainbow (dark violet through various colors to white).

of the anatomy as with plain-film radiographs. These presentation forms are postprocessing choices that present the stored 3D volume of echo information in different ways on the display.

> A 3D volume of echo data can be displayed in several ways, including 2D slices, surface renderings, and transparent views.

Digital-to-Analog Converter

After numbers are retrieved from the memory and postprocessed, they are converted into voltages that determine the brightnesses of echoes on the display. This task is accomplished by the **digital-to-analog converter**. The digital-to-analog converter converts the digital data received from the image memory to analog voltages that are fed to

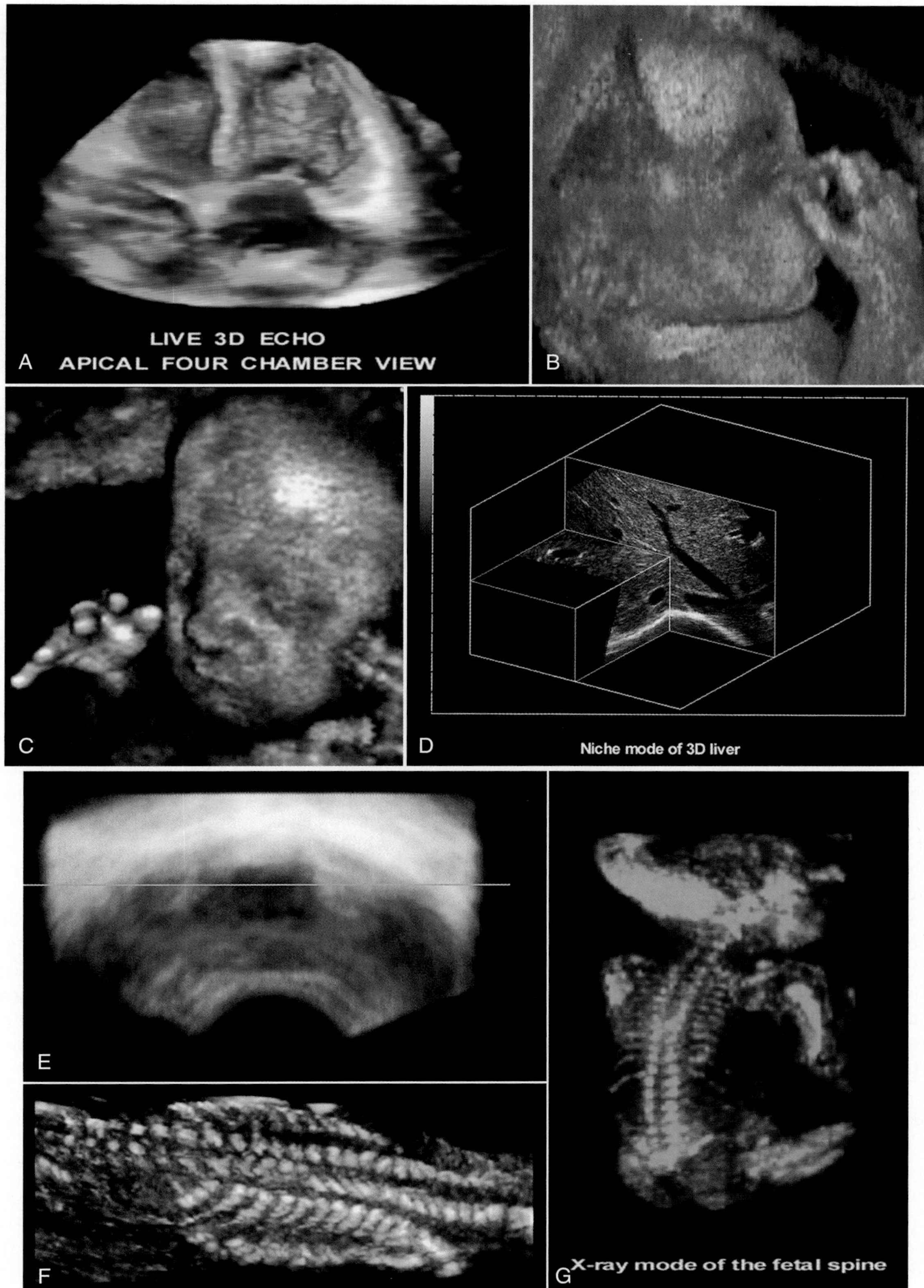

FIGURE 4-33 Various postprocessing choices for presenting three-dimensional images. Three-dimensional surface renderings. **A,** Cardiac image. **B,** Fetus holding nose. **C,** Fetal head and hands. **D,** Three orthogonal two-dimensional slices through the three-dimensional liver echo volume. **E-G,** Transparent (x-ray) mode. **E,** All echoes in the volume can be included, as in this image of the prostate, or **(F-G)** only the strongest ones.

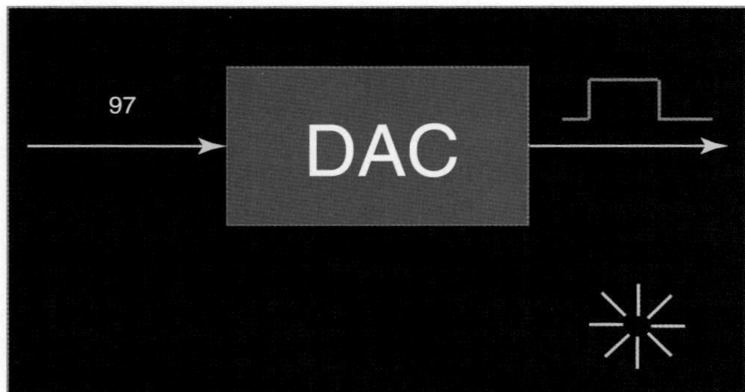

FIGURE 4-34 The digital-to-analog converter (DAC) converts the numbers (digital) stored in the memory to proportional (analog) voltages that control the brightness of each echo on the display.

the display to determine the echo brightnesses displayed (Figure 4-34).

Finally, although in this discussion we have recognized memory only as image memory in the image processor, various instruments may store echo information at various points along the processing chain, including storing radio frequency echo data before amplitude detection. We have simplified the discussion by dealing with memory only as image memory in the image processor.

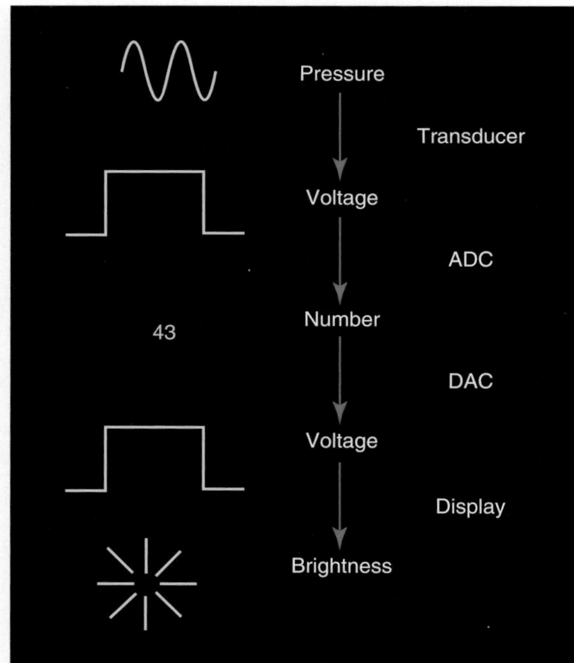

FIGURE 4-35 Information chain from the echo (pressure), through the transducer and electronics, to the display. The analog-to-digital converter (ADC) is part of the beam former. An echo is stored as a number in the image memory (part of the image processor). The digital-to-analog converter (DAC) is part of the image processor.

DISPLAY

The chain of events covered thus far in this chapter is illustrated in Figure 4-35. Gray-scale operation causes a brightening of the spot for each echo in memory. The brightness (gray scale) is proportional to the echo strength. The memory is filled with echoes from many pulses as the beam is scanned through the anatomy to be imaged. The 2D gray-scale scan is a brightness image that represents an anatomic cross-section in the scanning plane, as if the sound beam cuts a section through the tissue similar to a knife. Each individual image is called a *frame.* Because several frames can be acquired and presented every second, this is called *real-time display.* Several 2D scans can also be acquired to form a 3D volume of stored echo information.

Frame rate is the number of sonographic 2D or 3D images entered into the image memory per second, whereas **refresh rate** is the number of times per second that images are retrieved from the memory and presented on the display. These two rates can be, but are not necessarily, equal.

The information delivered to the display can be presented in several ways. Common to all clinical applications is brightness mode, also called **B mode**, **B scan**, or *gray-scale sonography.* Gray-scale anatomic displays can be in 2D or 3D forms. In echocardiography, motion mode (**M mode**) is also used. In ophthalmology, amplitude mode (**A mode**) is used as well.

Flat-Panel Display

Sonographic images are presented on computer displays because they represent the digital information stored in the image (computer) memory. Computer displays present image information in the form of horizontal lines (Figure 4-36, *A*). Each horizontal display scan line corresponds to a row of digital data in the image memory. The information is read out of the memory, row by row (much as we read a page of text), and is written on the display, line by line, similar to writing on a lined sheet of paper. Because the display includes more than the sonographic image (such as alphanumeric data, icons, and Doppler spectral display), the data in the memory are of various types. But whatever is stored in a given pixel in the memory (whether it is part of a gray-scale anatomic image, part of an alphabetic letter, or anything else) will appear at the corresponding pixel location on the display with the appropriate brightness and color. Because color is used in some cases, such as B color and color Doppler, color displays are common in sonographic instruments.

> The display is a flat-panel display that presents an image in horizontal lines from top to bottom.

Various standards are used in computer displays. An example is the SVGA (super-video-graphics array) standard, in which the pixel matrix can be, among other values, 1024 × 768 and the display refresh rate (the number of images per second extracted from image) is 60 Hz.

> A computer monitor is a display that presents data retrieved from the memory in a 2D pixel matrix, refreshing the display often (e.g., 60 times per second).

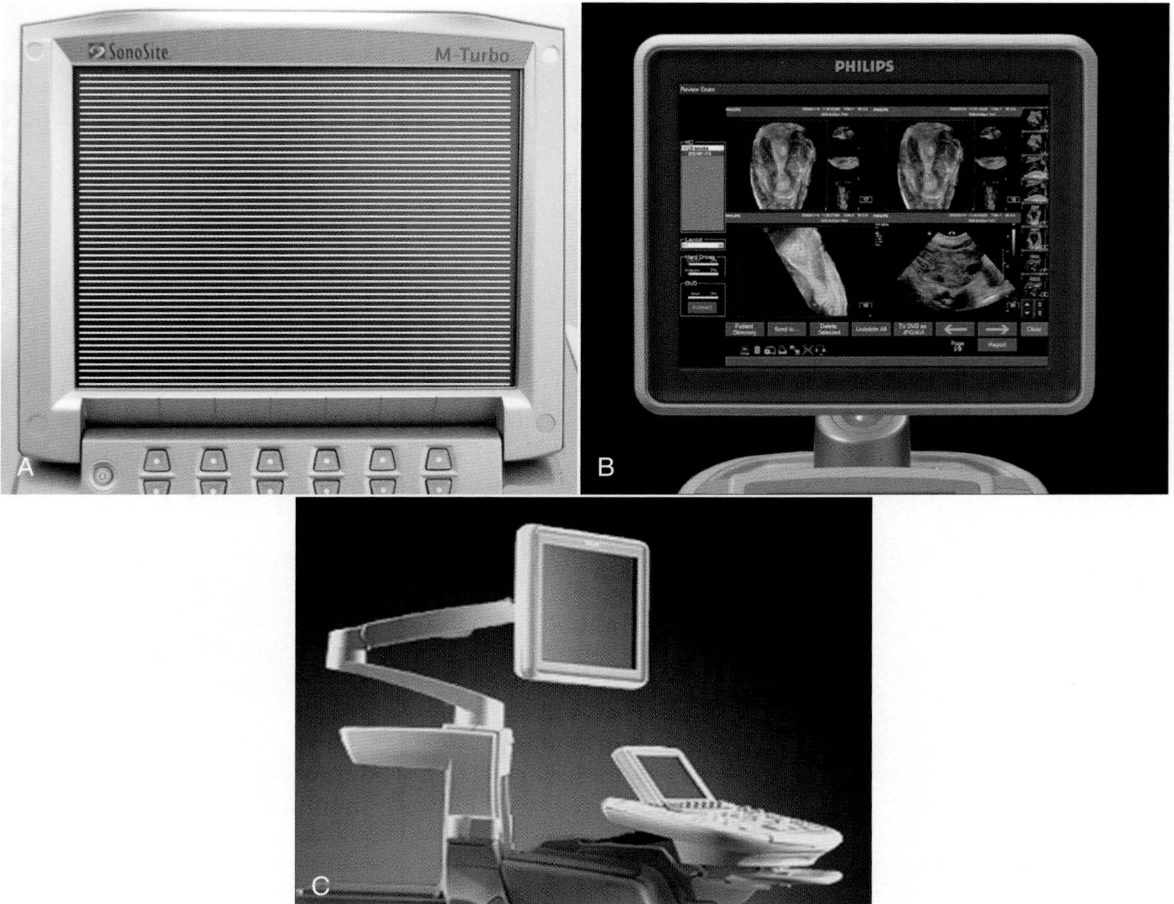

FIGURE 4-36 **A,** An image on a display is scanned from left to right, top to bottom in horizontal lines, each corresponding to a row of echo-amplitude numbers in image memory. **B-C,** Flat-panel displays.

Because we want to display pixels with proportional brightnesses, not the numbers that represent the echo intensities in the image memory, these numbers must be converted by the digital-to-analog converter to proportional voltages that control the brightness.

Flat-panel displays are common on computers, television sets, and sonographic instruments (see Figure 4-36, *B-C*). A **flat-panel display** is a back-lighted liquid crystal display (LCD). Such a display is composed of a rectangular matrix of thousands of LCD elements (e.g., a 1024 × 768 matrix contains 786,432 LCD elements). These elements can be electrically turned on or off individually and act as tiny light valves for blocking or passing the light from the light source underneath the matrix. More specifically, the elements can be turned on partially to allow a measured amount of light through, usually in 256 steps of luminance, that is, 256 displayed gray levels from black to white. Groups of red, green, and blue elements allow what is called *24-bit color* (8 bits or 256 luminance values for each primary color element) yielding 16,777,216 possible colors presented at each pixel location. Red, green, and blue (RGB) are known as *primary additive colors* because various combinations can produce nearly any color desired. For example, red and green, mixed equally, produce yellow. Green and blue produce *cyan,* the technical term for aqua. Red and blue produce magenta. Red, green, and blue, equally mixed, produce white (or gray, depending on brightness).

For measurement purposes, displays include range marker dots and calipers (Figure 4-37). Marker dots are presented as a series of dots in a line with a given separation (e.g., 1 cm). Calipers are two plus signs (or some other symbol) that can be placed anywhere on the display. The instrument calculates the distance between them and shows it on the display.

M Mode and A Mode

Another display mode (*M mode*) is used to show the motion of cardiac structures (Figure 4-38). M mode is a display form that presents depth (vertical axis) versus time (horizontal). An uncommon display (except in ophthalmologic sonography), which shows the amplitudes of echoes, is called the *A mode* (Figure 4-39). A mode is a depth versus amplitude display. The sound beam is stationary in these

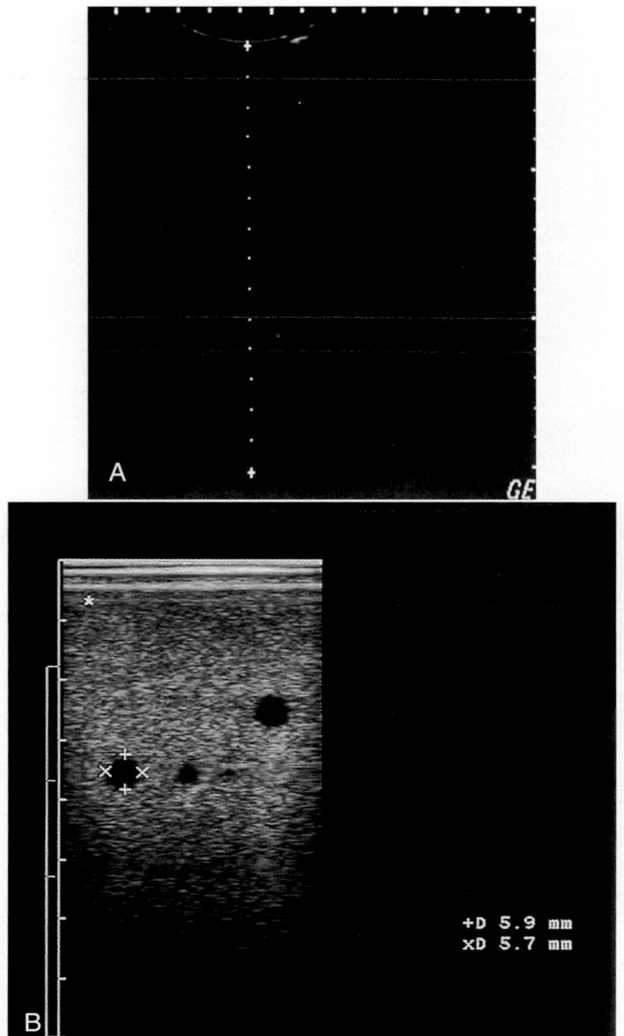

FIGURE 4-37 A, Range marker dots. B, Calipers with 5.7-mm and 5.9-mm separations.

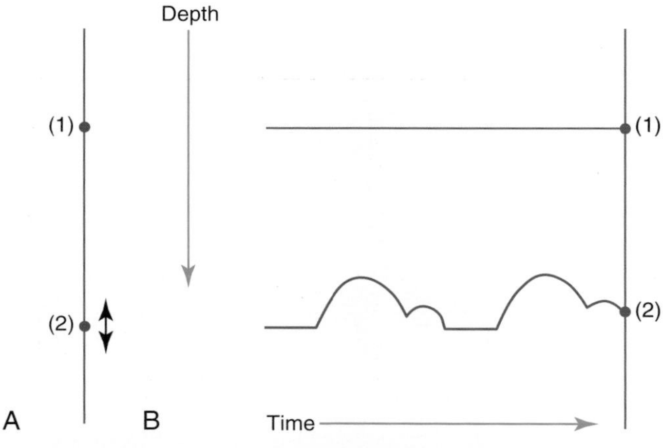

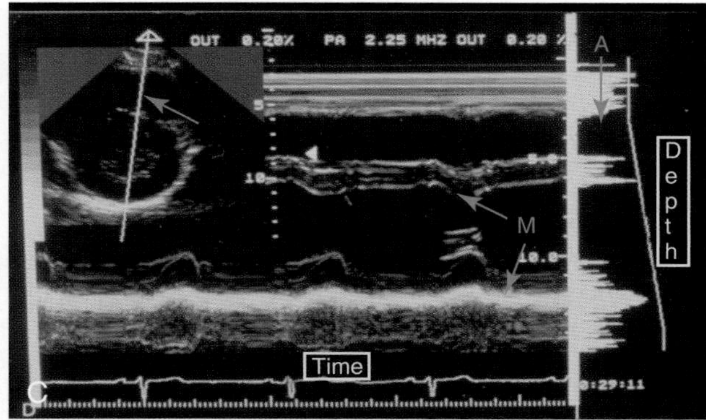

FIGURE 4-38 A, B mode presentation of echo depth with echoes from both a stationary structure *(1)* and a moving one *(2)*. B, If pulses are sent down the same path repeatedly, and vertical scan lines are placed next to each other, a display of depth-versus-time results. The pattern of motion of moving structures *(2)* is traced out on the display for evaluation. This is called *M mode display*. C, A mode and M mode presentations of moving cardiac structures. Depth is the vertical axis in both cases. For M mode, time increases to the right. The two-dimensional real-time anatomic cross-sectional image also is shown *(upper left)*. The green arrow indicates the repeating path of the ultrasound pulses used to generate the A and M mode displays.

presentations. Ultrasound pulses travel down the same path over and over. In the M mode display, the vertical scan lines are written next to each other across the horizontal time axis.

CONTRAST AND TEMPORAL RESOLUTIONS

Contrast Resolution

For linear assignment of echo intensities to numbers in the memory, the echo dynamic range is equally divided throughout the gray levels of the system. Table 4-5 gives, for 4- to 8-bit systems, the number of decibels of dynamic range covered by each shade (for two different echo dynamic range values, 40 dB and 60 dB, after attenuation compensation) and the average intensity difference between two echoes required for assignment to different shades (different numbers) in the memory. This relates to contrast resolution, which is the ability visually to observe subtle echo strength differences between adjacent tissues. An increase in the number of bits per pixel (more gray shades) improves contrast resolution. For a 4-bit, 40-dB dynamic range system, an echo must have nearly twice the intensity of another for it to be assigned a different shade. With a 60-dB dynamic range, more than twice the intensity would be required. For a 6-bit, 40-dB system, only a 15% difference is required. For an 8-bit, 60-dB system, a 5% difference is sufficient. Table 4-5 and Figure 4-40 show how a greater number of shades or a reduced dynamic range improves contrast resolution.

> Contrast resolution is the ability of a gray-scale display to distinguish between echoes of slightly different intensities. Contrast resolution depends on the number of bits per pixel in the image memory.

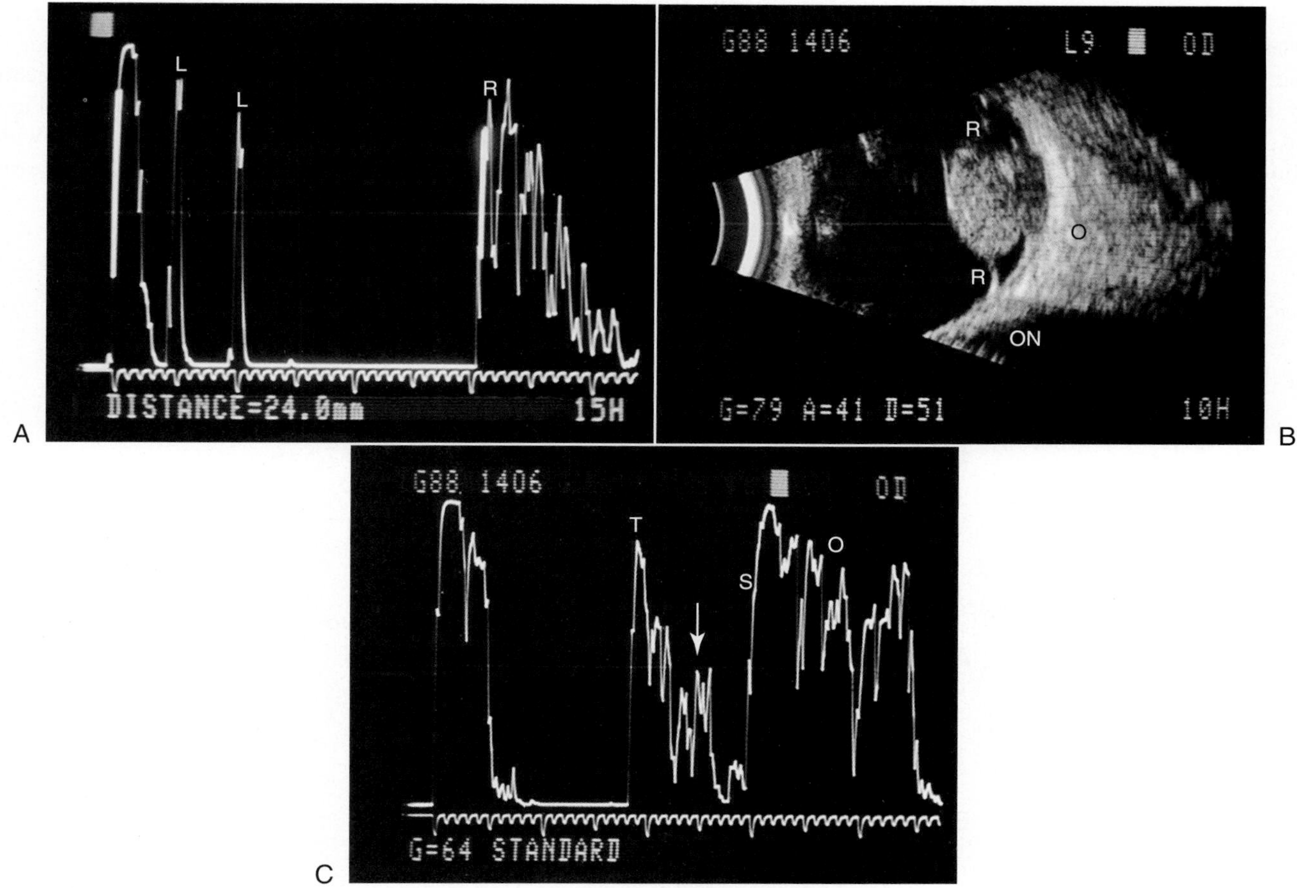

FIGURE 4-39 **A,** A normal ophthalmologic A mode presentation, where *L* represents lens echoes and *R* represents the retina. A longitudinal B scan (**B**) and standardized A mode presentation (**C**) demonstrate the typical acoustic appearance of a choroidal melanoma. The B scan shows a mushroom-shaped mass with exudative retinal detachment *(R)* at the tumor margins (*O,* orbital fat; *ON,* optic nerve). The A mode scan demonstrates a high spike from the tumor surface *(T)* and low to medium echogenicity within the lesion *(arrow)* (*S,* sclera; *O,* orbital fat). In this figure, the horizontal axis represents depth.

TABLE 4-5 Contrast Resolution of Digital Memories

	40-dB DYNAMIC RANGE		60-dB DYNAMIC RANGE	
Bits per Pixel	**Decibels per Shade**	**Intensity Difference (%)***	**Decibels per Shade**	**Intensity Difference (%)***
4	2.5	78	3.8	140
5	1.2	32	1.9	55
6	0.6	15	0.9	23
7	0.3	7	0.5	12
8	0.2	5	0.2	5

*The average difference required between two echoes for the echoes to be assigned different shades.

Liver metastases (Figure 4-41) illustrate the importance of contrast resolution because they can be slightly more or less echogenic than the surrounding normal liver tissue. The less difference in echogenicity, the more difficult it is to detect the masses. First, more gray shades (more bits per pixel) will be required to store the echoes emanating from metastases with different numbers in the memory than those for the surrounding liver. Even then, if a linear postprocessing assignment is used, these small number differences in the memory may not be observed in the display. For example, in Figure 4-41, *E,* in which more gray-scale range is assigned to the weaker echoes, if normal and abnormal tissue echoes differed by one digit in the memory (e.g., normal = 40 and abnormal = 41), there would be a 1.2%

difference in brightness (gray level) between the two on the display. This difference could be observed. However, with linear postprocessing (see Figure 4-41, *D*), there would be only a 0.4% brightness difference, which would go unnoticed. In Figure 4-41, *E*, the improvement in contrast resolution for weaker echoes (because of the steeper slope for echoes assigned values 0 to 64 in the memory) is accomplished at the cost of degraded contrast resolution for the remainder of the dynamic range (shallow slope for echoes that are assigned values 65 to 255 in the memory). Figure 4-32, *A-B*, shows a hemangioma, the presentation of which is enhanced by using a specially crafted, steep postprocessing

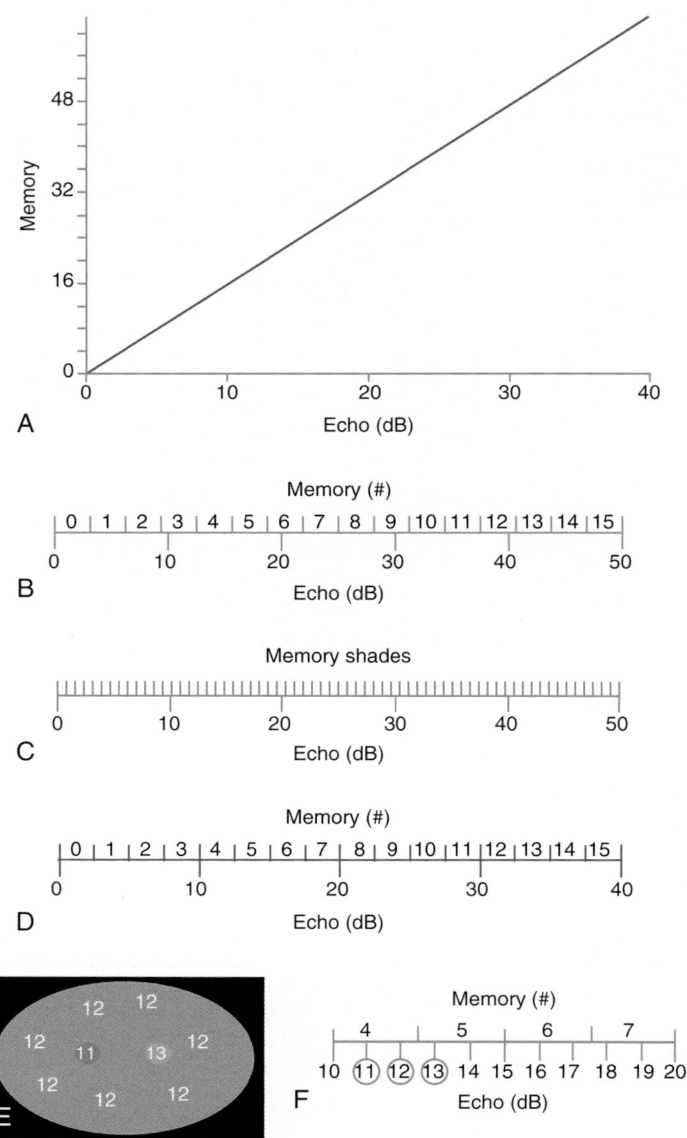

FIGURE 4-40 **A,** Assignment of numbers (to be stored in the memory) to echo intensities. Echo intensity is expressed in decibels in the form of a straight-line assignment (relative to the weakest echo, which is represented as 0 dB; the strongest echo is 40 dB, which is 10,000 times the intensity of the weakest). An instrument dynamic range of 40 dB and a 6-bit (64-shade) memory are assumed. **B,** With a 4-bit memory, a 50-dB dynamic range is divided into 16 regions (shades). **C,** With a 6-bit memory, a 50-dB dynamic range is divided into 64 regions, which are numbered 0 to 63. **D,** With a 4-bit memory, a 40-dB dynamic range is divided into 16 regions. **E,** Liver echoes are 12 dB in strength on the dynamic range scale, whereas two metastasic regions have strengths 11 and 13 dB, respectively. These regions should be displayed slightly darker and lighter as shown. **F,** The 10- to 20-dB dynamic range portion of **D** is expanded. If normal liver echoes were 12 dB (assigned 4 in the memory) and metastases were 13 dB (slightly hyperechoic; assigned 5), the normal and abnormal would be different in the memory and would appear with different brightnesses on the display. If the metastases were 11 dB (slightly hypoechoic), they would be assigned 4 in the memory, just as would the normal echoes, and the difference would be lost (identical displayed brightnesses).

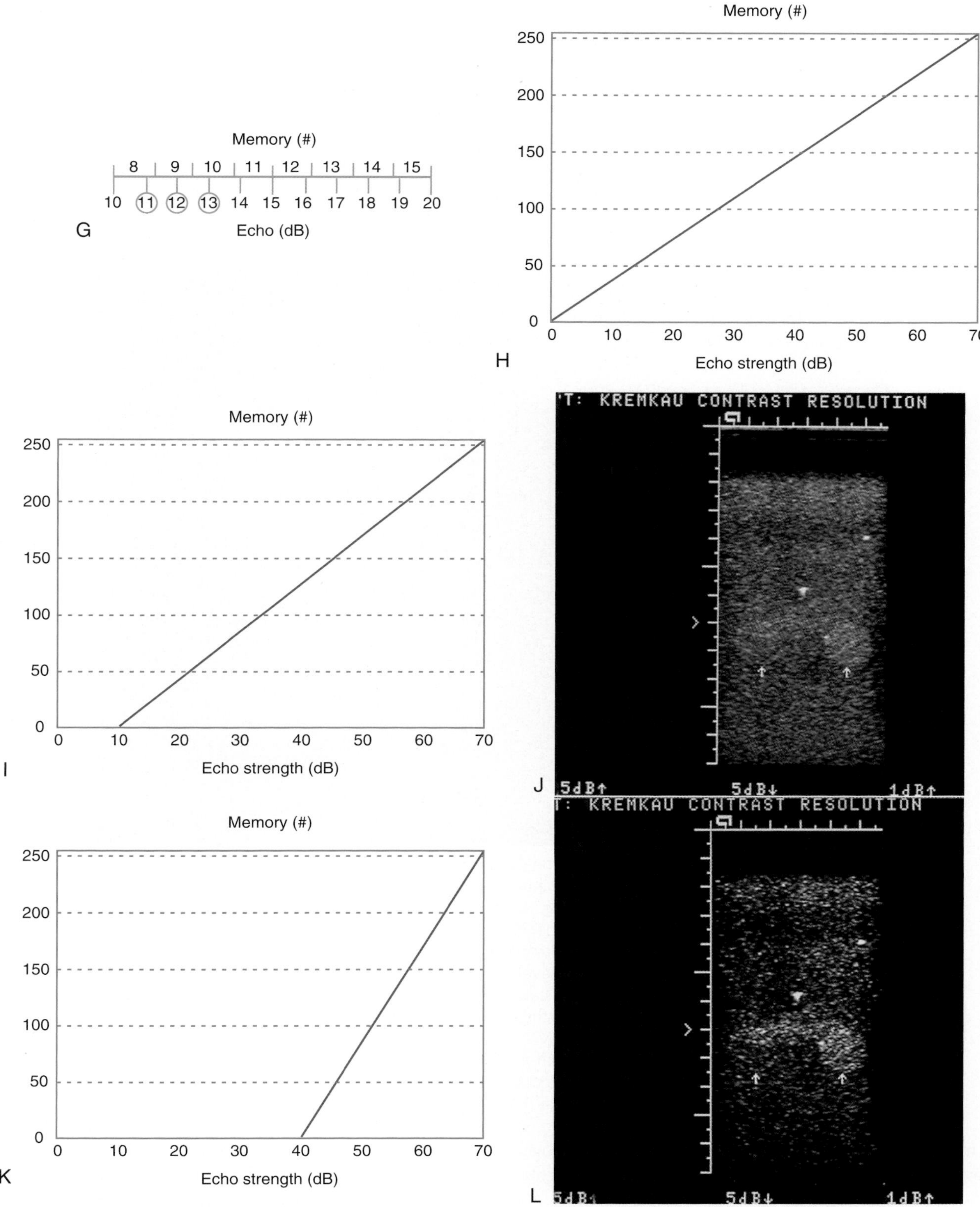

FIGURE 4-40, cont'd G, With a 5-bit (32-shade) memory, both metastatic regions in E would be assigned numbers different from those for normal liver and different from each other; that is, contrast resolution would be maintained for both. A dynamic range or compression (preprocessing) control reassigns echo intensities in memory, with the weaker portion as zeros and the remainder in linear fashion. The compression control is set at maximum (70 dB; H), 60 dB (**I-J**), and 30 dB (**K-L**). With decreasing dynamic range, more of the weaker portion is assigned to zero in memory (black on the display), and the contrast of the remainder (displayed) is enhanced with improved contrast resolution.

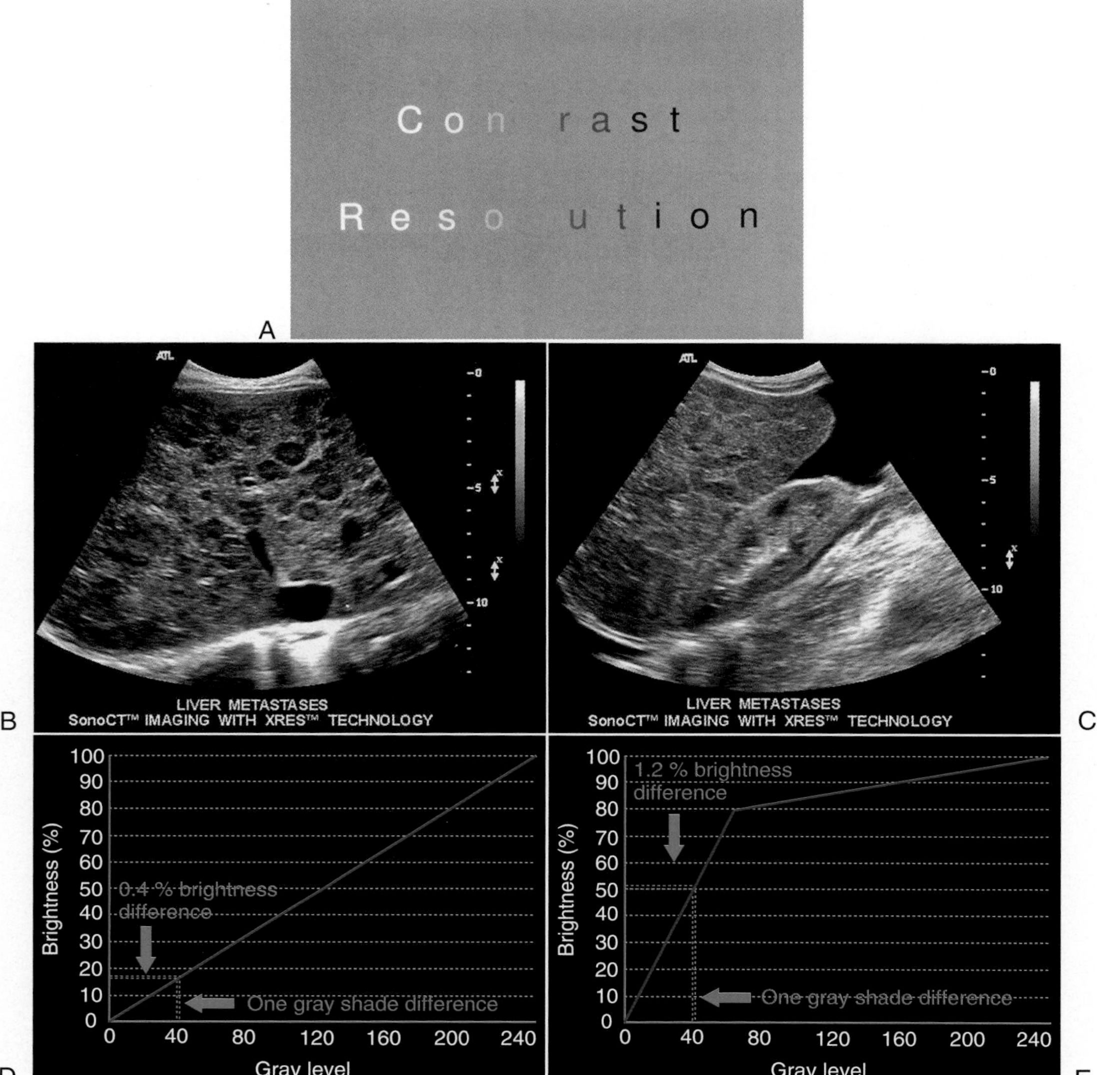

FIGURE 4-41 **A,** Contrast resolution is the ability of a gray-scale display to distinguish between echoes of slightly different amplitudes or intensities. **B,** Liver metastases that are less echogenic (and therefore darker) than the surrounding liver tissue. **C,** Liver metastases that are not easily visualized because they are only slightly hypoechoic compared with normal liver. Two tissue regions with slightly different echogenicities require good contrast resolution to be observed with different brightnesses. This requires enough gray levels so that echoes from the two regions are stored in the memory with different numbers to indicate their different strengths (echogenicities). Even then, the differences may not be observed on the display if they are minimal. **D,** In this example, one tissue region has echoes stored as gray level 40, whereas an adjacent region has echoes stored at gray level 41. These two regions would differ in brightness by 0.4% using a linear postprocessing assignment. This difference would not be noticed by a human observer. **E,** With a different postprocessing choice, the brightness difference is 1.2%, which could be observed.

assignment at the echo level that corresponds to the echogenicity of the hemangioma. The contrast between abnormal and normal tissues is greatly increased. If the mass were not obvious with linear postprocessing, the steep slope assignment likely would have made it visible.

Temporal Resolution

Sonographic instruments store several frames of echo information in the image memory per second. The number of sonographic images stored per second is called the *frame rate.* This is the rate at which the sound beam is scanned through the tissue cross-section by the transducer. A rapid sequence of frames yields what appears to be a continuously changing image. The effective frame rate observed on the display is limited by the refresh rate. For example, the echo information may be entering the image memory at a frame rate of 100 Hz, but if the refresh rate is 75 Hz, echo information is retrieved from the memory 75 times per second, and only 75 images per second

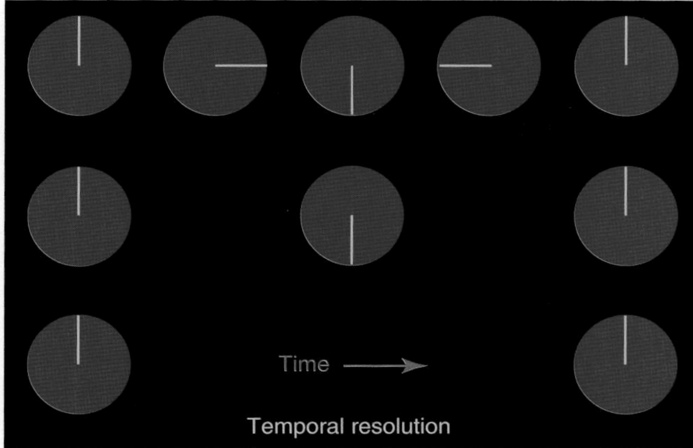

FIGURE 4-42 Temporal resolution improves with frame rate. *Top row,* A wheel is rotated in a clockwise direction. Four images are taken during one revolution; thus the frame rate is four per revolution. *Middle row,* With a frame rate of two per revolution, it can be seen that the wheel is rotating, but the direction is ambiguous: it could be clockwise or counterclockwise. *Bottom row,* The frame rate is one per revolution. The motion of the wheel is not observed; indeed, it appears to be stationary. A similar result would occur in echocardiography if one frame per cardiac cycle were acquired at the same instant in each cycle. The heart would appear to be inactive.

are then viewed on the display. However, there is an advantage to storing a frame rate that is higher than the refresh rate. When a frozen cine loop is displayed, the individual frames retain the temporal resolution achieved with the frame rate.

When the freeze-frame mode is activated, ultrasound beam scanning and echo data entry into the memory are halted, and the last frame entered is shown continuously on the display. Although the display continues to present what is in the memory at the refresh rate, it is the same image every time, thus it appears as a static, unchanging image.

Real-time imaging allows rapid and convenient acquisition of the desired image (with the display changing continuously while the scan plane is manually moved through tissues) and 2D imaging of the motion of moving structures (with the display changing continuously while the structures move). Temporal resolution is the ability of a display to distinguish closely spaced events in time and to present rapidly moving structures correctly. Temporal resolution is expressed in milliseconds, which is the time from the beginning of one frame to the beginning of the next one. This is also the time required to generate one complete frame. Temporal resolution improves while the frame rate increases (Figure 4-42) because less time elapses from one frame to the next.

Each frame is composed of many scan lines and may have more than one focus. For each focus on each scan line in each frame, a pulse is required. The required PRF, therefore, is determined by the required number of foci (n), lines per frame (LPF), and the frame rate (FR) in frames per second, that is, hertz (Hz). Indeed, the required PRF is equal to these three quantities multiplied together.

> For each focus on each scan line in each frame, a pulse is required.
>
> $$\mathrm{PRF\,(Hz)} = n \times \mathrm{LPF} \times \mathrm{FR\,(Hz)}$$

> To increase the number of foci, the PRF must increase.

> To increase the number of lines per frame, the PRF must increase.

> To increase the frame rate, the PRF must increase.

However, time is required for echoes to return while a pulse travels into the tissue. The greater the penetration, the longer it takes for all of the echoes to return (remember the "13 μs/cm rule"). To avoid misplacement of echoes on the display because of the late arrival of echoes, all echoes from one pulse must be received before the next pulse is emitted. To accomplish this, PRF must decrease while penetration increases. That is, if a lower operating frequency is used, penetration is increased and the PRF must decrease to avoid echo misplacement. This will occur as a FR reduction (Figure 4-43) for lower operating frequencies. The FR decreases when displayed depth is increased (see Figure 4-43, *C-D*). Likewise, wider images (requiring more scan lines) and multiple foci also reduce the FR (Figure 4-44) because more time is required, in both cases, to generate each frame. The relationship between these competing variables is as follows:

$$\mathrm{pen\,(cm)} \times n \times \mathrm{LPF} \times \mathrm{FR\,(Hz)} \leq 77{,}000\ \mathrm{cm/s}$$

> If penetration increases, the PRF must decrease.

> If penetration increases, the FR decreases.

> If the number of foci increases, the FR decreases.

> If the lines per frame increases, the FR decreases.

The symbol ≤ represents "less than or equal to." That is, when penetration is multiplied by the number of foci, the number of scan lines per frame, and the FR, the result must not exceed 77,000. Otherwise, the required PRF would not allow the return of all of the echoes before the emission of the next pulse (resulting in echo misplacement).

Table 4-6 lists the allowable PRFs and FRs for various penetration and lines-per-frame values. Multiple foci reduce permitted FRs inversely (e.g., two foci with a penetration of

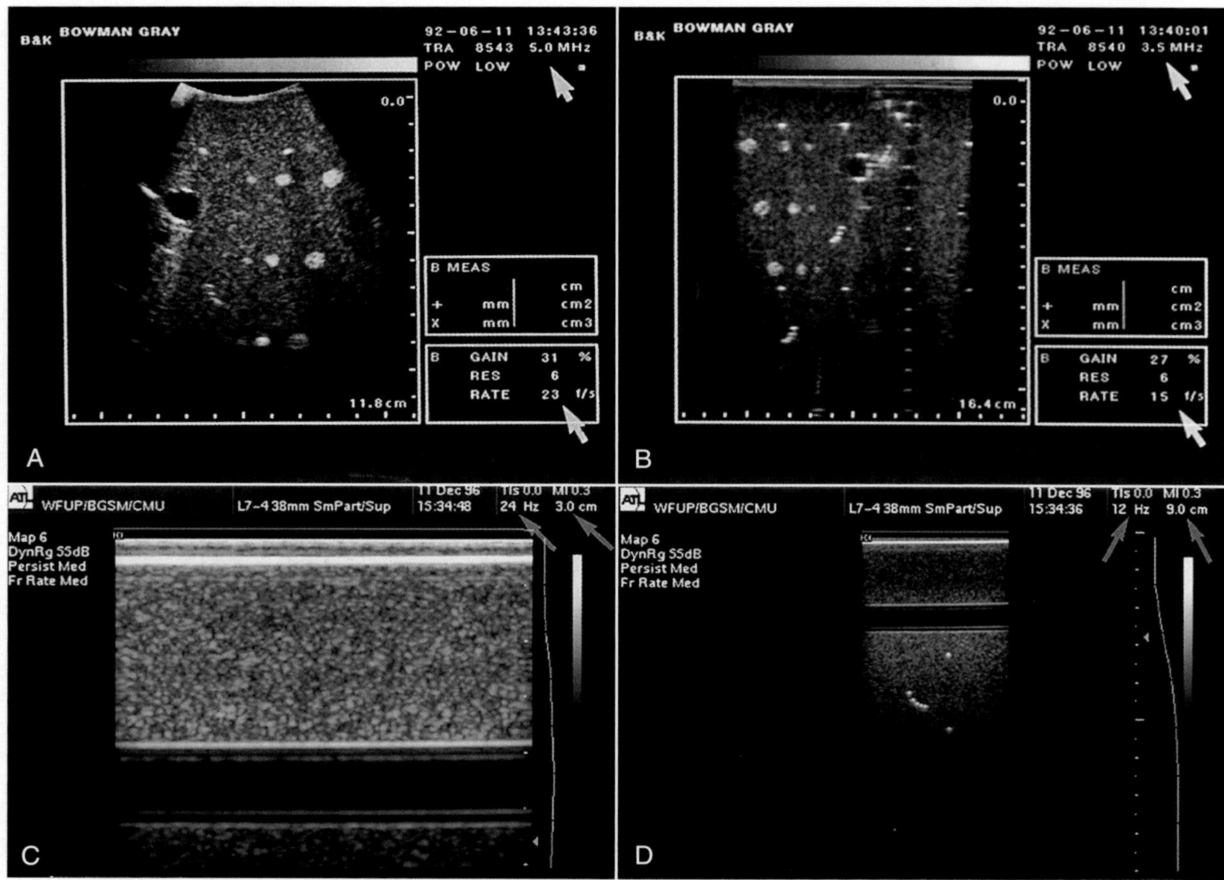

FIGURE 4-43 **A lower operating frequency allows greater penetration, thereby necessitating longer echo arrival time, which slows down the frame rate.** **A,** 5 MHz, penetration of 9 cm, 23 frames per second. **B,** 3.5 MHz, penetration of 13 cm, 15 frames per second. **C,** With a displayed depth of 3 cm, the frame rate is 24 frames per second (hertz; *arrow*). **D,** A displayed depth increase to 9 cm reduces the frame rate to 12 Hz. At first this seems surprising because the operating frequency (5.5 MHz) and therefore the penetration are the same in both cases. However, the effective penetration is reduced with the reduced displayed depth in **C** by increasing PRF. The echoes from beyond the displayed depth are weaker because of attenuation. When the next pulse is sent, the amplifier gain drops with the restarting of the time gain control. Thus the deeper echoes are not amplified enough to be seen (in incorrect locations, that is, range ambiguity artifact).

20 cm and 100 lines per frame are equivalent to one-half × 38, or 19 frames per second).

Temporal resolution in M and A modes is equal to pulse the repetition period because each the pulse produces a new line of echo information on these displays.

> Temporal resolution is the ability to follow moving structures in temporal detail. Temporal resolution depends on FR, which depends on depth, lines per frame, and number of foci.

CONTEMPORARY FEATURES

Coded Excitation

Earlier in this chapter, a single-cycle driving voltage was described (see Figure 4-3). Often, more complicated driving voltage-pulse forms called coded excitation are used. This approach accomplishes functions such as multiple transmission foci, separation of harmonic echo bandwidth from transmitted pulse bandwidth, increased penetration, reduction of speckle with improved contrast resolution, and gray-scale imaging of blood flow (called *B flow*). In straightforward pulsing, the pulser drives the transducer through the pulse delays with one voltage pulse per scan line. In coded excitation, ensembles of driving voltage pulses are applied to the transducer to generate a single scan line. For example, instead of a single pulse, a series (such as three pulses followed by a missing pulse [a gap], then two pulses followed by another gap, and then two pulses) could be used. Other examples are shown in Figure 4-45, *A-B*. A decoder in the reception portion of the beam former recognizes and disassembles the coded sequence in the returning echoes and stacks up the individual pulses in the sequence to make a short, high-intensity echo voltage out of them. The result

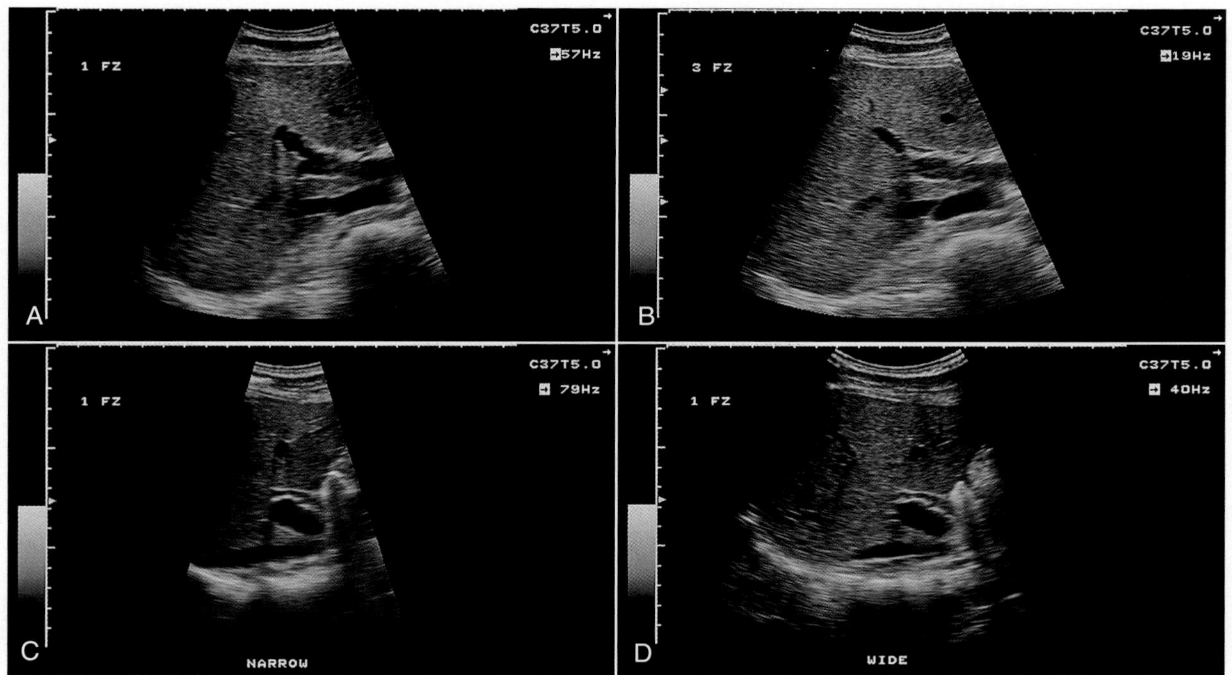

FIGURE 4-44 **A**, One focus; frame rate of 57. **B**, Multiple foci (3) reduce the frame rate to 19. **C**, Frame rate of 79. **D**, An increased frame width (doubling the number of scan lines) reduces the frame rate to 40.

TABLE 4-6 Pulse Repetition Frequency (PRF) and Frame Rate (FR) Permitted for Various Single-Focus Imaging Depths (Penetration) and 100 or 200 Scan Lines per Frame

Penetration (cm)	PRF (Hz)	FR	
		100 Lines	200 Lines
20	3850	38	19
15	5133	51	25
10	7700	77	38
5	15,400	154	77

is equivalent to having a much-higher-intensity driving pulse or a much more sensitive receiving system. Thus, for example, in the case of blood flow, weak echoes from blood are imaged and flow can be seen in gray scale along with the much stronger tissue echoes (see Figure 4-45, *C*).

> Coded excitation uses a series of pulses and gaps rather than a single driving pulse.

Coded excitation has been applied in radar for decades. A coded pulse is one that has internal amplitude, frequency, or phase modulation used for pulse compression. Pulse compression is the conversion, with use of a matched filter, of a relatively long coded pulse to one of short duration, excellent resolution, and equivalent high intensity and sensitivity. A matched filter maximizes the signal-to-noise ratio of the returning signal. The longer the coded pulse, the higher will be the signal-to-noise ratio in matched-filter implementations. Intrapulse coding is chosen to attain adequate axial resolution, and pulse duration is chosen to achieve the desired sensitivity. The matched-filter decoding process can be thought of as a sliding correlation of the parts of the coded pulse with the matched filter. The result of this process is, in effect, a shorter and stronger pulse yielding good resolution and sensitivity while conforming to the transmitted pulse amplitude and intensity limitations imposed by technologic and safety considerations. Such coding schemes are called *Barker codes*. An even better match can be achieved by Golay codes, which use pairs of transmitted pulses. The second pair is a bipolar sequence in which the latter portion of the pulse is the inverse of the first. This approach shortens the effective pulse length (improving axial resolution) and increases its amplitude (improving sensitivity). As a trade-off, the FR is reduced (degrading temporal resolution) because two pulses are required for each scan line.

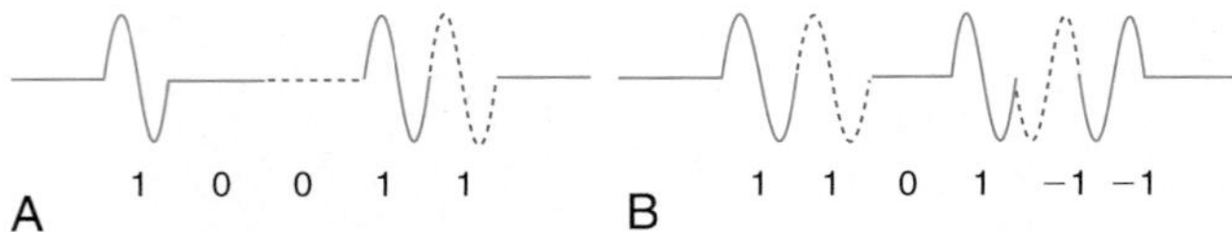

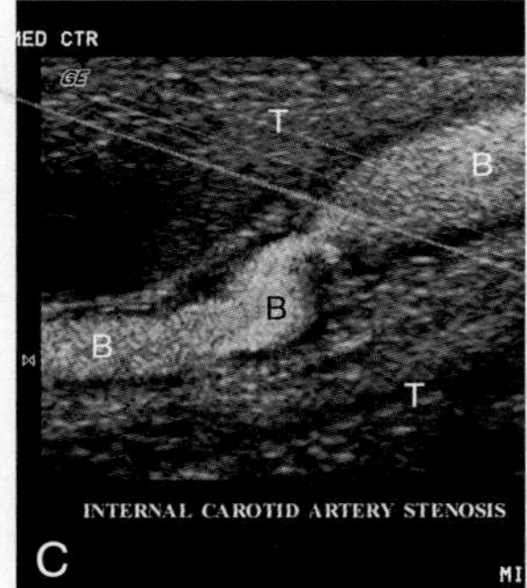

FIGURE 4-45 **Examples of coded pulse sequences.** Each pulse consists of a cycle of pressure variation. **A,** This sequence includes a pulse, two gaps, and two final pulses. **B,** This sequence includes two pulses, a gap, and one pulse followed by two inverted pulses. **C,** Blood flow imaging, in which weak echoes from flowing blood *(B)* are imaged along with much stronger tissue echoes *(T)*.

Harmonic Imaging

Earlier in this chapter, filtering in the signal processor was described (see Figures 4-14 and 4-15). A second type of filtering occurs with harmonic imaging, in which the fundamental (transmitted) frequency echoes are filtered out and the second harmonic frequency echoes are passed. (The generation of harmonic frequencies in tissue is discussed in Chapter 2.) At this point, the bandpass filter is centered at the second harmonic frequency with an appropriate bandwidth to include the bandwidth of the second harmonic echo signal (Figure 4-46, *A-D*). Harmonic imaging improves the image quality in three primary ways (see Figure 4-46, *E-F*):

- The harmonic beam is much narrower, improving lateral resolution, because harmonics are generated only in the highest-intensity portion of the beam.
- Grating lobe artifacts (discussed later) are eliminated because these extra beams are not sufficiently strong to generate the harmonics.
- Because the harmonic beam is generated at a depth beyond where some of the artifactual problems occur (e.g., superficial reverberation), the image degradation that they cause is reduced or eliminated.

Because the fundamental and second harmonic bandwidths must fit within the overall transducer bandwidth (see Figure 4-46, *A* and 4-47, *A*), they must be reasonably narrow. This means that the corresponding ultrasound pulses must be somewhat longer than otherwise, causing some degradation in axial resolution. A solution to this degradation in image quality is to use pulse inversion, a technique that uses two pulses per scan line rather than one. The second pulse is the inverse of the first. The echo sequences from the two pulses (see Figure 4-47, *B*) are combined to yield the resulting scan line. Fundamental frequency echoes are canceled (see Figure 4-47, *C*), and the second harmonic echoes remain (see Figure 4-47, *D*). This technique allows broad-bandwidth, short pulses to be used so that detail resolution is not degraded (see Figure 4-47, *E*). Instead, the FR is reduced, with some degradation of temporal resolution.

> Harmonic imaging improves image quality by sending pulses of some frequency into the body but then imaging echoes of frequency double those sent in.

Panoramic Imaging

Panoramic imaging provides a way to produce an image that has a wider field of view than what is available on an individual frame from a transducer. Panoramic imaging is an example of preprocessing that is achieved by manually sliding the transducer in a direction parallel to the scan plane, thus extending the scan plane. At the same time, the old echo information from previous frames is retained, whereas the new echoes are added to the image in the direction in which the scan plane is moving. The result is a larger field of view allowing presentation of large organs and regions of anatomy on one image (Figure 4-48). During the addition of new echoes, while the transducer is moved, it is important to properly locate the new echoes relative to the existing image. This is accomplished by correlating the locations of echoes common to adjacent frames (i.e., the overlap) so that the new information on the new frame is located properly (see Figure 4-48, *F-G*).

> Panoramic imaging expands the image beyond the normal limits of the field of view of the transducer.

Spatial Compounding

Spatial compounding is another example of preprocessing. It is a technique in which scan lines are directed in multiple directions by phasing so that structures are interrogated more than once by the ultrasound beam (Figure 4-49). Averaging sequential frames spatially, as many as nine typically, improves the quality of the image in several ways:

- As in persistence (which is temporal averaging), speckle is reduced.
- Clutter caused by artifacts is reduced.
- Smooth (specular) surfaces are presented more completely because they are interrogated at more than one angle, increasing the probability that close to 90-degree incidence is achieved (which is necessary to receive echoes from them).
- Structures previously hidden beneath highly attenuating objects can be visualized.

> Spatial compounding is the averaging of frames that view the anatomy from different angles.

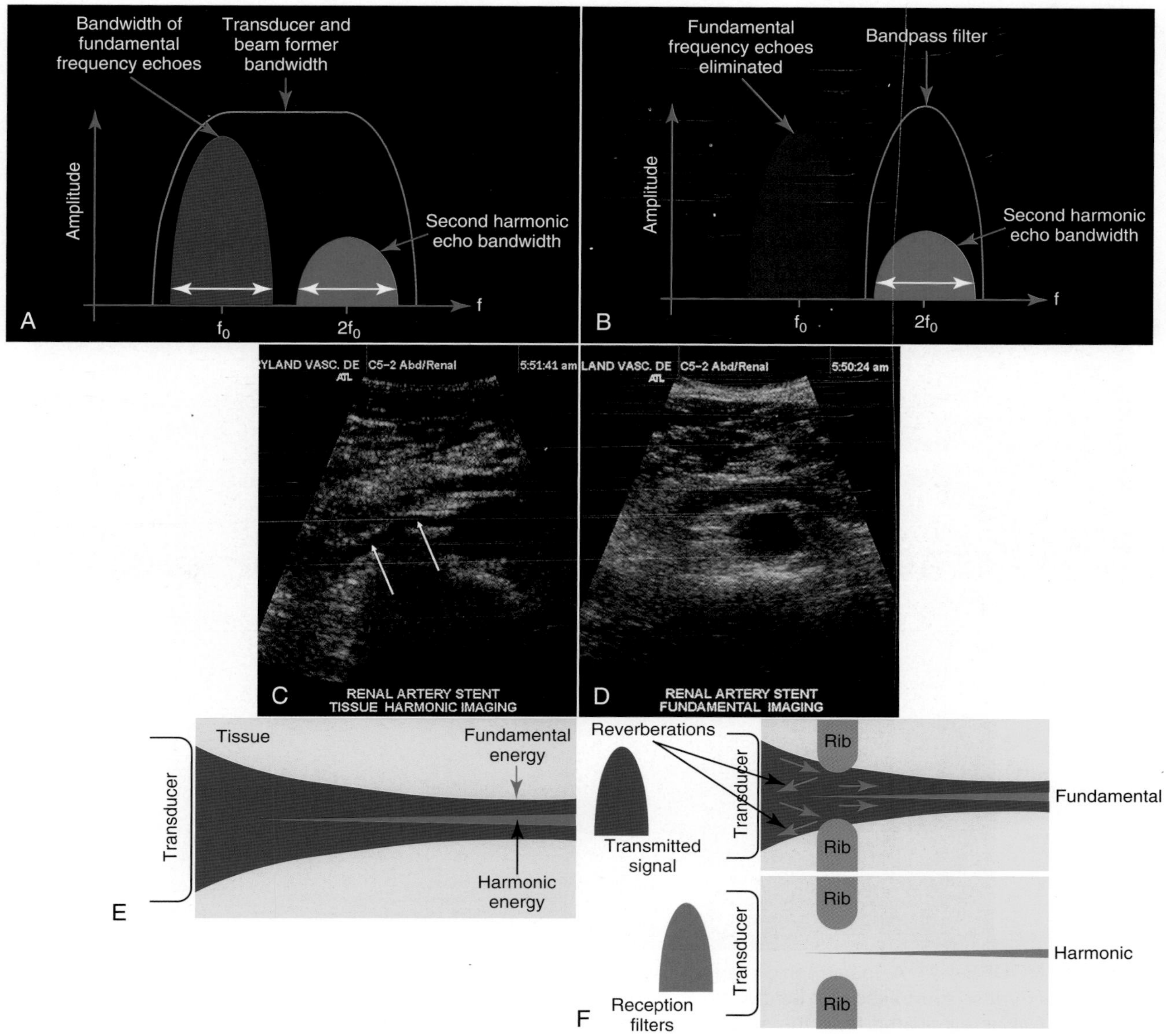

FIGURE 4-46 Harmonic imaging. **A,** Fundamental and second-harmonic echo bandwidths are shown. The beam former and transducer must pass both to generate the ultrasound beam and to accomplish harmonic imaging. **B,** For harmonic imaging, the bandpass filter eliminates the fundamental frequency echoes and passes the second harmonic echoes. The harmonic image (**C**) has improved quality compared with the fundamental-frequency image (**D**). **E,** The harmonic beam is much narrower than the fundamental. **F,** Reverberations are reduced with the harmonic beam.

Parallel Processing

Conventional sonography, as described to this point, forces interdependence on detail and temporal resolutions (previously discussed). For example, increasing multiple transmission focuses or increasing scan line density (lines per frame) to improve detail resolution decreases frame rate (degrading temporal resolution). This interdependence can be avoided by taking a different approach to the pulse-echo principle, namely by using all elements in the transducer to send a broad, unfocused beam of ultrasound into the anatomy simultaneously exposing the entire width of the image while the broad pulse travels down the path. Ultimately, this one wide pulse illuminates the entire field of view for the image. This means that echoes from all portions of the exposed image plane will arrive at various times at all the elements when in reception mode. Massive parallel processing (in all reception channels simultaneously), which is now feasible, then sorts out the echoes from all of this combined echo information, placing them in image memory in proper locations. Because one transmitted pulse provides all

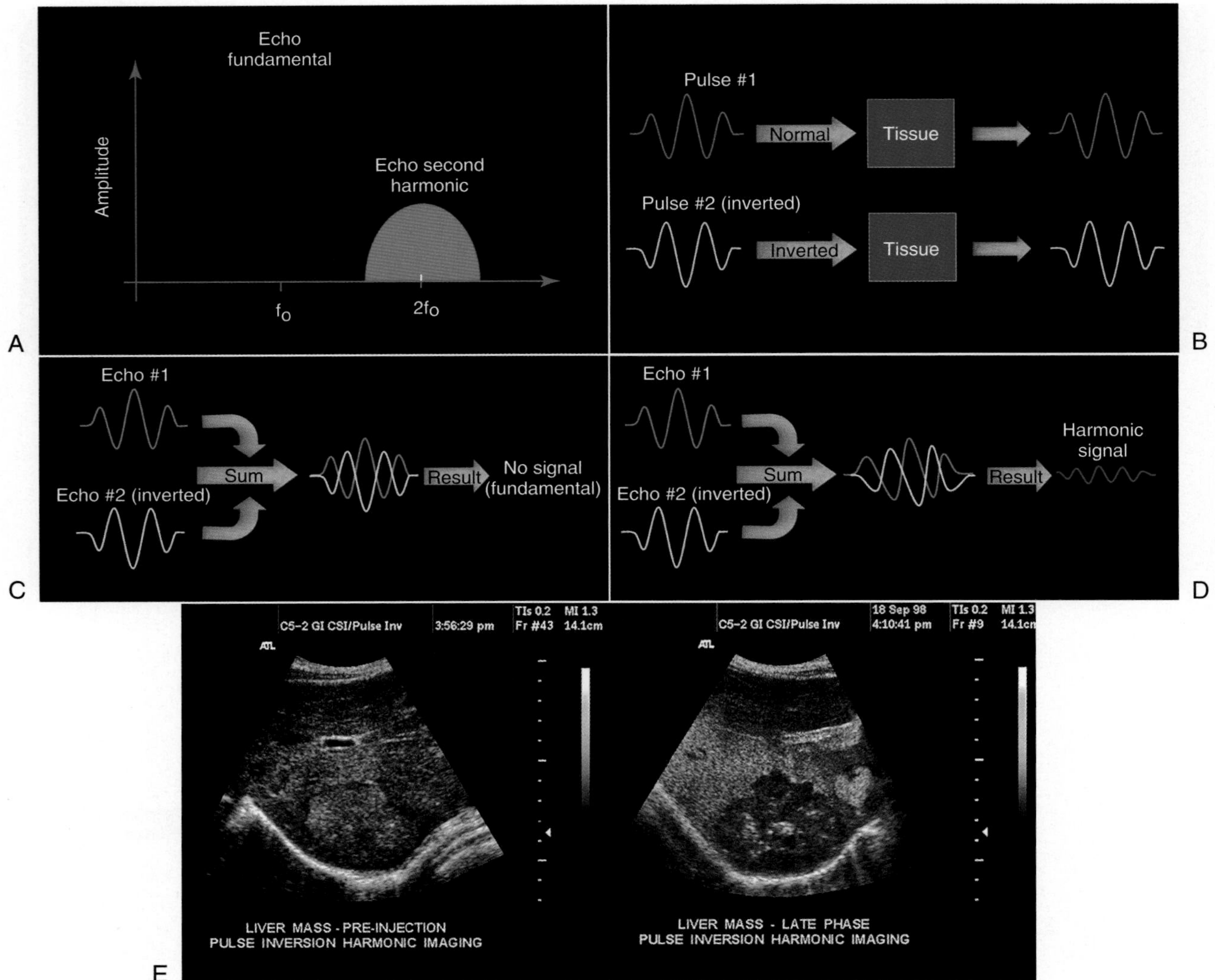

FIGURE 4-47 **A,** In harmonic imaging, two bandwidths (fundamental and second harmonic) must fit within the transducer bandwidth and not overlap, so that the fundamental frequency echoes can be eliminated from the second harmonic image. **B,** In pulse inversion harmonic imaging, a normal pulse of ultrasound is followed by an inverted pulse. Two series of echoes return from these two pulses (only one echo is shown for each pulse in this drawing). When the echoes from the two pulses are summed, the fundamental frequency echoes cancel **(C)**, whereas the second harmonic echoes are not canceled **(D)**. **E,** Preinjection and postinjection abdominal images with a contrast agent and pulse inversion harmonic imaging.

of the echo information for all portions of the image, rather than for just one scan line, the FR is increased by a factor of approximately 100 so that FRs in the hundreds or thousands can be achieved. This process can be described as a computed time-reversal approach that mimics backward propagation of the transmitted pulse, revealing the structures that produced all the echoes received. Synthetic focus is also achieved by sophisticated reception signal processing, so that effectively a narrow transmit beam is achieved through all portions of the image, rather than with multiple transmission focuses as previously implemented which reduced FRs.

> Parallel processing is a sophisticated processing technique that enables rapid image acquisition and very high FRs.

Elastography

Conventional sonographic anatomic images are presentations of the scattering properties of the imaged tissues. They do not provide any direct relation to mechanical tissue properties, but certainly have proven their value in diagnostic imaging over decades of implementation. A sonographic mode termed **elastography**[3] is available as an advanced feature

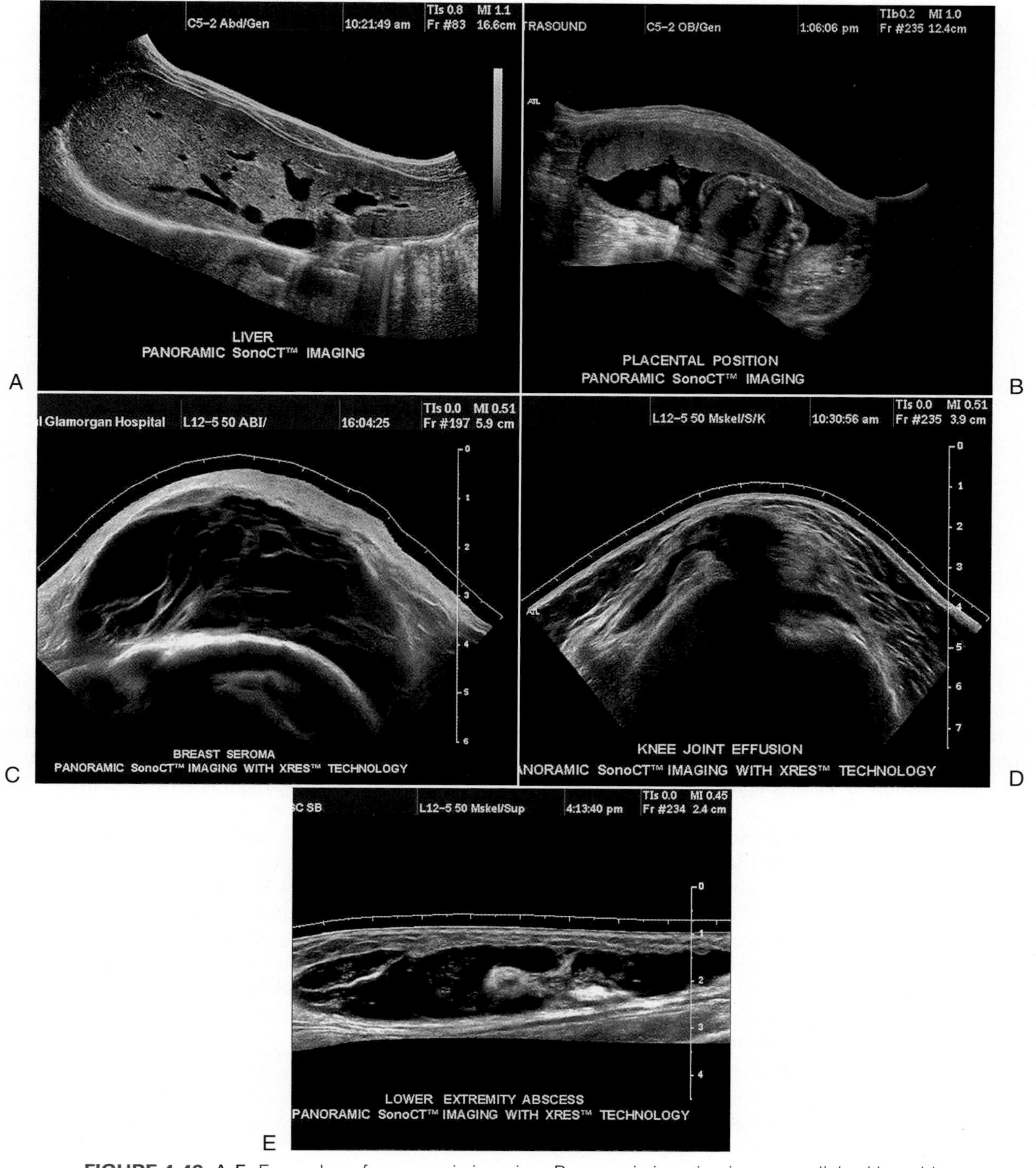

FIGURE 4-48 A-E, Examples of panoramic imaging. Panoramic imaging is accomplished by adding new information to one end of an image, spatially correlating the overlapping old echoes to properly locate the new ones.

Continued

on some instruments. Elastography presents qualitative or quantitative information regarding the stiffness, hardness, or softness of tissue. If a material, such as tissue, is subjected to a **stress** (a force per unit area) that compresses or stretches the material, the ratio of the applied stress to the resulting **strain** (the increase or decrease of the length of a segment of the material divided by its original length) is called **Young's modulus** and is a measure of the hardness or softness of the material. Thus soft materials have a small Young's modulus (i.e., a given stress results in a large strain), whereas a large Young's modulus corresponds to hard or stiff materials, for which a given stress results in little strain. As evidenced by the

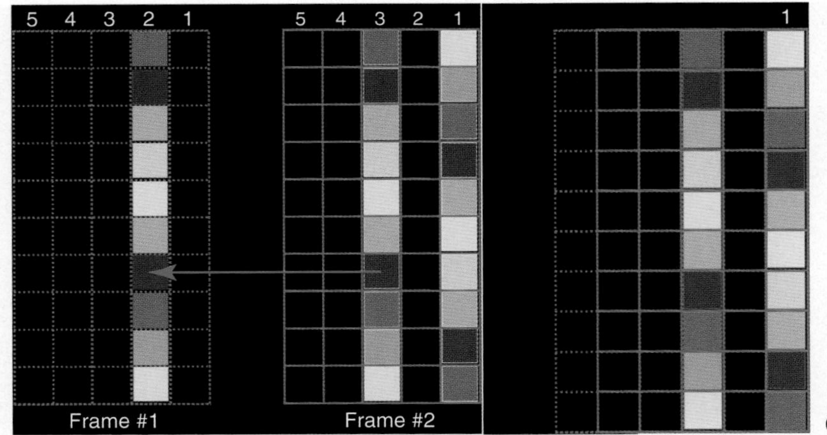

FIGURE 4-48, cont'd F, Two sequential frames are shown. Frame No. 2 temporally follows frame No. 1. Frame No. 2 is located slightly to the right of frame No. 1 in the anatomy by manual movement of the transducer by the sonographer. Thus a new scan line is added to frame No. 2. Scan line No. 3 in the new frame corresponds to scan line No. 2 in the previous frame. A spatial correlation process in the image processor identifies the equality of these two scan lines. Frame No. 2 then is slid to the left over the top of frame No. 1 so that the identical scan lines in the two frames overlap. **G,** The new scan line is thus added properly to the old frame. This process is repeated many times while the transducer is moved in a direction parallel to the scan plane. The old scan lines are retained while the new ones are added to the image.

success of manual palpation for centuries, hardness of tissue is a useful indicator of normality or abnormality. Elastography provides an imaging means of "palpation" and can even be quantitative in its evaluation of tissue hardness.

Various approaches to elastography have been implemented commercially. Static methods involve subjecting tissues to a manual force initiated by the sonographer physically pushing on the transducer and with the instrument tracking the movement of tissues by spatial correlation. It is then possible to estimate and depict tissue stiffness, because soft tissues will compress more than hard ones. Elastography is an imaging form of manual palpation. It is commonly shown as a color overlay on top of the gray-scale image (Figure 4-50) and has been used clinically for cancer detection, for characterization of small parts (breast, thyroid, and prostate), for assessment of the viability of the myocardium, and for monitoring of therapies that alter tissue composition, such as ablation procedures. This form of elastography is relatively simple to implement but is qualitative in that it shows relative hardness of various anatomic regions in relation to that of adjacent regions. It suffers from variability because it is operator dependent, and the Young's modulus cannot be calculated because the value of the applied stress is unknown.

Dynamic methods use a short-transient force or a time-varying repetitive force applied to the tissue. The force initially produces a compressional (transient or oscillatory) strain that travels with a high propagation speed, but through a phenomenon called *radiation force* can convert to **shear waves** (also called *transverse waves* as in Chapter 2) that travel at much slower speeds (0.5-10 m/s vs. 1440-1640 m/s for compressional waves) in directions perpendicular to the travel of the compressional wave. The small shear displacements of the slower propagating shear wave can be tracked by ultrafast means by using high frame rates to determine their propagation speed. Imaging the stiffness in this way is called *acoustic radiation force impulse (ARFI) imaging*. The shear wave propagation speed is quantitatively related to other material characteristics such as Young's modulus. Thus these dynamic methods provide the means to determine tissue hardness quantitatively. Recall that Young's modulus is stress divided by strain. Strain is unitless because it is a change in length divided by the original length. The unit for stress is the kilopascal (kPa). Thus the unit for Young's modulus is also the kilopascal. Young's modulus values in kPa for soft tissue range from approximately 1 for fat to 300 for fibrotic liver.

> Elastography is an imaging method that presents qualitative tissue stiffness information on the anatomic display and, in some cases, presents quantitative stiffness information.

Cardiac Strain Imaging

In elastography, the hardness (stiffness) of the tissue is imaged and/or quantitatively determined by producing a strain in the tissue by an external force or by radiation force. The heart is a four-chambered muscle that functions as a mechanical pump forcing blood circulation by contracting and relaxing. Therefore this is a case in which strain occurs in the contracting muscle (myocardium) because of its electrical stimulation rather than a strain that is a response to an external force (as discussed in the previous section). Strain and strain rate are indicators of the effectiveness of the myocardial function and

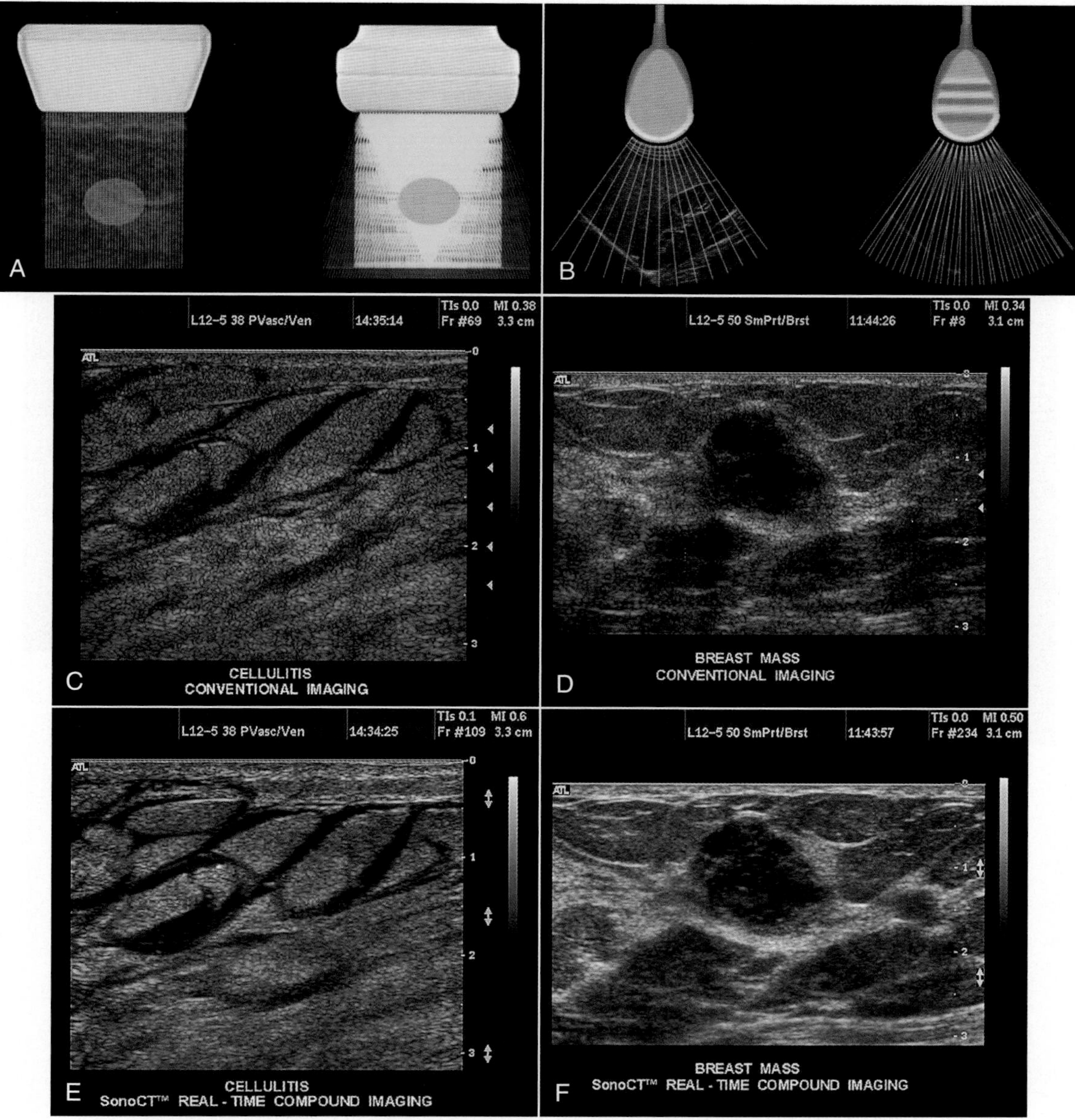

FIGURE 4-49 Conventional scan lines and spatial compounding with **(A)** linear array and **(B)** convex array. A comparison of conventional imaging **(C-D)** with compound imaging **(E-F)** shows improvement in image quality.

are useful diagnostic parameters. Strain and strain rate can be determined by 2D speckle-tracking techniques (which track the movement of specific portions of the myocardium) and from tissue-Doppler imaging techniques (discussed later). Examples of cardiac strain imaging are given in Figure 4-51.

> Cardiac strain imaging presents information regarding contraction and relaxation strain and strain rate information for the myocardium of the beating heart.

Output Devices

Sonographic instruments can export images and other information to external devices such as computer workstations (Figure 4-52). Figure 4-53 shows a diagram of the instrument with input and output devices. An internal hard disk in the instrument stores images and other information in digital form. Images also can be sent to a computer via a DVD drive (see Figure 4-52, *A*) or a USB connection (see Figure 4-52, *B*). Various standard protocols are used for communicating and storing digital images, for example, JPEG (joint photographic experts group), TIFF (tagged image file format), video clips (e.g., AVI [audio-video interweave]), and MPEG (moving picture experts group). Quality depends on the number of pixels per image and the amount of compression used (image compression is a process that reduces digital file size while retaining the data essential for acceptable image quality). Because sonographic images are not collections of random echo data,

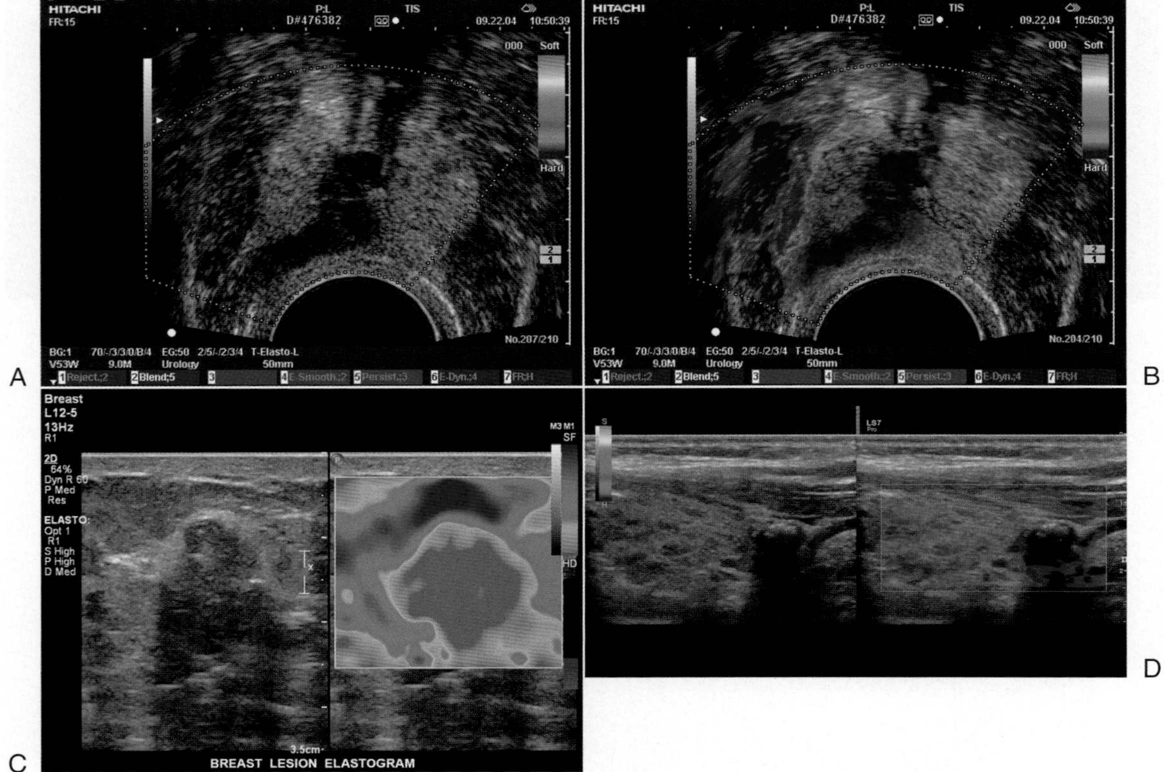

FIGURE 4-50 A, Large hypoechoic prostate tumor depicted in gray scale. **B,** The same tumor shown in elastography mode with red colors signifying soft tissues and blue colors signifying hard tissue. The designations "soft" and "hard" are relative to the maximum stiffness found in the image. Note the soft edges of the gland and the harder tumor. **C,** Gray-scale image of breast lesion *(left)* and elastogram of same lesion *(right)*. **D,** Gray-scale image of thyroid mass *(left)* and elastogram *(right)*. (C, Courtesy of Philips Healthcare; D Courtesy of GE Healthcare.)

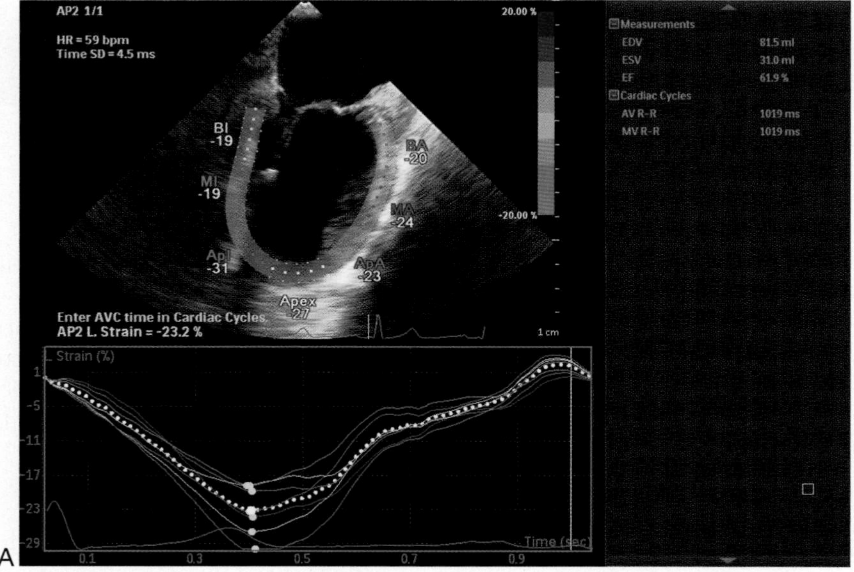

FIGURE 4-51 A-J. Cardiac strain examples. (I, Courtesy of GE Healthcare.)

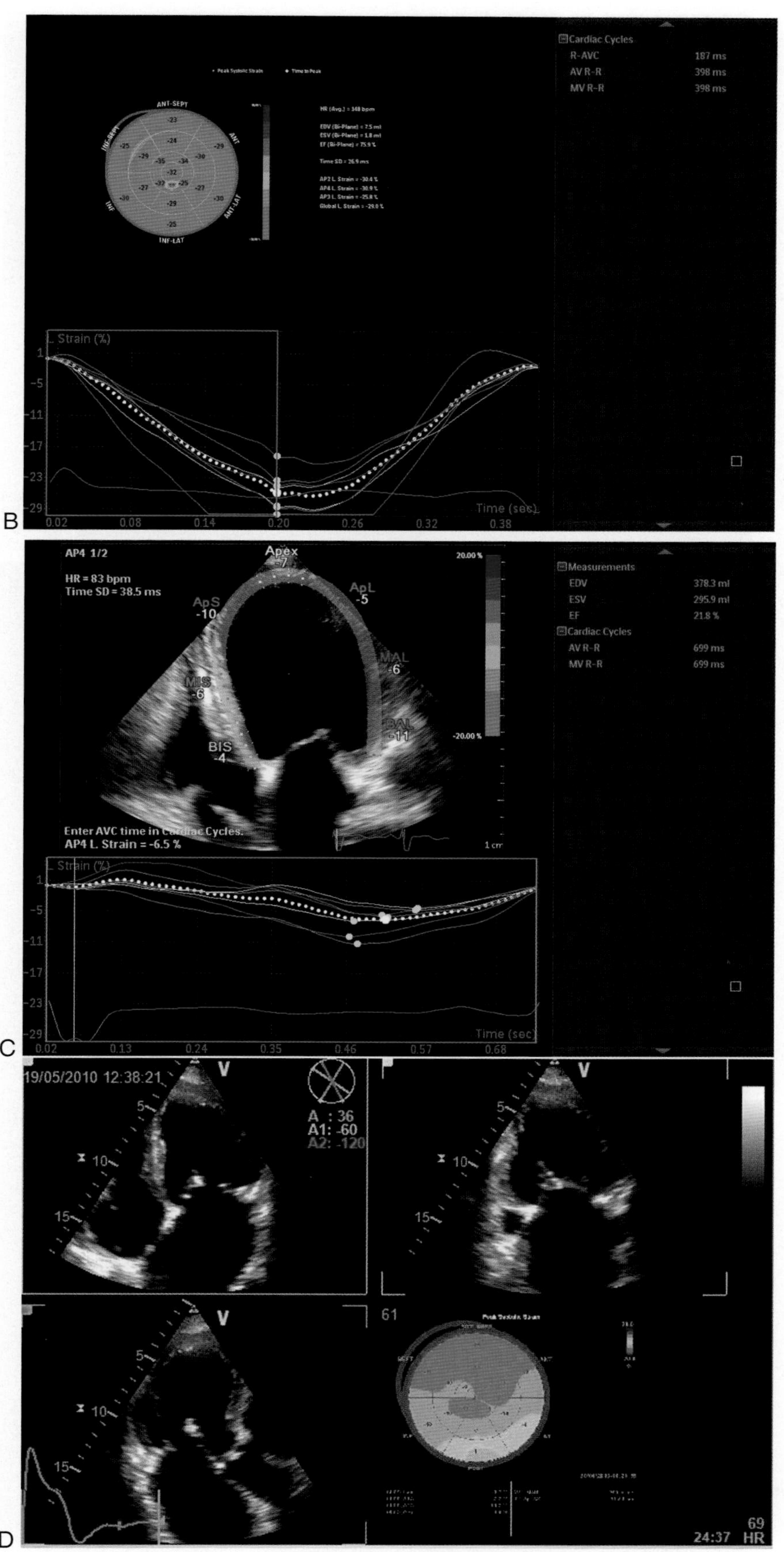

FIGURE 4-51, cont'd

Continued

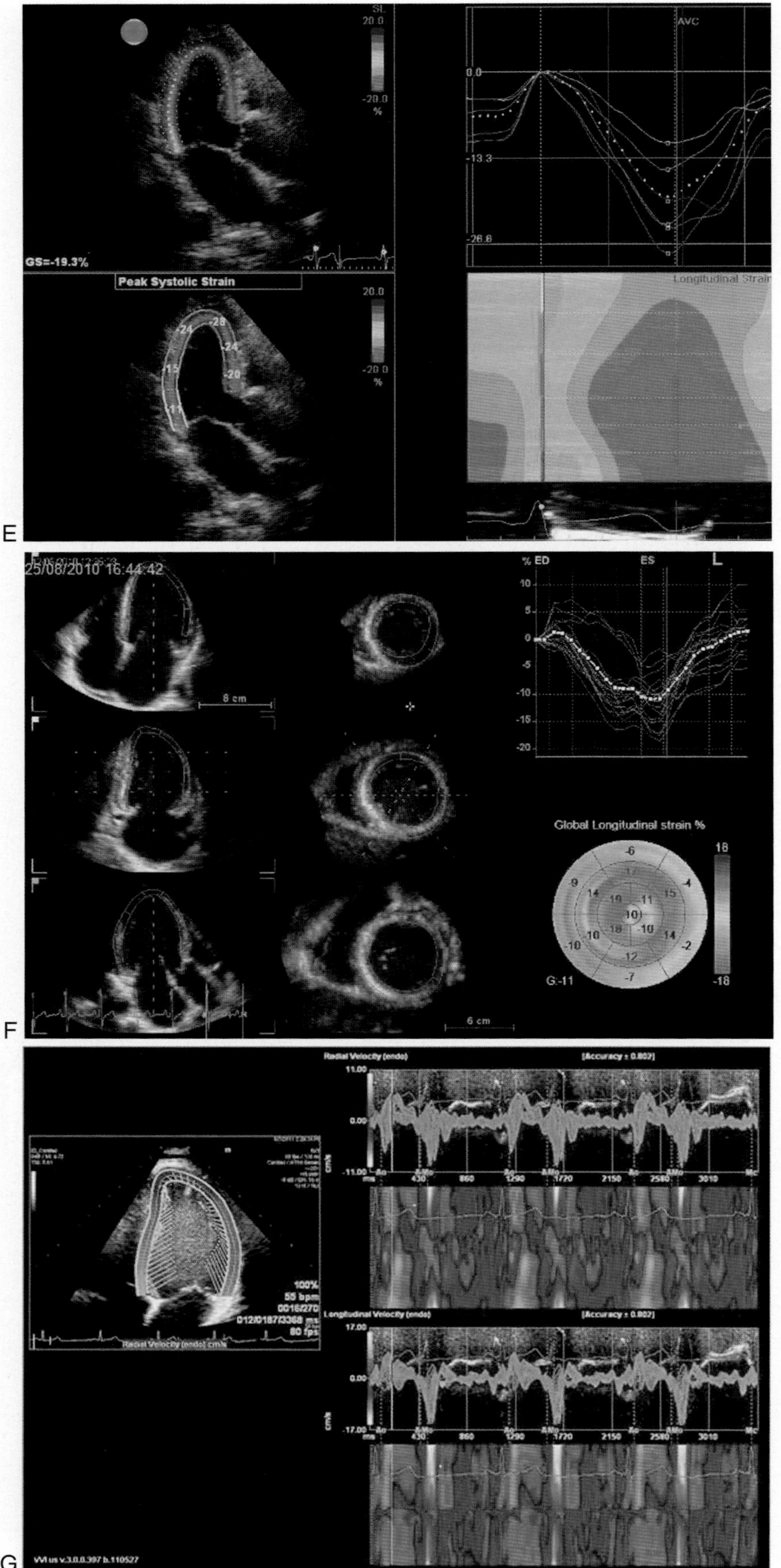

FIGURE 4-51, cont'd

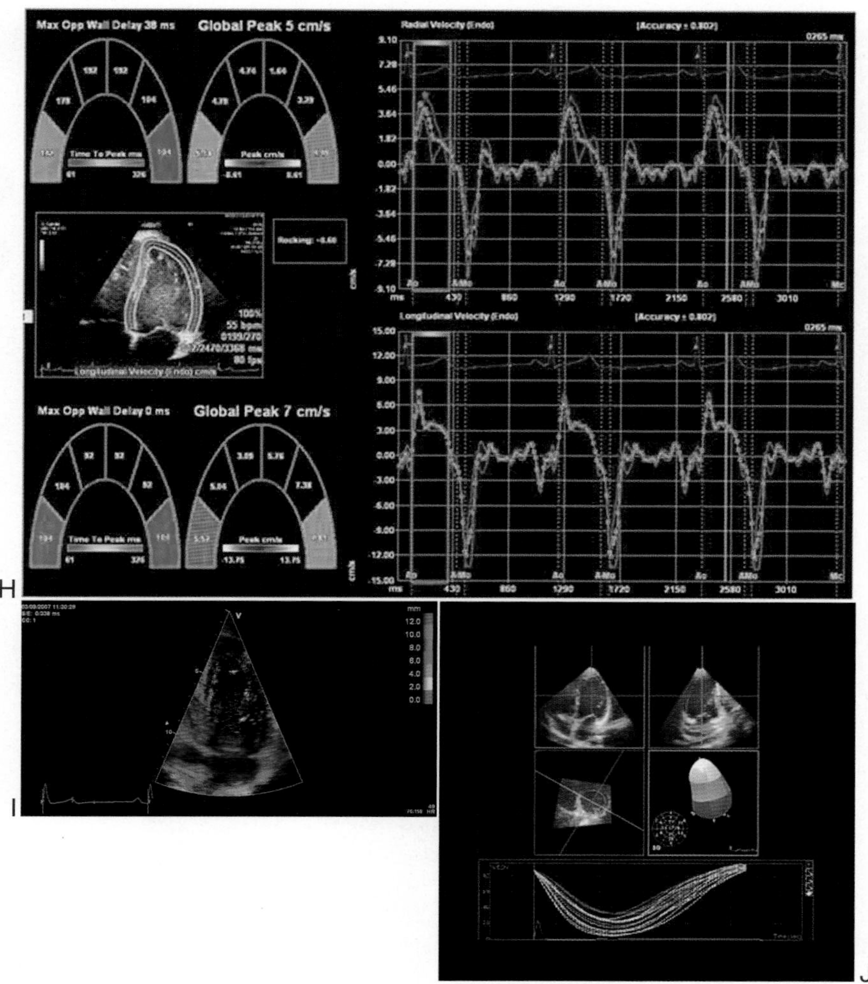

FIGURE 4-51, cont'd

their repeating patterns allow shortened coding, called *lossless compression,* to reduce file size. Lossless compression reduces file size to approximately one half its usual size without altering the image. *Lossy compression* involves visually similar, but not identical, images. The JPEG file is a compressed image file (file extension .jpg). File size is a trade-off with quality. The TIFF file (file extension .tif) has better quality than JPEG but has larger files. The same is true for MPEG (file extension .mpg) compared with AVI (file extension .avi). A single 8-bit (1 byte; 256 shade) uncompressed gray-scale image with 1024 × 768 pixels requires 768 kB of memory for the image data. Including the remaining data for proper handling of the image, the TIFF file size is 779 kB. A moderately compressed JPEG file size for the same image is 83 kB. A comparable color image would have a TIFF file size of 2.26 MB (three times the gray-scale file because data on three primary colors [red, green, blue] are stored rather than data on just one color [i.e., gray]). The compressed JPEG color file size is 95 kB. Communicating an uncompressed 256 gray-shade video clip of 30, 1024 × 768 pixel frames per second requires data transfer at 189 megabits per second (Mb/s) or 24 megabytes per second (MB/s). Compression, such as MPEG, reduces this requirement to a more manageable value.

Picture Archiving and Communications Systems

Picture archiving and communications systems (PACS) provide a means to electronically communicate images and associated information to workstations (see Figure 4-52, *C*) and devices external to the sonographic instrument, the examining room, and even the building in which the scanning is done. Indeed, through the Internet, these files can be transmitted to virtually anywhere in the world. PACS are used with all digital imaging modes, including ultrasound. The protocols for communicating images and associated information between imaging devices and workstations have been standardized in the Digital Imaging and Communications in Medicine (DICOM) standard.[4] This standard specifies a hardware interface, a minimum set of software commands, and a consistent set of data formats. This standard promotes communication of information, regardless of manufacturers of the linked devices, including the sonographic instrument, the PACS reading station, and other hospital/clinic information systems. The DICOM standard also enables the creation of diagnostic information bases that can be interrogated by a wide variety of devices geographically distributed.

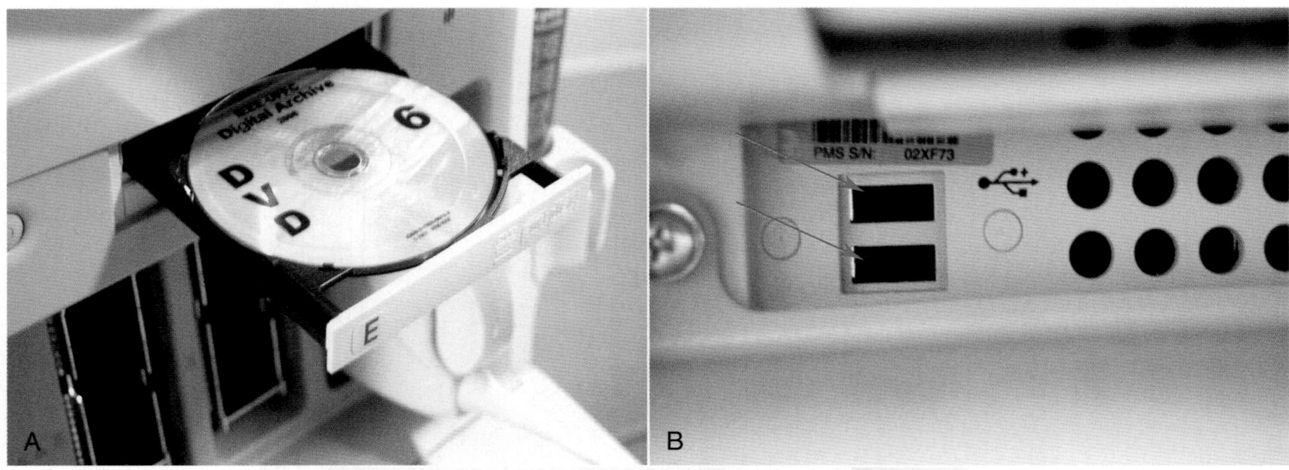

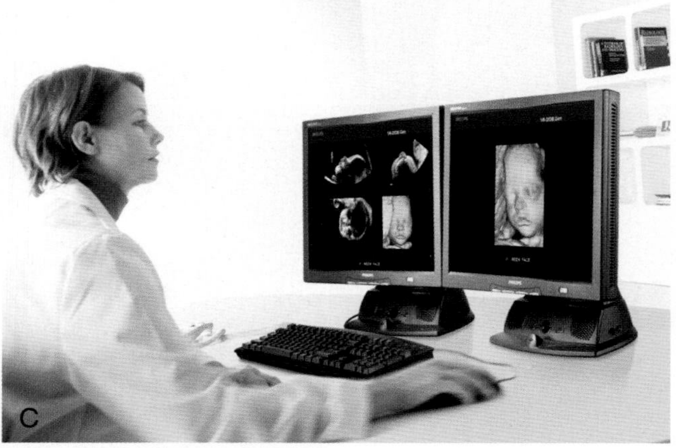

FIGURE 4-52 **A,** CD-DVD burner in a sonographic instrument. **B,** Universal serial bus (USB) ports *(arrows)* for connection to a flash memory device, other digital device, or a computer. **C,** Picture archiving and communications system workstation.

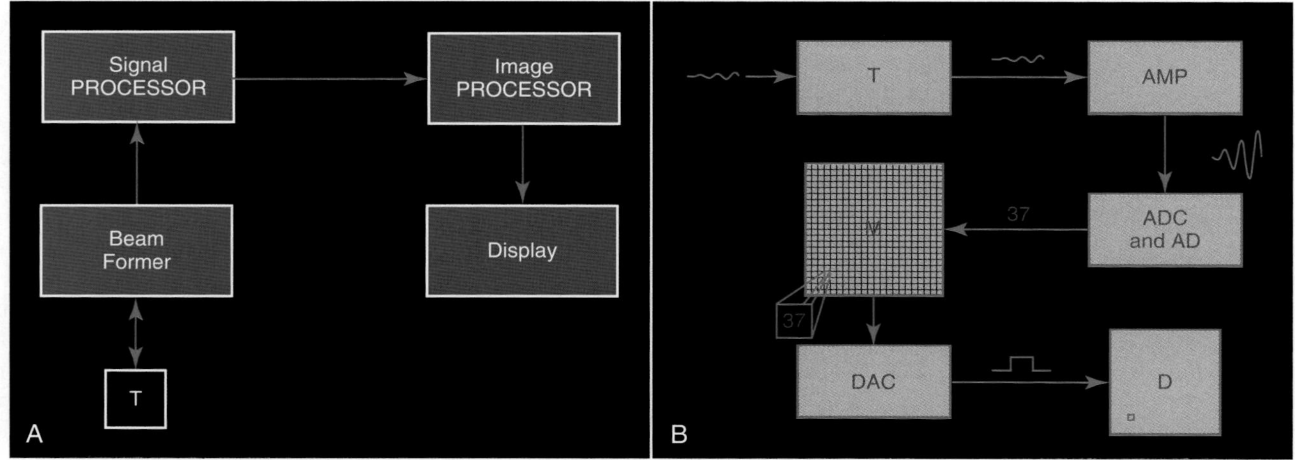

FIGURE 4-53 **A,** Major components of a sonographic instrument. **B,** The chain of events as an echo signal travels through the instrument. The transducer (T) converts the echo pressure variation to a voltage variation. The amplifier (AMP) increases the amplitude of the echo voltage. The analog-to-digital converter (ADC) converts the echo to a series of numbers, and the amplitude detector (AD) converts this series from radio frequency form to amplitude form. The echo amplitude is stored as a number in the image memory (M). The echo amplitude is retrieved from its pixel location in the memory. The digital-to-analog converter (DAC) converts the number to a corresponding voltage. The voltage determines the brightness of the echo presented on the display (D).

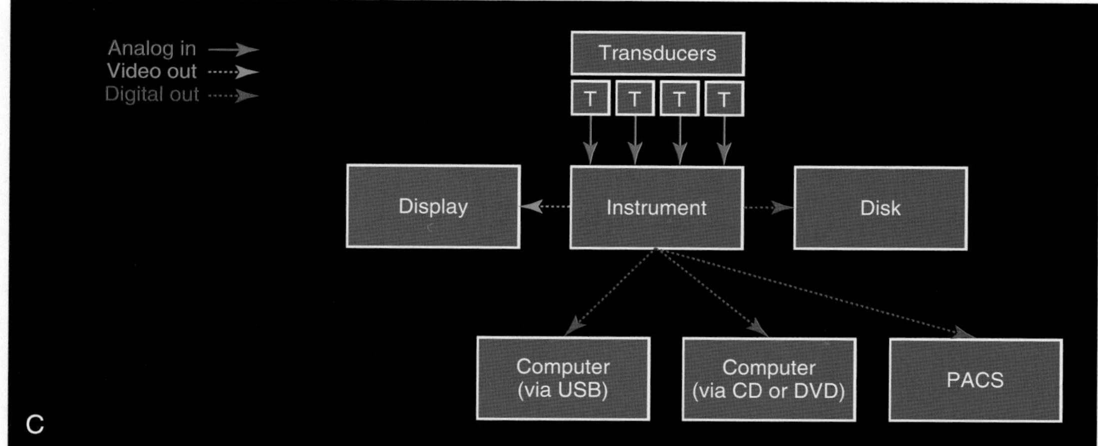

FIGURE 4-53, cont'd **C,** Echo information enters the instrument from the transducers in analog or digital form. Image information flows in digital form and then in video form to the internal display. Image information flows in digital form (numbers) to an internal disk and externally to a computer (via DVD or USB connection) and picture archiving and communications system (PACS) to be stored in digital format, just as it is in the image memory of the instrument. Such storage involves no loss of quality and allows postprocessing, measurements, and any other function that can be applied to a stored (frozen) image in the instrument memory.

REVIEW

The following key points are presented in this chapter:

- Sonographic instruments are of the pulse-echo type.
- These instruments use the strength, direction, and arrival time of received echoes to generate A, B, and M mode displays.
- Sonographic instruments include the beam former, signal processor, image processor, and display, and often these are attached to peripheral recording and display devices.
- The beam former is responsible for directing, focusing, and apodizing the ultrasound beam on transmission and reception. The beam former also amplifies the echo voltages, compensates for attenuation using time gain compensation, and digitizes the voltages.
- The signal processor filters, detects, and compresses the echo signal.
- The image processer converts the echo data in scan-line format to image format for storage and display.
- A mode presents depth-versus-echo amplitude display.
- B and M modes use a display of echo strength as brightness.
- M mode shows reflector motion in time. M mode is a presentation of echo depth versus time.
- B mode scans show anatomic cross-sections through the scanning plane.
- Image memories store echo intensity information as binary numbers in memory elements.
- Contrast resolution improves with increasing bits per pixel.
- Real-time imaging is the rapid sequential display of ultrasound images (frames), resulting in a moving presentation.
- Real-time imaging requires rapid, repeatable, sequential scanning of the sound beam through the tissue. This is accomplished with electronic transducer arrays.
- Increasing frame rate improves temporal resolution.
- Elastography is an imaging method that presents qualitative tissue stiffness information on the anatomic display and, in some cases, presents quantitative stiffness information.
- Cardiac strain imaging presents information regarding contraction and relaxation strain and strain rate information for the myocardium of the beating heart.

EXERCISES

Answers appear in the Answers to Exercises section at the back of the book.

1. The ultrasound PRF is equal to the voltage ____________ repetition frequency of the pulser.
   a. amplitude
   b. pulse
   c. period
   d. duration
2. Increased voltage amplitude produced by the pulser increases the ____________ and ____________ of ultrasound pulses produced by the transducer.
   a. amplitude, intensity
   b. amplitude, frequency
   c. frequency, period
   d. frequency, intensity

3. If a 6-MHz transducer images to a depth of 10 cm, to avoid range ambiguity, the maximum PRF permitted is ___________.
   a. 7.7 kHz
   b. 6.0 kHz
   c. 10.0 kHz
   d. 1.54 MHz
4. Functions performed by the signal processor include ___________, ___________, and ___________.
   a. amplification, digitizing, filtering
   b. amplification, filtering, digital-to-analog conversion
   c. amplification, filtering, compression
   d. filtering, detection, compression
5. Match the following functions with what they accomplish.
   a. Amplification
   b. Compression
   c. Filtering
   d. Detection
   e. Compression
      1. converts pulses from radio frequency to amplitude form.
      2. increases all amplitudes.
      3. decreases dynamic range.
      4. corrects for tissue attenuation.
      5. reduces noise.
6. If the input voltage to an amplifier is 1 mV and the output voltage is 10 mV, the voltage amplification ratio is ___________. The power ratio is ___________. The gain is ___________ dB.
   a. 10, 20, 30
   b. 10, 100, 100
   c. 10, 100, 20
   d. 10, 10, 10
7. An amplifier with a gain of 60 dB has 1 μW of power applied to the input. The output power is ___________ W.
   a. 60
   b. 1
   c. 10
   d. 1000
8. An amplifier with a gain of 60 dB has 10 μV of voltage applied to the input. The output voltage is ___________ mV.
   a. 10
   b. 100
   c. 1000
   d. 60
9. Time gain compensation is accomplished in the ___________.
   a. pulser
   b. beam former
   c. signal processor
   d. postprocessor
   e. image processor
10. Compensation takes into account reflector ___________.
    a. impedance
    b. size
    c. amplitude
    d. depth
11. Compensation amplifies echoes differently, according to their arrival ___________.
    a. times
    b. positions
    c. directions
    d. strengths
12. Compression decreases the ___________ range to a range that the ___________ and human ___________ can handle.
    a. frequency, instrument, intelligence
    b. dynamic, display, vision
    c. amplitude, display, hearing
    d. dynamic, pulser, vision
13. If a display has a dynamic range of 20 dB and the smallest voltage it can handle is 200 mV, then the largest voltage it can handle is ___________ V.
    a. 20
    b. 2.0
    c. 0.2
    d. 0.02
14. Detection converts voltage pulses from ___________ form to ___________ form.
    a. ultrasound, infrasound
    b. infrasound, ultrasound
    c. radio frequency, amplitude
    d. ultrasound, radio frequency
15. Filtering widens bandwidth. True or false?
16. Filtering is accomplished in the ___________.
    a. pulser
    b. beam former
    c. signal processor
    d. postprocessor
    e. image processor
17. The compression or dynamic range control reduces the range of echo amplitudes displayed by reducing the weakest to ___________ and/or the strongest ones to the ___________ value and assigning the others to increasing values. This produces a(n) ___________ contrast image with elimination of weakest and maximizing of strongest echoes.
    a. minimum, maximum, higher
    b. zero, 100, zero
    c. zero, maximum, higher
    d. 10, 100, optimum
18. An amplifier has a power output of 100 mW when the input power is 0.1 mW. The amplifier gain is ___________ dB.
    a. 10
    b. 20
    c. 30
    d. 40
19. If the beam-former output to the transducer is reduced by 3, 6, or 9 dB, the ultrasound pulse output intensity is reduced by ___________%, ___________%, or ___________%, respectively.
    a. 50, 75, 87.5
    b. 50, 25, 12.5
    c. 6, 12, 18
    d. 33, 66, 99

20. One watt is ___________ dB below 100 W.
   a. 1
   b. 2
   c. 10
   d. 20
21. One watt is ___________ dB above 100 mW.
   a. 1
   b. 2
   c. 10
   d. 20
22. If the input power is 1 mW and the output is 10,000 mW, the gain is ___________ dB.
   a. 10
   b. 20
   c. 30
   d. 40
23. If an amplifier has a gain of 15 dB, the ratio of output power to input power is ___________. (Refer to Table 4-1.)
   a. 15
   b. 22
   c. 30
   d. 32
24. If the output of a 22-dB gain amplifier is connected to the input of a 23-dB gain amplifier, the total gain is ___________ dB. The overall power ratio is ___________. (Refer to Table 4-1.)
   a. 22, 45
   b. 45, 23
   c. 45, 32,000
   d. 32,000, 45,000
25. If a 17-dB electric attenuator is connected to a 15-dB amplifier, the net gain is ___________ dB. The net attenuation is ___________ dB. For a 1-W input, the output is ___________ W. (Refer to Table 2-3.)
   a. 2, 2, 2
   b. 2, -2, -2
   c. -2, 2, 6.3
   d. -2, 2, 0.63
26. For the digital memory shown in Figure 4-54, enter the number stored in each pixel location.
   a. Lower right: ___________
   b. Middle right: ___________
   c. Upper right: ___________
   d. Upper middle: ___________
   e. Upper left: ___________
27. The contrast resolution for an instrument that has an echo dynamic range of 43 dB and 32 shades is ___________ dB per shade.
   a. 1.3
   b. 3.2
   c. 4.3
   d. 32
   e. 43
28. The contrast resolution for an instrument that has a 6-bit memory and a 45-dB echo dynamic range is ___________ dB per shade.
   a. 0.3
   b. 0.5
   c. 0.7
   d. 0.9
   e. 6
29. Match the following:
   a. Analog:
   b. Digital:
   c. Preprocessing:
   d. Postprocessing:
   e. Pixel:
   f. Bit:
      1. Picture element
      2. Assignment of stored numbers
      3. Discrete
      4. Binary digit
      5. Proportional
      6. Assignment of displayed brightness
30. Typical image pixel dimensions are ___________.
   a. 640 × 128
   b. 16 × 64
   c. 100 × 100
   d. 512 × 1540
   e. 512 × 384
31. How many bits per pixel are required for each number of shades?
   a. 16: ___________
   b. 32: ___________
   c. 64: ___________
   d. 128: ___________
   e. 256: ___________
32. ___________ total memory elements are required for a 100 × 100-pixel, 5-bit digital memory.
   a. 500
   b. 1000
   c. 5000
   d. 10,000
   e. 50,000

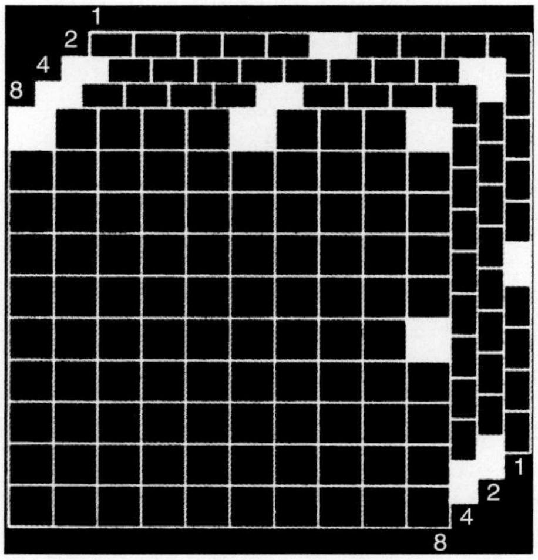

FIGURE 4-54 **Digital memory description.** Illustration to accompany Exercise 26. The white color indicates that the memory device is on.

33. Memories of __________ bits per pixel are common in ultrasound today.
a. 4 to 8
b. 4 to 6
c. 6 to 8
d. 5 to 7
e. 4 to 5

34. Digital memories store __________.
a. logarithms
b. electric magnetism
c. electric current
d. electric charge
e. numbers

35. __________ is commonly controllable by the operator.
a. Postprocessing
b. Pixel matrix
c. Bits per pixel
d. Digitization
e. All of the above

36. In binary numbers, how many symbols are used?
a. 0
b. 1
c. 2
d. 4

37. The term *binary digit* is commonly shortened into the single word __________.
a. bigit
b. binit
c. bidig
d. bit

38. Each binary digit in a binary number is represented in the memory by a memory element, which, at any time, is in one of __________ states that are __________ or __________.
a. 2, on, off
b. many, odd, even
c. 4, high, low
d. 10, odd, even

39. Match the following (See Figure 4-32, *E*)
Column in an 8-bit binary number hgfedcba:
Decimal number represented by a 1 in the column:

a. __________	**1.** 64
b. __________	**2.** 32
c. __________	**3.** 1
d. __________	**4.** 16
e. __________	**5.** 8
f. __________	**6.** 128
g. __________	**7.** 2
h. __________	**8.** 4

40. The binary number 10110 represents zero 1, one 2, one 4, zero 8, and one 16; that is, the decimal number 0 + 2 + 4 + 0 + 16 = 22. What decimal number does the binary number 11001 represent?
a. 15
b. 20
c. 25
d. 35

41. The decimal number 13 is made up of one 1, zero 2, one 4, and one 8 (8 + 4 + 0 + 1 = 13). The number therefore is represented by the binary number __________.
a. 1011
b. 1101
c. 1110
d. 0111

42. Match the following:

Decimal Number	Binary Number
a. 1 __________	**1.** 0001111
b. 5 __________	**2.** 0011001
c. 10 __________	**3.** 0001010
d. 15 __________	**4.** 0110010
e. 20 __________	**5.** 0000001
f. 25 __________	**6.** 1100100
g. 30 __________	**7.** 0101000
h. 40 __________	**8.** 0011110
i. 50 __________	**9.** 0010100
j. 100 __________	**10.** 0000101

43. How many binary digits are required in the binary numbers representing the following decimal numbers?
a. 0 __________
b. 1 __________
c. 5 __________
d. 10 __________
e. 25 __________
f. 30 __________
g. 63 __________
h. 64 __________
i. 75 __________
j. 100 __________

44. How many bits are required to represent each decimal number in binary form?
a. 7 __________
b. 15 __________
c. 3 __________
d. 511 __________
e. 1023 __________
f. 63 __________
g. 255 __________
h. 1 __________
i. 127 __________
j. 31 __________

45. How many bits are required to store numbers representing each number of different gray shades?
a. 2 __________
b. 4 __________
c. 8 __________
d. 15 __________
e. 16 __________
f. 25 __________
g. 32 __________
h. 64 __________
i. 65 __________
j. 128 __________

46. The primary formats of image presentation are called ___________ *mode,* ___________ *mode,* and ___________ *mode.* They are used in ___________, ___________, and ___________ types of clinical imaging, respectively.
   a. B (brightness), M (motion), A (amplitude), all, cardiac, ophthalmic
   b. A (amplitude), B (brightness), M (motion), all, cardiac, ophthalmic
   c. B (brightness), M (motion), A (amplitude), cardiac, all, ophthalmic
   d. B (brightness), M (motion), A (amplitude), ophthalmic, all, cardiac
47. ___________ mode is used for studying the motion of a structure such as a heart valve.
   a. A
   b. B
   c. M
   d. all of the above
48. A B scan presents a cross-section through the ___________ plane.
   a. longitudinal
   b. transverse
   c. elevational
   d. scan
49. A display that shows various echo strengths as different brightnesses is called a ___________-___________ or ___________ ___________ *display.*
   a. gray-scale, B mode
   b. cross-sectional, anatomic mode
   c. sono-scan, sectional mode
   d. gray-mode, square pixel
50. The ___________ ___________ stores the gray-scale image and allows it to be displayed on a computer monitor.
   a. signal processor
   b. preprocessor
   c. postprocessor
   d. image memory
51. Match the following:
   a. Linear array ___________ 1. Rectangular
   b. Convex array ___________ 2. Sector
   c. Phased array ___________
   d. Vector array ___________
52. If the PRF of an instrument is 1 kHz and it displays (single focus) 25 frames per second, there are ___________ lines per frame.
   a. 20
   b. 40
   c. 60
   d. 100
53. The PRF is ___________ Hz if 30 frames (40 lines each) are displayed per second (single focus).
   a. 600
   b. 1200
   c. 30
   d. 40
54. Imaging involving 10-cm penetration, a single focus, 100 scan lines per frame, and 30 frames per second can be accomplished without range ambiguity. True or false?
55. The maximum frame rate permitted for 15-cm penetration, three foci, and 200 scan lines per frame is ___________.
   a. 3.0
   b. 5.5
   c. 8.5
   d. 15
   e. 30
56. The primary components of a diagnostic ultrasound imaging system are the ___________, ___________ ___________, ___________ ___________, ___________ ___________, and ___________.
   a. transducer, beam former, signal processor, image processor, display
   b. transducer, image former, echo processor, scan convertor, output
   c. pulser, pulser delay, T/R switch, echo delays, summer
   d. amplifier, digital convertor, analog convertor, scan convertor, display
57. The information that can be obtained from an M mode display includes ___________.
   a. distance and motion pattern
   b. transducer frequency, reflection coefficient, and distance
   c. acoustic impedances, attenuation, and motion pattern
   d. none of the above
58. The time gain compensation control compensates for ___________.
   a. machine instability in the warm-up time
   b. attenuation
   c. transducer aging
   d. the ambient light in the examining area
   e. patient examination time
59. A gray-scale display shows ___________.
   a. gray color on a white background
   b. echoes with one brightness level
   c. white color on a gray background
   d. a range of echo amplitudes
60. The dynamic range of an ultrasound system is ___________.
   a. the speed with which ultrasound examination can be performed
   b. the range over which the transducer can be manipulated while an examination is performed
   c. the ratio of the maximum amplitude to the minimum echo strength that can be displayed
   d. the range of voltages applied to the transducer
61. A ___________ ___________ formats scan line data to image form.
   a. beam former
   b. scan convertor
   c. signal processor
   d. image formatter

62. Which of the following is *not* performed by a signal processor?
   a. Detection
   b. Filtering
   c. Digital-to-analog conversion
   d. Radio frequency–to–amplitude conversion
   e. Compression
63. In a digital memory, echo intensity is represented by ____________.
   a. positive charge distribution
   b. a number stored in the memory
   c. electron density of the display writing beam
   d. a and c
   e. all of the above
64. If there were no attenuation in tissue, ____________ would not be needed.
   a. filtering
   b. compression
   c. detection
   d. time gain compensation
65. Echo imaging includes ultrasound generation, propagation and reflection in tissues, and reception of returning ____________.
   a. echoes
   b. impedances
   c. propagations
   d. transmissions
66. The diagnostic ultrasound systems in common clinical use today are of the ____________-____________ type.
   a. transmit-receive
   b. pulse-echo
   c. through-transmission
   d. A-mode
67. Gray-scale instruments show echo amplitude as ____________ on the display.
   a. numbers
   b. color
   c. spikes
   d. brightness
68. Pulse-echo instruments look for three things: the ____________, ____________, and arrival ____________ of echoes returning from tissues.
   a. amplitude, frequency, location
   b. strength, direction, time
   c. focus, delay, direction
   d. frequency, duration, delay
69. An image memory stores image information in the form of ____________ numbers.
   a. electric charge
   b. binary
   c. decimal
   d. impedance
   e. none of the above
70. Imaging systems produce a visual ____________ from the electric ____________ received from the transducer.
   a. display, voltages
   b. map, numbers
   c. presentation, amplifiers
   d. display, numbers
71. The transducer is connected to the signal processor through the ____________ ____________.
   a. pulser delay
   b. image processor
   c. scan convertor
   d. beam former
72. The transducer receives voltages from the ____________ ____________ in pulse-echo systems.
   a. pulser delay
   b. image processor
   c. scan convertor
   d. beam former
73. The ____________ ____________ receives digitized echo voltages from the beam former.
   a. signal processor
   b. image processor
   c. scan convertor
   d. beam former
74. Increasing gain generally produces the same effect as ____________ ____________.
   a. decreasing attenuation
   b. increasing attenuation
   c. increasing compression
   d. increasing rectification
   e. b and c
75. The ADC is part of the ____________.
   a. beam former
   b. signal processor
   c. image processor
   d. display
   e. a and b
   f. c and e
76. Voltage pulses from the pulser are applied through delays to the ____________.
   a. digitizer
   b. transducer
   c. ADCs
   d. preprocessor
77. Detection is a function of the ____________.
   a. beam former
   b. signal processor
   c. image processor
   d. display
   e. a and b
78. If gain is reduced by one half, with input power unchanged, the output power is ____________ what it was before.
   a. equal to
   b. twice
   c. one half
   d. none of the above
79. If gain is 30 dB and output power is reduced by one half, the new gain is ____________ dB.
   a. 15
   b. 60

c. 33
d. 27
e. none of the above

80. If four shades of gray are shown on a display, each twice the brightness of the preceding one, the brightest shade is ____________ times the brightness of the dimmest shade.
a. 2
b. 4
c. 8
d. 16
e. 32

81. The dynamic range displayed in Exercise 80 is ____________ dB.
a. 10
b. 9
c. 5
d. 2
e. 0

82. In which units are gain and attenuation usually expressed?
a. dB
b. dB/cm
c. cm
d. cm/3 dB
e. None of the above

83. Time gain compensation makes up for the fact that reflections from deeper reflectors arrive at the transducer with greater amplitude. True or false?

84. The modes that show one-dimensional (depth) real-time images are ____________ and ____________ modes.
a. A, B
b. A, C
c. B, M
d. A, M

85. The mode that shows two-dimensional real-time images is the ____________ mode.
a. A
b. B
c. C
d. M

86. A real-time B mode display may be produced by rapid ____________ scanning of a transducer array.
a. electronic
b. manual
c. visual
d. reverse

87. Each complete scan of the sound beam produces an image on the display that is called a ____________.
a. picture
b. frame
c. window
d. movie

88. For a single focus, the number of lines in each frame is equal to the number of times the transducer is ____________ while the frame is produced; that is, while the sound beam is scanned.
a. quiet
b. focused
c. pulsed
d. delayed

89. In real-time scanning, the required PRF depends on the number of ____________ per frame and ____________ rate.
a. lines, frame
b. scans, scan
c. echoes, pulsing
d. focuses, propagation

90. Increasing the number of foci reduces ____________ ____________.
a. detail resolution
b. contrast resolution
c. pulse repetition
d. frame rate

91. To correct for attenuation, time gain compensation must ____________ the gain for increasing depth.
a. increase
b. decrease
c. correct
d. decelerate

92. If a higher frequency is used, resolution is ____________, imaging depth ____________, and the time gain compensation slope must be ____________.
a. improved, decreases, increased
b. degraded, increases, decreased
c. unchanged, increases, eliminated
d. improved, increased, increased

93. For pixel dimensions 256 × 512 and 512 × 512, calculate the number of image pixels.
a. 131,072, 262,144
b. 262,144, 524,288
c. 131,072, 524,288
d. 524,288, 262,144

94. Which type of array gives a wide view close to the transducer? ____________ Which of the following produce(s) a sector format image? ____________
a. Vector
b. Linear
c. Phased
d. Convex
e. More than one of the above

95. In elastography, the display presents qualitative or quantitative information on
a. stress
b. stiffness
c. strain rate
d. stress rate

96. In Figure 4-55, if two foci were used, the frame rate would be ____________.
a. 33
b. 22
c. 11
d. 6
e. 1

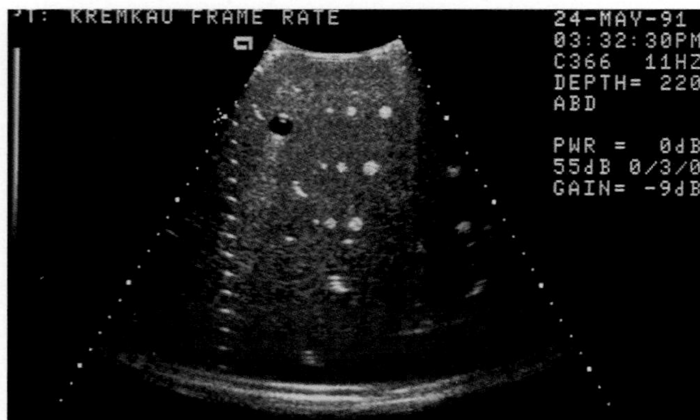

FIGURE 4-55 Illustration to accompany Exercise 96.

97. What is adjusted improperly in Figure 4-56?
    a. Gain
    b. Time gain compensation
    c. Compression
    d. Frame rate
    e. Rejection

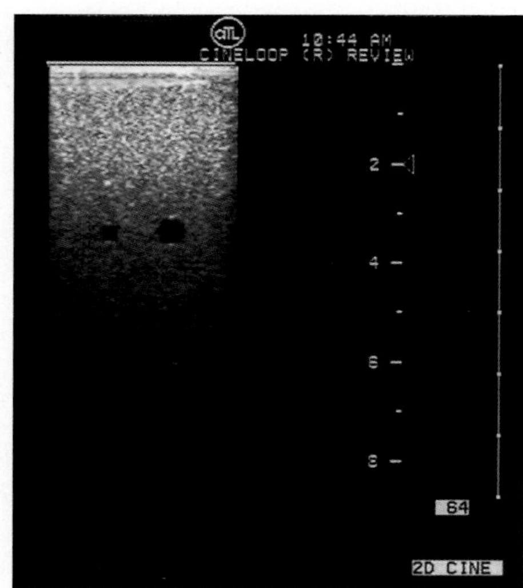

FIGURE 4-56 Illustration to accompany Exercise 97.

98. The *decreasing* gain of the time gain compensation curve (*arrows*) in Figure 4-57 is caused by ___________.
    a. weak attenuation
    b. refraction
    c. strong attenuation
    d. beam broadening
    e. beam narrowing

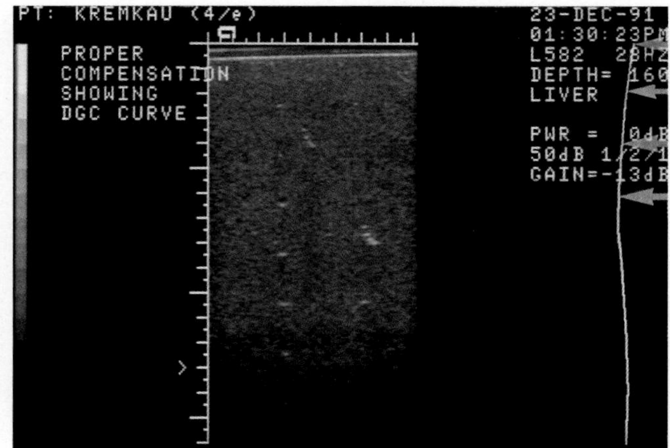

FIGURE 4-57 Illustration to accompany Exercise 98.

99. In the linear amplifier of Figure 4-58, the gain is ___________ dB.
    a. 1000
    b. 300
    c. 100
    d. 60
    e. 10

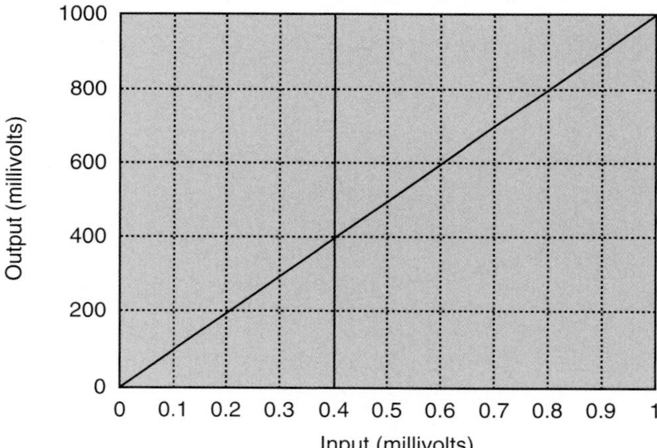

FIGURE 4-58 Illustration to accompany Exercise 99.

100. Compression is a function of the ___________.
    a. beam former
    b. signal processor
    c. image processor
    d. postprocessor

5

Doppler Principles

LEARNING OBJECTIVES

After reading this chapter, the student should be able to do the following:

- List and compare the various kinds of flow encountered in blood circulation.
- Explain how a stenosis affects flow.
- Define and discuss the Doppler effect, the Doppler shift, and the Doppler angle.
- Explain how two-dimensional flow information is color encoded on a sonographic display.
- Compare Doppler-shift with Doppler-power displays.
- Explain how flow detection is localized to a specific site in tissue by using pulsed Doppler techniques.
- Describe spectral analysis.
- Discuss examples of how spectral analysis is applied to evaluate flow conditions at the site of measurement and elsewhere.

OUTLINE

KEY TERMS

Autocorrelation
Baseline shift
Bernoulli effect
Bidirectional
Clutter
Color-Doppler display
Compliance
Continuous-wave Doppler
Cosine
Disturbed flow
Doppler angle
Doppler effect
Doppler equation
Doppler-power display
Doppler shift
Doppler spectrum
Duplex instrument
Eddies
Ensemble length
Fast Fourier transform
Filter
Flow
Fluid
Frequency spectrum
Gate
Hue
Inertia
Laminar flow
Luminance
Parabolic flow
Phase quadrature
Plug flow
Poise
Poiseuille equation
Priority
Pulsatile flow
Pulsed Doppler
Range gating
Resistance
Sample volume
Saturation
Spectral analysis
Spectral broadening
Spectral-Doppler display
Spectrum analyzer

KEY TERMS—cont'd

Stenosis
Streamlines
Turbulence
Variance
Viscosity
Volumetric flow rate
Wall filter
Window

In addition to anatomic imaging, ultrasound provides a means for detecting and presenting motion information. Motions of interest diagnostically include (cardiac) motion of the beating mechanical heart and the motion of the resulting blood **flow** in circulation. Motion is detected by using the **Doppler effect** with ultrasound. In this chapter we first consider characteristics of blood flow in the human circulatory system, the flow that will be detected, quantified, and evaluated with Doppler ultrasound. Next, we discuss details of the Doppler effect and how the motion information is presented in audible and visual forms called *color Doppler* and *spectral Doppler*.

FLOW

The circulatory system consists of the heart, arteries, arterioles, capillaries, venules, and veins, altogether containing approximately 5 L of blood. The heart is the pump that produces blood flow through the circulatory system. It is a contracting and relaxing muscle (the myocardium) with four chambers: two atria and two ventricles. Blood flows from the superior and inferior vena cava and pulmonary veins into the right and left atria, respectively, and from there into the ventricles. From the left and right ventricles, blood flows into the aorta and pulmonary artery, respectively. When the heart contracts, the intended result is forward flow into the aorta and pulmonary artery. Valves are present in the heart to permit forward flow and prevent reverse flow. Malfunctioning valves can restrict forward flow by not opening sufficiently (**stenosis**) or allow reverse flow by not closing completely (insufficiency or regurgitation). Doppler ultrasound is useful to detect both of these conditions.

Flow in the heart, arteries, and veins can be detected with Doppler ultrasound. The capillaries are the tiniest vessels, measuring a few micrometers in diameter. The human body has approximately one billion capillaries. Across the capillary walls, the exchange of gases, nutrients, and waste products within the cells takes place, sustaining their life. This is the role of the circulatory system.

Fluid

Matter generally is classified into three categories: gas, liquid, and solid. Gases and liquids are **fluids**; that is, they are substances that flow and conform to the shape of their containers. To flow is to move in a stream, continually changing position and, possibly, direction. Rivers flow downstream. Water flows through a garden hose. Air flows through a fan. Blood flows through the heart, arteries, capillaries, and veins.

 Gases and liquids are fluids, materials that flow.

Viscosity is the **resistance** to flow offered by a fluid in motion. Viscosity is given in units of **poise** or kilogram per meter-second (kg/m-s). One poise is 1 g/cm-s or 0.1 kg/m-s. Water has a relatively low viscosity compared with molasses, for example, which has a high viscosity. The viscosity of blood plasma is approximately 50% greater than that of water. The viscosity of normal blood is 0.035 poise at 37° C, approximately five times that of water. Blood viscosity (poise) can vary from approximately 0.02 (with anemia) to approximately 0.10 (with polycythemia). Blood viscosity also varies with flow speed.

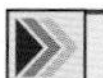 Viscosity is the resistance of a fluid to flow.

Pressure, Resistance, and Volumetric Flow Rate

Pressure is the driving force behind fluid flow. Pressure is force per unit area. Pressure is equally distributed throughout a static fluid and exerts its force in all directions (Figure 5-1). A pressure difference is required for flow to occur. Equal pressure applied at both ends of a liquid-filled tube will result in no flow. If the pressure is greater at one end than at the other, the liquid will flow from the higher-pressure end to the lower-pressure end. This pressure difference can be generated by a pump (e.g., the heart in the circulatory system) or by the force of gravity (e.g., by raising one end of a tube higher than the other). (Because this is the situation in the lower-extremity veins in a standing person, these vessels have valves to prevent reverse flow.) The greater the pressure difference, the greater the flow rate. This pressure difference is sometimes called the *pressure gradient,* although, strictly defined, pressure gradient is the pressure difference *divided by the distance between the two pressure locations.* The term *gradient* comes from the Latin *gradus* and refers to the upward or downward sloping of something. While the pressure decreases from one end of the tube to the other, this decrease can be thought of as a slope (i.e., the pressure difference divided by the distance over which the pressure drop occurs; Figure 5-2). A constant driving pressure produces a steady (unchanged with time) flow. The driving pressure produced by the heart varies with time. This concept is considered later in this section.

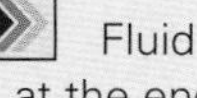 Fluid flows in a tube in response to a pressure difference at the ends.

Volumetric flow rate (Q) (sometimes simply called *flow,* although that term has other uses) refers to the volume of blood passing a point per unit of time. Volumetric flow rate is usually expressed in milliliters per minute or per second.

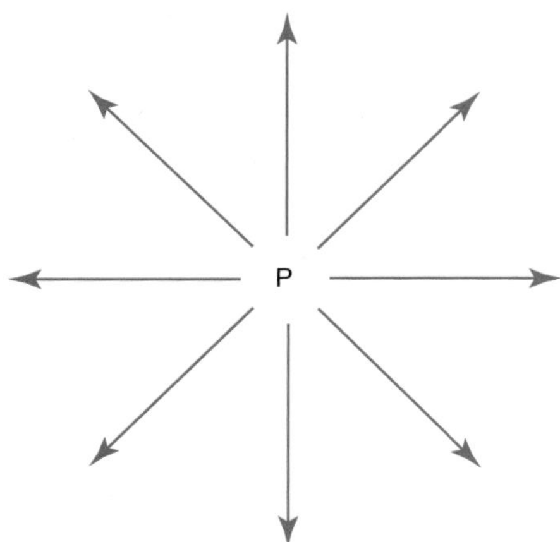

FIGURE 5-1 Pressure *(P)* is distributed uniformly throughout a static fluid and exerts its force in all directions.

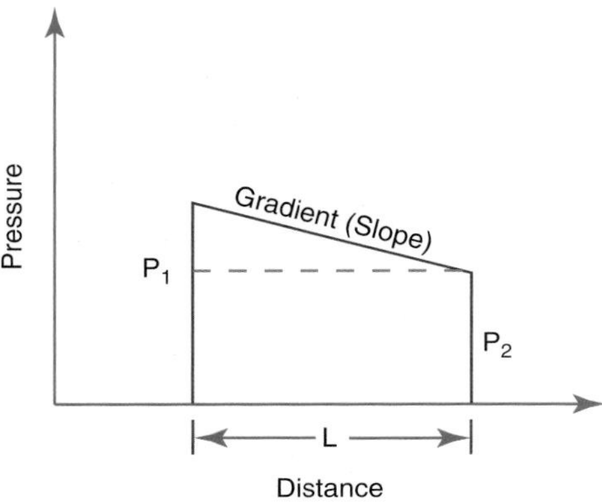

FIGURE 5-2 The pressure gradient or slope is the pressure difference *(P_1 – P_2)* divided by the separation *(L)* between the two pressure locations.

The total adult blood flow rate (cardiac output) is approximately 5000 mL/min (i.e., the total blood volume circulates in approximately 1 minute). The volumetric flow rate in a long straight tube is determined not only by the pressure difference *(ΔP)* but also by the resistance *(R)* to flow.

$$Q(\text{mL/s}) = \frac{\Delta P(\text{dyne/cm}^2)}{R(\text{poise})}$$

If pressure difference increases, volumetric flow rate increases.

If flow resistance increases, volumetric flow rate decreases.

The flow resistance in a long, straight tube depends on the fluid viscosity (η) and the tube length (L) and radius (r), as follows:

$$R(\text{g/cm}^4\text{-s}) = 8 \times L(\text{cm}) \times \frac{\eta(\text{poise})}{\pi \times [r^4(\text{cm}^4)]}$$

 If tube length increases, flow resistance increases.

 If tube radius increases, flow resistance decreases.

 If viscosity increases, flow resistance increases.

As expected, an increase in viscosity or tube length increases resistance, whereas an increase in the radius or diameter of the tube decreases resistance. The latter effect is particularly strong, with resistance depending on radius to the fourth power (r^4). Thus doubling the radius of a tube decreases its resistance to one sixteenth its original value. From experience, we know that a longer- or smaller-diameter garden hose reduces water flow rate. We can presume that if we tried to force molasses through a hose, we would not get nearly the flow rate that we would with water.

Poiseuille Equation

Use of the flow resistance equation in the flow rate equation and tube diameter (d) instead of radius yields the **Poiseuille equation** for volumetric flow rate:

$$Q(\text{mL/s}) = \frac{\Delta P(\text{dyne/cm}^2) \times \pi \times d^4(\text{cm}^4)}{128 \times L(\text{cm}) \times \eta(\text{poise})}$$

Recall that this equation is for steady flow in long, straight tubes. Thus the equation serves only as a rough approximation of the conditions in blood circulation. The equation is useful, however, in making qualitative conclusions and predictions.

 If pressure difference increases, flow rate increases.

 If diameter increases, flow rate increases.

 If length increases, flow rate decreases.

 If viscosity increases, flow rate decreases.

The resistance of the arterioles accounts for approximately half of the total resistance in systemic circulation. The muscular walls of arterioles can constrict or relax, producing dramatic changes in flow resistance. The walls thus can control blood flow to specific tissues and organs in response to their needs.

The volumetric flow rate in a tube depends on the pressure difference, the length and diameter of the tube, and the viscosity of the fluid.

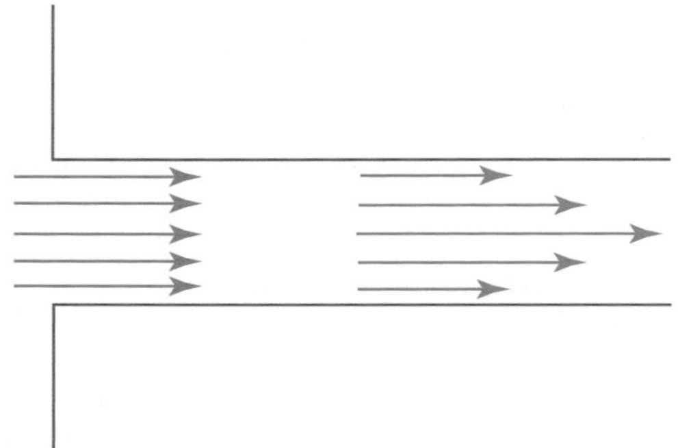

FIGURE 5-3 At the entrance to a tube or vessel, plug flow exists. After some distance, laminar flow is achieved.

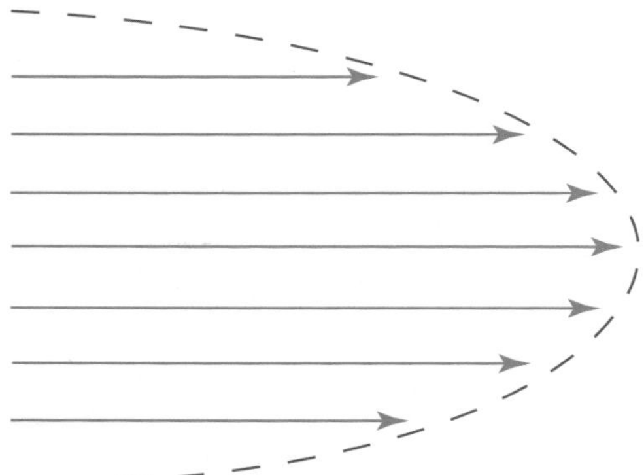

FIGURE 5-4 Parabolic flow profile. The *dashed line* is a parabola.

Types of Flow

Flow can be divided into five spatial categories: (1) plug, (2) laminar, (3) parabolic, (4) disturbed, and (5) turbulent. At the entrance to a tube, the speed of the fluid is essentially constant across the tube (Figure 5-3). This is called **plug flow** because it is similar to the motion of a solid object (a plug, for example) that does not flow but moves as a unit. Plug flow is a form of **laminar flow**. Laminar flow (from the Latin term for "layer") is a flow condition in which **streamlines** (which describe the motion paths of fluid particles) are straight and parallel. While the fluid flows down the tube, **parabolic flow** develops (Figure 5-4). Flow speed is maximum at the center of the tube and minimum or zero at the tube walls. A decreasing profile of flow speeds from the center to the wall is present. Successive layers of fluid slide over each other with relative motion. The pressure difference at each end of the tube overcomes the viscous resistance of the layers sliding over each other, maintaining the laminar flow through the tube. Steady flow in a long, straight tube results in a parabolic flow profile. Parabolic flow is a particular pattern of laminar flow in which varying flow speeds across the tube are described by a parabola (see the curved dashed line in Figure 5-4). In the case of parabolic flow, the average flow speed across the vessel is equal to one half of the maximum flow speed (at the center). Parabolic flow is not commonly seen in blood circulation because blood vessels generally are not long and straight. However, nonparabolic laminar flow is commonly seen; indeed, its absence is often an indicator of abnormal flow conditions at a site where there is vascular or cardiac-valvular disease.

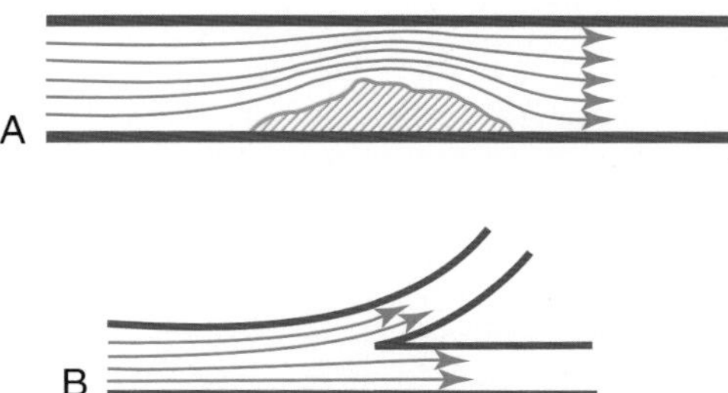

FIGURE 5-5 Disturbed flow at a stenosis (A) and at a bifurcation (B).

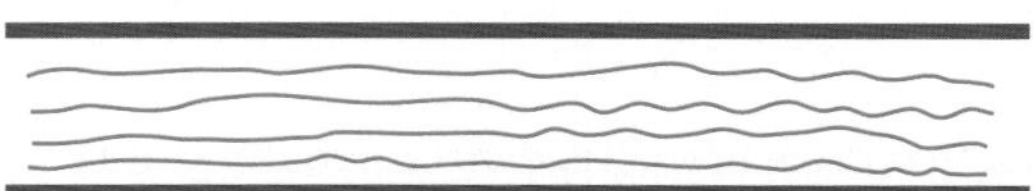

FIGURE 5-6 Turbulent flow in a vessel may result from too great a flow speed.

> Laminar flow is flow in which layers of fluid slide over each other in straight lines.

Disturbed flow occurs when the parallel streamlines describing the flow (see Figure 5-3) are altered from their straight form (Figure 5-5). This occurs, for example, in the region of a stenosis or at a bifurcation (the point at which a vessel splits into two). In disturbed flow, particles of fluid still flow in the forward direction. Parabolic and disturbed flows are forms of laminar flow.

In the final category, turbulent flow, or **turbulence**, the flow pattern is random and chaotic, with particles moving at different speeds in many directions, even in circles called **eddies**, with forward *net* flow still maintained. While flow speed increases in a tube, turbulent flow eventually will occur (Figure 5-6). Turbulence also occurs in the transition from high flow speed in a narrow channel to slow flow in a broad stream (Figure 5-7).

> *Disturbed flow* is a form of laminar flow in which streamlines are not straight. *Turbulent flow* is nonlaminar flow with random and chaotic speeds and directions.

Pulsatile Flow

Thus far, we have considered steady flow in which pressures, flow speeds, and flow patterns do not change with time. This is generally the situation on the venous side of the circulatory system, although cardiac pulsations or respiratory cycles can influence venous flow in some locations. However, in the heart and in arterial circulation, flow is pulsatile, being directly influenced by the effects of the

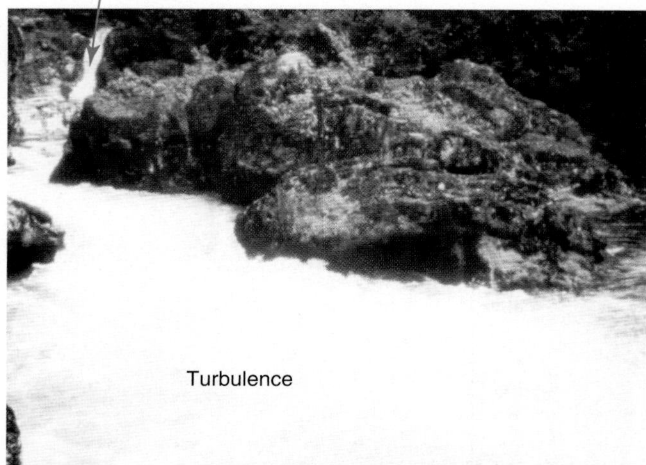

FIGURE 5-7 In a narrow gorge, flow speeds are high; beyond the narrow region, there is abundant turbulence.

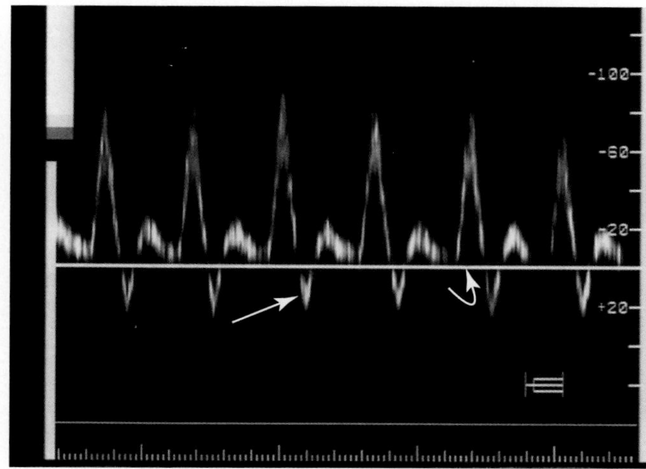

FIGURE 5-8 Flow reversal *(straight arrow)* below the baseline *(curved arrow)* is seen in the superficial femoral artery in diastole.

beating heart with pulsatile variations of increasing and decreasing pressure and flow speed. For steady flow, volumetric flow rate is simply related to pressure difference and flow resistance. With **pulsatile flow**, the relationship between the varying pressure and flow rate depends on flow impedance, which includes resistance, as discussed earlier; the **inertia** of the fluid as it accelerates and decelerates; and the **compliance** (expansion and contraction) of the nonrigid vessel walls. The mathematic analysis is complex and is not presented here. Two dominant characteristics of interest in this type of flow are the Windkessel effect and flow reversal. When the pressure pulse forces a fluid into a compliant vessel, such as the aorta, the vessel expands and increases the volume within. (This is why it is easy to feel the pulse on the wrist or neck.) Later in the cycle, when the driving pressure is reduced, the compliant vessel is able to contract, producing extended flow later in the pressure cycle. This process is known as the *Windkessel effect.* In the aorta, the Windkessel effect results in continued flow in the forward direction because aortic valve closure prevents backward flow into the heart. In the distal circulation, the expansion of distensible vessels results in the reversal of flow in diastole while the pressure decreases and the distended vessels contract. Flow reversal occurs where there are no valves to prevent it (Figure 5-8). This is a normal occurrence in these locations. Pulsatile flow in compliant vessels thus includes added forward flow and/or flow reversal in diastole, depending on location within arterial circulation. Arterial diastolic flow (absence, presence, direction, quantity) reveals much information concerning the state of downstream arterioles, where flow cannot be measured directly with ultrasound.

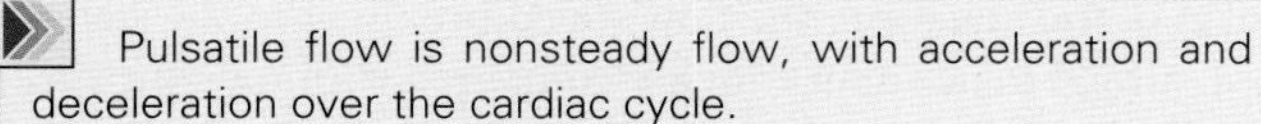
Pulsatile flow is nonsteady flow, with acceleration and deceleration over the cardiac cycle.

Pulsatile flow in distensible vessels includes added forward flow and/or flow reversal over the cardiac cycle in some locations in circulation.

Continuity Rule

A narrowing of the lumen of a vessel, or stenosis, produces disturbed (see Figure 5-5, *A*) and possibly turbulent flow (see Figure 5-7). The average flow speed in the stenosis must be greater than the average flow speed proximal and distal to the stenosis so that the volumetric flow rate is constant throughout the vessel. Examples of increased flow speed at a stenosis and turbulence beyond it are given later in this chapter. Volumetric flow rate must be constant in all three regions—proximal to the stenosis, at the stenosis, and distal to the stenosis—because blood is neither created nor destroyed while it flows through a vessel. This concept is called the *continuity rule.* Volumetric flow rate is equal to the average flow speed across the vessel, multiplied by the cross-sectional area of the vessel. Therefore, if the stenosis has an area measuring one half of the area of the proximal and distal vessel, the average flow speed within the stenosis is twice the average flow speed proximal and distal to the stenosis. If a stenosis has a diameter that is one half the diameter of the adjacent area, the area at the stenosis is one fourth that of the adjacent area, so the average flow speed in the stenosis must quadruple.

Flow speed increases at a stenosis, and turbulence can occur distal to it.

The apparent contradiction of Poiseuille's law and the continuity rule for a stenosis is sometimes puzzling to students. Poiseuille's law states that flow speed decreases with smaller diameters, whereas the continuity rule says that flow speed increases with smaller diameters. How can this be so? The answer is that the two situations are different.

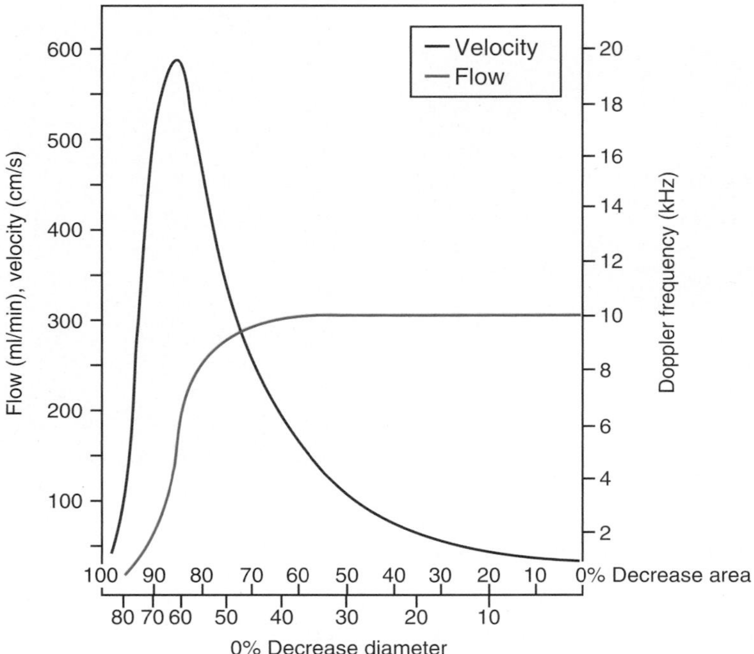

FIGURE 5-9 As the diameter of the stenosis is reduced (moving to the left on the horizontal axis; tighter stenosis), volumetric flow rate (Q) is unaffected initially because the stenosis does not contribute substantially to the total vessel resistance. While the diameter continues to decrease, however, the vessel resistance increases, reducing the volumetric flow rate (eventually to zero at occlusion). Flow rate and, thus, distal pressure begin to drop significantly beyond a diameter reduction of approximately 50% (area reduction of 75%). While the diameter of the stenosis decreases, the flow speed increases (because of the flow continuity requirement), reaches a maximum, and then decreases to zero as the increasing flow resistance effect dominates. (Modified from Spencer MP, Reid JM: Quantitation of carotid stenosis with continuous-wave (C-W) Doppler ultrasound, *Stroke* 10:326–330, 1979. Reprinted with permission. Copyright © 1979, American Heart Association.)

Poiseuille's law deals with a long, straight vessel with no stenosis. The diameter in Poiseuille's law refers to the diameter of the *entire vessel.* By contrast, the diameter in the continuity rule refers to the diameter of a short portion of a vessel (the stenosis). If the diameter of the entire vessel is reduced (as in vasoconstriction), flow speed is reduced. If the diameter of only a short segment of a vessel is reduced (stenosis), the flow speed in the vessel is unaffected, except at the stenosis, where it is increased. Flow speed increases because the stenosis has little effect on the overall flow resistance of the entire vessel if the stenosis length is small compared with the vessel length, and if the lumen in the stenosis is not too small (does not approach occlusion). Figure 5-9 illustrates these dependencies of volumetric flow rate and flow speed at the stenosis with increasing stenosis. The maximum normal flow speed in circulation is approximately 100 cm/s. However, in stenotic regions, flow speeds can increase to a few meters per second. Doppler ultrasound is useful for detecting flow speed increases that are associated with vascular disease.

The increased flow speed within a stenosis can cause turbulence distal to the stenosis. Sounds produced by turbulence, which can be heard with a stethoscope, are called *bruits.* The ultimate stenosis is called an *occlusion,* in which the vessel is blocked and there is no flow. Using our garden hose analogy again, we can compress the hose (not near the nozzle) and see little effect on the flow at the nozzle until the hose is compressed to near-occlusion. At that point, turbulence may occur, and vibration can be felt on the surface of the hose.

Bernoulli Effect

At the stenosis, the pressure is less than it is proximal and distal to the stenotic area (Figure 5-10). This pressure difference is necessary to allow the fluid to accelerate into the stenosis and decelerate out of it and also to maintain energy balance. (Pressure energy is converted to flow energy upon entry, and then vice versa upon exit.) This decreased pressure in regions of high flow speed is known as the **Bernoulli effect** and is described by the Bernoulli equation, a description of the constant energy of the fluid flow through a stenosis, ignoring viscous loss. As flow energy increases, pressure energy decreases. The magnitude of the decrease in pressure (ΔP) that results from the increasing flow speed (v) at the stenosis can be found from the Bernoulli equation. In a simplified form of the equation, the flow speed proximal to the stenosis is assumed to be small enough, compared with the flow speed in the stenosis, to be ignored. Pressure drop from a stenotic

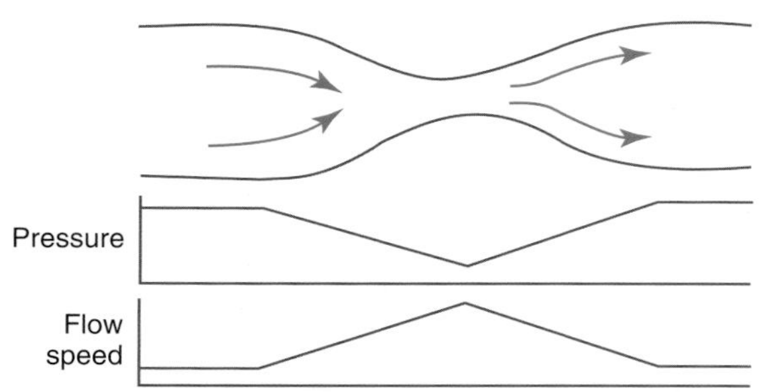

FIGURE 5-10 To maintain flow continuity, flow speed must increase through a stenosis. In conjunction with this, the pressure drops (the Bernoulli effect) in the stenosis. (From Kremkau FW: Fluid flow III, *J Vasc Technol* 17:153-154, 1993. Reprinted with permission.)

heart valve can reduce cardiac output. To calculate pressure drop across a stenotic valve, the following form of the equation is used in Doppler echocardiography:

$$\Delta P = 4(v_2)^2$$

In this equation, v_2 is the flow speed (meters/second) in the jet and ΔP (millimeters of mercury) is the pressure drop across the valve. For example, if the flow speed in the jet is 5 m/s, the pressure drop is 100 mm Hg. Thus pressure drop can be calculated from a measurement of flow speed at the stenotic valve by using Doppler ultrasound.

> If flow speed increases, the magnitude of the pressure drop increases.

> The Bernoulli effect is a drop in pressure associated with high flow speed at a stenosis.

DOPPLER EFFECT

The Doppler effect is a change in frequency (and wavelength) caused by the motion of a sound source, receiver, or reflector. If a reflector is moving toward the source and receiver, the received echo has a higher frequency than would occur without the motion. Conversely, if the motion is away (receding), the received echo has a lower frequency. The amount of increase or decrease in frequency depends on the speed of reflector motion, the angle between the wave propagation direction and the motion direction, and the frequency of the wave emitted by the source.

A quantitative description of the Doppler effect is provided by the **Doppler equation**. Three forms of the Doppler equation deal with three situations: (1) moving source, (2) receiver, or (3) reflector. Only the moving reflector result will be given because it is the relevant situation of interest for diagnostic Doppler ultrasound.

A moving reflector (Figure 5-11) or scatterer of a wave is a combination of a moving receiver and a source. For a moving reflector approaching a stationary source, more cycles of a wave are encountered in 1 second than if the reflector were stationary. Additionally, the reflected cycles are compressed in front of the reflector while it moves into its own reflected wave. Both effects increase the frequency of the reflected wave (echo).

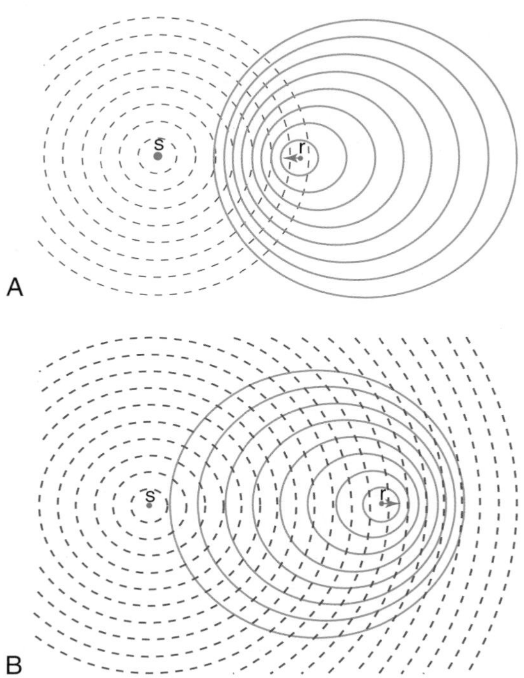

FIGURE 5-11 A moving reflector *(r)* returns a higher frequency echo if it is approaching the source and receiver *(s)* **(A)** and a lower frequency echo if it is moving away from the source and receiver **(B)**.

Doppler Shift

The change in frequency caused by motion is called the *Doppler-shift frequency* or, more commonly, the **Doppler shift** (f_D). The Doppler shift is equal to the received frequency (f_R) minus the source frequency (f_o). For an approaching reflector (scatterer), the Doppler shift is positive; that is, the received frequency is greater than the source frequency. For a receding reflector, the Doppler shift is negative; that is, the received frequency is smaller than the source frequency. The relationship between the Doppler shift and the reflector speed *(v)* is expressed by the Doppler equation:

$$f_D\,(\text{kHz}) = f_R\,(\text{kHz}) - f_o(\text{kHz}) = f_o(\text{kHz}) \times \frac{[2 \times v(\text{cm/s})]}{c\,(\text{cm/s})}$$

> If the scatterer speed increases, the Doppler shift increases. If source frequency increases, the Doppler shift increases.

> The Doppler shift is the difference between the emitted frequency and the echo frequency returning from moving scatterers.

TABLE 5-1 Doppler Frequency Shifts for Various Scatterer Speeds toward* the Sound Source at a Zero Doppler Angle

Incident Frequency (MHz)	Scatterer Speed (cm/s)	Reflected Frequency (MHz)	Doppler Shift (kHz)
2	50	2.0013	1.3
5	50	5.0032	3.2
10	50	10.0065	6.5
2	200	2.0052	5.2
5	200	5.013	13.0
10	200	10.026	26.0

*Motion away from the source would yield negative Doppler shifts.

Take, for example, a source frequency of 5 MHz, a scatterer speed of 50 cm/s (0.5 m/s), and a propagation (sound) speed of 1540 m/s. The scatterer is approaching the source, so the received frequency is greater than the source frequency, with a positive Doppler shift of 0.0032 MHz or 3.2 kHz. For a scatterer moving away from a receiver, the Doppler shift is −3.2 kHz. Other examples that use various source frequencies and scatterer speeds are given in Table 5-1.

The Doppler shift is detected by the instruments described in this chapter. However, we are interested in the speed of tissue motion or blood flow, not the Doppler shift itself. To facilitate this, the Doppler equation is rearranged to place the speed of motion alone on the left side of the equation. Substituting the speed of sound in tissues (154,000 cm/s) and by using units as indicated for the various quantities, the equation is in the following form implemented by the instrument:

$$v(\text{cm/s}) = \frac{77(\text{cm/ms}) \times f_D(\text{kHz})}{f_0(\text{MHz})}$$

> The Doppler equation relates the Doppler shift to flow speed and frequency.

The fact that the Doppler shift is proportional to the blood flow speed explains why the Doppler effect is so useful in medical diagnosis. Doppler instruments measure the Doppler shift. Blood flow is what interests us. The measured shifts are proportional to flow speed, which is the information we seek. The Doppler shift is measured by the instrument and the Doppler equation is solved to yield calculated flow-speed information.

Doppler Ultrasound

With diagnostic medical ultrasound, stationary transducers are used to emit and receive the ultrasound. The Doppler effect is a result of the motion of blood, the flow of which we wish to measure, or the motion of tissue that we wish to evaluate. Physiologic flow speeds, even in highly stenotic jets, do not exceed a few meters per second. Table 5-1 gives Doppler shifts resulting from typical physiologic flow speeds. The minimum detectable blood flow speed with Doppler ultrasound is a few millimeters per second. The maximum is determined by *aliasing* (discussed in Chapter 6).

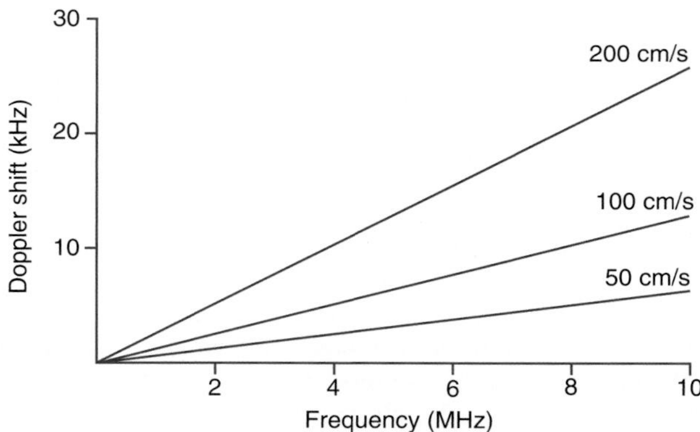

FIGURE 5-12 The Doppler shift as a function of operating frequency, as determined by the Doppler equation for various flow speeds (at a zero Doppler angle).

> The Doppler shift is proportional to flow speed.

Operating Frequency

For a given flow in a vessel, the Doppler shift measured by an instrument is proportional to the operating frequency of the instrument (Figure 5-12; also see Table 5-1). Thus measurement of Doppler shifts from flow in the same vessel by using two transducers operating at 2 MHz and 4 MHz will yield two Doppler shifts. The higher-frequency transducer will have a Doppler shift that is twice that of the lower-frequency transducer. Therefore, when comparing Doppler shifts, one must consider the frequency of the devices. The operating frequency is incorporated into the calculation of flow speed with use of the Doppler equation. Thus comparisons of flow speeds between different instruments and transducers have taken this variable into account.

> The Doppler shift is proportional to the operating frequency.

Doppler frequencies used in vascular studies are slightly less than those used for anatomic imaging, because echoes from blood are weaker than echoes from soft tissues.

Doppler Angle

If the direction of sound propagation is exactly opposite the flow direction, the maximum positive Doppler shift is obtained. If the flow speed and propagation speed directions are the same (parallel), the maximum negative Doppler shift is obtained. If the angle between these two directions (Figure 5-13) is nonzero (nonparallel), lesser Doppler shifts will occur. The Doppler shift depends on the **cosine** of the **Doppler angle** (θ):

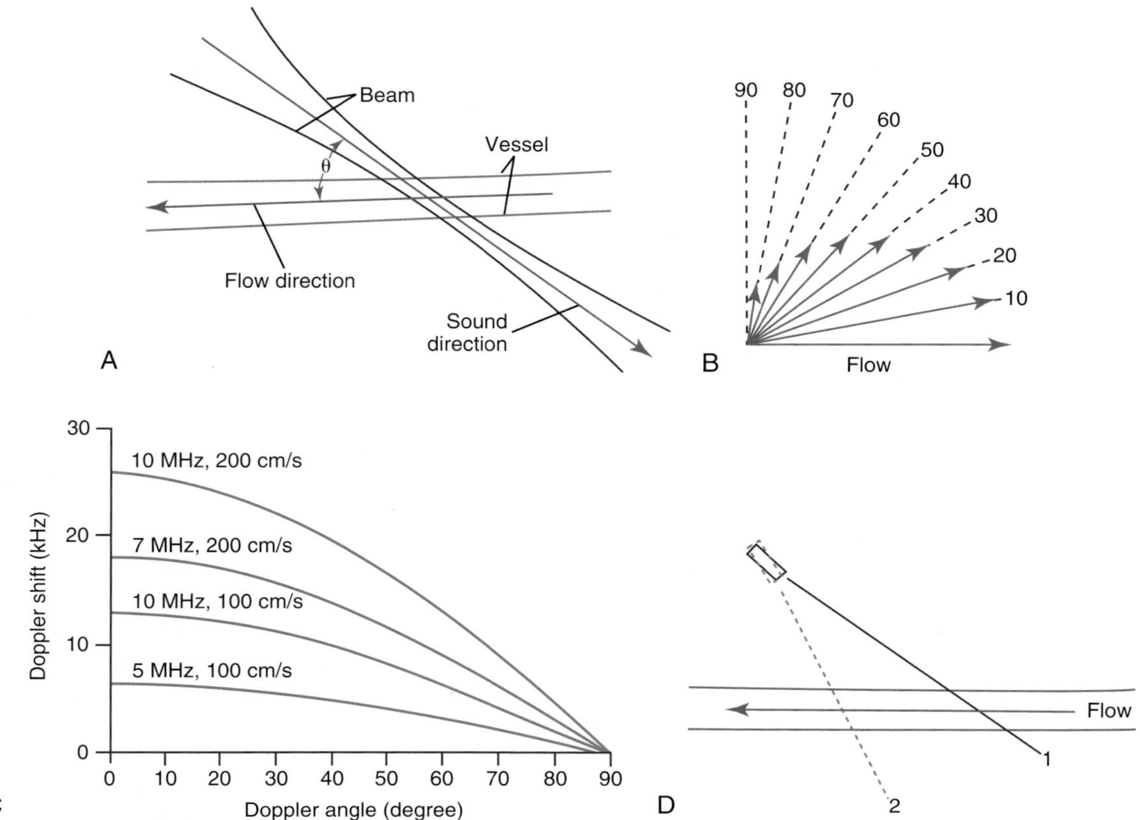

FIGURE 5-13 **A,** The Doppler angle θ is the angle between the direction of flow and the sound propagation direction. **B,** With constant flow, while the Doppler angle increases, echo Doppler shift frequency decreases. The length of the arrows indicates the magnitude of the Doppler shift as the Doppler angle increases. **C,** The Doppler shift as a function of angle, as determined by the Doppler equation for various incident frequencies and scatterer speeds. **D,** The same flow in a vessel, viewed at different angles, yields different Doppler shifts.

$$f_D(\text{kHz}) = \frac{[f_o(\text{kHz}) \times 2 \times v(\text{cm/s}) \times (\cos\theta)]}{c(\text{cm/s})}$$

$$v(\text{cm/s}) = \frac{[77(\text{cm/ms}) \times f_D(\text{kHz})]}{[f_o(\text{MHz}) \times \cos\theta]}$$

Table 5-2 gives cosine values for various angles. Only the portion of the motion direction that is parallel to the sound beam contributes to the Doppler effect. The cosine gives the component of the flow velocity vector that is parallel to the sound beam (Figure 5-14). For a given flow, the larger the Doppler angle, the less the Doppler shift (see Figure 5-13, *B-C*). Table 5-3 lists examples of Doppler shifts for various angles.

> If the Doppler shift increases, the calculated scatterer speed increases.

> If the source frequency increases, the calculated scatterer speed decreases.

TABLE 5-2 Cosines for Various Angles

Angle A (degrees)	Cosine A
0	1.000
5	0.996
10	0.98
15	0.97
20	0.94
25	0.91
30	0.87
35	0.82
40	0.77
45	0.71
50	0.64
55	0.57
60	0.50
65	0.42
70	0.34
75	0.26
80	0.17
85	0.09
90	0.00

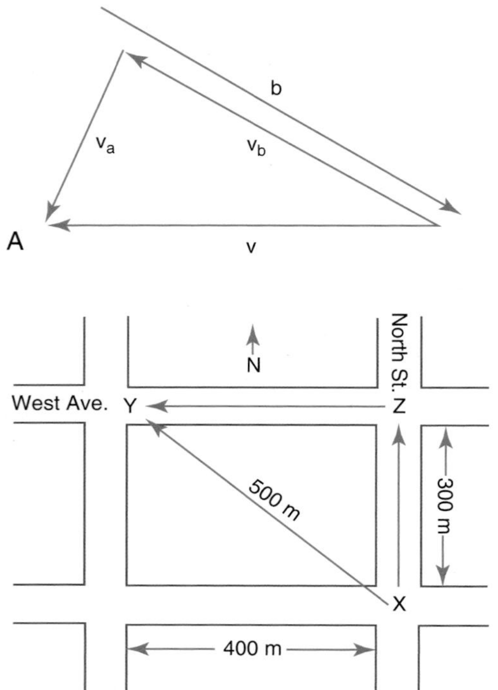

FIGURE 5-14 **A,** The flow velocity vector *(v)* can be broken into two components: one (v_b) that is parallel to the sound beam *(b)* direction and one (v_a) that is perpendicular to the sound beam direction. Only the component parallel to the beam contributes to the Doppler effect. **B,** A city block can be used as an analogy to the vector components in **A.** To get from point X to point Y, one could walk diagonally across the block, a distance of 500 m. However, if buildings blocked that path, an alternative route would be 300 m north on North Street and then 400 m west on West Avenue. The 500-m northwest vector from X to Y is equivalent to a 300-m north vector plus a 400-m west vector (i.e., the result is the same: depart from X and arrive at Y). In this example, the component of the XY vector parallel to North Street is the XZ vector, and the component parallel to West Avenue is the ZY vector.

TABLE 5-3 Doppler Frequency Shifts for Various Angles and Scatterer Speeds toward the Sound Source of Frequency 5 MHz

Scatterer Speed (cm/s)	Angle (degrees)	Doppler Shift (kHz)
100	0	6.5
100	30	5.6
100	60	3.2
100	90	0.0
300	0	19.0
300	30	17.0
300	60	9.7
300	0	0.0

If the cosine increases, the calculated scatterer speed decreases.

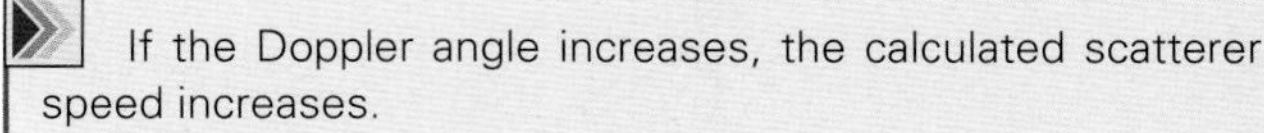
If the Doppler angle increases, the calculated scatterer speed increases.

Angle Accuracy

Flow speed calculations based on Doppler shift measurements can be accomplished correctly only with proper incorporation of the Doppler angle. The calculations, therefore, are only as good as the accuracy of the measurement, estimate, or guess of that angle. Estimation of the angle is usually done by orienting an indicator line on the anatomic display so that it is parallel to the presumed direction of flow (e.g., parallel to the vessel wall for a straight vessel with no flow obstruction). This is a subjective operation performed by the instrument operator. Error in this estimation of the Doppler angle is more critical at large angles than at small ones, because the cosine changes rapidly at large angles. Table 5-4 gives error values for various angles. For example, if the correct Doppler angle is 60 degrees but the estimation is 5 degrees in error (the angle estimate is 55 or 65 degrees), the error in the cosine value is approximately 15%, yielding a calculated speed that is in error by approximately 18%. Figure 5-15 shows how the error in the calculated flow speed increases with angle. For this reason, and because Doppler shift frequencies become very small at large angles, thereby reducing the system sensitivity, Doppler measurements (and particularly the calculated flow speeds) are not reliably achieved at Doppler angles greater than approximately 60 degrees. In principle, if the angle is incorporated correctly, the calculated flow speed in the vessel should be the same, regardless of the Doppler angle; that is, the actual flow speed is certainly not altered by the Doppler angle used in detecting it (Table 5-5). Not surprisingly, however, inaccuracies in angle estimation do occur. Flow is also often not parallel to vessel walls, even in unobstructed vessels.

At Doppler angles less than approximately 30 degrees, the sound no longer enters the blood at all but is reflected totally at the wall–blood boundary. One generally achieves success, then, at angles greater than this. However, in Doppler echocardiography, Doppler angles of near-zero are useful, and zero is commonly assumed (i.e., angle correction is not incorporated in this application as it is in vascular work). The angle between the beam and the heart wall is large, which avoids the total reflection problem (Figure 5-16).

In this discussion, we have considered the Doppler angle only in the scan plane. One must remember that the flow may not be parallel to the imaging scan plane, which includes the Doppler beam, thus there may be a component of Doppler angle between flow direction and scan plane. Thus one must keep in mind the three-dimensional character of the components involved in the process (vessel anatomy, flow direction, and ultrasound image scan plane).

COLOR-DOPPLER DISPLAYS

Doppler instruments present information on the presence, direction, speed, and character of blood flow (Box 5-1) and on the presence, direction, and speed of tissue motion. This information is present in audible, color-Doppler, and spectral-Doppler forms (Box 5-2). Color-Doppler imaging

TABLE 5-4 Cosine and Calculated-Speed Errors for Angle Errors of 2 and 5 Degrees

	COSINE ERROR (%)		SPEED ERROR (%)	
True Angle (degrees)	+2 Degrees	+5 Degrees	+2 Degrees	+5 Degrees
0	−0.1	−0.4	+0.1	+0.4
10	−0.7	−1.9	+0.7	+2.0
20	−1.3	−3.6	+1.3	+3.7
30	−2.1	−5.4	+2.1	+5.7
40	−3.0	−7.7	+3.1	+8.3
50	−4.2	−10.8	+4.4	+12.1
60	−6.1	−15.5	+6.5	+18.3
70	−9.6	−24.3	+10.7	+32.1
80	−19.9	−49.8	+24.8	+99.2

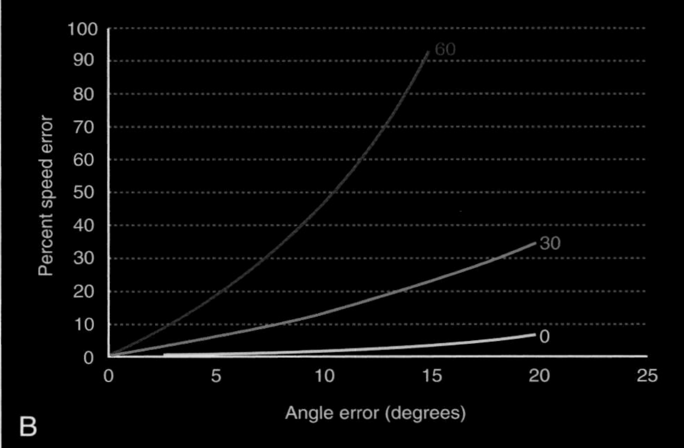

FIGURE 5-15 **A,** Percentage calculated speed error versus correct Doppler angle for 5-, 10-, 15-, and 20-degree angle errors. **B,** Percentage calculated speed error versus angle error for three values (0, 30, and 60 degrees) of the correct Doppler angle.

TABLE 5-5 Doppler Shifts (for 4 MHz) at Various Doppler Angles for the Same Flow Yielding a Consistent Calculated Flow Speed

Doppler Shift (kHz)	Angle (degrees)	Calculated Flow Speed (cm/s)
2.25	30	50
1.99	40	50
1.84	45	50
1.67	50	50
1.30	60	50

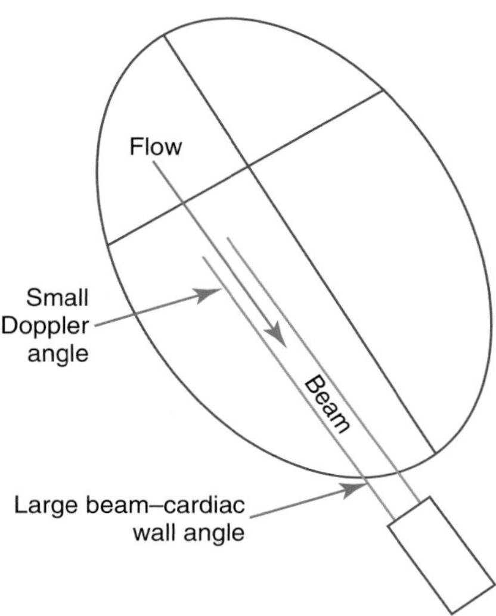

FIGURE 5-16 In cardiac Doppler work, Doppler angles are usually small, whereas the angle between the beam and the cardiac wall is usually large.

BOX 5-1 Types of Flow Information Provided by Doppler Ultrasound

- Presence of flow
  - Yes
  - No
- Direction of flow
  - →
  - ←
- Speed of flow
  - Slow
  - Fast
- Character of flow
  - Laminar
  - Turbulent

BOX 5-2 Various Forms of Presentation of Doppler Information

- Audible sounds
- Strip-chart recording
- Spectral display
- Color-Doppler display

presents two-dimensional, cross-sectional, real-time blood flow, or tissue motion information along with two-dimensional, cross-sectional, gray-scale anatomic imaging. Two-dimensional real-time presentations of flow information allow the observer to readily locate regions of abnormal flow for further evaluation by using spectral analysis. The direction of flow is appreciated readily, and disturbed or turbulent flow is presented dramatically in two-dimensional form. Color Doppler presents anatomic information in the conventional gray-scale form, but also rapidly detects Doppler shift frequencies at several locations along each scan line, presenting them in color at appropriate locations in the cross-sectional image.

Color-Doppler Principle

Color-Doppler imaging (sometimes called *color-flow imaging*) extends the use of the pulse-echo imaging principle to include Doppler-shifted echoes that indicate blood flow or tissue motion. Echoes returning from stationary tissues are detected and presented in gray scale in appropriate locations along scan lines. Depth is determined by echo arrival time, and brightness is determined by echo intensity. If a returning echo has a different frequency from that emitted, a Doppler shift has occurred because the echo-generating object was moving. Depending on whether the motion is toward or away from the transducer, the Doppler shift is positive or negative. At locations along scan lines where Doppler shifts are detected, arbitrary colors are assigned to the display pixels according to a chosen color-assignment map.

Doppler-shifted echoes can be recorded and presented in color at many locations along each scan line (Figure 5-17, *A-B*). As in all sonography, many such scan lines make up one cross-sectional image (see Figure 5-17, *C–D*). Several of these images (frames) are presented each second, yielding real-time color-Doppler sonography.

> Color Doppler imaging is an extension of conventional gray-scale sonography, showing regions of blood flow or tissue motion in color.

Linear array presentation of color-Doppler information is sometimes inadequate when the vessel runs parallel to the skin surface because the pulses (and scan lines) run perpendicular to the transducer surface (and therefore to the skin surface), resulting in a 90-degree Doppler angle where the pulses

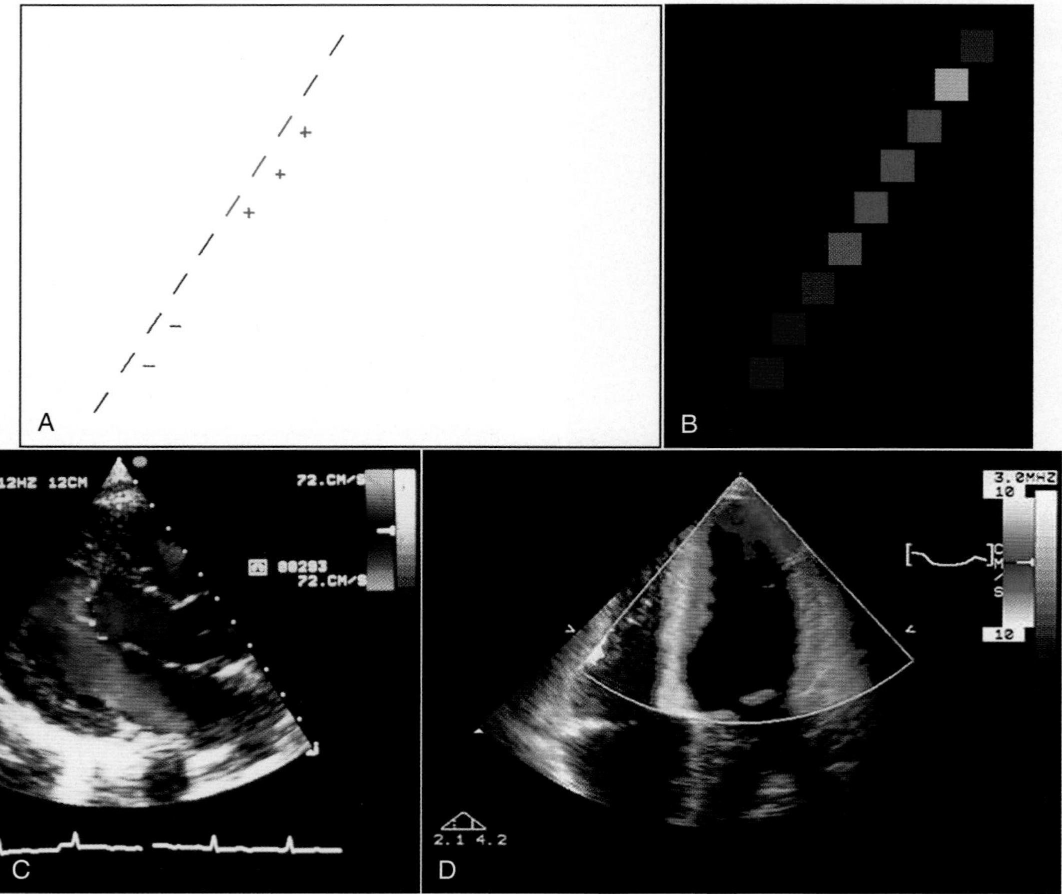

FIGURE 5-17 **A,** Ten echoes are received as a pulse travels through tissues. Three *(red)* have positive Doppler shifts, and two *(blue)* have negative shifts. **B,** These echoes are shown (in this example) as red and blue pixels, respectively, on the color-Doppler display. As in gray-scale sonography, a two-dimensional cross-sectional image is made up of many scan lines. **C,** A parasternal long-axis image of normal mitral valve blood flow. **D,** A parasternal short-axis view of myocardial tissue motion (color kinesis).

intersect the flow in the vessel. If the flow is parallel to the vessel walls, the 90-degree Doppler angle would yield no Doppler shift, and hence no color within the vessel. To solve this problem, phasing is used to steer each emitted pulse from the array in a given direction (e.g., 20 degrees away from perpendicular).

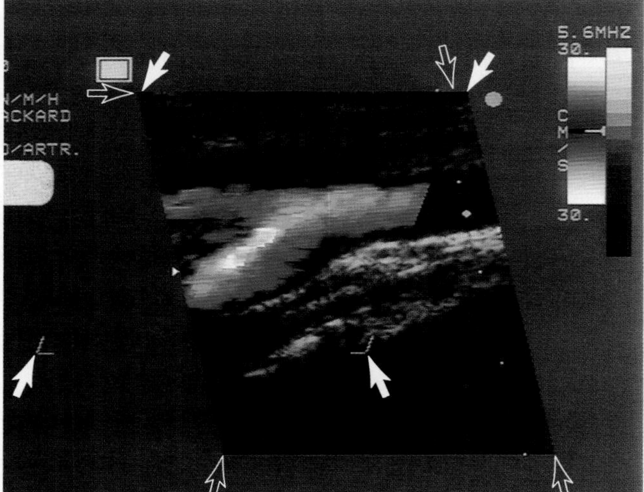

FIGURE 5-18 A perpendicular Doppler angle is avoided in this image by electronically steering the color-producing Doppler pulses to the left of vertical. The corners of the resulting parallelogram in which color can be displayed are shown by the solid arrows. Note that on this instrument, the gray-scale anatomic imaging pulses can also be steered (in this case, to the right of vertical). The corners of the resulting gray-scale parallelogram are shown by the open arrows. (From Kremkau FW: Principles and pitfalls of real-time color-flow imaging. In Bernstein EF, editor: *Vascular diagnosis,* 4th ed, St. Louis, 1993, Mosby.)

All the color pulses and color scan lines are steered at the same angle, resulting in a parallelogram presentation of color-Doppler information on the display (Figure 5-18).

Instruments

The **color-Doppler display** is part of a sonographic instrument (see Figure 4-1, *A*). The beam former, signal processor, image processor, and display perform the same functions as in anatomic imaging. In addition, the signal processor has the ability to detect Doppler shifts, and the display is capable of presenting Doppler-shifted echoes in color.

> Color Doppler uses conventional sonographic instruments with the ability to detect Doppler shifts and present them on the display in color.

Doppler-Shift Detection

The signal processor receives the digitized voltages from the beam former that represent the echoes returning from the tissue. Non–Doppler-shifted echoes are processed conventionally, as in any sonographic instrument. Doppler-shifted echoes are commonly detected in the signal processor by using a mathematic technique called **autocorrelation**, which rapidly determines the mean and **variance** of the Doppler-shift signal (Figure 5-19) at each location along the scan line (at each selected echo arrival time during pulse travel). The autocorrelation technique is a mathematic process that yields Doppler-shift information for each sample time (and corresponding depth down the scan line) following pulse emission. The sign, mean, and variance of the Doppler signal are stored at appropriate locations in the memory corresponding to anatomic sites where the Doppler

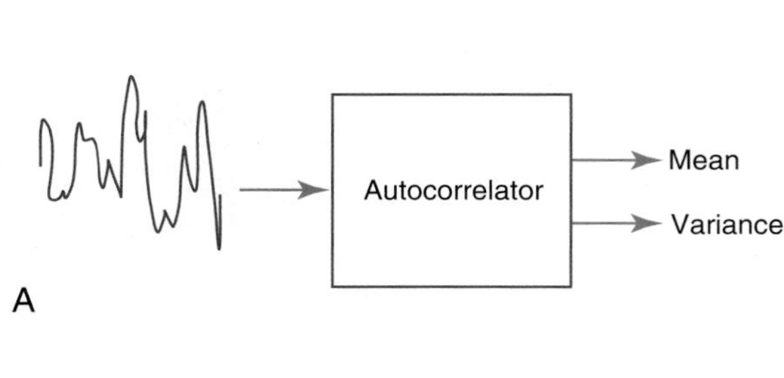

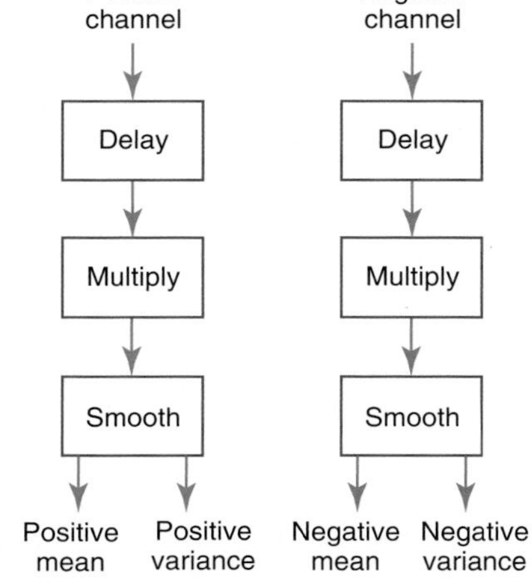

FIGURE 5-19 A, The autocorrelator rapidly performs Doppler demodulation on the complicated echo signal (entering at left). The outputs of the autocorrelator yield the magnitude of the mean and the variance of Doppler shifts at each location in the scanned cross-section. These items of information are stored in each pixel location in the memory. Color assignments are selected appropriately to indicate these items of information two-dimensionally on the display. **B,** After division of the Doppler signal into positive and negative Doppler-shift channels, each signal is multiplied by a version of itself delayed by one pulse repetition period. High-frequency variations are filtered out (smoothed) to yield the mean and variance of Doppler shifts. Variance is a measure of data spread around a mean. Variance is equal to the standard deviation squared.

Continued

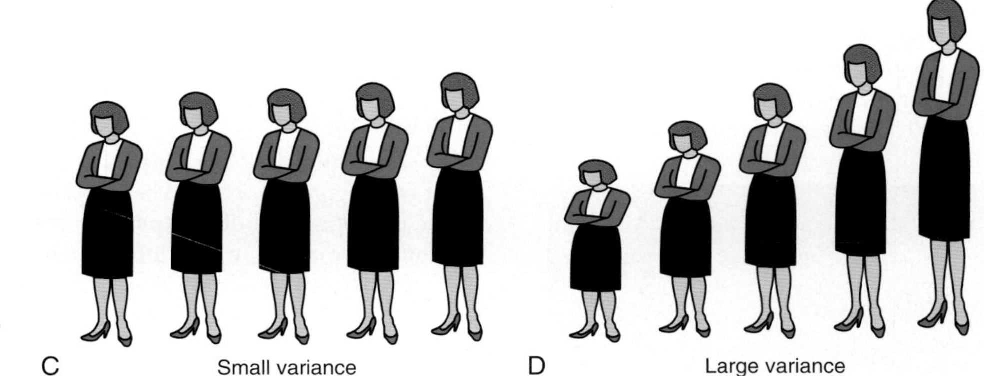

FIGURE 5-19, cont'd C-D, Two groups of women with equal mean heights but unequal variances.

shifts have been found. Typically 100 to 400 Doppler samples (locations) per scan line are shown on a color-Doppler display. Depending on the depth and width of the color presentation, typically 5 to 50 frames per second can be shown. Recall that for gray-scale sonography, a single pulse produces one scan line. For multiple foci, multiple pulses per scan line are required. In color-Doppler instruments, multiple pulses are involved in all images because they are required in the autocorrelation process. A three-pulse minimum is required for one speed estimate. More pulses are required for improved accuracy of the estimates, for variance determinations, or to improve detection of lower-frequency mean Doppler shifts (slower flows).

> Autocorrelation is the mathematic process commonly used to detect Doppler shifts in color-Doppler instruments.

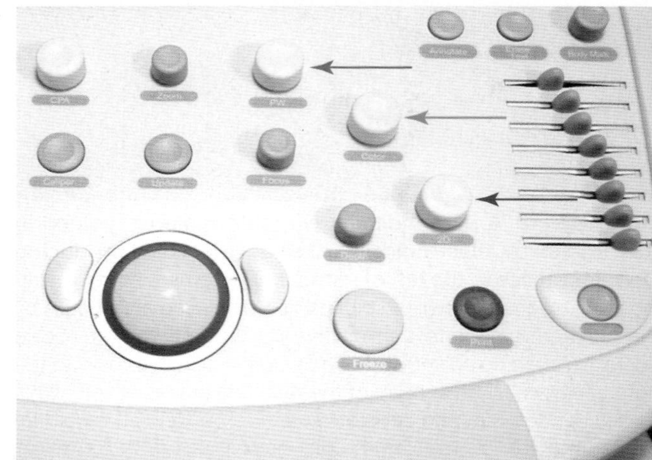

FIGURE 5-20 Color-Doppler gain control *(green arrow).* The gray-scale *(blue arrow)* and spectral-Doppler *(red arrow)* gain controls also are indicated.

Color Controls

Color controls (Figure 5-20) include gain, color **window** location, width and depth, steering angle, color-map inversion, **wall filter**, **priority**, **baseline shift**, velocity range (pulse repetition frequency [PRF]), color map selection, variance, smoothing, and **ensemble length**. Steering angle control permits avoidance of 90-degree angles (Figure 5-21). Color inversion alternates the color assignments on either side of the zero-Doppler-shift baseline on the color map (see Figure 5-21, *D-E*). The wall filter allows elimination of clutter caused by tissue and wall motion (Figure 5-22). However, one must take care not to set the wall filter too high, or slower blood flow signals will be removed (see Figure 5-22, *C*). The operator of a gray-scale sonographic instrument does not have direct control of PRF. But in Doppler operation, the operator controls PRF with the scale control. This control sets the PRF and the limit at the color bar extremes. Decreasing the value permits observation of slower flows (smaller Doppler shifts) (see Figure 5-22, *F*) but increases the probability of an artifact, called *aliasing,* for faster flows (aliasing is described in Chapter 6). Priority selects the gray-scale echo strength below which color, instead of gray level, will be shown at each pixel location (Figure 5-23). Baseline control allows shifting the baseline up or down to correct aliasing. Smoothing (also called *persistence*) provides frame-to-frame averaging to reduce noise (Figure 5-24). Ensemble length is the number of pulses used for each color scan line. The minimum is 3, with 10 to 20 being common. Greater ensemble lengths provide more accurate estimates of mean Doppler shift, improved detection of slow flows, and complete representation of flow within a vessel (see Figure 5-24) but at the expense of longer time per frame and therefore lower frame rates. Wider color windows (viewing areas) also reduce frame rates because more scan lines are required for each frame (Figure 5-25).

Color-Doppler Limitations

Several aspects of color-Doppler imaging are, by their nature, limiting. These aspects include angle dependence, lower frame rates, and lack of detailed spectral information. Spectral Doppler presents the entire range of Doppler shift frequencies received while they change over the cardiac cycle. Color-Doppler displays present only a statistical representation of the complete spectrum at each pixel location on the display. The sign, mean value, and, if chosen, the power or the variance of the spectrum are color coded into combinations of **hue**, **saturation**, and **luminance** that are presented at each display pixel location. Some Doppler displays are able to read the quantitative digital values for mean Doppler shifts (sometimes converted to angle-corrected equivalent flow speed) at chosen pixel locations (Figure 5-26). One must realize that these are mean values that must be compared carefully with the peak systolic values, which are used commonly to evaluate spectral displays. Because color-Doppler techniques require several pulses per scan line (as opposed to one pulse per scan line for single-focus, gray-scale anatomic imaging), frame rates are lower than those for gray-scale anatomic imaging. Therefore multiple foci are not used in color-Doppler imaging. The relationship between penetration (*pen*), line density, and frame rate is the same as that presented in Chapter 4, except that ensemble length (*n*) replaces the number of foci. The maximum permissible frame rate (FR_m) is as follows:

$$FR_m\,(Hz) = \frac{77{,}000\,(cm/s)}{[pen\,(cm) \times lines\ per\ frame\ (LPF) \times n]}$$

If ensemble length increases, frame rate decreases.

Doppler-Shift Displays

Where Doppler-shifted echoes have been stored, hue, saturation, and luminance appropriate to the shift information are presented according to a choice of schemes. The selected scheme is presented on the display as a color map (Figure 5-27). The map allows the observer to interpret the meaning of the hue, saturation, and luminance at each location in terms of the sign, magnitude, and variance of Doppler shifts. Hue indicates the sign of the Doppler shift. Changes in hue, saturation, or luminance up or down the map from the center indicate increasing Doppler shift magnitude. When selected, variance is shown as a change in hue from left to right across the map.

The color map, always shown on the display, is the key to understanding how image colors are related to Doppler characteristics.

Angle

As with any Doppler technique, angle is important. Figure 5-28 shows convex array and linear array views of vascular flow. Note that the images are similar in appearance, with red on the left and blue on the right. But note that the relative position of the color bars is inverted. How is this inconsistency explained? In fact, why does the color change at all, considering that there is no reason not to expect unidirectional flow in these vessels? The color changes in the vessel in Figure 5-28, *A*, because, with the sector image format, pulses and scan lines travel in different directions away from the transducer. Thus they have different Doppler angles with the flow in a straight vessel. Some pulses view the flow upstream and some downstream (see Figure 5-28, *B*). At the 90-degree Doppler angle point,

Text continued on p. 153

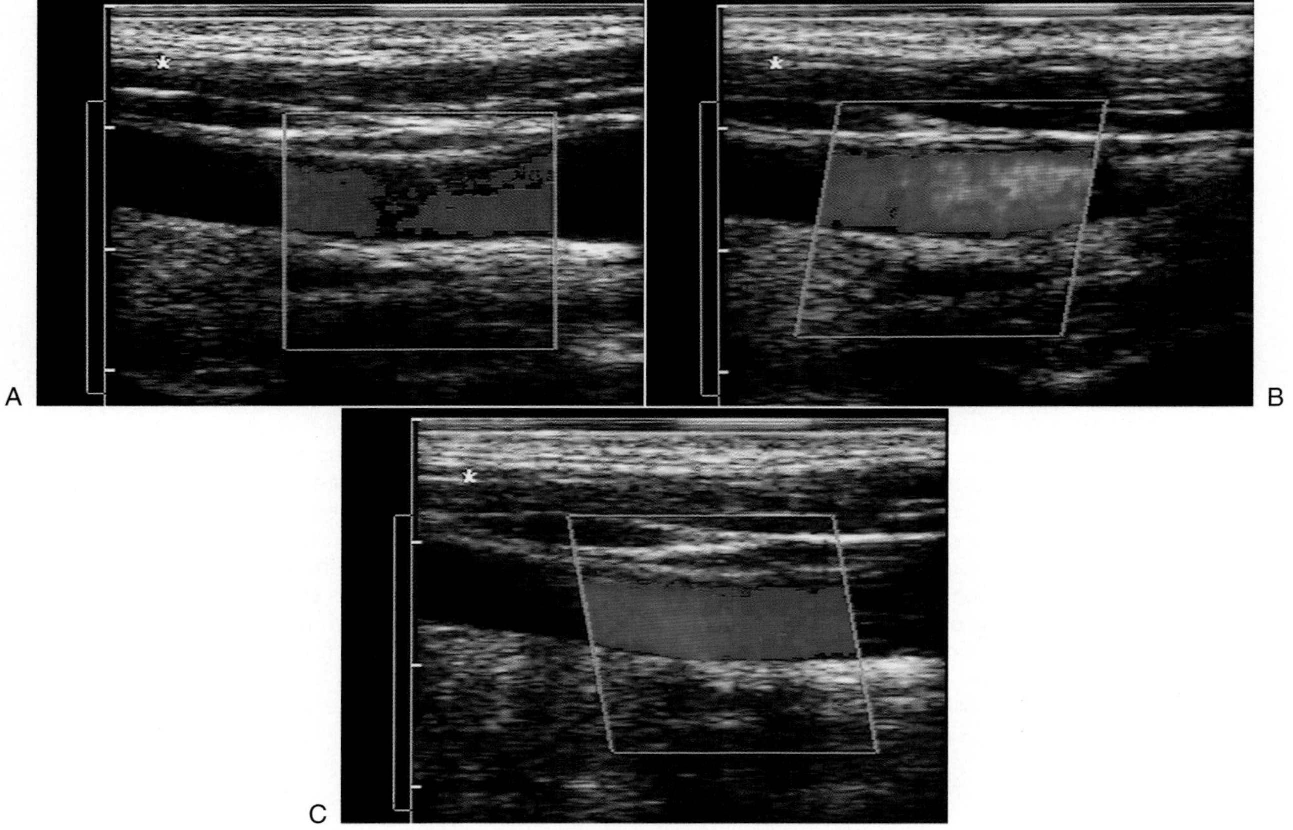

FIGURE 5-21 Color scan lines are directed down vertically **(A)**, to the left of vertical **(B)**, and to the right of vertical **(C)**. Flow is from left to right, producing positive *(red)* or negative *(blue)* Doppler shifts, depending on the relationship between scan lines and flow (i.e., viewing upstream or downstream).

Continued

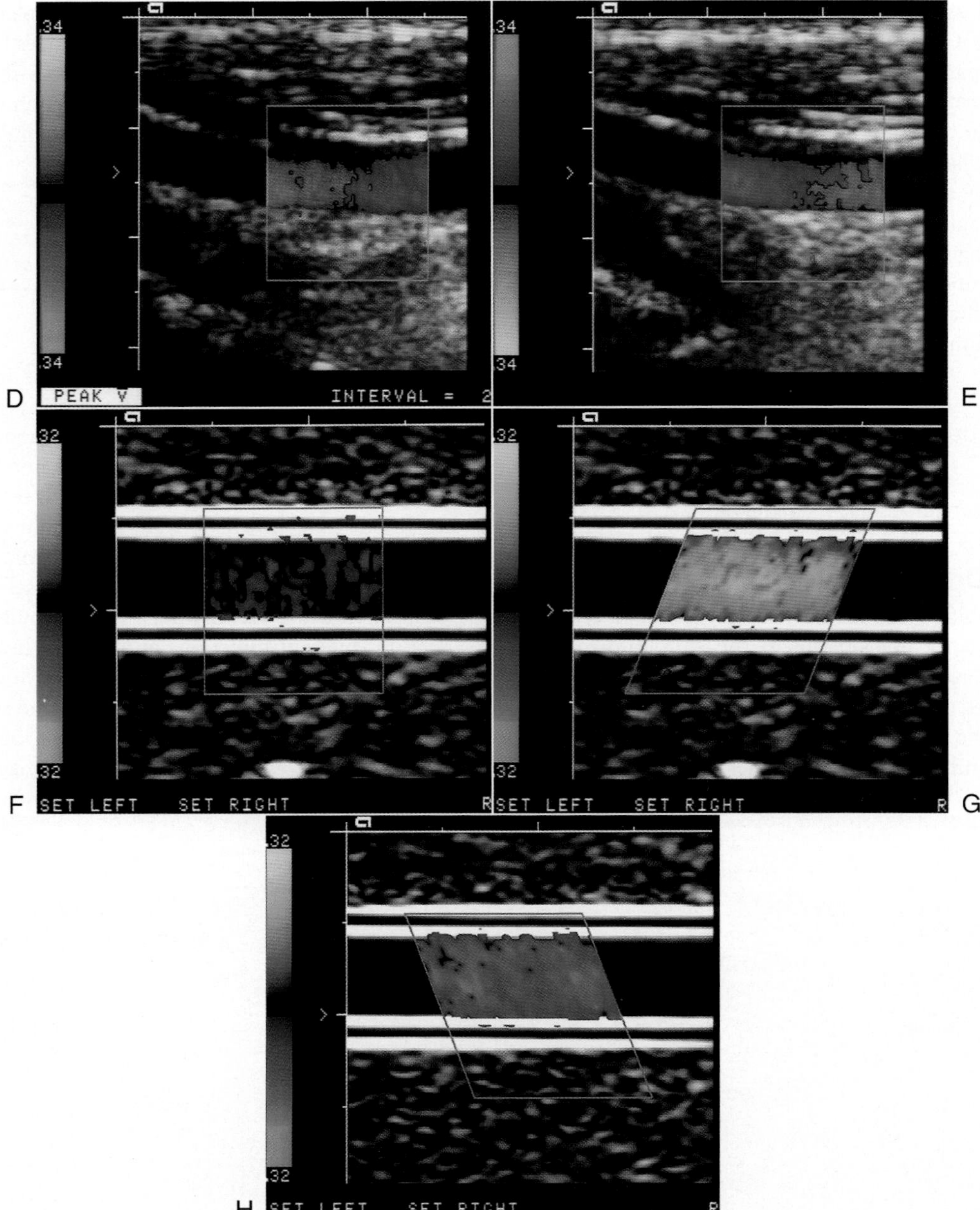

FIGURE 5-21, cont'd D, In this hue map, red and blue are assigned to positive and negative Doppler shifts, respectively, progressing to yellow and cyan (by the addition of green) at the map limits. **E,** In this map, the color assignments are inverted from those presented in *D* (i.e., blue and red are assigned to positive and negative Doppler shifts, respectively). Note the color change occurring within each color window. This is caused by vessel curvature. **F,** With flow in a straight tube, positive and negative Doppler shifts are distributed equally throughout the color window with a Doppler angle of 90 degrees. **G,** Uniform positive Doppler shifts are observed with the color window steered 20 degrees to the left (70-degree Doppler angle). **H,** Uniform negative Doppler shifts are observed with the color window steered to the right. (**A-C** from Kremkau FW: Doppler principles, *Semin Roentgenol* 27:6-16, 1992; **D-E** from Kremkau FW: Principles and pitfalls of real-time color-flow imaging. In Bernstein EF, editor: *Vascular diagnosis*, 4th ed, St. Louis, 1993, Mosby.)

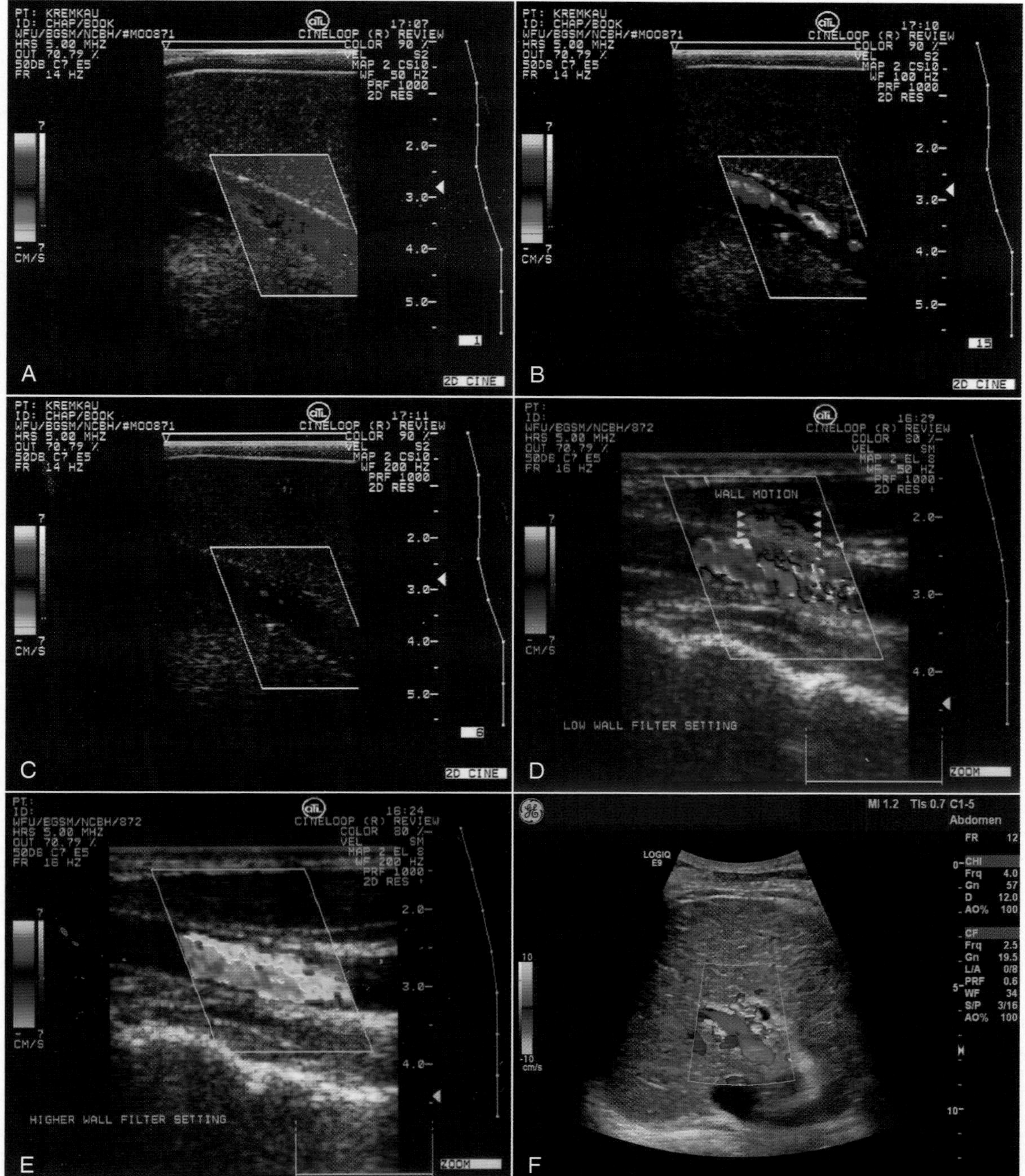

FIGURE 5-22 A, Tissue motion causes clutter, obscuring the flow in the vessel and clouding the gray-scale tissue with color-Doppler information. B, Wall filter has been increased to 100 Hz, thereby eliminating the color clutter. C, Wall filter has been increased (too much) to 200 Hz, eliminating virtually all the color-Doppler information derived from the vessel. D, With a low wall filter setting (50 Hz), wall motion appears in color on the image. E, With a higher wall filter setting (200 Hz), this motion no longer appears in color. F, Slow portal flow imaged with low pulse repetition frequency. (A-C from Kremkau FW: Principles and pitfalls of real-time color-flow imaging. In Bernstein EF, editor: *Vascular diagnosis*, 4th ed, St. Louis, 1993, Mosby; D–E from Kremkau FW: Principles and instrumentation. In Merritt CRB, editor: *Doppler color imaging*, New York, 1992, Churchill Livingstone.)

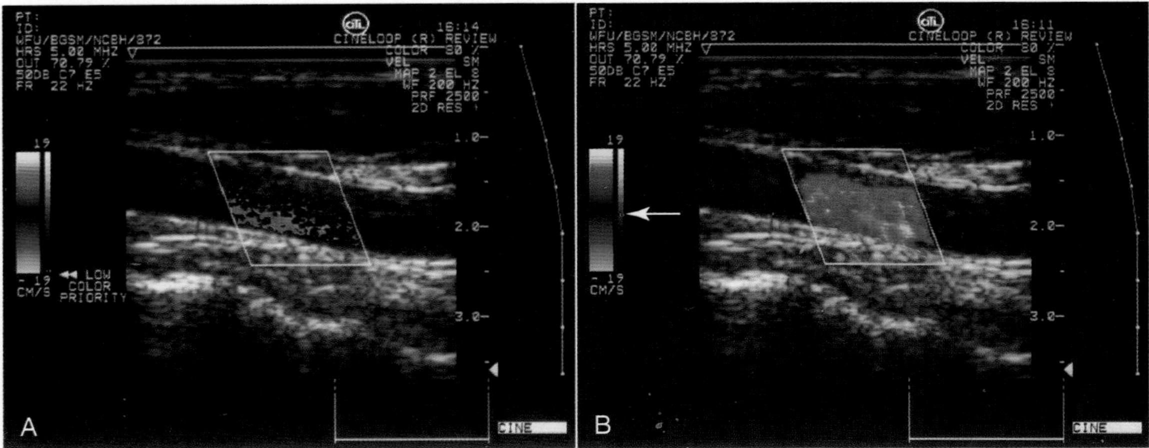

FIGURE 5-23 **A,** With the color priority set low *(at the bottom of the gray bar)*, weak, non–Doppler-shifted reverberation and off-axis echoes within the vessel take precedence over the Doppler-shifted echoes, and little color is displayed. **B,** With a higher color priority setting *(halfway up the gray bar [arrow])*, the Doppler-shifted echoes *(color)* take precedence over the weaker gray-scale echoes. (From Kremkau FW: Principles and instrumentation. In Merritt CRB, editor: *Doppler color imaging,* New York, 1992, Churchill Livingstone.)

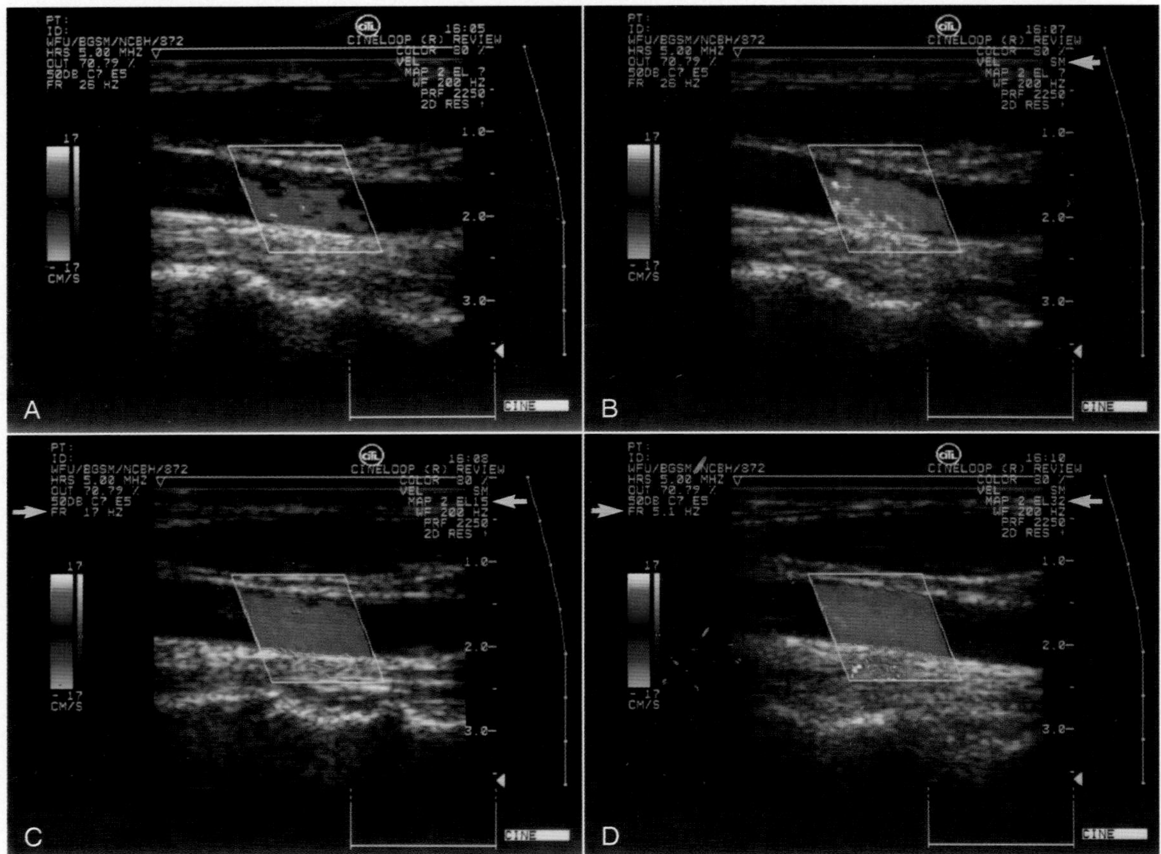

FIGURE 5-24 **A,** With no smoothing (persistence), only the Doppler-shifted echoes received from the pulses generating an individual frame are shown. **B,** With smoothing, consecutive frames are averaged, filling gaps in the presentation and presenting a smoother but less detailed representation of flow. **C–D,** More accurate and complete detection of flow information is obtained with increasing ensemble lengths. The ensemble lengths shown are 7 (see **B**), 15 (see **C**), and 32 (see **D**). Note the decrease in frame rate from 26 to 17 to 5.1 frames per second. (From Kremkau FW: Principles and instrumentation. In Merritt CRB, editor: *Doppler color imaging,* New York, 1992, Churchill Livingstone.)

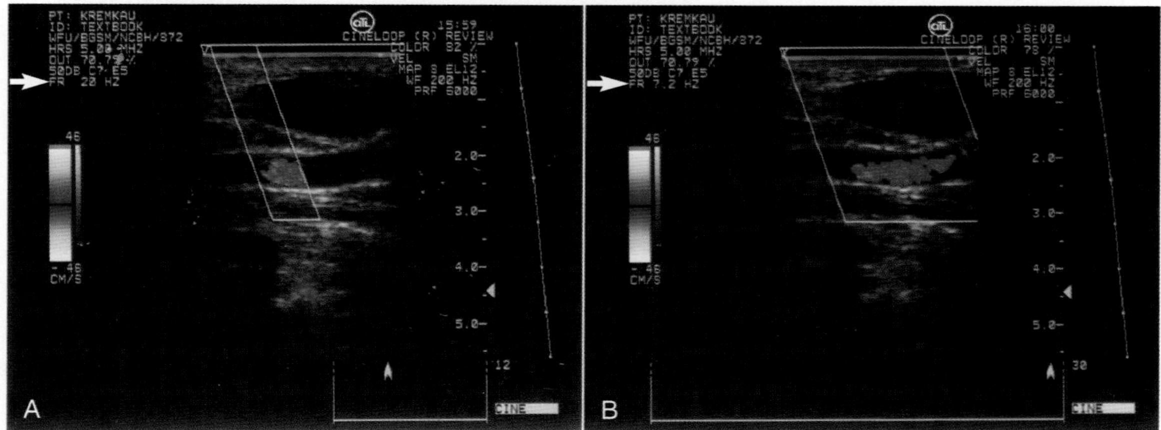

FIGURE 5-25 Tripling the color window width decreases the frame rate from 20 Hz **(A)** to 7.2 Hz **(B)**. (From Kremkau FW: Principles and instrumentation. In Merritt CRB, editor: *Doppler color imaging*, New York, 1992, Churchill Livingstone.)

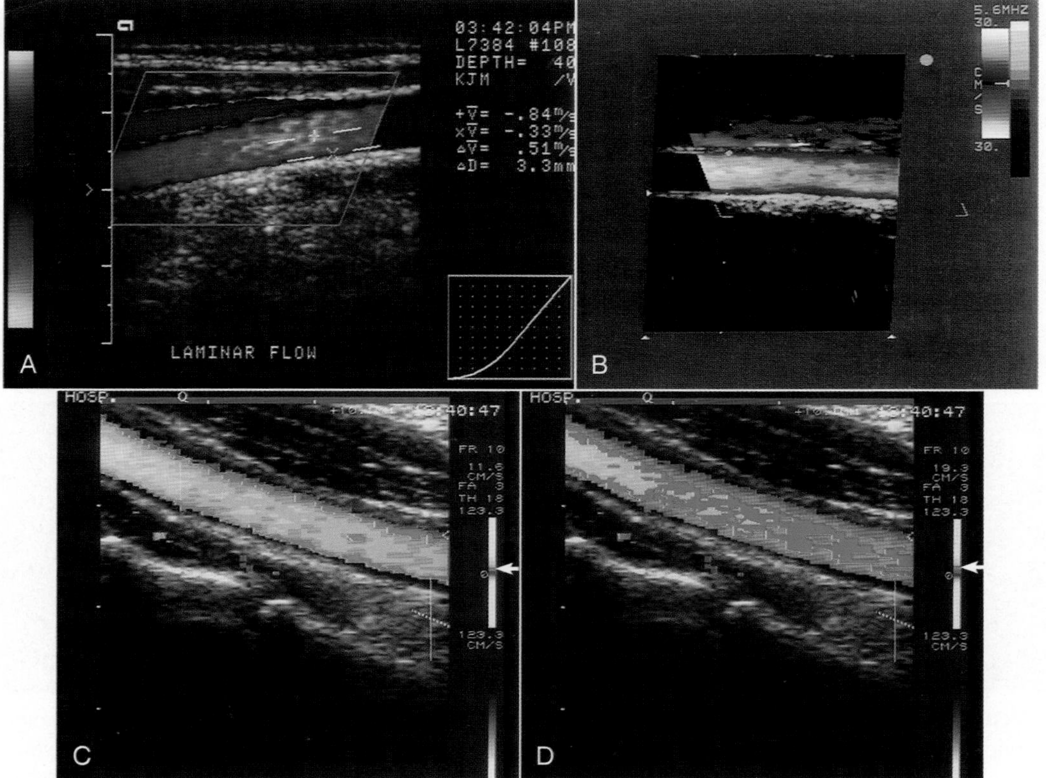

FIGURE 5-26 **A,** Digital readout of stored mean Doppler shift (converted to mean flow speed) at specific pixel locations. Conversion to speed requires angle correction. The value at the vessel center (84 cm/s) is greater than at the edge (33 cm/s), as expected for laminar flow. **B,** Laminar flow. The color bar used in this scan progresses from dark red and dark blue to bright white (indicating decreasing saturation and increasing luminance). The regions near the vessel wall are dark, with progressive brightening and decreasing saturation to white at the center left. This corresponds to the low flow speeds at the vessel wall and high flow speeds at the vessel center that are characteristic of laminar flow. **C,** The green tag is set at a specific level (11.6; *arrow*) on an angle-corrected, calibrated color bar. The green region on the display, therefore, indicates areas where that specific flow speed exists. **D,** The green tag is set at 19.3. As the set flow speed value increases, the indicated region *(green)* moves to the center, where higher speeds are expected. (**A** from Kremkau FW: Doppler principles, *Semin Roentgenol* 27:6–16, 1992; **B-D** from Kremkau FW: Principles and instrumentation. In Merritt CRB, editor: *Doppler color imaging,* New York, 1992, Churchill Livingstone.)

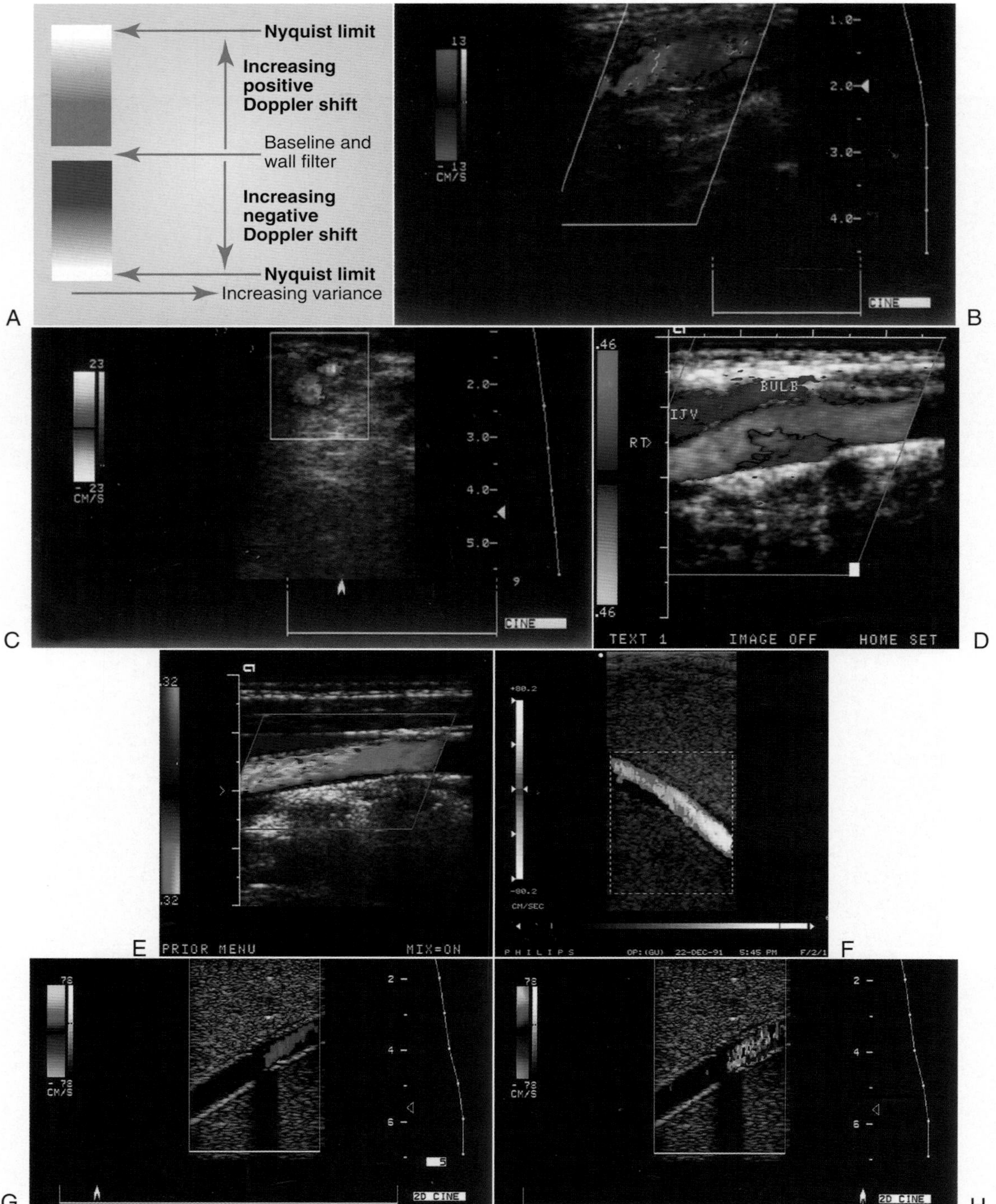

FIGURE 5-27 **Color map information. A,** Diagram describing the information contained in a color map or color bar. **B,** A luminance map. Increasing luminance of red or blue indicates, respectively, increasing positive or negative mean Doppler shifts. **C,** A saturation map is used to show flow transversely in two vessels. Flow in the upper vessel is toward the transducer, yielding positive Doppler shifts *(red).* Flow in the lower vessel is away from the transducer, yielding negative Doppler shifts *(blue).* On this color map, red and blue progress to white (decreasing saturation, increasing luminance) with increasing positive and negative Doppler shift means, respectively. **D,** A hue map showing flow in the carotid artery (with reversal in the bulb) and jugular vein. Increasingly positive Doppler shifts progress from dark blue to bright cyan *(blue plus green).* Increasingly negative Doppler shifts progress from dark red to bright yellow *(red plus green).* **E,** A luminance *(dark blue and red to bright blue and red)* map with variance included. Increasing variance adds green to red or blue *(producing yellow or cyan),* progressing from left to right across the map. **F,** A saturation map. Red and blue progress toward white. **G,** A stenosis in a tube *(located at the shadow)* increases the flow speed. Proximal to (left of) the stenosis, flow speed is too slow to be detected, whereas distal to (right of) the stenosis, positive Doppler shifts are seen. **H,** The variance map shows spectral broadening *(green)* in the turbulent flow region distal to the stenosis. (**A** from Kremkau FW: Principles and instrumentation. In Merritt CRB, editor*: Doppler color imaging,* New York, 1992, Churchill Livingstone; **B-F** from Kremkau FW: Principles of color flow imaging, *J Vasc Technol* 15:104–111, 1991.)

the color changes because the situation changes from upstream to downstream. However, this is not the case in Figure 5-28, *C*. All the pulses travel in the same direction (straight down) from this linear-array transducer. If the color change is not due to changing scan line directions, then it must be due to changing flow direction. Careful inspection of Figure 5-28, *C*, reveals that the vessel is not perfectly straight but curves up. Flow is from right to left in the vessel, so flow is away from the transducer on the right (negative Doppler shift is blue on this map) and toward the transducer on the left (positive Doppler shift is red; see Figure 5-28, *D*). A view further to the left reveals a second color change caused by the curve downward (see Figure 5-28, *E*). Figure 5-28, *F*, shows an example of lack of color in a vessel. This lack of Doppler shift could be caused by lack of flow or flow viewed with a 90-degree Doppler angle. With an acceptable angle (see Figure 5-28, *G*), flow is revealed.

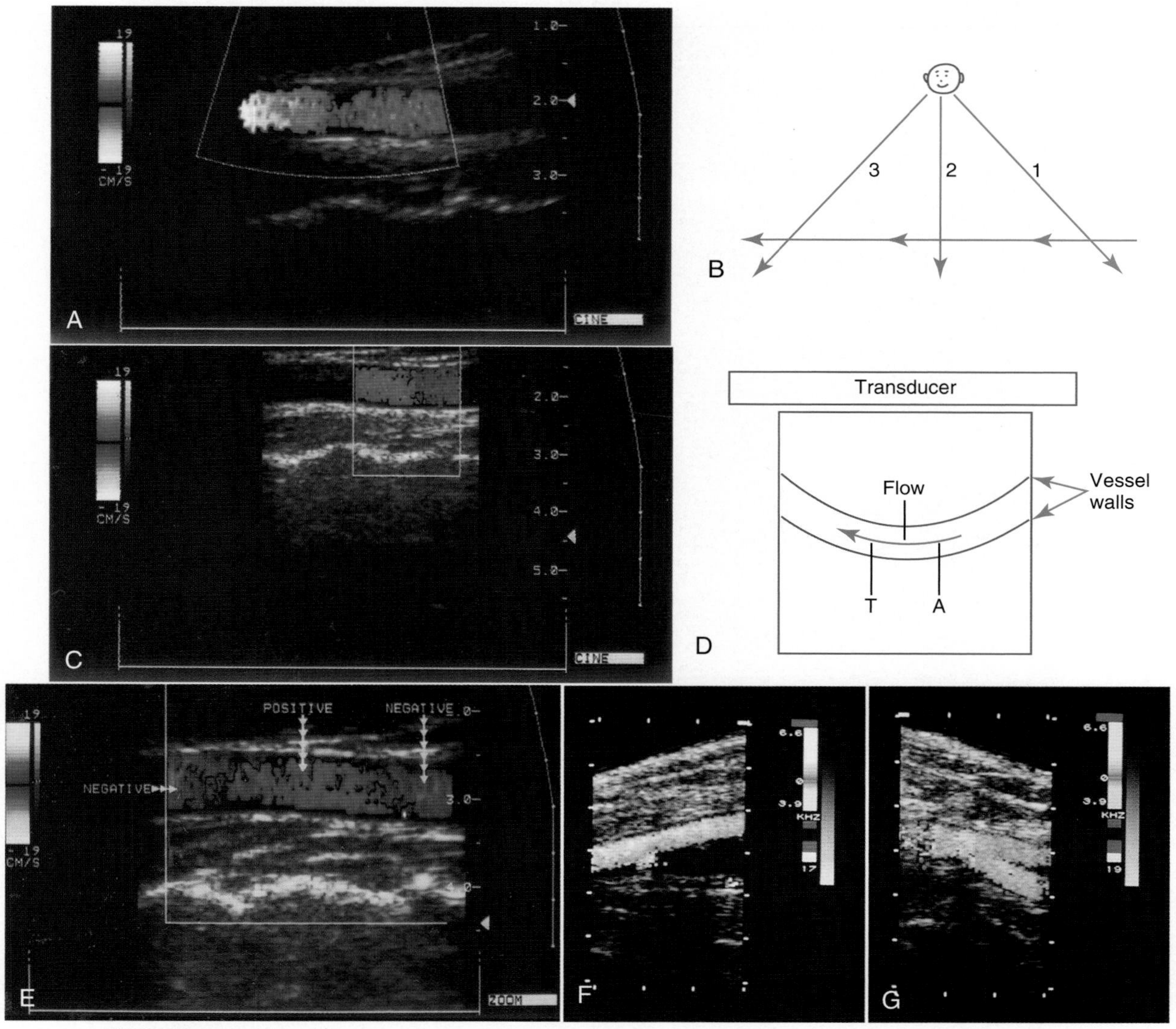

FIGURE 5-28 **A,** In this saturation map, blue and red are assigned to positive and negative Doppler shifts, respectively, progressing to white at the extremes. **B,** With flow moving from right to left, an observer looking to the right *(1)* is looking upstream; when looking to the left *(3)*, the observer has a downstream view. The perpendicular view *(2)* is neither upstream nor downstream. **C,** In this map, the color assignments are reversed from those in **A** (i.e., red and blue are assigned to positive and negative Doppler shifts, respectively). **D,** Exaggerated representation of the image in **C** in which point A represents flow away from the transducer and point T represents flow toward the transducer. **E,** Extension to the left of the color box in **C** reveals another color change caused by vessel curvature (concave-down). **F,** The profunda branch off the femoral artery appears to have no flow (no color within it). **G,** This view of the profunda shows color within it. The 90-degree Doppler angle in **F** causes no Doppler shift, and therefore color is lacking. (**A-C** from Kremkau FW: Principles of color flow imaging, *J Vasc Technol* 15:104–111, 1991; **E** from Kremkau FW: Color flow color assignments, *J Vasc Technol* 15:265–266, 1991.)

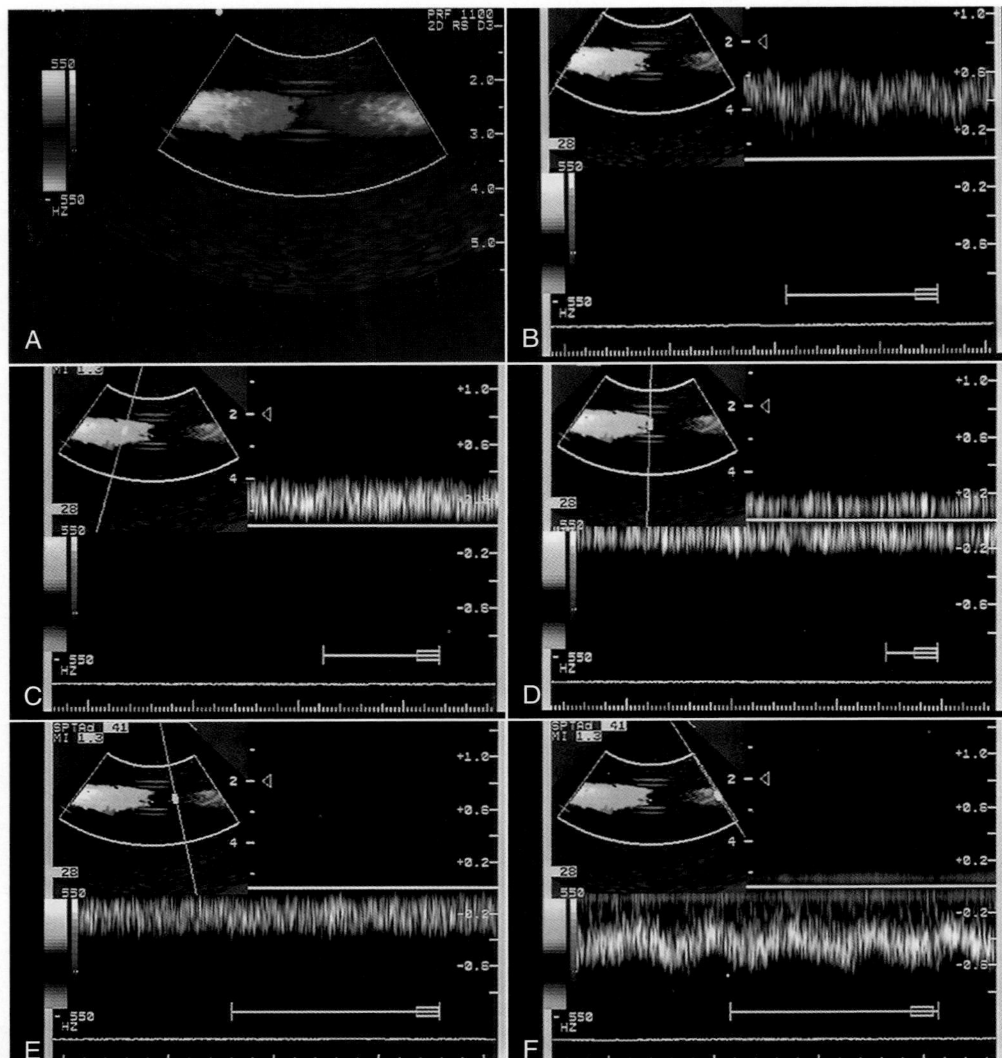

FIGURE 5-29 **Sector format, color-Doppler presentation of flow from left to right in a straight tube. A,** Approximate Doppler shifts (from the color map) are yellow (500 Hz), red (200 Hz), black (0 Hz), blue (−200 Hz), and cyan (−500 Hz). Spectra from these five regions (shown in **B–F**) confirm these estimates. Doppler shifts decrease while Doppler angles increase toward the center of the color window.

> A changing Doppler angle in an image produces various colors in different locations.

Figure 5-29, *A*, shows various Doppler shifts while the Doppler angle changes across the display in the sector format. Yellow corresponds to a large positive shift, red to a small positive shift, black to a zero shift, blue to a small negative shift, and cyan to a large negative shift. Flow is from left to right. Figure 5-29, *B–F*, confirms all this by spectral displays, which are discussed later in this chapter.

In Figure 5-30, some interesting questions arise. First, in *A*, what is the blood flow direction? According to the color map in the upper left-hand corner of the figure, negative Doppler shifts are coded in red and yellow, whereas positive Doppler shifts are coded in blue and cyan. The color scan lines (and pulses) are steered to the left, and negative Doppler shifts (red and yellow) are received from the blood flowing within the vessel in the upper and lower portions of the figure. If we are looking to the left and seeing blood flowing away from us (negative Doppler shifts), the blood must be flowing from right to left in the upper and lower horizontal portions of the vessel. What about the central portion of the vessel? Clearly, the blood would have to be flowing from left to right there, but why are negative Doppler shifts also seen in this portion? The answer is that this portion of the vessel is not horizontal but is angled down, so even though the blood is flowing from left to right, it is also flowing away from the transducer because of the downward direction (more precisely, it is flowing from upper left to lower right). Thus negative Doppler shifts are found throughout the vessel in this

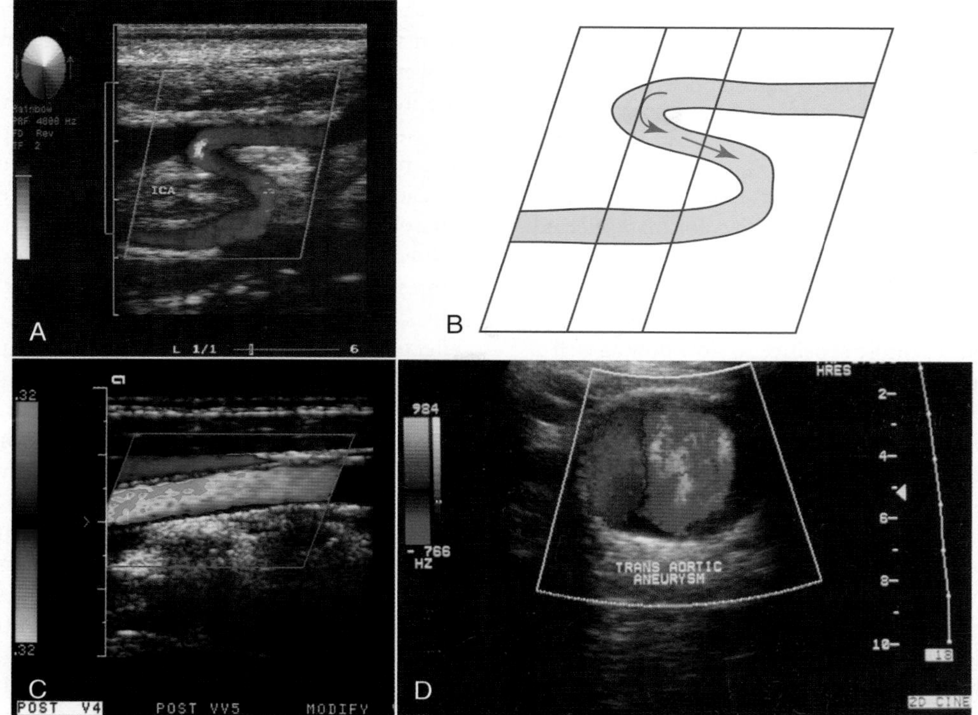

FIGURE 5-30 **A,** A tortuous artery. **B,** This drawing shows the angle relationships depicted in **A**. **C** shows an almost straight artery. **D,** Circular flow in an aneurysm. The black area between the red and blue areas indicates true flow reversal. (**A-C** from Kremkau FW: Color interpretation, *J Vasc Technol* 16:215–216, 1992.)

scan. In other words, the flow direction gets close to, but never crosses, the perpendicular to the scan lines (see Figure 5-30, *B*).

Another intriguing question arises with respect to Figure 5-30, *A*. Does the yellow region in the bend at the upper left indicate where the blood flows the fastest? According to the color map, this region is where the highest negative Doppler shifts are generated. Does that mean, however, that this is where the highest flow speeds are encountered? The answer in this case is no. The highest negative Doppler shifts are found in this region because the smallest Doppler angles are encountered there, and not because high flow speeds are found there. In this region, the flow is approximately parallel to the scan lines (see Figure 5-30, *B*), yielding Doppler angles of around zero. No evidence of vessel narrowing is present to explain increased flow speed. The increased Doppler shift can be explained purely on grounds of angle.

In Figure 5-30, *C*, the region shown in cyan (aqua or blue-green) indicates positive Doppler shifts according to the color map, whereas the blood flow in the rest of the vessel is generating negative Doppler shifts (red and yellow). Again, the scan lines are steered to the left, so negative Doppler shifts indicate that we are looking downstream, seeing flow away from the transducer. Therefore blood flow is from right to left in this carotid artery, with the head oriented to the left as usual. How then can we explain the positive Doppler shifts found in the upper left-hand portion of the vessel? Possibilities include turbulent flow, flow reversal, and flow speed exceeding 32 cm/s in this region, producing aliasing. Flow reversal and turbulent flow can be eliminated because the region between the negative (red and yellow) and positive (cyan) Doppler shift regions contains no dark or black region (baseline indicating flow reversal). One can easily distinguish between true flow reversal (which involves dark regions, as shown around the baseline of the color bar) (see Figure 5-30, *D*) and aliasing (which involves bright colors, as indicated at the bar extremes). Thus the aqua region is a region of flow away from the transducer that has exceeded the negative aliasing limit of 32 cm/s and has become an aliased positive Doppler shift (cyan).

Does this mean that the flow speed in the aliased aqua region exceeds 32 cm/s? In this case the answer is no. The aliasing limit, which is one half the PRF, has been exceeded. This aliasing limit has been converted, using the Doppler equation, to an equivalent flow speed of 32 cm/s, as indicated at the map extremes. However, because there is no angle correction in this scan, an angle of zero was assumed in the conversion from the Doppler shift to flow speed. Therefore aliased flow exceeds 32 cm/s only when it is parallel to the scan lines. Because the Doppler angle in this example is approximately 60 degrees, the Doppler shifts are only about one-half what they would be at zero degrees. Therefore the flow in the aliased region has exceeded approximately 64 cm/s. One must exercise care in estimating flow speeds with tagging (see Figure 5-26, *C–D*) or aliasing limits that are converted to flow speed units without correcting for angle.

> Proper understanding of the effects of angle on the Doppler shift and of how color is related to the Doppler shift is necessary to interpret complex images properly.

Doppler-Power Displays

Doppler shift displays encode mean Doppler shifts in a two-dimensional matrix according to the color map selected. **Doppler-power displays** (also called power Doppler) present two-dimensional Doppler information by color-encoding the *strength* of Doppler shifts. This approach is free of aliasing and angle dependence and is more sensitive to slow flow as well as flow in small or deep vessels. Names applied to this technique include *color power Doppler, ultrasound angio, color-Doppler energy,* and *color power angio.* Rather than assigning various hue, saturation, and luminance values to mean Doppler shift frequency values, as in Doppler shift displays, this technique assigns these color values to Doppler shift *power* values. The power of Doppler shifts is determined by the *concentration* of moving scatterers producing the Doppler shifts and is independent of Doppler shift frequency and Doppler angle. In addition to the colors already encountered, magenta (a combination of red and blue) is used on some Doppler-power maps.

> Doppler-power displays color-encode Doppler shift power values on the display.

The Doppler detector in color-Doppler imaging instruments yields the sign, mean, variance, and amplitude and power of the **Doppler spectrum** (Figure 5-31, *A*) at each of the hundreds of **sample volume** locations in an anatomic cross-section. Traditionally, in color-Doppler imaging, sign and mean Doppler shift, and sometimes variance (usually in cardiac applications), are color-encoded and displayed. These parameters depend on the Doppler angle and are subject to aliasing (Figure 5-32, *A*). Power Doppler integrates the area under the spectrum (see Figure 5-31, B). This area is independent of angle and aliasing, displaying the effects of neither (see Figure 5-32, *B*). Thus an advantage of Doppler-power displays is the uniform (angle-independent and alias-free) presentation of flow information, although this is accomplished with a loss in direction, speed, and flow character information. This extends even through regions of 90-degree Doppler angle (see Figure 5-32, *B–C*) because the Doppler-shift spectrum there has a nonzero area (see Figure 5-31, *B*), even though its mean is zero, yielding a black region in color-Doppler imaging displays (see Figure 5-32, *A,C*). Power Doppler is also essentially free of variations in flow speed (as in the cardiac cycle) and thus can be frame averaged to improve the signal-to-noise ratio and sensitivity substantially (Figure 5-33). Because aliasing is not a problem in power Doppler, lower PRFs can be used to detect slow flows. Box 5-3 lists the advantages and disadvantages of Doppler-power displays. In general, Doppler

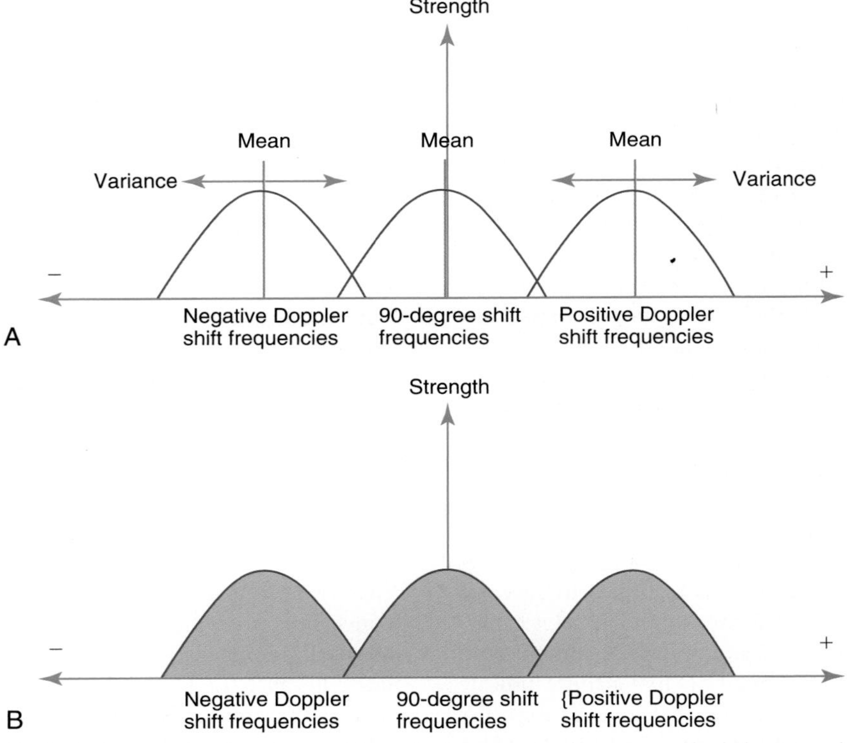

FIGURE 5-31 **A,** Spectra for flow toward (positive) and away from (negative) the transducer and perpendicular (90 degrees) to the sound beam. Conventional color-Doppler imaging determines and displays, in color-coded form, the sign and mean (and sometimes the variance) of the Doppler shift frequency spectrum. **B,** Doppler power determines and displays, in color-coded form, the size of the area under the spectral curve. The axes of the spectral graph represent strength (amplitude, power, energy, or intensity) versus frequency.

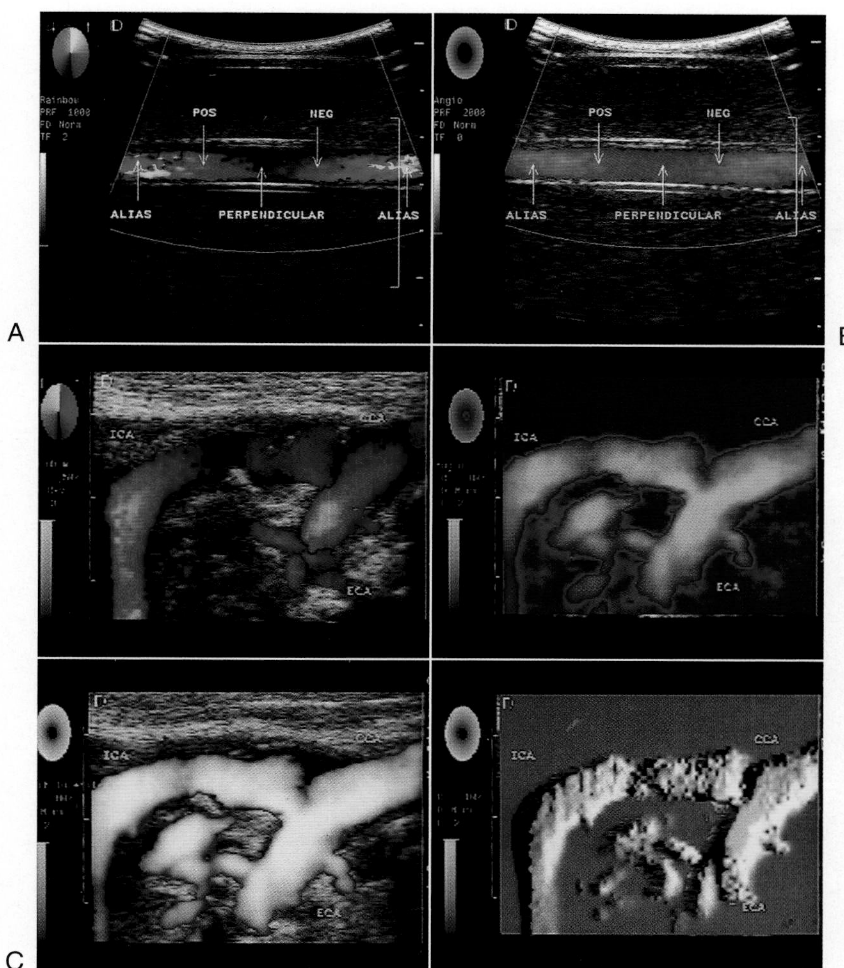

FIGURE 5-32 **A,** A color-Doppler shift image of flow in a straight tube, acquired in sector format. The varying Doppler angle from left to right yields aliasing and positive, negative, and zero Doppler-shift regions. **B,** A Doppler-power presentation of the situation shown in **A** yields a uniform image, free of angle dependence and aliasing. However, it contains no directional, speed, or dynamic information. **C,** Angle independence is seen in the Doppler-power images of the carotid artery; compare them with the Doppler shift display *(upper left)*. Doppler-power imaging is shown in color, topographic, and gray-scale forms *(clockwise from upper right)*. (See also Figure 1-13, *B–C*.)

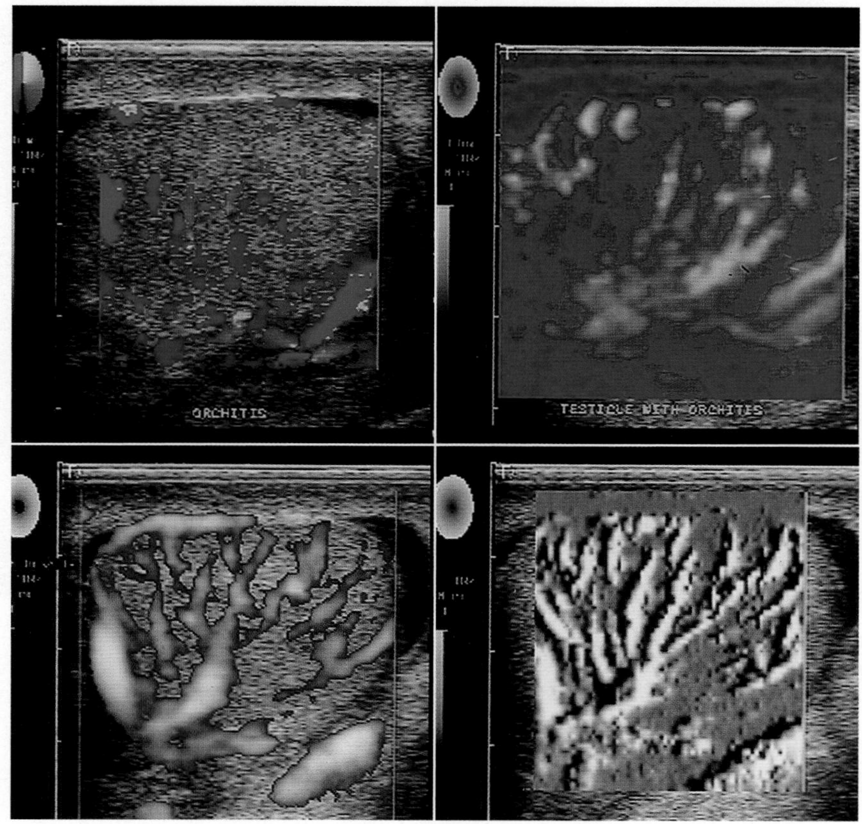

FIGURE 5-33 **A,** Improved sensitivity to testicular flow compared with Doppler shift imaging *(upper left)*. Small vessel flow is imaged in fetal pulmonary vasculature

Continued

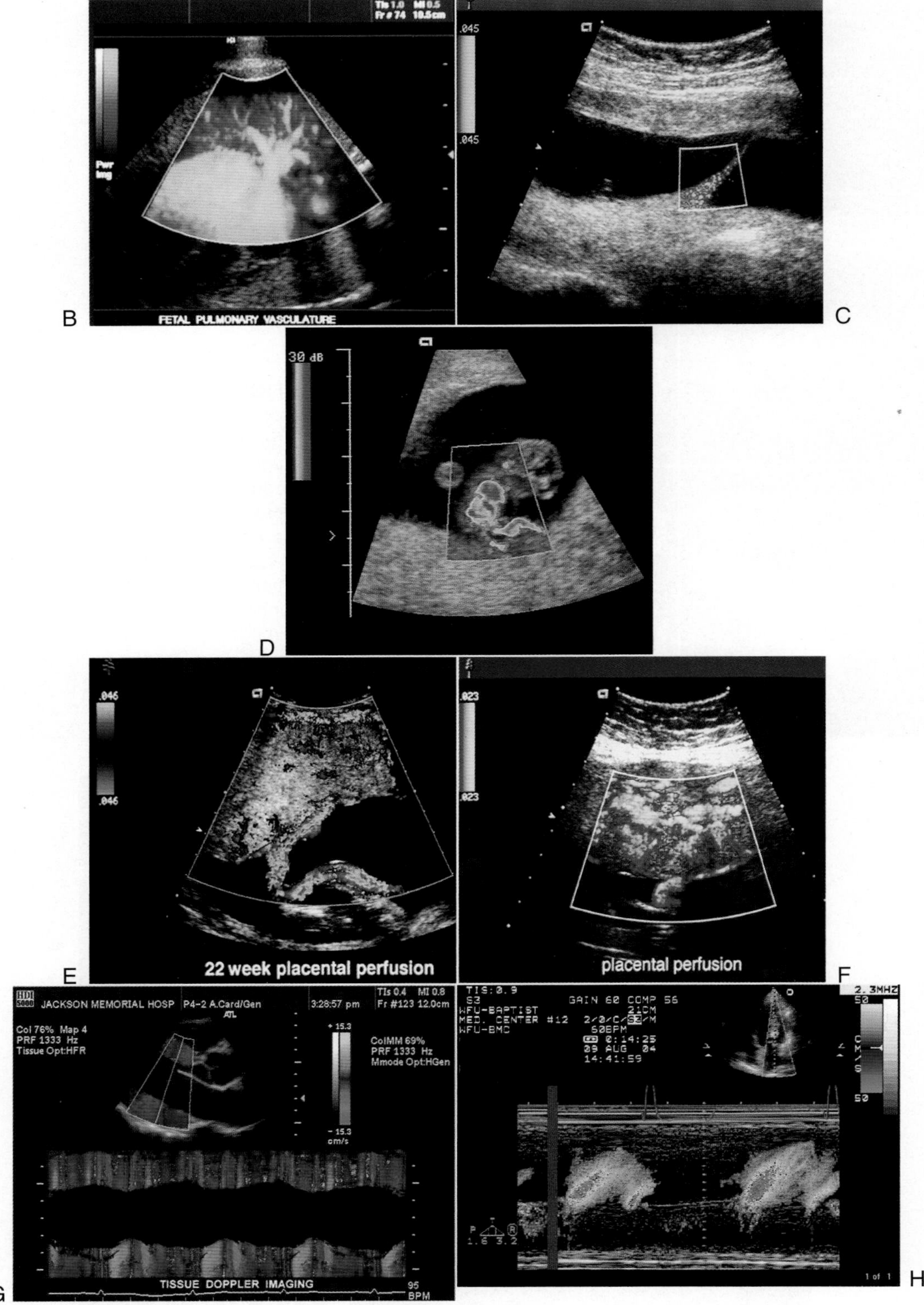

FIGURE 5-33, cont'd (B) and within the membrane separating a twin gestation (C). D, First-trimester fetal circulation. A comparison of placental Doppler shift imaging (E) and Doppler-power imaging (F) reveals improved flow detection with the latter. M-mode color-Doppler displays of myocardial motion (G) and ventricular inflow in the heart (H).

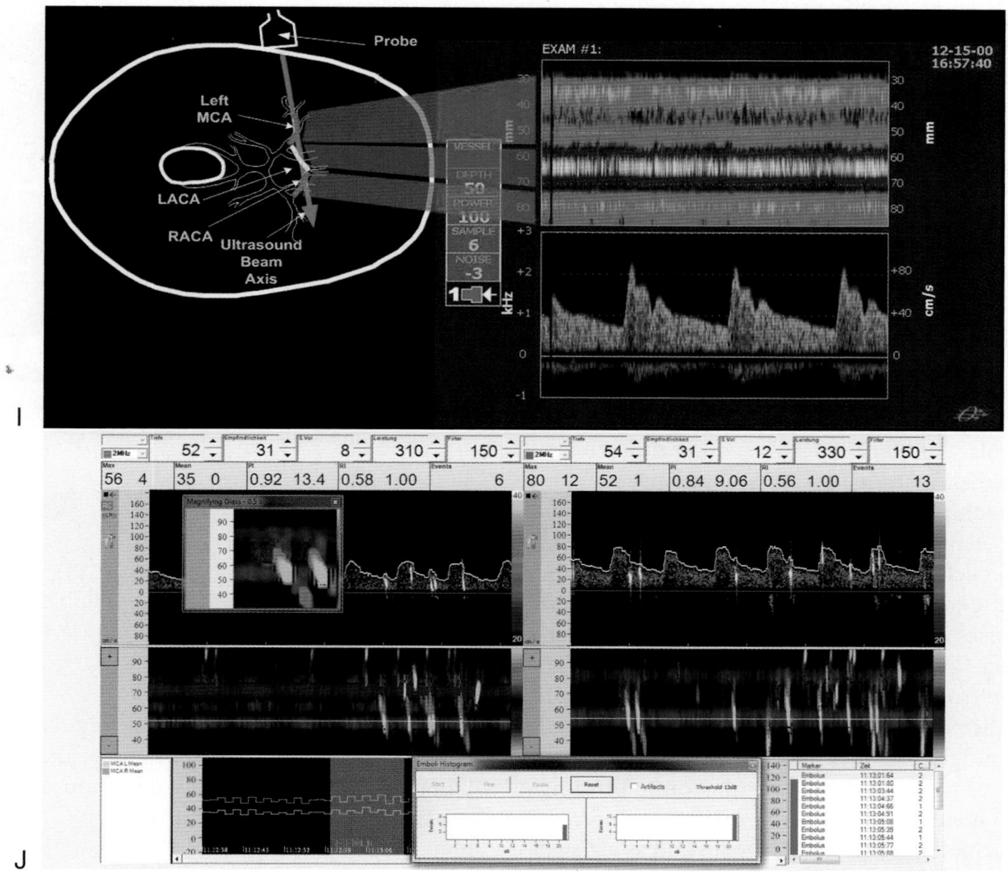

FIGURE 5-33, cont'd I, Power-Doppler M mode in transcranial Doppler. Red indicates flow toward and blue flow away from the transducer. The horizontal line at the 50-mm depth on the M-mode presentation indicates the depth from which the spectral display below is obtained. **J,** Power-Doppler M-mode transcranial Doppler shows traveling emboli (the bright slanted Doppler shifts in the lower half of the display). (Courtesy John Bennett, PhD; **I,** courtesy of Spencer Technologies.)

BOX 5-3 Advantages and Disadvantages of Doppler-Power Displays with Respect to Doppler-Shift Displays

Advantages

- Angle independence
- No aliasing
- Improved sensitivity (deeper penetration, smaller vessels, slower flows)

Disadvantages

- No directional information
- No flow speed information
- No flow character information

ultrasound can determine (1) the presence or absence of flow, (2) the direction and (3) speed of flow, and (4) the character of flow. Power Doppler is superior in terms of the first, but at the expense of the other three. Table 5-6 compares color-Doppler displays.

> Doppler-power displays do not have direction, speed, or flow character information included and are insensitive to angle effects and aliasing. They are more sensitive than Doppler-shift displays in that they can present slower flows as well as flows in deeper or tinier vessels.

Recall that motion mode (M mode) presents a depth versus time display to record motion of moving structures (see Figure 4-38). With a stationary beam, color-Doppler presents a motion versus time display of Doppler shifts produced by moving tissue or blood flow (see Figure 5-33, *G-H*). Power-Doppler M-mode displays have been applied to transcranial Doppler (TCD) imaging to assist in navigating the intracranial vasculature (see Figure 5-33, *I*) and confirm the presence of emboli (see Figure 5-33, *J*).

SPECTRAL-DOPPLER DISPLAYS

In addition to color-Doppler operation, two types of spectral-Doppler operation—continuous-wave (CW) and pulsed-wave (PW)—are used for Doppler presentation of flow

TABLE 5-6 Comparison of Doppler-Shift Display and Doppler-Power Display

Presentation	Doppler Shift Display	Doppler Power Display
Quantitative	No	No
Global	Yes	Yes
Perfusion	No	Yes

in the heart and in blood vessels. All three are combined into one multipurpose instrument (Figure 5-34). CW operation detects Doppler-shifted echoes in the region of overlap between the beams of the transmitting and receiving transducer elements. Differences between other transducers and those designed exclusively for CW Doppler use are that the latter are not damped and that they have separate sending and receiving elements. PW operation emits ultrasound pulses and receives echoes using a single element transducer or an array. Because of the required Doppler frequency shift detection, the pulses are longer than those used in imaging. Through **range gating**, PW Doppler has the ability to select information from a particular depth along the beam. To use PW Doppler effectively, it commonly is combined with gray-scale sonography. Such operation is called *duplex scanning* because of the dual functions (anatomic imaging and flow measurement). CW and PW operations present Doppler shift information in an audible form and as a visual display.

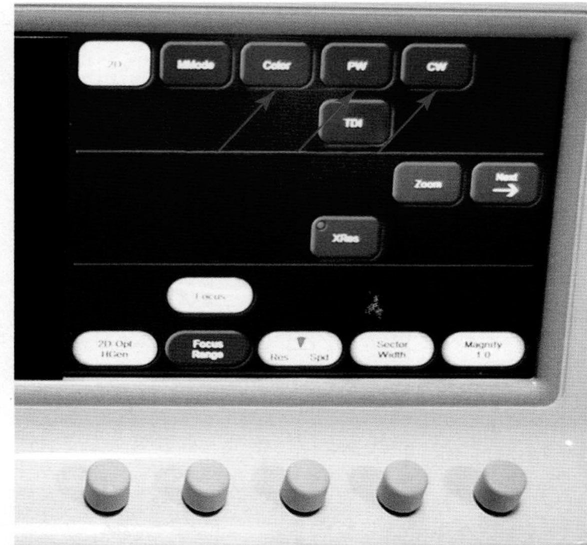

FIGURE 5-34 Continuous-wave (CW), pulsed-wave (PW), and color-Doppler modes are available in one instrument, with each mode selectable from the control panel *(arrows)*.

Continuous-Wave Operation

Spectral-Doppler operation provides continuous or pulsed voltages to the transducer and converts echo voltages received from the transducer to audible and visual information corresponding to scatterer motion. If an instrument distinguishes between positive and negative Doppler shifts, it is called **bidirectional**. **Continuous-wave Doppler** instruments include a CW oscillator and a Doppler detector that detects the changes in frequency (Doppler shifts) resulting from scatterer motion and presents them as audible sounds and as a visual display corresponding to the motion.

Components of a Continuous-Wave Doppler System

A diagram of the components of a CW Doppler system is presented in Figure 5-35, *A*. The oscillator produces a continuously alternating voltage with a 2- to 10-MHz frequency, which is applied to the source transducer element. The ultrasound frequency is determined by the oscillator and is set to equal the operating frequency of the transducer. In the transducer assembly there is a separate receiving transducer element that produces voltages with frequencies equal to the frequencies of the returning echoes. If there is scatterer motion, the reflected ultrasound and the ultrasound produced by the source transducer will have different frequencies. The Doppler detector detects the difference between these two frequencies, which is the Doppler shift, and drives a loudspeaker at this frequency. Doppler shifts are typically one thousandth of the operating frequency, which puts them in the audible range. Doppler shifts also are commonly sent through a **spectrum analyzer** to a **spectral-Doppler display** for visual observation and evaluation.

The detector (see Figure 5-35, *B*) amplifies the echo voltages it receives from the receiving element, detects the Doppler shift information in the returning echoes, and determines the motion direction from the sign of the Doppler shift. Doppler shifts are determined by mixing the returning voltages with the CW voltage from the oscillator. This produces the sum and difference of the oscillator and echo frequencies (see Figure 5-35, *B*). The difference is the desired Doppler shift. The sum is a much higher frequency (approximately double the operating frequency) and is filtered out. The difference is zero for echoes returning from stationary structures. In the case of echoes from moving structures or flowing blood, this difference is the Doppler shift, which provides information about motion and flow (positive or negative).

> The Doppler detector detects Doppler shifts and determines their sign (positive or negative).

Positive and negative shifts indicate motion toward and away from the transducer, respectively. The detector shown in Figure 5-35, *B*, does not provide this directional information. Determining direction and separating Doppler shift voltages into separate forward and reverse channels is accomplished by the **phase quadrature** detector. The forward and reverse channel signals are sent to separate

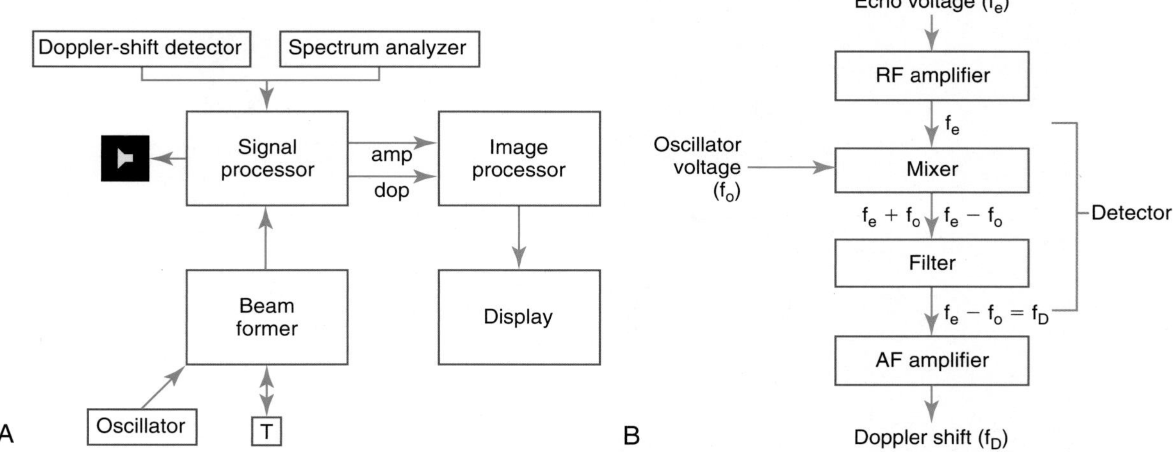

FIGURE 5-35 **A,** Block diagram of a sonographic instrument functioning in continuous-wave Doppler mode. The oscillator (part of the beam former) produces a continuously alternating voltage that drives the source transducer element *(T)*. The receiving transducer element *(T)* produces a continuous voltage in response to echoes it is continuously receiving. The signal processor includes a Doppler shift detector that detects differences in frequency between the voltages produced by the oscillator and by the receiving element. The Doppler shifts produce voltages that drive the loudspeakers and a visual display. The frequency of the audible sound is equal to the Doppler shift and is proportional to the reflector speed and to the cosine of the angle between the sound propagation direction and the boundary motion. **B,** Block diagram of a continuous-wave Doppler detector. The radio frequency *(RF)* amplifier increases the echo voltage amplitude. The frequency of the echo voltage is f_e. In the mixer, this frequency is combined with the oscillator voltage, the frequency of which is f_o. The mixer yields the sum and difference of these two frequency inputs ($f_e + f_o$ and $f_e - f_o$). The low-pass (high-frequency rejection) filter removes $f_e + f_o$, leaving $f_e - f_o$, which is the Doppler shift frequency (f_D). This frequency then is strengthened in the audio frequency *(AF)* amplifier. The mixer and filter together constitute the Doppler detector.

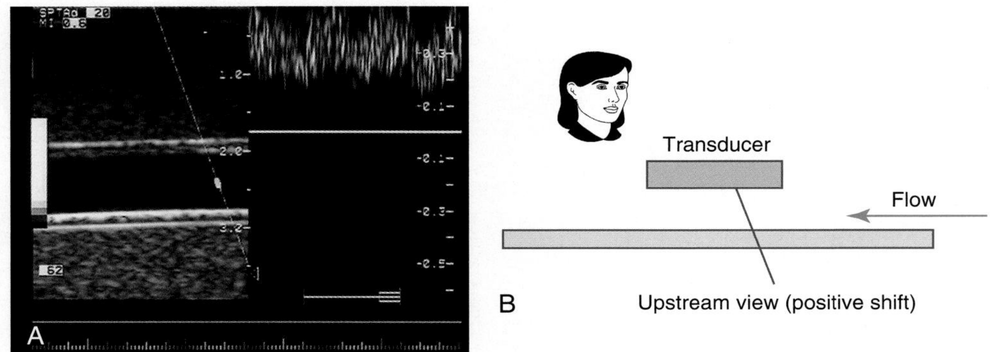

FIGURE 5-36 The beam is steered to the right and positive Doppler shifts are received **(A)**. Thus this is an upstream view **(B)**, and flow is from right to left. Therefore steering the beam to the left

Continued

loudspeakers so that forward and reverse Doppler shifts can be heard separately. The signals also are sent to a visual display to show positive and negative Doppler shifts above and below the display baseline, which represents zero Doppler shift (Figure 5-36).

Continuous-Wave Sample Volume

CW operation detects flow that occurs anywhere within the intersection of the transmitting and receiving beams of the dual-transducer assembly (Figure 5-37). The sample volume is the region from which Doppler-shifted echoes return and are presented audibly or visually. In this case the sample volume is the overlapping region of the transmitting and receiving beams. Because the sample volume is large, CW Doppler systems can give complex and confusing presentations if two or more different motions or flows are included in the sample volume (e.g., two blood vessels viewed simultaneously). **Pulsed-Doppler** systems solve this problem by detecting motion or flow at a selected depth with a relatively small sample volume. However, the large sample volume of a CW system is helpful when searching for a Doppler maximum associated with a vascular or valvular stenosis.

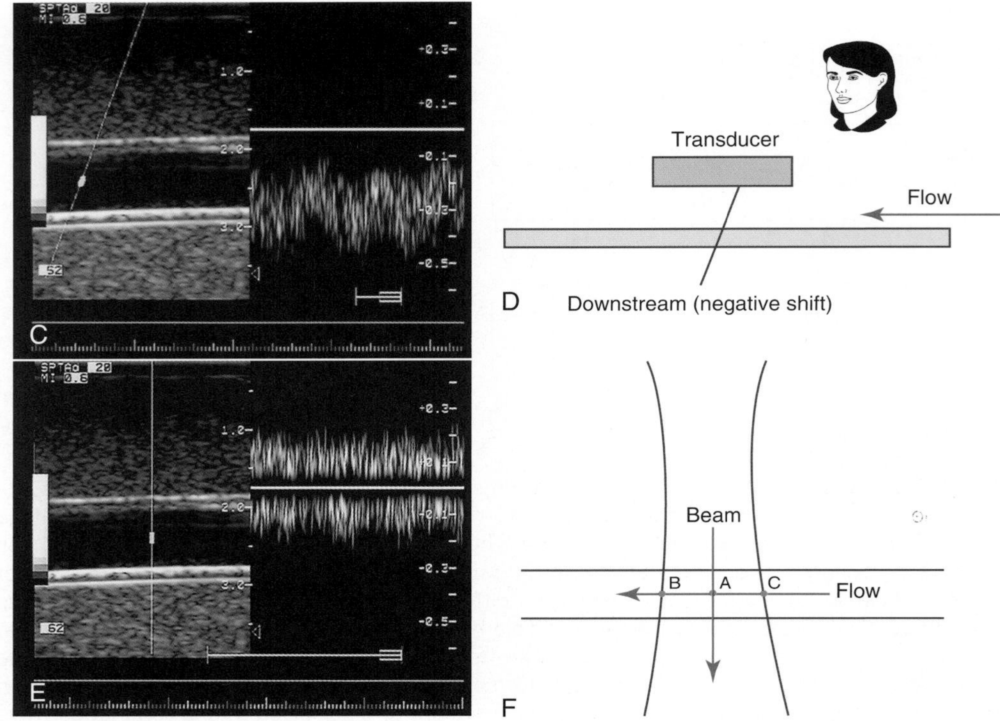

FIGURE 5-36, cont'd (C) would provide a downstream view (D) with negative Doppler shifts. With the beam perpendicular to the flow (E), Doppler shifts are received, both positive and negative, because of beam spreading (F); that is, a portion of the beam views upstream while a portion views downstream. The beam axis portion (90-degree angle) yields a zero Doppler shift.

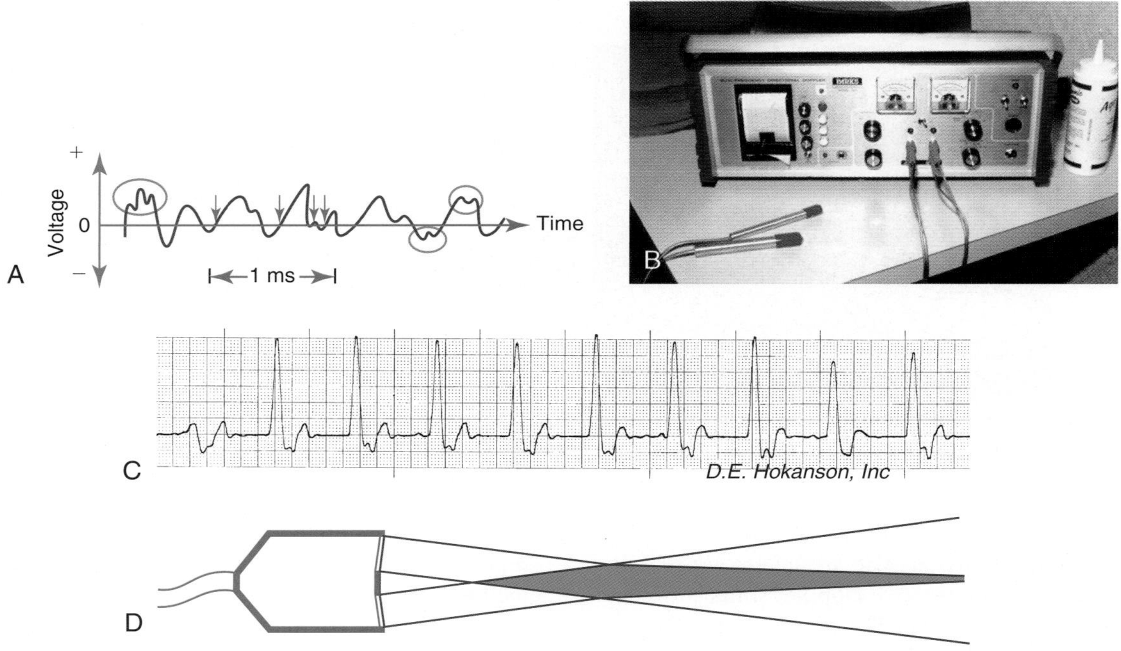

FIGURE 5-37 **A,** A zero-crossing detector counts the number of zero crossings per second in the positive or negative direction. In the 1-ms period shown, four zero crossings (negative to positive) occurred *(arrows),* corresponding to a mean frequency of 4 kHz. Higher frequencies that are missed by the zero-crossing technique are circled. **B,** A zero-crossing continuous-wave Doppler instrument. **C,** Chart output from a zero-crossing instrument shows a time-varying average Doppler shift. **D,** Continuous-wave Doppler systems have dual-element transducer assemblies, one for transmitting and one for receiving. The region over which Doppler information can be acquired (Doppler sample volume) is the region of overlap between the transmitting and receiving beams *(green region).*

Because a distribution of flow velocities is encountered by the beam as it traverses a vessel, a distribution of many Doppler-shifted frequencies returns to the transducer and the instrument. In arterial circulation or in the heart, these Doppler shifts are changing continually over the cardiac cycle and are displayed as a function of time with appropriate real-time frequency-spectrum processing (Figure 5-38). These displays provide quantitative data for evaluating Doppler-shifted echoes. The display device is, again, the flat-panel display. The displayed Doppler information is stored in the digital memory before it is displayed so that it can be frozen and backed through the last few seconds of preceding information.

Angle Incorporation or Correction

To convert a display correctly from Doppler shift versus time to flow speed versus time, the Doppler angle must be incorporated accurately into the calculation process (Figure 5-39). This incorporation is commonly called *angle correction* Either term is appropriate because lack of angle incorporation leaves the instrument to assume that the Doppler angle is zero, which is incorrect unless the angle is, in fact, zero. Figure 5-39, *B*, illustrates the importance of accurate angle correction. Figure 5-39, *C-F*, shows errors encountered when the Doppler angle is handled incorrectly. Recall that as angle increases, the Doppler shift decreases. Thus, when the

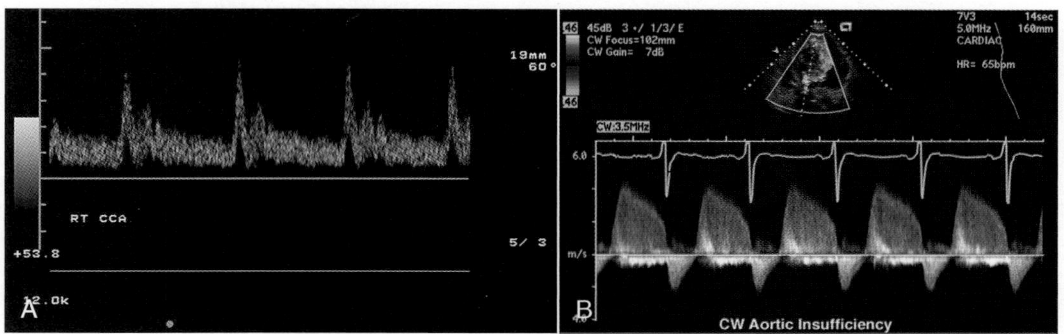

FIGURE 5-38 **A,** A display of vascular Doppler shift frequencies as a function of time. This is a pulsed-wave Doppler spectral display. **B,** A cardiac continuous-wave Doppler spectral display.

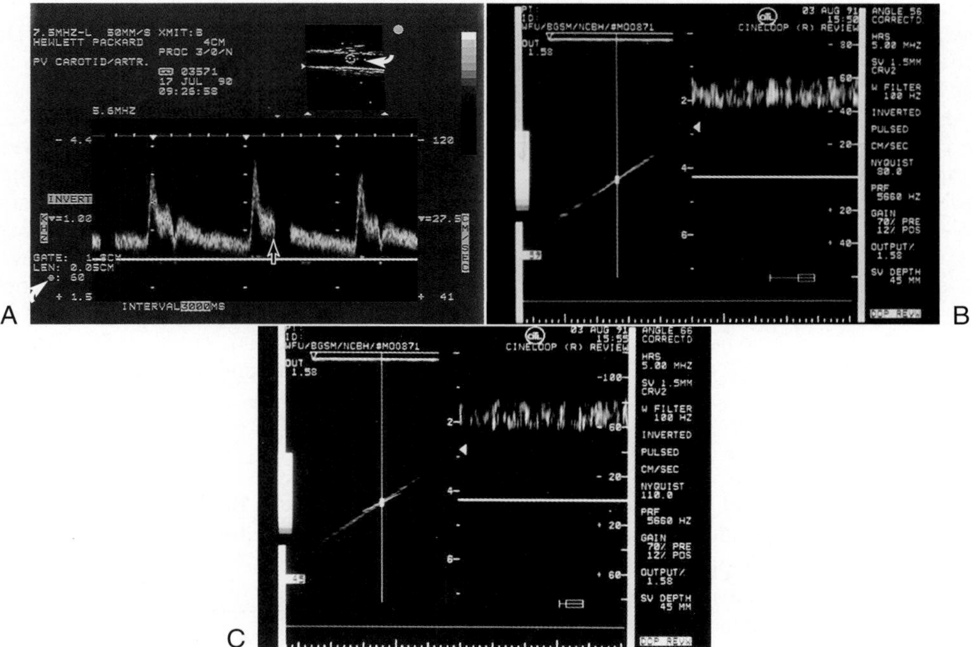

FIGURE 5-39 **A,** A spectral display with Doppler-shift (kilohertz) calibration of the vertical axis on the left and flow speed (cm/s, centimeters per second) calibration on the right. Conversion from the former to the latter requires angle incorporation *(curved arrows)*. The Doppler angle in this example is 60 degrees. The gap in Doppler information *(open arrow)* occurs when the instrument takes time to generate a frame of the anatomic image *(upper right)*. **B–C,** A moving-string test object is imaged, resulting in the Doppler spectral display shown. With proper angle incorporation (56 degrees) the 50 cm/s string speed is shown correctly **(B)**. With improper angle incorporation (66 degrees), an incorrect string speed of 70 cm/s is shown **(C)**. This is a 40% error.

Continued

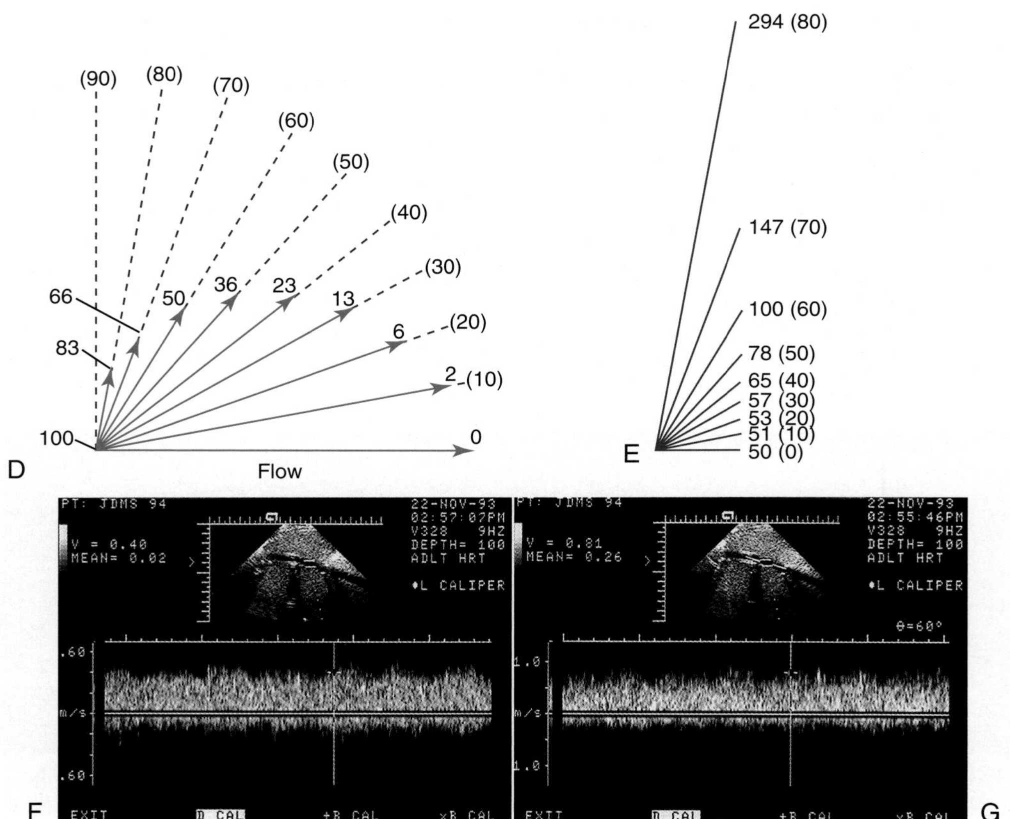

FIGURE 5-39, cont'd D, If a zero Doppler angle is assumed correctly, there is zero error in the calculated flow speed. However, if the angle is actually nonzero, error results. The error in flow speed increases as the angle error (in parentheses) increases. For example, if the Doppler angle is 10 degrees but is assumed to be zero, the calculated flow speed will be 2% less than the correct value. At 60 and 80 degrees, the errors are 50% and 83%, respectively. At 90 degrees, there is zero Doppler shift. The calculated flow speed is zero (100% error). **E,** If the Doppler angle is zero but is assumed to be some other value, the calculated flow speeds are too large. Here, the correct value is 50 cm/s. The error increases with angle *(in parentheses).* For example, at 60 and 80 degrees, the calculated values are 100 and 294 cm/s, respectively. **F,** No angle correction is used in this display. The instrument assumes a Doppler angle of zero and calculates flow speed (*v*) at 40 cm/s. However, the Doppler angle is actually 60 degrees, yielding half the Doppler shift that a zero-degree angle would. **G,** When the cosine of 60 degrees (0.5) is incorporated into the Doppler equation, the result is 81 cm/s. (**B-C** from Kremkau FW: Doppler principles, *Semin Roentgenol* 27:6–16, 1992; **F–G** from Kremkau FW: Doppler, *J Diagn Med Sonogr* 10:337–338, 1994. Reprinted by permission of Sage Publications, Inc.)

angle indicator on the instrument is set at 60 degrees, the instrument responds by doubling the calculated flow speed from what it would have been at a Doppler angle of zero. In other words, the Doppler equation, arranged to have the calculated flow speed alone on one side of the equal sign, has the cosine Doppler angle in the denominator on the other side. As the angle indicator is increased, the cosine decreases, increasing the calculated speed value. This compensates for the reduction in the Doppler shift caused by the Doppler angle actually involved in the ultrasound beam and flow intersection. For example, if the actual Doppler angle is 60 degrees, the Doppler shift is half what it would have been at zero degrees. If the angle is set properly on the instrument at 60, the cosine in the denominator of the Doppler equation is set at 0.5. This doubles the calculated flow speed to the correct value.

> The Doppler sample volume of a continuous-wave Doppler instrument is relatively large, being the overlapping region of the transmission and reception beams.

Wall Filter

In Doppler studies, a wall filter that rejects frequencies below an adjustable value is used to eliminate the high-intensity, low-frequency Doppler shift echoes, called **clutter**, caused by

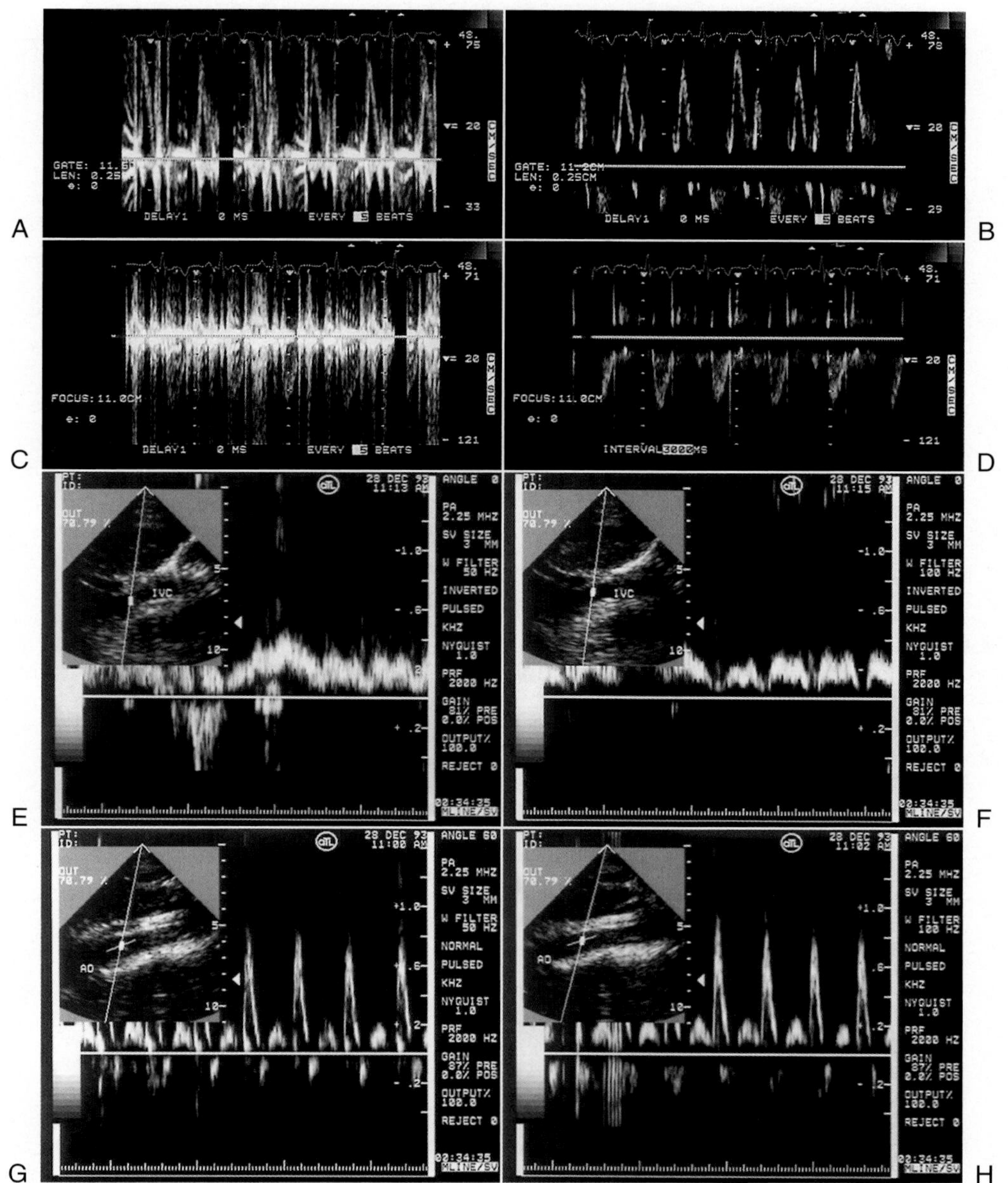

FIGURE 5-40 A, Clutter in the spectrum of inflow at the mitral valve is shown. **B,** The clutter in A is removed by increasing the wall filter setting. **C,** Clutter in the spectrum of the left ventricular outflow tract. **D,** The clutter in C is removed with an increase in the wall filter setting. **E,** Clutter in the display of inferior vena caval flow. **F,** The clutter shown in E is removed by adjusting the wall filter from 50 to 100 Hz. **G,** Clutter in the display of aortic flow. **H,** The clutter shown in **G** is removed by adjusting the wall filter.

Continued

heart or vessel wall or cardiac valve motion with pulsatile flow (Figure 5-40). Sometimes called *wall-thump filter,* the filter rejects these strong echoes that otherwise would overwhelm the weaker echoes from blood. These strong echoes have low Doppler shift frequencies because the tissue structures do not move as fast as blood does. The upper limit of the filter is adjustable over a range of approximately 25 to 3200 Hz. However, the **filter**, if not properly used, can erroneously alter conclusions with regard to diastolic flow and distal flow resistance by eliminating legitimate lower-frequency Doppler shifts.

> Wall filters remove clutter (low-frequency Doppler shifts from moving tissue).

Pulsed-Wave Operation

A diagram of the components of pulsed-wave Doppler operation is given in Figure 5-41, *A*. The pulser (in the beam former) functions as it does in sonographic imaging, except that it generates pulses of several cycles of voltage that drive the transducer where ultrasound pulses are

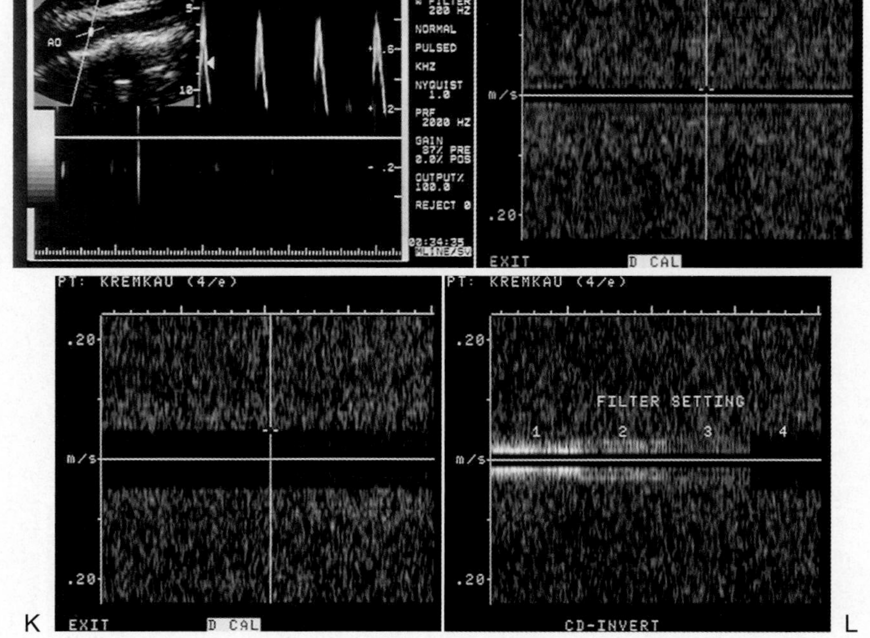

FIGURE 5-40, cont'd **I,** The wall filter is set too high (200 Hz), eliminating all but the peak systolic portion of the spectrum. **J,** Using electronic noise on the spectrum (with high Doppler gain), a low wall filter setting eliminates Doppler shifts corresponding to flow speeds of less than 1 cm/s. **K,** A higher setting eliminates speeds of less than 5 cm/s. **L,** Four wall filter settings reduce or eliminate frequencies as shown.

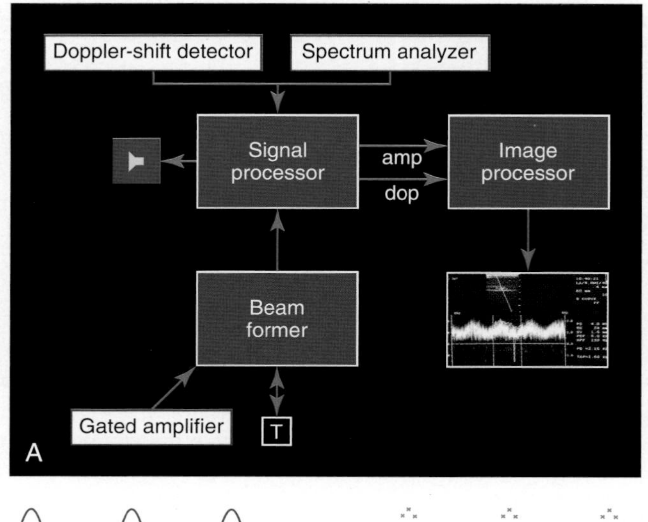

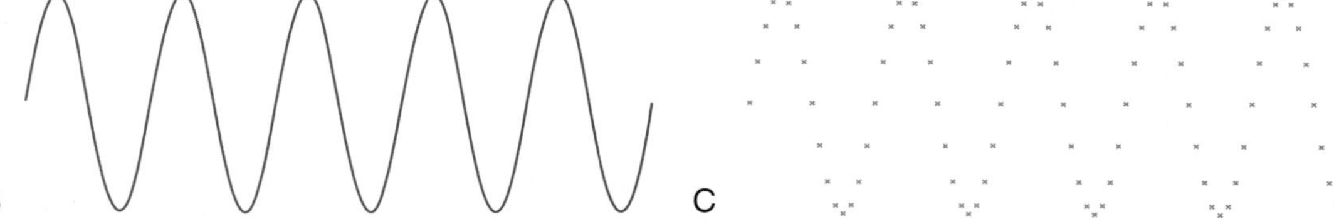

FIGURE 5-41 **A,** Block diagram of a sonographic instrument functioning in pulsed-wave Doppler mode. The beam former produces voltage pulses of several cycles each, which drive the transducer (T). The signal processor includes a Doppler-shift detector, where shift frequencies are compared with the frequency of the outgoing pulses. The difference (the Doppler shift) is sent to the loudspeakers and, through the spectrum analyzer and image processor, to the display. The beam former also contains a gate that selects echoes from a given depth according to arrival time and thus gives motion information from a selected depth. **B,** Five cycles of a 500-Hz Doppler shift frequency occurring in 10 ms of time. **C,** In a pulsed-wave Doppler instrument, each pulse yields echoes from the sample volume. These echoes, after Doppler detection, yield samples (x) of the Doppler shift from the sample volume. In this example, 80 samples are determined in a 10-ms time period. Therefore the pulse repetition frequency of the instrument is 8 kHz (with each pulse yielding one sample of the Doppler shift).

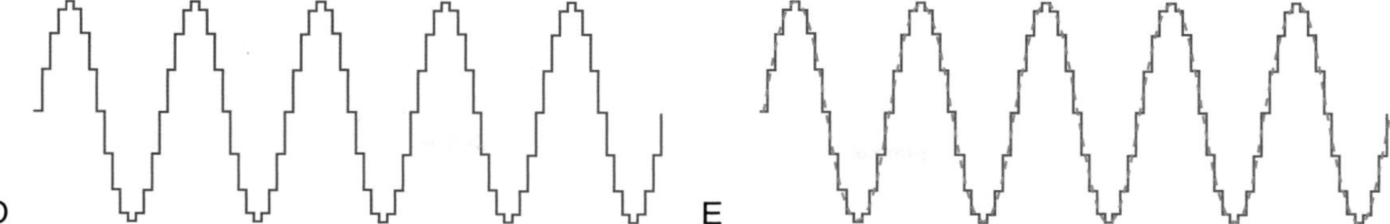

FIGURE 5-41, cont'd D, The pulsed-wave Doppler gate is also called a *sample-and-hold amplifier.* It samples the returning stream of echoes (resulting from one emitted pulse of ultrasound) at the appropriate time for the desired depth (see Table 5-7) and holds the value until the next pulse and sample are accomplished. **E,** Low-pass filtering (which removes higher frequencies) smooths the sampled result *(solid line),* yielding the desired Doppler shift waveform *(dashed line)* comparable with that shown in **B.**

produced. Recall that imaging pulses are two or three cycles long. Pulses used in Doppler instruments, however, have pulse lengths of approximately 5 to 30 cycles. This is necessary to determine the Doppler shifts of returning echoes accurately. Echo voltages from the transducer are processed in the detector. In the detector, echo voltages are amplified, their frequency is compared with the pulser frequency, and Doppler shifts are determined. Doppler shifts are sent to loudspeakers for audible output and to the display for visual observation. Based on their arrival time (recall the 13 μs/cm rule), echoes coming from reflectors at a given depth may be selected by the amplifier gate. Thus motion information may be obtained from a specific depth. This is called *range gating.* The operator controls the gate length and location.

Range gating enables depth selectivity and a small Doppler sample volume.

A PW Doppler instrument does not detect the complete Doppler shift in the same way as a CW instrument but, rather, obtains samples of it because the PW instrument is a sampling system. Each pulse yields a sample of the Doppler shift signal. The Doppler shifts are determined as described previously, except that the mixer does not receive a continuous input echo voltage but, rather, a sampled one. Echoes arrive from the sample volume depth in pulsed form at a rate equal to PRF. Each of these returning echoes yields a sample of the Doppler shift from the Doppler detector. These samples are connected and smoothed (filtered) to yield the sampled waveform (see Figure 5-41, *B–E*).

A pulsed wave Doppler system is a sampling system.

Range Gate

The gate selects the sample volume location from which returning Doppler-shifted echoes are accepted (Table 5-7 and Figures 5-42 to 5-44). The width of the sample volume is equal to the beam width. The gate has some length over which it permits reception (Table 5-8). For example (applying the 13 μs/cm rule), a gate that passes echoes arriving from 13 to 15 μs after pulse generation is listening over a depth range of 10.0 to 11.5 mm. In this case the gate is located at a depth of 10.8 mm with a length (depth range) of ± 0.8 mm. Longer gate lengths are used when searching for the desired vessel and flow location, and shorter gate lengths are used for spectral analysis and evaluation. The shorter gate length improves the quality of the spectral display.

TABLE 5-7 Echo Arrival Time for Various Reflector Depths (Gate Locations)

Depth (mm)	Time (μs)
10	13
20	26
30	39
40	52
50	65
60	78
70	91
80	104
90	117
100	130
150	195
200	260

The Doppler sample volume is determined by beam width, gate length, and emitted pulse length. One half of the pulse length (the same as axial resolution in sonography) is added to gate length to yield effective sample volume length (Table 5-9). Thus the pulse length must shorten while the gate length is reduced. The sample volume width is equal to the beam width at the sample volume depth.

Duplex Instrument

Including PW Doppler capability in a gray-scale sonographic instrument yields what is commonly called a duplex instrument (see Figure 5-44, *G*). The duplex instrument has the capacity to image anatomic structures and to analyze motion and flow at a known point in the anatomic field. Imaging allows intelligent positioning of the gate and angle correction in a PW Doppler system.

Duplex systems must be time shared; that is, imaging and Doppler flow measurements cannot be done simultaneously. Electronic scanning with arrays permits rapid switching between imaging and Doppler functions (several times per second), allowing what can appear to be simultaneous acquisition of real-time image and Doppler flow information. Imaging frame rates are slowed to allow for the acquisition of Doppler information between frames. Similarly, a time-out from the spectral display is taken to present a sonographic frame (see Figure 5-39, *A*, *open arrow*).

> Duplex instruments enable intelligent use of the Doppler sample volume by showing its location in the gray-scale anatomic display.

Spectral Analysis

The Doppler shift voltage from the detector does not go directly to the display but undergoes further processing, otherwise it would resemble Figure 5-45, *A*. This is the visual picture of what a listener hears from the loudspeaker. Spectral analysis (see Figure 5-45, *B*) provides a more meaningful and

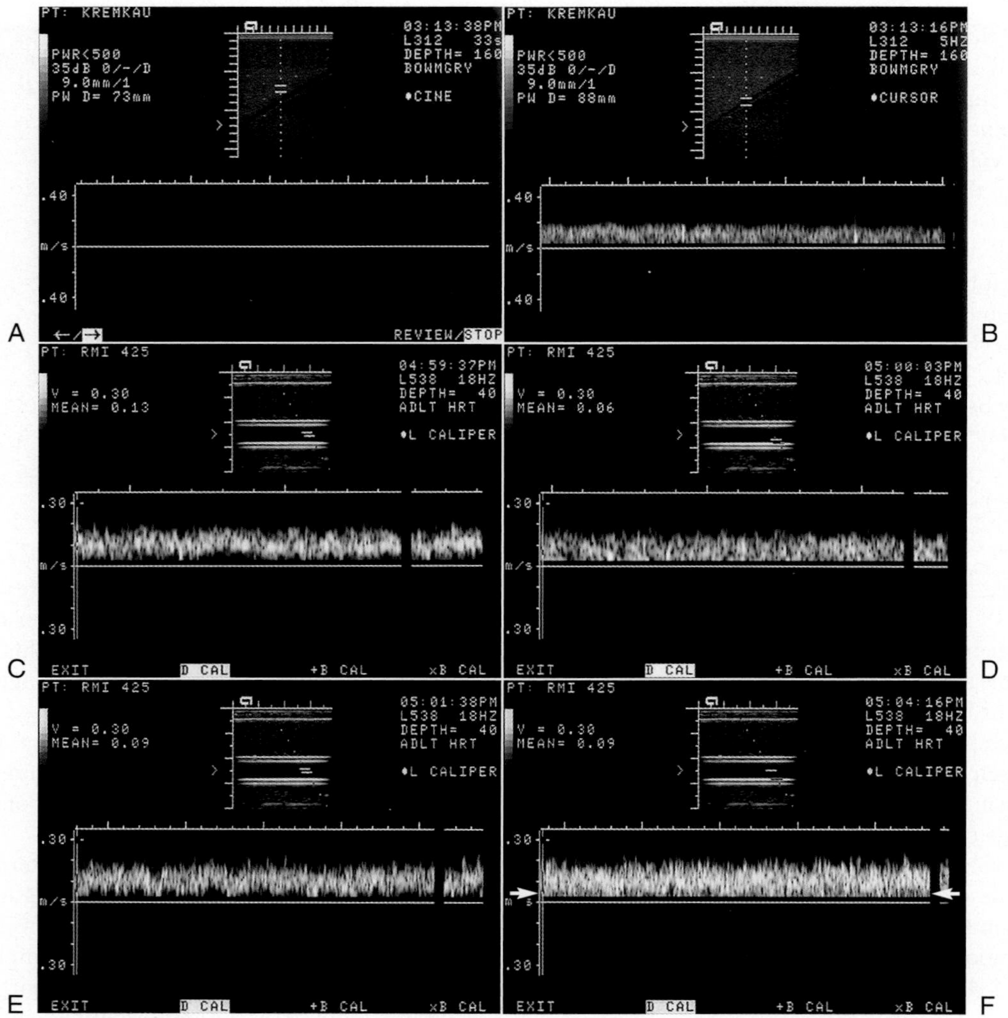

FIGURE 5-42 **A,** The pulsed-wave Doppler sample volume is located at 73 mm of depth (95 μs arrival time). No Doppler shift is seen on the lower display because Doppler-shifted echoes from within the tube arrive at about 114 μs. **B,** When the gate is open later (corresponding to a depth of 88 mm), Doppler shifts are received and displayed (indicating a constant flow rate in the tube). **C,** The gate is located in the center of the tube. **D,** The gate is located near the tube wall. Mean flow speed is 6 cm/s compared with 13 cm/s in **C.** This is the expected result with laminar flow. **E,** The gate is again located at the center of the tube. **F,** The gate length is extended to include the flow from the center, out to the tube wall. Note the strengthening of the lower flow speeds (Doppler shifts) *(arrows)* compared with **E,** where the slower flow is not included in the sample volume.

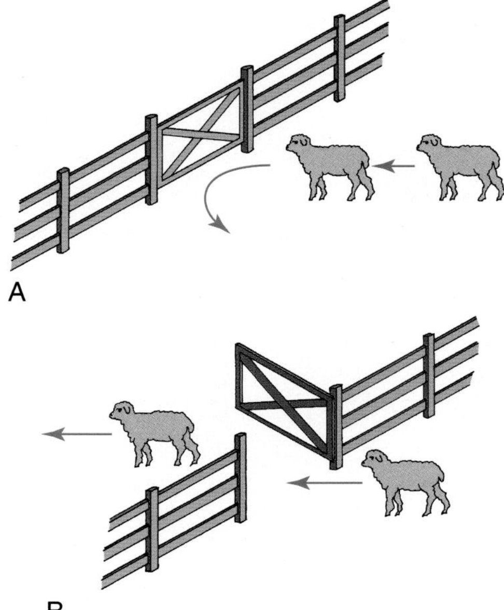

FIGURE 5-43 **A,** Two sheep arrive at a closed gate and are not received into the pen. **B,** Two sheep arrive later at the gate, when it is open, and are received into the pen. In a Doppler detector the gate accepts and rejects echoes in a similar manner.

TABLE 5-8 Spatial Gate Length for Various Temporal Gate Lengths

Length (mm)	Time (μs)
1	1.3
2	2.6
3	3.9
4	5.2
5	6.5
10	13.0
15	19.5
20	26.0

TABLE 5-9 Amount Added to Effective Gate Length by Pulse Length for Various Cycles per Pulse and Frequencies

Amount Added (mm)	Cycles	f (MHz)
1.9	5	2
3.8	10	2
7.7	20	2
0.8	5	5
1.5	10	5
3.1	20	5
0.4	5	10
0.8	10	10
1.5	20	10

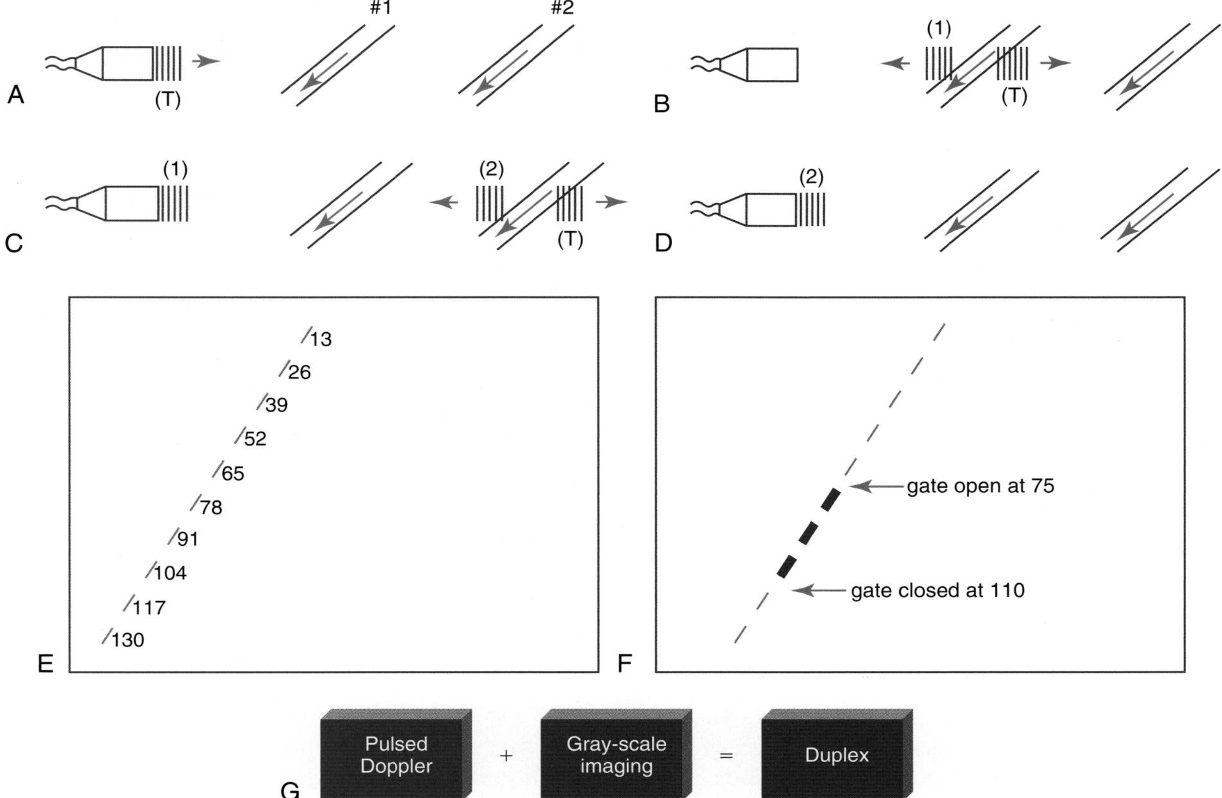

FIGURE 5-44 **A,** A pulse (T) leaves the transducer. **B,** An echo *(1)* is generated in vessel number *1*. **C,** Echo *1* arrives at the transducer. At the same time, another echo *(2)* is generated at vessel number *2*. **D,** Echo *2* arrives at the transducer after echo *1*. These echoes will be processed by the instrument if the gate is open when they arrive. **E,** Echoes from 1-, 2-, 3-, 4-, 5-, 6-, 7-, 8-, 9-, and 10-cm depths arrive at the times (microseconds) indicated. **F,** If the gate is open from 75 to 110 μs after pulse emission, only the echoes in **E,** arriving at 78, 91, and 104 μs, will be accepted. The others will be rejected. **G,** A duplex instrument is a sonographic instrument with pulsed-wave Doppler capability incorporated.

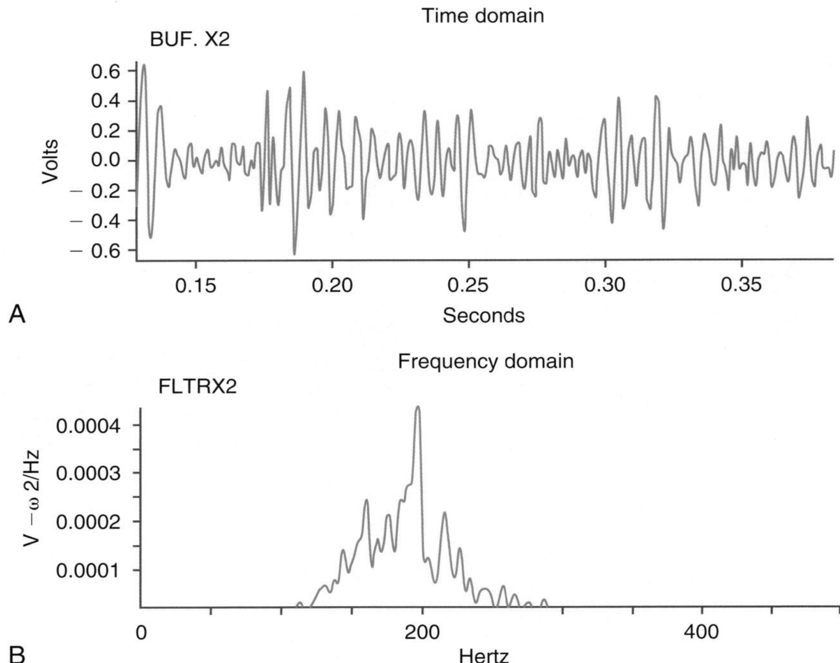

FIGURE 5-45 **A,** Demodulated Doppler shift signal for microspheres flowing at nearly uniform speed. When applied to a loudspeaker, a mix of many frequencies is heard. Approximately 10 cycles occur during a period of 0.20 to 0.25 second. Thus the fundamental period of this signal is approximately 50 ms, yielding a fundamental frequency of 200 Hz. **B,** After the Fourier transform is applied, a frequency spectrum is obtained. The center frequency is approximately 200 Hz. This is what was predicted in **A.** (From Burns PN: The physical principles of Doppler and spectral analysis, *J Clin Ultrasound* 15:567–590, 1987. Reprinted by permission of John Wiley & Sons, Inc.)

useful way to present the Doppler information visually. The presentation is in the form of a Doppler **frequency spectrum**.

Frequency Spectrum

The term *spectral* means "relating to a spectrum." A spectrum is an array of the components of a wave, separated and arranged in order of increasing frequency. The term *analysis* comes from the Greek word meaning "to break up" or "to take apart." Thus spectral analysis is the breaking up of the frequency components of a complex wave or signal and spreading them out in order of increasing frequency.

> Spectral analysis presents Doppler shift frequencies in frequency order.

The human auditory system analyzes sound. The ear and brain break down the complex sounds we receive into the component frequencies contained in the sounds. Thus we can listen to a Doppler signal and recognize normal and abnormal flow sounds. Visual presentation of these sounds provides additional capability for recognition of flow characteristics and for diagnosis of disease.

Various kinds of flow occur in blood vessels. Changes in vessel size, turns, and abnormalities such as the presence of plaque or stenoses can alter the flow character. We have seen that flow can be characterized as *plug, laminar, parabolic, disturbed,* and *turbulent.* Portions of the blood flowing within a vessel are moving at different speeds (even for normal flow) and sometimes in different directions. Thus while the ultrasound beam intersects this flow and produces echoes, many different Doppler shifts are received from the vessel by the system, even from a small sample volume. These Doppler shifts are called the *Doppler frequency spectrum.* The extent of the range of generated Doppler shift frequencies depends on the character of the flow. For near-plug flow, a narrow range of Doppler shift frequencies is received. In disturbed and turbulent flows, broader and much broader ranges of Doppler shift frequencies, respectively, can be received.

> Different flow conditions produce various spectral presentations.

Fast Fourier Transform

The **fast Fourier transform** is the mathematic technique the instrument uses to derive the Doppler spectrum from the returning echoes of various frequencies (Figure 5-46). Fast Fourier transform displays can show **spectral broadening**, which is widening of the Doppler shift spectrum (i.e., an increase in the range of Doppler shift frequencies present) caused by a broader range of flow speeds and directions encountered by the sound beam with disturbed or turbulent flow.

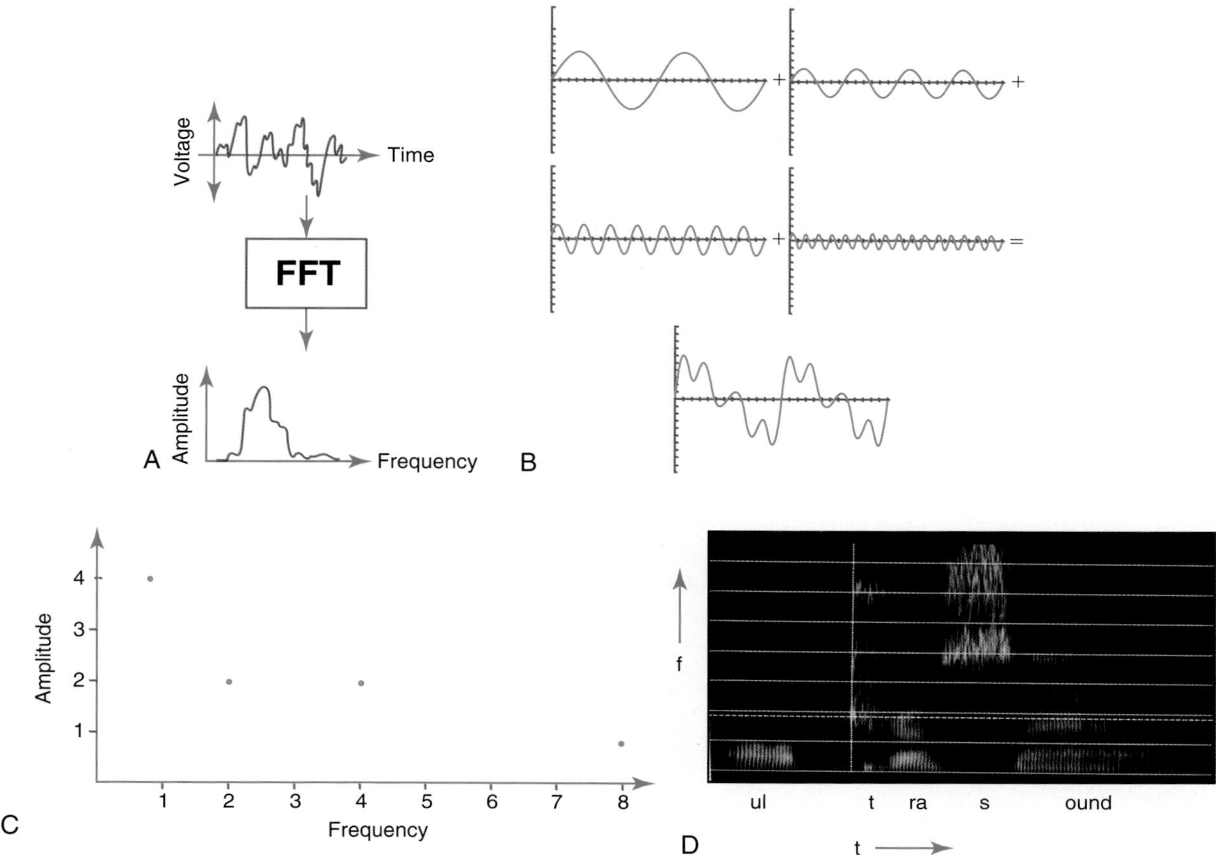

FIGURE 5-46 Fast Fourier transform (FFT). **A,** The Doppler shift signal (containing many frequencies) is transformed by the FFT into a spectrum. (See Figure 5-45 for an example of the Doppler signal before [A] and after [B] FFT processing.) **B,** Four voltages of different frequencies are combined to give the complex result. **C,** The FFT analysis of this combined voltage yields this spectrum of four frequency components (a frequency of 1 with amplitude 4, two frequencies [2 and 4] with amplitude 2, and one frequency of 8 with amplitude of 1). **D,** Spectral analysis of the word *ultrasound.* Time progresses to the right while the word is uttered, and approximately 100 FFTs are performed. The vertical axis represents frequency. The low frequencies of the *ul, ra,* and *ound* syllables are seen, along with the high frequencies of the *t* and *s* sounds.

> The fast Fourier transform is used to generate Doppler shift spectral displays.

Spectral Displays

The received Doppler signal is a combination of many Doppler shift frequencies, yielding a complex waveform (see Figures 5-45, *A*, and 5-46, *B*). With the fast Fourier transform, these frequencies are separated into a spectrum that is presented on a two-dimensional display as Doppler shift frequency on the horizontal axis and power or amplitude of each frequency component on the vertical axis (see Figures 5-45, *B*, and 5-46, *A, C*). Depending on the speed of the processor, approximately 100 to 1000 spectra can be generated per second. In the case of venous flow, such a spectral display usually would be rather constant. However, in the case of the pulsatile flow in arterial circulation, such a presentation changes continually, shifting to the right in systole as the blood accelerates and Doppler shifts increase, shifting to the left in diastole, and changing in amplitude distribution over the cardiac cycle. Interpretation of this changing presentation is difficult; indeed, the character of the changes over the cardiac cycle could be important. Therefore presentation of this changing spectrum as a function of time is valuable and useful. Such a trace is shown in Figures 5-46, *D*, 5-47, and 5-48. In these presentations the vertical axis represents Doppler shift frequency and the horizontal axis represents time (Figure 5-49). The amplitude or power of each Doppler shift frequency component at any instant is now presented as brightness (gray scale; see Figure 5-38, *A*) or color (see Figure 1-14). Doppler signal power is proportional to blood cell concentration (number of cells per unit volume). A bright spot on a spectral display means that a strong Doppler shift frequency component was received at that instant of time (see Figure 5-38). A dark spot means that a Doppler shift frequency component was weak or nonexistent at that point in time. Intermediate values of gray shade or brightness indicate intermediate amplitudes or powers of frequency components at the given times.

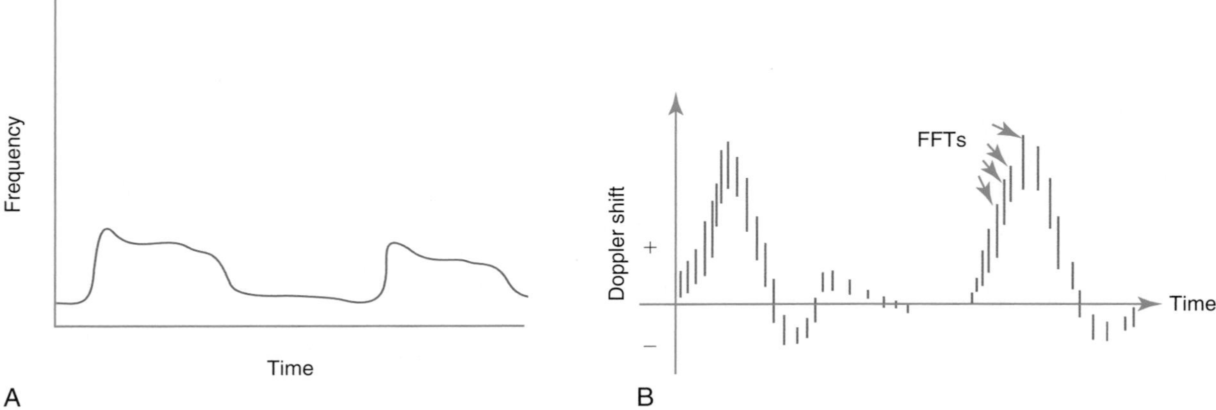

FIGURE 5-47 **A,** A display of Doppler shift as a function of time for pure plug flow. The Doppler shift frequency is represented on the vertical axis. The amplitude of the Doppler shift frequency at each instant of time is represented by gray level or color. In this example, there is only a single shift frequency at each instant of time (i.e., no spectrum). **B,** A spectral display for nonplug flow is composed of several (100–1000 per second) fast Fourier transform (FFT) spectra arranged vertically next to each other across the time (horizontal) axis.

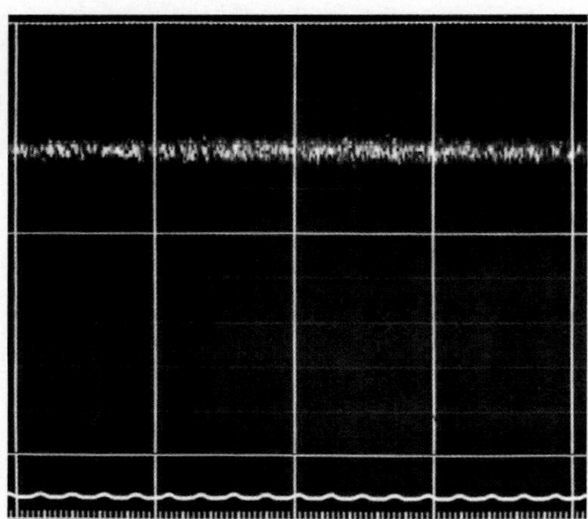

FIGURE 5-48 **A spectral display of the signal shown in Figure 5-45.** The flow is constant, yielding Doppler shift frequencies of approximately 200 Hz. (The horizontal markers represent 100 Hz.) (From Burns PN: The physical principles of Doppler and spectral analysis, *J Clin Ultrasound* 15:567–590, 1987. Reprinted by permission of John Wiley & Sons, Inc.)

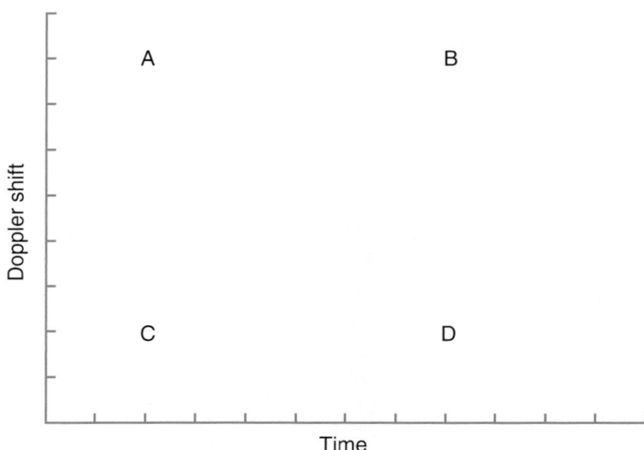

FIGURE 5-49 **Four points on a spectral display.** Points *A* and *C* occur at an earlier time, compared with points *B* and *D,* which occur later. Points *A* and *B* represent higher Doppler shift frequencies than points *C* and *D.*

A strong signal at a particular frequency and time means that many scattering blood cells are moving at speeds and directions corresponding to that Doppler shift. A weak frequency means that few cells are traveling at speeds and directions corresponding to that Doppler shift at that point in time.

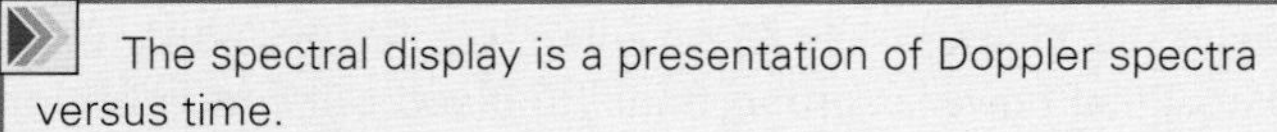

The spectral display is a presentation of Doppler spectra versus time.

Spectral Broadening

Spectral trace presentations provide information about flow that can be used to discern conditions at the site of measurement and at sites proximal or distal to it. Peak flow speeds and spectral broadening are indicative of the degrees of stenosis. Spectral "broadening" is a vertical thickening of the spectral trace (Figure 5-50). If all the cells were moving at the same speed, the spectral trace would be a thin line (see Figure 5-47, *A*). As stated previously, though, this is not the case in practice. However, narrow spectra can be observed, particularly in large vessels (Figure 5-51, *A*). The apparent narrowing of the spectrum while the blood accelerates in systole can be misinterpreted. A spectrum of consistent width appears to be thinner in a steep-rise portion of a curve (Figure 5-52). While flow is disturbed or becomes turbulent, greater variation in velocities of various portions of the flowing blood produce a greater range of Doppler shift frequencies. This results in a broadened spectrum presented on the spectral display

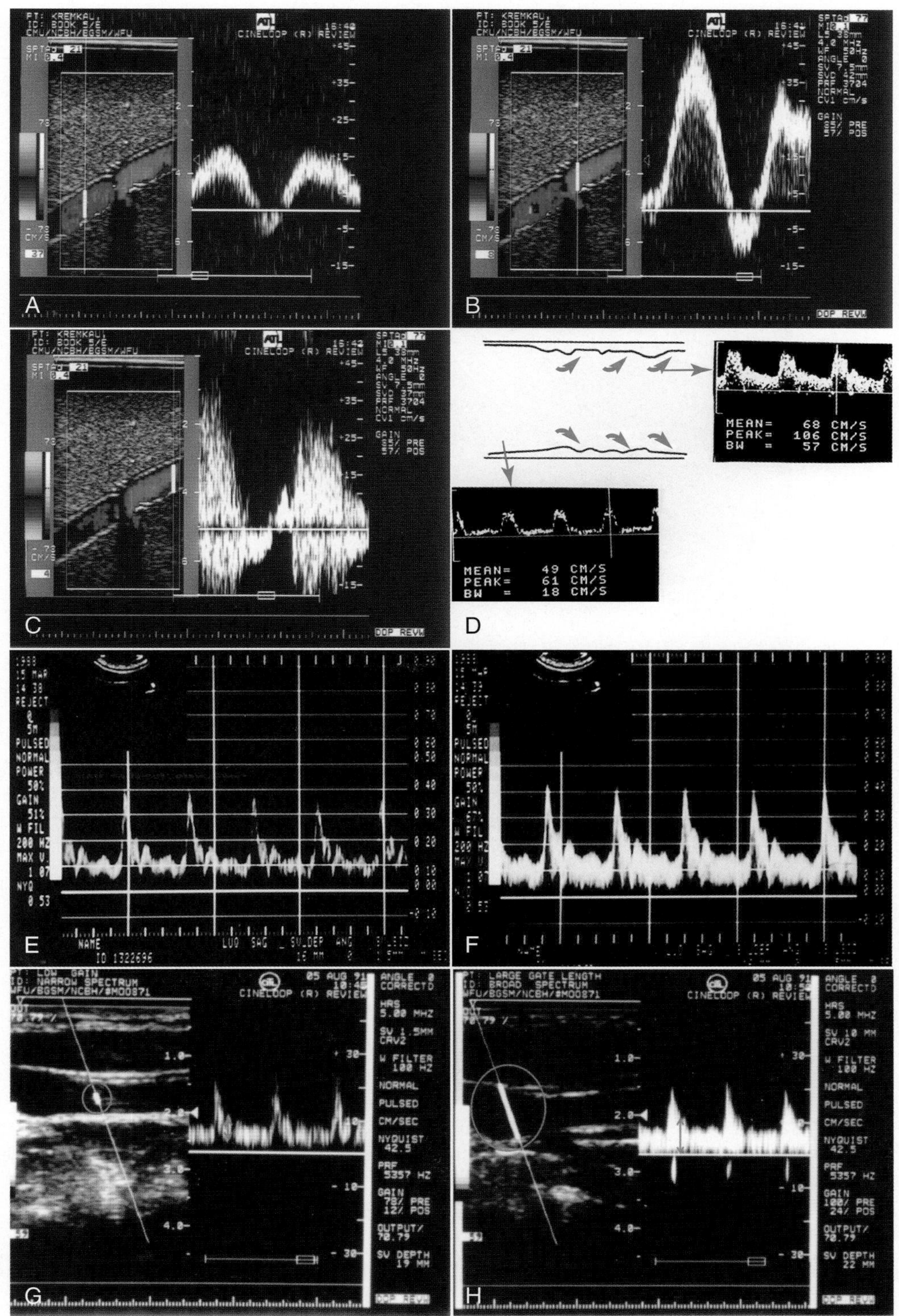

FIGURE 5-50 Flow (*lower left to upper right*) in a tube with a stenosis in tissue-equivalent material. **A,** Proximal to the stenosis, a narrow spectrum is observed (indicating approximately plug [i.e., blunted] flow). **B,** At the stenosis, a reasonably narrow spectrum still is seen, but the Doppler shifts have tripled because of the high flow speed through the stenosis. **C,** Distal to the stenosis, a broad spectrum is observed, along with negative Doppler shifts, both of which are caused by turbulent flow. Compare these observations with the flow conditions in and beyond a narrow gorge (see Figure 5-7). **D,** Spectral broadening produced by atheroma. **E,** Display produced at a correct Doppler gain setting. **F,** Artifactual spectral broadening caused by excessive gain. **G,** Display produced at a correct sample volume length. **H,** Artifactual spectral broadening caused by excessive sample volume length. (**D-F** from Taylor KJW, Holland S: Doppler US. Part I. Basic principles, instrumentation, and pitfalls, *Radiology* 174:297–307, 1990.)

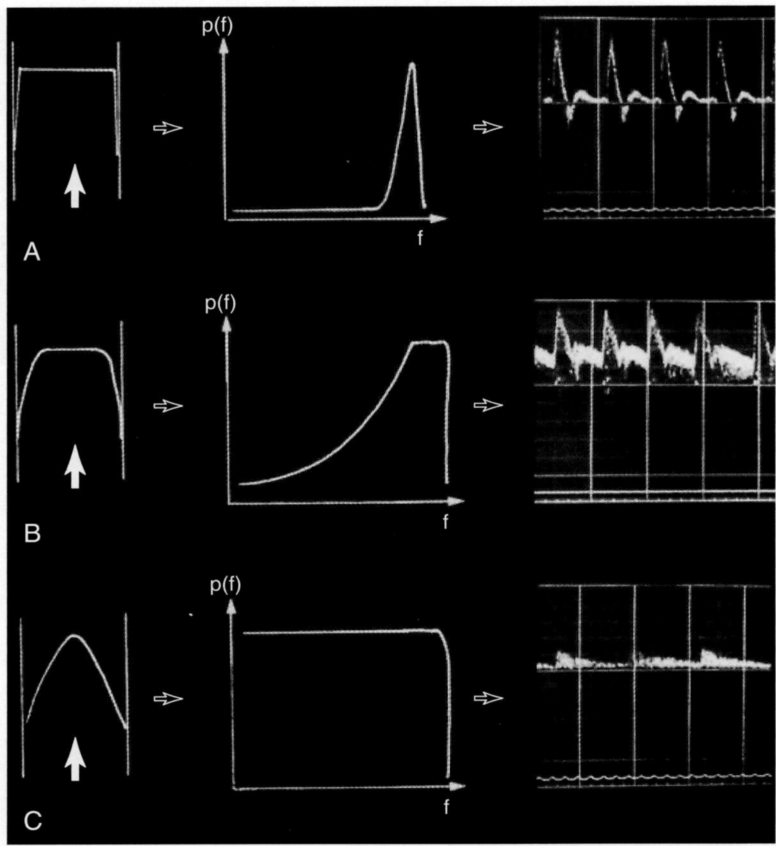

FIGURE 5-51 Flow speed profiles *(left),* Doppler spectra (power versus frequency; *center*), and spectral displays *(right)* are shown for nearly plug flow in the aorta **(A)**, blunted parabolic flow in the celiac trunk **(B)**, and parabolic flow in the ovarian artery **(C)**. (From Burns PN: The physical principles of Doppler and spectral analysis, *J Clin Ultrasound* 15:567–590, 1987. Reprinted by permission of John Wiley & Sons, Inc.)

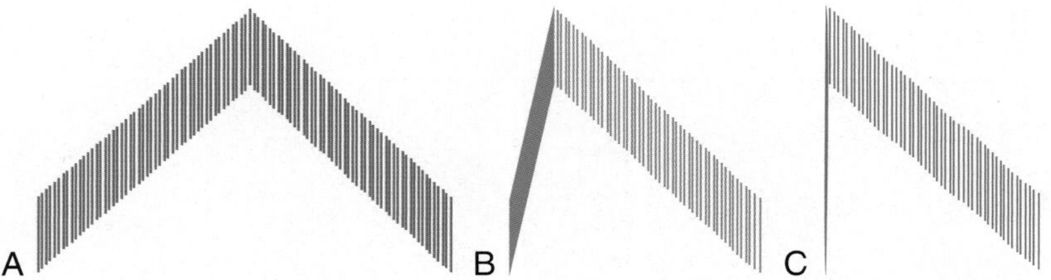

FIGURE 5-52 Apparent spectral narrowing in rapidly accelerating flow. **A,** Slowly accelerating and decelerating flow shows that the spectral widths (bandwidths) are all equal. **B-C,** While the acceleration phase becomes steeper, the bandwidths appear to narrow. However, the vertical lines representing bandwidth in all cases are the same.

(see Figure 5-50, *C,D*). Thus spectral broadening is indicative of disturbed or turbulent flow and can be related to a pathologic condition. However, spectral broadening can also be produced artificially by excessive Doppler gain (see Figure 5-50, *E–F*) or excessive sample volume length (see Figure 5-50, *G–H*), and some broadening is produced by beam spreading (see Figure 5-36, *F*), particularly with wide-aperture arrays.

> Disturbed or turbulent flow conditions produce spectral broadening

Downstream (Distal) and Upstream (Proximal) Conditions

Doppler flow measurements can yield information about downstream (distal) conditions. Flow reversal in early diastole and lack of flow in late diastole (see Figures 5-8 and 5-51, *A*) indicate high resistance to flow downstream (e.g., because of vasoconstriction of arterioles). If flow resistance is reduced because of vasodilation, significant differences in the spectral display are observed (Figure 5-53). A comparison between low-resistance and high-resistance flow spectra is given in Figure 5-54.

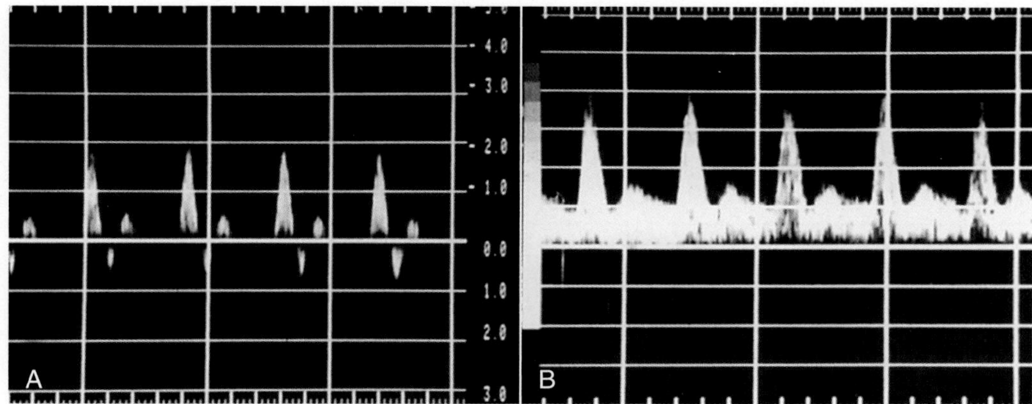

FIGURE 5-53 **A,** High distal resistance flow in the popliteal artery with the patient's leg at rest. **B,** Low distal resistance flow is observed after exercise. (From Taylor KJW, Holland S: Doppler US. Part I. Basic principles, instrumentation, and pitfalls, *Radiology* 174:297–307, 1990.)

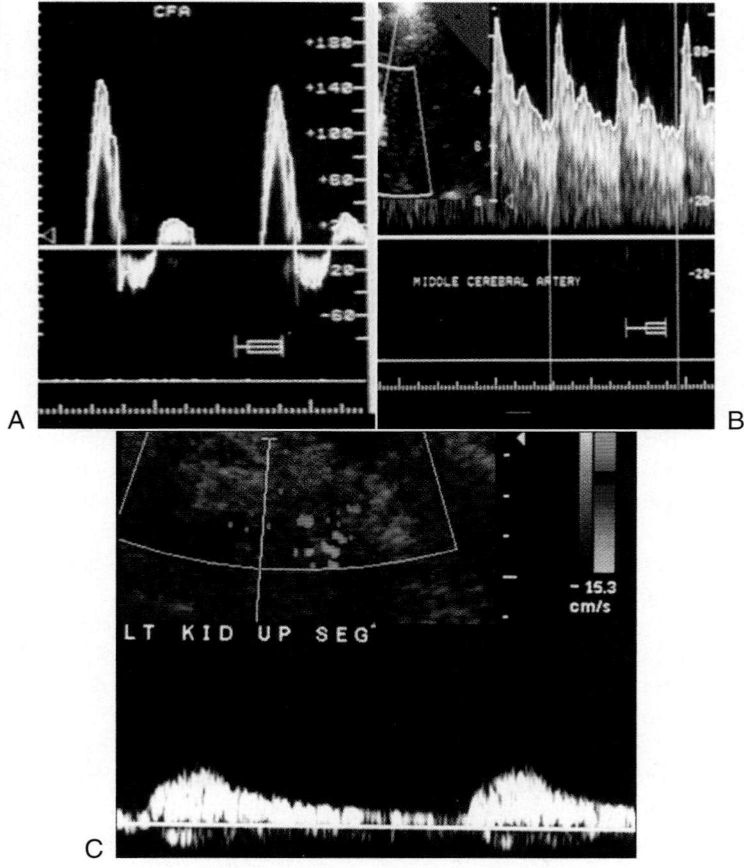

FIGURE 5-54 **A,** High distal resistance flow is seen in the common femoral artery of the resting lower limb. **B,** Low distal resistance flow is seen in the middle cerebral artery. Although these spectral displays are very different, they are both normal for the locations and conditions given. **C,** *Tardus-parvus* waveform typical of flow with proximal stenosis.

Stenoses upstream (proximal) produce spectral displays that have the so-called *tardus-parvus* character (see Figure 5-54, *C*).

Normal vessels can be occluded in diastole when pressure drops below the critical value for flow. When this happens, no diastolic Doppler shift is detected.

> High- and low-impedance conditions upstream and downstream give rise to various spectral displays.

Table 5-10 compares the three types of Doppler displays: (1) color-Doppler shift, (2) color-Doppler power, and (3) spectral displays.

TABLE 5-10 Comparison of Doppler-Shift Display, Doppler-Power Display, and Spectral Display

Presentation	Color Doppler–Shift Display	Color Doppler–Power Display	Spectral Display
Quantitative	No	No	Yes
Global	Yes	Yes	No
Perfusion	No	Yes	No

REVIEW

The following key points are presented in this chapter.

- The heart provides the pulsatile pressure necessary to produce blood flow.
- Volumetric flow rate is proportional to the pressure difference at the ends of a tube.
- Volumetric flow rate is inversely proportional to flow resistance.
- Flow resistance increases with viscosity and tube length and decreases strongly with increasing tube diameter.
- Flow classifications include steady, pulsatile, plug, laminar, parabolic, disturbed, and turbulent.
- In a stenosis, flow accelerates, pressure drops (Bernoulli effect), and flow is disturbed or turbulent.
- Pulsatile flow is common in arterial circulation.
- Diastolic flow and/or flow reversal occur in some locations within the arterial system.
- The Doppler effect is a change in frequency resulting from motion.
- In sonographic applications, blood flow and tissue motion are the sources of the Doppler effect.
- The change in frequency of the returning echoes with respect to the emitted frequency is called the *Doppler shift.*
- For flow toward the transducer, the Doppler shift is positive.
- For flow away from the transducer, the Doppler shift is negative.
- The Doppler shift depends on the speed of the scatterers of sound, the Doppler angle, and the operating frequency of the Doppler system.
- Greater flow speeds and smaller Doppler angles produce larger Doppler shifts but not stronger Doppler-shifted echoes.
- Higher operating frequencies produce larger Doppler shifts.
- Typical ranges of flow speeds (10 to 100 cm/s), Doppler angles (30 to 60 degrees), and operating frequencies (2 to 10 MHz) yield Doppler shifts in the range of 100 Hz to 11 kHz for vascular studies.
- In Doppler echocardiography, in which zero angle and speeds of a few meters per second can be encountered, Doppler shifts can be as high as 30 kHz.
- Color-Doppler imaging acquires Doppler-shifted echoes from a two-dimensional cross-section of tissue scanned by an ultrasound beam.
- Doppler-shifted echoes are presented in color and superimposed on the gray-scale anatomic image of nonshifted echoes that were received during the scan.
- Flow echoes are assigned colors according to the color map chosen.
- Several pulses (the number is called *ensemble length*) are needed to generate a color scan line.
- Color controls include gain, map selection, variance on/off, persistence, ensemble length, color/gray priority, scale (PRF), baseline shift, wall filter, and color window angle, location, and size.
- Doppler-shift displays are subject to Doppler angle dependence and aliasing.
- Doppler-power displays color-coded Doppler-shift strengths into angle-independent, aliasing-independent, more sensitive presentations of flow information.
- CW Doppler systems provide motion and flow information without depth selection capability.
- PW Doppler systems provide the ability to select the depth from which Doppler information is received.
- Spectral analysis provides visual information on the distribution of Doppler-shift frequencies resulting from the distribution of the scatterer speeds and directions encountered.
- The Doppler spectrum is generated by the range of scatterer velocities encountered by the ultrasound beam.
- The spectrum is derived electronically using the fast Fourier transform and is presented on the display as Doppler shift versus time, with brightness indicating power.
- Flow conditions at the site of measurement are indicated by the width (vertical thickness) of the spectrum, with spectral broadening being indicative of disturbed and turbulent flows.
- Flow conditions downstream, especially distal flow impedance, are indicated by the relationship between peak systolic and end diastolic flow speeds.

EXERCISES

Answers appear in the Answers to Exercises section at the back of the book.

1. Which of the following are parts of the circulatory system? (More than one correct answer.)
   a. Heart
   b. Cerebral ventricle
   c. Artery
   d. Arteriole
   e. Capillary
   f. Bile duct
   g. Venule
   h. Vein

2. The ___________ are the tiniest vessels in the circulatory system.
   a. arteries
   b. arterioles
   c. capillaries
   d. bile ducts
   e. venules
   f. veins
3. In which of the following can Doppler ultrasound detect flow? (More than one correct answer.)
   a. The heart
   b. Arteries
   c. Arterioles
   d. Capillaries
   e. Venules
   f. Veins
4. To flow is to move in a ___________.
   a. direction
   b. container
   c. stream
   d. reversal
5. The characteristic of a fluid that offers resistance to flow is called ___________.
   a. resistance
   b. viscosity
   c. inertia
   d. impedance
   e. density
6. Poise is a unit of ___________.
   a. resistance
   b. viscosity
   c. inertia
   d. impedance
   e. density
7. Pressure is ___________ per unit area.
   a. resistance
   b. viscosity
   c. inertia
   d. force
8. Pressure is ___________.
   a. nondirectional
   b. unidirectional
   c. omnidirectional
   d. all of the above
   e. none of the above
9. Flow is a response to pressure ___________ or ___________.
   a. difference, gradient
   b. increase, decrease
   c. fore, aft
   d. presence, absence
10. If the pressure is greater at one end of a liquid-filled tube or vessel than it is at the other, the liquid will flow from the ___________-pressure end to the ___________-pressure end.
    a. higher, lower
    b. lower, higher
    c. depends on the liquid
    d. all of the above
    e. none of the above
11. The volumetric flow rate in a tube is determined by ___________ difference and ___________.
    a. resistance, pressure
    b. pressure, resistance
    c. diameter, length
    d. pressure, length
12. Flow increases if ___________ increase(s).
    a. pressure difference
    b. pressure gradient
    c. resistance
    d. a and b
    e. all of the above
13. While flow resistance increases, volumetric flow rate ___________.
    a. increases
    b. decreases
    c. is unchanged
    d. depends on pressure
14. If pressure difference is doubled, volumetric flow rate is ___________.
    a. unchanged
    b. quartered
    c. halved
    d. doubled
    e. quadrupled
15. If flow resistance is doubled, volumetric flow rate is ___________.
    a. unchanged
    b. quartered
    c. halved
    d. doubled
    e. quadrupled
16. Flow resistance in a vessel depends on ___________.
    a. vessel length
    b. vessel radius
    c. blood viscosity
    d. all of the above
    e. none of the above
17. Flow resistance decreases with an increase in ___________.
    a. vessel length
    b. vessel radius
    c. blood viscosity
    d. all of the above
    e. none of the above
18. Flow resistance depends most strongly on _________.
    a. vessel length
    b. vessel radius
    c. blood viscosity
    d. all of the above
    e. none of the above

19. Volumetric flow rate decreases with an increase in ___________.
   a. pressure difference
   b. vessel radius
   c. vessel length
   d. blood viscosity
   e. c and d
20. When the speed of a fluid is constant across a vessel, the flow is called ___________ flow.
   a. volume
   b. parabolic
   c. laminar
   d. viscous
   e. plug
21. The type of flow (approximately) seen in Figure 5-55, *A*, is ___________.
   a. volume
   b. steady
   c. parabolic
   d. viscous
   e. plug
22. The type of flow seen in Figure 5-55, *B*, is ___________.
   a. volume
   b. steady
   c. parabolic
   d. viscous
   e. plug

A

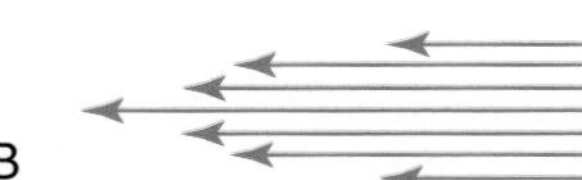

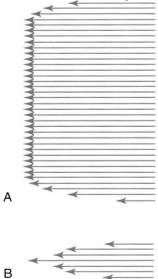

FIGURE 5-55 Two types of flow patterns. Illustration to accompany Exercises 21 and 22.

23. ___________ flow occurs when straight parallel streamlines describing the flow are altered.
   a. Volume
   b. Turbulent
   c. Parabolic
   d. Disturbed
24. ___________ flow involves random and chaotic flow patterns, with particles flowing in all directions.
   a. Volume
   b. Turbulent
   c. Parabolic
   d. Disturbed
25. Turbulent flow is more likely ___________ to a stenosis.
   a. proximal
   b. distal
26. A narrowing of the lumen of a tube is called a ___________.
   a. stenosis
   b. gorge
   c. titer
   d. kink
27. Proximal to, at, and distal to a stenosis, ___________ must be constant.
   a. laminar flow
   b. disturbed flow
   c. turbulent flow
   d. volumetric flow rate
   e. none of the above
28. For the answer to Exercise 27 to be true, flow speed at the stenosis must be ___________ that proximal and distal to it.
   a. greater than
   b. less than
   c. less turbulent than
   d. less disturbed than
   e. none of the above
29. Poiseuille equation predicts a(n) ___________ in flow speed with a decrease in vessel radius.
   a. increase
   b. decrease
30. The continuity rule predicts a(n) ___________ in flow speed with a localized decrease (stenosis) in vessel diameter.
   a. increase
   b. decrease
31. In a stenosis, the pressure is ___________ the proximal and distal values.
   a. less than
   b. equal to
   c. greater than
   d. depends on the fluid
   e. none of the above
32. Added forward flow and flow reversal in diastole can occur with ___________ flow.
   a. volume
   b. turbulent
   c. laminar
   d. disturbed
   e. pulsatile

33. While stenosis diameter decreases, ___________ pass(es) through a maximum.
   a. flow speed at the stenosis
   b. flow speed proximal to the stenosis
   c. volumetric flow rate
   d. the Doppler shift at the stenosis
   e. a and d
34. In Figure 5-56, at which point is pressure the lowest?
   a. P
   b. S
   c. D
   d. P and D
   e. None of the above

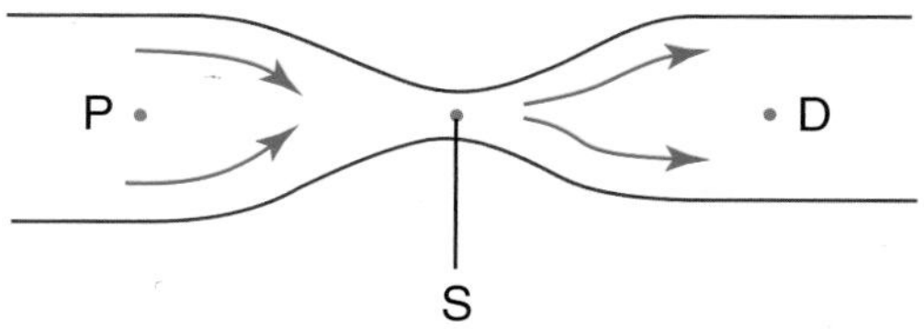

FIGURE 5-56 **Proximal to** *(P)*, **at** *(S)*, **and distal to** *(D)* **a stenosis.** Illustration to accompany Exercises 34 to 37. (From Kremkau FW: Fluid flow, *J Vasc Technol* 17:153–154, 1993. Reproduced with permission.)

35. In Figure 5-56, at which point is flow speed the lowest?
   a. P
   b. S
   c. D
   d. P and D
   e. None of the above
36. In Figure 5-56, at which point is volumetric flow rate the lowest?
   a. P
   b. S
   c. D
   d. P and D
   e. None of the above
37. In Figure 5-56, at which point is pressure energy the greatest?
   a. P
   b. S
   c. D
   d. P and D
   e. None of the above
38. The ___________ effect is used to detect and measure ___________ in vessels.
   a. Bernoulli, blood
   b. Poiseuille, pressure
   c. Poiseuille, flow
   d. Doppler, flow
39. Motion of an echo-generating structure causes an echo to have a different ___________ from that of the emitted pulse.
   a. form
   b. strength
   c. amplitude
   d. frequency
40. If the incident frequency is 1 MHz, the propagation speed is 1600 m/s, and the reflector speed is 16 m/s toward the source, the Doppler shift is ___________ MHz, and the reflected frequency is ___________ MHz.
   a. −0.02, 1.02
   b. 0.02, 1.02
   c. 0.026, 1.026
   d. −0.026, 1.026
41. If 2-MHz ultrasound is reflected from a soft tissue boundary moving at 10 m/s toward the source, the Doppler shift is ___________ MHz.
   a. −0.02, 1.02
   b. 0.02, 1.02
   c. 0.026
   d. −0.026
42. If 2-MHz ultrasound is reflected from a soft tissue boundary moving at 10 m/s away from the source, the Doppler shift is ___________ MHz.
   a. −0.02, 1.02
   b. 0.02, 1.02
   c. 0.026
   d. −0.026
43. The Doppler shift is the difference between ___________ and ___________ frequencies.
   a. operating, emitted
   b. echo, received
   c. fundamental, harmonic
   d. received, emitted
44. When incident sound direction and reflector motion are not parallel, calculation of the reflected frequency involves the ___________ of the angle between these directions.
   a. sine
   b. cosine
   c. tangent
   d. cotangent
45. If the angle between incident sound direction and reflector motion is 60 degrees, the Doppler shift and reflected frequency in Exercise 40 are ___________ MHz and ___________ MHz.
   a. 0.02, 1.02
   b. 0.01, 1.01
   c. −0.02, 1.02
   d. −0.026, 1.026
46. If the angle between incident sound direction and reflector motion is 90 degrees, the cosine of the angle is ___________, and the reflected frequency in Exercise 40 is ___________ MHz.
   a. 0.02, 1.02
   b. 0.01, 1.01
   c. 0.0, 1.00
   d. 0.0, −1.00

47. For an operating frequency of 2 MHz, a flow speed of 10 cm/s, and a Doppler angle of 0 degrees, calculate the Doppler shift (kHz).
   a. −0.026
   b. 0.026
   c. −0.26
   d. 0.26
48. For an operating frequency of 6 MHz, a flow speed of 50 cm/s, and a Doppler angle of 60 degrees, calculate the Doppler shift (kHz).
   a. 1.95
   b. 9.15
   c. 5.91
   d. 5.19
49. For blood flowing in a vessel with a plug flow profile, the Doppler shift is __________ across the vessel.
   a. constant
   b. variable
   c. parabolic
   d. circular
50. Which Doppler angle yields the greatest Doppler shift?
   a. −90
   b. −45
   c. 0
   d. 45
   e. 90
51. To proceed from a measurement of Doppler shift frequency to a calculation of flow speed, __________ __________ must be known or assumed.
   a. pressure amplitude
   b. peak frequency
   c. Doppler angle
   d. average intensity
52. If operating frequency is doubled, the Doppler shift is __________.
   a. halved
   b. unchanged
   c. doubled
   d. quadrupled
53. If flow speed is doubled, the Doppler shift is __________.
   a. halved
   b. unchanged
   c. doubled
   d. quadrupled
54. If Doppler angle is doubled, the Doppler shift is __________.
   a. doubled
   b. halved
   c. increased
   d. decreased
55. Color-Doppler instruments present two-dimensional, color-coded images representing __________ that are superimposed on gray-scale images representing __________.
   a. flow, anatomy
   b. motion, flow
   c. anatomy, frequency
   d. amplitude, frequency
56. Which of the following on a color-Doppler display is (are) presented in real time?
   a. Gray-scale anatomy
   b. Flow direction
   c. Doppler spectrum
   d. a and b
   e. All of the above
57. Color-Doppler instruments use an __________ technique to yield Doppler information in real time.
   a. automatic
   b. autocorrelation
   c. autonomic
   d. autocratic
58. The information in Exercise 57 includes __________ Doppler shift, __________, __________, and __________.
   a. peak, sine, variables, intensity
   b. mean, sign, variance, power
   c. median, direction, deviation, amplitude
   d. mean, sine, tangent, variance
59. The angle dependencies of Doppler-shift displays and Doppler-power displays are different. True or false?
60. Do the different colors appearing in Figure 5-28, *A* and *C*, indicate that flow is going in two different directions in the vessel? Yes or no?
61. In color-Doppler instruments, color is used only to represent flow direction. True or false?
62. In practice, approximately __________ pulses are required to obtain one line of color-Doppler information.
   a. 1
   b. 10
   c. 100
   d. 1000
63. About __________ frames per second are produced by a color-Doppler instrument.
   a. 10
   b. 20
   c. 40
   d. 80
   e. More than one of the above
64. Doppler-shift displays are not dependent on Doppler angle. True or false?
65. If a color-Doppler instrument shows two colors in the same vessel, it always means flow is occurring in opposite directions in the vessel. True or false?
66. A region of bright color on a Doppler-shift display always indicates the highest flow speeds. True or false?
67. Increasing the ensemble length __________ the frame rate.
   a. increases
   b. decreases
   c. doubles
   d. triples

68. The ___________ technique is commonly used to detect echo Doppler shifts in color-Doppler instruments.
a. automatic
b. autocorrelation
c. autonomic
d. autocratic

69. Which of the following reduce the frame rate of a color-Doppler image? (More than one correct answer.)
a. Wider color window
b. Longer color window
c. Increased ensemble length
d. Higher transducer frequency
e. Higher priority setting

70. Lack of color in a vessel containing blood flow may be attributable to ___________. (More than one correct answer.)
a. low color gain
b. a high wall filter setting
c. a low priority setting
d. baseline shift
e. aliasing

71. Increasing ensemble length ___________ color sensitivity and accuracy and ___________ frame rate.
a. improves, increases
b. degrades, increases
c. degrades, decreases
d. improves, decreases
e. none of the above

72. Which control can be used to help with clutter?
a. Wall filter
b. Gain
c. Baseline shift
d. PRF
e. Smoothing

73. Color map baselines are always represented by ___________.
a. white
b. black
c. red
d. blue
e. cyan

74. Doubling the width of a color window produces a(n) ___________ frame rate.
a. doubled
b. quadrupled
c. unchanged
d. halved
e. quartered

75. Steering the color window to the right or left produces a(n) ___________ frame rate.
a. doubled
b. quadrupled
c. unchanged
d. halved
e. quartered

76. Autocorrelation produces ___________. (More than one correct answer.)
a. the color of the Doppler shift
b. the mean value of the Doppler shift
c. variance
d. spectrum
e. peak Doppler shift

77. Steering the color window to the right or left changes ___________.
a. frame rate
b. PRF
c. the Doppler angle
d. the Doppler shift
e. more than one of the above

78. Color-Doppler frame rates are ___________ gray-scale rates.
a. equal to
b. less than
c. more than
d. depends on color map
e. depends on priority

79. In a single frame, color can change in a vessel because of ___________.
a. vessel curvature
b. sector format
c. helical flow
d. diastolic flow reversal
e. all of the above

80. Angle is not important in transverse color-Doppler views through vessels. True or false?

81. Compared with Doppler-shift imaging, Doppler-power imaging is ___________.
a. more sensitive
b. angle independent
c. aliasing independent
d. speed independent
e. all of the above

82. Doppler-power imaging indicates (with color) the ___________ of flow.
a. presence
b. direction
c. speed
d. character
e. more than one of the above

83. Doppler-shift imaging indicates (with color) the ___________ of flow.
a. presence
b. direction
c. speed
d. character
e. more than one of the above

84. The functions of a Doppler detector include ___________.
a. amplification
b. phase quadrature detection
c. Doppler shift detection
d. sign determination
e. all of the above

85. An earlier gate time means ___________ sample volume depth.
   a. a later
   b. a shallower
   c. a deeper
   d. a stronger
   e. none of the above
86. Doppler signal power is proportional to ___________.
   a. volume flow rate
   b. flow speed
   c. the Doppler angle
   d. cell concentration
   e. more than one of the above
87. Doppler ultrasound provides information about flow conditions only at the site of measurement. True or false?
88. Stenosis affects ___________.
   a. peak systolic flow speed
   b. end diastolic flow speed
   c. spectral broadening
   d. window
   e. all of the above
89. Spectral broadening is a ___________ of the spectral trace.
   a. vertical thickening
   b. horizontal thickening
   c. brightening
   d. darkening
   e. horizontal shift
90. If all the cells in a vessel were moving at the same constant speed, the spectral trace would be a ___________ line.
   a. thin horizontal
   b. thin vertical
   c. thick horizontal
   d. thick vertical
   e. none of the above
91. Disturbed flow produces a narrower spectrum. True or false?
92. Turbulent flow produces a narrower spectrum. True or false?
93. As stenosis progresses, which of the following increase(s)?
   a. Lumen diameter
   b. Systolic Doppler shift
   c. Diastolic Doppler shift
   d. Spectral broadening
   e. More than one of the above
94. Higher flow speed always produces a higher Doppler shift on a spectral display. True or false?
95. Flow reversal in diastole indicates ___________.
   a. a stenosis
   b. an aneurysm
   c. high distal resistance
   d. low distal resistance
   e. more than one of the above
96. Decreased distal resistance normally causes end diastolic flow to ___________.
   a. increase
   b. decrease
   c. be disturbed
   d. become turbulent
   e. more than one of the above
97. If angle correction is set at 60 degrees but should be zero degrees, the display indicates a flow speed of 100 cm/s. The correct flow speed is ___________ cm/s.
   a. 25
   b. 50
   c. 100
   d. 200
   e. 400
98. If angle correction is set at zero degrees but should be 60 degrees, the display indicates a flow speed of 100 cm/s. The correct flow speed is ___________ cm/s.
   a. 25
   b. 50
   c. 100
   d. 200
   e. 400
99. If a 5-kHz Doppler shift corresponds to 100 cm/s, then a 2.5-kHz shift corresponds to ___________ cm/s.
   a. 100
   b. 75
   c. 50
   d. 25
100. Which of the following is increased if Doppler angle is increased?
   a. Aliasing
   b. Doppler shift
   c. Effect of angle error
   d. b and c
   e. None of the above

6

Artifacts

LEARNING OBJECTIVES

After reading this chapter, the student should be able to do the following:

- List reasons for incorrect presentation of anatomic structures by sonographic gray-scale images.
- List reasons for incorrect presentation of motion and flow information by spectral and color-Doppler displays.
- Describe how specific artifacts can be recognized.
- Explain how to deal with artifacts to avoid the pitfalls and misdiagnoses they can cause.

OUTLINE

KEY TERMS

Aliasing
Anechoic
Comet tail
Cross-talk
Enhancement
Hypoechoic
Mirror image
Nyquist limit
Range ambiguity
Reverberation
Shadowing
Slice thickness
Speckle
Speed error

In previous chapters we have covered the principles relevant to sonographic imaging and Doppler ultrasound. We have seen how these techniques are intended to function. However, things can go wrong. In imaging, an artifact is anything that does not correctly display the structures or functions (such as blood flow and motion) that are imaged. An artifact is caused by some problematic aspect of the imaging technique. In addition to helpful artifacts, several hinder correct interpretation and diagnosis. One must avoid these artifacts or handle them properly when they are encountered.

Artifacts are incorrect representations of anatomy or function. Artifacts in sonography occur as apparent structures that have one of the following characteristics:

1. Not real
2. Missing
3. Misplaced
4. Of incorrect brightness, shape, or size

Some artifacts are produced by improper equipment operation or settings (e.g., incorrect gain and compensation settings). Other artifacts are inherent in the sonographic and Doppler methods of today's scanners and can occur even with proper equipment and technique. Artifacts that occur in sonography are listed in Box 6-1, in which they are grouped as they are considered in the following sections.

The assumptions inherent in the design of sonographic instruments include the following:

- Sound travels in straight lines.
- Echoes originate only from objects located on the beam axis.
- The amplitude of returning echoes is related directly to the reflecting or scattering properties of distant objects.
- The distance to reflecting or scattering objects is proportional to the round-trip travel time (13 μs/cm of depth).

If any of these assumptions are violated, an artifact occurs.

Several artifacts are encountered in Doppler ultrasound, including incorrect display of Doppler flow information, either in color Doppler or in spectral format. The most common of these is **aliasing**. Other artifacts include **range ambiguity** and spectrum **mirror image**.

PROPAGATION

Slice Thickness

Limited detail resolution can introduce artifacts, because a failure to resolve means a loss of detail, and two adjacent structures may be visualized as one structure. The beam width perpendicular to the scan plane (the third dimension; Figure 6-1, *A*) results in slice-thickness artifacts. For example, the appearance of false debris in a simple echo-free cyst (see Figure 6-1, B). These artifacts occur because of the finite thickness of the interrogating beam used to scan the patient. Echoes originate not only from the center of the main beam, but also from off-center (the **slice thickness**). These echoes are all collapsed into a zero-thickness, two-dimensional image that is composed of echoes that have come from a not-so-thin tissue volume scanned by the beam. The slice-thickness artifact is also called the *section-thickness* or *partial-volume* artifact. It may be possible to resolve this artifact by using tissue harmonic imaging, because the sound beam in this mode is narrower than in the regular gray-scale mode (see Figure 6-1, *C*).

BOX 6-1 Sonographic Artifacts

Propagation Group
- Comet tail
- Grating lobe
- Mirror image
- Range ambiguity
- Refraction
- Reverberation
- Ring-down
- Slice (section) thickness
- Speckle
- Speed error

Attenuation Group
- Enhancement
- Focal enhancement
- Refraction (edge) shadowing
- Shadowing

> Beam width perpendicular to the scan plane causes slice thickness artifact.

Speckle

Apparent detail resolution can be deceiving. The detailed echo pattern often is not related directly to the scattering properties of tissue (called *tissue texture*) but is a result of the interference effects of the scattered sound from the distribution of all the scatterers within the tissue. There are many small scatterers (smaller than the wavelength) included in the ultrasound pulse at any instant while it travels through the tissue. Their echoes can combine constructively or destructively, which produces the familiar pattern of bright and dark spots in a gray-scale image. This phenomenon is called acoustic **speckle** (Figure 6-2) and may obstruct the detection of low-contrast objects in an

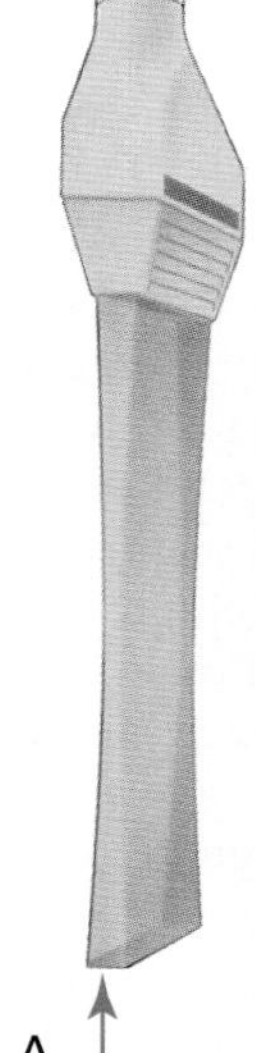

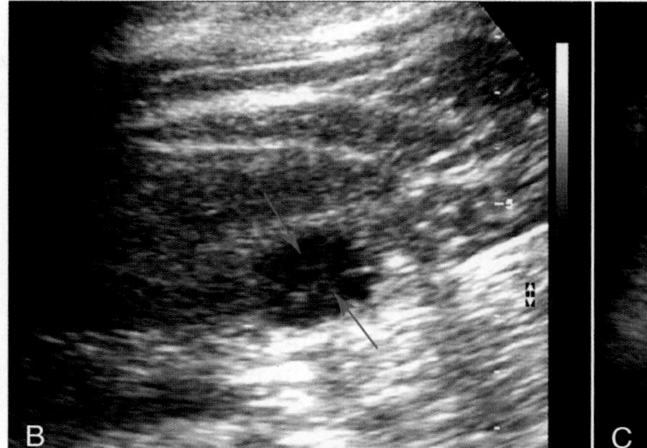

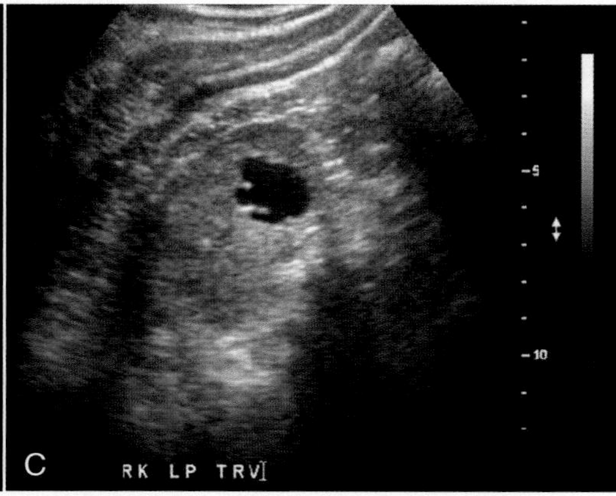

FIGURE 6-1 **A,** The scan "plane" through the tissue is really a three-dimensional volume. Two dimensions (axial and lateral) are in the scan plane, but there is a third dimension (called *slice thickness* or *section thickness*). The third dimension *(arrow)* is collapsed to zero thickness when the image is displayed in two-dimensional format. **B,** A simple renal cyst that should be echo-free is filled with echoes *(arrows),* which could indicate a solid renal lesion. These off-axis echoes are a result of scan-plane slice thickness. **C,** When tissue harmonic imaging is activated (resulting in a narrower beam-profile), the slice-thickness artifact disappears.

otherwise homogenous background (e.g., liver lesions). Strictly speaking, speckle is not an artifact because it results from the underlying distribution of scatterers. Given how difficult it is to predict speckle patterns in practice, most modern instruments have implemented some form of speckle reduction technique (see Figure 6-2).

> *Speckle* is the granular appearance of images that is caused by the interference of echoes from the distribution of scatterers in tissue.

Reverberation

Multiple reflections (**reverberations**) can occur between two strong reflectors or between the transducer and a strong reflector (Figure 6-3, *A*). When these multiple echoes are received by the scanner, they may be sufficiently strong to be detected by the instrument and then displayed. This may cause confusion in the interpretation of the displayed image. The process by which they are produced is shown in Figure 6-3, *B*. Reverberations are shown in the sonographic image as additional reflectors that do not represent real structures (Figure 6-4). The multiple reflections are displayed beneath the real reflector at intervals equal to the distance between the transducer and the real reflector. Each subsequent reflection is weaker than the one before, but this drop in echo strength is counteracted (at least partially) by the attenuation compensation (TGC) function. The **comet tail** artifact is a particular case of reverberation, in which two closely spaced surfaces generate a series of closely spaced, discrete echoes (Figure 6-5).

> Reverberations are multiple reflections between a structure and the transducer, between structures, or within a structure.

Mirror Image

The mirror-image artifact, also a form of reverberation, shows structures that exist on one side of a strong reflector as being present on the other side as well. Figure 6-6 explains how

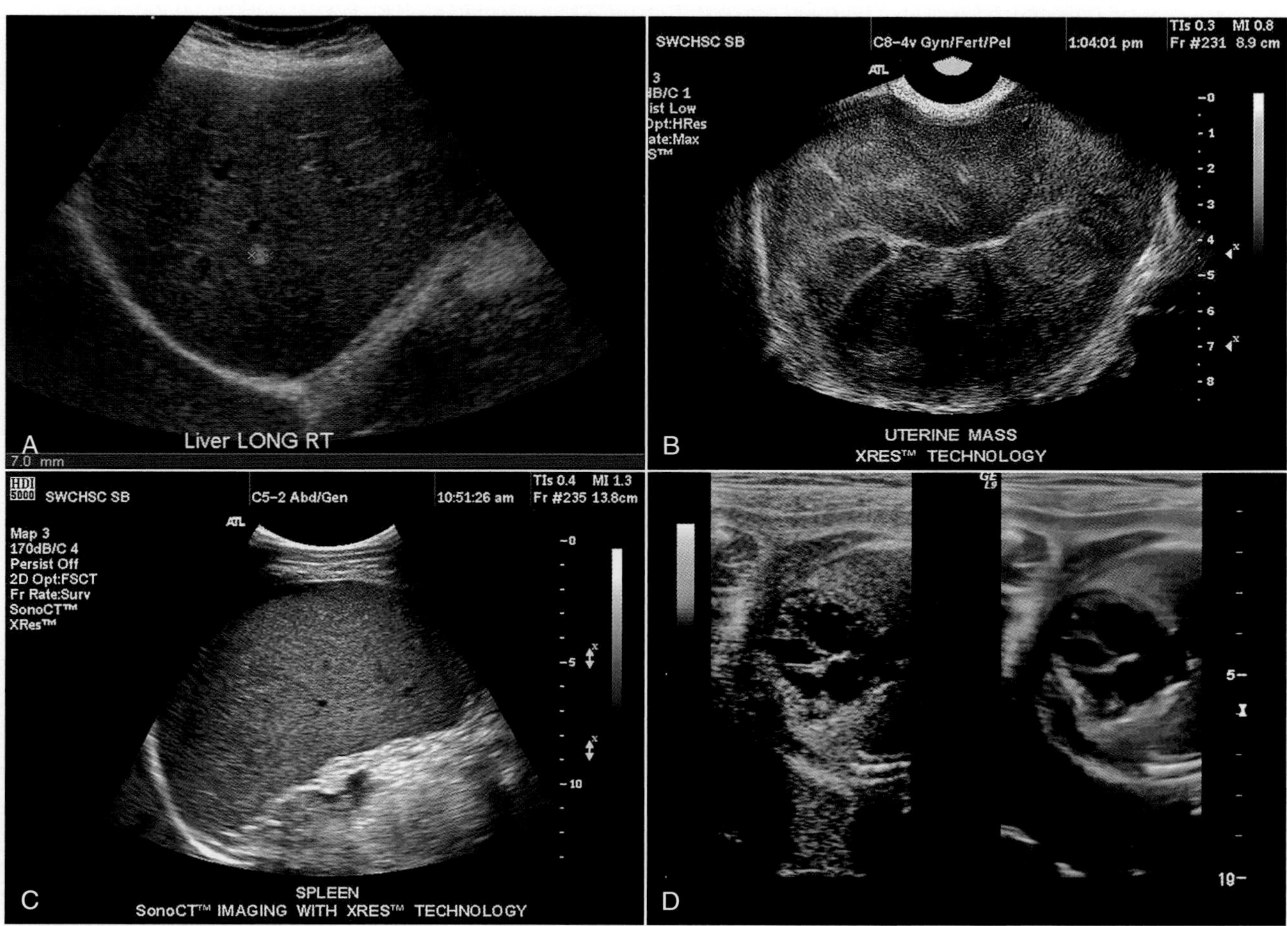

FIGURE 6-2 **A–C,** Three examples of the typically grainy appearance of ultrasound images that is not primarily the result of detail resolution limitations but rather of speckle. Speckle is the interference pattern resulting from constructive and destructive interference of echoes returning simultaneously from many scatterers within the propagating ultrasound pulse at any instant. **D,** Approaches to speckle reduction (right image compared with the left) are implemented in modern instruments.

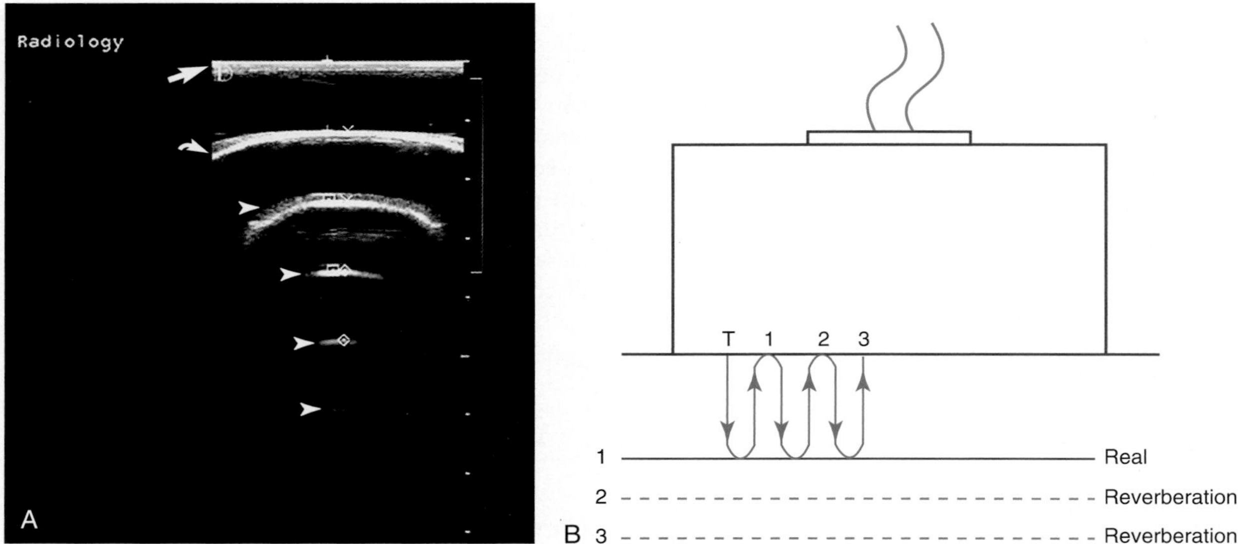

FIGURE 6-3 **A,** Reverberation *(arrowheads)* resulting from multiple reflection through a water path between a linear array transducer *(straight arrow)* and the surface of an apple *(curved arrow)*. **B,** The behavior in **A** is explained as follows: A pulse *(T)* is transmitted from the transducer. A strong echo is generated at the real reflector and is received *(1)* at the transducer, allowing correct imaging of the reflector. However, the echo is reflected partially at the transducer so that a second echo *(2)* is received, as well as a third *(3)*. Because these echoes arrive later, they appear deeper on the display, where there are no reflectors. The lateral displacement of the reverberating sound path is for figure clarity. In fact, the sound repeatedly travels down and back on the same path.

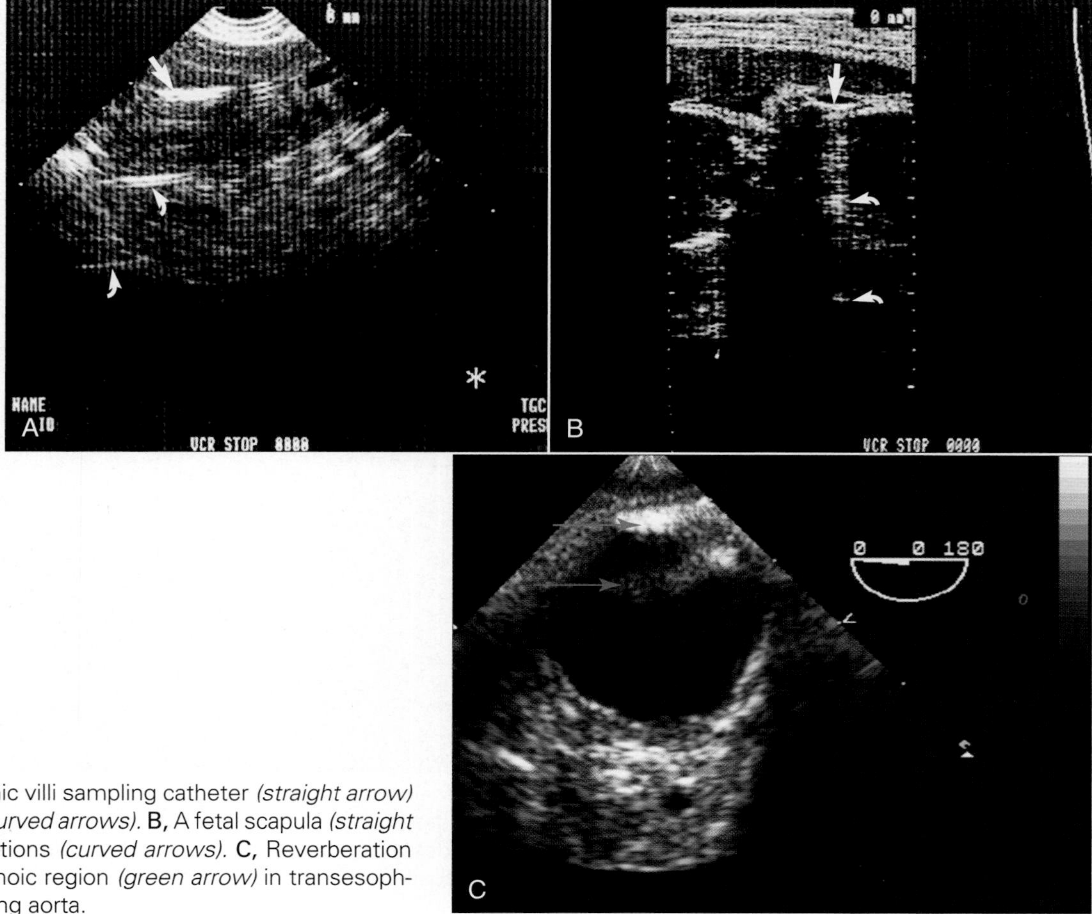

FIGURE 6-4 **A,** A chorionic villi sampling catheter *(straight arrow)* and two reverberations *(curved arrows)*. **B,** A fetal scapula *(straight arrow)* and two reverberations *(curved arrows)*. **C,** Reverberation *(red arrow)* from hyperechoic region *(green arrow)* in transesophageal scan of the ascending aorta.

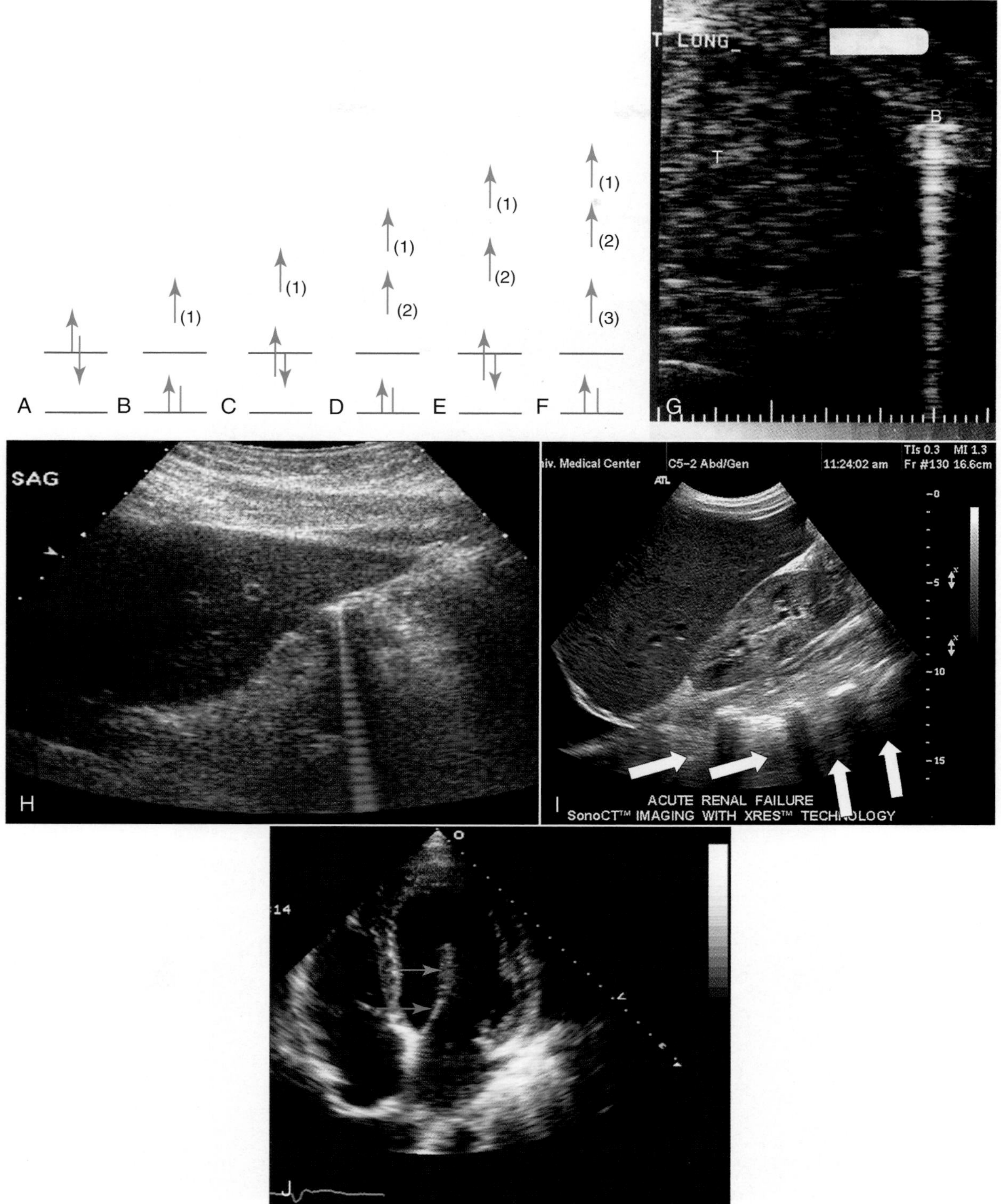

FIGURE 6-5 Generation of comet-tail artifact (closely spaced reverberations). Action progresses in time from left to right. **A,** An ultrasound pulse encounters the first reflector, is reflected partially, and is transmitted partially. **B,** Reflection and transmission at the first reflector are complete. Reflection at the second reflector is occurring. **C,** Reflection at the second reflector is complete. Partial transmission and partial reflection are again occurring at the first reflector as the second echo passes through. **D,** The echoes from the first *(1)* and second *(2)* reflectors are traveling toward the transducer. A second reflection (repeat of **B**) is occurring at the second reflector. **E,** Partial transmission and reflection are again occurring at the first reflector. **F,** Three echoes are now returning—the echo from the first reflector *(1),* the echo from the second reflector *(2),* and the echo from the second reflector *(3)*—that originated from the back side of the first reflector (**C**) and reflected again from the second reflector (**D**). A fourth echo is being generated at the second reflector (**F**). **G,** Comet-tail artifact from an air rifle BB shot pellet *(B)* adjacent to the testicle *(T).* The front and rear surface of the BB shot are the two reflecting surfaces involved in this example. **H,** Comet-tail artifact from gas bubbles in the duodenum. **I,** Comet tail *(arrows)* from diaphragm. **J,** Apical four-chamber view of comet tail artifact *(green arrow)* in the left ventricle. The artifact is connected to anterior mitral leaflet *(red arrow).* (**G** from Kremkau FW, Taylor KJW: Artifacts in ultrasound imaging, *J Ultrasound Med* 5:227, 1986.)

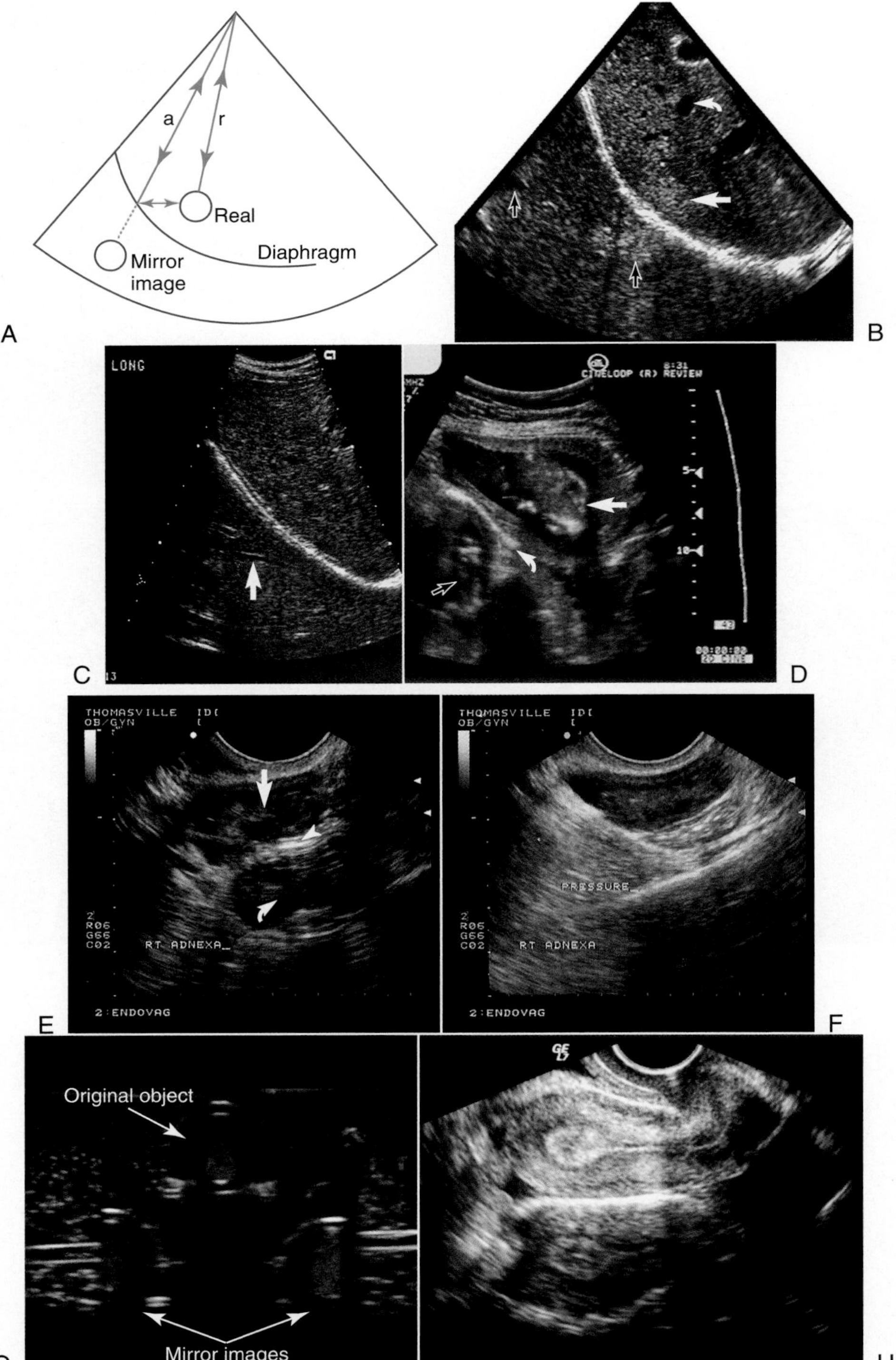

FIGURE 6-6 **A,** When pulses encounter a real hepatic structure directly *(scan line r),* the structure is imaged correctly. If the pulse first reflects off the diaphragm *(scan line a)* and returns along the same path, the structure is displayed on the other side of the diaphragm. **B,** A hemangioma *(straight arrow)* and vessel *(curved arrow)* with their mirror images *(open arrows).* **C,** A vessel is mirror-imaged *(arrow)* superior to the diaphragm but does not appear inferior because it is outside the unmirrored scan plane. **D,** A fetus *(straight arrow)* also appears as a mirror image *(open arrow).* The mirror *(curved arrow)* is probably echogenic muscle. **E,** Ovary *(arrow)* with mirror image *(curved arrow)* that could be mistaken for an adnexal mass or ectopic pregnancy. Bowel gas *(arrowhead)* is apparently the mirror in this case. **F,** Applying external abdominal pressure displaces the gas, eliminating the mirror image. **G,** Mirror image of a thick-walled vessel in a tissue-equivalent phantom. The echoes are being reflected from the echogenic scatterers used in the circulating fluid and the vessel wall resulting in two mirror images split on either side of the center line *(arrows).* **H,** Uterus with its mirror image below it.

this happens and shows examples. Mirror-image artifacts are common around the diaphragm and pleura because of the total reflection from air-filled lung, and they occasionally occur in other locations. Sometimes the mirrored structure is not in the unmirrored scan plane (see Figure 6-6, *C*).

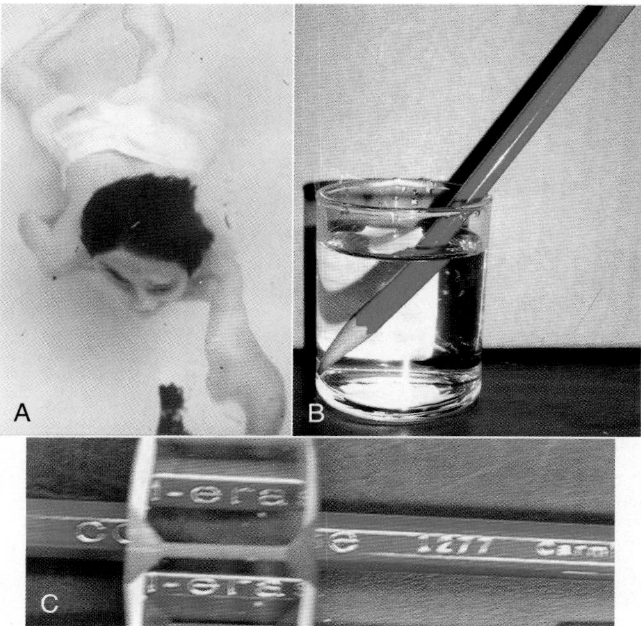

FIGURE 6-7 **A,** Refracted light from a child in a swimming pool distorts his appearance. We see a thin arm and a thick one, a large eye and a small one, a thin leg, a thick one, and even a third lower limb emerging. **B,** A pencil in water appears to be broken. **C,** A pencil beneath a prism appears to be split in two.

> A mirror-image artifact duplicates a structure on the opposite side of a strong reflector.

Refraction

Refraction of light enables lenses to focus and distorts the presentation of objects, as shown in Figure 6-7. Refraction can cause a reflector to be positioned improperly (laterally) on a sonographic display (Figure 6-8). This is likely to occur, for example, when the transducer is placed on the abdominal midline (see Figure 6-8, *C*, and Figure 6-9), producing doubling of single objects. Beneath are the rectus abdominis muscles, which are surrounded by fat. These tissues present refracting boundaries because of their different propagation speeds.

> Refraction displaces structures laterally from their correct locations.

Grating Lobes

Side lobes are beams that propagate from a single element in directions different from the primary or main beam. Grating lobes are additional beams emitted from an array transducer that are stronger than the side lobes of individual elements (Figure 6-10). Side and grating lobes are weaker than the primary beam and normally do not produce echoes that are displayed in the image, particularly if they fall on a normally echogenic region of the scan. However, if grating lobes encounter a strong reflector (e.g., bone or gas), their echoes may well be displayed, particularly if they fall within an anechoic region. If so, they appear in incorrect locations, such as in these obstetric examples (Figure 6-11). Note that the grating lobe artifact

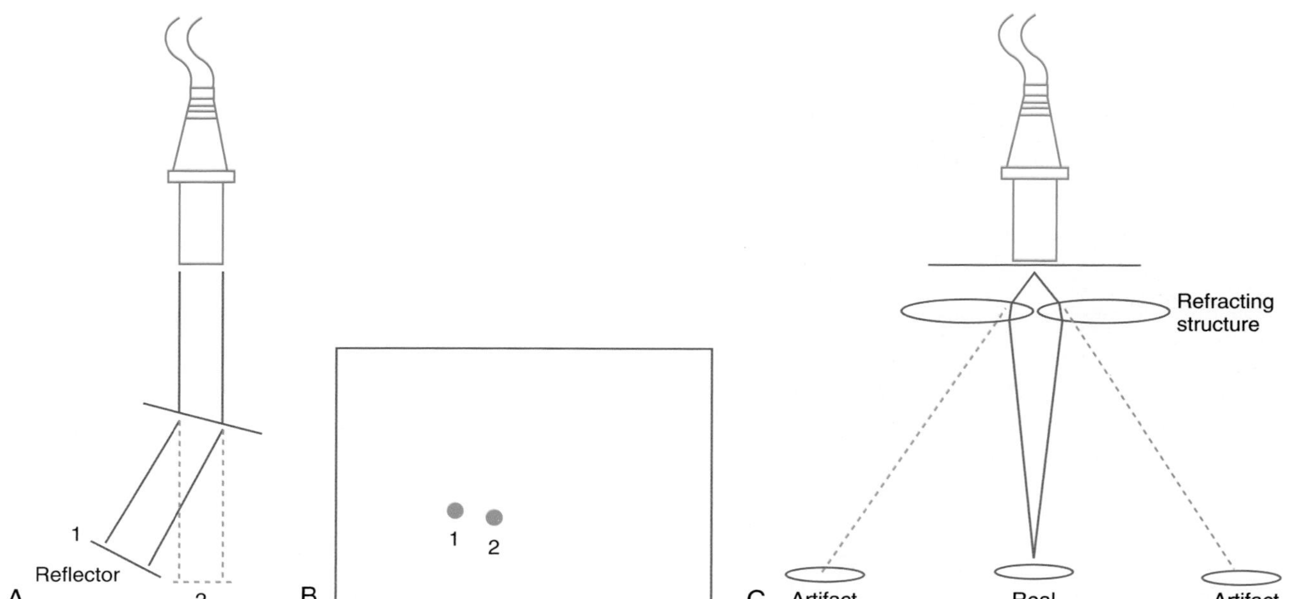

FIGURE 6-8 Refraction **(A)** results in improper positioning of a reflector on the display **(B).** The system places the reflector at position 2 (because that is the direction from which the echo was received), when in fact the reflector is actually at position 1. **C,** One real structure is imaged as two artifactual objects because of the refracting structure close to the transducer. If unrefracted pulses can propagate to the real structure, a triple presentation (one correct, two artifactual) will result.

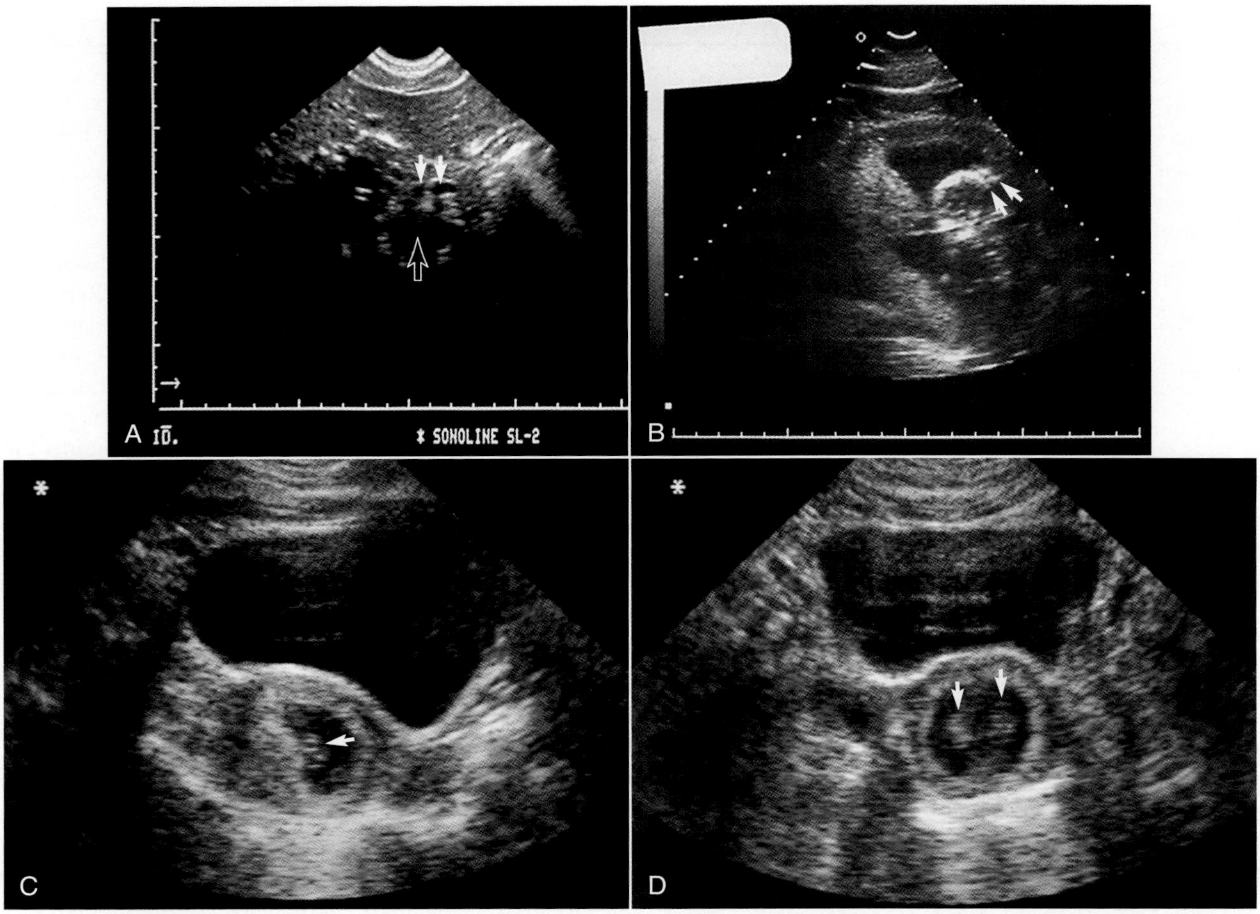

FIGURE 6-9 **A,** Refraction (probably through the rectus abdominis muscle) has widened the aorta *(open arrow)* and produced a double image of the celiac trunk *(arrows).* **B,** Refraction has produced a double image of a fetal skull *(arrows).* Refraction also may cause a single gestation (**C**) to appear as a double gestation (**D**).

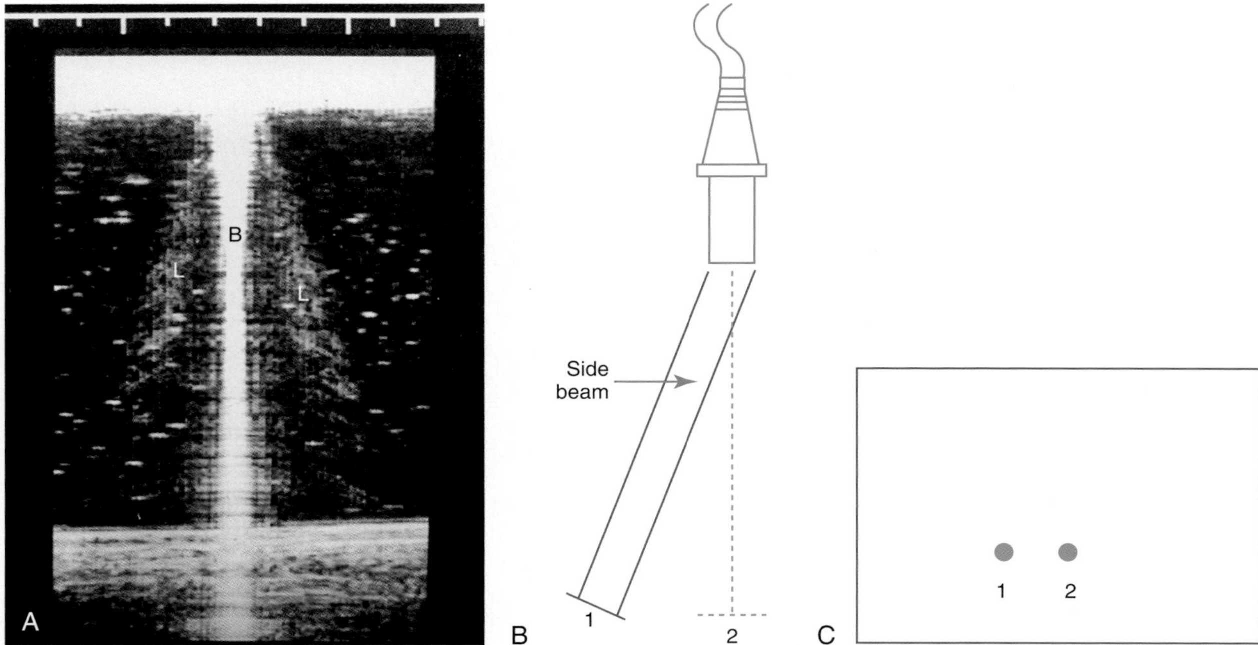

FIGURE 6-10 **A,** The primary beam *(B)* and grating lobes *(L)* from a linear array transducer. **B,** A side lobe or grating lobe can produce and receive a reflection from a "side view." **C,** This will be placed on the display at the proper distance from the transducer but in the wrong location (direction) because the instrument assumes that echoes originate from points along the main beam axis. The instrument shows the reflector at position 2 because that is the direction in which the main beam travels. The reflector is actually in position 1.

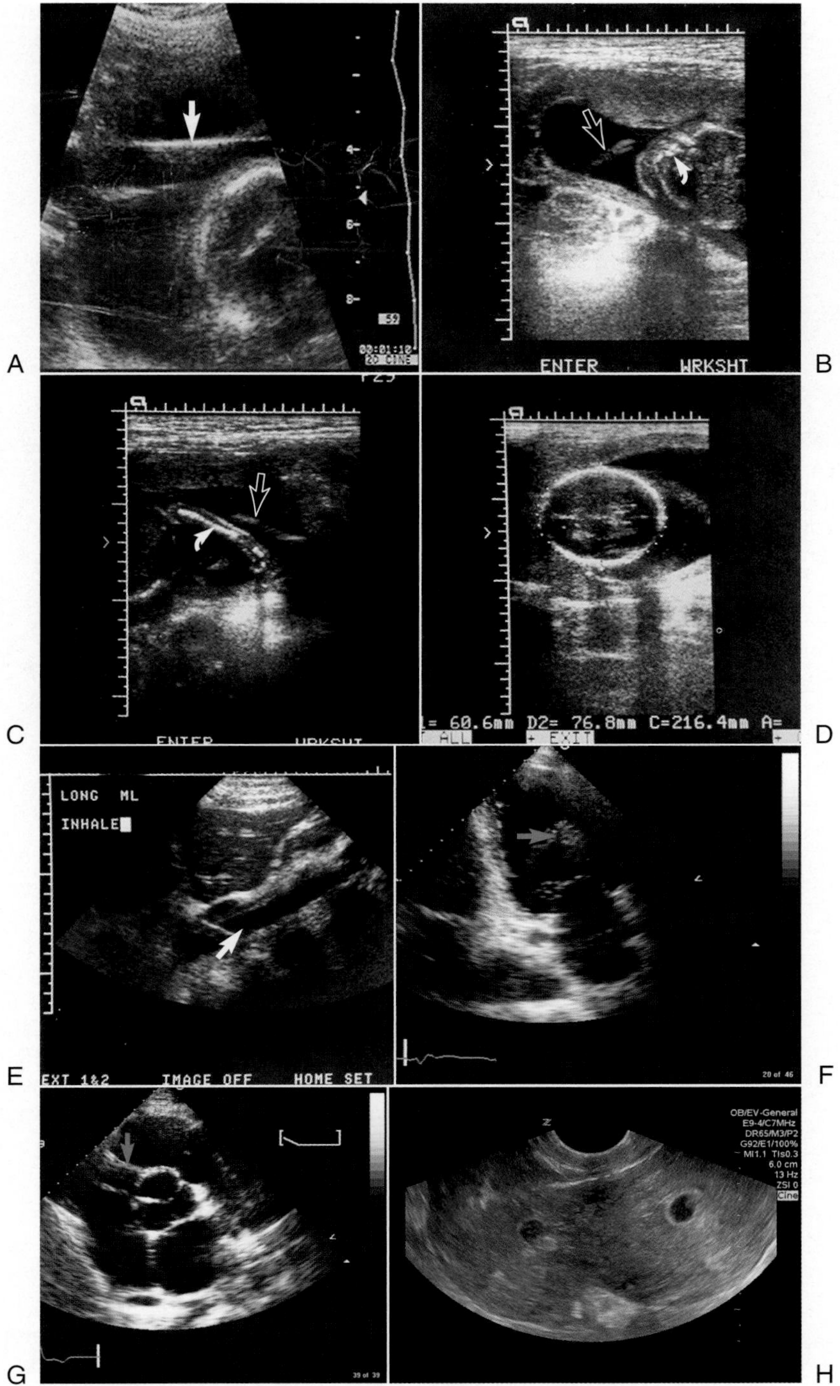

FIGURE 6-11 Grating lobe examples. A, A real amniotic sheet *(arrow)*. **B–C,** Grating lobe duplication *(open arrows)* of fetal bones *(curved arrows)* resembles amniotic bands or sheets. **D,** Grating lobe duplication of a fetal skull. **E,** Artifactual grating lobe echoes *(arrow)* cross the aorta. In these examples, we observe that the grating lobe artifact is always weaker than the correct presentation of the structure. **F,** Apical two-chamber view of grating-lobe artifact *(arrow)* in left ventricle. **G,** Short-axis view of aortic and tricuspid valves with grating lobe artifact *(arrow)*. **H,** At first glance, this seems to be a mirror image artifact, similar to what is seen in abdominal imaging (see Figure 6-6, *A-C*). However, it is not for two reasons: (1) There is no apparent echogenic mirror, and (2) The repeat on the left side is not horizontally reversed as would be the case with mirroring. Rather, it is a less echogenic repeat of what is on the right. Therefore this is a grating-lobe duplication. Such duplications appear laterally and with less brightness than the correct presentation. (Courtesy of David Bahner, MD, RDMS, College of Medicine, Ohio State University.)

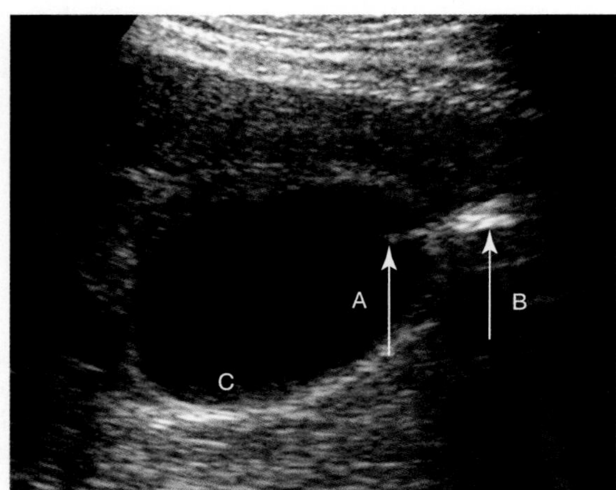

FIGURE 6-12 Needle tip *(A arrow)* is correctly seen in a cyst for aspiration, whereas grating lobes show the out-of-plane body of the needle *(B arrow)*. In this example, there is also a slice thickness artifact depicting nonexistent sludge in the cyst *(C)*.

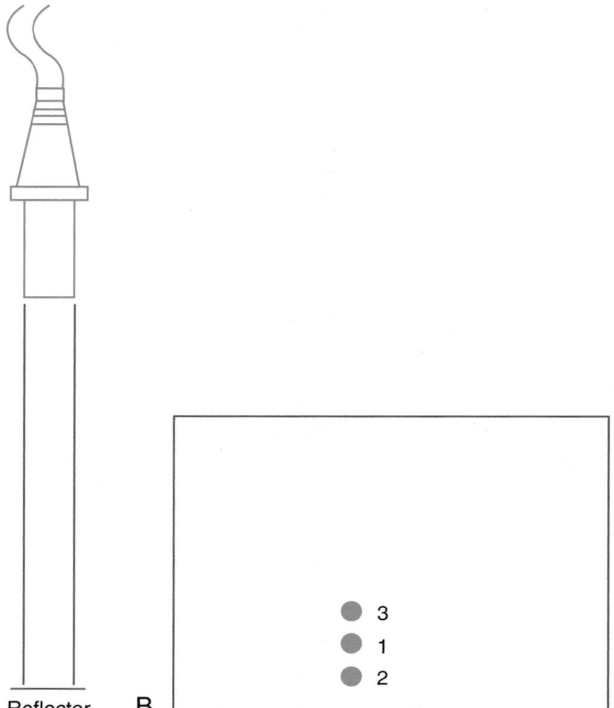

FIGURE 6-13 The propagation speed over the traveled path (**A**) determines the reflector position on the display (**B**). The reflector is actually in position 1. If the actual propagation speed is less than that assumed, the reflector will appear in position 2. If the actual speed is more than that assumed, the reflector will appear in position 3.

is normally weaker than the correct presentation of the structure. However, that may not always be the case with very strong reflectors, such as metallic needles (Figure 6-12).

Grating lobes duplicate structures laterally to the true ones.

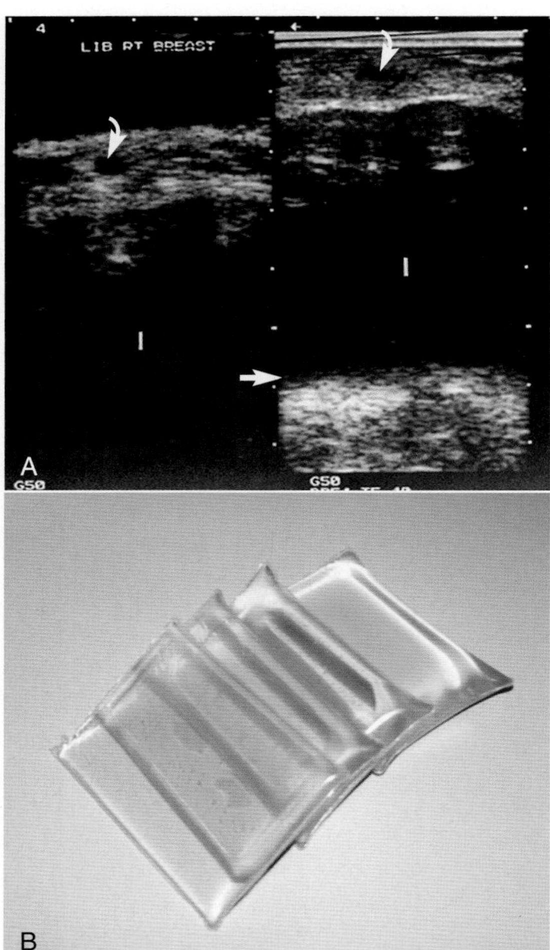

FIGURE 6-14 The low propagation speed in a silicone breast implant *(I)* causes the chest wall *(straight arrow)* to appear deeper than it should (**A**). Note that a cyst *(curved arrow)* is shown more clearly on the left image than on the right because a gel standoff pad (**B**) has been placed between the transducer and the breast, moving the beam focus closer to the cyst.

Speed Error

Propagation **speed error** occurs when the assumed value for the speed of sound in soft tissues (1.54 mm/μs, leading to the 13 μs/cm rule) is incorrect. If the propagation speed that exists over a path traveled is greater than 1.54 mm/μs, the calculated distance to the reflector is too small, and the display will place the reflector too close to the transducer (Figure 6-13). This occurs because the increased speed causes the echoes to arrive sooner. If the actual speed is less than 1.54 mm/μs, the reflector will be displayed too far from the transducer (Figure 6-14) because the echoes arrive later. Refraction and propagation speed error can also cause a structure to be displayed with an incorrect shape.

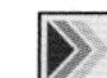
Propagation speed error displaces structures axially.

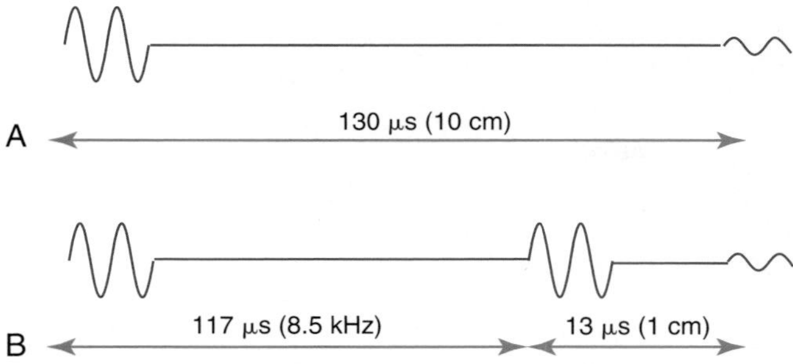

FIGURE 6-15 **A,** An echo (from a 10-cm depth) arrives 130 μs after pulse emission. **B,** If the pulse repetition period were 117 μs (corresponding to a pulse repetition frequency of 8.5 kHz), the echo in **A** would arrive 13 μs after the next pulse was emitted. The instrument would place this echo at a 1-cm depth rather than the correct value. This range location error is known as the *range-ambiguity artifact.*

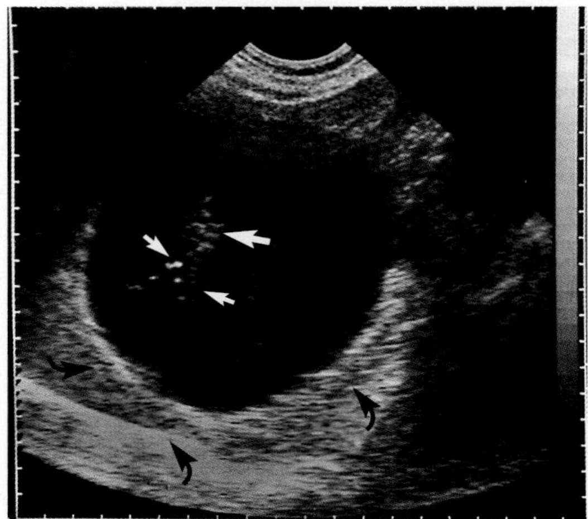

FIGURE 6-16 **A large renal cyst (diameter approximately 10 cm) contains artifactual range-ambiguity echoes *(white arrows).*** They are generated from structures below the display. These deep echoes arrive after the next pulse is emitted. Because the time from the emission of the last pulse to echo arrival is short, the echoes are placed closer to the transducer than they should be. Echoes arrive from much deeper (later) than usual in this case because the sound passes through the long, low-attenuation paths in the cyst. These echoes may have come from bone or a far body wall. Low attenuation in the cyst is indicated by the enhancement below it *(curved black arrows).*

Range Ambiguity

In sonographic imaging, it is assumed that for each pulse all echoes are received before the next pulse is emitted. If this were not the case, error could result (Figures 6-15 and 6-16). The maximum depth imaged correctly by an instrument is determined by its pulse repetition frequency (PRF). To avoid range ambiguity, PRF automatically is reduced in deeper imaging situations. This also causes a reduction in frame rate.

> The range-ambiguity artifact places structures much closer to the surface than they should be.

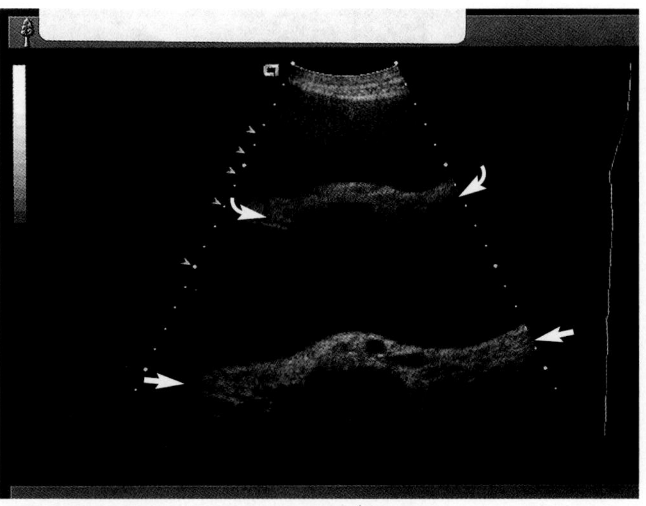

FIGURE 6-17 **Abdominal ascites produces a large echo-free region in this scan.** A structure is located at a depth of approximately 13 cm *(straight arrows).* Located in the anechoic region at a depth of approximately 6 cm is a structure *(curved arrows)* shaped like the structure at 13 cm. How could this artifact appear closer than the actual structure, implying that these echoes arrived earlier than those from the correct location? It turns out that the artifact is actually a combination of two: reverberation and range ambiguity. The artifact seen is a reverberation from the deep structure and the transducer. But a reverberation should appear at twice the depth of the actual structure, that is, at about 26 cm. However, the arrival of the reverberation echoes occurs approximately 78 μs after the next pulse is emitted, so that they are placed at a 6-cm depth. Single artifacts are difficult enough. Fortunately, combinations like this occur infrequently.

Sometimes two artifacts combine to present even more challenging cases. An example involving range ambiguity is shown in Figure 6-17.

ATTENUATION

Shadowing

Shadowing is the reduction in echo amplitude from reflectors that lie behind a strongly reflecting or attenuating structure (Figure 6-18). A strongly attenuating or reflecting structure weakens the sound distal to it, causing echoes from the distal region to be weak and thus to appear darker, like a shadow. Of course, the returning echoes also must pass through the attenuating structure, adding to the shadowing effect. Examples of shadowing structures include calcified plaques (see Figure 6-18, *A*), stiff breast lesions (see Figure 6-18, *B*), and stones (Figure 6-19, *A*). Shadowing also can occur behind the edges of objects that are not necessarily strong attenuators (Figure 6-20). In this case the cause may be the defocusing action of a refracting curved surface. Alternatively, it may be attributable to destructive interference caused by portions of an ultrasound pulse passing through tissues with different propagation speeds and subsequently getting out of phase. In either

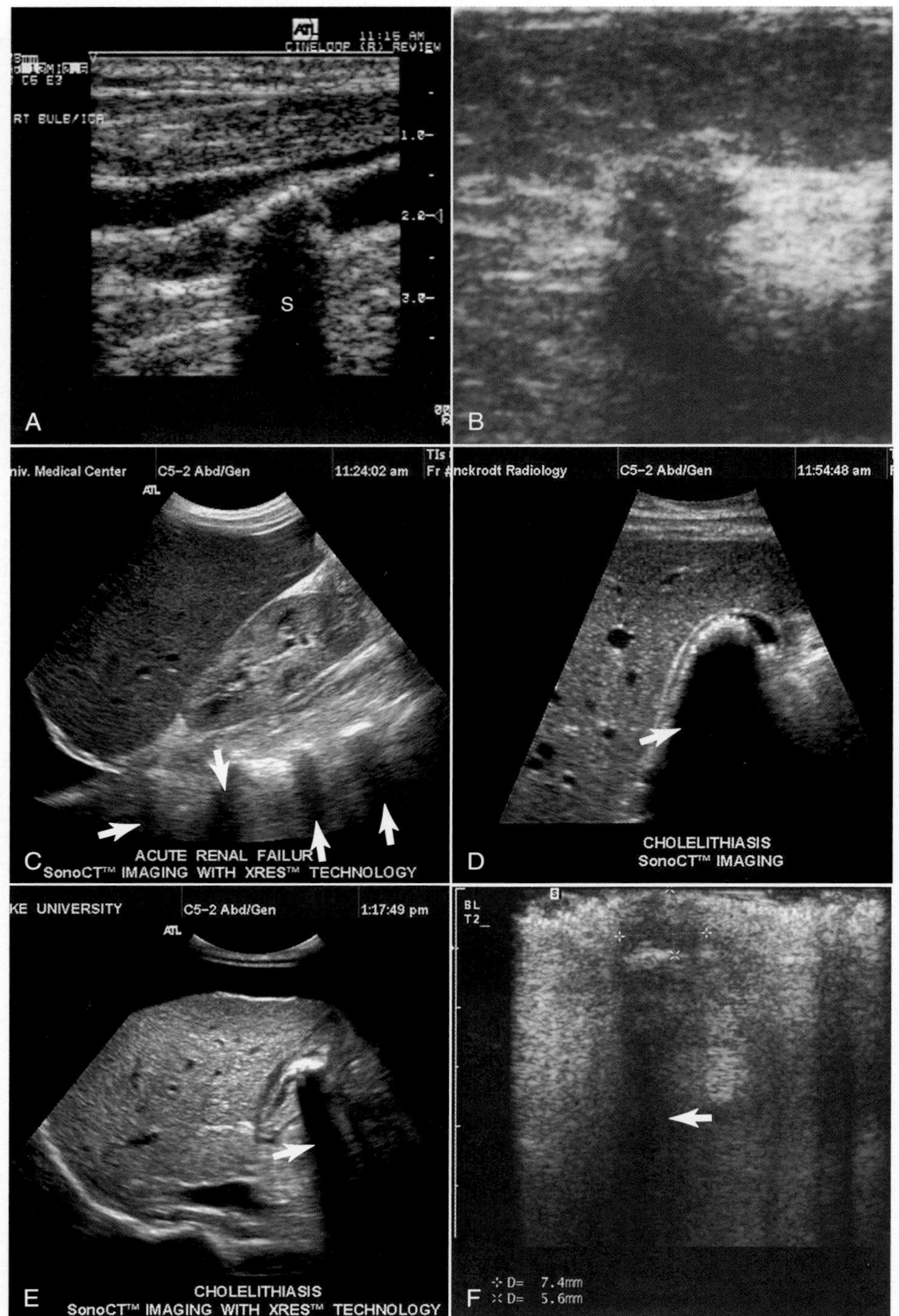

FIGURE 6-18 A, Shadowing *(S)* from a high-attenuation calcified plaque in the common carotid artery. B, Shadowing from a stiff breast lesion. C–F, Examples of shadowing *(arrows).*

case the intensity of the beam decreases beyond the edge of the structure, causing echoes to be weakened.

> Shadowing is the weakening of echoes distal to a strongly attenuating or reflecting structure or from the edges of a refracting structure.

Enhancement

Enhancement is the strengthening of echoes from reflectors that lie behind a weakly attenuating structure (see Figures 6-16 and 6-19). Shadowing and enhancement result in reflectors being displayed on the image with amplitudes that are too low and too high, respectively. Brightening of echoes also can be caused by the increased intensity in the focal region of a beam because the beam is narrow there. This is called

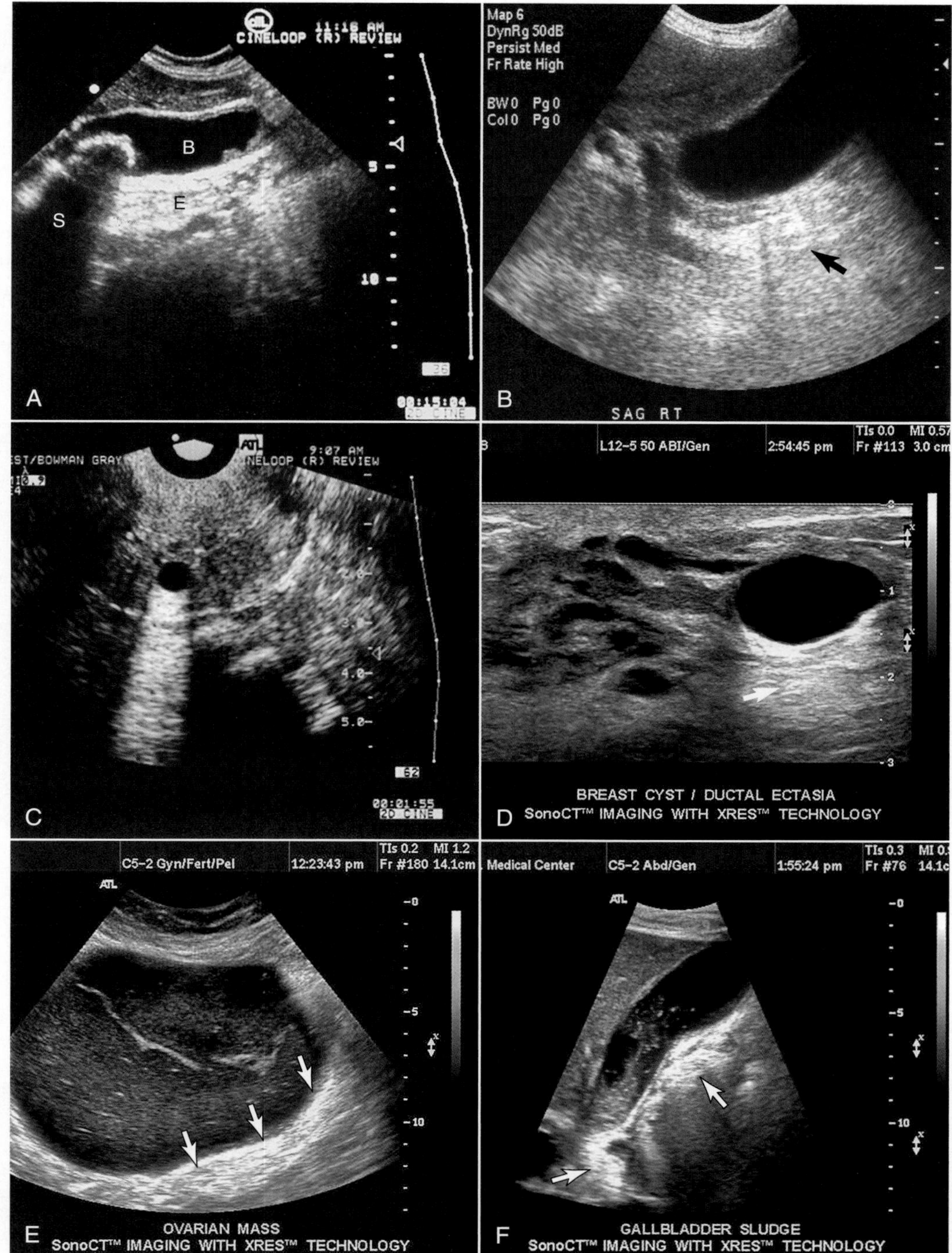

FIGURE 6-19 **A**, Shadowing *(S)* from a gallstone and enhancement *(E)* caused by the low attenuation of bile *(B)*. **B**, Enhancement *(arrow)* from the low attenuation of bile in the gallbladder. **C**, Enhancement beyond a cervical cyst. **D–F**, Examples of enhancement *(arrows)*.

focal enhancement or *focal banding* (Figure 6-21). Shadowing and enhancement artifacts are often useful for determining the nature of masses and structures. Shadowing and enhancement are reduced with spatial compounding (and other speckle reduction techniques), because several directional approaches to each anatomic site are used to form the final image, allowing the beam to "get around" the attenuating or enhancing structure. This may be useful with shadowing because it can uncover structures (especially pathologic ones) that were not imaged because they were located in the shadow.

> Enhancement is the strengthening of echoes distal to a weakly attenuating structure.

External influences also can produce artifacts. As an example, interference from electronic equipment adds unwanted noise to the image (Figure 6-22).

SPECTRAL DOPPLER

Aliasing

Aliasing is the most common artifact encountered in Doppler ultrasound. The word *alias* comes from the Middle English *elles,* the Latin *alius,* and the Greek *allos,* which all mean "other" or "otherwise." Contemporary meanings for the word include (as an adverb) "otherwise called" or "otherwise known as" and (as a noun) "an assumed or additional name." Aliasing in its technical use indicates improper representation of information that has been sampled insufficiently. The sampling can be spatial or temporal. Inadequate spatial sampling can result in improper conclusions about the object or population sampled. For example, we could assemble 10 families, each composed of a father, a mother, and a child, and line all of the families up in that order—father, mother, child, father, mother, child. If we wanted to sample the contents of these families by taking 10 photographs, we could choose to photograph one of every three persons (e.g., the first, fourth, and seventh persons in the line). However, if we did this, we would conclude that all families are composed of three adult males, no women,

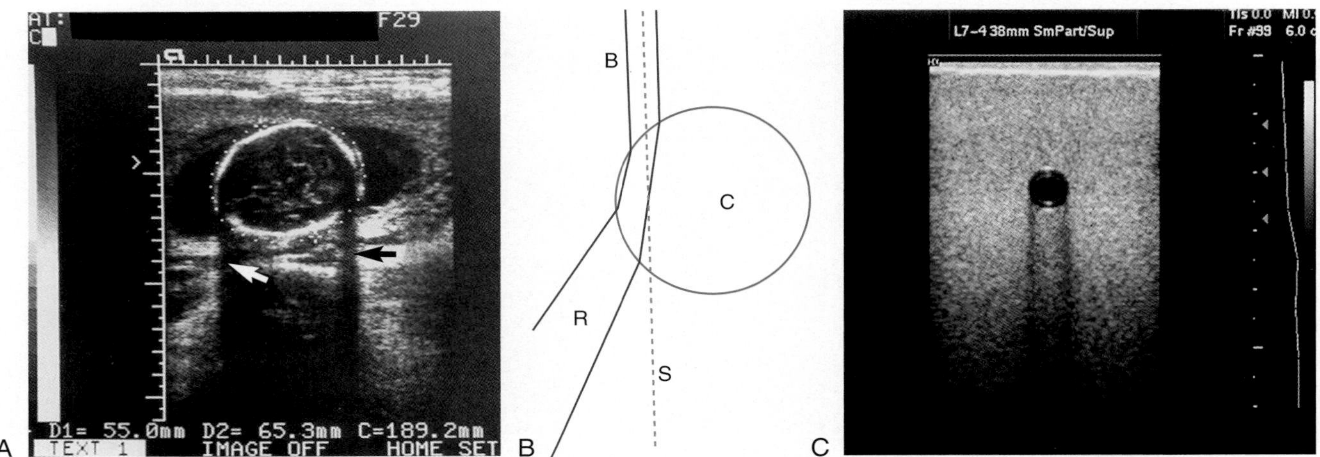

FIGURE 6-20 A, Edge shadows *(arrows)* from a fetal skull. **B,** While a sound beam *(B)* enters a circular region *(C)* of higher propagation speed, it is refracted, and refraction occurs again while it leaves. This causes spreading of the beam with decreased intensity. The echoes from region *R* are presented deep to the circular region in the neighborhood of the dashed line. Because of beam spreading, these echoes are weak and thus cast a shadow *(S).* **C,** Edge shadows from a tube (shown in transverse view) embedded in tissue-equivalent material in a flow phantom.

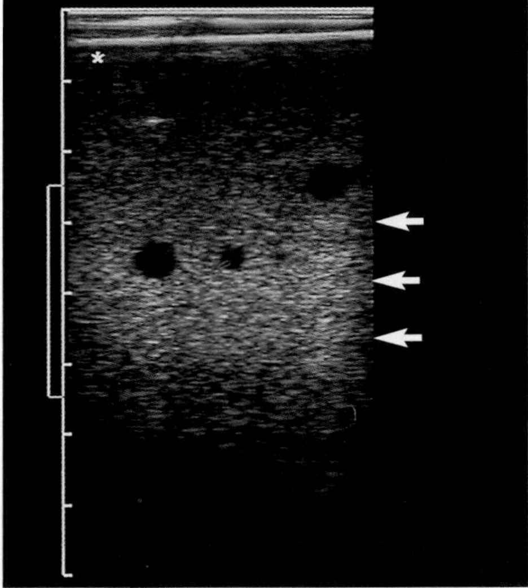

FIGURE 6-21 Focal banding *(arrows)* is the brightening of echoes around the focus, where intensity is increased by the narrowing of the beam.

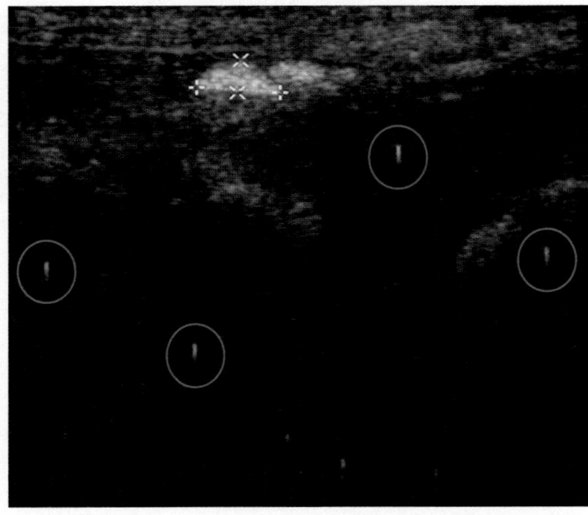

FIGURE 6-22 Interference *(circled random white specks)* from nearby electronic equipment seen below a small lymph node.

and no children. In this example, spatial undersampling of one third of the population would result in an incorrect conclusion regarding the total population.

An optical form of temporal aliasing occurs in motion pictures when wagon wheels appear to rotate at various speeds and in reverse direction. Similar behavior is observed when a fan is lighted with a strobe light. Depending on the flashing rate of the strobe light, the fan may appear stationary or to rotate clockwise or counterclockwise at various speeds.

TABLE 6-1 Aliasing and Range-Ambiguity Artifact Values

Pulse Repetition Frequency (kHz)	Doppler Shift Above Which Aliasing Occurs (kHz)	Range Beyond Which Ambiguity Occurs (cm)
5.0	2.5	15
7.5	3.7	10
10.0	5.0	7
12.5	6.2	6
15.0	7.5	5
17.5	8.7	4
20.0	10.0	3
25.0	12.5	3
30.0	15.0	2

BOX 6-2 Methods of Correcting or Eliminating Aliasing

1. Shift the baseline.
2. Increase the pulse repetition frequency.
3. Increase the Doppler angle.
4. Use a lower operating frequency.
5. Use a continuous wave device.

Nyquist Limit

Pulsed-wave Doppler instruments are sampling instruments. Each emitted pulse yields a sample of the desired Doppler shift. The upper limit to Doppler shift that can be detected properly by pulsed instruments is called the **Nyquist limit** (NL). If the Doppler-shift frequency exceeds one half of the PRF (which is typically in the 5- to 30-kHz range for pulsed Doppler instruments), temporal aliasing occurs:

$$NL\,(kHz) = \frac{1}{2} \times PRF\,(kHz)$$

Improper Doppler shift information (improper direction and improper value) results. Higher PRFs (Table 6-1) permit higher Doppler shifts to be detected, but also increase the chance that the range-ambiguity artifact will occur. Continuous-wave Doppler instruments do not experience aliasing. However, recall that neither do they provide depth localization (localized sample volume).

> Aliasing is the appearance of Doppler spectral information on the wrong side of the baseline.

Figures 6-23 and 6-24 illustrate aliasing in the carotid artery and in the aorta of a normal individual. Also illustrated is how aliasing can be corrected or eliminated (Box 6-2) by increasing PRF, increasing Doppler angle (which decreases the Doppler shift for a given flow), or shifting the baseline. The latter is an electronic cut-and-paste technique that moves the misplaced aliasing peaks to their proper location. The technique is successful as long as there are no legitimate Doppler shifts in the region of the aliasing. If there are legitimate Doppler shifts, they will be moved to an inappropriate location along with the aliasing peaks. Baseline shifting is not helpful if the desired information (e.g., peak systolic Doppler shift) is buried in another portion of the spectral display (see Figure 6-23, *G*).

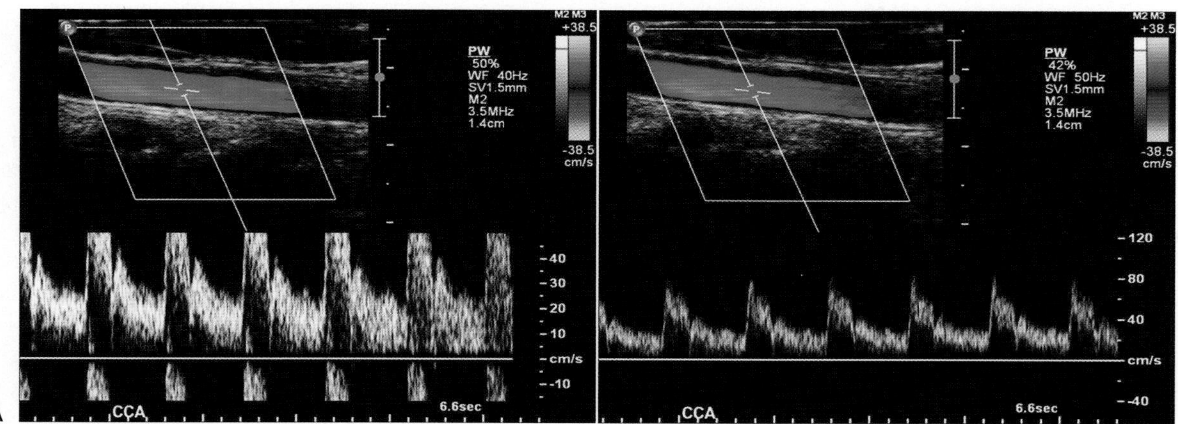

FIGURE 6-23 **A,** Aliasing in the common carotid artery (CCA). **B,** Pulse repetition frequency (scale control) is increased to eliminate the aliasing.

Continued

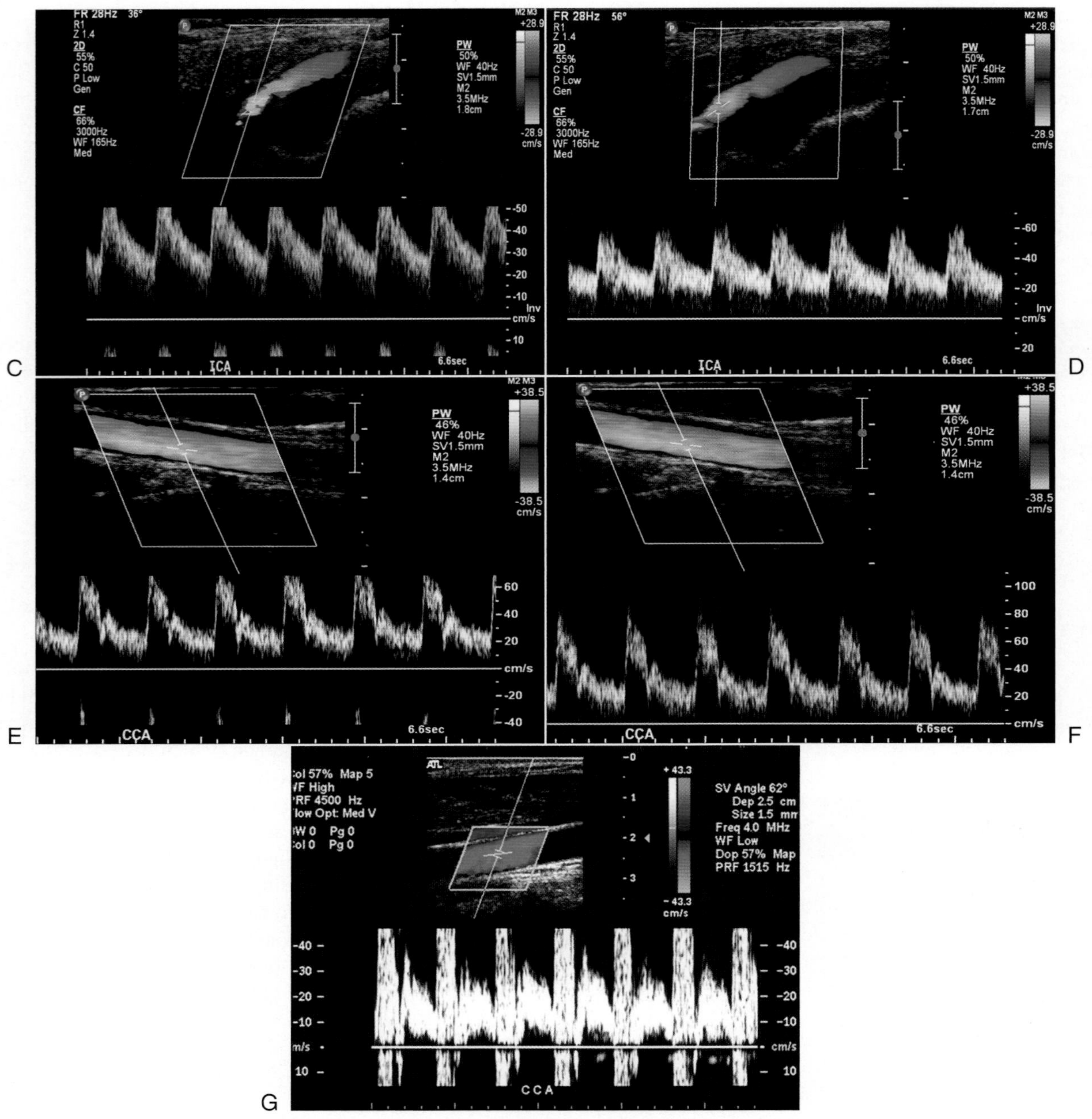

FIGURE 6-23, cont'd **C,** Aliasing in the internal carotid artery at a 36-degree Doppler angle. **D,** When the Doppler angle is increased to 56 degrees, the aliasing is resolved. **E–F,** Baseline is shifted down to correct for aliasing in the CCA. **G,** This is an example in which baseline shifting would not be helpful.

Other approaches to eliminating aliasing include changing to a lower-frequency (see Figure 6-24) or switching to continuous-wave operation. The common and convenient solutions to aliasing are shifting the baseline, increasing PRF, or, in extreme cases, both.

> Aliasing is caused by undersampling of the Doppler shifts.

Aliasing occurs with a pulsed Doppler system because it is a sampling system; that is, a pulsed Doppler system acquires samples of the desired Doppler shift frequency from which it must be synthesized (see Figure 5-41). If samples are taken often enough, the correct result is achieved. Figure 6-25 shows temporal sampling of a signal. Sufficient sampling yields the correct result. Insufficient sampling yields an incorrect result.

The NL, or Nyquist frequency, describes the minimum number of samples required to avoid aliasing. At least two samples per cycle of the desired Doppler shift must be made for the image to be obtained correctly. For a complicated signal, such as a Doppler signal containing many frequencies, the sampling rate must be such that at least two samples occur for each cycle of the highest frequency present. To restate this

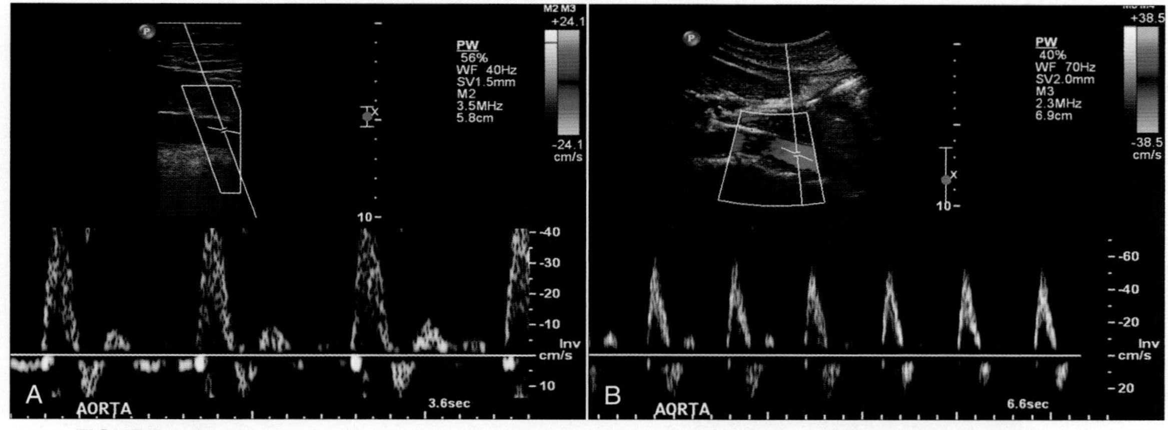

FIGURE 6-24 Aliasing in the aorta when imaged at 3.5 MHz **(A)** can be eliminated by imaging at a lower frequency of 2.3 MHz **(B)** in which the Doppler shifts are reduced to less than the Nyquist limit.

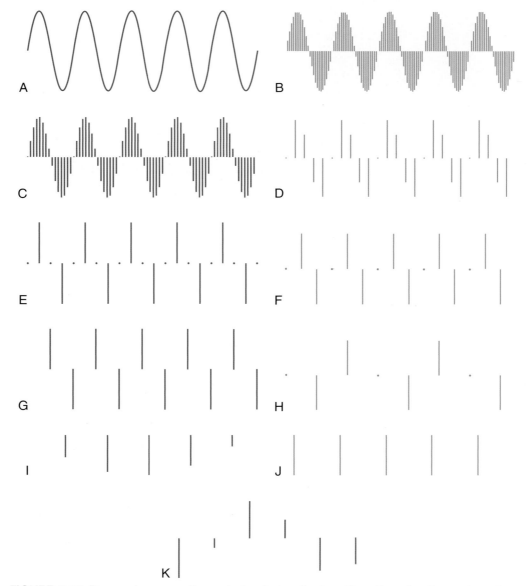

FIGURE 6-25 Decreasing sampling rate leads to aliasing. Sampling of a five-cycle voltage **(A)** is progressively decreased from 25 samples per cycle **(B)**, to 15 samples per cycle **(C)**, to five samples per cycle **(D)**, to four samples per cycle **(E)**, to three samples per cycle **(F)**, to two samples per cycle **(G)**, and finally to successive sampling of one sample per cycle **(H–K)**. In the last four cases, aliasing occurs.

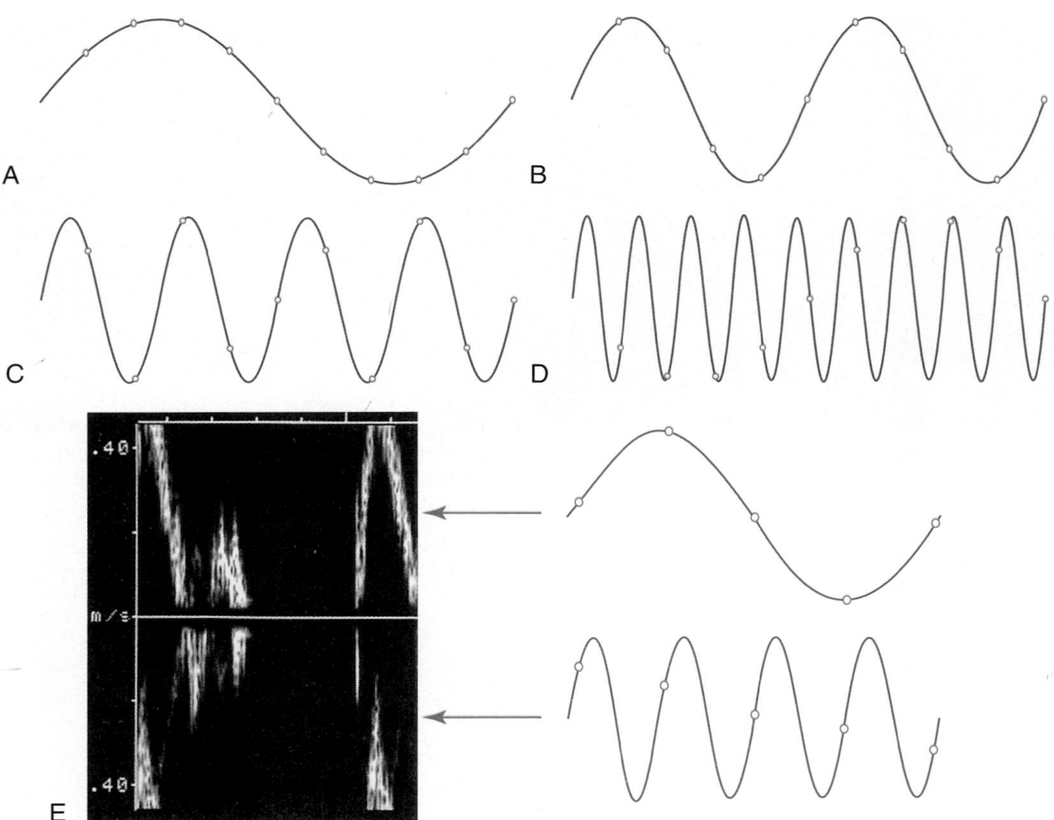

FIGURE 6-26 Increasing frequency leads to aliasing. Signal voltages are sampled at 10 points *(red circles):* **(A)** one cycle, **(B)** two cycles, **(C)** four cycles, and **(D)** nine cycles. As signal frequency is increased, aliasing occurs when the Nyquist limit is exceeded (in this case, beyond five cycles). Thus **D** is an example of aliasing. It can be seen that connecting the circles would yield a one-cycle representation of what is actually a nine-cycle signal voltage. **E,** In this spectral display the presentation above the baseline is correct (unaliased, five samples per cycle), whereas the systolic peaks appear incorrectly below the baseline (aliased, one sample per cycle).

rule, if the highest Doppler-shift frequency present in a signal exceeds one half of the PRF, aliasing will occur (Figure 6-26).

> Aliasing is corrected by shifting the baseline, increasing the PRF, or both.

Two correction methods used less often are reduction of the operating frequency and switching to continuous-wave mode. Operating frequency reduction reduces the Doppler shift. Continuous-wave operation, because it is not pulsed, is not a sampling mode and is thus not subject to aliasing. However, it does not provide range discrimination.

Range Ambiguity

In attempting to solve the aliasing problem by increasing the PRF, one can encounter the range-ambiguity artifact described previously. This artifact occurs when a pulse is emitted before all the echoes from the previous pulse have been received. When this happens, early echoes from the last pulse are received simultaneously with late echoes from the previous pulse. The system is unable to determine whether an echo is an early one (superficial) from the last pulse or a late one (deep) from the previous pulse (Figure 6-27). To deal with this problem, the instrument simply assumes that all echoes are derived from the last pulse and that these echoes originate from depths determined by the 13 μs/cm rule. As long as all echoes are received before the next pulse is sent out, this is true. However, with high PRFs, this may not be the case. Therefore Doppler flow information may come from locations other than the assumed one (the gate location). In effect, multiple gates or sample volumes are operating at different depths. Table 6-1 lists, for various PRFs, the ranges beyond which ambiguity occurs. Table 6-2 lists, for various depths, the maximum Doppler-shift frequency (NL) that avoids aliasing and the range-ambiguity artifact. Maximum flow speeds that avoid aliasing for given angles also are listed. Instruments sometimes increase PRF (to avoid aliasing) into a range in which range ambiguity occurs. Multiple sample volumes are shown on the display to indicate this situation.

> High PRF causes Doppler-range ambiguity. Multiple sample volumes appear as a result.

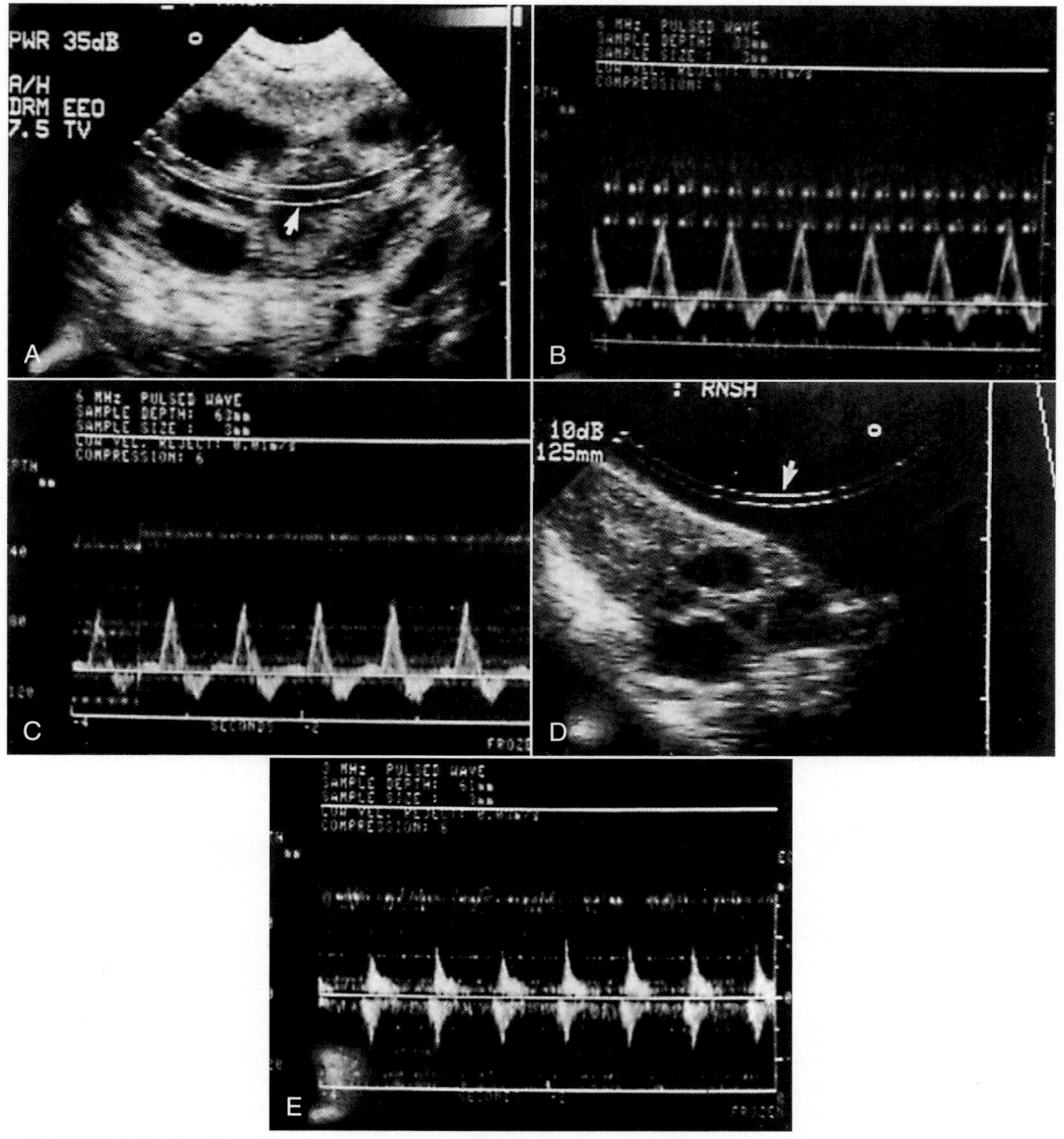

FIGURE 6-27 **Ambiguity is caused by sending out a pulse before all echoes from the previous pulse are received. A,** This transvaginal image shows the pulsed Doppler range gate *(arrow)* set at 33 mm within an ovary. **B,** The resulting Doppler spectrum shows a waveform typical of the external iliac artery. **C,** A signal identical to that shown in **B** was obtained when the range was increased to 63 mm, proving that the signal actually originated from the external iliac artery at this depth. **D,** A strong arterial Doppler signal was obtained when the range gate *(arrow)* was placed within the urinary bladder at a depth of 31 mm. **E,** A signal identical to that obtained in **D** was detected when the range gate depth was increased to 61 mm, indicating that the signal actually arose from an artery at this depth.

Continued

Mirror Image

The mirror-image artifact described previously can also occur with Doppler systems. This means that an image of a vessel and a source of Doppler-shifted echoes can be duplicated on the opposite side of a strong reflector. The duplicated vessel containing flow could be misinterpreted as an additional vessel that has a spectrum identical to that of the real vessel. Figure 6-28 shows an example of image and spectrum duplication of the subclavian artery. The strong reflector in this case is the air at the pleural boundary.

A mirror image of a Doppler spectrum can appear on the opposite side of the baseline when, indeed, flow is unidirectional and should appear only on one side of the baseline. This is an electronic duplication of the spectral information. The duplication can occur when Doppler gain is set too high (causing overloading in the amplifier and leakage, called **cross-talk**, of the signal from the proper channel into the other channel; Figure 6-29). Duplication can also occur when the Doppler angle is near 90 degrees (Figure 6-30). In this situation the duplication is usually

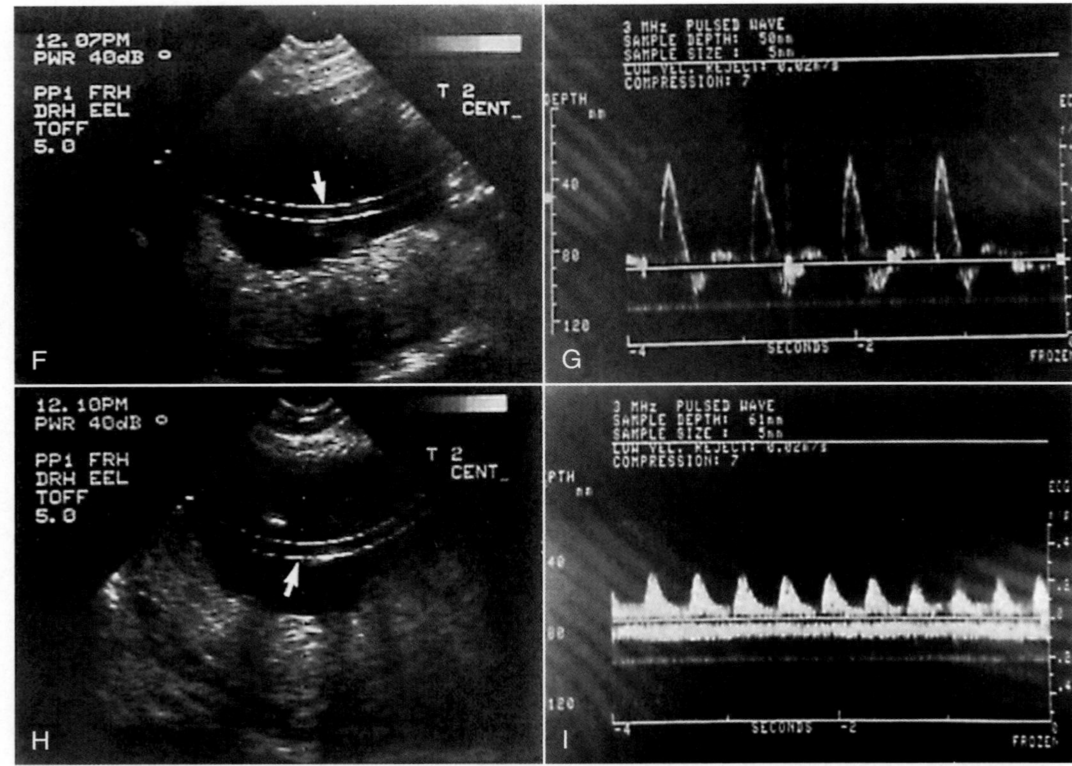

FIGURE 6-27, cont'd **F,** The range gate *(arrow)* placed at a depth of 50 mm in the uterus of a pregnant woman (16 weeks' gestation). Range gate *(arrow)* from **F** produces signals typical of the external iliac artery **(G). H,** In the same patient, a slight adjustment of the range gate *(arrow)* produced the desired umbilical artery signal **(I),** eliminating the artifactual iliac artery signal caused by range ambiguity. (From Gill RW et al: New class of pulsed Doppler US ambiguity at short ranges, *Radiology* 173:272, 1989.)

TABLE 6-2 Aliasing and Range-Ambiguity Limits*

			Maximum Flow Speed (cm/s)		
Depth (cm)	**PRF (kHz)**	**Nyquist Limit (kHz)**	**0**	**30**	**60**
1	77.0	38.5	593	685	1186
2	38.5	19.2	296	342	593
4	19.2	9.6	148	171	296
8	9.6	4.8	74	86	148
16	4.8	2.4	37	43	74

*For various depths the maximum pulse repetition frequency (PRF) that avoids range ambiguity and the corresponding maximum Doppler shift frequency (Nyquist limit) that avoids aliasing are listed. Maximum flow speeds corresponding to the maximum Doppler shift also are listed for three Doppler angles (0, 30, and 60 degrees), assuming a 5-MHz operating frequency.

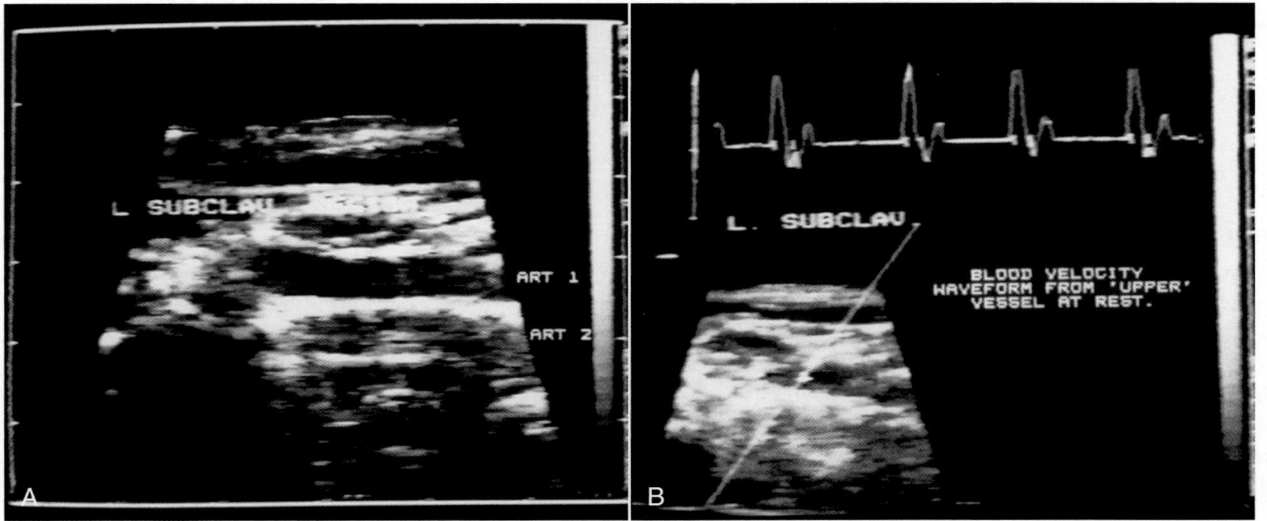

FIGURE 6-28 **A,** The subclavian artery *(ART 1)* and its mirror image *(ART 2).* **B,** Flow signal from artery.

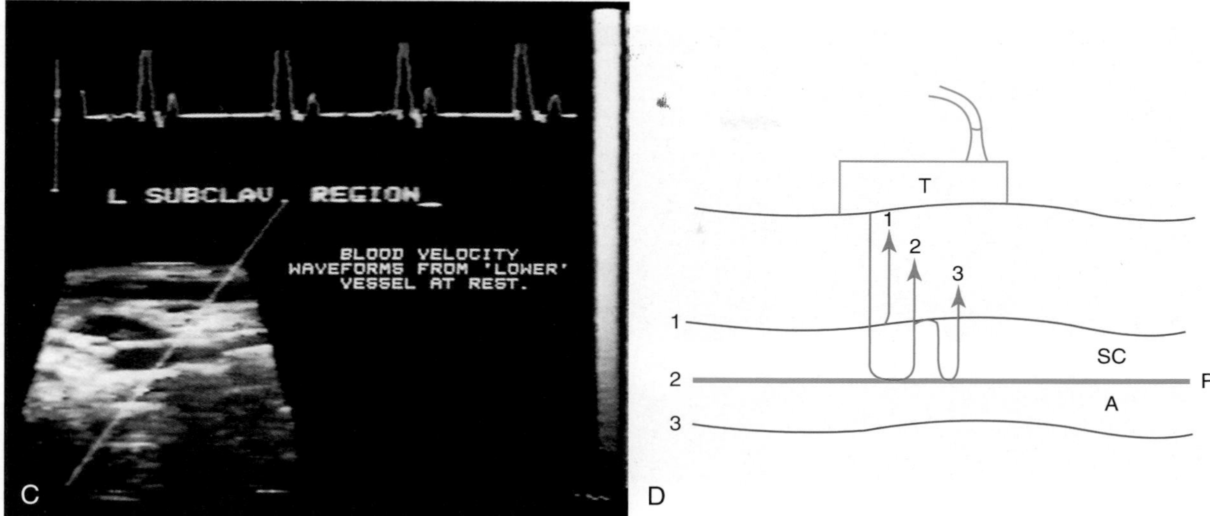

FIGURE 6-28, cont'd **C,** Flow signal from the mirror image of the artery. **D,** Multiple reflections produce a mirror image. Paths *1* and *2* are legitimate, but path 3 arrives late, producing the artifactual deep arterial wall. *T,* Transducer; *SC,* subclavian artery; *P,* pleura; *A,* artifactual artery; *(D* from Kremkau FW: Principles and pitfalls of real-time color-flow imaging. In Bernstein EF, editor: *Vascular diagnosis, ed 4,* St. Louis, 1993, Mosby.*)*

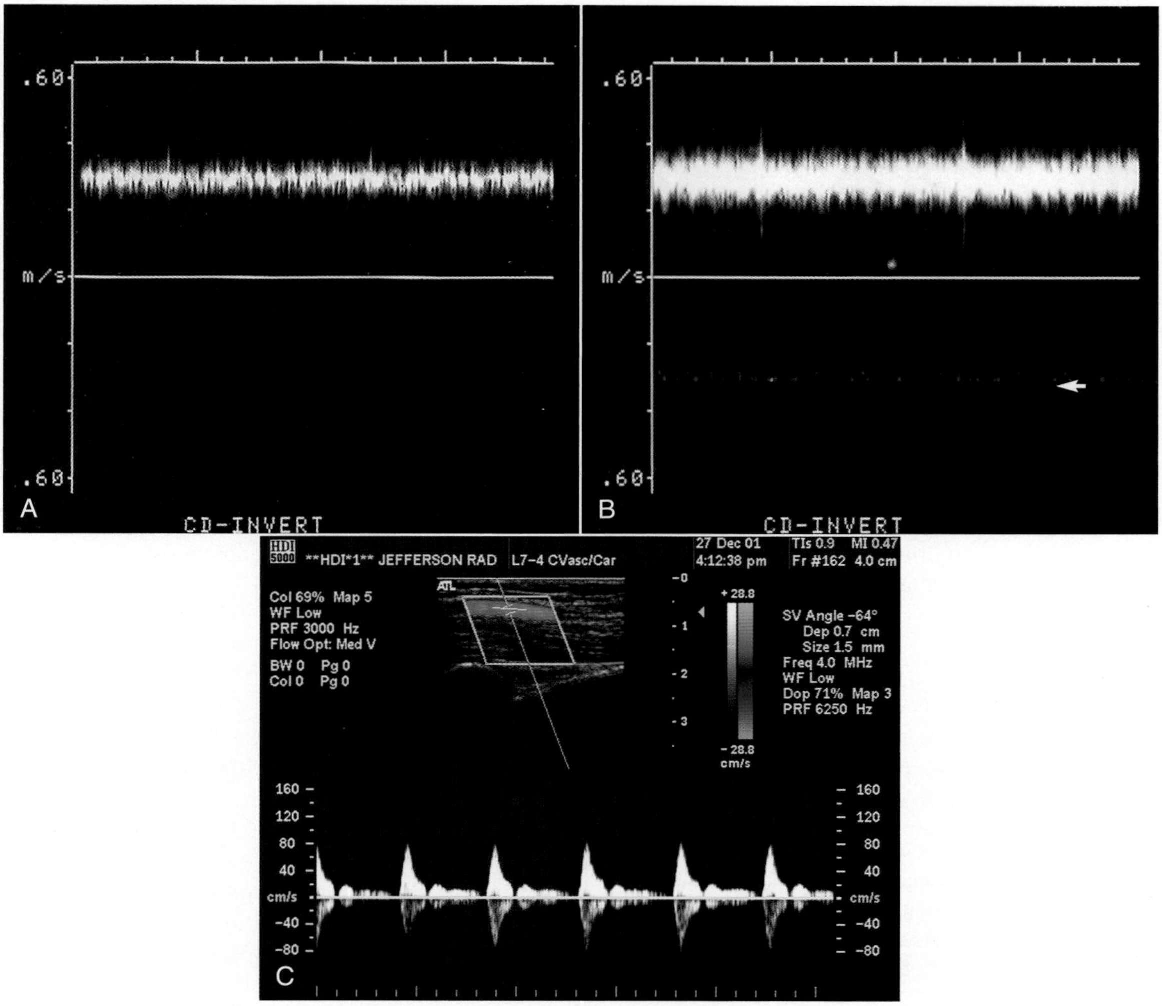

FIGURE 6-29 **A,** Spectrum produced by a string moving at 30 cm/s. **B,** An increase in gain produces spectral broadening and a mirror image *(arrow).* **C,** High gain produces a mirror image of the carotid artery spectrum below the baseline.

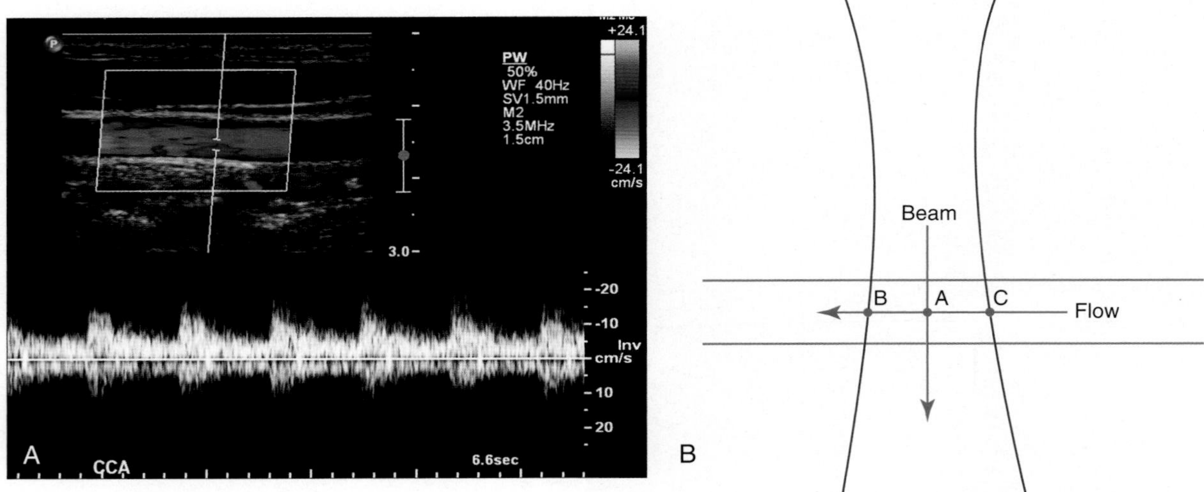

FIGURE 6-30 **A,** The Doppler angle is nearly 90 degrees in the common carotid artery, which produces a spectral mirror image with flow on both sides of the baseline. **B,** Because beams are focused and not cylindrical, portions of the beam (**C**) can experience flow toward the transducer, whereas other portions (**B**) can experience flow away when the beam axis intersects (**A**) the flow at 90 degrees.

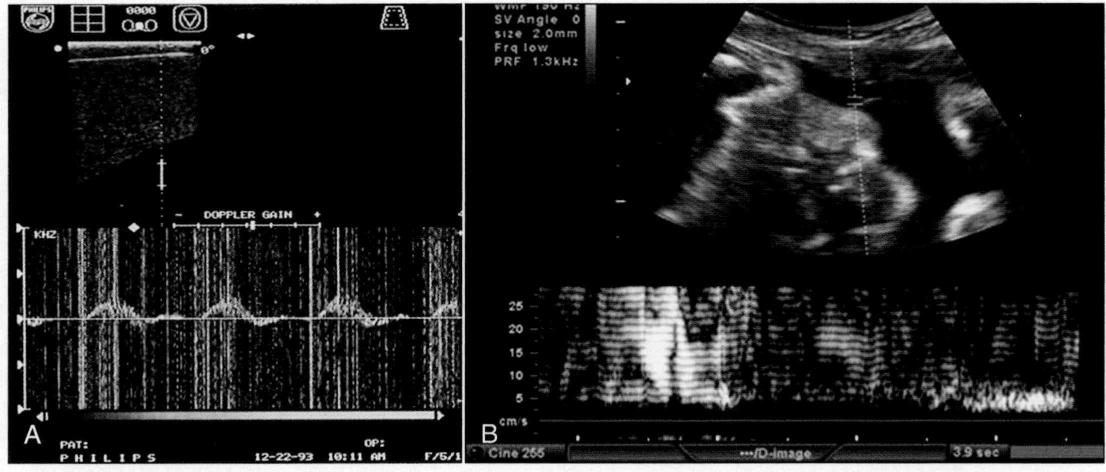

FIGURE 6-31 **A,** Interference from nearby electrical equipment clouds the spectral display with electric noise (the vertical "snow" lines). **B,** External interference produces bands of frequency that are fairly constant with time.

legitimate because beams are focused and not cylindrical. Thus while the beam axis is perpendicular to the flow direction, one edge of the beam is angled upstream and the other edge downstream.

> *Spectral mirror image* is the appearance of spectral information on both sides of the baseline. It occurs at high Doppler gains and Doppler angles near 90 degrees.

Doppler spectra have a speckle quality similar to that observed in gray-scale sonography, discussed previously. Electromagnetic interference from nearby equipment can cloud the spectral display with lines or "snow" (Figure 6-31).

COLOR DOPPLER

Artifacts observed with color-Doppler imaging are two-dimensional color presentations of artifacts that are seen in gray-scale sonography or Doppler-spectral displays. They are incorrect presentations of two-dimensional motion information, the most common of which is aliasing. However, others occur, including anatomic mirror image, Doppler angle-effects, shadowing, and clutter.

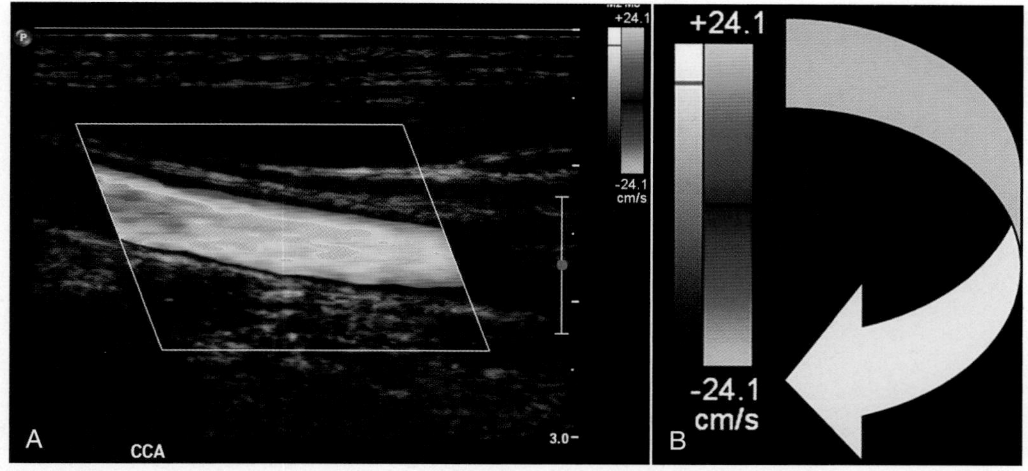

FIGURE 6-32 A, Negative *(blue)* Doppler shifts are shown in the arterial flow in this image. These are actually positive Doppler shifts that have exceeded the higher Nyquist limit (converted here to the equivalent flow speed: +24.1 cm/s) and are wrapped around to the negative portion of the color bar (B). (Similarly, negative shifts that exceed the –24.1 cm/s limit would alias to the positive side.)

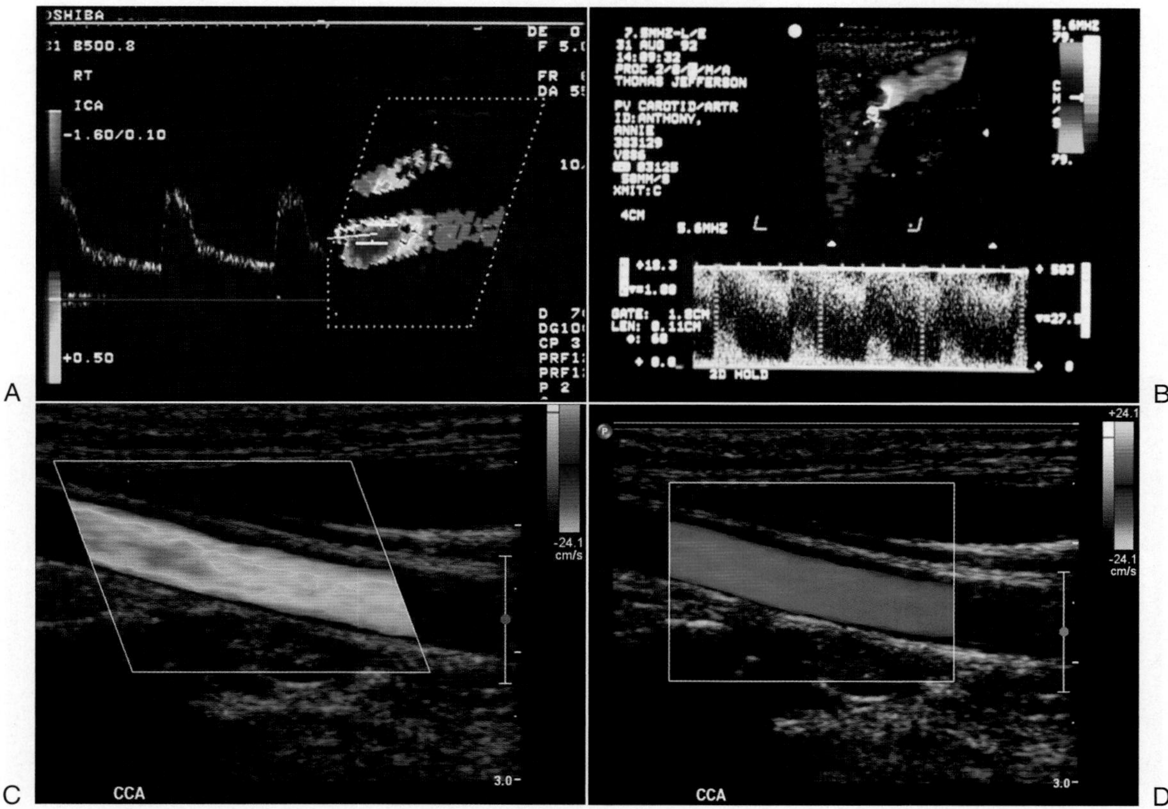

FIGURE 6-33 A, A color-Doppler image with aliasing. The blue colors demonstrate aliasing, whereas the higher pulse repetition frequency (PRF) associated with the spectral Doppler ensures that the spectral display is not aliased. B, An example in which both the color and spectral displays of the carotid are aliasing. C, Aliasing in the common carotid artery with a color box angled incorrectly. D, Adjusting the angle of the color box eliminates the aliasing.

Continued

Aliasing

Aliasing occurs when the Doppler shift exceeds the NL (Figure 6-32), which happens more often in color Doppler than in spectral Doppler due to the reduced PRFs used in the former relative to the latter. The result is incorrect flow direction displayed on the color-Doppler image (Figure 6-33). Increasing the flow speed range (which is actually an increase in PRF) can solve the problem (see Figures 6-33, *E–F*, and 6-34). However, a too-high range can cause loss of flow information, particularly if the wall filter is set high. This artifact can also

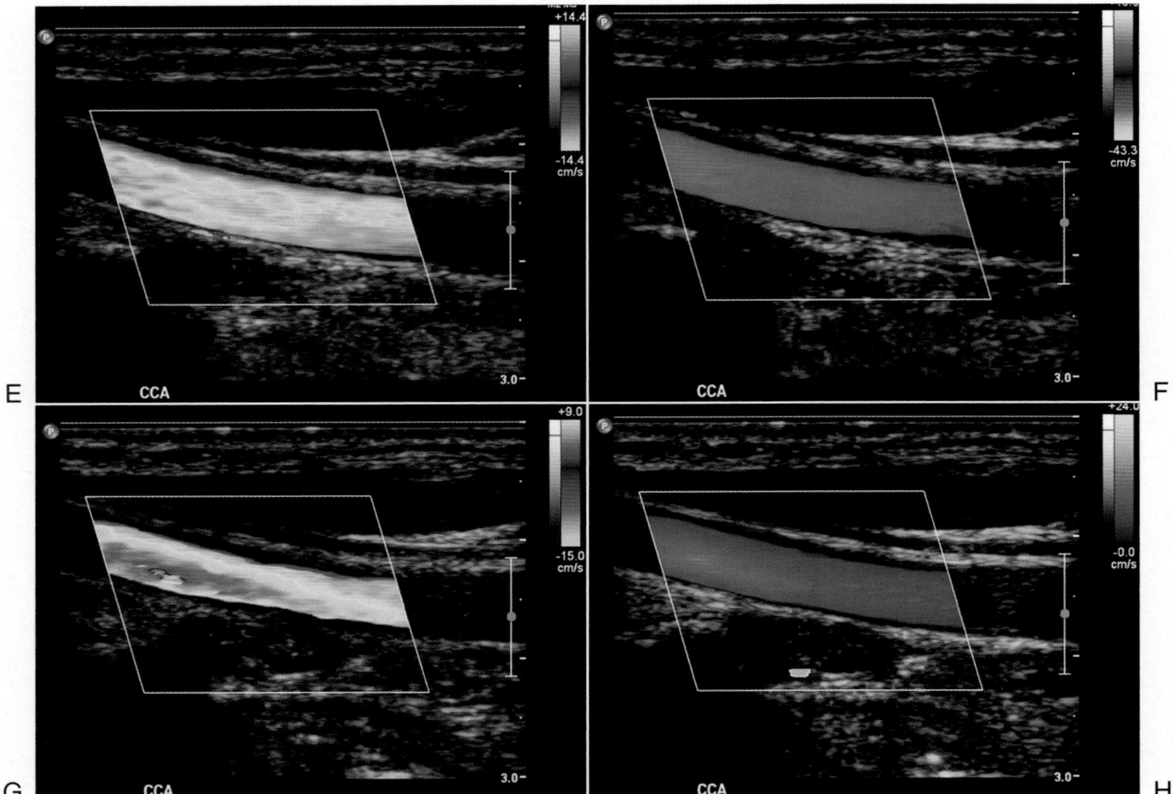

FIGURE 6-33, cont'd E–F, Increasing the color scale from 14.4 cm/s to 43.3 cm/s resolves the aliasing. G–H, Color correction can be achieved by changing the baseline from covering –15 to 9.0 cm/s to covering the 0 to 24 cm/s range.

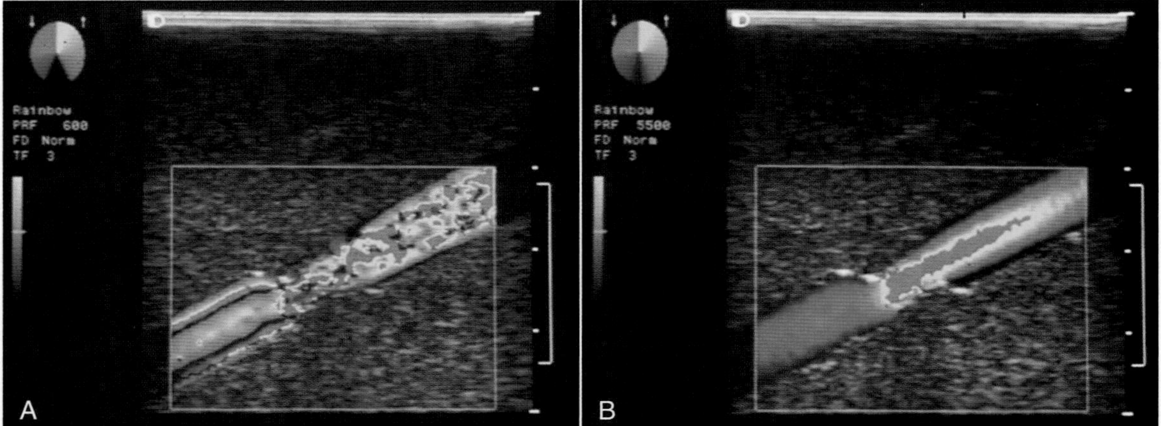

FIGURE 6-34 A, Flow in this phantom with an 80% stenosis is toward the upper right, producing positive Doppler shifts. The pulse repetition frequency (600 Hz) and Nyquist limit (300 Hz) are too low, resulting in aliasing (negative Doppler shifts) at the edge of the vessel as well as at the center of the flow in the vessel (positive Doppler shifts). B, With the pulse repetition frequency increased to 5500 Hz, the aliasing has been eliminated except for right in the stenosis, where the aliasing outlines the stenotic jet.

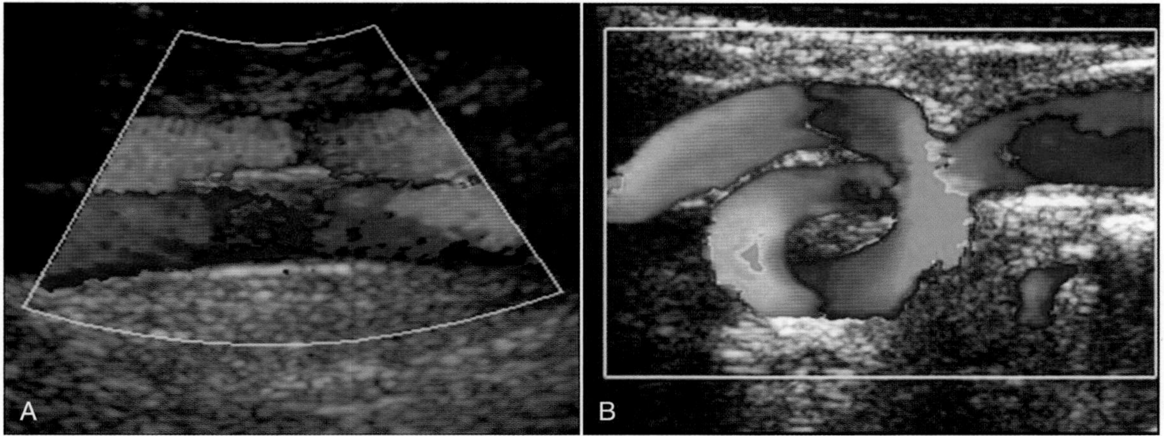

FIGURE 6-35 **A,** Two vessels with the anterior having flow from the left to the right and vice versa in the posterior vessel. Thus the flow in the anterior vessel is upstream from the transducer in the left half of the image (thus coded *red*) and down stream in the right half of the image (color coded *blue*). The posterior vessel has flow in the opposite direction and, hence, is color coded blue followed by red. **B,** The same effect can be observed in a tortuous carotid artery.

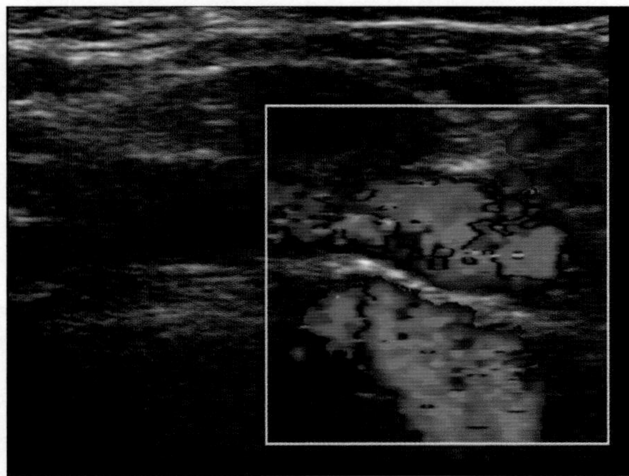

FIGURE 6-36 **Longitudinal color Doppler image of the subclavian vein.** The pleura causes the mirror image. The diagram in Figure 6-28, *D* shows how this artifact occurs.

be eliminated (or at least reduced) by angling the color-box (see Figure 6-33, *C–D*). Baseline shifting can decrease or eliminate the effect of aliasing (see Figure 6-33, *G–H*), as in spectral displays.

> Aliasing in color-Doppler imaging appears as an incorrect color from the opposite side of the baseline on the color map.

A related artifact is the multiple angle artifact—the Doppler angle in color-Doppler displays is assumed (unrealistically) to be zero. Hence the color overlay is coded relative to the location of the transducer, which can lead to somewhat confusing displays (Figure 6-35).

Mirror Image, Shadowing, Refraction, Clutter, and Noise

In the mirror (or ghost) artifact (Figure 6-36), an image of a vessel and source of Doppler-shifted echoes can be duplicated on the opposite side of a strong reflector (e.g., pleura or diaphragm). This is a color-Doppler extension of the gray-scale artifact of Figure 6-28. Shadowing is the weakening or elimination of Doppler-shifted echoes beyond a shadowing object, just as occurs with non–Doppler-shifted (gray-scale) echoes (Figure 6-37, *A*). Refraction can confuse the interpretation

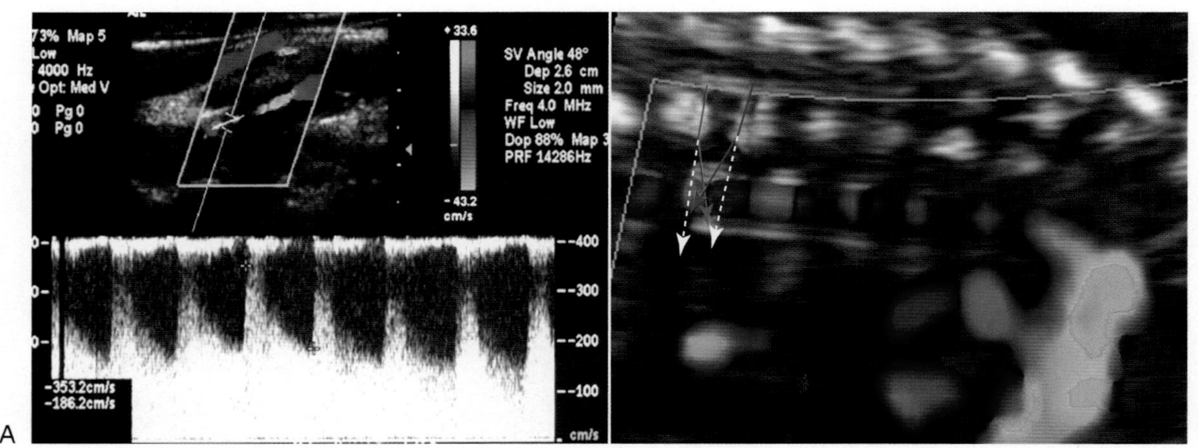

FIGURE 6-37 **A,** Shadowing from calcified plaque follows the gray-scale scan lines straight down. Notice how the color aliases. **B,** Refraction from ribs produces alternating positive and negative Doppler-shift regions in this fetal aorta. Positive Doppler shift is red. Flow is from right to left. The red sound path is refracted to an upstream view and presented red on the dashed scan line. The blue path is refracted to a downstream view and presented blue on its dashed scan line.

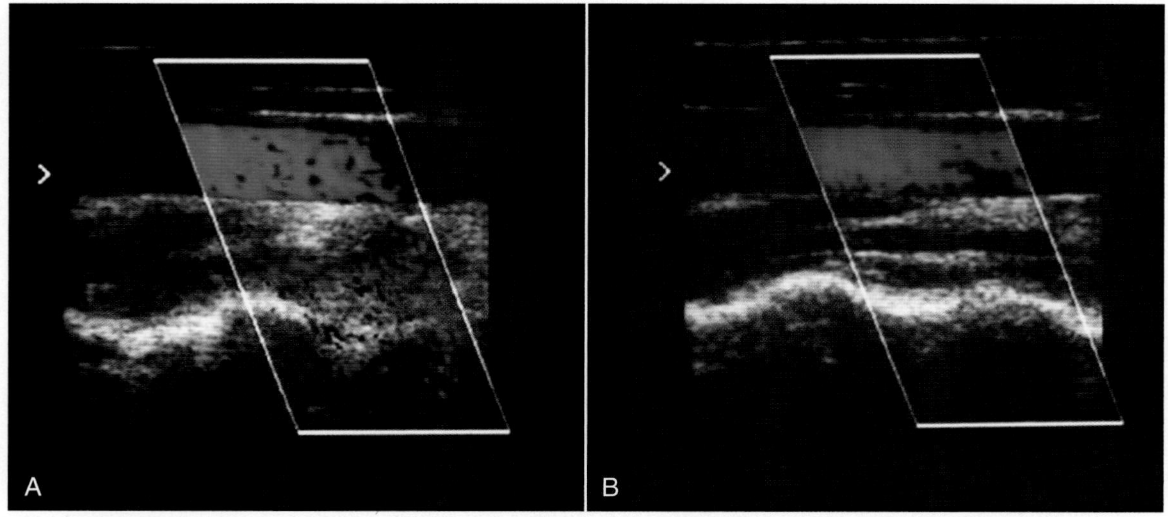

FIGURE 6-38 **A,** Clutter from tissue motion (i.e., flash artifact) in the neck (caused by speaking) appears as color Doppler below the common carotid artery. **B,** When the speaking stops the clutter is gone, revealing the underlying tissue.

of color-Doppler presentations (see Figure 6-37, *B*). Clutter, also known as the flash artifact, results from tissue, heart wall or valve, or vessel wall motion (Figure 6-38). Such clutter is eliminated by wall filters. Doppler angle effects include zero Doppler shift when the Doppler angle is 90 degrees (see Figure 5-28, *F*), as well as the change of color in a straight vessel viewed with a sector transducer (see Figure 5-28, *A*). Noise in the color-Doppler electronics can mimic flow, particularly in **hypoechoic** or anechoic regions with gain settings too high (Figure 6-39).

This chapter has discussed several ultrasound imaging and flow artifacts, all of which are listed in Table 6-3, along with their causes. In some cases the names of the artifacts are identical to their causes. Shadowing and enhancement are useful in interpretation and diagnosis. Other artifacts can cause confusion and error. Artifacts seen in two-dimensional imaging are evidenced in three-dimensional imaging also, sometimes in unusual ways.[5] All of these artifacts can hinder proper interpretation and diagnosis, and this must be avoided or handled properly when encountered. A proper understanding of artifacts and how to deal with them when they are encountered enables sonographers and sonologists to use them to advantage while avoiding the pitfalls they can cause.

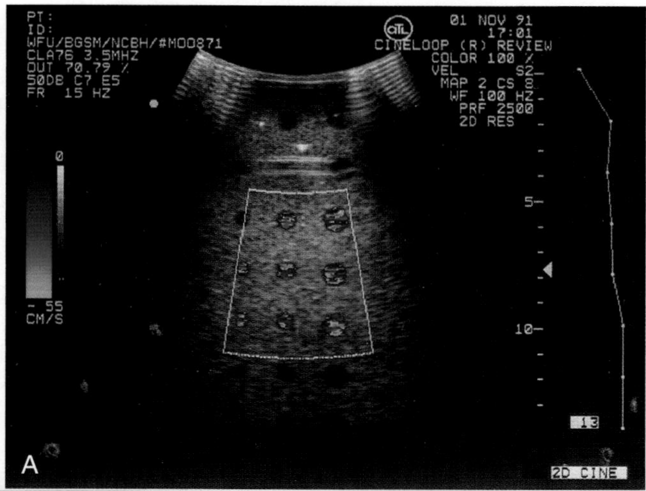

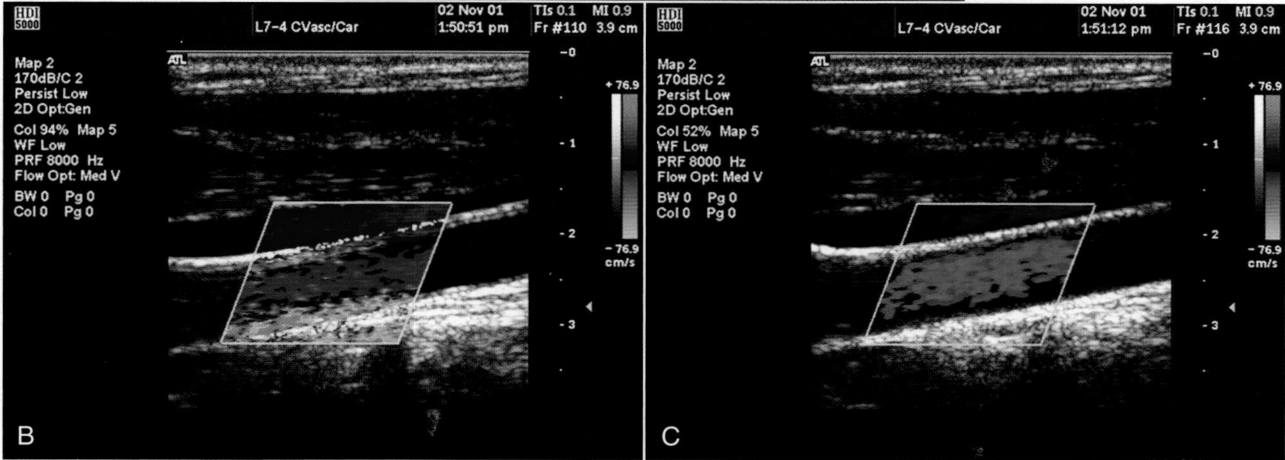

FIGURE 6-39 **A,** Color appears in echo-free (cystic) regions of a tissue-equivalent phantom. The color gain has been increased sufficiently to produce this effect. The instrument tends to write color noise preferentially in areas where non–Doppler-shifted echoes are weak or absent. **B–C,** A tissue can also be overwritten when the color gain is too high and reducing it (here from 94% to 52%) eliminates the artifact. (**A** from Kremkau FW: Principles and pitfalls of real-time color-flow imaging. In Bernstein EF, editor: *Vascular diagnosis,* ed 4, St. Louis, 1993, Mosby.)

TABLE 6-3 Artifacts and Their Causes

Artifact	Cause
Axial resolution	Pulse length
Comet tail	Reverberation
Grating lobe	Grating lobe
Lateral resolution	Pulse width
Mirror image	Multiple reflection
Refraction	Refraction
Reverberation	Multiple reflection
Slice thickness	Pulse width
Speckle	Interference
Speed error	Speed error
Range ambiguity	Finite speed of sound in tissue
Shadowing	High attenuation
Edge shadowing	Refraction or interference
Enhancement	Low attenuation
Focal enhancement	Focusing
Aliasing	Exceeding the Nyquist limit
Spectrum mirror	High Doppler gain

REVIEW

The following key points are presented in this chapter:

- The beam width perpendicular to the scan plane causes slice thickness artifacts.
- Apparent fine-image details are not related directly to tissue texture but are a result of interference effects from a distribution of scatterers in the tissue, called *speckle.*
- Reverberation produces a set of equally spaced artifactual echoes distal to the real reflector.
- In the mirror-image artifact, objects that are present on one side of a strong reflector are displayed on the other side as well.
- Refraction displaces echoes laterally.
- Propagation speed error and refraction can cause objects to be displayed in improper locations or incorrect sizes or both.
- Shadowing is caused by high-attenuation objects in the sound path.
- Refraction also can cause edge shadowing.
- Enhancement results from low-attenuation objects in the sound path.
- Aliasing occurs when the Doppler shift frequency exceeds one half of the PRF.
- Aliasing can be reduced or eliminated by using baseline shift, increasing the PRF or Doppler angle, reducing operating frequency, or using continuous-wave operation.

EXERCISES

Answers appear in the Answers to Exercises section at the back of the book.

1. The pulser of an instrument automatically reduces the PRF for deeper imaging to avoid the ___________ ___________ artifact.
   a. comet tail
   b. grating lobe
   c. mirror image
   d. range ambiguity
2. If an echo arrives 143 μs after the pulse that produced it was emitted, it should be located at a depth of ___________ cm. If a second pulse was emitted 13 μs before the arrival of this echo, it will be placed incorrectly at a depth of ___________ cm.
   a. 11, 1
   b. 14, 13
   c. 13, 14
   d. 13, 13
3. If the propagation speed in a soft tissue path is 1.60 mm/μs, a diagnostic instrument assumes a propagation speed too ___________ and will show reflectors too ___________ the transducer.
   a. high, close to
   b. high, far from
   c. low, close to
   d. low, far from
4. Mirror image can occur with only one reflector. True or false?
5. The most common artifact encountered in Doppler ultrasound is _________.
   a. aliasing
   b. range ambiguity
   c. spectrum mirror image
   d. location mirror image
   e. electromagnetic interference
6. Which of the following can reduce or eliminate aliasing?
   a. Increased PRF
   b. Increased Doppler angle
   c. Increased operating frequency
   d. Use of continuous wave mode
   e. More than one of the above
7. The fine texture in soft tissue indicates the excellent resolution that actually exists there. True or false?
8. The fact that a beam, as it scans through tissue, has some nonzero width perpendicular to the scan plane results in the ___________ ___________ artifact.
   a. mirror image
   b. range ambiguity
   c. slice thickness
   d. speed error
9. Which of the following can cause improper location of objects on a display? (More than one correct answer.)
   a. Shadowing
   b. Enhancement
   c. Speed error
   d. Mirror image
   e. Refraction
   f. Grating lobe
10. Refraction can cause shadowing. True or false?
11. The transducer face is one of the reflectors involved in reverberations in which illustration, Figure 6-40, *A* or *B*?
12. Match these artifact causes with their result: (More than one correct answer.)

a. Reverberation	**1.** Unreal structure displayed
b. Shadowing	**2.** Structure missing on the display
c. Enhancement	**3.** Structure displayed with improper brightness
d. Propagation speed error	**4.** Structure improperly positioned
e. Refraction	**5.** Structure improperly shaped

13. Reverberation results in added reflectors being imaged with equal ___________.
    a. depth
    b. separation
    c. width
    d. brightness

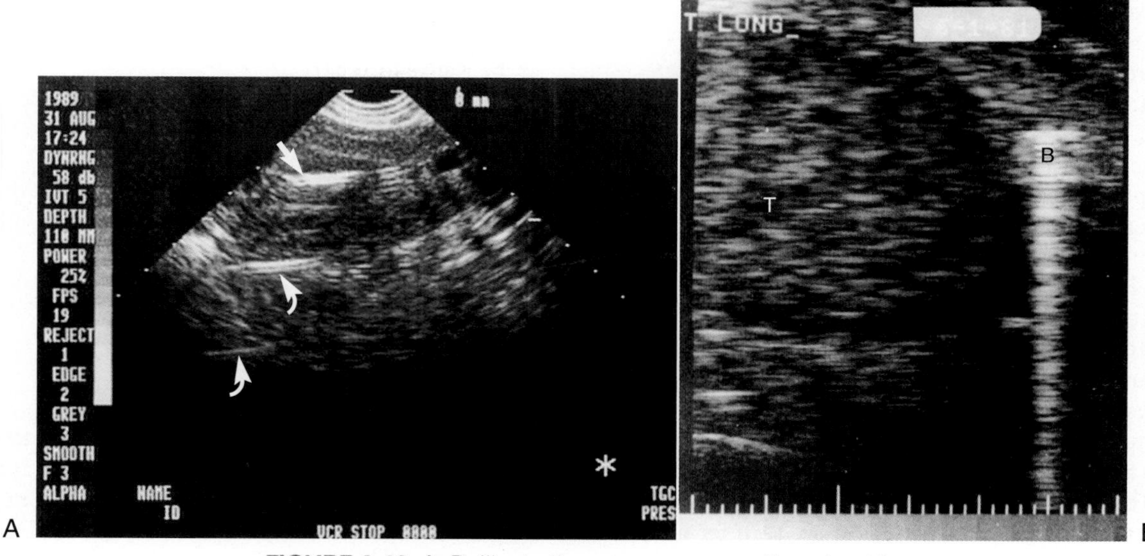

FIGURE 6-40 A–B, Illustrations to accompany Exercise 11.

14. In reverberation, subsequent reflections are ____________ than previous ones.
    a. shallower
    b. brighter
    c. weaker
    d. stronger
15. Enhancement is caused by a ____________.
    a. strongly reflecting structure
    b. weakly attenuating structure
    c. strongly attenuating structure
    d. refracting boundary
    e. propagation speed error
16. Which of the following can correct or eliminate aliasing?
    a. Decreased PRF
    b. Decreased Doppler angle
    c. Increased operating frequency
    d. Baseline shifting
    e. More than one of the above
17. Shadowing results in decreased echo amplitudes. True or false?
18. Propagation speed error results in improper ____________ position of a reflector on the display.
    a. lateral
    b. axial
19. To avoid aliasing, a signal voltage must be sampled at least ____________ time(s) per cycle.
    a. 1
    b. 2
    c. 3
    d. 4
    e. 5
20. If the highest Doppler-shift frequency present in a signal exceeds ____________ the PRF, aliasing will occur.
    a. one tenth
    b. one half
    c. two times
    d. five times
    e. ten times
21. When Doppler gain is set too high, which artifact is likely to occur?
    a. Aliasing
    b. Range ambiguity
    c. Spectrum mirror image
    d. Location mirror image
    e. Speckle
22. Which artifact should be suspected if one observes twin gestational sacs when scanning through the rectus abdominis muscle?
    a. Refraction
    b. Reverberation
    c. Speckle
    d. Enhancement
23. Range ambiguity can occur in which of the following?
    a. Imaging instruments
    b. Duplex instruments
    c. Pulsed wave Doppler instruments
    d. Color flow instruments
    e. All of the above
24. If the PRF is 4 kHz, which of the following Doppler shifts will cause aliasing?
    a. 1 kHz
    b. 2 kHz
    c. 3 kHz
    d. 4 kHz
    e. More than one of the above
25. If the PRF is 10 kHz, which of the following Doppler shifts will cause aliasing?
    a. 1 kHz
    b. 2 kHz
    c. 3 kHz
    d. 4 kHz
    e. None of the above

26. There is no problem with aliasing as long as the Doppler shifts are ___________ half the PRF.
   a. less than
   b. approximately equal to
   c. greater than
   d. all of the above
   e. none of the above
27. If Doppler shift is 2.6 kHz, no aliasing would result with a PRF of 10 kHz. True or false?
28. If there were a problem in Exercise 27, ___________ Doppler ultrasound could be used to avoid it.
   a. pulsed
   b. continuous-wave
   c. color
   d. power
29. If red represents a positive Doppler shift and blue represents a negative one, what color is seen for normal flow toward the transducer? What color is seen for aliasing flow toward the transducer? What colors are seen for normal flow away and for aliasing flow away from the transducer?
   a. red, red, blue, blue
   b. red, blue, red, blue
   c. blue, red, blue, red
   d. red, blue, blue, red
30. When a pulse is emitted before all the echoes from the previous pulse have been received, which artifact occurs?
   a. Mirror image
   b. Range ambiguity
   c. Slice thickness
   d. Speed error
31. When a strong reflector is located in the scan plane, which of the following artifacts is likely to occur?
   a. Aliasing
   b. Range ambiguity
   c. Spectrum mirror image
   d. Location mirror image
   e. Speckle
32. Increasing PRF to avoid aliasing can cause the following:
   a. Baseline shift
   b. Range ambiguity
   c. Spectrum mirror image
   d. Location mirror image
   e. Speckle
33. Which of the following decreases the likelihood of range-ambiguity artifact?
   a. Decreasing operating frequency
   b. Decreasing PRF
   c. Decreasing Doppler angle
   d. Baseline shift
   e. Increasing pulser output
34. Range ambiguity produces which error in spectral-Doppler studies?
   a. Incorrect spectral peaks
   b. Incorrect gate location
   c. Intensity too high
   d. Intensity too low
   e. All of the above
35. Range ambiguity produces which error in anatomic imaging?
   a. Range too long
   b. Range too short
   c. Intensity too high
   d. Doppler shift too high
   e. Doppler shift too low
36. If a pulse is emitted 65 μs after the previous one, echoes returning from beyond ___________ cm will produce range ambiguity.
   a. 1
   b. 2
   c. 3
   d. 4
   e. 5
37. If the maximum imaging depth is 5 cm, the frequency is 2 MHz, and the Doppler angle is zero, what is the maximum flow speed that will avoid aliasing and range ambiguity?
   a. 100 cm/s
   b. 200 cm/s
   c. 300 cm/s
   d. 400 cm/s
   e. 500 cm/s
38. Solving aliasing by decreasing operating frequency increases the possibility of range-ambiguity artifact. True or false?
39. If operating frequency is increased to decrease the possibility of range ambiguity (by increasing attenuation), the possibility of aliasing increases. True or false?
40. If a pulsed wave Doppler sample volume is located at a depth of 8 cm, the sampled echoes arrive at what time following the emission of the pulse?
   a. 25 μs
   b. 50 μs
   c. 75 μs
   d. 104 μs
   e. 117 μs
41. In Exercise 40, if the PRF is set at 11 kHz, a second gate would be located at what depth?
   a. 1 cm
   b. 2 cm
   c. 3 cm
   d. 4 cm
   e. 5 cm
42. Connect the dots (samples) in Figure 6-41 to determine the Doppler shift frequency. How many cycles are in each example?
   a. ___________
   b. ___________
   c. ___________
   d. ___________
   e. ___________
43. The frequencies that were sampled in Exercise 42 are shown in Figure 6-42. In which example(s) has aliasing occurred?

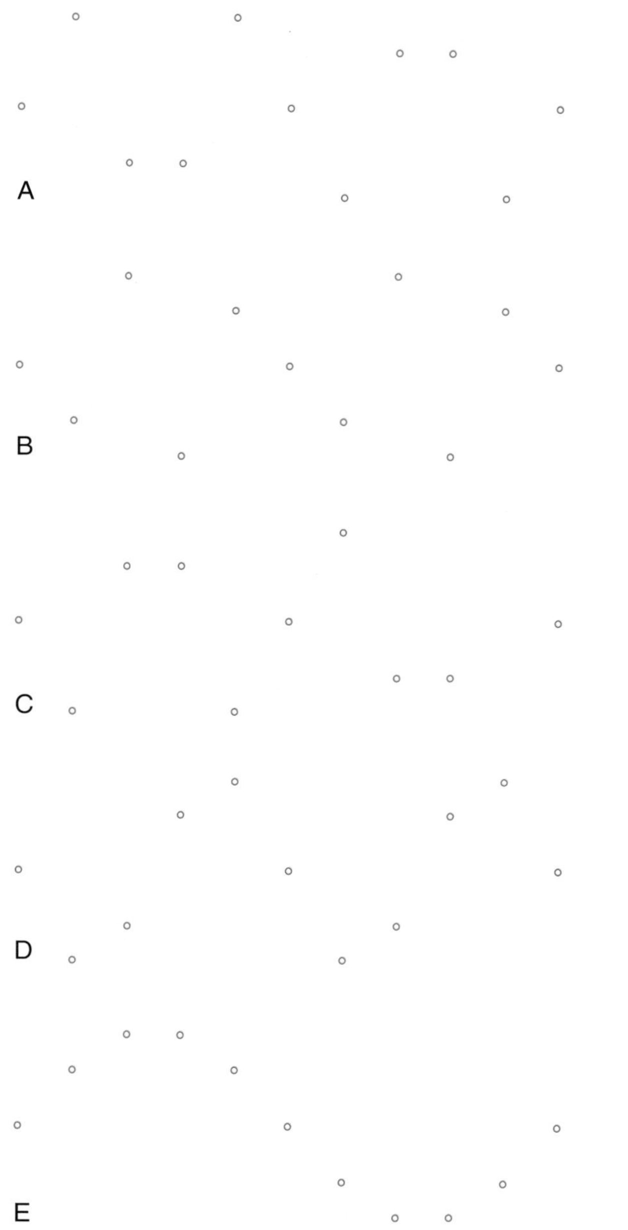

FIGURE 6-41 A–E, Illustrations to accompany Exercise 42.

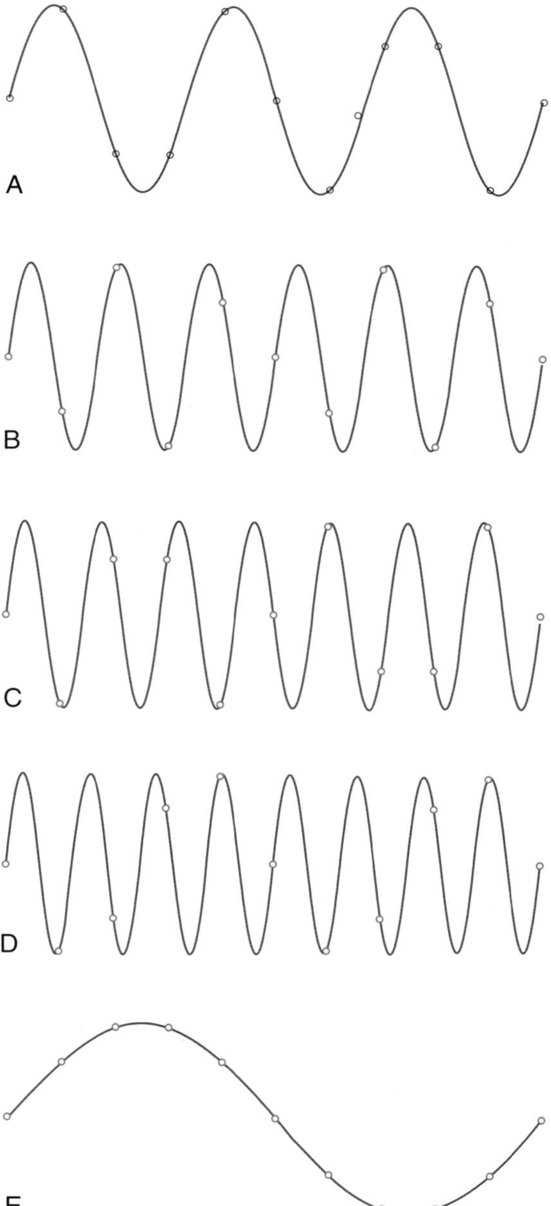

FIGURE 6-42 A–E, Illustrations to accompany Exercise 43.

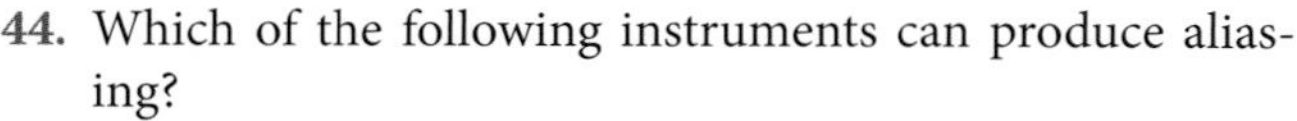

44. Which of the following instruments can produce aliasing?

a. Continuous-wave Doppler
b. Pulsed-wave Doppler
c. Duplex
d. Color Doppler
e. More than one of the above

45. In Figure 6-43 the solid line shows the Doppler shift. The dashed line shows the ___________ result of connecting samples of the shift. To avoid aliasing in this signal, at least __________ samples would be required.

a. correct, 5
b. correct, 10
c. aliased, 5
d. aliased, 10

46. In Figure 6-44 (*R*, red; *B*, blue), assume the color bar shown in G and give the direction of blood flow (*R* for from right to the left; *L* for from left to the right) in each case.

47. Figure 6-45 shows five regions of different colors in the flow. Match each of the following with the proper region.

a. ____________	**1.** 90-degree Doppler angle
b. ____________	**2.** Unaliased flow toward
c. ____________	**3.** Unaliased flow away
d. ____________	**4.** Aliased flow toward
e. ____________	**5.** Aliased flow away

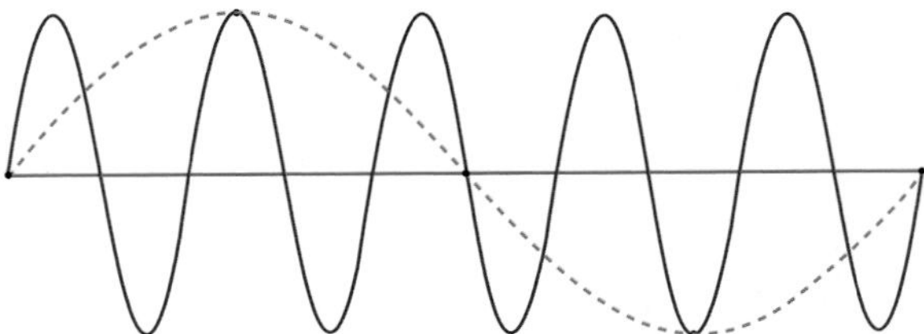

FIGURE 6-43 Illustration to accompany Exercise 45.

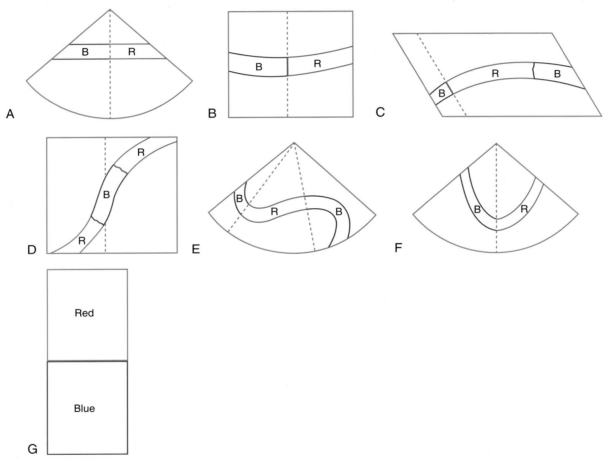

FIGURE 6-44 A–G, Illustrations to accompany Exercise 46. (From Kremkau FW: Is it coming or going? Color flow interpretation. *J Vasc Technol* 18:365–366, 1994.)

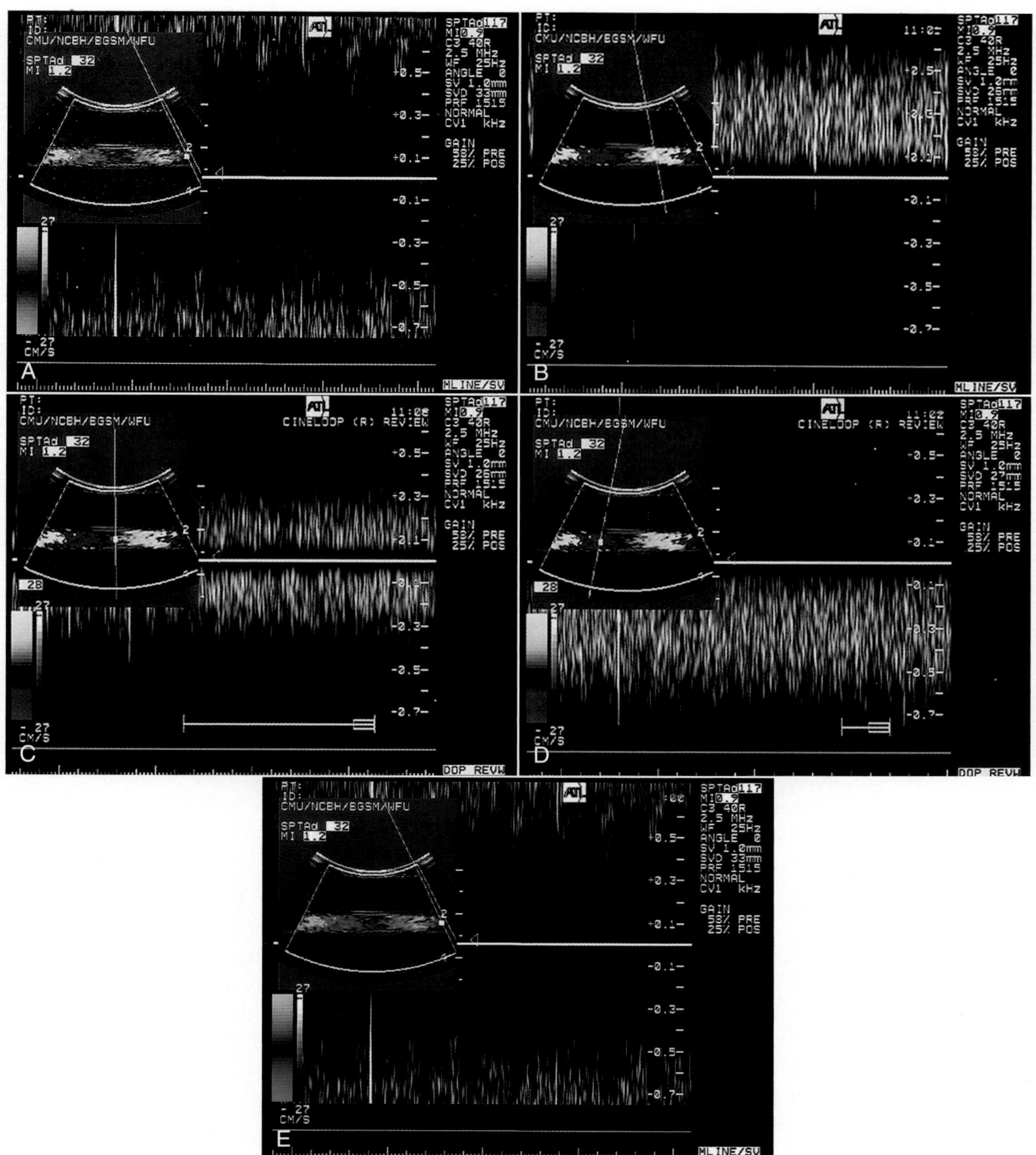

FIGURE 6-45 A–E, Illustrations to accompany Exercise 47.

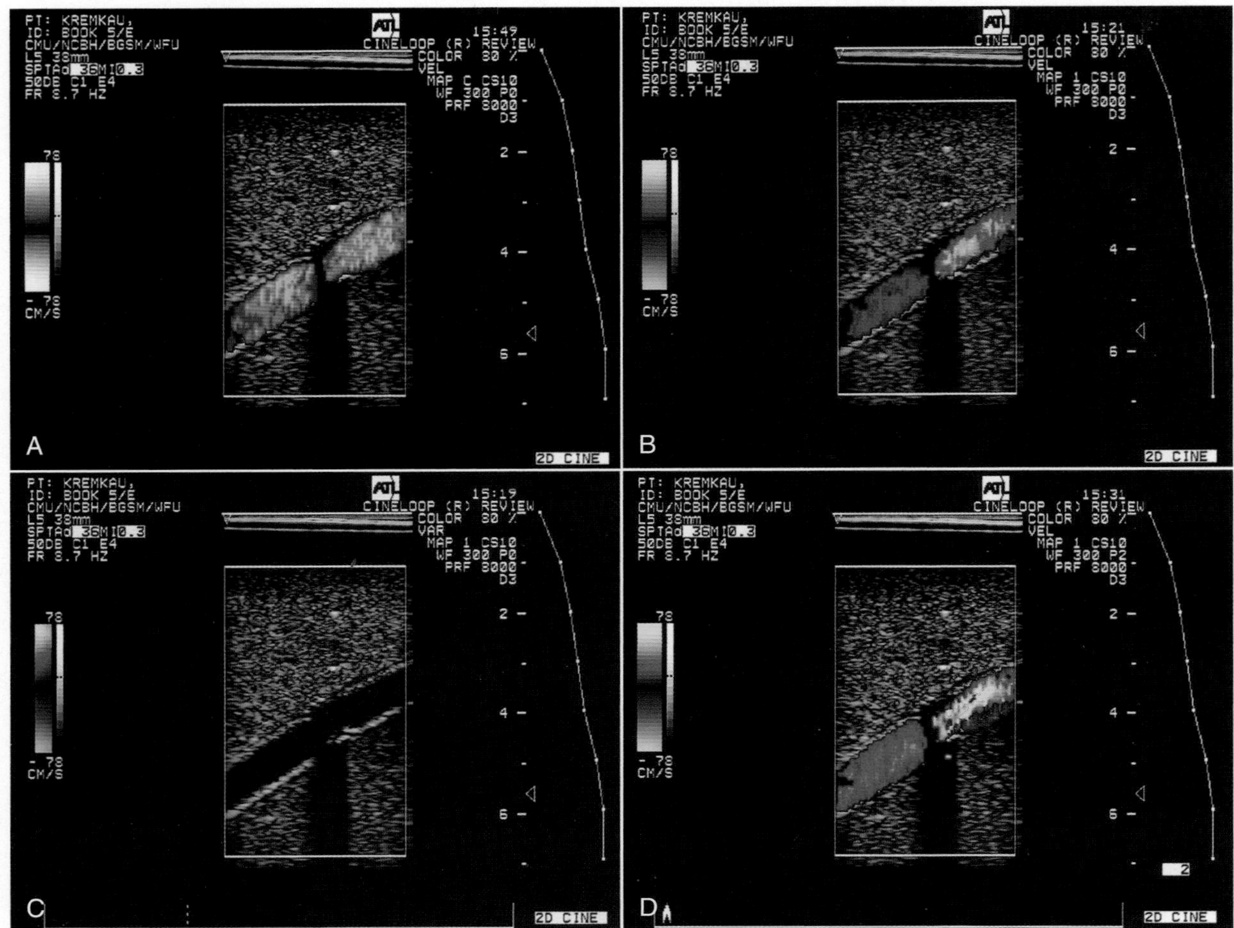

FIGURE 6-46 A–D, Illustrations to accompany Exercises 48 to 50.

48. Which part of Figure 6-46 shows a Doppler-power display?
  a. A
  b. B
  c. C
  d. D

49. Referring to Figure 6-46, *B-D,* what is the order of figure parts when they are arranged according to increasing flow speed?
  a. B, C, D
  b. D, C, B
  c. C, B, D
  d. B, D, C

50. What artifact appears in all parts of Figure 6-46? What is the additional artifact that appears in Figure 6-46, *D*?
  a. shadowing, aliasing
  b. aliasing, shadowing
  c. enhancement, shadowing
  d. enhancement, aliasing

7

Performance and Safety

LEARNING OBJECTIVES

After reading this chapter, the student should be able to do the following:

- Explain how to determine whether a sonographic or Doppler instrument is working properly.
- List the devices that are available to test various performance characteristics of instruments.
- Compare a test object with a phantom.
- Describe how instrument output is measured.
- List typical instrument output values.
- Explain what is known about bioeffects in cells, animals, and human beings.
- Describe what is known about risk in the use of sonography or Doppler ultrasound.
- Explain how an operator of an ultrasound instrument can implement the ALARA principle by minimizing exposure of the patient to ultrasound during diagnostic scanning.

OUTLINE

KEY TERMS

ALARA
Cavitation
Hydrophone
Mechanical index
Phantom
Polyvinylidene fluoride
Radiation force
Test object
Thermal index

Now that we have covered the principles of sonography and Doppler ultrasound and the artifacts that can and do occur, we turn to four important topics:

1. The evaluation of the performance of sonographic instruments.
2. The acoustic outputs of sonographic instruments.
3. The bioeffects that can be caused by ultrasound.
4. Risk and safety considerations in the use of sonographic instruments.

Several devices (Figure 7-1) are available to determine whether sonographic and Doppler ultrasound instruments are operating correctly and consistently. These devices can be divided into two groups:

1. Those that measure the acoustic output of the instrument. This group considers only the beam former and the transducer acting together as a source of ultrasound.
2. Those that test the operation of the instrument (anatomic imaging and flow evaluation performance). This group takes into account the operation of the entire instrument. Imaging and Doppler performance are important to evaluate the instrument as a diagnostic tool. The acoustic output of an instrument is important when considering bioeffects and safety.

Bioeffects are useful in the therapeutic applications of ultrasound, a subject not considered in this book.[6] Of interest here is what the known bioeffects of ultrasound indicate about the safety or risk of diagnostic ultrasound. We desire knowledge about the probability of damage or injury and under what conditions this probability is maximized (to avoid those conditions) or minimized (to seek those conditions while obtaining useful diagnostic information).

PERFORMANCE MEASUREMENTS

Imaging performance is determined primarily by measuring the following parameters:

- Detail resolution
- Contrast resolution
- Penetration and dynamic range
- Time gain compensation operation
- Accuracy of depth and distance measurement

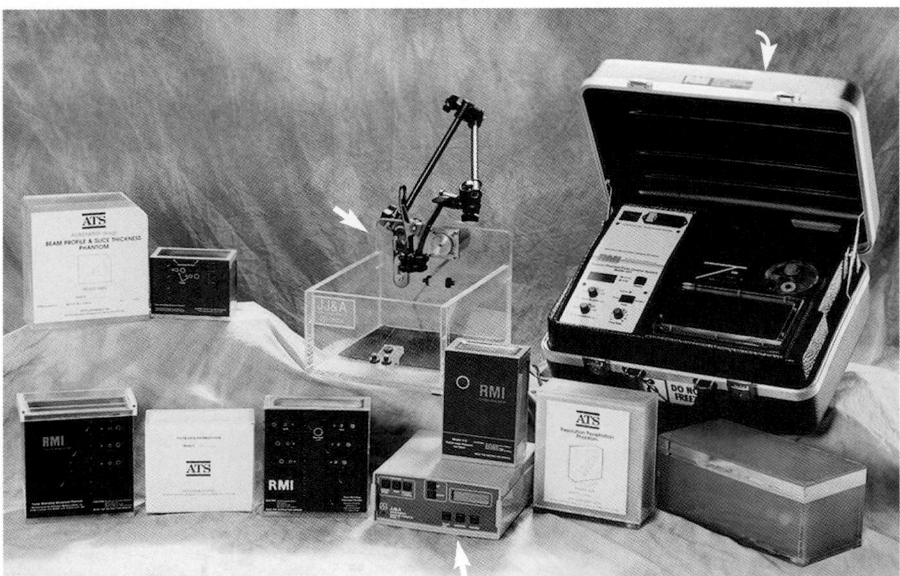

FIGURE 7-1 Several test objects and phantoms. Those intended for Doppler applications are indicated by arrows. The other devices are used to evaluate imaging performance.

Several devices are commercially available to test imaging performance. These devices fall into two categories: (1) tissue-equivalent **phantoms** and (2) **test objects**. Tissue-equivalent phantoms have some characteristics representative of tissues (such as scattering and attenuation properties); test objects do not. Some devices are combinations of the two (e.g., tissue-equivalent phantoms that contain resolution targets). Phantoms and test objects can be used not only by service personnel but also by instrument operators. The American College of Radiology Ultrasound Accreditation Program requires that routine quality control testing must occur regularly. The minimum requirement is semiannual testing. The American Institute of Ultrasound in Medicine (AIUM; *www.aium.org*) Practice Accreditation program requires that equipment maintenance and calibration be regularly performed on all ultrasound equipment. The AIUM has published a manual on quality assurance, available for purchase.[7]

Gray-Scale Test Objects and Tissue-Equivalent Phantoms

Tissue-equivalent phantoms are made of graphite-filled aqueous gels or urethane rubber materials. Graphite particles act as ultrasound scatterers (echo producers) in materials. Graphite is the soft carbon that is used in pencils and as a lubricant. Attenuation in these materials is similar to that for soft tissue, and propagation speed is 1.54 mm/μs in gels and 1.45 mm/μs in rubber. Compensation for the latter speed error is accomplished by positioning targets in the rubber material to closer locations. However, errors can still occur because of speed error. Tissue-equivalent phantoms typically contain echo-free (cystic) regions of various diameters and thin nylon lines (approximately 0.2 mm in diameter) to measure detail resolution and distance accuracy. Some phantoms contain cones or cylinders containing material of various scattering strengths (various graphite concentrations) that are hyperechoic or hypoechoic compared with the surrounding material. Figures 7-2 to 7-8 give examples of several phantoms.

> Tissue-equivalent phantoms simulate tissue properties, allowing assessment of detail and contrast resolutions, penetration, dynamic range, and time gain compensation operation.

Test objects do not simulate tissue characteristics but do provide some specific measure of instrument performance. The beam-profile slice-thickness test object (Figure 7-9) contains a thin, scattering layer in an echo-free material. The object can be used to show beam width in the scan plane or perpendicular to it (section thickness).

> Test objects contain nylon lines and scattering layers to allow evaluation of detail resolution and beam profiles.

Doppler Test Objects and Tissue-Equivalent Phantoms

Test objects and tissue- and blood-mimicking phantoms are commercially available for the evaluation of Doppler instruments (Figures 7-10 and 7-11). These objects are useful for testing the effective penetration of the Doppler beam, the ability to discriminate between different flow directions, the accuracy of sample volume location, and the accuracy of the measured flow speed. Doppler flow phantoms use a flowing blood-mimicking liquid. Doppler test objects use a moving solid object (usually a string) for scattering the ultrasound. They can be calibrated and can produce pulsatile and reverse motions.

Doppler phantoms have some disadvantages, such as the presence of bubbles and nonuniform flow, but can simulate

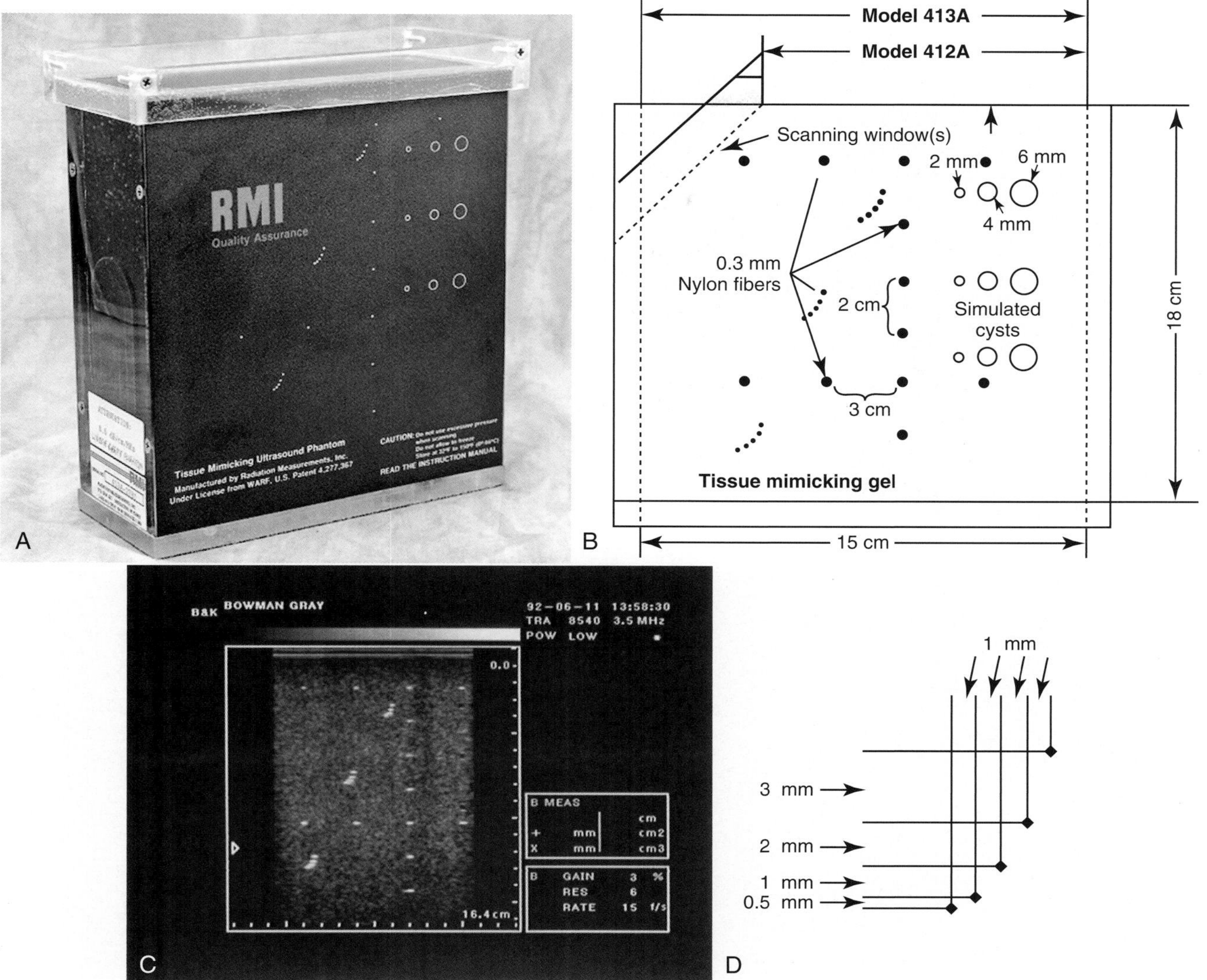

FIGURE 7-2 **A,** A tissue-equivalent phantom containing groups of nylon lines and cystic regions of various sizes. **B,** Diagram detailing the construction of such a phantom. **C,** Scan of a phantom. **D,** Arrangement of the axial resolution line set in this phantom and in that pictured in Figure 7-3. This set was used in Figure 3-29, *D–F,* to illustrate axial resolution at three frequencies.

clinical conditions, such as tissue attenuation (see Figure 7-11). These phantoms are calibrated with an electromagnetic flow meter or by fluid volume collection over time. Refer to Figure 5-39, *B-C,* which illustrates the use of a string test object in the evaluation of Doppler angle correction; Figure 6-29, *A-B,* which shows the use of a string test object in evaluating spectral mirror image; Figure 5-42, which illustrates the use of a flow phantom in determining the accuracy of the gate location indicator on the anatomic display; and Figure 5-29, which shows the use of a flow phantom to illustrate the effect of Doppler angle on Doppler shift.

> Doppler test objects and flow phantoms enable the evaluation of spectral calibration and gate location and penetration of spectral and color-Doppler instruments.

OUTPUT MEASUREMENTS

Several devices can measure the acoustic output of ultrasound instruments.[8] These devices are normally used by engineers and physicists rather than by instrument operators. Only the **hydrophone** is discussed here. The hydrophone sometimes is called a *microprobe.* It is used in two forms (Figures 7-12 and 7-13):

1. A small transducer element (with a diameter of 1 mm or less) mounted on the end of a hollow needle.
2. A large piezoelectric membrane with small metallic electrodes centered on both sides.

The membrane is made of **polyvinylidene fluoride.** Polyvinylidene fluoride is used in both types of hydrophones because of its wide bandwidth. Various construction approaches, not considered here, are used for hydrophones.

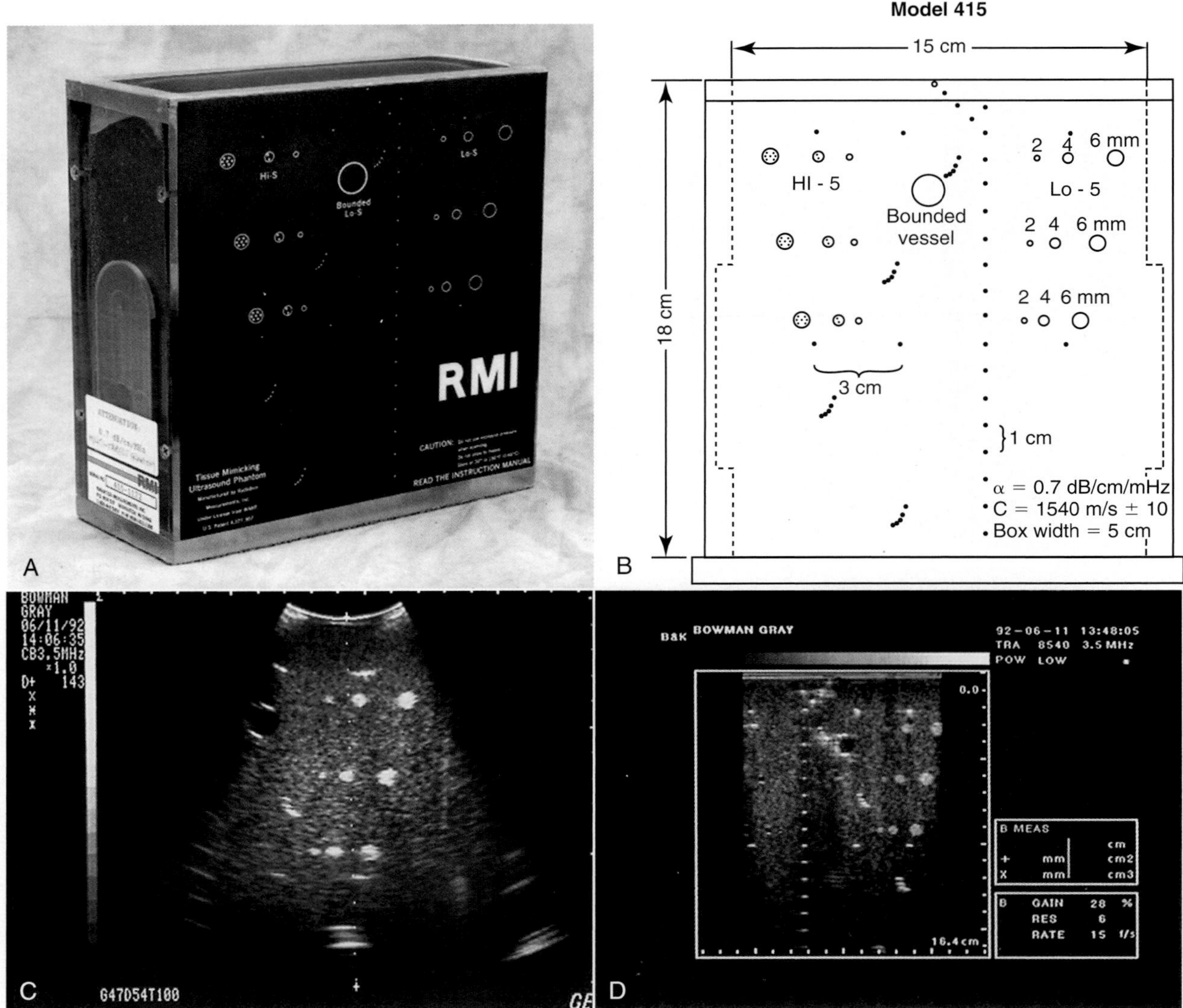

FIGURE 7-3 **A,** A tissue-equivalent phantom containing nylon lines, simulated cysts, a cystic region with an echogenic rim (simulated bounded vessel), and hyperechoic-simulated lesions of various sizes. **B,** Diagram detailing the construction of such a phantom. **C–D,** Scans of phantom.

Hydrophones receive sound reasonably well from all directions without altering the sound by their presence. In response to the varying pressure of the sound, they produce a varying voltage that can be displayed on an oscilloscope. This produces a picture, from which period, pulse repetition period, and pulse duration (PD) can be determined. From these quantities, frequency, pulse repetition frequency, and duty factor can be calculated. Using the hydrophone calibration (relationship between voltage and acoustic pressure), pressure amplitude may also be determined. In addition, wavelength, spatial pulse length, and intensities can be calculated as well.

With the use of hydrophones, acoustic pressure output levels have been measured, and intensities and output indexes have been calculated for various diagnostic ultrasound instruments and transducers. Generally, sonographic outputs are the lowest and pulsed spectral Doppler outputs are the highest, with M mode and color-Doppler imaging outputs falling between the two.

> Needle and membrane hydrophones are used to measure pressure amplitude and period, from which several other acoustic pulse parameters can be calculated.

BIOEFFECTS

The biologic effects and safety of diagnostic ultrasound have received considerable attention. Several review articles, textbooks, and institutional documents have been published. Comprehensive, authoritative publications have been produced by the Bioeffects Committee of the American Institute of Ultrasound in Medicine (AIUM).[9,10]

In the remainder of this chapter, we review knowledge regarding bioeffects in cells, plants, and experimental animals, mechanisms of interaction between ultrasound and biologic cells and tissues, regulatory activities, epidemiology, risk and safety considerations, and elements of prudent practice.

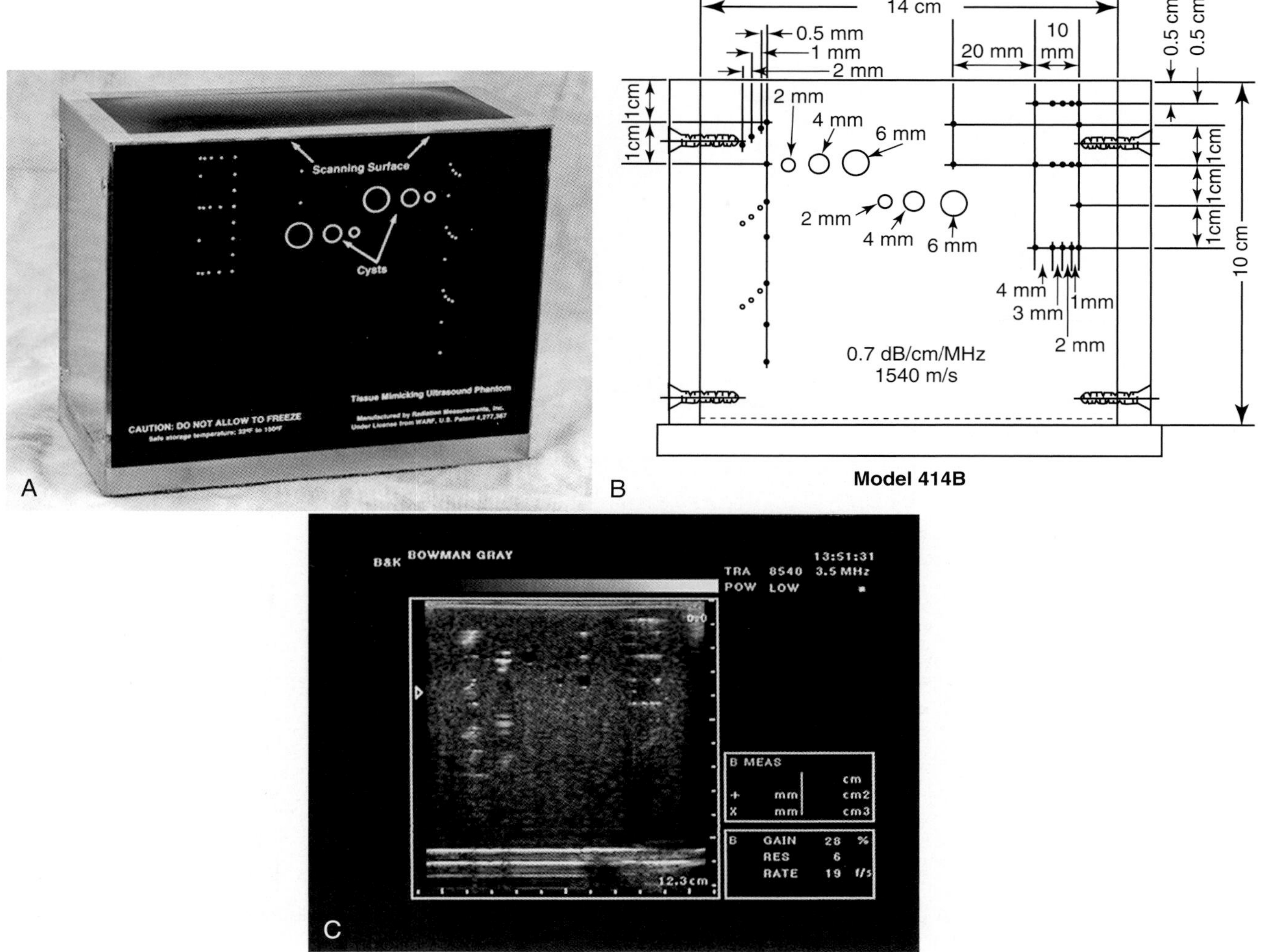

FIGURE 7-4 **A,** A smaller phantom designed for higher-frequency "small parts" applications. **B,** Diagram detailing the construction of such a phantom. **C,** Scan of phantom.

As with any diagnostic test, there may be some risk, that is, some probability of damage or injury, with the use of diagnostic ultrasound. This risk, if known, must be weighed against the benefit to determine the appropriateness of the diagnostic procedure. Knowledge of ways to minimize the risk, even if the risk is unidentified, is useful to everyone involved in diagnostic ultrasound. Sources of information used in developing policy regarding the use of diagnostic ultrasound are diagrammed in Figure 7-14, *A*. These sources include (1) bioeffects data from experimental systems, (2) output data from diagnostic instruments, and (3) knowledge and experience with regard to how the diagnostic information obtained is of benefit in patient management. Comparison of the first two components allows an assessment of risk, whereas the combination of the latter two components yields an awareness of the benefit. It seems reasonable to assume that there is some risk (however small) in the use of diagnostic ultrasound because ultrasound is a form of energy and has at least the potential to produce a biologic effect that could constitute risk. Even if this risk is so minimal that it is difficult to identify, prudent practice dictates that routine measures be implemented to minimize the risk while obtaining the necessary information to achieve the diagnostic benefit. This is the ALARA (As Low As Reasonably Achievable) principle of prudent scanning.

Our knowledge of bioeffects resulting from ultrasound exposure comes from several sources (see Figure 7-14, *B*). These sources include experimental observations in cell suspensions and cultures, plants, and experimental animals; epidemiologic studies in human beings; and studies of interaction mechanisms, such as heating and cavitation.

> Knowledge of bioeffects is important for the safe and prudent use of sonography.

Cells

Because cells in suspension or in culture are so different from those in the intact patient in a clinical environment, one must exercise restraint in extrapolating in vitro results

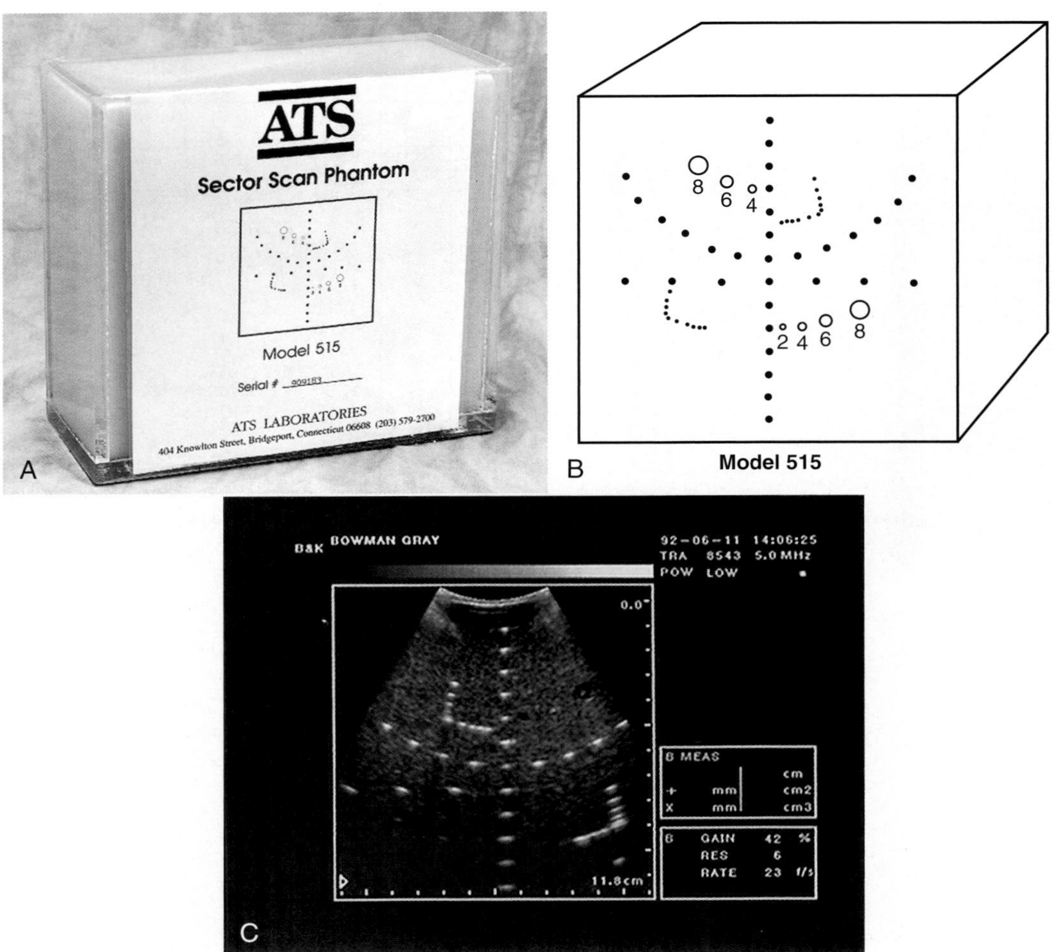

FIGURE 7-5 **A,** A phantom designed for sector scan applications. **B,** Diagram detailing the construction of such a phantom. **C,** Scan of phantom.

to clinical significance. Cellular studies are useful in determining mechanisms of interaction and guiding the design of experimental animal studies and epidemiologic studies. The American Institute of Ultrasound in Medicine (AIUM) *(www.aium.org/resources/statements.aspx)* issued the following statement on in vitro biologic effects in 2012:

> *It is often difficult to evaluate reports of ultrasonically induced in vitro effects with respect to their clinical significance. An in vitro effect can be regarded as a real biological effect. However, the predominant physical and biological interactions and mechanisms involved in an in vitro effect may not pertain to the in vivo situation. Results from in vitro experiments suggest new endpoints and serve as a basis for design of in vivo experiments. In vitro studies provide the capability to control experimental variables that may not be controllable in vivo and thus offer a means to explore and evaluate specific mechanisms and test hypotheses. Although they may have limited applicability to in vivo biological effects, such studies can disclose fundamental intercellular or intracellular effects of ultrasound. While it is valid for authors to place their results in context and to suggest further relevant investigations, reports which do more than that should be viewed with caution.*

Plants

The primary components of plant tissues—stems, leaves, and roots—contain gas-filled channels between the cell walls. Thus plants have served as useful biologic models for studying the effects of cavitation.

Through this mechanism, normal cellular organization and function can be disturbed. Irreversible effects appear to be limited to cell death. Reversible effects include chromosomal abnormalities, mitotic index reductions, and growth rate reduction. Membrane damage induced by microstreaming shear stress appears to be the cause of cell death in leaves. Intensity thresholds for lysis of leaf cells are much higher with pulsed ultrasound than with continuous wave ultrasound. Apparently, the response of the bubbles within tissues to continuous and pulsed fields is different.

> Plant studies are useful primarily to understand cavitational effects in living tissue.

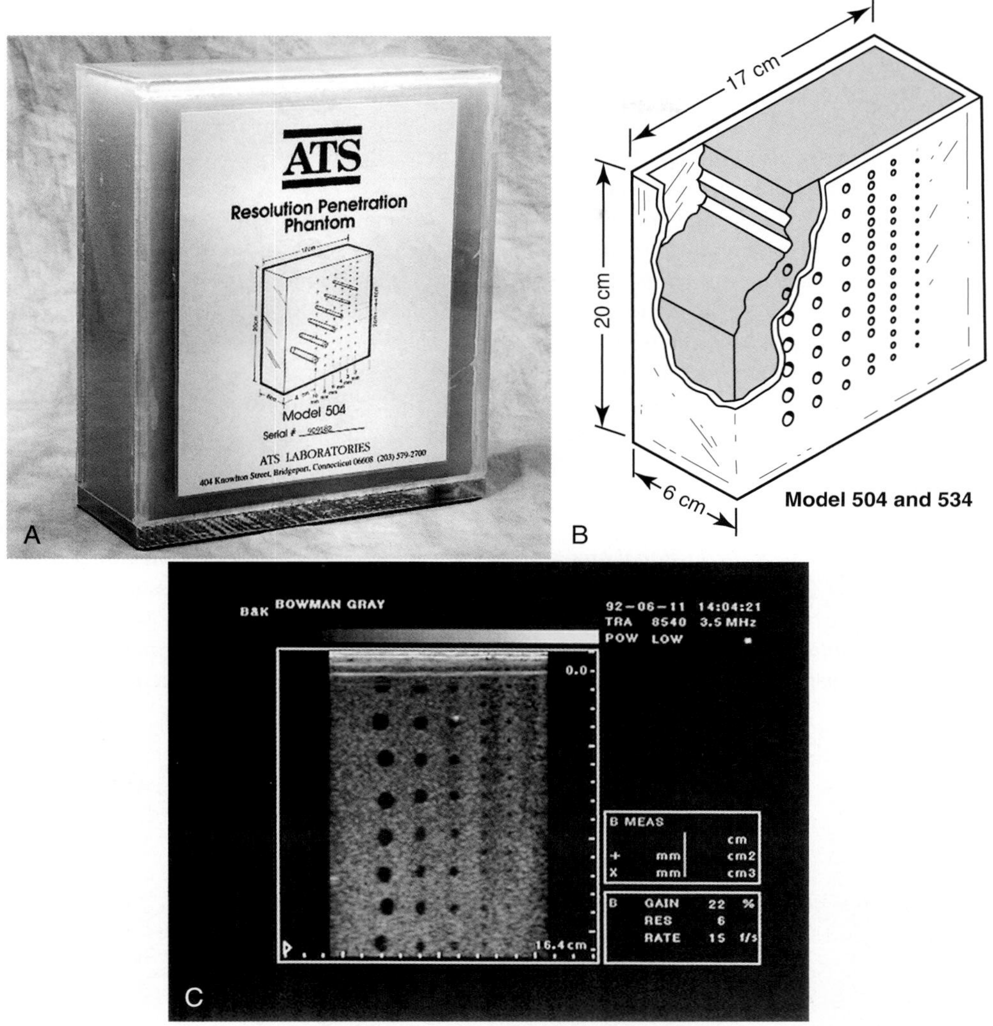

FIGURE 7-6 **A**, A resolution penetration phantom that contains columns of simulated cysts of various sizes. **B**, Diagram detailing the construction of such a phantom. **C**, Scan of phantom. This phantom was used to illustrate resolution and penetration at two frequencies in Figure 3-34.

Animals

With experimental animals, reported in vivo effects include fetal weight reduction, postpartum mortality, fetal abnormalities, tissue lesions, hind limb paralysis, blood flow stasis, wound repair enhancement, and tumor regression. Many studies on fetal weight reduction in mice and rats have been performed. All rat studies and several mouse studies yielded negative results. Focal lesion production is a well-documented bioeffect that has been observed over a wide range of intensity and exposure duration (ED) conditions (Figure 7-15).

In 2008, the AIUM *(www.aium.org/resources/statements.aspx)* issued the following statement on mammalian in vivo biologic effects:

Information from experiments using laboratory mammals has contributed significantly to our understanding of ultrasonically induced biological effects and the mechanisms that are most likely responsible. The following statement summarizes observations relative to specific diagnostic ultrasound parameters and indices.

In the low-megahertz frequency range there have been no independently confirmed adverse biological effects in mammalian tissues exposed in vivo under experimental ultrasound conditions, as follows:

1. **Thermal Mechanisms:** *No effects have been observed for an unfocused beam having free-field spatial-peak temporal-average (SPTA) intensities* below 100 mW/cm², or a focused† beam having intensities below 1 W/cm², or thermal index values of less than 2.*

   For fetal exposures, no effects have been reported for a temperature increase above the normal physiologic

*Free-field SPTA intensity for continuous wave and pulsed exposures.
†Quarter-power (–6 dB) beam width smaller than 4 wavelengths or 4 mm, whichever is less at the exposure frequency.

temperature, ΔT, when $\Delta T < 4.5 - (\log_{10}t/0.6)$, where t is exposure time ranging from 1 to 250 minutes, including off time for pulsed exposure.

For postnatal exposures producing temperature increases of 6° C or less, no effects have been reported when $\Delta T < 6 - (\log_{10}t/0.6)$, including off time for pulsed exposure. For example, for temperature increases of 6.0° C and 2.0° C, the corresponding limits for the exposure durations t are 1 and 250 minutes.

For postnatal exposures producing temperature increases of 6° C or more, no effects have been reported when $\Delta T < 6 - (\log_{10}t/0.3)$, including off time for pulsed exposure. For example, for a temperature increase of 9.6° C, the corresponding limit for the exposure duration is 5 seconds (= 0.083 minutes).

2. **Nonthermal Mechanisms:** *In tissues that contain well-defined gas bodies, for example, lung, no effects have been observed for in situ peak rarefactional pressures below approximately 0.4 MPa or mechanical index values less than approximately 0.4.*

   In tissues that do not contain well-defined gas bodies, no effects have been reported for peak rarefactional pressures below approximately 4.0 MPa or mechanical index values less than approximately 4.0.

> Studies of bioeffects in experimental animals have allowed determination of conditions under which thermal and nonthermal bioeffects occur.

Mechanisms of action by which ultrasound could produce biologic effects can be divided into two groups: (1) heating and (2) mechanical. The mechanical mechanism is also called *nonthermal.*

Heat

Recall that attenuation in tissue is primarily due to absorption, that is, conversion of ultrasound to heat. Thus ultrasound produces a temperature rise while it propagates through tissues. The extent of the temperature rise produced depends on the applied intensity and frequency (because the absorption coefficient is approximately proportional to frequency) of sound and on beam focusing and tissue perfusion. Heating increases while intensity or frequency is increased. For a given transducer output intensity, with increasing tissue depths, heating is decreased at higher frequencies because of the increased

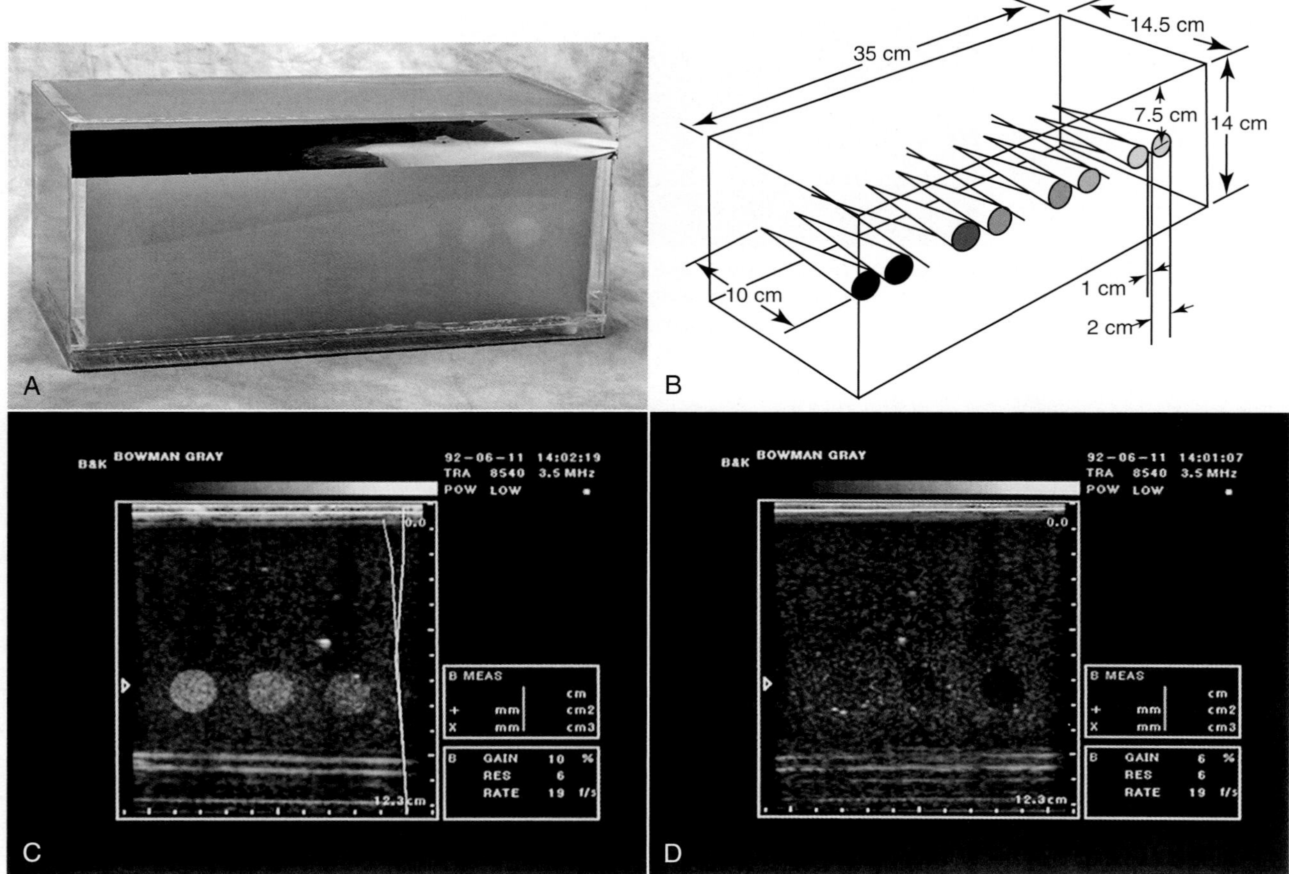

FIGURE 7-7 **A,** A contrast-detail phantom containing cones of material of various echogenicities. **B,** Diagram detailing the construction of such a phantom. **C,** Scan of hyperechoic sections of phantom. **D,** Scan of hypoechoic sections of phantom.

attenuation that reduces the intensity arriving at depth. Temperature rises are considered significant if they exceed 2° C. Intensities greater than a few hundred milliwatts per square centimeter (mW/cm^2) can produce such temperature rises. Absorption coefficients are higher in bone than they are in soft tissues. Therefore bone heating, particularly in the fetus, receives special consideration.

Heating has been shown to be an important consideration in some reports on bioeffects. Mathematic models have been developed for calculating temperature rises in tissues. These models have been used to calculate estimated intensities required for a given temperature rise. In 2009 the AIUM (*www.aium.org/resources/statements.aspx*) issued the following conclusions regarding heat:

1. *Excessive temperature increase can result in toxic effects in mammalian systems. The biological effects observed depend on many factors, such as the exposure duration, the type of tissue exposed, its cellular proliferation rate, and its potential for regeneration.*

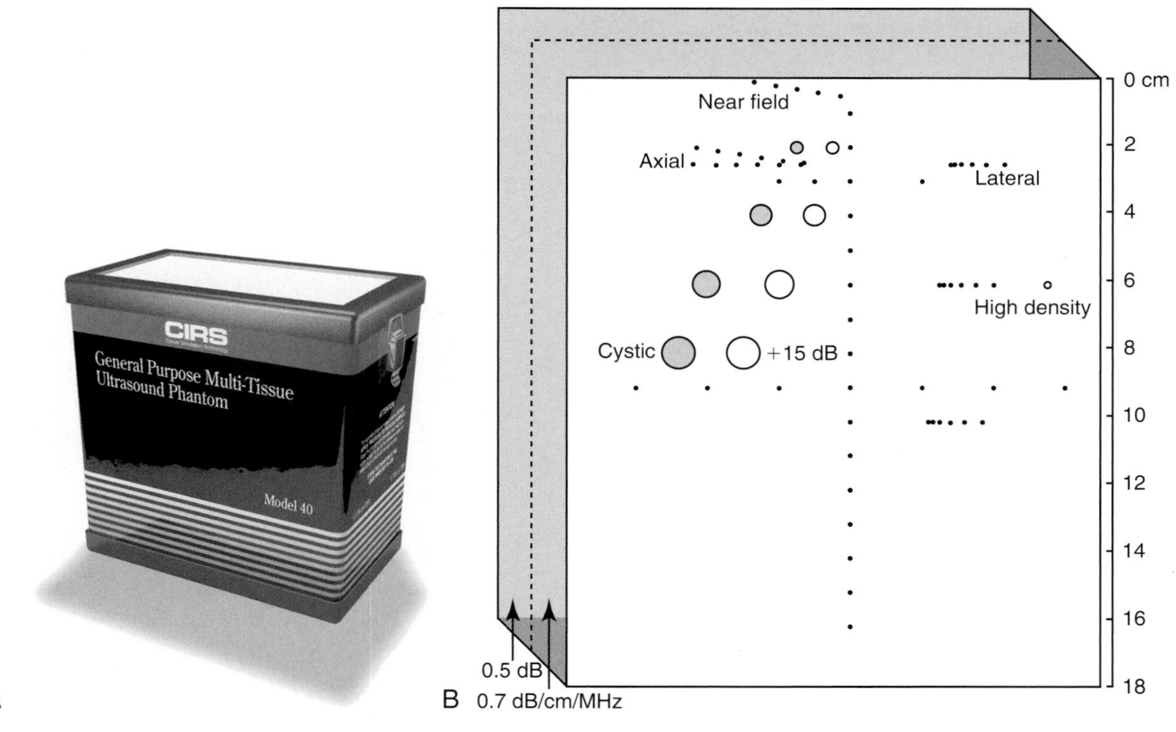

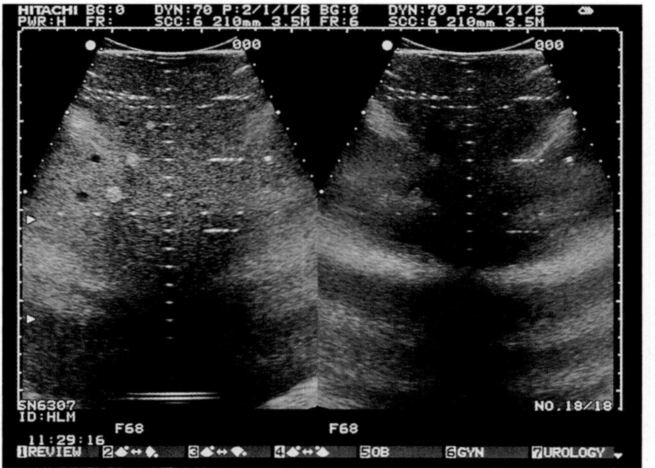

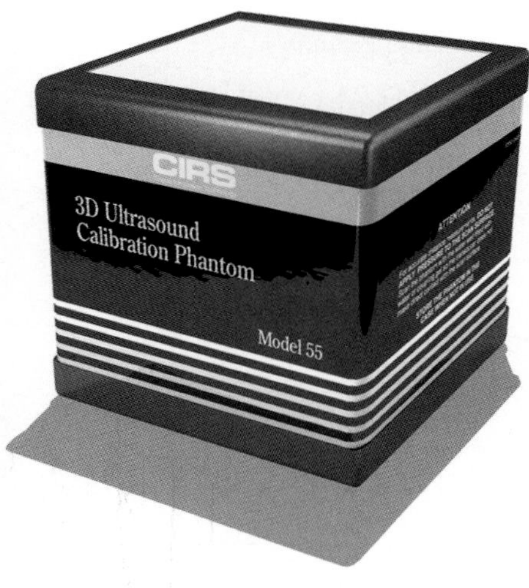

FIGURE 7-8 A, General purpose phantom with two background tissue materials (0.5 and 0.7 dB/cm-MHz). **B,** Construction diagram for the phantom in **A. C,** Image scanned with phantom in **A. D,** Three-dimensional calibration phantom for the assessment of volumetric measurement accuracy. **E,** Construction diagram for **D. F,** Images obtained by scanning **D. G,** Fetal-training phantom. **H,** Two-dimensional image from **G. I,** Three-dimensional image from **G.**

Continued

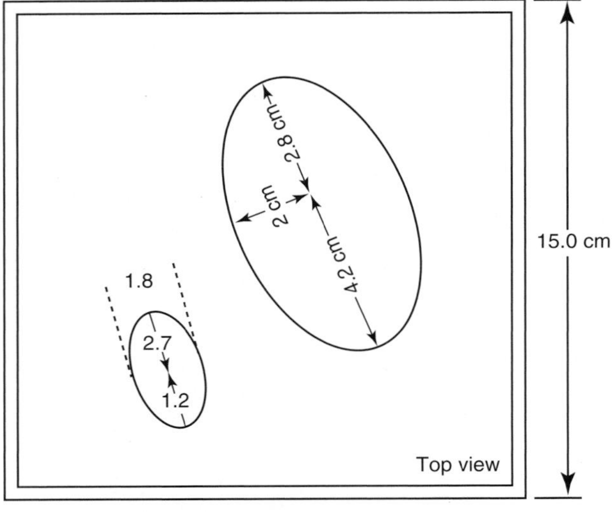

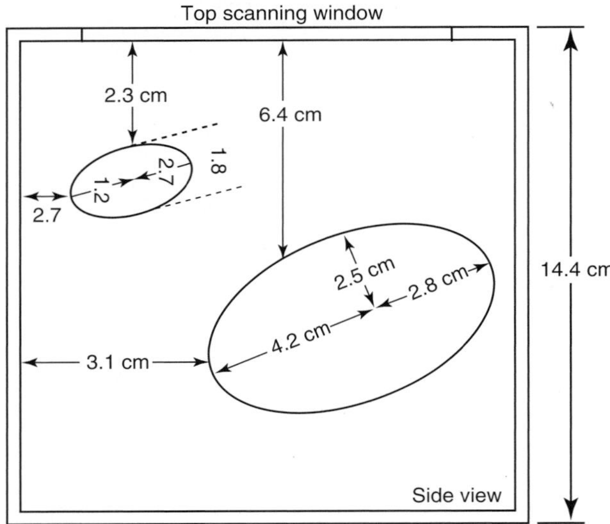

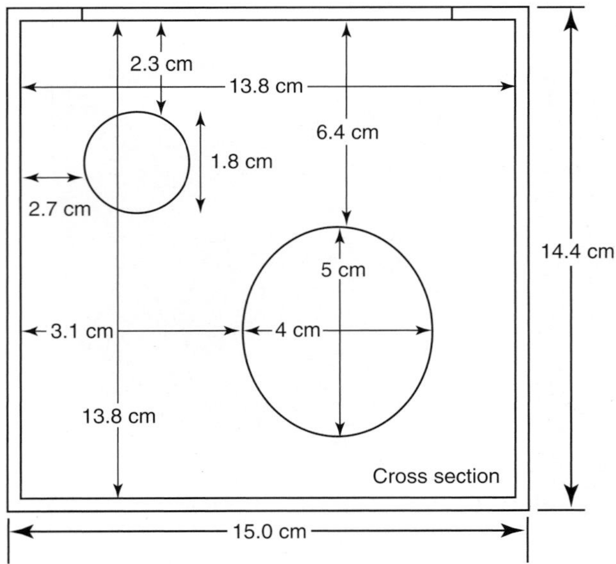

FIGURE 7-8, cont'd

Age and stage of development are important factors when considering fetal and neonatal safety. Temperature increases of several degrees Celsius above the normal core range can occur naturally. The probability of an adverse biological effect increases with the duration of the temperature rise.

2. *In general, adult tissues are more tolerant of temperature increases than fetal and neonatal tissues. Therefore, higher temperatures and/or longer exposure durations would be required for thermal damage. The considerable data available on the thermal sensitivity of adult tissues support the following inferences:*

   For exposure durations up to 50 hours, there have been no significant, adverse biological effects observed due to temperature increases less than or equal to 2° C above normal.

   For temperature increases between 2° C and 6° C above normal, there have been no significant, adverse biological effects observed due to temperature increases less than or equal to $6 - \log_{10}(t/60)/0.6$*, where t is the exposure duration in seconds. For example, for temperature increases of 4° C and 6° C, the corresponding limits for the exposure durations t are 16 min and 1 min, respectively.*

   For temperature increases greater than 6° C above normal, there have been no significant, adverse biological effects observed due to temperature increases less than or equal to $6 - \log_{10}(t/60)/0.3$*, where t is the exposure duration in seconds. For example, for temperature increases of 9.6° C and 6.0° C, the corresponding limits for the exposure durations t are 5 and 60 seconds, respectively.*

   For exposure durations less than 5 seconds, there have been no significant, adverse biological effects observed due to temperature increases less than or equal to $9 - \log_{10}(t/60)/0.3$*, where t is the exposure duration in seconds. For example, for temperature increases of 18.3° C, 14.9° C, and 12.6° C, the corresponding limits for the exposure durations t are 0.1, 1 and 5 seconds, respectively.*

3. *Acoustic output from diagnostic ultrasound devices is sufficient to cause temperature elevations in fetal tissue. Although fewer data are available for fetal tissues, the following conclusions are justified:*

   In general, temperature elevations become progressively greater from B-mode to color-Doppler to spectral-Doppler applications.

   For identical exposure conditions, the potential for thermal bioeffects increases with the dwell time during examination.

   For identical exposure conditions, the temperature rise near bone is significantly greater than in soft tissues, and it increases with ossification development throughout gestation. For this reason, conditions where an acoustic beam impinges on ossifying fetal bone deserve special attention due to its close proximity to other developing tissues.

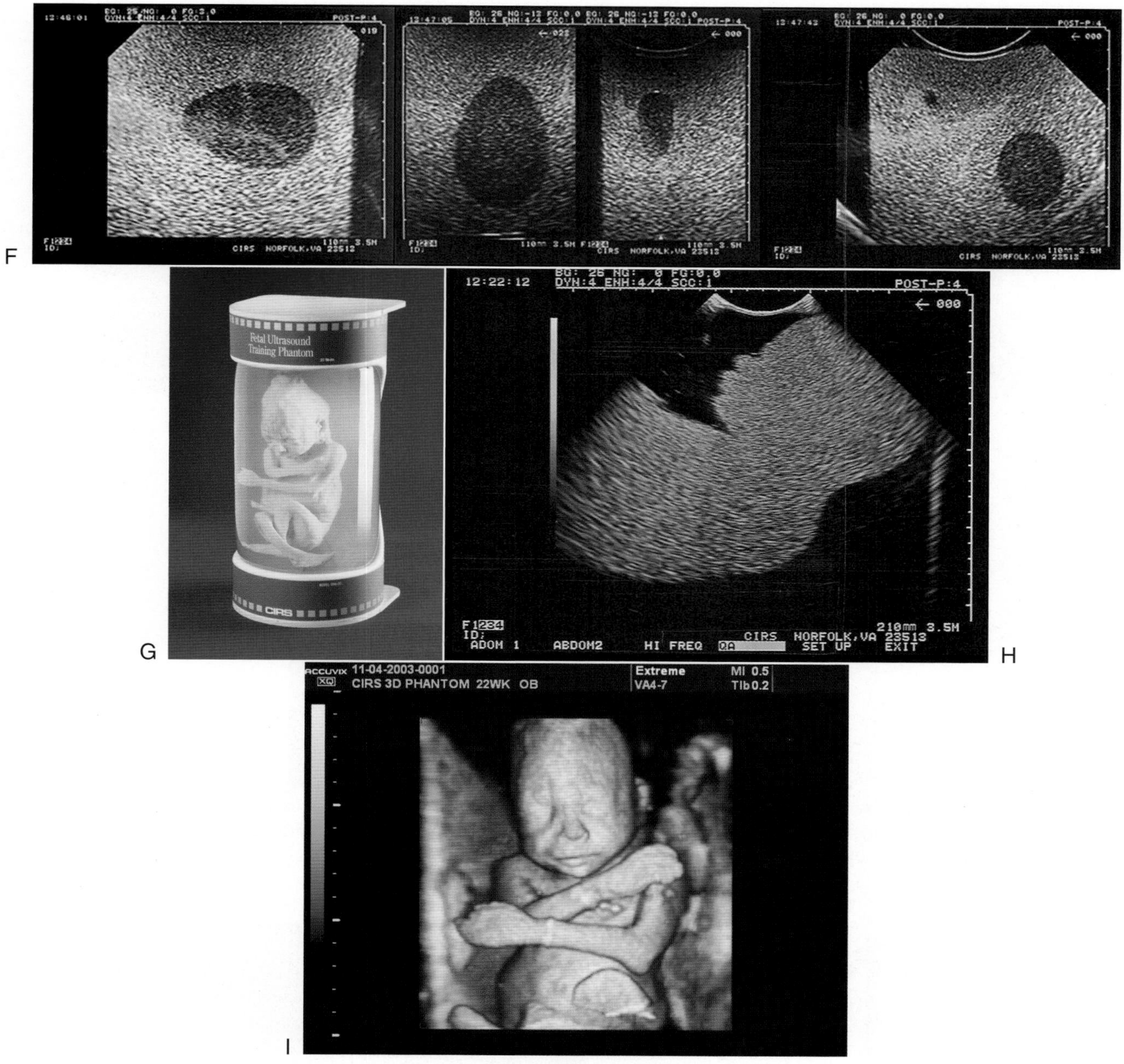

FIGURE 7-8, cont'd

The current FDA regulatory limit for $I_{SPTA.3}$ is 720 mW/cm^2. For this, and lesser intensities, the theoretical estimate of the maximum temperature increase in the conceptus can exceed 2°C.

Although, in general, an adverse fetal outcome is possible at any time during gestation, most severe and detectable effects of thermal exposure in animals have been observed during the period of organogenesis. For this reason, exposures during the first trimester should be restricted to the lowest outputs consistent with obtaining the necessary diagnostic information.

Ultrasound exposures that elevate fetal temperature by 4° C above normal for 5 minutes or more have the potential to induce severe developmental defects. Thermally induced congenital anomalies have been observed in a large variety of animal species. In current clinical practice, using commercially available equipment, it is unlikely that such thermal exposure would occur at a specific fetal anatomic site.

Transducer self-heating is a significant component of the temperature rise of tissues close to the transducer. This may be of significance in transvaginal scanning, but no data for the fetal temperature rise are available.

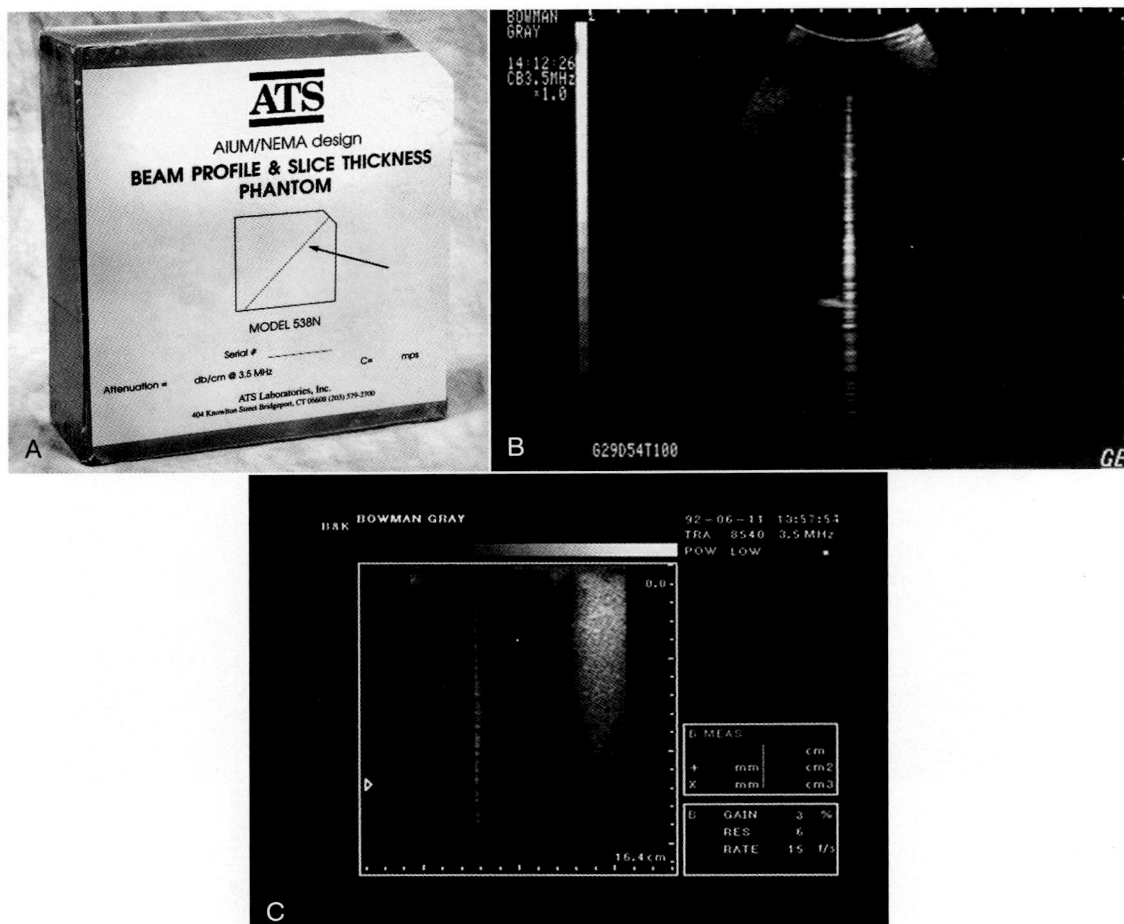

FIGURE 7-9 **A,** A beam profile and section thickness test object. It contains a thin, scattering layer *(arrow)* in an anechoic material. **B–C,** Scans of beam profiles. Shown in Figure 3-22, *D–F* are beam profiles obtained using this test object.

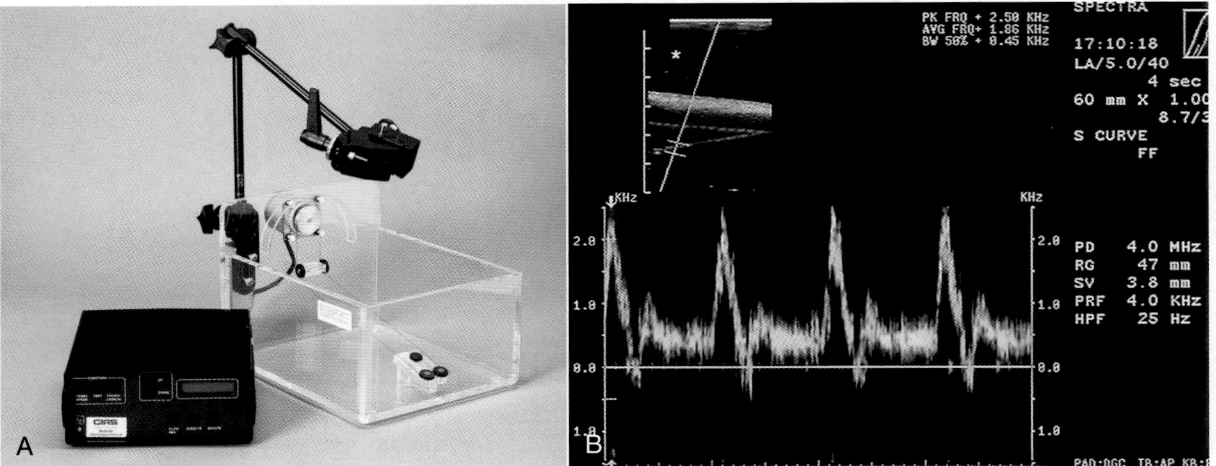

FIGURE 7-10 **A,** A moving-string test object and controller. **B,** Spectral display of a moving string (operating in pulsatile mode).

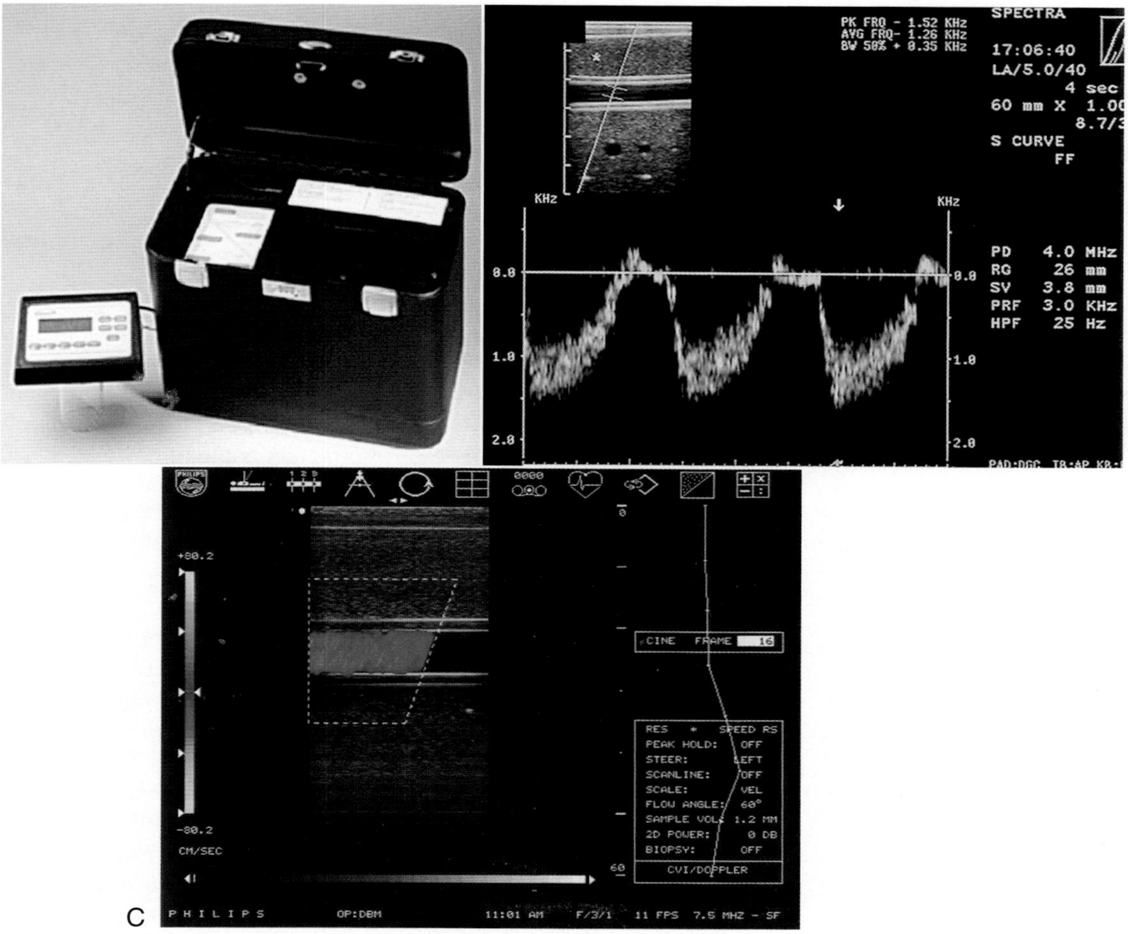

FIGURE 7-11 **A,** Doppler flow phantom. **B,** Spectral display from a flow phantom. **C,** Color-Doppler image from a flow phantom.

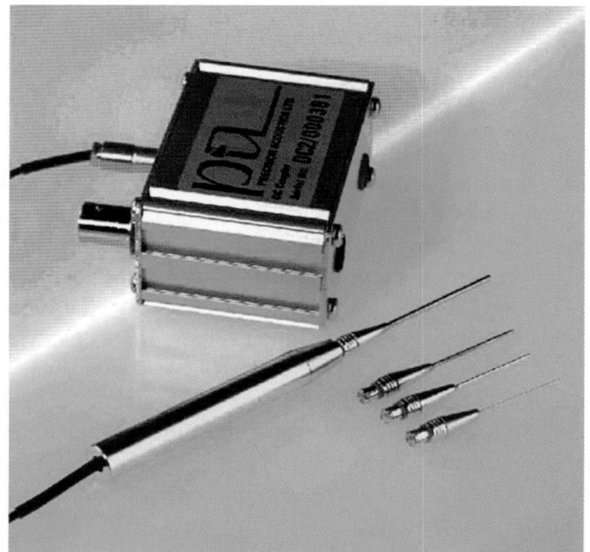

FIGURE 7-12 A hydrophone consisting of a small transducer element mounted on the end of a needle.

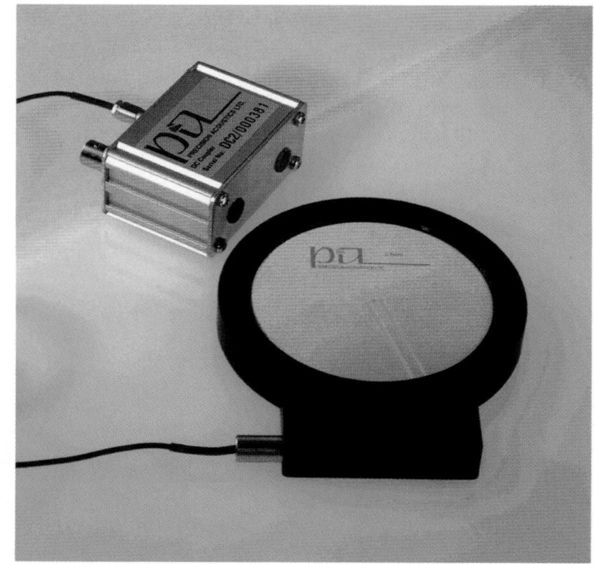

FIGURE 7-13 A hydrophone consisting of a thin membrane with metal electrodes.

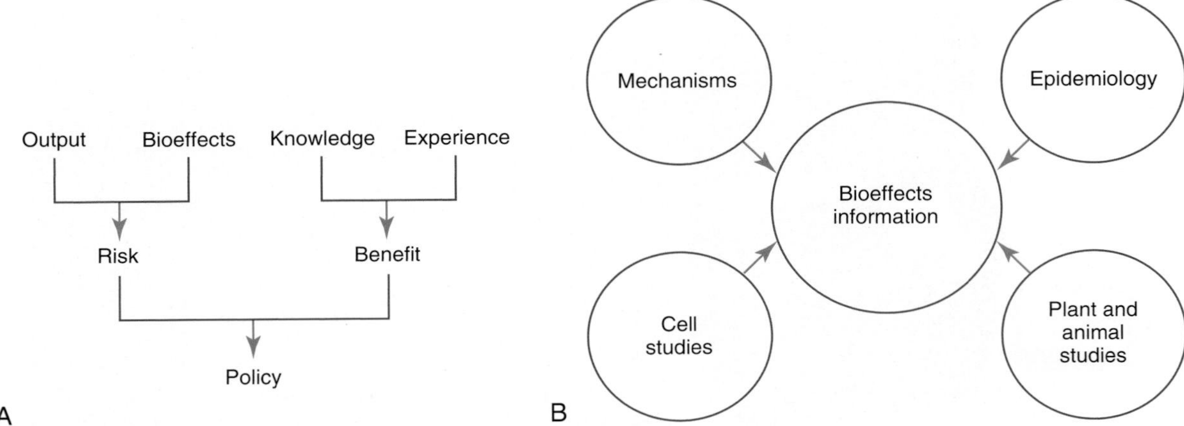

FIGURE 7-14 A, Ultrasound risk and benefit information. Risk information comes from experimental bioeffects (including epidemiology) and instrument output data. Benefit information is derived from knowledge and experience in diagnostic ultrasound use and efficacy. Together, they lead to a policy on the prudent use of ultrasound imaging in medicine. **B,** Bioeffects information sources.

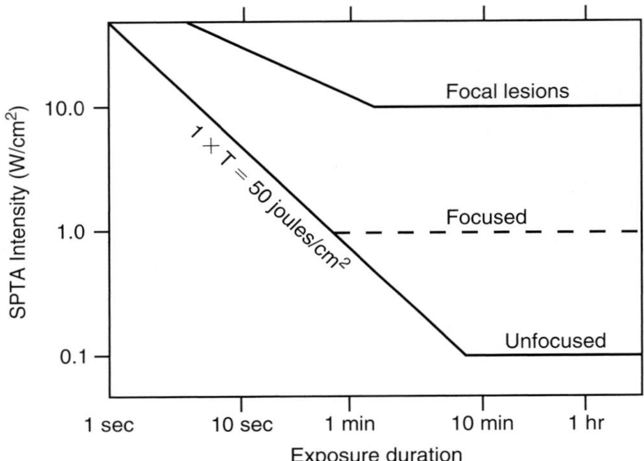

FIGURE 7-15 Comparison of the minimum spatial peak–temporal average (SPTA) intensities required for ultrasonic bioeffects specified in the American Institute of Ultrasound in Medicine (AIUM) Statement on Mammalian Bioeffects. The minimum levels required for focal lesions also are shown in the figure for comparison. Note that logarithmic scaling has been used for the axes of this figure, so the horizontal lines are separated by factors of 10 in intensity. (From the American Institute of Ultrasound in Medicine: *Bioeffects and safety of diagnostic ultrasound,* Laurel, 1993, The Institute.)

4. *The temperature increase during exposure of tissues to diagnostic ultrasound fields is dependent upon (a) output characteristics of the acoustic source such as frequency, source dimensions, scan rate, power, pulse repetition frequency, pulse duration, transducer self-heating, exposure time and wave shape and (b) tissue properties such as attenuation, absorption, speed of sound, acoustic impedance, perfusion, thermal conductivity, thermal diffusivity, anatomic structure and nonlinearity parameter.*

5. *Calculations of the maximum temperature increase resulting from ultrasound exposure* in vivo *are not exact because of the uncertainties and approximations associated with the thermal, acoustic, and structural characteristics of the tissues involved. However, experimental evidence shows that calculations are generally capable of predicting measured values within a factor of 2. Thus, such calculations are used to obtain safety guidelines for clinical exposures where direct temperature measurements are not feasible. These guidelines, called* Thermal Indices,* *provide a real-time display of the relative probability that a diagnostic system could induce thermal injury in the exposed subject. Under most clinically relevant conditions, the soft-tissue thermal index, TIS, and the bone thermal index, TIB, either overestimate or closely approximate the best available estimate of the maximum temperature increase (Δ Tmax). For example, if TIS = 2, then Δ Tmax ≤ 2°C.*

Experimental measurements have shown reasonable confirmation of the mathematical calculations. The biologic consequences of hyperthermia include fetal absorption or abortion, growth restriction, microphthalmia, cataract formation, abdominal wall defects, renal agenesis, palatal defects, reduction in brain waves, microencephaly, anencephaly, spinal cord defects, amyoplasia, forefoot hypoplasia, tibial and fibular deformations, and abnormal tooth genesis. Approximately 80 known biologic effects are due to hyperthermia. None has occurred at temperatures of less than 39° C. Above that, the occurrence of a biologic effect depends on temperature and exposure time, as shown in Figure 7-16.

*Thermal indices are nondimensional ratios of estimated temperature increases to 1° C for specific tissue models (see the Standard for Real-Time Display of Thermal and Mechanical Acoustic Output Indices on Diagnostic Ultrasound Equipment, Revision 1, AIUM/NEMA, 2001).

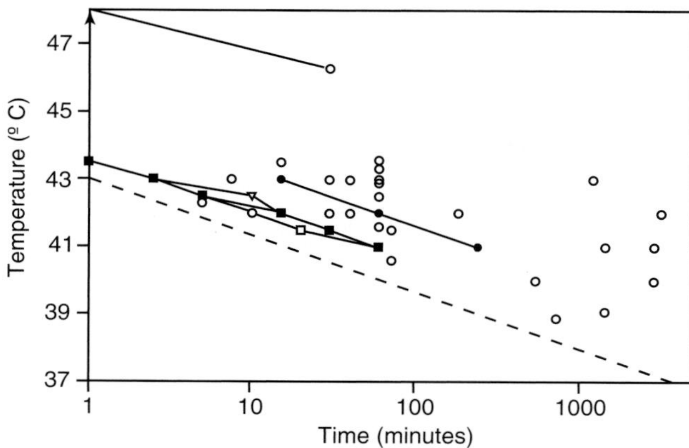

FIGURE 7-16 Thermal bioeffects. A plot of thermally produced biologic effects that have been reported in the literature, in which the temperature elevation and exposure durations are provided. Each data point represents the lowest temperature reported for any duration or the shortest duration for any temperature reported for a given effect. *Solid lines* represent multiple data points relating to a single effect. The *dashed line* represents a lower boundary (t_{43} = 1) for observed, thermally induced biologic effects. (From Miller MV, Ziskin MC: Biological consequences of hyperthermia, *Ultrasound Med Biol* 15:707–722, *1989*. Copyright 1989 by World Federation of Ultrasound in Medicine and Biology.)

> Ultrasound is absorbed by tissue, producing a temperature rise. If critical time–temperature values are exceeded, tissue damage occurs.

Mechanical

Nonthermal or mechanical mechanisms of interaction include radiation force, streaming, and cavitation. **Radiation force** is the force exerted by a sound beam on an absorber or a reflector. This force can deform or disrupt structures. Radiation force also can cause flow in an absorbing fluid. This flow can cause shear stresses that can deform or disrupt structure. Some bioeffects observed in experimental studies have been attributed to these nonthermal, noncavitational mechanisms of interaction.

Cavitation is the production and behavior of bubbles in a liquid medium. A propagating sound wave is one means by which cavitation can occur. Two types of cavitation are recognized to occur. *Stable cavitation* is the term used to describe bubbles that oscillate in diameter with the passing pressure variations of the sound wave. Streaming of surrounding liquid can occur in this situation, resulting in shear stresses on suspended cells or intracellular organelles. Detection of cavitation in tissues under continuous wave, high-intensity conditions has been reported. *Transient (collapse) cavitation* occurs when bubble oscillations are so large that the bubble collapses, producing pressure discontinuities (shock waves), localized extremely high temperatures, and light emission in clear liquids. Transient cavitation has the potential for significant destructive effects. Transient cavitation is the means by which laboratory cell disruptors operate. One theory predicts that ultrasound could produce transient cavitation under diagnostically relevant conditions in water. Another theory incorporates a range of bubble sizes that yields a predictable dependence of the cavitation threshold on pressure and frequency. Experimental verification of this dependence has been carried out using stabilized microbubbles in water. Thresholds for cavitation in soft tissue and body liquids have been determined recently.

The AIUM *(www.aium.org/resources/statements.aspx)* has summarized information on the cavitation mechanism in its conclusions regarding gas bodies, which were approved in 2008:

> *Biologically significant, adverse, nonthermal effects have only been identified with certainty for diagnostically relevant exposures in tissues that have well-defined populations of stabilized gas bodies. Such gas bodies either may occur naturally or may be injected from an exogenous source such as an ultrasound contrast agent. This statement concerns the former, while a separate statement deals with contrast agents.*
>
> 1. *The outputs of some currently available diagnostic ultrasound devices can generate levels that produce hemorrhage in the lungs and intestines of laboratory animals.*
> 2. *A mechanical index (MI)* has been formulated to assist users in evaluating the likelihood of cavitation-related adverse biological effects for diagnostically relevant exposures. The MI is a better indicator than single-parameter measures of exposure, for example, derated spatial-peak pulse-average intensity (ISPPA.3) or derated peak rarefactional pressure (pr.3), for known adverse nonthermal biological effects of ultrasound.*
> 3. *The threshold value of the current MI for lung hemorrhage in the mouse is approximately 0.4. The corresponding threshold for the intestine is MI = 1.4. The implications of these observations for human exposure are yet to be determined.*
> 4. *Thresholds for adverse nonthermal effects depend upon tissue characteristics, exposure duration (ED), and ultrasound parameters such as frequency (fc), pulse duration (PD), and pulse repetition frequency (PRF). For lung hemorrhage in postnatal laboratory animals, an empirical relation for the threshold value of* in situ *acoustic pressure is*
>
> $$P\wedge r = (2.4\ f_c^{0.28} PRF^{0.04})/(PD^{0.27} ED^{0.23}) MPa,$$
>
> *where the ranges and units of the variables investigated are (fc) = 1 to 5.6 MHz, PRF = 0.017 to 1.0 kHz, PD = 1.0 to 11.7 μs, and ED = 2.4 to 180 s. The above relationship differs significantly from the corresponding form used for the MI, and a lung-specific MI is in development.*

*The MI is equal to the derated peak rarefactional pressure (in MPa) at the point of the maximum derated pulse intensity integral divided by the square root of the ultrasonic center frequency (in MHz) (see the Standard for Real-Time Display of Thermal and Mechanical Acoustic Output Indices on Diagnostic Ultrasound Equipment, Revision 2, AIUM/NEMA, 2004).

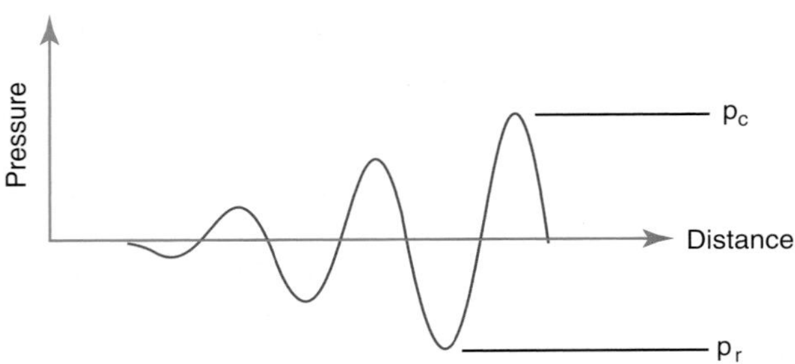

FIGURE 7-17 Pressure versus distance for a three-cycle pulse of ultrasound. p_c, Peak compressional pressure; p_r, peak rarefactional pressure.

5. *The worst-case theoretical threshold for bubble nucleation and subsequent inertial cavitation in soft tissue is MI = 3.9 at 1 MHz. The threshold decreases to MI approximately 1.9 at 5 MHz and above, a level equal to the maximum output permitted by the U.S. Food and Drug Administration for diagnostic ultrasound devices. Experimental values for the cavitation threshold correspond to MI >4 for extravasation of blood cells in mouse kidneys, and MI >5.1 for hind limb paralysis in the mouse neonate.*
6. *For diagnostically relevant exposures (MI≤1.9), no independently confirmed, biologically significant adverse nonthermal effects have been reported in mammalian tissues that do not contain well-defined gas bodies.*

Peak rarefactional pressure is illustrated in Figure 7-17. Experimental measurements have been performed that have shown reasonable confirmation of theoretical calculations (Figure 7-18). The only well-documented mammalian biologic consequence of gas bodies in an ultrasound beam is blood cell extravasation in inflated lung. It has not occurred at acoustic pressure amplitudes of less than 0.3 MPa. Above that, its occurrence depends on frequency, exposure time, and pulsing conditions.

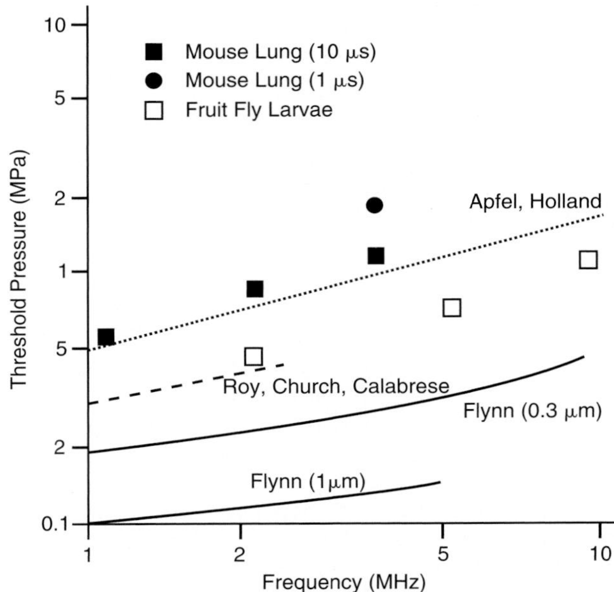

FIGURE 7-18 Threshold (in situ) rarefactional pressures for biologic effects in vivo of low-temporal-average intensity, pulsed ultrasound. Pulse durations are shown in parentheses in the legend. In all cases, the tissues contain identifiable, small, stabilized gas bodies. As in diagnostic ultrasound, all exposures consist of repetitive pulses (at 10 μs). Total exposure times were less than 5 minutes. (Adapted from the American Institute of Ultrasound in Medicine: *Bioeffects and safety of diagnostic ultrasound*, Laurel, MD, 1993, The Institute.)

Cavitation can occur in tissues containing gas bubbles with sufficient pressure amplitude and frequency conditions. Damage can result from cavitational activity in tissue.

The development of contrast agents in diagnostic ultrasound introduces a new consideration regarding cavitation effects; that is, these agents introduce bubbles (that normally would not be there) into circulation and into tissues. This decreases the acoustic pressure threshold for, and increases the severity of, cavitation bioeffects. The AIUM (*www.aium.org/resources/statements.aspx*) issued the following statement on contrast agents in 2008:

Presently available ultrasound contrast agents consist of suspensions of gas bodies (stabilized gaseous microbubbles). The gas bodies have the correct size for strong echogenicity with diagnostic ultrasound and also for passage through the microcirculation. Commercial agents undergo rigorous clinical testing for safety and efficacy before Food and Drug Administration approval is granted, and they have been in clinical use in the United States since 1994. Detailed information on the composition and use of these agents is included in the package inserts. To date, diagnostic benefit has been proved in patients with suboptimal echocardiograms to opacify the left ventricular chamber and to improve the delineation of the left ventricular endocardial border. Many other diagnostic applications are under development or clinical testing.

Contrast agents carry some potential for nonthermal bioeffects when ultrasound interacts with the gas bodies. The mechanism for such effects is related to the physical phenomenon of acoustic cavitation. Several published reports describe adverse bioeffects in mammalian tissue in vivo *resulting from exposure to diagnostic ultrasound with gas body contrast agents in the circulation. Induction of premature ventricular contractions by triggered contrast echocardiography in humans has been reported for a noncommercial agent and in laboratory animals for commercial agents. Microvascular leakage, killing of cardiomyocytes, and glomerular capillary hemorrhage, among other bioeffects, have been reported in animal studies. Two medical ultrasound societies have examined this potential risk of bioeffects in diagnostic ultrasound with contrast agents and provide extensive reviews of the topic: the World Federation for Ultrasound in Medicine and Biology (WFUMB) Contrast Agent Safety Symposium and the American Institute of Ultrasound in Medicine 2005 Bioeffects Consensus Conference. Based on review of these reports and of recent literature, the Bioeffects Committee issues the following statement:*

Statement on Bioeffects of Diagnostic Ultrasound with Gas Body Contrast Agents

Induction of premature ventricular contractions, microvascular leakage with petechiae, glomerular capillary hemorrhage, and local cell killing in mammalian tissue in vivo *have been reported and independently confirmed for diagnostic ultrasound exposure with a mechanical index (MI) above about 0.4 and a gas body contrast agent present in the circulation.*

Although the medical significance of such microscale bioeffects is uncertain, minimizing the potential for such effects represents prudent use of diagnostic ultrasound. In general, for imaging with contrast agents at an MI above 0.4, practitioners should use the minimal agent dose, MI, and examination time consistent with efficacious acquisition of diagnostic information. In addition, the echocardiogram should be monitored during high-MI contrast cardiac-gated perfusion echocardiography, particularly in patients with a history of myocardial infarction or unstable cardiovascular disease. Furthermore, physicians and sonographers should follow all guidance provided in the package inserts of these drugs, including precautions, warnings and contraindications.

SAFETY

Information derived from in vitro and in vivo experimental studies has not included any known risks in the use of diagnostic ultrasound. Thermal and mechanical mechanisms have been considered but do not appear to operate significantly at diagnostic intensities. Currently, there is no known risk associated with the use of diagnostic ultrasound. Experimental animal data have helped define the intensity-exposure time region in which bioeffects can occur. However, physical and biologic differences between the two situations make it difficult to apply the results from one to the risk assessment in the other. In the absence of any known risk—but recognizing the possibility that subtle, low-incidence, or delayed bioeffects could occur—a conservative approach to the medical use of ultrasound is recommended. This approach is described in more detail later in this section.

Instrument Outputs

Several reports and compilations of output data have been published.[11] Instrument output may be expressed in many ways. Intensity has been the most popular quantity presented to describe instrument output. Several intensities may be used. Spatial peak–temporal average (SPTA) intensity is used in the AIUM statement on mammalian bioeffects, and it relates reasonably well to a thermal mechanism of interaction. The SPTA is the output intensity most commonly presented. Imaging instruments dominate the lower portion of the range, whereas spectral-Doppler instruments dominate the higher portion. In general, spectral-Doppler outputs are the highest, gray-scale imaging outputs are the lowest, and outputs of M mode and color Doppler fall between the two.

These output intensity measurements usually are made with hydrophones located in the beam in a water bath. Attenuation in water is low compared with that in tissues, so an intensity at a comparable location within tissues would be considerably less than that in water. Models have been applied to account for the tissue attenuation. The AIUM *(www.aium.org/resources/statements.aspx)* issued the following statement on these models in 2012:

1. *Tissue models are necessary to estimate attenuation and acoustic exposure levels in situ from measurements of acoustic output made in water. Presently available models are limited in their ability to represent clinical conditions because of varying tissue paths during diagnostic ultrasound exposures and uncertainties in acoustical properties of soft tissues. No single tissue model is adequate for predicting in vivo exposures in all situations from measurements made in water, and continued improvement and verification of these models is necessary for making improved exposure assessments for specific applications.*
2. *A homogeneous tissue model with an attenuation coefficient of 0.3 dB/cm-MHz throughout the beam path is commonly used when estimating exposure levels. The model is conservative in that it overestimates the in situ acoustic exposure when the path between the transducer and the site of interest is composed entirely of soft tissue with or without bone. When the path contains significant amounts of fluid, as in many first- and second-trimester pregnancies scanned transabdominally, this model may underestimate the in situ acoustical exposure. The amount of underestimation depends on each specific situation.*
3. *"Fixed-path" tissue models, in which soft tissue thickness is held constant, sometimes are used to estimate in situ acoustical exposures when the beam path is greater than 3 cm and consists largely of fluid. When this model is used to estimate maximum exposure to the fetus during transabdominal scans, a value of 1 dB/MHz may be used as a conservative estimate of total attenuation during all trimesters.*
4. *Existing tissue models that are based on linear propagation may not be adequate when nonlinear acoustic distortion is present.*

> Instrument output data are available that allow comparison with conditions necessary for bioeffects to occur.

U.S. Food and Drug Administration

Manufacturers are required to submit premarket notifications to the U.S. Food and Drug Administration (FDA) before marketing a device for a specific application in the United States. The FDA then reviews this notification to determine whether the device is substantially equivalent, with regard to safety and effectiveness, to instruments on the market before the enactment of the relevant act (1976). If the device is determined to be substantially equivalent, the manufacturer then may market it for that application. Part of the FDA evaluation involves output data for the instrument, which then are compared with maximum values determined for pre-1976 devices. These values are given in the FDA *510(k) Guide for Measuring and Reporting Acoustic Output of Diagnostic Ultrasound Medical Devices* and are presented in Table 7-1. Some of the values have been updated since the 1985 publication of this guide. The current values are shown in the table. To facilitate another path to device approval, a voluntary output display standard was developed by a joint committee involving the AIUM, the FDA, the National Electrical Manufacturers Association, and several other ultrasound-related professional societies. The goal of this activity was to develop a voluntary standard that would provide a parallel pathway to the current regulatory 510(k) process. The process would allow exemption from the upper limits given in the 510(k) guide (except that an overall upper limit of 720 mW/cm^2 SPTA still would apply) in exchange for presenting output information on the display. The standard includes two indices that would be displayed: thermal and mechanical. The **thermal index** (TI) is defined as the transducer acoustic output power divided by the estimated power required to raise tissue temperature by 1° C. The estimated power calculation for the TI involves frequency, aperture, and intensity. Three variations exist on the TI. The TIS (thermal index for soft tissues) applies when the beam travels through soft tissue and does not encounter bone. The TIB (thermal index for bone) applies for bone at or near the beam focus after passing through soft tissue. The TIC (thermal index for cranial tissues) applies when the transducer is close to bone. The **mechanical index** (MI) is equal to the peak rarefactional pressure (see Figure 7-17) divided by the square root of the center frequency of the pulse bandwidth:

$$MI = \frac{p_r(MPa)}{\left[f(MHz)\right]^{1/2}}$$

where p_r is pressure amplitude and f is frequency.

Display of any of these indexes would not be required if the instrument were incapable of exceeding index values of 1. Modern instruments incorporate this output display standard (Figure 7-19).

> The Food and Drug Administration regulates ultrasound instruments according to application and output intensities and thermal and mechanical indices.

TABLE 7-1 510(k) Guide Spatial Peak: Temporal Average In Situ Intensity Upper Limits

Diagnostic Application	ISPTA (mW/cm^2)
Cardiac	430
Peripheral vessel	20
Ophthalmic	17
Fetal imaging and other*	94

ISPTA, Spatial-peak, temporal-average intensity.
*Abdominal, intraoperative, pediatric, small organ (breast, thyroid, testes), neonatal cephalic, adult cephalic.

Epidemiology

A dozen or so epidemiologic studies have been conducted and their results published, but these and other surveys in widespread clinical usage during a period of many years have yielded no evidence of any adverse effect from diagnostic ultrasound. One study included 806 children, approximately half of whom had been exposed to diagnostic ultrasound in utero. The study measured Apgar scores, gestational age, head circumference, birth weight and length, congenital abnormalities, neonatal infection, and congenital infection at birth; it also included conductive and nerve measurements of hearing, visual acuity, and color vision; cognitive function and behavioral assessments; and complete and detailed neurologic examinations in children aged 7 to 12 years. No biologically significant differences between exposed and unexposed children were found. Another study measured the

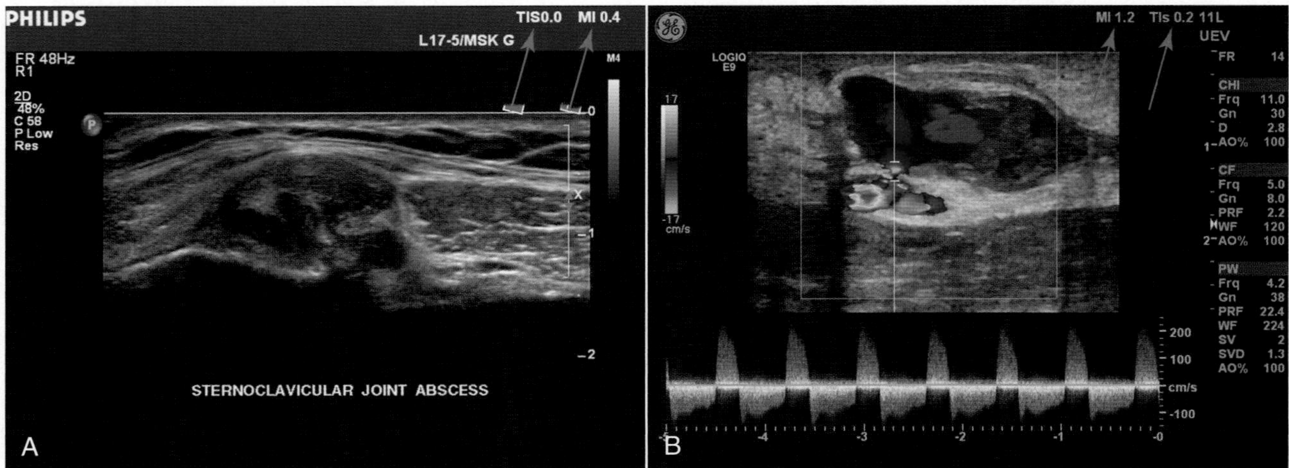

FIGURE 7-19 Displays showing thermal and mechanical indices *(arrows)*.

head circumference, height, and weight of 149 sibling pairs of the same sex, one of whom had been exposed to diagnostic ultrasound in utero. No statistically significant differences of head circumference at birth or of height and weight between birth and 6 years were found between ultrasound-exposed and unexposed siblings.

Although these studies have some limitations and flaws, they have not revealed any risk associated with the clinical use of diagnostic ultrasound. The AIUM *(www.aium.org/resources/statements.aspx)* developed and approved in 2010 the following statement regarding epidemiology:

> *Based on the epidemiologic data available and on current knowledge of interactive mechanisms, there is insufficient justification to warrant conclusion of a causal relationship between diagnostic ultrasound and recognized adverse effects in humans. Some studies have reported effects of exposure to diagnostic ultrasound during pregnancy, such as low birth weight, delayed speech, dyslexia, and non-right-handedness. Other studies have not demonstrated such effects. The epidemiologic evidence is based primarily on exposure conditions prior to 1992, the year in which acoustic limits of ultrasound machines were substantially increased for fetal/obstetric applications.*

> Epidemiologic studies have revealed no known risk to the use of diagnostic ultrasound.

Prudent Use

As discussed previously, epidemiologic studies have revealed no known risk associated with the use of diagnostic ultrasound. Experimental animal studies have shown bioeffects to occur only at intensities higher than those expected at relevant tissue locations during ultrasound imaging and flow measurements with most equipment. Thus a comparison of instrument output data, adjusted for tissue attenuation, with experimental bioeffects data does not indicate any risk. We must be open, however, to the possibility that unrecognized risk may exist. Such risk, if it does exist, may have eluded detection up to this point because it is subtle or delayed, or has incidence rates close to normal values. While more sensitive endpoints are studied during longer periods or with larger populations, such risk may be identified. However, future studies might not reveal any positive effects either, which strengthens the possibility that medical ultrasound imaging has no detectable risk.

In the meantime, with no known risk and with known benefit to the procedure, a conservative approach to imaging should be used; that is, ultrasound imaging should be used when medically indicated, with minimum exposure of the patient and fetus (Figure 7-20). Exposure is limited by minimizing instrument output and exposure time during a study. Instrument outputs for spectral-Doppler studies can be significantly higher than those for other applications. It thus seems most likely that the greatest potential for risk in ultrasound diagnosis (although no specific risk has been identified even in this case), is with fetal spectral-Doppler studies. These studies involve potentially high-output intensities with stationary beams and a presumably more sensitive fetus.

The AIUM *(www.aium.org/resources/statements.aspx)* first issued its statement on clinical safety in 1982. The statement was last updated in 2012 to the following:

> *Diagnostic ultrasound has been in use since the late 1950s. Given its known benefits and recognized efficacy for medical diagnosis, including use during human pregnancy, the American Institute of Ultrasound in Medicine herein addresses the clinical safety of such use: No independently confirmed adverse effects caused by exposure from present diagnostic ultrasound instruments have been reported in human patients in the absence of contrast agents. Biological effects (such as localized pulmonary bleeding) have been reported in mammalian systems at diagnostically relevant exposures but the clinical significance of such effects is not yet known. Ultrasound should be used by qualified health professionals to provide medical benefit to the patient. Ultrasound exposures during examinations should be as low as reasonably achievable (ALARA).*

> Prudent practice of sonography involves application of the ALARA principle. By requiring medical indication and by using minimum output and exposure time in diagnostic examinations, exposure and risk are minimized.

In conclusion, extensive mechanistic, in vitro, in vivo, and epidemiologic studies have revealed no known risk devolving with the current ultrasound instrumentation used in medical diagnosis. However, a prudent and conservative approach to ultrasound safety is to assume that there may be unidentified risk, which should be minimized in medically indicated ultrasound studies by minimizing exposure time and output. This is known as the ALARA principle (see Figure 7-20). The AIUM *(www.aium.org/resources/statements.aspx)* issued a statement on this principle in 2014:

> *The potential benefits and risks of each examination should be considered. The ALARA (As Low As Reasonably Achievable) Principle should be observed when adjusting controls that affect the acoustical output and by considering transducer dwell times. Further details on ALARA may be found in the AIUM publication "Medical Ultrasound Safety."*[10]

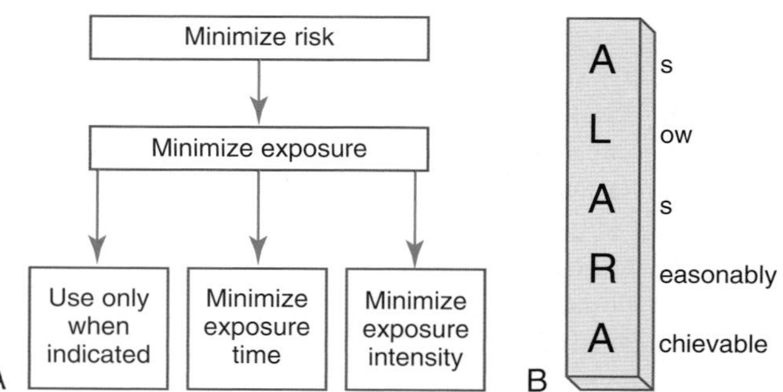

FIGURE 7-20 Minimizing risk by minimizing exposure (**A**) is the cornerstone of the ALARA principle (**B**).

It is difficult to make a firm statement about the clinical safety of diagnostic ultrasound. The experimental and epidemiologic bases for risk assessment are incomplete. However, much work has been done, and no evidence of clinical harm has been revealed. Patients should be informed that there currently is no basis for concluding that diagnostic ultrasound produces any harmful effects in patients. However, unobserved effects could be occurring. Thus ultrasound should not be used indiscriminately. The AIUM Clinical Safety Statement forms an excellent basis for formulating a response to patient questions and concerns. Prudence in practice is exercised by minimizing exposure time and output. Display of instrument outputs in the forms of thermal and mechanical indices facilitates such prudent use.

In more than five decades of use, there has been no report of injury to patients or to operators from medical ultrasound equipment. Those working in the ultrasound community want to maintain that level of safety. In the past, application-specific output limits and the user's knowledge of equipment controls and patient body characteristics were the means to minimize exposure. Now, more information is available. The mechanical and thermal indices provide users with information that can be applied specifically to the ALARA principle. Values of mechanical and thermal indices eliminate some of the guesswork and provide an indication of what actually may be happening within the patient and what occurs when control settings are changed. These values make it possible for the user to obtain the best image possible while following the ALARA principle and thus maximizing the benefit-risk ratio.

REVIEW

The following key points are presented in this chapter:

- Phantoms and test objects provide a means for measuring the detail resolution, distance accuracy, compensation, sensitivity, and dynamic range of diagnostic instruments.
- Hydrophones are used to measure the acoustic output of diagnostic instruments.
- The AIUM has stated that there have been no independently confirmed, significant bioeffects reported to occur in mammalian tissues exposed to focused SPTA intensities of less than 1 W/cm. Furthermore, no risk has been identified with the use of diagnostic ultrasound in human beings.
- Because there is limited specific knowledge, a conservative approach is justified. Such an approach calls for diagnostic ultrasound to be used, with minimum exposure, when medical benefit is expected to be derived from the procedure.

EXERCISES

Answers appear in the Answers to Exercises section at the back of the book.

1. A tissue-equivalent __________ has an attenuation of approximately 0.5 dB/cm-MHz and a propagation speed of 1.54 mm/μs. A __________ does not mimic tissue but provides a means for measuring some aspect of instrument performance.
   - **a.** phantom, test object
   - **b.** hydrophone, phantom
   - **c.** transducer, phantom
   - **d.** transducer, test object
2. Match the parameters measured with the items used (answers may be used more than once):
   1. Nylon fibers
   2. Attenuating scattering material
   3. Simulated cysts
   4. Hyperechoic- and hypoechoic-simulated lesions
   5. Thin scattering layer
   - **a.** Axial resolution
   - **b.** Lateral resolution
   - **c.** Range accuracy
   - **d.** Caliper accuracy
   - **e.** Contrast resolution
   - **f.** Compensation
   - **g.** Sensitivity
   - **h.** Dynamic range
   - **i.** Beam profile
   - **j.** Section thickness
3. Match the parameters measured with the correlating types of observation modes (answers may be used more than once):
   1. Gain settings
   2. Deepest scattering material imaged
   3. Fiber distances from the transducer or from each other on the display
   4. Minimum spacing of separately displayed fibers
   5. Lateral smearing of fibers
   - **a.** Axial resolution
   - **b.** Lateral resolution
   - **c.** Range accuracy
   - **d.** Caliper accuracy
   - **e.** Compensation
   - **f.** Sensitivity
   - **g.** Dynamic range
4. Test objects and phantoms are available commercially. True or false?
5. Test objects and phantoms can be used by the instrument operator. True or false?
6. A moving __________ test object is useful in checking the accuracy of Doppler spectral displays.
   - **a.** spectral
   - **b.** string
   - **c.** water
   - **d.** fluid

7. A __________ phantom is useful in simulating physiologic __________ conditions for a Doppler instrument.
   a. tissue, flow
   b. flow, equilibrium
   c. tissue, equilibrium
   d. flow, flow
8. Which of the following is used for Doppler sensitivity measurements?
   a. Cyst phantom
   b. Profile test object
   c. String test object
   d. Contrast phantom
   e. None of the above
9. Tissue-equivalent phantoms attempt to represent some acoustic property of __________.
   a. tissues
   b. blood
   c. cancer
   d. skin
10. The string test object measures volumetric flow rate. True or false?
11. With use of a hydrophone, which of the following can be measured or calculated? (There is more than one correct answer.)
   a. Impedance
   b. Amplitude
   c. Period
   d. Pulse duration
   e. Pulse repetition period
12. All hydrophones consist of a small element mounted on the end of a needle. True or false?
13. A needle hydrophone contains a small __________ element.
   a. transducer
   b. piezoelectric
   c. neither a nor b
   d. both a and b
14. Because of its small size, a hydrophone can measure spatial details of a sound beam. True or false?
15. A hydrophone __________.
   a. interacts with light
   b. produces a voltage
   c. measures intensity directly
   d. measures total energy
   e. none of the above
16. Match the items in column **A** with those in **B** and **C** (answers may be used more than once). (Note: Items in **A** can be calculated from **B** if **C** is known.)

   A
   a. Frequency: __________, __________
   b. Pulse repetition frequency: __________, __________
   c. Duty factor: __________, __________
   d. Wavelength: __________, __________
   e. Spatial pulse length: __________, __________
   f. Energy: __________, __________
   g. Intensity: __________, __________

   B
   1. Wavelength
   2. Period
   3. Pulse repetition period
   4. Frequency
   5. Energy
   6. Power

   C
   7. Number of cycles in the pulse
   8. Pulse duration
   9. Propagation speed
   10. Exposure time
   11. Beam area
   12. Nothing else
17. The piezoelectric material commonly used in hydrophones is __________.
   a. quartz
   b. PZT
   c. PVDF
   d. PDQ
   e. PVC
18. The important characteristic of the material used in hydrophones (*see Exercise 17*) is __________.
   a. impedance
   b. propagation speed
   c. efficiency
   d. density
   e. bandwidth
19. Heating depends most directly on __________.
   a. SATA intensity
   b. SATP intensity
   c. SPTP intensity
   d. pressure
20. Conditions under which cavitation may occur are best described by __________.
   a. SATA intensity
   b. SATP intensity
   c. SPTP intensity
   d. peak rarefactional pressure
21. Bioeffects have been observed in experimental animals with intensities greater than __________.
   a. 100 mW/cm^2 SPTA
   b. 1 W/cm^2 SPTA
   c. 10 W/cm^2 SPTA
   d. 1 mW/cm^2 SPTP
   e. 10 mW/cm^2 SPTP
22. Bioeffects have been observed in experimental animals with focused intensities greater than __________.
   a. 100 mW/cm SPTA
   b. 1 W/cm SPTA
   c. 10 W/cm SPTA
   d. 1 mW/cm SPTP
   e. 10 mW/cm SPTP
23. Focal lesions have been observed in experimental animals with intensities greater than __________.
   a. 100 mW/cm SPTA
   b. 1 W/cm SPTA
   c. 10 W/cm SPTA
   d. 1 mW/cm SPTP
   e. 10 mW/cm SPTP

24. The available epidemiologic data are sufficient to make a final judgment on the safety of diagnostic ultrasound. True or false?
25. Exposure is minimized by using diagnostic ultrasound ___________.
   a. only when indicated
   b. with minimum intensity
   c. with minimum time
   d. all of the above
   e. none of the above
26. Which of the following is (are) used currently to indicate output on the display?
   a. Percent
   b. Decibel
   c. SPTA intensity
   d. Mechanical index
   e. All of the above
27. Which of the following affect(s) exposure of a fetus?
   a. Intensity at the transducer
   b. Distance to the fetus
   c. Frequency
   d. Gain
   e. More than one of the above
   f. All of the above
28. There is no possible hazard involved in the use of diagnostic ultrasound. True or false?
29. Ultrasound should not be used as a diagnostic tool because of the bioeffects it can produce. True or false?
30. No independently confirmed, significant bioeffects in mammalian tissues have been reported at intensities below ___________.
   a. 10 W/cm^2 SPTP
   b. 100 mW/cm^2 SPTA
   c. 10 mW/cm^2 SPTA
   d. 10 mW/cm^2 SATA
   e. 1 mW/cm^2 SATP
31. Is there any known risk with the current use of diagnostic ultrasound? Yes or no?
32. Are there any bioeffects that ultrasound produces in small animals under experimental conditions? Yes or no?
33. Which of the following are mechanisms by which ultrasound can produce bioeffects? (More than one correct answer.)
   a. Direction ionization
   b. Absorption
   c. Photoelectric effect
   d. Cavitation
   e. Compton effect
34. Which of the following relates to heating?
   a. Impedance
   b. Sound speed
   c. Absorption
   d. Refraction
   e. Diffraction
35. Which of the following endpoints is documented well enough in the scientific literature to allow a risk assessment for diagnostic ultrasound to be based on it?
   a. Fetal weight
   b. Sister-chromatid exchange
   c. Fetal abnormalities
   d. Carcinogenesis
   e. None
36. On which of the following endpoints has more than one epidemiologic study shown a statistically significant effect of ultrasound exposure?
   a. Fetal activity
   b. Birth weight
   c. Fetal abnormalities
   d. Dyslexia
   e. None
37. Which of the following acoustic parameters has (have) been documented in ultrasound epidemiologic studies published thus far?
   a. Frequency
   b. Exposure time
   c. Intensity and pulsing conditions
   d. Scanning patterns
   e. None
38. A device commonly used to measure the output of diagnostic ultrasound instruments is a(n) ___________.
   a. hydrophone
   b. optical interferometer
   c. Geiger counter
   d. photoelectric cell
   e. absorption radiometer
39. A typical output intensity (SPTA) for an ultrasound imaging instrument is ___________.
   a. 1540 W
   b. 13 kW/mm^2
   c. 3.5 MHz
   d. 1 mW/cm^2
   e. 2 dB/cm
40. Which of the following typically has the highest output intensity?
   a. Fetal monitor Doppler
   b. Duplex pulsed Doppler
   c. Color-Doppler shift
   d. Color power Doppler
   e. Phase array, gray scale
41. As far as we know now, which of the following is the most correct and informative response to a patient's question, "Will this hurt me or my baby?"
   a. No.
   b. Yes.
   c. We don't know.
   d. The risks are well understood, but the benefits always outweigh them.
   e. There is no known risk with ultrasound imaging as it is applied currently.
42. To minimize whatever risk there may be with ultrasound imaging, which of the following should be done? (More than one correct answer.)
   a. Scan to produce pictures for the family album.
   b. Scan to determine fetal sex.

c. Minimize exposure time.
d. Scan for medical indication(s) only.
e. Minimize exposure intensity.

43. Which of the following controls affect instrument output intensity?
a. Dynamic range, compression
b. Transmit, output
c. Near gain, far gain
d. Overall gain
e. Slope, time gain compensation

44. Which of the following are correct for a duplex, pulsed-wave Doppler instrument? (More than one correct answer.)
a. Tissue anywhere in the Doppler beam is exposed to ultrasound.
b. Tissue anywhere in the imaging plane is exposed to ultrasound.
c. Imaging intensities are higher than for conventional gray-scale instruments.
d. Doppler intensities are higher than for continuous-wave fetal monitoring.

45. The tissue of greatest concern regarding bioeffects in an abdominal scan is the ____________.
a. spleen
b. pancreas
c. liver
d. kidney
e. fetus

46. Would it be wise to substitute a duplex, pulsed-wave Doppler device for an inoperative fetal monitor for long-term (e.g., 24-hour) monitoring in labor?
a. Yes
b. No
c. Depends on frame rate of the image
d. Depends on frequency of the Doppler beam
e. Depends on gate location

47. Which of the following is (are) likely to be exposed to ultrasound during a diagnostic study?
a. Patient
b. Sonographer
c. Sonologist
d. Observers in the room
e. More than one of the above

48. No bioeffects have been observed in nonhuman mammalian tissues at thermal index values of less than ____________.
a. 5
b. 4
c. 3
d. 2
e. 1

49. No bioeffects have been observed in nonhuman mammalian tissues at mechanical index values of less than ____________.
a. 0.5
b. 0.4
c. 0.3
d. 0.2
e. 0.1

50. No bioeffects have been observed in nonhuman mammalian tissues at peak rarefactional pressure values (megapascals) of less than ____________.
a. 0.5
b. 0.4
c. 0.3
d. 0.2
e. 0.1

8

Review

OUTLINE

ARDMS SPI Examination Content Outline

Comprehensive Examination

Diagnostic sonography is medical cross-sectional and three-dimensional anatomic and flow imaging that uses pulse-echo ultrasound. Pulses of ultrasound are generated by a transducer and are sent into the patient, where they produce echoes at organ boundaries and within tissues. These echoes return to the transducer, where they are detected and then presented on the display of a sonographic instrument. Each pulse produces a series of echoes that is displayed as a scan line. An anatomic image is composed of many scan lines. If flowing blood or moving tissues produce echoes, a frequency change, called *Doppler shift,* occurs. Doppler shifts provide motion information that can be presented audibly or as a spectral or two- or three-dimensional color-Doppler display.

Ultrasound is sound (a wave of traveling acoustic variables that include pressure, density, and particle motion) with a frequency greater than 20 kHz. Ultrasound is described by frequency, period, wavelength, propagation speed, amplitude, intensity, and attenuation. Pulsed ultrasound is described by additional terms: pulse repetition frequency (PRF), pulse repetition period, pulse duration, duty factor, and spatial pulse length. Propagation speed and impedance are characteristics of the medium that are determined by density and stiffness. Attenuation increases with frequency and path length. Imaging depth decreases with increasing frequency. The soft tissue propagation speed is 1.54 mm/μs, and the attenuation coefficient is 0.5 dB/cm for each megahertz of frequency. When sound encounters boundaries between media with different impedances, part of the sound is reflected (echo) and part is transmitted. With perpendicular incidence, if the two media have the same impedance, there is no reflection. With oblique incidence, the sound is refracted at a boundary between the media where propagation speeds are different. Incidence and reflection angles are always equal. Scattering occurs at rough media boundaries and within heterogeneous media. The range equation is used to determine distance to reflectors. Pulse-echo round-trip travel time is 13 μs/cm. The use of harmonic echoes improves image quality, and contrast media enhance echo generation and detection.

Ultrasound transducers convert electric energy to ultrasound energy, and vice versa. They operate on the piezoelectric principle. The preferred operating frequency depends on element thickness. Axial resolution is equal to one half of the spatial pulse length. Pulsed transducers have damping material to shorten the spatial pulse length for acceptable resolution. Transducers produce sound in the form of beams with near and far zones. Lateral resolution is equal to beam width. Beam width is reduced by focusing to improve resolution. *Linear* and *convex* are types of array construction. *Sequenced, phased,* and *vector* are types of array scanning operations. Phasing also enables electronic control of focus.

Diagnostic ultrasound imaging (sonographic) systems are of the pulse-echo type. They use the strength, direction, and arrival time of received echoes to generate A-, B-, and M-mode displays. Imaging systems consist of the transducer, beam former, signal processor, image processor, and display. Beam formers direct the transmitted beam through the imaged tissue cross-section, direct and focus the reception beam, amplify the received echo voltages, compensate for attenuation, and digitize the echo voltages. Signal processors filter, detect, and compress echo signals. Image processors convert scan line signals to image formats, store images in digital form, and perform preprocessing and postprocessing on images. Preprocessing includes persistence, panoramic imaging, spatial compounding, and three-dimensional acquisition. A mode shows echo amplitudes. B and M modes use a brightness display. M mode shows reflector motion in time. B scans show anatomic cross-sections in gray scale through the scanning plane. Image memories store echo amplitude information as numbers in the memory elements. Contrast resolution improves with increasing bits per pixel (layers of memory). Real-time imaging is the rapid sequential display of ultrasound images resulting in a moving presentation. Such imaging requires automatic, rapid, repeatable, sequential scanning of the sound beam through the tissue. This scanning is accomplished by electronic transducer arrays. Rectangular or sector display formats result from such scanning techniques. Displays are flat panel liquid-crystal displays (LCDs). Instruments often are connected to peripheral recording devices and to picture archiving and communications systems (PACS).

Fluids (gases and liquids) are substances that flow. Blood is a liquid that flows through the vascular system under the influence of pulsatile pressure provided by the beating heart. Volume flow rate is proportional to pressure difference at the ends of a tube and inversely proportional to flow resistance. Flow resistance increases with viscosity and tube length and decreases (strongly) with increasing tube diameter. Seven (two temporal and five spatial) flow classifications include *steady, pulsatile, plug, laminar, parabolic, disturbed,* and *turbulent.* In a stenosis, flow speeds up, pressure drops (Bernoulli effect), and flow is disturbed. If flow speed exceeds a critical value, turbulence occurs. Pulsatile flow is common in arterial circulation. Diastolic flow, flow reversal, or both may occur in some locations within the arterial system. Fluid inertia and vessel compliance are characteristics that are important in determining flow with pulsatile driving pressure.

The Doppler effect is a change in frequency resulting from motion. In most medical ultrasound applications, the motion is that of blood flow in circulation. The change in frequency of the returning echoes with respect to the emitted frequency is called the *Doppler shift.* For flow toward the transducer, the Doppler shift is positive; for flow away, it is negative. The Doppler shift depends on the speed of the scatterers of sound, the angle between their direction and that of the sound propagation, and the operating frequency of the Doppler system. A moving scatterer of sound produces a double Doppler shift. Greater flow speeds and smaller Doppler angles produce larger Doppler shifts but not stronger echoes. Higher operating frequencies produce larger Doppler shifts. Typical ranges of flow speeds (10 to 100 cm/s), Doppler angles (30 to 60 degrees), and operating frequencies (2 to 10 MHz) yield Doppler shifts in the range of 100 Hz to 11 kHz for vascular studies. In Doppler echocardiography, in which zero angle and speeds of a few meters per second can be encountered, Doppler shifts can be as high as 30 kHz.

Doppler instruments make use of the Doppler shift to yield information regarding motion and flow. Color-Doppler imaging acquires Doppler-shifted echoes from a cross-section of tissue scanned by an ultrasound beam. These echoes then are presented in color and are superimposed on the gray-scale anatomic image of nonshifted echoes that were received during the scan. The flow echoes are assigned colors according to the selected color map. Red, orange, yellow, blue, cyan, and white indicate positive or negative Doppler shifts (i.e., approaching or receding flow). Yellow, cyan, or green is used to indicate variance (disturbed or turbulent flow). Several pulses (the number is called *ensemble length*) are needed to generate a color scan line. Color controls include gain, color map selection, variance on/off, persistence, ensemble length, color/gray priority, scale (PRF), baseline shift, wall filter, and color window angle, location, and size. Color-Doppler instruments are pulsed-wave Doppler instruments and are subject to the same limitations—Doppler angle dependence and aliasing—as are other Doppler instruments. Doppler-power displays color encode the strength of the Doppler shifts into a sensitive presentation of flow information that is angle-independent and aliasing-independent .

Continuous-wave systems provide motion and flow information without depth selection capability. Pulsed-wave Doppler systems have the capability of selecting a depth from which Doppler information is received. Spectral analysis provides quantitative information on the distribution of received Doppler-shift frequencies that result from the distribution of scatterer velocities (speeds and directions) encountered. In addition to audible output, visual presentation of flow spectra is possible in Doppler systems. Combined (duplex) systems that use real-time sonography and continuous-wave and pulsed-wave Doppler are available commercially. The Doppler spectrum is generated by the range of scatterer velocities encountered by the ultrasound beam. The Doppler spectrum is derived electronically using the fast Fourier transform (FFT) and is presented on the display as Doppler shift versus time, with brightness indicating power. Flow conditions at the site of measurement are indicated by the width of the spectrum; spectral broadening indicates disturbed and turbulent flow. Flow conditions downstream, particularly distal flow resistance, are indicated by the relationship between peak systolic and end diastolic flow speeds. Various indexes for quantitatively presenting this information have been developed.

Axial resolution is determined by spatial pulse length, whereas lateral resolution is determined by beam width. The beam width perpendicular to the scan plane causes section thickness artifacts. Apparent resolution close to the transducer is not related directly to tissue texture but is a result of interference effects from a distribution of scatterers in the tissue (speckle). Reverberation produces a set of equally spaced artifactual echoes distal to the real reflector. Refraction displaces echoes laterally. In the mirror-image artifact, objects that are present on one side of a strong reflector are displayed on the other side as well. Shadowing is caused by high-attenuation objects in the sound path. Enhancement results from low-attenuation objects in the sound path. Propagation speed error and refraction can cause objects to be displayed in improper locations or incorrect sizes or both. Refraction also can cause edge shadowing. Artifacts that can occur with Doppler ultrasound include aliasing, range ambiguity, color-Doppler image and Doppler signal mirroring, and spectral trace mirroring. Aliasing is the most common artifact. Aliasing occurs when the Doppler-shift frequency exceeds one half the PRF (the Nyquist limit). Aliasing can be reduced or eliminated by increasing the PRF or Doppler angle, shifting the baseline, reducing operating frequency, or switching to continuous-wave operation.

Phantoms and test objects provide means for measuring the detail and contrast resolutions, distance accuracy, compensation, penetration, and dynamic range of diagnostic instruments. Hydrophones are used to measure the acoustic output of diagnostic instruments.

The American Institute of Ultrasound in Medicine (AIUM) has stated that no independently confirmed, significant bioeffects have been reported to occur in mammalian tissues exposed to focused spatial peak–temporal average intensities of less than 1 W/cm^2. Furthermore, no risk has been identified with the use of diagnostic ultrasound in human beings.

Because there is limited specific knowledge, a conservative approach is justified; that is, diagnostic ultrasound should be used, with minimum exposure, when medical benefit is expected to be derived from the procedure (ALARA [As Low As Reasonably Achievable] principle).

ARDMS SPI EXAMINATION CONTENT OUTLINE

This American Registry of Diagnostic Medical Sonographers (ARDMS) *Sonography Principles and Instrumentation* (SPI) Examination Content Outline is available at *www.ardms.org*. It is reproduced here (by permission), indicating chapters in this textbook that cover each topic.

1. **Patient care, safety and communication** [5%]
   A. Patient identification/documentation
   B. Patient interaction
   C. Verification of requested examination
   D. Emergency situations
   E. Universal precautions
   F. Bioeffects and ALARA [Chapter 7]
2. **Physics principles** [20%] [Chapter 2]
   A. Properties of ultrasound waves
   B. Interactions of sound with tissue
   C. Power, intensity, and amplitude
   D. Units of measurement
3. **Ultrasound transducers** [20%] [Chapter 3]
   A. Transducer construction and characteristics
   B. Transducer types (sector, linear, phased arrays, etc.)
   C. Spatial resolution
   D. Transducer selection
4. **Pulse-echo instrumentation** [30%] [Chapter 4]
   A. Display modes and their formation (A mode, B mode, M mode, 3-D, etc.)
   B. Transmission of ultrasound
   C. Reception of ultrasound (preprocessing)
   D. Beam former
   E. Postprocessing of ultrasound signals
   F. Pulse-echo imaging artifacts [Chapter 6]
   G. Tissue harmonic imaging
   H. Realtime ultrasound instrumentation
   I. Recording and storage devices
5. **Doppler instrumentation and hemodynamics** [20%] [Chapter 5]
   A. Ability to acquire color flow image
   B. Ability to acquire a Doppler spectral image
   C. Ability to take measurements from the spectral waveform
   D. Hemodynamics
6. **Quality assurance/quality control of equipment** [5%]
   A. Preventive maintenance
   B. Malfunctions
   C. Performance testing with phantoms [Chapter 7]

COMPREHENSIVE EXAMINATION

Answers appear in the Answers to Exercises section at the back of the book.

1. Which of the following frequencies is in the ultrasound range?
   a. 15 Hz
   b. 15 kHz
   c. 15 MHz
   d. 17,000 Hz
   e. 17 km
2. The average propagation speed in soft tissues is ____________.
   a. 1.54 mm/μs
   b. 0.501 m/s
   c. 1540 dB/cm
   d. 37.0 km/min
   e. 1 to 10 km/min
3. The propagation speed is greatest in ____________.
   a. lung
   b. liver
   c. bone
   d. fat
   e. blood
4. Which of the following has a significant dependence on frequency in soft tissues?
   a. Propagation speed
   b. Density
   c. Stiffness
   d. Attenuation
   e. Impedance
5. The frequencies used in diagnostic ultrasound imaging ____________.
   a. are much lower than those used in Doppler measurements
   b. determine imaging depth in tissue
   c. determine detail resolution
   d. all of the above
   e. b and c
6. An echo from a 5-cm deep reflector arrives at the transducer ____________ μs after pulse emission.
   a. 13
   b. 154
   c. 65
   d. 5
   e. 77
7. A small (relative to the wavelength) reflector is said to ____________ an incident sound beam.
   a. focus
   b. speculate
   c. scatter
   d. shatter
   e. amplify
8. Which of the following determines the operating frequency of an ultrasound transducer?
   a. Element diameter
   b. Element thickness
   c. Speed of sound in tissue
   d. Element impedance
   e. All of the above

9. The fundamental operating principle of medical ultrasound transducers is ____________.
   a. Snell's law
   b. Doppler law
   c. magnetostrictive effect
   d. piezoelectric effect
   e. impedance effect
10. The axial resolution of a transducer is primarily determined by ____________.
   a. spatial pulse length
   b. the near-field limit
   c. the transducer diameter
   d. the acoustic impedance of tissue
   e. density
11. The lateral resolution of a transducer is primarily determined by ____________.
   a. spatial pulse length
   b. the near-field limit
   c. the aperture
   d. the acoustic impedance of tissue
   e. applied voltage
12. Increasing frequency ____________.
   a. improves resolution
   b. increases penetration
   c. increases refraction
   d. a and b
   e. a and c
13. Ultrasound bioeffects ____________.
   a. do not occur
   b. do not occur with diagnostic instruments
   c. are not confirmed below a spatial peak–temporal average intensity of 100 mW/cm^2
   d. b and c
   e. none of the above
14. Diagnostic ultrasound frequency range is ____________.
   a. 2 to 10 mHz
   b. 2 to 10 kHz
   c. 2 to 20 MHz
   d. 5 to 15 kHz
   e. none of the above
15. What determines the lower and upper limits of frequency range useful in diagnostic ultrasound?
   a. Resolution and penetration
   b. Intensity and resolution
   c. Intensity and propagation speed
   d. Scattering and impedance
   e. Impedance and wavelength
16. Reverberation causes us to think there are reflectors that are too great in ____________.
   a. impedance
   b. attenuation
   c. range
   d. size
   e. number
17. A flat panel display is composed of a back-lighted rectangular matrix of thousands of ____________ display elements.
   a. plasma
   b. television
   c. fluorescent
   d. liquid-crystal
   e. piezo-crystal
18. In an ultrasound imaging instrument, a flat panel display may be used as a ____________.
   a. pulser
   b. digitizer
   c. memory
   d. display
   e. preprocessor
19. The compensation (time gain compensation) control ____________.
   a. compensates for machine instability in the warm-up time
   b. compensates for attenuation
   c. compensates for transducer aging and the ambient light in the examining area
   d. decreases patient examination time
   e. none of the above
20. A image processor changes signals from ____________ to ____________ format.
   a. gray scale, color
   b. radio frequency, amplitude
   c. B mode, M mode
   d. scan line, image
   e. none of the above
21. Enhancement is caused by a ____________.
   a. strongly reflecting structure
   b. weakly attenuating structure
   c. strongly attenuating structure
   d. frequency error
   e. propagation speed error
22. Echo intensity is represented in image memory by ____________.
   a. positive charge distribution
   b. a number
   c. electron density of the display writing beam
   d. a and c
   e. all of the above
23. Which of the following is (are) performed in a signal processor?
   a. Filtering
   b. Detection
   c. Compression
   d. All of the above
   e. None of the above
24. Increasing the pulse repetition frequency ____________.
   a. improves detail resolution
   b. increases maximum unambiguous depth
   c. decreases maximum unambiguous depth
   d. both a and b
   e. both a and c
25. Attenuation is corrected by ____________.
   a. demodulation
   b. desegregation
   c. decompression
   d. compensation
   e. remuneration

26. What must be known to calculate distance to a reflector?
 a. Attenuation, speed, density
 b. Attenuation, impedance
 c. Attenuation, absorption
 d. Travel time, speed
 e. Density, speed
27. Which of the following improve(s) sound transmission from the transducer element into the tissue?
 a. Matching layer
 b. Doppler effect
 c. Damping material
 d. Coupling medium
 e. a and d
28. Lateral resolution is improved by ___________.
 a. damping
 b. pulsing
 c. focusing
 d. reflecting
 e. absorbing
29. Axial resolution is improved by ___________.
 a. damping
 b. pulsing
 c. focusing
 d. reflecting
 e. absorbing
30. An image memory divides the cross-sectional image into ___________.
 a. frequencies
 b. bits
 c. pixels
 d. binaries
 e. wavelengths
31. In general, as a reflector approaches a transducer at constant speed, the positive Doppler-shift frequency ___________.
 a. increases
 b. decreases
 c. remains constant
 d. b or c
 e. none of the above
32. A reduction in vessel diameter produces a(n) ___________.
 a. increase in flow resistance
 b. decrease in area
 c. increase in flow speed
 d. decrease in flow speed
 e. all of the above
33. Which of the following increases vascular flow resistance?
 a. Decreasing vessel length
 b. Decreasing viscosity
 c. Decreasing vessel diameter
 d. Decreasing pressure
 e. Decreasing flow speed
34. The Doppler effect occurs as ___________.
 a. leukocytes move through plasma
 b. erythrocytes move through plasma
 c. erythrocytes move through serum
 d. blood moves relative to the vessel wall
 e. all of the above
35. When a reflector is moving toward the transducer, ___________.
 a. propagation speed increases
 b. propagation speed decreases
 c. the Doppler shift is positive (higher frequency)
 d. the Doppler shift is negative (lower frequency)
 e. none of the above
36. Doppler sample volume is determined by ___________.
 a. beam width
 b. pulse length
 c. frequency
 d. amplifier gate length
 e. all of the above
37. Doppler shift frequencies ___________.
 a. are generally in the audible range
 b. are usually higher than 1 MHz
 c. can be applied to a loudspeaker
 d. a and b
 e. a and c
38. The quantitative presentation of frequencies contained in echoes is called ___________.
 a. preamplification
 b. digitizing
 c. optical encoding
 d. spectral analysis
 e. all of the above
39. The Doppler frequency shift is caused by ___________.
 a. relative motion between the transducer and the reflector
 b. the patient shivering in a cool room
 c. a high transducer frequency and real-time scanner
 d. small reflectors in the transducer beam
 e. changing transducer thickness
40. The Doppler effect is a change in ___________.
 a. intensity
 b. wavelength
 c. frequency
 d. all of the above
 e. b and c
41. The Doppler shift is zero when the angle between the sound direction and the movement (flow) direction is ___________ degrees.
 a. 30
 b. 60
 c. 90
 d. 45
 e. none of the above
42. The duplex Doppler presents ___________.
 a. anatomic (structural) data
 b. physiologic (flow) data
 c. impedance data
 d. more than one of the above
 e. all of the above
43. The Doppler shift frequencies are usually in a relatively narrow range above 20 kHz. True or false?

44. Continuous wave sound is used in ____________.
   a. all ultrasound imaging instruments
   b. only bistable instruments
   c. all Doppler instruments
   d. some Doppler instruments
   e. some M-mode instruments
45. An advantage of continuous-wave Doppler over pulsed Doppler is ____________.
   a. depth information
   b. bidirectionality
   c. no aliasing
   d. b and c
   e. all of the above
46. In color-Doppler instruments, hue can represent ____________.
   a. sign (+ or –) of Doppler shift
   b. flow direction
   c. magnitude of the Doppler shift
   d. amplitude of the Doppler shift
   e. all of the above
47. The Doppler effect for a scatterer moving toward the sound source causes the scattered sound (compared with incident sound) received by the transducer to have ____________.
   a. increased intensity
   b. decreased intensity
   c. increased impedance
   d. increased frequency
   e. decreased impedance
48. Duplex Doppler instruments include ____________.
   a. pulsed-wave Doppler
   b. continuous-wave Doppler
   c. B-scan imaging
   d. dynamic imaging
   e. more than one of the above
49. If the Doppler shifts from normal and stenotic arteries are 4 kHz and 10 kHz, respectively, for which will there be aliasing with a pulse repetition frequency of 7 kHz?
   a. Normal artery
   b. Stenotic artery
   c. Both
   d. Neither
50. The signal processor in a Doppler system compares the ____________ of the output with the returning echo voltage from the transducer.
   a. wavelength
   b. intensity
   c. impedance
   d. frequency
   e. all of the above
51. In the Doppler equation that follows, which can normally be ignored?

$$f_D = \frac{2fv}{(c - v)}$$

   a. *v* in the denominator
   b. *v* in the numerator
   c. *f*
   d. *D*
   e. b and c
52. For which of the following is the reflected frequency less than the incident frequency?
   a. Advancing flow
   b. Receding flow
   c. Perpendicular flow
   d. Laminar flow
   e. All of the above
53. Doppler ultrasound can measure flow speed in the ____________.
   a. heart
   b. veins
   c. arterioles
   d. capillaries
   e. a and b
54. Which of the following are fluids?
   a. Gas
   b. Liquid
   c. Solid
   d. a and b
   e. All of the above
55. The mass per unit volume of a fluid is called its ____________.
   a. resistance
   b. viscosity
   c. kinematic viscosity
   d. impedance
   e. density
56. The resistance to flow offered by a fluid is called ____________.
   a. resistance
   b. viscosity
   c. kinematic viscosity
   d. impedance
   e. density
57. Viscosity divided by density is called ____________.
   a. resistance
   b. viscosity
   c. kinematic viscosity
   d. impedance
   e. density
58. If the following is increased, flow increases.
   a. Pressure difference
   b. Pressure gradient
   c. Resistance
   d. a and b
   e. All of the above
59. Flow resistance depends most strongly on________.
   a. vessel length
   b. vessel radius
   c. blood viscosity
   d. all of the above
   e. none of the above

60. Proximal to, at, and distal to a stenosis, ___________ must be constant.
a. laminar flow
b. disturbed flow
c. turbulent flow
d. volume flow rate
e. none of the above

61. Added forward flow and flow reversal in diastole are results of ___________ flow.
a. volume
b. turbulent
c. laminar
d. disturbed
e. pulsatile

62. A broad spectrum indicates ___________ flow.
a. pulsatile
b. laminar
c. constant
d. turbulent
e. a and b

63. While diameter at a stenosis decreases, the following pass(es) through a maximum.
a. Flow speed at the stenosis
b. Flow speed proximal to the stenosis
c. Volume flow rate
d. Doppler shift at the stenosis
e. a and d

64. The Doppler shift (kilohertz) for 4 MHz, 50 cm/s, and 60 degrees is ___________.
a. 0.5
b. 1.0
c. 1.3
d. 2.6
e. 5.0

65. Physiologic flow speeds can be as much as ___________% of the propagation speed in soft tissues.
a. 0.01
b. 0.3
c. 5
d. 10
e. 50

66. Which Doppler angle yields the greatest Doppler shift?
a. −90
b. −45
c. 0
d. 45
e. 90

67. Doppler shift frequency does not depend on ___________.
a. amplitude
b. flow speed
c. operating frequency
d. Doppler angle
e. propagation speed

68. The Fourier transform technique is not used in color-Doppler operation because it is not ___________ enough.
a. slow
b. fast
c. bright
d. cheap
e. none of the above

69. Which of the following on a color-Doppler display is (are) presented in real time?
a. Gray-scale anatomy
b. Flow direction
c. Doppler spectrum
d. a and b
e. All of the above

70. For a 5-MHz instrument and a 60-degree Doppler angle, a 100-Hz filter eliminates flow speeds below ___________.
a. 1 cm/s
b. 2 cm/s
c. 3 cm/s
d. 4 cm/s
e. 5 cm/s

71. For a 7.5-MHz instrument and a 0-degree Doppler angle, a 100-Hz filter eliminates flow speeds below ___________.
a. 1 cm/s
b. 2 cm/s
c. 3 cm/s
d. 4 cm/s
e. 5 cm/s

72. The functions of a Doppler detector include ___________.
a. amplification
b. phase quadrature detection
c. demodulation
d. all of the above
e. none of the above

73. A later amplifier gate time means a(n) ___________ sample volume depth.
a. earlier
b. shallower
c. deeper
d. stronger
e. none of the above

74. The Doppler shift is typically ___________ the source frequency.
a. one thousandth
b. one hundredth
c. one tenth
d. 10 times
e. 100 times

75. Approximately ___________ pulses are required to obtain one line of color-Doppler information.
a. 1
b. 10
c. 100
d. 1000
e. 1,000,000

76. There are approximately ___________ samples per line on a color-Doppler display.
   a. 2
   b. 20
   c. 200
   d. 2000
   e. 2,000,000
77. Which of the following Doppler instruments can produce aliasing?
   a. Continuous wave
   b. Pulsed
   c. Duplex
   d. Color
   e. More than one of the above
78. For normal flow in a large vessel, a ___________ range of Doppler shift frequencies is received.
   a. narrow
   b. broad
   c. steady
   d. disturbed
   e. all of the above
79. Doppler signal power is proportional to ___________.
   a. the volume flow rate
   b. flow speed
   c. the Doppler angle
   d. cell density
   e. more than one of the above
80. Stenosis affects ___________.
   a. peak systolic flow speed
   b. end diastolic flow speed
   c. spectral broadening
   d. window
   e. all of the above
81. Spectral broadening is a ___________ of the spectral trace.
   a. vertical thickening
   b. horizontal thickening
   c. brightening
   d. darkening
   e. horizontal shift
82. While stenosis is increased, ___________ increase(s).
   a. vessel diameter
   b. systolic Doppler shift
   c. diastolic Doppler shift
   d. spectral broadening
   e. more than one of the above
83. Flow reversal in diastole (normal flow) indicates ___________.
   a. stenosis
   b. aneurysm
   c. high distal flow resistance
   d. low distal flow resistance
   e. more than one of the above
84. Approximately ___________ fast Fourier transforms are performed per second on a spectral display.
   a. 3
   b. 10
   c. 100 to 1000
   d. 700 to 7000
   e. 17,000
85. Each fast Fourier transform appears on a spectral display as a ___________.
   a. dot
   b. circle
   c. horizontal line
   d. vertical line
   e. none of the above
86. Hue is ___________.
   a. color seen
   b. light frequency
   c. brightness
   d. mix with white
   e. more than one of the above
87. A component not included in a continuous-wave Doppler instrument is a(n) ___________.
   a. loudspeaker
   b. wall filter
   c. oscillator
   d. demodulator
   e. gate
88. On a spectral display, amplitude is indicated by ___________.
   a. brightness
   b. horizontal position
   c. vertical position
   d. b and c
   e. none of the above
89. Doppler shift can change because of changes in ___________.
   a. velocity
   b. speed
   c. direction
   d. frequency
   e. all of the above
90. A gate-open time of 10 μs corresponds to a sample volume length (millimeters) of ___________.
   a. 10.0
   b. 7.7
   c. 3.8
   d. 3.3
   e. 2.0
91. Sample volume width is determined by ___________.
   a. gate-open time
   b. pulse duration
   c. pulse repetition frequency
   d. pulse repetition period
   e. beam width
92. What problem(s) is (are) encountered if pulse repetition frequency is 10 kHz, sample volume is located at 10-cm depth, and the Doppler shift is 4 kHz?
   a. Aliasing
   b. Mirror image
   c. Refraction
   d. Range ambiguity
   e. More than one of the above

93. What problem(s) is (are) encountered if pulse repetition frequency is 10 kHz, sample volume is located at a 5-cm depth, and the Doppler shift is 6 kHz?
a. Aliasing
b. Mirror image
c. Refraction
d. Range ambiguity
e. More than one of the above

94. What problem(s) is (are) encountered if pulse repetition frequency is 10 kHz, sample volume is located at a 10-cm depth, and the Doppler shift is 6 kHz?
a. Aliasing
b. Mirror image
c. Refraction
d. Range ambiguity
e. More than one of the above

95. The functions of a color-Doppler signal processor include ___________.
a. amplification
b. phase quadrature detection
c. demodulation
d. autocorrelation
e. all of the above

96. If all cells in a vessel were moving at the same constant speed, the spectral trace would be a ___________ line.
a. thin horizontal
b. thick horizontal
c. thin vertical
d. thick vertical
e. none of the above

97. Doppler power displays ___________.
a. are independent of Doppler angle
b. are more sensitive than Doppler-shift displays
c. are independent of aliasing
d. show uniform flow presentations
e. all of the above.

98. For a physiologic flow speed, a 5-MHz beam could produce a Doppler shift of about ___________.
a. 5 kHz
b. 5 MHz
c. 5 Hz
d. depends on the mode (continuous-wave or pulsed-wave)
e. none of the above

99. Spectral analysis is performed in a Doppler instrument ___________.
a. electronically
b. mathematically
c. acoustically
d. mechanically
e. more than one of the above

100. The Doppler shift is proportional to ___________.
a. the volume flow rate
b. flow speed
c. the Doppler angle
d. cell density
e. more than one of the above

101. Which of the following can be used to evaluate the performance of a Doppler instrument?
a. Contrast detail phantom
b. String test object
c. Flow phantom
d. b and c
e. All of the above

102. Place the following instruments in general order of increasing acoustic output: (1) spectral Doppler, (2) sonographic, (3) color Doppler.
a. 1, 2, 3
b. 2, 3, 1
c. 3, 1, 2
d. 3, 2, 1
e. 2, 1, 3

103. If operating frequency is 5 MHz, Doppler angle is 60 degrees, pulse repetition frequency is 9 kHz, and the Doppler shift is 2 kHz, what problem is encountered if the angle is changed to zero?
a. Aliasing
b. Range ambiguity
c. Mirror image
d. Refraction
e. None

104. When angle correction is applied on a color-Doppler display, the Nyquist limits (in centimeters per second) on the color map ___________.
a. increase
b. decrease
c. do not change
d. are irrelevant
e. are ambiguous

105. When angle correction is applied on a color-Doppler display, the Nyquist limits (in kilohertz) on the color map ___________.
a. increase
b. decrease
c. do not change
d. are irrelevant
e. are ambiguous

106. Flow is ___________ if it appears red on a color-Doppler display.
a. approaching
b. receding
c. turbulent
d. disturbed
e. undetermined (depends on color map)

107. Two different colors in the same vessel indicate ___________.
a. flow reversal
b. sector scan
c. vessel curvature
d. aliasing
e. any of the above

108. The following increase(s) the amount of color appearing in a vessel.
a. Increased color gain
b. Increased wall filter
c. Increased priority
d. Increased pulse repetition frequency
e. More than one of the above

109. The following decrease(s) the amount of color appearing in a vessel.
a. Increased wall filter
b. Increased pulse repetition frequency
c. Increased ensemble length
d. Baseline shift
e. More than one of the above

110. Which of the following on a color-Doppler display is (are) presented as a two-dimensional, cross-sectional display?
a. Gray-scale anatomy
b. Flow direction
c. Doppler spectrum
d. a and b
e. All of the above

111. Comparing gray with white is an example of ___________.
a. hue
b. luminance
c. saturation
d. b and c
e. all of the above

112. Comparing red with green is an example of ___________.
a. hue
b. luminance
c. saturation
d. b and c
e. all of the above

113. There are about ___________ frames per second produced by a color-Doppler instrument.
a. 10
b. 20
c. 40
d. 80
e. more than one of the above

114. The autocorrelation technique yields ___________.
a. the mean Doppler shift
b. a sign of the Doppler shift
c. a spread around the mean (variance)
d. all of the above
e. none of the above

115. Increasing ensemble length ___________ color sensitivity and accuracy and ___________ frame rate.
a. improves, increases
b. degrades, increases
c. degrades, decreases
d. improves, decreases
e. none of the above

116. Which control can be used to help with clutter?
a. Wall filter
b. Gain
c. Baseline shift
d. Pulse repetition frequency
e. Smoothing

117. Doubling the width of a color window produces a(n) ___________ frame rate.
a. doubled
b. quadrupled
c. unchanged
d. halved
e. quartered

118. Steering the color window to the right or left changes the ___________.
a. frame rate
b. pulse repetition frequency
c. the Doppler angle
d. the Doppler shift
e. more than one of the above

119. Lack of color in a vessel may be due to___________.
a. low color gain
b. low wall filter setting
c. small Doppler angle
d. low baseline shift
e. more than one of the above

120. Which control(s) can help with aliasing?
a. Wall filter
b. Gain
c. Smoothing
d. Pulse repetition frequency
e. More than one of the above

121. Pulse duration is the ___________ for a pulse to occur.
a. space
b. time
c. delay
d. pressure
e. reciprocal

122. Spatial pulse length equals the number of cycles in the pulse multiplied by ___________.
a. period
b. impedance
c. beam width
d. resolution
e. wavelength

123. If pulse duration is 1 μs and the pulse repetition period is 100 μs, duty factor is ___________.
a. 1%
b. 10%
c. 50%
d. 90%
e. 100%

124. The attenuation of 5-MHz ultrasound in 4 cm of soft tissue is ___________.
a. 5 dB/cm
b. 10 dB
c. 2.5 MHz/cm
d. 2 cm
e. 5 dB/MHz

125. If the maximum value of an acoustic variable in a sound wave is 10 units and the normal (no sound) value is 7 units, the amplitude is ____________ units.
   a. 1
   b. 3
   c. 7
   d. 10
   e. 17

126. Impedance equals propagation speed multiplied by ____________.
   a. density
   b. stiffness
   c. frequency
   d. attenuation
   e. path length

127. Which of the following cannot be determined from the others?
   a. Frequency
   b. Amplitude
   c. Intensity
   d. Power
   e. Beam area

128. For perpendicular incidence, in medium 1, density equals 1 and propagation speed equals 3; in medium 2, density equals 1.5 and propagation speed equals 2. What is the intensity reflection coefficient?
   a. 0
   b. 1
   c. 2
   d. 3
   e. 4

129. For perpendicular incidence, if the intensity transmission coefficient is 96%, what is the intensity reflection coefficient?
   a. 2%
   b. 4%
   c. 6%
   d. 8%
   e. 10%

130. The colors presented on a Doppler-power display represent the ____________ of the spectrum.
   a. mean Doppler shift
   b. variance
   c. area
   d. angle
   e. all of the above

131. For oblique incidence and a medium 2 speed that is equal to twice the speed of medium 1, the transmission angle will be about ____________ times the incidence angle.
   a. 0.5
   b. 17
   c. 2
   d. 4
   e. 5

132. The range equation describes the relationship of ____________.
   a. reflector distance, propagation time, and sound speed
   b. distance, propagation time, and reflection coefficient
   c. number of cows and sheep on a ranch
   d. propagation time, sound speed, and transducer frequency
   e. dynamic range and system sensitivity

133. Axial resolution in a system equals ____________.
   a. four times the spatial pulse length
   b. the ratio of reflector size to transducer frequency
   c. the maximum reflector separation expected to be displayed
   d. the minimum reflector separation expected to be displayed
   e. spatial pulse length

134. In soft tissue, two boundaries that generate reflections are separated in axial distance (depth) by 1 mm. With a two-cycle pulse of ultrasound, the minimum frequency that will axially resolve these boundaries is ____________.
   a. 1.0 MHz
   b. 2.0 MHz
   c. 3.0 MHz
   d. 4.0 MHz
   e. 5.0 MHz

135. Transducers operating properly in pulse-echo imaging systems have a quality factor of approximately ____________.
   a. 1 to 3
   b. 7 to 10
   c. 25 to 50
   d. 100
   e. 500

136. Which of the following quantities varies most with distance from the transducer face?
   a. Axial resolution
   b. Lateral resolution
   c. Frequency
   d. Wavelength
   e. Period

137. The near-zone length for an unfocused, 5-MHz, circular transducer with a 13-mm diameter is greater than that for a 5-MHz transducer with a diameter of ____________.
   a. 19 mm
   b. 15 mm
   c. 9 mm
   d. depends on impedance
   e. none of the above

138. If the near-zone length of an unfocused transducer that is 13 mm in diameter extends (in soft tissue) 6 cm from the transducer face, at which of the following distances from the face can the lateral resolution be improved by focusing the sound from this transducer?
   a. 13 cm
   b. 8 cm
   c. 3 cm
   d. 9 cm
   e. none of the above

139. The lateral resolution of an ultrasound system depends on ____________.
  a. the aperture
  b. the transducer frequency
  c. the speed of sound in soft tissue
  d. the memory and the display
  e. all of the above

140. Which of the following is a characteristic of a medium through which sound is propagating?
  a. Impedance
  b. Intensity
  c. Amplitude
  d. Frequency
  e. Period

141. Which of the following cannot be determined from the others?
  a. Frequency
  b. Period
  c. Amplitude
  d. Wavelength
  e. Propagation speed

142. For perpendicular incidence, if the impedances of two media are the same, there will be no ________.
  a. inflation
  b. reflection
  c. refraction
  d. calibration
  e. b and c

143. What is the transmitted intensity if the incident intensity is 1 and the impedances are 1.00 and 2.64?
  a. 0.2
  b. 0.4
  c. 0.6
  d. 0.8
  e. 1.0

144. Increasing the intensity produced by the transducer ____________.
  a. is accomplished by increasing pulser voltage
  b. increases the sensitivity of the system
  c. increases the possibility of biologic effects
  d. all of the above
  e. none of the above

145. If the propagation speeds of two media are equal, incidence angle equals ____________.
  a. the reflection angle
  b. the transmission angle
  c. the Doppler angle
  d. a and b
  e. b and c

146. If no reflection occurs at a boundary, it always means that media impedances are equal in the case of ____________.
  a. perpendicular incidence
  b. oblique incidence
  c. refraction
  d. a and b
  e. b and c

147. Increasing spatial pulse length ____________.
  a. accompanies increased transducer damping
  b. is accompanied by decreased pulse duration
  c. improves axial resolution
  d. all of the above
  e. none of the above

148. Place the following media in order of increasing sound propagation speed.
  a. Gas, solid, liquid
  b. Solid, liquid, gas
  c. Gas, liquid, solid
  d. Liquid, solid, gas
  e. Solid, gas, liquid

149. What is the wavelength of 1-MHz ultrasound in tissue with a propagation speed of 1540 m/s?
  a. 1×10^6 m
  b. 1.54 mm
  c. 1540 m
  d. 1.54 cm
  e. 0.77 cm

150. What is the spatial pulse length for two cycles of ultrasound having a wavelength of 2 mm?
  a. 4 cm
  b. 4 mm
  c. 7 mm
  d. 1.5 mm
  e. 3 mm

151. Increased damping produces ____________.
  a. increased bandwidth
  b. shorter pulses
  c. decreased efficiency
  d. all of the above
  e. none of the above

152. If no refraction occurs as an oblique sound beam passes through the boundary between two materials, what is unchanged as the boundary is crossed?
  a. Impedance
  b. Propagation speed
  c. Intensity
  d. Sound direction
  e. b and d

153. If the spatial average intensity in a beam is 1 W/cm² and the transducer is 5 cm² in area, what is the total acoustic power?
  a. 1 W
  b. 2 W
  c. 3 W
  d. 4 W
  e. 5 W

154. How does the propagation speed in bone compare with that in soft tissue?
  a. Lower
  b. The same
  c. Higher
  d. Cannot say unless soft tissue is specified
  e. b and c

155. Attenuation along a sound path is a decrease in ____________.

a. frequency
b. amplitude
c. intensity
d. b and c
e. impedance

156. A focused transducer that is 13 mm in diameter has a lateral resolution at the focus of better than (i.e., smaller than) ____________.

a. 26 mm
b. 13 mm
c. 6.5 mm
d. depends on frequency
e. none of the above

157. An important factor in the selection of a transducer for a specific application is the ultrasonic attenuation of tissue. Because of this attenuation, a 7.5-MHz transducer generally should be used for ____________.

a. imaging deep structures
b. imaging superficial structures
c. imaging deep and shallow structures
d. imaging adult intracranial structures
e. all of the above

158. A real-time scan ____________.

a. consists of many frames produced per second
b. depends on how short a time the sonographer takes to make a scan
c. is made only between 8 AM and 5 PM
d. yields a gray-scale image, whereas other scans yield only an M-mode display
e. none of the above

159. Which of the following is determined by the pulser in an instrument?

a. Amplitude
b. Pulse repetition frequency
c. Length of time required for a pulse to reach a specific reflector and return to the instrument
d. More than one of the above
e. None of the above

160. If the power at the output of an amplifier is 1000 times the power at the input, the gain is ____________.

a. 60 dB
b. 30 dB
c. 1000 dB
d. 1000 volts
e. none of the above

161. The dynamic range of an ultrasound system is defined as ____________.

a. the speed with which ultrasound examination can be performed
b. the range over which the transducer can be manipulated
c. the ratio of the maximum to the minimum intensity that can be displayed
d. the range of pulser voltages applied to the transducer
e. none of the above

162. The display generally will have a dynamic range ____________ than other portions of the ultrasound instrument.

a. larger
b. smaller

163. The number 30 in the binary system is ____________.

a. 0110
b. 1110
c. 1001
d. 1111
e. none of the above

164. An ultrasound instrument that could represent 64 shades of gray would require an 8-bit memory. True or false?

165. Imaging systems consist of a beam former, display, and ____________ and ____________ processors.

a. beam, digitizer
b. image, amplifier
c. signal, pulser
d. amplifier, digitizer
e. signal, image

166. Phased array systems involve the sequential switching of a small group of elements along the array. True or false?

167. For a two-cycle pulse of 5 MHz in soft tissue, the axial resolution is ____________.

a. 0.1 mm
b. 0.3 mm
c. 0.5 mm
d. 0.7 mm
e. 0.9 mm

168. Postprocessing is the process of assigning numbers to be placed in the memory. True or false?

169. The minimum displayed axial dimension of a reflector is approximately equal to ____________.

a. the beam diameter
b. half the beam diameter
c. twice the beam diameter
d. the spatial pulse length
e. half the spatial pulse length
f. twice the spatial pulse length

170. The minimum displayed lateral dimension of a reflector is approximately equal to ____________.

a. the beam diameter
b. half the beam diameter
c. twice the beam diameter
d. the spatial pulse length
e. half the spatial pulse length
f. twice the spatial pulse length

171. M-mode recordings have ____________ dimension(s).

a. two spatial
b. one spatial and one temporal
c. one Doppler and one temporal
d. one Doppler and one spatial
e. b and c

172. Nonlinear propagation of ultrasound in tissue generates ____________.
a. speckle
b. attenuation
c. harmonics
d. refraction
e. reverberations

173. The operation in the signal processor that reduces noise is ____________.
a. filtering
b. time gain compensation
c. scan conversion
d. compression
e. detection

174. The binary number 01001 is ____________ in the decimal system.
a. 1
b. 3
c. 5
d. 7
e. 9

175. Reflectors may be added to the display because of ____________.
a. reverberation
b. propagation speed error
c. enhancement
d. oblique reflection
e. the Doppler shift

176. If the propagation speed in a soft tissue path is 1.60 mm/μs, a diagnostic instrument assumes a propagation speed too ____________ and will show reflectors too ____________ the transducer.
a. high, close to
b. high, far from
c. low, close to
d. low, far from
e. none of the above

177. The reflector information that can be obtained from an M-mode display includes ____________.
a. distance and motion pattern
b. transducer frequency, reflection coefficient, and distance
c. acoustic impedance, attenuation, and motion pattern
d. all of the above
e. none of the above

178. Increasing gain generally produces the same effect as ____________.
a. decreasing attenuation
b. increasing compression
c. increasing rectification
d. both b and c
e. all of the above

179. A gray-scale display shows ____________.
a. gray color on a white background
b. reflections with one brightness level
c. a white color on a gray background
d. a range of reflection amplitudes or intensities
e. none of the above

180. Electric pulses from the pulser are applied through the delays and transmit/receive switch to the ____________.
a. pulser
b. transducer
c. demodulator
d. display
e. memory

181. Peak detection is part of ____________.
a. amplipression
b. rejection
c. a and b
d. compression
e. amplitude demodulation

182. Multiple focus is not used with color-Doppler instruments because of ____________.
a. ensemble length
b. wall filter
c. priority
d. low frame rate
e. a and d

183. If the gain of an amplifier is reduced by 3 dB and input power is unchanged, the output power of the amplifier is ____________ what it was before.
a. equal to
b. twice
c. one half
d. greater than
e. none of the above

184. If gain was 30 dB and output power is reduced by one half, the new gain is ____________ dB.
a. 15
b. 60
c. 33
d. 27
e. none of the above

185. If four shades of gray are shown on a display, each twice the brightness of the preceding one, the brightest shade is ____________ times the brightness of the dimmest shade.
a. 2
b. 4
c. 8
d. 16
e. 32

186. The dynamic range displayed in Exercise 185 is ____________ dB.
a. 100
b. 9
c. 5
d. 2
e. 0

187. Phantoms with nylon lines measure ____________.
a. resolution
b. pulse duration
c. spatial average–temporal average intensity
d. wavelength
e. all of the above

188. The following may be used to measure acoustic output.
  a. Hydrophone
  b. Optical encoder
  c. 100-mm test object
  d. All of the above
  e. None of the above
189. Real-time imaging is made possible by ____________.
  a. preprocessors
  b. single-element transducers
  c. gray-scale display
  d. transmit/receive switches
  e. arrays
190. Gain and attenuation are usually expressed in ____________.
  a. decibels
  b. decibels per centimeter
  c. centimeters
  d. centimeters per decibel
  e. none of the above
191. Gray-scale display requires ____________.
  a. array transducers
  b. cathode-ray storage tubes
  c. more than one bit per pixel
  d. b and c
  e. all of the above
192. With which of the following is time represented on one axis?
  a. B mode
  b. B scan
  c. M mode
  d. A la mode
  e. None of the above
193. Analog voltages occur at the output of the ____________.
  a. beam former
  b. transducer
  c. signal processor
  d. display
  e. a and b
194. Digital signals occur at the output of the ____________.
  a. beam former
  b. transducer
  c. signal processor
  d. display
  e. a and c
195. Which of the following produce(s) a rectangular image format?
  a. Vector array
  b. Convex array
  c. Phased array
  d. Linear array
  e. All of the above
196. The piezoelectric effect describes how ____________ is converted into ____________ by a ____________.
  a. electricity, an image, display
  b. incident sound, reflected sound, boundary
  c. ultrasound, electricity, transducer
  d. ultrasound, heat, tissue
  e. none of the above
197. Propagation speed in soft tissues ____________.
  a. is directly proportional to frequency
  b. is inversely proportional to frequency
  c. is directly proportional to intensity
  d. is inversely proportional to intensity
  e. none of the above
198. Doppler-power imaging indicates (with color) the ____________ of flow.
  a. presence
  b. direction
  c. speed
  d. character
  e. more than one of the above
199. While frequency is increased, ____________.
  a. wavelength increases
  b. a three-cycle ultrasound pulse decreases in length
  c. imaging depth decreases
  d. propagation speed decreases
  e. b and c
200. Focusing ____________.
  a. improves lateral resolution
  b. improves axial resolution
  c. increases beam width in the focal region
  d. shortens pulse length
  e. increases duty factor

GLOSSARY

All of the key terms that were listed at the beginning of the individual chapters are compiled and defined here. More detailed and complete compilations of terminology are available.[12]

A

A mode Mode of operation in which the display presents echo amplitude versus depth (used in ophthalmology).

absorption Conversion of sound to heat.

acoustic Having to do with sound.

acoustic variables Pressure, density, and particle vibration; sound wave quantities that vary in space and time.

ALARA as **l**ow **a**s **r**easonably **a**chievable. The principle that it is prudent to obtain diagnostic information with the least amount possible of energy exposure to the patient.

aliasing Improper Doppler-shift information from a pulsed spectral-Doppler or color-Doppler instrument when the true Doppler shift exceeds one-half the pulse repetition frequency.

amplification The process by which small voltages are increased to larger ones.

amplifier A device that accomplishes amplification.

amplitude Maximum variation of an acoustic variable or voltage.

analog Related to a procedure or system in which data are represented by proportional, continuously variable, physical quantities (e.g., electric voltage).

analog-to-digital converter A device that converts voltage amplitude to a number. Abbreviated ADC.

anechoic Echo free.

aperture Size of a transducer element (for a single-element transducer) or group of elements (for an array).

apodization Nonuniform (i.e., involving different voltage amplitudes) driving of elements in an array to reduce grating lobes.

array A transducer assembly containing several piezoelectric elements.

attenuation Decrease in amplitude and intensity with distance as a wave travels through a medium.

attenuation coefficient Attenuation per centimeter of wave travel.

autocorrelation A rapid technique, used in most color-Doppler instruments, to obtain mean Doppler-shift frequency.

axial In the direction of the transducer axis (sound travel direction).

axial resolution The minimum reflector separation along the sound path that is required to produce separate echoes (i.e., to distinguish between two reflectors).

B

B mode Mode of operation in which the display presents a spot of appropriate brightness for each echo received by the transducer.

B scan A B-mode image that represents an anatomic cross-section through the scanning plane.

backscatter Sound scattered back in the direction from which it originally came.

bandwidth Range of frequencies contained in an ultrasound pulse; range of frequencies within which a material, device, or system can operate.

baseline shift Movement of the zero Doppler-shift frequency or zero flow speed line up or down on a spectral display.

beam Region containing continuous wave sound; region through which a sound pulse propagates.

beam former The part of an instrument that accomplishes electronic beam scanning, apodization, steering, focusing, and aperture with arrays.

Bernoulli effect Pressure reduction in a region of high-flow speed.

bidirectional Indicating Doppler instruments capable of distinguishing between positive and negative Doppler shifts (approaching and receding flow).

bistable Having two possible states (e.g., on or off, white or black, one or zero).

bit Binary digit; one or zero.

C

cavitation Production and dynamics of bubbles in sound.

channel A single one- or two-way path for transmitting electric signals, in distinction from other parallel paths; an independent transmission delay line and transducer element path; an independent reception transducer element, amplifier, analog-to-digital converter, and delay line path.

cine loop Sequential display of all the frames stored in memory at a controllable frame rate.

clutter Noise in the Doppler signal that generally is caused by high-amplitude, Doppler-shifted echoes from the heart or vessel walls.

coded excitation A sophisticated form of transmission in which the driving voltage pulses have intrapulse variations in amplitude, frequency, and/or phase.

color-Doppler display The presentation of two-dimensional, real-time Doppler-shift information in color superimposed on a real-time, gray-scale, anatomic, cross-sectional image. Flow directions toward and away from the transducer (i.e., positive and negative Doppler shifts) are presented as different colors on the display.

comet tail A series of closely spaced reverberation echoes.

compensation Equalization of received echo amplitude differences caused by different attenuations for different reflector depths; also called *depth gain compensation* or *time gain compensation.*

compliance Distensibility; nonrigid stretchability of vessels.

composite Combination of a piezoelectric ceramic and a nonpiezoelectric polymer.

compression Reduction in differences between small and large amplitudes. Region of high density and pressure in a compressional wave.

constructive interference Combination of positive or negative pressures.

continuous wave A wave in which cycles repeat indefinitely; not pulsed. Abbreviated CW.

continuous-wave Doppler A Doppler device or procedure that uses continuous-wave ultrasound.

contrast agent A suspension of bubbles or particles introduced into circulation to enhance the contrast between anatomic structures, thereby improving their imaging.

contrast resolution Ability of a gray-scale display to distinguish between echoes of slightly different intensities.

convex array Curved linear array.

cosine The cosine of angle A in Figure C-1 is the length of side b divided by the length of side c. Abbreviated cos.

coupling medium A gel used to provide a good sound path between a transducer and the skin by eliminating the air between the two.

critical Reynolds number The Reynolds number above which turbulence occurs.

cross-talk Leakage of strong signals in one direction channel of a Doppler receiver into the other channel; can produce the spectral-Doppler mirror-image artifact.

crystal Element.

Curie point Temperature at which an element material loses its piezoelectric properties.

cycle One complete variation of an acoustic variable.

D

damping Material attached to the rear face of a transducer element to reduce pulse duration; the process of pulse duration reduction.

decibel Unit of power or intensity ratio; the number of decibels is 10 times the logarithm (to the base 10) of the power or intensity ratio. Abbreviated dB.

demodulation Detection.

density Mass divided by volume.

depth gain compensation See *compensation.* Abbreviated DGC.

destructive interference Combination of positive and negative pressures.

detail resolution The ability to image fine detail and to distinguish closely spaced reflectors. (See *axial resolution* and *lateral resolution.*)

detection Conversion of voltage pulses from radio frequency to video form. Also called *demodulation, amplitude detection,* and *envelope detection.*

digital Related to a procedure or system in which data are represented by numeric digits.

digital-to-analog converter A device that converts a number to a proportional voltage amplitude. Abbreviated DAC.

disk A thin, flat, circular object.

display A device that presents a visual image derived from voltages received from an image processor.

disturbed flow Flow that cannot be described by straight, parallel streamlines.

Doppler angle The angle between the sound beam and the flow direction.
Doppler effect A change in frequency caused by reflector motion.
Doppler equation The mathematical description of the relationship between the Doppler shift, frequency, Doppler angle, propagation speed, and reflector speed.
Doppler-power display Color-Doppler display in which colors are assigned according to the strength (amplitude, power, intensity, energy) of the Doppler-shifted echoes.
Doppler shift Reflected frequency minus incident frequency; the change in frequency caused by motion.
Doppler spectrum The range of frequencies present in Doppler-shifted echoes.
duplex instrument An ultrasound instrument that combines gray-scale sonography with pulsed Doppler and, possibly, continuous-wave Doppler.
duty factor Fraction of time that pulsed ultrasound is on.
dynamic aperture Aperture that increases with increasing focal length (to maintain constant focal width).
dynamic focusing Continuously variable reception focusing that follows the increasing depth of the transmitted pulse as it travels.
dynamic range Ratio (in decibels) of largest to smallest power that a system can handle; ratio of the largest to smallest intensity of echoes encountered.

E

echo Reflection.
eddies Regions of circular flow patterns present in turbulence.
elastography Imaging tissue stiffness by tracking movement under mechanical stress.
element The piezoelectric component of a transducer assembly.
elevational resolution The detail resolution in the direction perpendicular to the scan plane. It is equal to the section thickness and is the source of section thickness artifact.
energy Capability of doing work.
enhancement Increase in echo amplitude from reflectors that lie behind a weakly attenuating structure.
ensemble length Number of pulses used to generate one color-Doppler image scan line.

F

far zone The region of a sound beam in which the beam diameter increases as the distance from the transducer increases; also called *far field.*
fast Fourier transform Digital computer implementation of the Fourier transform.
filter An electric circuit that passes frequencies within a defined range.
flat-panel display A back-lighted rectangular matrix of thousands of liquid crystal display elements.
flow To move in a stream; volume flow rate.
fluid A material that flows and conforms to the shape of its container; a gas or liquid.
focal length Distance from a focused transducer to the center of a focal region or to the location of the spatial peak intensity.
focal region Region of minimum beam diameter and area.
focal zone Length of the focal region.
focus The concentration of the sound beam into a smaller beam area than would exist otherwise.
Fourier transform A mathematical technique for obtaining a Doppler frequency spectrum.
fractional bandwidth Bandwidth divided by operating frequency.
frame A single image produced by one complete scan of the sound beam.
frame rate Number of frames of echo information stored each second.
Fraunhofer zone Far zone.
freeze-frame Constant display of one of the frames in memory.
frequency Number of cycles per second.
frequency spectrum The range of Doppler-shift frequencies present in the returning echoes.
Fresnel zone Near zone.
fundamental frequency The primary frequency in a collection of frequencies that can include odd and even harmonics and subharmonics.

G

gain Ratio (in decibels) of amplifier output to input electric power.
gate A device that allows only echoes from a selected depth (arrival time) to pass.
grating lobes Additional weaker beams of sound traveling out in directions different from the primary beam as a result of the multi-element structure of transducer arrays.
gray scale Range of brightnesses (gray levels) between white and black.

H

harmonics Frequencies that are even and odd multiples of another, commonly called *fundamental* or *operating frequency.*
hertz Unit of frequency, one cycle per second; unit of pulse repetition frequency, one pulse per second. Abbreviated Hz.
hue The color perceived based on the frequency of light.
hydrophone A small transducer element mounted on the end of a narrow tube; a piezoelectric membrane with small metallic electrodes.
hypoechoic Having relatively weak echoes. Opposite of hyperechoic (having relatively strong echoes).

I

image A reproduction, representation, or imitation of the physical form of a person or thing.
image memory The part of the image processor where echo information is stored in image format.
image processor An electronic device that manipulates and prepares images for visual presentation.
impedance Density multiplied by the sound propagation speed.
incidence angle Angle between incident sound direction and a line perpendicular to the boundary of a medium.
inertia Resistance to acceleration.
instrument An electronic system that electrically drives a transducer, receives returning echoes, and presents them on a visual display as an anatomic image, Doppler spectrum, or color-Doppler presentation.
intensity Power divided by area.
intensity reflection coefficient Reflected intensity divided by incident intensity; the fraction of incident intensity reflected.
intensity transmission coefficient Transmitted intensity divided by incident intensity; the fraction of incident intensity transmitted into the second medium.
interference Combinations of positive and/or negative pressures.

K

kilohertz One thousand hertz. Abbreviated kHz.

L

laminar flow Flow in which fluid layers slide over each other in a smooth, orderly manner, with no mixing between layers.
lateral Perpendicular to the direction of sound travel.
lateral gain control Gain controls that enable different gain values to be applied laterally across an image to compensate for differing attenuation values in different anatomic regions.
lateral resolution Minimum reflector separation perpendicular to the sound path that is required to produce separate echoes.
lead zirconate titanate A ceramic piezoelectric material. Abbreviated PZT.
lens A curved material that focuses a sound or light beam.
linear Adjectival form of *line.*
linear array Array made of rectangular elements arranged in a straight line.
linear image An anatomic image presented in a rectangular format.
linear phased array Linear array operated by applying voltage pulses to all elements, but with small time differences (phasing) to direct ultrasound pulses out in various directions.
linear sequenced array Linear array operated by applying voltage pulses to groups of elements sequentially.
longitudinal wave Wave in which the particle motion is parallel to the direction of wave travel (compressional wave).
luminance Brightness of a presented hue and saturation.

M

M mode A B-mode presentation of changing reflector position (motion) versus time (used in echocardiography).
mass Measure of the resistance of an object to acceleration.
matching layer Material attached to the front face of a transducer element to reduce the reflections at the transducer surface.
mechanical index An indicator of nonthermal mechanism activity; equal to the peak rarefactional pressure divided by the square root of the center frequency of the pulse bandwidth.

medium Material through which a wave travels.

megahertz One million hertz. Abbreviated MHz.

mirror image An artifactual gray-scale, color flow, or Doppler signal appearing on the opposite side (from the real structure or flow) of a strong reflector.

multiple reflection Several reflections produced by a pulse encountering a pair of reflectors; reverberation.

N

natural focus The narrowing of a sound beam that occurs with an unfocused flat transducer element.

near zone The region of a sound beam in which the beam diameter decreases as the distance from the transducer increases; also called *near field.*

nonlinear propagation Sound propagation in which the propagation speed depends on pressure causing the wave shape to change and harmonics to be generated.

Nyquist limit The Doppler-shift frequency above which aliasing occurs; one half of the pulse repetition frequency.

O

oblique incidence Sound direction that is not perpendicular to media boundaries.

operating frequency Preferred (maximum efficiency) frequency of operation of a transducer. (See *resonance frequency.*)

P

panoramic imaging The extension of the field of view beyond the normal limits of a transducer scan plane.

parabolic flow Laminar flow with a profile in the shape of a parabola.

penetration Imaging depth.

period Time per cycle.

perpendicular Geometrically related by 90 degrees.

perpendicular incidence Sound direction that is perpendicular to the boundary between media.

persistence Averaging sequential frames together.

phantom Tissue-equivalent device that has characteristics that are representative of tissues (e.g., scattering, propagation speed, and attenuation).

phase A description of progress through a cycle; one full cycle is divided into 360 degrees of phase.

phase quadrature Two signals differing by one fourth of a cycle.

phased array An array that steers and focuses the beam electronically (with short time delays).

phased linear array Linear sequenced array with phased focusing added; linear sequenced array with phased steering of pulses to produce a parallelogram-shaped display.

picture archiving and communications system The system provides means for electronically communicating images and associated information to work stations and devices external to the sonographic instrument, the examining room, and even the building in which the scanning is done. Abbreviated PACS.

piezoelectricity Conversion of pressure to electric voltage.

pixel Picture element; the unit into which imaging information is divided for storage and display in a digital instrument.

plug flow Flow with all fluid portions traveling with the same flow speed and direction.

poise Unit of viscosity.

Poiseuille equation The mathematical description of the dependence of volume flow rate on pressure, vessel length and radius, and fluid viscosity.

polyvinylidene fluoride A piezoelectric thin-film material.

postprocessing Image processing done after storage in the memory.

power Rate at which work is done; rate at which energy is transferred.

preprocessing Signal and image processing accomplished before storage in the memory.

pressure Force divided by the area in a fluid.

priority The gray-scale echo strength below which color-Doppler information is shown preferentially on a display.

probe Transducer assembly.

propagation Progression or travel.

propagation speed Speed at which a wave moves through a medium.

pulsatile flow Flow that accelerates and decelerates with each cardiac cycle.

pulsatility index A description of the relationship between peak systolic and end diastolic flow speeds or Doppler shifts.

pulse A brief excursion of a quantity from its normal value; a few cycles.

pulse duration Interval of time from beginning to end of a pulse.

pulse repetition frequency Number of pulses per second; sometimes called *pulse repetition rate.* Abbreviated PRF.

pulse repetition period Interval of time from the beginning of one pulse to the beginning of the next.

pulsed Doppler A Doppler device or procedure that uses pulsed-wave ultrasound.

pulsed ultrasound Ultrasound produced in pulsed form by applying electric pulses or voltages of one or a few cycles to the transducer.

pulse-echo technique Ultrasound imaging in which pulses are reflected and used to produce a display.

R

radiation force The force exerted by a sound beam on an absorber or a reflector.

radio frequency Voltages representing echoes in cyclic form. Abbreviated RF.

range ambiguity An artifact produced when echoes are placed too close to the transducer because a second pulse was emitted before they were received from the first pulse.

range equation Relationship between round-trip pulse travel time, propagation speed, and distance to a reflector.

range gating Selection of the depth from which echoes are accepted based on echo arrival time.

rarefaction Region of low density and pressure in a compressional wave.

rayl Unit of impedance.

real time Imaging with a rapid frame sequence display.

real-time display A display that, with a sufficient frame rate, appears to image moving structures or a changing scan plane continuously.

reflection Portion of sound returned from a media boundary; echo.

reflection angle Angle between the reflected sound direction and a line perpendicular to the media boundary.

reflector Media boundary that produces a reflection; reflecting surface.

refraction Change of sound direction on passing from one medium to another.

refresh rate The number of times each second that information is sent from the image memory to the display. The number of times per second that a computer monitor redraws the information found in the memory.

resistance Pressure difference divided by volume flow rate for steady flow.

resolution The ability to distinguish echoes in terms of space, time, or strength (called *detail, temporal,* and *contrast resolutions,* respectively).

resonance The condition in which a driven mechanical vibration is of a frequency similar to a natural vibration frequency of the structure, yielding maximum response.

resonance frequency Operating frequency.

reverberation Multiple reflection.

Reynolds number A number that depends on flow speed and viscosity to predict the onset of turbulence.

S

sample volume The anatomic region from which pulsed Doppler echoes are accepted.

saturation The amount of hue present in a mix with white.

scan line A line produced on a display that represents ultrasonic echoes returning from the body. A sonographic image is composed of many such lines.

scanhead Transducer assembly.

scanning The sweeping of a sound beam through the anatomy to produce an image.

scatterer An object that scatters sound in many directions because of its small size or its surface roughness.

scattering Diffusion or redirection of sound in several directions upon encountering a particle suspension or a rough surface.

sector A geometric figure bounded by two radii and the arc of the circle included between them.

sector image An anatomic image presented in a pie slice–shaped format.

sensitivity Ability of an imaging system to detect weak echoes.

shadowing Reduction in echo amplitude from reflectors that lie behind a strongly reflecting or attenuating structure.

shear wave See *transverse wave*.

side lobes Weaker beams of sound traveling out from a single element in directions different from those of the primary beam.

signal Information-bearing voltages in an electric circuit; an acoustic, visual, electric, or other conveyance of information. The physical representation of a message or information.

signal processor An electronic device that manipulates electric signals in preparation for appropriate presentation of information contained in them.

slice thickness Thickness of the scanned tissue volume perpendicular to the scan plane; also called *section thickness.*

sonography Medical two-dimensional, cross-sectional, and three-dimensional anatomic and flow imaging using ultrasound.

sound Traveling wave of acoustic variables.

sound beam The region of a medium that contains virtually all of the sound produced by a transducer.

source An emitter of ultrasound; transducer.

spatial compounding Averaging of frames that view the anatomy from different angles.

spatial pulse length Length of space over which a pulse occurs.

speckle The granular appearance of images and spectral displays that is caused by the interference of echoes from the distribution of scatterers in tissue.

spectral analysis Separation of frequencies in a Doppler signal for display as a Doppler spectrum; the application of the Fourier transform to determine the frequency components present in a Doppler signal.

spectral broadening The widening of the Doppler-shift spectrum; that is, the increase in the range of Doppler-shift frequencies present that occurs because of a broadened range of flow velocities encountered by the sound beam. This occurs for disturbed and turbulent flow.

spectral-Doppler display The presentation of Doppler information in a quantitative form of Doppler shift versus time. Visual display of a Doppler spectrum.

spectrum analyzer A device that derives a frequency spectrum from a complex signal.

specular reflection Reflection from a large (relative to wavelength), flat, smooth boundary.

speed error Propagation speed that is different from the assumed value (1.54 mm/μs).

stenosis Narrowing of a vessel lumen.

stiffness Property of a medium; applied pressure divided by the fractional volume change produced by the pressure.

streamline A line representing the path of motion of a particle of fluid.

strength Nonspecific term referring to amplitude or intensity.

stress A force per unit area applied to a material that compresses or stretches it.

strain The increase or decrease of the length of a segment of a material, subjected to a stress, divided by its original length.

T

temporal resolution Ability to distinguish closely spaced events in time; improves with increased frame rate.

test object A device without tissue-like properties that is designed to measure some characteristic of an imaging system.

thermal index An indicator of thermal mechanism activity (estimated temperature rise); a value equal to transducer acoustic output power divided by the estimated power required to raise tissue temperature by 1° C.

time gain compensation Equalization of echo amplitude differences caused by different attenuations for different reflector depths; also called *depth gain compensation.* Abbreviated TGC.

transducer A device that converts energy from one form to another.

transducer assembly Transducer element(s) with damping and matching materials assembled in a case.

transmission angle Angle between the transmitted sound direction and a line perpendicular to the media boundary.

transverse wave A sound wave in which the particle motion is perpendicular to the direction of wave travel. (See *shear wave.*)

turbulence Random, chaotic, multidirectional flow of a fluid with mixing between layers; flow that is not laminar.

U

ultrasound Sound having a frequency greater than what humans can hear, that is, greater than 20 kHz.

ultrasound transducer A device that converts electric energy to ultrasound energy, and vice versa.

V

variance Square of standard deviation; one of the outputs of the autocorrelation process; a measure of spectral broadening (i.e., spread around the mean).

vector array Linear sequenced array that emits pulses from different starting points and (by phasing) in different directions.

viscosity Resistance of a fluid to flow.

volume imaging Three-dimensional imaging.

volumetric flow rate Volume of fluid passing a point per unit of time (i.e., per second or minute).

W

wall filter An electric filter that passes frequencies above a set level and eliminates strong, low-frequency Doppler shifts from pulsating heart or vessel walls or tissue motion.

wave Traveling variation of one or more quantities.

wavelength Length of space over which a cycle occurs.

window An anechoic region appearing beneath echo frequencies presented on a Doppler spectral display.

Y

Young's modulus A measure of the hardness (stiffness) of a material. It is the ratio of the applied stress to the resulting strain in a material subjected to the stress.

Z

zero-crossing detector An analog detector that yields mean Doppler shift as a function of time.

ANSWERS TO EXERCISES

CHAPTER 1

1. d
2. a
3. a
4. c
5. c
6. d
7. a
8. b
9. c
10. a
11. c
12. a
13. b
14. d
15. d
16. b
17. d
18. d
19. a
20. c
21. a
22. d
23. e
24. c
25. b

CHAPTER 2

1. b
2. d
3. c
4. d
5. d
6. b
7. a
8. a
9. c
10. c
11. b
12. a
13. a
14. d
15. d
16. b
17. d
18. c
19. c
20. b
21. a
22. c
23. d (fastest in solids)
24. b
25. a
26. d (mechanical, longitudinal, or compressional)
27. b
28. d (determined by the medium)
29. b
30. a (information or energy)
31. c
32. True
33. c
34. d
35. c
36. d
37. c
38. d
39. True
40. True
41. a
42. c
43. b
44. d
45. b
46. b
47. b
48. c
49. b
50. c
51. 1 (100%)
52. a
53. b (Soft tissue propagation speed is 1.54 mm/μs; wavelength is 0.3 mm.)
54. c (Period is 0.2 μs; soft tissue is irrelevant.)
55. d (1000 pulses per second; 1⁄1000 second from one pulse to the next)
56. a (0.04%)
57. d
58. e (50,000)
59. c
60. a
61. a
62. b
63. d
64. a (also W/cm^2)
65. d
66. c
67. b
68. a
69. d
70. d
71. a
72. c

73. b
74. a
75. d
76. c
77. a
78. a
79. d
80. c
81. False (Attenuation = absorption + scattering)
82. True
83. b
84. b (Attenuation is 8 dB, and intensity ratio is 0.16.)
85. d (Attenuation is 80 dB, and intensity ratio is 0.00000001.)
86. c (0.5 × 7.5 MHz × 0.8 cm = 3 dB)
87. a
88. c
89. d
90. d
91. True, for perpendicular incidence
92. d (difference in numerator; sum in denominator)
93. b
94. a
95. c
96. d
97. True
98. d
99. a
100. False

CHAPTER 3

1. a
2. d
3. b
4. c
5. d
6. a
7. b
8. c
9. d
10. b
11. d
12. a
13. d
14. b
15. e
16. d
17. a
18. False
19. False
20. Back
21. Front
22. c
23. a
24. f (a, b, c)
25. d
26. a
27. c
28. No (because these frequencies are outside the bandwidth [4.5 to 5.5 MHz])
29. No (because these frequencies are outside the 2.5-MHz bandwidth [3.75 to 6.25 MHz])
30. a
31. b
32. a
33. c
34. c
35. a
36. b
37. False (can focus only in the near zone)
38. c
39. d (all of the above)
40. False (See Figure 3-14.)
41. a
42. a
43. d
44. a (the lateral dimension in the scan plane)
45. c
46. d
47. a, 1; b, 2; c, 1
48. b
49. c
50. a, e
51. b, c, d
52. c
53. d
54. b
55. d
56. a
57. c
58. True
59. b
60. a
61. b
62. d
63. a
64. False
65. False
66. b
67. d (less than 20 MHz in many applications)
68. c
69. d
70. c
71. a
72. e
73. True
74. True
75. False, in general (only true near the transducer)
76. b, c, e, f
77. a, 4; b, 3; c, 2; d, 1
78. a, d
79. a, 10; b, 0.15; c, 14; d, 6.5; e, 13; f, 14
80. c

81. b
82. d
83. d (frequency not needed)
84. a (size not needed)
85. True
86. False
87. d
88. True
89. False
90. a, 1, 2, 3; b. 2; c. 2; d. 1
91. e
92. a
93. b, c, d
94. True (axial resolution 0.3 mm)
95. c
96. b
97. d
98. c
99. d
100. a, 1; b, 4; c, 3; d, 5; e, 2

CHAPTER 4

1. b
2. a
3. a (A minimum echo reception time of 130 μs is required.)
4. d
5. a, 2; b, 4; c, 5; d, 1; e, 3
6. c
7. b
8. a
9. b
10. d
11. a
12. b
13. b
14. c
15. False
16. c
17. c
18. c
19. a
20. d
21. c
22. d
23. d
24. c
25. d
26. a, 6; b, 9; c, 10; d, 13; e, 14
27. a (43/32)
28. c (45/64)
29. a, 5; b, 3; c, 2; d, 6; e, 1; f, 4
30. e
31. a, 4; b, 5; c, 6; d, 7; e, 8
32. e
33. c
34. e
35. a
36. c (0 and 1)
37. d
38. a
39. a, 3; b, 7; c, 8; d, 5; e, 4; f, 2; g, 1; h, 6
40. c
41. b
42. a, 5; b, 10; c, 3; d, 1; e, 9; f, 2; g, 8; h, 7; i, 4; j, 6
43. a, 1 (0); b, 1 (1); c, 3 (101); d, 4 (1010); e, 5 (11001); f, 5 (11110); g, 6 (111111); h, 7 (1000000); i, 7 (1001011); j, 7 (1100100)
44. a, 3 (111); b, 4 (1111); c, 2 (11); d, 9 (111111111); e, 10 (1111111111); f, 6 (111111); g, 8 (11111111); h, 1 (1); i, 7 (1111111); j, 5 (11111)
45. a, 1 (0, 1); b, 2 (00, 01, 10, 11); c, 3 (000, 001, 010, 011, 100, 101, 110, 111); d, 4; e, 4; f, 5; g, 5; h, 6; i, 7; j, 7
46. a
47. c
48. d
49. a
50. d
51. a, 1; b, 2; c, 2; d, 2
52. b
53. b
54. True ($10 \times 1 \times 100 \times 30 = 30{,}000 < 77{,}000$)
55. c
56. a
57. a
58. b
59. d
60. c
61. b
62. c
63. b
64. d
65. a
66. b
67. d
68. b
69. b
70. a
71. d
72. d
73. a
74. a
75. a
76. b
77. b
78. c
79. d
80. c
81. b
82. a
83. False
84. d
85. b
86. a

87. b
88. c
89. a
90. d
91. a
92. a
93. a
94. b; e (a, c, d)
95. b
96. d
97. b
98. e (approaching the focus)
99. d
100. b

CHAPTER 5

1. a, c, d, e, g, h
2. c
3. a, b, f
4. c
5. b
6. b
7. d
8. c
9. a
10. a
11. b
12. d
13. b
14. d
15. c
16. d
17. b
18. b
19. e
20. e
21. e
22. c
23. d
24. b
25. b
26. a
27. d
28. a
29. b
30. a
31. a
32. e
33. e
34. b
35. d
36. e
37. d
38. d
39. d
40. b
41. c
42. d
43. d
44. b
45. b (The Doppler shift is cut in half.)
46. c (There is no Doppler shift at 90 degrees.)
47. d
48. a
49. a
50. c
51. c
52. c
53. c
54. d
55. a
56. d
57. b
58. b
59. True (Power displays have no angle dependence.)
60. No
61. False
62. b
63. e (a, b, or c)
64. False
65. False (It also can mean aliasing or changing Doppler angle.)
66. False (Remember the Doppler angle.)
67. b
68. b
69. a and c
70. a, b, c
71. d
72. a
73. b
74. d
75. c
76. b, c
77. e (c and d)
78. b
79. e
80. False
81. e
82. a
83. e (a, b, c, d)
84. e
85. b
86. d
87. False
88. e
89. a
90. a
91. False
92. False
93. e (b, c, d)
94. False (Remember the Doppler angle.)
95. c
96. a

97. b
98. d
99. c
100. c

CHAPTER 6

1. d
2. a
3. c (assumes 1.54 mm/μs, lower than the actual speed)
4. False
5. a
6. e (a, b, d)
7. False (This is the display of the interference pattern [speckle] of scattered sound from the distribution of scatterers within the ultrasound pulse in the tissue.)
8. c (also called section thickness)
9. c, d, e, f
10. True (edge shadowing)
11. Figure 6-40, *A*. Figure 6-40, *B*, shows a comet tail artifact originating as reverberations within a structure.
12. a, 1; b, 2, 3; c, 3; d, 4, 5; e, 4, 5
13. b
14. c
15. b
16. d
17. True
18. b
19. b
20. b
21. c
22. a (double image)
23. e
24. e (c and d)
25. e
26. a
27. True
28. b
29. d
30. b
31. d
32. b
33. b
34. b
35. b
36. e
37. c
38. True (less attenuation, greater penetration, later echoes)
39. True (Doppler shift increases with increasing frequency.)
40. d
41. a
42. a, 3; b, 4; c, 3; d, 2; e, 1
43. b, c, d
44. e (b, c, d)
45. d
46. a, R (Color changes at a 90-degree angle because scan lines go in different directions. They are heading upstream on the right and downstream on the left.); b, L (Vessel curvature causes flow to be away from the transducer on the left and toward the transducer on the right.); c, R (The blue area at right is aliasing.); d, L (The blue in the center is aliasing.); e, L; f, L (The color changes because the vessel is curved; flow is away from the transducer on the left and toward the transducer on the right.)
47. a, 4; b, 2; c, 1; d, 3; e, 5
48. a
49. c, b, d
50. a

CHAPTER 7

1. a
2. a, 1, 3; b, 1, 3; c, 1; d, 1; e, 4; f, 2; g, 2; h, 2; i, 5; j, 5
3. a. 4; b. 5; c. 3; d. 3; e. 1; f. 2; g. 1, 2
4. True
5. True
6. b
7. d
8. e
9. a
10. False
11. b, c, d, e
12. False
13. d
14. True
15. b
16. a, 2, 12; b, 3, 12; c, 3, 8; d, 4 or 2, 9; e, 1, 7; f, 6, 10; g, 6, 11
17. c
18. e
19. a
20. d
21. a
22. b
23. c
24. False
25. d
26. e
27. e (a, b, c)
28. False
29. False
30. b
31. No
32. Yes
33. b and d
34. c
35. e
36. e
37. e
38. a
39. d
40. b
41. e
42. c, d, e
43. b

44. a, b, d
45. e (pregnancy possibility in fertile female)
46. b
47. a
48. d
49. b
50. b

CHAPTER 8

After each answer is the chapter number in which the subject is discussed. Most answers also have explanatory comments.

1. c. Ultrasound is sound of frequency greater than 20 kHz (0.02 MHz). (Chapter 2)
2. a. Propagation speeds in soft tissues are in the range of approximately 1.4 to 1.6 mm/μs. Answer c is not in speed units. (Chapter 2)
3. c. Solid; high stiffness. (Chapter 2)
4. d. Propagation speed and impedance increase only slightly with frequency. (Chapter 2)
5. e. (Chapters 2 and 3)
6. c. Round-trip travel time is 13 μs/cm. (Chapter 2)
7. c. Scattering occurs with rough surfaces and with heterogeneous media (made up of small particles relative to the wavelength). Large, flat, smooth surfaces produce specular reflections. (Chapter 2)
8. b. The operating frequency of a transducer is such that its thickness is equal to one half of the wavelength in the transducer element material. (Chapter 3)
9. d. Transducer elements expand and contract when a voltage is applied; conversely, when returning echoes apply pressure to the element, a voltage is generated. (Chapter 3)
10. a. Axial resolution is equal to one half of the spatial pulse length. (Chapter 3)
11. c. Lateral resolution is equal to beam width. Beam width depends on the aperture (size of the element or group of elements generating the beam). (Chapter 3)
12. a. Penetration decreases with increasing frequency, and frequency has no effect on refraction. (Chapters 2 and 3)
13. c. This is part of the American Institute of Ultrasound in Medicine's "Statement on Mammalian In Vivo Ultrasonic Biological Effects." (Chapter 7)
14. c. Frequencies lower than this range do not provide the needed resolution, whereas frequencies higher than this range do not allow for adequate penetration for medical purposes. (Chapters 2 and 3)
15. a. See answer to question 14. (Chapters 2 and 3)
16. e. Reverberation adds additional reflectors on the display that are deeper than the true ones. (Chapter 6)
17. d. (Chapter 4)
18. d. (Chapter 4)
19. b. (Chapter 4)
20. d. (Chapter 4)
21. b. (Chapter 6)
22. b. (Chapter 4)
23. d. (Chapter 4)
24. c. Pulse repetition frequency has no direct effect on detail resolution. (Chapters 4 and 6)
25. d. (Chapter 4)
26. d. Distance equals one half of the speed multiplied by the round-trip time. (Chapter 2)
27. e. The matching layer improves sound transmission by reducing the reflection at the transducer–skin boundary. The coupling medium improves it by removing the air layer between the transducer and the skin. (Chapter 3)
28. c. (Chapter 3)
29. a. (Chapter 3)
30. c. (Chapter 4)
31. d. If the transducer is in the path of the reflector, answer c is correct because the Doppler angle is zero. If this is not the case, then b is correct because the Doppler angle will increase (decreasing the Doppler shift) while the reflector approaches. (Chapter 5)
32. e. The diameter referred to can be the entire vessel diameter or the diameter of a small portion of it (stenosis). For the former, d is correct. For the latter, c is correct at the stenosis. In either case, both a and b are correct. (Chapter 5)
33. c. Poiseuille equation shows that resistance increases with increasing vessel length, increasing fluid viscosity, or decreasing vessel diameter. (Chapter 5)
34. d. The blood cells move along with the plasma, not through it. (Chapter 5)
35. c. Propagation speed is determined by the medium, not by motion. (Chapters 2 and 5)
36. e. (Chapter 5)
37. e. (Chapter 5)
38. d. Spectral comes from spectrum, referring to color spectrum. A prism is an optical spectrum analyzer that breaks down white light into its component colors. (Chapter 5)
39. a. (Chapter 5)
40. e. If frequency changes, wavelength changes also. (Chapters 2 and 5)
41. c. (Chapter 5)
42. d. Answers a and b are correct. Anatomic data are provided by the real-time B scan, and physiologic data are provided by the pulsed Doppler portion of the operation. (Chapter 5)
43. False. Physiologic Doppler-shift frequencies are usually in the audible frequency range. (Chapter 5)
44. d. All imaging instruments and some Doppler instruments use pulsed ultrasound. (Chapter 4)
45. c. (Chapter 5)
46. e. (Chapter 5)
47. d. (Chapter 5)
48. e. They include pulsed Doppler (and sometimes continuous-wave Doppler) and dynamic B-scan imaging. (Chapter 5)
49. c. Both Doppler shifts exceed one half of the pulse repetition frequency. (Chapter 5)

50. d. (Chapter 5)
51. a. This is because physiologic speeds (v) are small compared with the speed of sound (c) in tissues. (Chapter 5)
52. b. (Chapter 5)
53. e. Arterioles and capillaries are too small. (Chapter 5)
54. d. (Chapter 5)
55. e. (Chapter 5)
56. b. (Chapter 5)
57. c. (Chapter 5)
58. d. This is the Poiseuille law. Increasing resistance decreases flow. (Chapter 5)
59. b. It depends on radius to the fourth power. (Chapter 5)
60. d. This is the continuity rule. (Chapter 5)
61. e. (also the results of distensible vessels) (Chapter 5)
62. d. (Chapter 5)
63. e. See Figure 5-9. (Chapter 5)
64. c. (assuming a reflector moving at 50 cm/s) (Chapter 5)
65. b. (that is, about 5 m/s) (Chapter 5)
66. c. (smaller angle, larger cosine, larger shift) (Chapter 5)
67. a. (Chapter 5)
68. e. Spectrum is not needed; it cannot be displayed in a pixel. (Chapter 5)
69. d. The spectrum can be shown in addition to the color-Doppler display. (Chapter 5)
70. c. (Chapter 5)

$$\upsilon = \frac{77 \times 0.100}{(5 \times 0.5)} = 3.08$$

71. a. (Chapter 5)

$$\upsilon = \frac{77 \times 0.100}{7.5} = 1.03$$

72. d. (Chapter 5)
73. c. (13 μs of delay per centimeter of depth) (Chapter 5)
74. a. This is because flow speeds are typically one thousandth the speed of sound in tissues. (Chapter 5)
75. b. The range is about 4 to 32. (Chapter 5)
76. c. The range is about 40 to 400. (Chapter 5)
77. e. Any pulsed instrument (b, c, d) can. (Chapter 5)
78. a. This is called near-plug flow. (Chapter 5)
79. d. (Chapter 5)
80. e. A stenosis generally increases a, b, and c and decreases d. (Chapter 5)
81. a. (that is, a widening of the spectrum) (Chapter 5)
82. e. Items b, c, and d are increased; a is decreased. (Chapter 5)
83. c. The blood flows back out of the high-impedance vascular bed during the low-pressure portion of the cardiac cycle. (Chapter 5)
84. c. (Chapter 5)
85. d. (Chapter 5)
86. e. (a resulting from b) (Chapter 5)
87. e. (Chapter 5)
88. a. (gray level or, sometimes, color) (Chapter 5)
89. e. (a = b + c) (Chapter 5)
90. b. (Chapter 5)
91. e. Items a and b determine sample volume length. (Chapter 5)
92. d. Echoes from the sample volume arrive after another pulse is emitted. (Chapter 5)
93. a. The shift exceeds the Nyquist limit (5 kHz). (Chapter 5)
94. e. (a and d) (Chapter 5)
95. e. (Chapter 5)
96. a. (Chapter 5)
97. e. (Chapter 5)
98. a. Because physiologic flow speeds are about one thousandth the ultrasound propagation speed (1540 m/s), Doppler shifts are about one thousandth the operating frequency. (Chapter 5)
99. e. (a and b) (Chapter 5)
100. b. (also proportional to the cosine of the Doppler angle) (Chapter 5)
101. d. Item a is for gray-scale instruments. (Chapter 5)
102. b. (Chapter 7)
103. e. Shift increases to 4 kHz, which is still less than the Nyquist limit (4.5 kHz). (Chapter 5)
104. a. A nonzero Doppler angle increases calculated equivalent flow speed. (Chapter 5)
105. c. The Nyquist limit is still one half of the pulse repetition frequency. (Chapter 5)
106. e. (Chapter 5)
107. e. (Chapters 5 and 6)
108. e. (a and c) (Chapter 5)
109. e. (a and b; c increases the amount of color) (Chapter 5)
110. d. Item c is not strictly part of the color flow display. Also, it is not a cross-sectional display but rather a frequency-versus-time presentation. (Chapter 5)
111. b. White is brighter than gray. (Chapter 5)
112. a. Red and green are different hues, representing different light wave frequencies. (Chapter 5)
113. e. (a, b, c; about 5 to 50 frames per second are displayed) (Chapter 5)
114. d. (Chapter 5)
115. d. (Chapter 5)
116. a. The wall filter removes the lower-frequency clutter Doppler shifts. (Chapter 5)
117. d. (twice as many scan lines per frame) (Chapter 5)
118. e. Items c and d change because the scan line (pulse path) orientation changes. (Chapter 5)
119. a. Items b and c increase the amount of color. (Chapter 5)
120. d. Increasing pulse repetition frequency increases the Nyquist limit, reducing aliasing. (Chapter 5)
121. b. (Chapter 2)
122. e. The wavelength is the length of each cycle in a pulse. (Chapter 2)
123. a. Duty factor is pulse duration divided by pulse repetition period. (Chapter 2)
124. b. The attenuation coefficient of 5-MHz ultrasound is approximately 2.5 dB/cm. The attenuation coefficient multiplied by the path length yields the attenuation (in decibels). Only answer b is given in attenuation (decibel) units. (Chapter 2)
125. b. Amplitude is the maximum amount that an acoustic variable varies from the normal value (in this case, 10−7=3 units). (Chapter 2)

126. a. (Chapter 2)
127. a. Amplitude, intensity, power, and beam area are related to one another. If two of these are known, the others can be found. Frequency is independent of these. All four of them can be known, and yet frequency remains undetermined. (Chapter 2)
128. a. Impedance 1 equals 3, which equals impedance 2; thus there is no reflection. (Chapter 2)
129. b. If 96% of the intensity is transmitted, 4% is reflected because what is not reflected is transmitted (i.e., the two must add up to 100%). (Chapter 2)
130. c. (Chapter 5)
131. c. If the second speed is twice the first speed, then the transmission angle is approximately twice the incidence angle. (Chapter 2)
132. a. Reflector distance × speed × time. (Chapter 2)
133. d. If reflectors are separated by less than the axial resolution, they are not separated on the display. (Chapter 3)
134. b. Axial resolution is equal to one half the spatial pulse length. Spatial pulse length is equal to the number of cycles in the pulse multiplied by wavelength. Wavelength is equal to propagation speed divided by frequency. For 1 MHz, wavelength is 1.54 mm, spatial pulse length is 2 × 1.54, and axial resolution is 1.54 mm, so two reflectors separated by 1 mm would not be resolved. For 2 MHz, the resolution is 0.77, and the reflectors would be resolved. (Chapter 3)
135. a. For highly damped transducers the quality factor (Q) is approximately equal to the number of cycles in the pulse. (Chapter 3)
136. b. Beam width changes with distance from transducer and thus so does lateral resolution. (Chapter 3)
137. c. Near-zone length increases with transducer diameter so that the only transducer that would have a shorter near-zone length would be a transducer of smaller diameter. (Chapter 3)
138. c. Focusing can be accomplished only in the near zone of a beam. (Chapter 3)
139. e. Answers a, b, and c affect the beam. Resolution of the system also is affected by the electronics of the instrument. (Chapter 3)
140. a. All the others are characteristics of the sound. (Chapter 2)
141. c. Frequency, period, wavelength, and propagation speed are related to one another. However, all four of these can be known, and yet the amplitude is undetermined. (Chapter 2)
142. e. For perpendicular incidence, there is no refraction. For equal impedances, there is no reflection. (Chapter 2)
143. d. (Chapter 2)

$$\text{IRC} = \left(\frac{2.64-1.00}{2.64+1.00}\right)^2 = \left(\frac{1.64}{3.64}\right)^2 = (0.45)^2 = 0.2$$

For an intensity reflection coefficient (IRC) of 0.2 and an incident intensity of 1, the reflected intensity is 0.2 and the transmitted intensity is 0.8. (Chapter 2)
144. d. (Chapters 4 and 7)
145. d. Incidence angle always equals the reflection angle. For equal propagation speeds, incidence angle equals the transmission angle as well. (Chapter 2)
146. a. For oblique incidence, it is possible to have no reflection, even if the media impedances are unequal. (Chapter 2)
147. e. Increased transducer damping decreases the spatial pulse length. Increasing spatial pulse length is accompanied by increased pulse duration and degraded axial resolution. (Chapters 2 and 3)
148. c. (Chapter 2)
149. b. Wavelength is equal to propagation speed divided by frequency. (Chapter 2)
150. b. Spatial pulse length is equal to wavelength multiplied by the number of cycles in the pulse. (Chapter 2)
151. d. (Chapter 3)
152. e. No refraction means that there is no change in sound direction. This is a result of no change in propagation speed (i.e., equal propagation speeds on both sides of the boundary). (Chapter 2)
153. e. If there is 1 W in each square centimeter of area, then there are 5 W in 5 cm^2 of area. (Chapter 2)
154. c. Speeds in solids are higher than in liquids. Soft tissue behaves acoustically as a liquid (as it is mostly water). (Chapter 2)
155. d. (Chapter 2)
156. c. An unfocused 13-mm transducer has a beam width of 6.5 mm at the near-zone length. Focusing would reduce the lateral resolution below this value (i.e., improve it). (Chapter 3)
157. b. A 7.5-MHz transducer can image to a depth of only a few centimeters in tissue. (Chapter 2)
158. a. The other answers make little sense. (Chapter 4)
159. d. (a and b) (Chapter 4)
160. b. For each 10 dB, there is a factor of 10 increase in power. (Chapter 4)
161. c. (Chapter 4)
162. b. (Chapter 4)
163. e. Decimal numbers greater than 15 require at least five bits in a binary number. The number 30 in binary is 11110. (Chapter 4)
164. False. Sixty-four shades require a 6-bit memory. (Chapter 4)
165. e. (Chapter 4)
166. False. This is a description of a linear sequenced array rather than a phased array. (Chapter 3)
167. b. (Chapter 3)

$$\text{AR} = \frac{1}{2}\text{SPL} = 0.5 \times n \times c/f = \left(\frac{1}{2}\right)(2)(1.54/5) = 0.3$$

168. False. Postprocessing is the assignment of display brightness to numbers coming out of memory. (Chapter 4)
169. e. (Chapter 3)
170. a. (Chapter 3)
171. b. In M mode, echo depth is displayed as a function of time. (Chapter 4)
172. c. (Chapter 2)
173. a. (Chapter 4)

174. e. (1 + 8 = 9) (Chapter 4)
175. a. (Chapter 6)
176. c. The instrument assumes a speed of 1.54 mm/μs. Echoes will arrive sooner because of their higher propagation speed and will be placed closer to the transducer than they should be. (Chapters 2 and 6)
177. a. (Chapter 4)
178. a. Increasing gain or decreasing attenuation increases echo intensity. (Chapters 2 and 4)
179. d. (Chapter 4)
180. b. (Chapters 3 and 4)
181. e. (Chapter 4)
182. e. Multiple pulses per scan line (ensemble length) are required for color-Doppler imaging. More pulses per scan line for multiple foci would make the frame rate unacceptably low. (Chapter 5)
183. c. A reduction of 3 dB is a 50% reduction. (Chapter 4)
184. d. See answer to Exercise 183. (Chapter 4)
185. c. (Chapter 4)
186. b. A factor of 8 is three doublings (i.e., 3 + 3 + 3 dB). (Chapter 4)
187. a. (Chapter 7
188. a. (Chapter 7)
189. e. (Chapter 3)
190. a. (Chapters 2 and 4)
191. c. (Chapter 4)
192. c. (Chapter 4)
193. e. Transmission output side (to the transducer) of a beam former is analog. (Chapters 3 and 4)
194. e. Reception output side of a beam former (to the signal processor) is digital. (Chapter 4)
195. d. (Chapter 3)
196. c. (Chapter 3)
197. e. Propagation speed is independent of frequency and intensity. (Chapter 2)
198. a. (Chapter 5)
199. e. (Chapter 2)
200. a. (Chapter 3)

A APPENDIX

Lists of Symbols

TABLE A-1 Listed by Symbol

Symbol	Represents
A	area
a	attenuation
a_c	attenuation coefficient
a_p	aperture
AR	axial resolution
c	propagation speed
cos	cosine
c_t	element propagation speed
d	diameter; distance to reflector; distance from transducer
DF	duty factor
d_f	focal beam diameter
f	frequency
f_D	Doppler-shift frequency
fl	focal length
f_o	operating frequency
FR	frame rate
f_R	received (echo) frequency
FR_m	maximum frame rate
I	intensity
I_i	incident intensity
I_r	reflected intensity
IRC	intensity reflection coefficient
I_t	transmitted intensity
ITC	intensity transmission coefficient
L	path length; tube length
LPF	lines per frame
LR	lateral resolution
n	number of cycles per pulse; number of foci; ensemble length
NL	Nyquist limit
P	power
p	pressure amplitude
PD	pulse duration
pen	penetration
PRF	pulse repetition frequency
PRP	pulse repetition period
Q	volumetric flow rate
R	flow resistance
r	radius
SPL	spatial pulse length
T	period
th	element thickness
v	flow speed, scatterer speed
v_a	average flow speed
w_b	beam width
z	impedance
ΔP	pressure difference; pressure drop
η	viscosity
θ_D	Doppler angle
θ_i	incidence angle
θ_r	reflection angle
θ_t	transmission angle
λ	wavelength
ρ	density

TABLE A-2 Listed by Parameter

Parameter	Represented by
aperture	a_p
area	A
attenuation	a
attenuation coefficient	a_c
average flow speed	v_a
axial resolution	AR
beam width	w_b
cosine	cos
density	ρ
diameter	d
distance from transducer	d
distance to reflector	d
Doppler angle	θ_D
Doppler-shift frequency	f_D
duty factor	DF
element propagation speed	c_t
element thickness	th
ensemble length	n
flow resistance	R
flow speed	v
focal beam diameter	d_f
focal length	fl
frame rate	FR
frequency	f
impedance	z
incidence angle	θ_i
incident intensity	I_i
intensity	I
intensity reflection coefficient	IRC
intensity transmission coefficient	ITC
lateral resolution	LR
lines per frame	LPF
maximum frame rate	FR_m
number of cycles per pulse	n
number of foci	n
Nyquist limit	NL
operating frequency	f_o
path length	L
penetration	pen
period	T
power	P
pressure amplitude	p
pressure difference	ΔP
pressure drop	ΔP
propagation speed	c
pulse duration	PD
pulse repetition frequency	PRF
pulse repetition period	PRP
radius	r
received (echo) frequency	f_R
reflected intensity	I_r
reflection angle	θ_r
scatterer speed	v
spatial pulse length	SPL
transmission angle	θ_t
transmitted intensity	I_t
tube length	L
viscosity	η
volumetric flow rate	Q
wavelength	λ

B APPENDIX

Compilation of Equations

For convenient reference, the equations in this book, except for those in the Advanced Concepts sections on the accompanying Evolve site, are compiled here.

Chapter 2

$$T\ (\mu s) = \frac{1}{f\ (MHz)}$$

$$\lambda\ (mm) = \frac{c\ (mm/\mu s)}{f\ (MHz)}$$

$$PRP\ (ms) = \frac{1}{PRF\ (kHz)}$$

$$PD\ (\mu s) = n \times T\ (\mu s)$$

$$DF = \frac{PD\ (\mu s)}{PRP\ (\mu s)} = \frac{PD\ (\mu s) \times PRF\ (kHz)}{1000}$$

$$SPL\ (mm) = n \times \lambda\ (mm)$$

$$I\ (mW/cm^2) = \frac{P\ (mW)}{A\ (cm^2)}$$

$$a\ (dB) = a_c\ (dB/cm) \times L\ (cm)$$

$$a\ (dB) = \frac{1}{2}(dB/cm\text{-}MHz) \times f\ (MHz) \times L\ (cm)$$

$$z\ (rayls) = \rho\ (kg/m^3) \times c\ (m/s)$$

$$IRC = \frac{I_r\ (W/cm^2)}{I_i\ (W/cm^2)} = \left[\frac{(z_2 - z_1)}{(z_2 + z_1)}\right]^2$$

$$ITC = \frac{I_t\ (W/cm^2)}{I_i\ (W/cm^2)} = 1 - IRC$$

$$\theta_i\ (degrees) = \theta_r\ (degrees)$$

$$d\ (mm) = \frac{1}{2}[c\ (mm/\mu s) \times t\ (\mu s)]$$

Chapter 3

$$f_o\ (MHz) = \frac{c_t\ (mm/\mu s)}{2 \times th\ (mm)}$$

$$AR\ (mm) = \frac{SPL\ (mm)}{2}$$

$$LR\ (mm) = w_b\ (mm)$$

Chapter 4

$$pen\ (cm) \times PRF\ (kHz) \leq 77\ (cm/ms)$$

$$PRF\ (Hz) = n \times LPF \times FR\ (Hz)$$

$$pen\ (cm) \times n \times LPF \times FR\ (Hz) \leq 77{,}000\ cm/s$$

Chapter 5

$$Q\ (mL/s) = \frac{\Delta P\ (dyne/cm^2)}{R\ (poise)}$$

$$R\ (g/cm^4\text{-}s) = 8 \times L\ (cm) \times \frac{\eta\ (poise)}{\pi \times [r^4 (cm^4)]}$$

$$Q\ (mL/s) = \frac{\Delta P\ (dyne/cm^2) \times \pi \times d^4\ (cm^4)}{128 \times L\ (cm) \times \eta\ (poise)}$$

$$\Delta P = 4(v_2)^2$$

$$f_D\ (kHz) = f_R\ (kHz) - f_o\ (kHz) = f_o\ (kHz) \times \frac{[2 \times v\ (cm/s)]}{c\ (cm/s)}$$

$$v\ (cm/s) = \frac{77\ (cm/ms) \times f_D\ (kHz)}{f_o\ (MHz)}$$

$$f_D\ (kHz) = \frac{[f_o\ (kHz) \times 2 \times v\ (cm/s) \times (\cos\theta)]}{c\ (cm/s)}$$

$$v\ (cm/s) = \frac{[77\ (cm/ms) \times f_D\ (kHz)]}{[f_o\ (MHz) \times \cos\theta]}$$

$$FR_m\ (Hz) = \frac{77{,}000\ (cm/s)}{pen\ (cm) \times LPF \times n}$$

Chapter 6

$$NL\ (kHz) = \frac{1}{2} \times PRF\ (kHz)$$

Chapter 7

$$MI = \frac{p_r\ (MPa)}{[f\ (MHz)]^{1/2}}$$

APPENDIX C

Mathematics Review

Algebra and trigonometry are used in the discussion of ultrasound and Doppler principles. Logarithms are involved in decibels, and binary numbers are involved in digital electronics. Mathematic concepts that are applicable to the material in this book are reviewed in this appendix. Relevant aspects of algebra, trigonometry, logarithms, scientific notation, binary numbers, units, and statistics are covered.

First, we review some mathematic terminology. In algebraic equations such as

$$x + y = z$$

$$x - y = z$$

x and *y* are called *terms.* Terms are connected with each other by addition or subtraction. With addition, the result is called the *sum.* With subtraction, the result is called the *difference.*

In the equations,

$$x \times y = z$$

$$\frac{x}{y} = z$$

x and *y* are called *factors.* Factors are connected with each other by multiplication or division. When multiplied, the result is called the *product.* When divided, the result is called the *quotient.*

The inverse or reciprocal of x is 1/x, sometimes described as "one over" x.

Algebra

Transposition of quantities in algebraic equations is accomplished by performing identical mathematical operations on both sides.

Example C-1

For the equation,

$$x + y = z$$

transpose to get x alone (solve for x). To do this, subtract y from both sides:

$$x + y - y = z - y$$

Because y − y = 0, the left-hand side of the equation is

$$x + y - y = x + 0 = x$$

so that

$$x = z - y$$

Example C-2

For the equation,

$$x - y = z$$

solve for x. Add y to both sides:

$$x - y + y = z + y$$

$$x + 0 = z + y$$

$$x = z + y$$

Example C-3

For the equation,

$$xy = z$$

solve for x. Divide both sides by y:

$$\frac{xy}{y} = \frac{z}{y}$$

Because y/y = 1

$$\frac{xy}{y} = x(1) = x$$

and

$$x = \frac{z}{y}$$

Example C-4

For the equation,

$$\frac{x}{y} = z$$

solve for x. Multiply both sides by y:

$$\left(\frac{x}{y}\right)y = zy$$

$$x(1) = zy$$

$$x = zy$$

Example C-5

Using some numbers, and combining the previous examples, consider the equation

$$\left(\frac{5x+3}{2}\right) - 3 = 1$$

and solve for x. First, add 3 to both sides:

$$\left(\frac{5x+3}{2}\right) - 3 + 3 = 1 + 3$$

$$\frac{5x+3}{2} = 4$$

Multiply by 2:

$$\left(\frac{5x+3}{2}\right)\times 2=4\times 2$$

$$5x+3=8$$

Subtract 3:

$$5x+3-3=8-3$$

$$5x=5$$

Divide by 5:

$$x=1$$

Substitution of the answer into the original equation shows that the equality is satisfied and the answer is correct:

$$\left[\frac{5(1)+3}{2}\right]-3=1$$

$$\left(\frac{8}{2}\right)-3=1$$

$$4-3=1$$

$$1=1$$

Example C-6

For the equation,

$$c=f\times\lambda$$

solve for wavelength. Divide by frequency:

$$\frac{c}{f}=\frac{f\times\lambda}{f}$$

$$\frac{c}{f}=\lambda$$

Example C-7

If the intensity reflection coefficient (IRC) is 0.1 and the reflected intensity (I_r) is 5 mW/cm^2, find the incident intensity (I_i), given that

$$IRC=\frac{I_r}{I_i}$$

Multiply by incident intensity:

$$IRC\times I_i=\frac{I_r}{I_i}\times I_i$$

Divide by intensity reflection coefficient:

$$\frac{IRC\times I_i}{IRC}=\frac{I_r}{IRC}$$

$$I_i=\frac{I_r}{IRC}=\frac{5\,mW/cm^2}{0.1}=50\,mW/cm^2$$

Example C-8

If the intensity reflection coefficient (IRC) is 0.01 and the impedance for medium 1 (z_1) is 4.5, find the medium 2 impedance (z_2), given that

$$IRC=\left(\frac{z_2-z_1}{z_2+z_1}\right)^2$$

Take the square root of each side:

$$IRC^{1/2}=\frac{z_2-z_1}{z_2+z_1}$$

Multiply by the sum of z_2 and z_1:

$$IRC^{1/2}\times(z_2+z_1)=(z_2-z_1)$$

Add z_1:

$$IRC^{1/2}\times(z_2+z_1)+z_1=z_2$$

Subtract $IRC^{1/2}\times z_2$:

$$(IRC^{1/2}\times z_1)+z_1=z_2-(IRC^{1/2}\times z_2)$$

$$z_1(1+IRC^{1/2})=z_2(1-IRC^{1/2})$$

Divide by (1 − $IRC^{1/2}$) and interchange sides of the equation:

$$z_2=z_1\left[\frac{(1+IRC^{1/2})}{(1-IRC^{1/2})}\right]$$

$$=4.5\left[\frac{1+(0.01)^{1/2}}{1-(0.01)^{1/2}}\right]$$

$$=4.5\left(\frac{1+0.1}{1-0.1}\right)=4.5\left(\frac{1.1}{0.9}\right)=4.5(1.22)=5.5$$

Trigonometry

If the sides and angles of a right triangle ("right" means one of the angles equals 90 degrees) are labeled as in Figure C-1, the sine of angle A (sin A), the cosine of angle A (cos A), and the tangent of angle A (tan A) are defined as follows:

$$\sin A=\frac{\text{length of side a}}{\text{length of side c}}$$

$$\cos A=\frac{\text{length of side b}}{\text{length of side c}}$$

$$\tan A=\frac{\text{length of side a}}{\text{length of side b}}$$

Example C-9

If the lengths of the sides a, b, and c are 1, $\sqrt{3}$, and 2, respectively, what are sin A and cos A?

$$\sin A=\frac{1}{2}=0.5$$

$$\cos A=\frac{\sqrt{3}}{2}=0.87$$

If the sine or cosine is known, angle A may be found using a calculator or a table such as Table C-1.

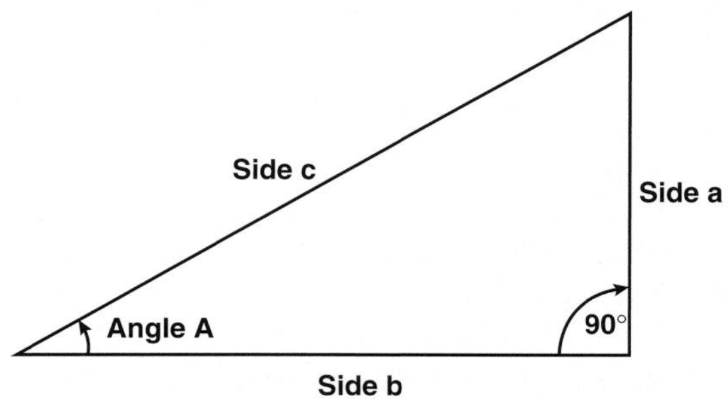

FIGURE C-1 If the sides and angles of a right triangle are labeled as in this figure, the cosine of angle A (cos A) is equal to the length of side b divided by the length of side c. Sine A is equal to the length of side a divided by the length of side c.

Example C-10

If sin A is 0.5, what is A? From Table C-1, A = 30 degrees.

Example C-11

If cos A is 0.87, what is A? From Table C-1, A = 30 degrees.

If angle A is known, sin A or cos A may be found by using a calculator or a table such as Table C-1.

Example C-12

If A = 45 degrees, what are the sin A and cos A? From Table C-1, sin A = 0.71 and cos A = 0.71.

Logarithms. The logarithm to the base 10 (log) of a number is equal to the number of tens that must be multiplied together to result in that number. More generally, the logarithm is the power to which 10 must be raised to give a particular number.

Example C-13

What is the logarithm of 1000? To obtain 1000, three tens must be multiplied together:

$$10 \times 10 \times 10 = 1000$$

Three tens then yield the logarithm (log) of 1000.

$$\log 1000 = 3$$

The logarithm of the reciprocal of a number is equal to the negative of the logarithm of the number.

Example C-14

What is the logarithm of 0.01?

$$0.01 = \frac{1}{100}$$

$$\log 100 = 2$$

$$\log 0.01 = \log \frac{1}{100} = -2$$

Decibels are quantities that result from taking 10 times the logarithm of the ratio of two powers or intensities.

Example C-15

Compare the following two powers in decibels: power 1 = 1 W; power 2 = 10 W.

$$10\log\left(\frac{\text{power 1}}{\text{power 2}}\right) = 10\log\left(\frac{1}{10}\right) = 10(-\log 10) = 10(-1) = -10\text{ dB}$$

TABLE C-1 Trigonometric Functions			
Angle (°)	**Sine**	**Cosine**	**Tangent**
0	0	1.00	0
30	0.50	0.87	0.58
45	0.71	0.71	1.00
60	0.87	0.50	1.73
90	1.00	0	∞

Note: The symbol ∞ indicates infinity or indeterminate; that is, dividing by zero can be executed an unlimited number of times.

Power 1 is 10 dB less than power 2, or power 1 is 10 dB below power 2. Also

$$10\log\left(\frac{\text{power 2}}{\text{power 1}}\right) = 10\log\left(\frac{10}{1}\right) = 10(\log 10) = 10(1) = 10\text{ dB}$$

Power 2 is 10 dB more than power 1, or power 2 is 10 dB above power 1.

Example C-16

An amplifier has a power output of 100 mW when the input power is 0.1 mW. What is the amplifier gain in decibels?

$$\text{amplifier gain (dB)} = 10\log\left(\frac{\text{power out}}{\text{power in}}\right)$$
$$= 10\log\left(\frac{100}{0.1}\right) = 10\log 1000 = 10(3) = 30\text{ dB}$$

Example C-17

An electric attenuator has a power output of 0.01 mW when the input power is 100 mW. What is the attenuation of the attenuator in decibels?

$$\text{attenuator attenuation (dB)} = -10\log\left(\frac{\text{power out}}{\text{power in}}\right)$$
$$= -10\log\left(\frac{0.01}{100}\right) = -10\log\left(\frac{1}{10{,}000}\right)$$
$$= -10(-\log 10{,}000)$$
$$= -10(-4) = 40\text{ dB}$$

The first minus sign is used in the equation to give the attenuation as a positive number. If the minus number had not been used, the "gain" of the attenuator would have been calculated, which would have turned out to be −40 dB. A gain of −40 dB is the same as an attenuation of 40 dB.

Example C-18

Compare intensity 2 with intensity 1; intensity 1 = 10 mW/cm^2; intensity 2 = 0.01 mW/cm^2.

$$10\log\left(\frac{\text{intensity 2}}{\text{intensity 1}}\right) = 10\log\left(\frac{0.01}{10}\right)$$
$$= 10\log\left(\frac{1}{1000}\right) = 10(-\log 1000)$$
$$= 10(-3) = -30\text{ dB}$$

Intensity 2 is 30 dB less than or below intensity 1.

Example C-19

As sound passes through a medium, its intensity at one point is 1 mW/cm^2 and at a point 10 cm farther along is 0.1 mW/cm^2. What are the attenuation and attenuation coefficient? (See Chapter 2.)

$$\text{attenuation (dB)} = -10\log\left(\frac{\text{intensity at second point}}{\text{intensity at first point}}\right)$$
$$= -10\log\left(\frac{0.1}{1}\right) = -10\log\left(\frac{1}{10}\right)$$
$$= -10(-\log 10) = -10(-1) = 10\text{ dB}$$

See Example C-17 for comment on the first minus sign. The attenuation coefficient is the attenuation (dB) divided by the separation between the two points:

$$\text{attenuation coefficient (dB/cm)} = \frac{\text{attenuation (dB)}}{\text{separation (cm)}} = \frac{10 \text{ dB}}{10 \text{ cm}} = 1 \text{ dB/cm}$$

Example C-20

Show by example that log x^2 is equal to 2 log x.

Let x = 5.

Then log x = 0.70 and 2 log x = 1.40.

Thus x = 5^2 = 25 and log 25 = 1.40.

Example C-21

Power and intensity are proportional to amplitude squared. A power or intensity ratio expressed in decibels is calculated using the definition

$$10\log\left(\frac{\text{power 1}}{\text{power 2}}\right)$$

This is equivalent to

$$20\log\left(\frac{\text{amplitude 1}}{\text{amplitude 2}}\right)$$

as seen with the following values:

Amplitude 1 = 4

Amplitude 2 = 3

Power 1 = 4^2 = 16

Power 2 = 3^2 = 9

$$\text{power ratio (dB)} = 10\log\left(\frac{\text{power 1}}{\text{power 2}}\right) = 10\log\left(\frac{16}{9}\right) = 2.5$$

$$\text{amplitude ratio (dB)} = 20\log\left(\frac{\text{amplitude 1}}{\text{amplitude 2}}\right) = 20\log\left(\frac{4}{3}\right) = 2.5$$

Table C-2 lists various values of power or intensity ratio with corresponding decibel values of gain or attenuation.

Some authors put output or end-of-path values in the numerator of the equation used for calculating decibels. If the numerator value is less than the denominator value (e.g., attenuation), a negative decibel value is calculated. For example, if the input and output powers for an electrical attenuator were 2 W and 1 W, respectively, −3 dB results; that is, this attenuator has −3 dB of gain. In this book, only positive decibel values are considered with clarification regarding whether attenuation or gain is considered. In this example, the result would be given as 3 dB of attenuation.

Scientific Notation

Scientific notation uses factors of 10, expressed in exponential form, to shorten the expression of very large or very small numbers. For example, 1,540,000 mm/s can be expressed as 1.54×10^6. In the expression x^y, x is called the base and y is called the exponent. When multiplying factors in scientific notation, the exponents are added. When dividing, the exponents are subtracted.

TABLE C-2 Decibel Values of Attenuation or Gain for Various Values of Power or Intensity Ratio*

Decibel Gain or Attenuation	Attenuation	Gain
1	0.79	1.3
3	0.50	2.0
6	0.25	4.0
10	0.10	10.0
30	0.001	1000
100	0.0000000001	10,000,000,000

*The ratio is output power or intensity divided by input power or intensity.

Example C-22

$$\frac{(1.54\times10^6 \text{ mm/s})\times(3.60\times10^3 \text{ s/hr})}{(1.61\times10^6 \text{ mm/mile})} = 3.44\times10^3 \text{ mph}$$

Here, the multiplication result is 5.54×10^9. Then the division by 1.61×10^6 yields 3.44×10^3.

Binary Numbers

The use of digital memories in ultrasound imaging instruments presents a need for understanding the binary numbering system. Digital (computer) memories and data processors use binary numbers in carrying out their functions because they contain electronic components that operate in only two states, off (0) and on (1).

Binary digits (bits) consist of only zeros and ones, represented by the symbols 0 and 1. As in the decimal numbering system, with which we are so familiar, other numbers must be represented by moving these symbols to different positions (columns). In the decimal system, where there are ten symbols (0 through 9), there is no symbol for the number ten (nine is the largest number for which there is a symbol). To represent ten in symbolic form, the symbol for one is used, moving it to the second (from the right) column. A zero is placed in the right column to clarify this so that ten is, symbolically, 10. The symbol for one has been used in such a way that it no longer represents one, but rather ten.

A similar procedure is used in the binary numbering system. The symbol 1 represents the largest number (one) for which there is a symbol in the system. To represent the next number (2), the same thing is done as in the decimal system; that is, the symbol 1 is placed in the next column to represent the number 2. Columns in the two systems represent values as follows:

....	millions	hundred-thousands	ten-thousands	thousands	hundreds	tens	ones

Decimal

....	sixty-fours	thirty-twos	sixteens	eights	fours	twos	ones

Binary

In the decimal system, each column represents 10 times the column to the right. In the binary system each column represents two times the column to the right.

The decimal number 1234 represents (reading from right to left) four ones, three tens, two hundreds, and one thousand; that is, 4 + 30 + 200 + 1000 = 1234. Likewise, the decimal number 10,110 represents zero ones, one ten, one hundred, zero thousands, and one ten thousand. The binary number 10110 represents zero ones, one two, one four, zero eights, and one sixteen, or 0 + 2 + 4 + 0 + 16 = 22 in decimal form. This represents a straightforward way of converting a number from the binary system to the decimal system.

Example C-23

Convert the binary number 101010 to decimal form. This number represents 0 + 2 + 0 + 8 + 0 + 32, or 42 in decimal form.

To convert a number from decimal to binary form, one must successively subtract the largest possible multiples of 2, which are the binary column values, in succession from the decimal number.

Example C-24

Convert the decimal number 60 to binary form:

a. Can 64 be subtracted from 60? No. (Enter 0 in the 64 column of the binary number.)

b. Can 32 be subtracted from 60? Yes. (Enter 1 in the 32 column.)
60 − 32 = 28 (the difference)

c. Can 16 be subtracted from 28? Yes. (Enter 1 in the 16 column.)
28 − 16 = 12 (the difference)

d. Can 8 be subtracted from 12? Yes. (Enter 1 in the 8 column.)
12 − 8 = 4 (the difference)

e. Can 4 be subtracted from 4? Yes. (Enter 1 in the 4 column.)
4 − 4 = 0 (the difference)

f. Can 2 be subtracted from 0? No. (Enter 0 in the 2 column.)

g. Can 1 be subtracted from 0? No. (Enter 0 in the 1 column.)

Therefore the decimal 60 equals 0111100 in the binary system. As in the decimal system, we normally drop leading zeroes, that is, those to the left of the first nonzero digit. The result is 111100. To check this answer, convert it back to decimal form. This number, 111100, reading from the right, represents 0 + 0 + 4 + 8 + 16 + 32, or 60 in decimal form.

TABLE C-3 Binary and Decimal Number Equivalents

Decimal	Binary	Decimal	Binary
0	000000	32	100000
1	000001	33	100001
2	000010	34	100010
3	000011	35	100011
4	000100	36	100100
5	000101	37	100101
6	000110	38	100110
7	000111	39	100111
8	001000	40	101000
9	001001	41	101001
10	001010	42	101010
11	001011	43	101011
12	001100	44	101100
13	001101	45	101101
14	001110	46	101110
15	001111	47	101111
16	010000	48	110000
17	010001	49	110001
18	010010	50	110010
19	010011	51	110011
20	010100	52	110100
21	010101	53	110101
22	010110	54	110110
23	010111	55	110111
24	011000	56	111000
25	011001	57	111001
26	011010	58	111010
27	011011	59	111011
28	011100	60	111100
29	011101	61	111101
30	011110	62	111110
31	011111	63	111111

Table C-3 lists the binary forms of the decimal numbers 0 to 63. Numbers 64 to 127 would have one additional digit, and so forth with higher multiples of 2.

TABLE C-4 Units and Unit Symbols for Physics and Acoustic Quantities

Quantity	Unit	Unit Symbol or Abbreviation
Acceleration	meters/second^2	m/s^2
Angle	degrees	°
Area	meters^2	m^2
Attenuation	decibels	dB
Attenuation coefficient	decibels/meter	dB/m
Beam area	meters^2	m^2
Current	amperes	A
Density	kilograms/meter^3	kg/m^3
Displacement	meters	m
Doppler shift	hertz	Hz
Energy	joules	J
Force	newtons	N
Frequency	hertz	Hz
Gain	decibels	dB
Heat	joules	J
Impedance	rayls	—
Intensity	watts/meter^2	W/m^2
Mass	kilograms	kg
Period	seconds	s
Power	watts	W
Pressure	newtons/meter^2	N/m^2
Propagation speed	meters/second	m/s
Pulse duration	seconds	s
Pulse repetition frequency	hertz	Hz
Pulse repetition period	seconds	s
Resistance	ohms	Ω
Spatial pulse length	meters	m
Speed	metes/second	m/s
Stiffness	newtons/meter^2	N/m^2
Temperature	degrees Kelvin	K
Time	seconds	s
Velocity	meters/second	m/s
Voltage	volts	V
Volume	meters^3	m^3
Wavelength	meters	m
Work	joules	J

Units

Units for the physics and acoustics quantities discussed in this book are presented in this section. They are drawn primarily from the international system of units (SI).

Table C-4 lists units for the quantities discussed in this book. Table C-5 gives equivalent units. Table C-6 lists prefixes for units, and Table C-7 gives conversion factors between common units.

In algebraic equations involving these units, the units for the quantity solved for are determined by manipulation of the units for the other quantities in the equation.

Example C-25

Determine the unit for frequency in the equation

$$\text{frequency} = \frac{\text{propagation speed (m/s)}}{\text{wavelength (m)}}$$

TABLE C-5 Equivalent Units for Physics and Acoustics Quantities

Unit Given in Table C-4	Equivalent Unit	Equivalent Unit Abbreviation
Hertz	1/second	1/s
Joules	newton-meters	N-m
Joules	watt-seconds	W-s
Rayls	kilograms/meter^2-second	kg/m^2-s
Newtons	kilogram-meters/second^2	kg-m/s^2
Newtons/meter	pascals	Pa
Watts	joules/second	J/s

TABLE C-6 Unit Prefixes

Prefix	Factor*	Symbol or Abbreviation
mega	1,000,000	M
kilo	1,000	k
centi	0.01	c
milli	0.001	m
micro	0.000001	μ

*Factor is the number of unprefixed units in a unit with the prefix. For example, there are 1000 Hz in 1 kHz, and there is 0.001 m in 1 mm.

TABLE C-7 Conversion Factors Among Common Units

To Convert	From	To	Multiply by
Area	m^2	cm^2	10,000
	cm^2	m^2	0.0001
Displacement	m	mm	1,000
	m	cm	100
	m	km	0.001
	mm	m	0.001
	mm	km	0.000001
	km	mm	1,000,000
Frequency	Hz	kHz	0.001
	Hz	MHz	0.000001
	kHz	MHz	0.001
	MHz	kHz	1,000
	kHz	Hz	1,000
	MHz	Hz	1,000,000
Intensity	W/cm^2	W/m^2	10,000
	W/cm^2	kW/m^2	10
	W/cm^2	mW/cm^2	1,000
	W/m^2	W/cm^2	0.0001
	W/m^2	mW/cm^2	0.1
	W/m^2	kW/m^2	0.001
Speed	m/s	km/s	0.001
	km/s	m/s	1,000
	km/s	mm/μs	1

The units on the right-hand side of the equation are

$$\frac{m/s}{m} = \frac{1}{s}$$

From Table C-5, it can be found that

$$\frac{1}{s} = Hz$$

Therefore the frequency unit is hertz.

Example C-26

Determine the unit for frequency in the equation

$$\text{frequency} = \frac{\text{propagation speed (m/s)}}{\text{wavelength (mm)}}$$

The units on the right-hand side of the equation are

$$\frac{m/s}{mm}$$

From Table C-6, it can be found that 1 mm equals 0.001 m, so that

$$\frac{m/s}{0.001\,m} = 1000\,1/s$$

and from Tables C-5 and C-6,

$$1000\ 1/s = 1000\ Hz = 1\,kHz$$

Therefore the frequency unit is kilohertz. To convert a frequency given in kilohertz to megahertz, multiply by 0.001. To convert a frequency given in kilohertz to hertz, multiply by 1000.

Example C-27

Determine the unit for intensity in the equation

$$\text{intensity} = \frac{\text{power (W)}}{\text{area (cm}^2\text{)}}$$

The units on the right-hand side of the equation are W/cm^2; therefore the intensity unit is watts per centimeter squared.

Example C-28

Determine the unit for impedance in the equation

$$\text{impedance} = \text{density (kg/m}^3\text{)} \times \text{propagation speed (km/s)}$$

The units on the right-hand side of the equation are

$$kg/m^3 \times km/s$$

From Table C-6,

$$kg/m^3 \times km/s = kg/m^3 \times 1000\,m/s = 1000\,kg/m^2{\cdot}s$$

From Table C-5,

$$1000\,kg/m^2{\cdot}s = 1000\ \text{rayls}$$

From Table C-6,

$$1000\ \text{rayls} = 1\ \text{krayl}$$

Therefore the impedance unit is kilorayl. Because this is uncommon, it would be better to keep the result in rayls.

TABLE C-8 Definitions of Numbers in Groups Tested*

Test Result	Disease	Nondiseased	Total
Positive	TPV	FPV	TP
Negative	FNV	TNV	TN
Total	TD	TND	TOT

*A positive test indicates disease. A negative test indicates disease-free. FNV (false-negative value), the number of diseased persons testing negative; FPV (false-positive value), the number of nondiseased persons who tested positive; TD, the total number of diseased persons; TN, the total number of persons testing negative; TND, the total number of nondiseased persons; TNV (true-negative value), the number of disease-free persons testing negative; TOT, the total number of persons in the study; TP, the total number of persons testing positive; TPV (true-positive value), the number of diseased persons (in the study) testing positive.

Statistics

Several concepts are used in evaluating the usefulness of diagnostic tests. These tests can be qualitative, as in the case of interpreting an anatomic image, or they can be quantitative, as with Doppler flow values. Diagnoses are positive and negative; that is, the test indicates the presence or absence of disease. Table C-8 defines the various groups involved in testing for disease.

The sensitivity (SENS) of a test is the proportion of those having the disease (TD) who test positive (TPV):

$$SENS = \frac{TPV}{TD}$$

The specificity (SPEC) of a test is the proportion of those who are disease-free (TND) who test negative (TNV):

$$SPEC = \frac{TNV}{TND}$$

The positive predictive value (PPV) of a test is the proportion of all positive (TP) test results that are correct, that is, the number of true positive results (TPV):

$$PPV = \frac{TPV}{TP}$$

The positive predictive value is the probability that a person who tests positive actually has the disease.

The negative predictive value (NPV) of a test is the proportion of all negative (TN) test results that are correct, that is, the number of true negative results (TNV):

$$NPV = \frac{TNV}{TN}$$

The negative predictive value is the probability that a person who tests negative is actually disease-free.

The accuracy (ACC) of a test is the proportion of all tests in the study (TOT) that have the correct result

$$ACC = \frac{(TPV + TNV)}{TOT}$$

Example C-29

Given the following table, calculate TD, TND, TP, TN, TOT, SENS, SPEC, PPV, NPV, and ACC.

Test Result	Disease	Nondiseased	Total
Positive	8	2	TP
Negative	5	85	TN
Total	TD	TND	TOT
Test Result	**Disease**	**Nondiseased**	**Total**
Positive	8	2	10
Negative	5	85	90
Total	13	87	100

$$\text{SENS} = \frac{8}{13} = 0.62$$

$$\text{SPEC} = \frac{85}{87} = 0.98$$

$$\text{PPV} = \frac{8}{10} = 0.80$$

$$\text{NPV} = \frac{85}{90} = 0.94$$

$$\text{ACC} = \frac{(8+85)}{100} = 0.93$$

EXERCISES

1. Solve each of the following for x:
   a. $x + y + 2 = z$
   b. $x - y = z - 1$
   c. $2xy = z$
   d. $\frac{x}{y} = 3z$
   e. $\frac{(x+5)}{4} - 2 = 4$
   f. $\frac{(3x+3)}{2} - 2 = 4$
2. Solve each of the following for the quantity with the asterisk:
   a. propagation speed = frequency* × wavelength
   b. $\text{intensity} = \frac{\text{power}}{\text{beam area}^*}$
   c. $\text{period} = \frac{1}{\text{frequency}^*}$
3. The age of an ultrasound instrument is equal to 3 times its age 3 years from now minus 3 times its age 3 years ago. What is its present age?
4. Let

$$y + x = \frac{1}{2}(7y - 3x)$$

   a. Subtract 2x from both sides so that

$$y - x = \frac{1}{2}(7y - 3x) - 2x$$

   b. Divide both sides by (y − x):

$$\frac{(y-x)}{(y-x)} = \frac{(7y-3x)}{2(y-x)} - \frac{2x}{(y-x)}$$

   c. Combine right side into single fraction:

$$\frac{(y-x)}{(y-x)} = \frac{(7y-3x-4x)}{2(y-x)} = \frac{7(y-x)}{2(y-x)}$$

   d. Multiply both sides by 2:

$$2\left[\frac{(y-x)}{(y-x)}\right] = 7\left[\frac{(y-x)}{(y-x)}\right]$$

   Therefore 2 = 7. What went wrong?
5. If side a, b, and c in Figure C-1 have lengths of 3, 4, and 5, respectively, then sin A is ___________ and cos A is___________.
6. If angle A is 90 degrees, sin A is ___________ and cos A is ___________.
7. If sin A is 0.17, angle A is ___________ degrees.
8. If cos A is 0.94, angle A is ___________ degrees.
9. Give the logarithms of the following numbers:
   a. 10 ___________
   b. 0.1 ___________
   c. 100 ___________
   d. 0.001 ___________
10. One watt is ___________ dB below 100 W.
11. One watt is ___________ dB above 100 mW.
12. If the input power is 1 mW and the output is 10,000 mW, the gain is ___________ dB.
13. If the input power is 1 W and the output is 100 mW, the gain is ___________ dB. The attenuation is ___________ dB.
14. If the intensities of traveling sound are 10 mW/cm^2 and 0.1 mW/cm^2 at two points 5 cm apart, the attenuation between the two points is ___________ dB. The attenuation coefficient is ___________ dB/cm.
15. If an amplifier has a gain of 33 dB, the ratio of output power to input power is ___________. (Use Table C-2.)
16. If an attenuator has an attenuation of 26 dB, the ratio of output power to input power is ___________. (Use Table C-2.)
17. If the intensity at the start of a path is 3 mW/cm^2 and the attenuation over the path is 13 dB, the intensity at the end of the path is ___________ mW/cm^2. (Use Table C-2.)
18. If the output of a 22-dB gain amplifier is connected to the input of a 24-dB gain amplifier, the total gain is ___________ dB. The overall power ratio is___________. (Use Table C-2.)
19. If a 17-dB attenuator is connected to a 14-dB amplifier, the net gain is ___________ dB. The net attenuation is ___________ dB. For a 1-W input, the output is ___________ W. (Use Table C-2.)
20. In binary numbers, how many symbols are used? ___________

21. The term binary digit commonly is shortened into the single word ___________.
22. Each binary digit in a binary number is represented in memory by a memory element, which at any time is in one of ___________ states.
23. Match the following:
Column in a binary number hgfedcba:
a. ___________
b. ___________
c. ___________
d. ___________
e. ___________
f. ___________
g. ___________
h. ___________
Decimal number represented by a 1 in the column:
1. 64
2. 32
3. 1
4. 16
5. 8
6. 128
7. 2
8. 4
24. The binary number 10110 represents zero ones, one two, one four, zero eights, and one sixteen, that is, 0 + 2 + 4 + 0 + 16 = 22. What decimal number is represented by the binary number 11001? ___________
25. The decimal number 13 is made up of one one, zero twos, one four, and one eight (8 + 4 + 0 + 1 = 13). The decimal number therefore is represented by the binary number ___________.
26. Match the following:

a. 1 ___________	1. 0001111
b. 5 ___________	2. 0011001
c. 10 ___________	3. 0001010
d. 15 ___________	4. 0110010
e. 20 ___________	5. 0000001
f. 25 ___________	6. 1100100
g. 30 ___________	7. 0101000
h. 40 ___________	8. 0011110
i. 50 ___________	9. 0010100
j. 100 ___________	10. 0000101

27. How many binary digits are required in the binary numbers representing the following numbers?
a. 0 ___________
b. 1 ___________
c. 5 ___________
d. 10 ___________
e. 25 ___________
f. 30 ___________
g. 63 ___________
h. 64 ___________
i. 75 ___________
j. 100 ___________
28. Match the following:
Largest decimal number that can be represented by a binary number with this many bits:

a. 7 ___________	1. 1
b. 15 ___________	2. 2
c. 3 ___________	3. 3
d. 511 ___________	4. 4
e. 1023 ___________	5. 5
f. 63 ___________	6. 6
g. 255 ___________	7. 7
h. 1 ___________	8. 8
i. 127 ___________	9. 9
j. 31 ___________	10. 10

29. How many bits are required to store numbers representing each number of different gray shades?
a. 2 ___________
b. 4 ___________
c. 8 ___________
d. 15 ___________
e. 16 ___________
f. 25 ___________
g. 32 ___________
h. 64 ___________
i. 65 ___________
j. 128 ___________
30. The unit of frequency in the equation

$$\text{frequency} = \frac{\text{propagation speed(km/s)}}{\text{wavelength (mm)}}$$

is ___________. To convert frequency in this unit to frequency in kilohertz, multiply by ___________.
31. A frequency of 50 kHz is equal to ___________ MHz and ___________ Hz.
32. A speed of 1.5 mm/μs is equal to ___________ km/s, ___________ m/s, ___________ cm/s, and ___________ mm/s.
33. If the frequency is 2 MHz and

$$\text{period} = \frac{1}{\text{frequency}}$$

the period is ___________ μs, ___________ ms, or ___________ s.
34. Mass is given in units of ___________.
a. megahertz
b. kilogram
c. degrees Kelvin
d. watt
e. none of the above
35. Displacement is given in ___________.
a. megahertz
b. decibel
c. ohm
d. meter
e. all of the above

36. Attenuation is given in ____________.
   a. decirayl
   b. deciwatt
   c. decibel
   d. decimeter
   e. decihertz
37. Given the following table, calculate TD, TND, TP, TN, TOT, SENS, SPEC, PPV, NPV, and ACC.

Test Result	Disease	Nondiseased	Total
Positive	80	20	TP
Negative	50	850	TN
Total	TD	TND	TOT

38. Solve the following for x and y:

$$x + y = 1 \quad x - y = 2$$

ANSWERS

1. a. z − y − 2; b. y + z − 1; c. z/2y; d. 3yz; e. 19; f. 3
2.
   a. $\frac{\text{propagation speed}}{\text{wavelength}}$
   b. $\frac{\text{power}}{\text{intensity}}$
   c. $\frac{1}{\text{period}}$
3. 18
4. Division by zero is what went wrong. Note that

$$y + x = \frac{1}{2}(7y - 3x)$$

yields

$$2(y + x) = 7y - 3x$$
$$2y + 2x = 7y - 3x$$
$$5x = 5y$$
$$x = y$$

so that dividing by (y − x) is dividing by zero (not allowed in algebra).
5. 0.6, 0.8
6. 1, 0
7. 10
8. 20
9. a, 1; b, −1; c, 2; d, −3
10. 20
11. 10
12. 40
13. −10, 10
14. 20, 4
15. 2000
16. 0.0025
17. 0.15
18. 46, 40,000
19. −3, 3, 0.50
20. Two (0, 1)
21. Bit
22. Two (off, on)
23. a, 3; b, 7; c, 8; d, 5; e, 4; f, 2; g, 1; h, 6
24. 25
25. 1101
26. a, 5; b, 10; c, 3; d, 1; e, 9; f, 2; g, 8; h, 7; i, 4; j, 6
27. a, 1 (0); b, 1 (1); c, 3 (101); d, 4 (1010); e, 5 (11001); f, 5 (11110); g, 6 (111111); h, 7 (1000000); i, 7 (1001011); j, 7 (1100100)
28. a, 3 (111); b, 4 (1111); c, 2 (11); d, 9 (111111111); e, 10 (1111111111); f, 6 (111111); g, 8 (11111111); h, 1 (1); i, 7 (1111111); j, 5 (11111)
29. a, 1 (0, 1); b, 2 (00, 01, 10, 11); c, 3 (000, 001, 010, 011, 100, 101, 110, 111); d, 4; e, 4; f, 5; g, 5; h, 6; i, 7; j, 7
30. Megahertz, 1000
31. 0.05, 50,000
32. 1.5, 1500, 150,000, 1,500,000
33. 0.5, 0.0005, 0.0000005
34. b
35. d
36. c
37.

Test Result	Disease	Nondiseased	Total
Positive	80	20	100
Negative	50	850	900
Total	130	870	1000

$$\text{SENS} = \frac{80}{130} = 0.62$$

$$\text{SPEC} = \frac{850}{870} = 0.98$$

$$\text{PPV} = \frac{80}{100} = 0.80$$

$$\text{NPV} = \frac{850}{900} = 0.94$$

$$\text{ACC} = \frac{(80 + 850)}{1000} = 0.93$$

38. $x = +3/2$

$y = -1/2$

Insertions of these values into the original equations verifies their correctness.

REFERENCES

1. Goldberg BB, Raichlen JS: *Ultrasound contrast agents*, London, 2001, Martin Dunitz.
2. Burns PN: Contrast agents for ultrasound. In Rumack CM, et al, editors: *Diagnostic ultrasound*, ed 4, St Louis, 2011, Elsevier/Mosby.
3. Gennisson JL, Deffieux T, Fink M, et al: Ultrasound elastography: principles and techniques, *Diagn Interv Imaging* 94: 487–496, 2013.
4. National Electrical Manufacturers Association: Digital Imaging and Communications in Medicine (DICOM) Set, Standards PS 3.1–3.16, Rosslyn, VA, 2003, National Electrical Manufacturers Association. Website: *http://medical.nema.org/dicom/*.
5. Nelson TR, Pretorius DH, Hull A, et al: Sources and impact of artifacts on clinical three-dimensional ultrasound imaging, *Ultrasound Obstet Gynecol* 16:374–383, 2000.
6. Baker KG, Robertson VJ, Duck FA: A review of therapeutic ultrasound, *Phys Ther* 81:1339–1350, 2001.
7. American Institute of Ultrasound in Medicine: *Routine quality assurance for diagnostic ultrasound equipment*, Laurel, MD, 2008, American Institute of Ultrasound in Medicine.
8. Harris GR: Progress in medical ultrasound exposimetry, *IEEE Trans Ultrason Ferroelectr Freq Control* 52:717–736, 2005.
9. AIUM bioeffects consensus report, *J Ultrasound Med* 27:499–644, 2008.
10. American Institute of Ultrasound in Medicine: *Medical ultrasound safety*, ed 3, Laurel, MD, 2014, American Institute of Ultrasound in Medicine.
11. Cibull SL, Harris GR, Nell DM: Trends in diagnostic ultrasound acoustic output from data reported to the US Food and Drug Administration for device indications that include fetal applications, *J Ultrasound Med* 32:192–193, 2013.
12. American Institute of Ultrasound in Medicine: *Recommended ultrasound terminology*, ed 3, Laurel, MD, 2008, American Institute of Ultrasound in Medicine.

INDEX

Pages followed by *b*, *t*, or *f* refer to boxes, tables, or figures, respectively.

Highlights from our research activities: Connect® French and McGraw-Hill LearnSmart®

- Over the last several years, we've brought together over 250 language professors from around the country to symposia and small-group forums in order to brainstorm new ideas and workshop solutions to the discipline's biggest challenges. The result is our new platform **Connect French**!

- Over 1,600 students, professors, and graduate teaching assistants beta-tested the **LearnSmart** platform for World Languages. The results were astounding: 91% of students said that **LearnSmart** led to success in their course and 97% said they would use **LearnSmart** in the future.

Special thanks to the instructors and students at **Boston College, College of Charleston, Florida Atlantic University, Boca Raton, Kennesaw State University, Portland State University, Texas State University, San Marcos, University of Minnesota, Twin Cities, and University of Rhode Island, Kingston,** for piloting **LearnSmart** for French during the Fall 2013 semester.

Key findings from the *Vis-à-vis* pre-revision reviews

We surveyed more than 100 introductory French instructors to find out how we could address the specific needs of the *Vis-à-vis* users. This is what we discovered:

- Reduced class hours and the demand for more hybrid and online courses limit the opportunities for meaningful instructor-student interaction in the target language. Instructors and students wanted more opportunities for oral communication, pronunciation practice, in and outside the classroom.

- Student engagement is a crucial factor in student success.

- More effective technology resources are needed to address the new course formats.

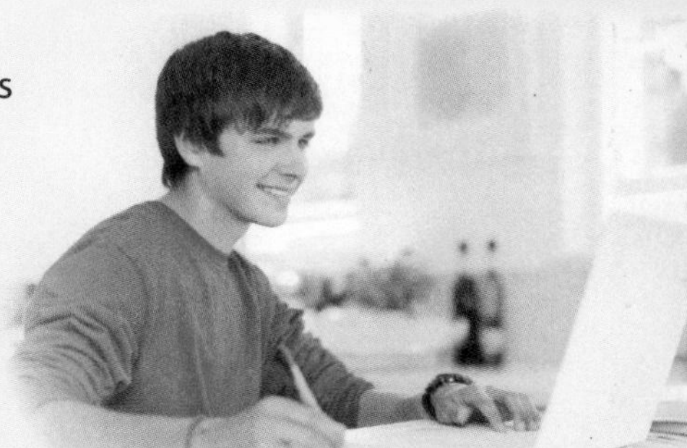

with more opportunities to listen, speak, record, and practice!

Mc Graw Hill Education | LEARNSMART®

Developed specifically for *Vis-à-vis*, **LearnSmart** for French is an intelligent learning system that uses a series of adaptive questions to pinpoint the unique knowledge gaps of each individual student. **LearnSmart** then provides them with an individualized learning path so that students spend less time in areas they already know and more time in areas they don't. The result is that students retain more knowledge, learn faster, study more efficiently, and come to French class better prepared to participate.

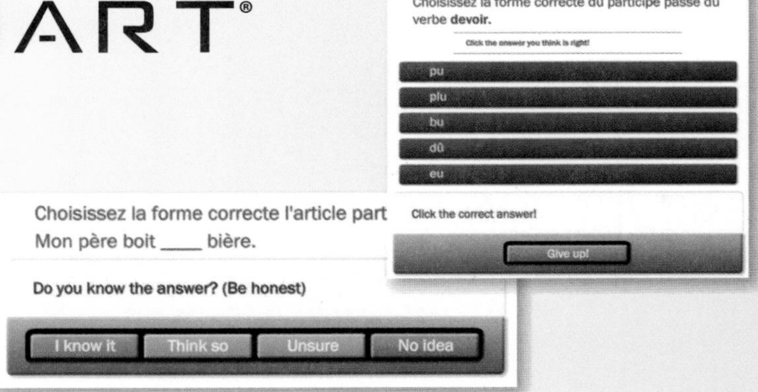
Choisissez la forme correcte du participe passé du verbe **devoir**.
pu
plu
bu
dû
eu
Click the correct answer!
Give up!
Choisissez la forme correcte l'article part
Mon père boit ____ bière.
Do you know the answer? (Be honest)
I know it
Think so
Unsure
No idea

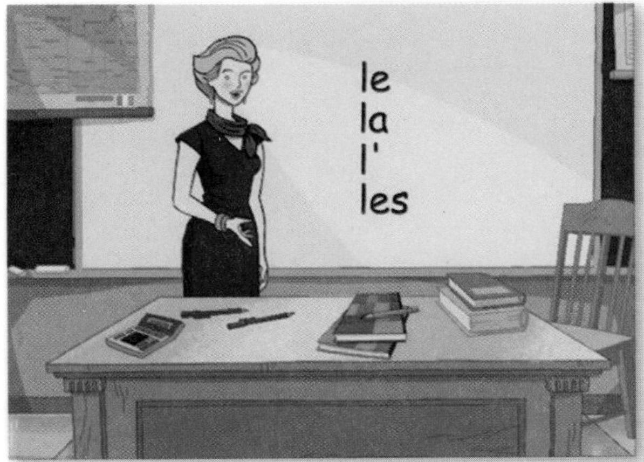
le
la
l'
les

Grammaire interactive tutorials

The **Grammaire interactive** tutorials work hand-in-hand with **LearnSmart** to provide students with the latest digital tools to improve their course outcomes. These tutorials, taught by an animated French instructor, are now available to students in **Connect French** as an alternative resource for reviewing and practicing core concepts. The practice quizzes that follow test students' mastery of the material.

What's New in the Sixth Edition?

- **Powerful digital tools: Connect® French** is McGraw-Hill's digital platform, which houses the eBook, the Workbook / Laboratory Manual activities, integrated audio and video, peer-editing writing tools, and voice tools, all of which vastly improve the quality of students' out-of-class work.

- **McGraw-Hill LearnSmart®** is the only super-adaptive learning tool on the market that is proven to significantly improve students' learning and course outcomes. As students work on each chapter's grammar and vocabulary modules, **LearnSmart** identifies the areas that students are struggling with most and provides them with the practice they need to master them. **LearnSmart** gives each student a unique learning experience tailored just for them. The **LearnSmart** mobile app allows students to study anytime and anywhere!

- **Contemporary language:** The **64 mini-dialogues** that introduce the grammar points in context have been completely rewritten and now feature the blog characters from the video and **Le blog de**… readings. The line art has been replaced by beautiful photos and the dialogues are presented in appealing, student-friendly formats: text messages, Blackboard IM video messages, and Facebook instant messages, in addition to face-to-face conversations. As in prior editions, the activity following each dialogue prompts students to use the structure in context before they delve into the explanation.

- **More pronunciation practice:** In response to reviewer feedback, the sixth edition offers a more robust treatment of pronunciation. These contextualized activities, which focus on the recognition and production of key sounds in French, build on the **Prononcez bien!** explanations that appear in the margins of each chapter. Both the explanations and the activities have been recorded and may be accessed and assigned in **Connect**.

- **Updated culture:** The **Reportage** readings between **Leçons 2** and **3** have been updated in **Chapitres 6, 9, 10,** and **11** to reflect the interests of today's students. The **Lecture** section of **Leçon 4** has also been revised. Among the five completely new readings in **Chapitres 1, 3, 9, 11,** and **13** are two literary texts, an article on Vélib' and Autolib', and a text with practical information on shopping in France.

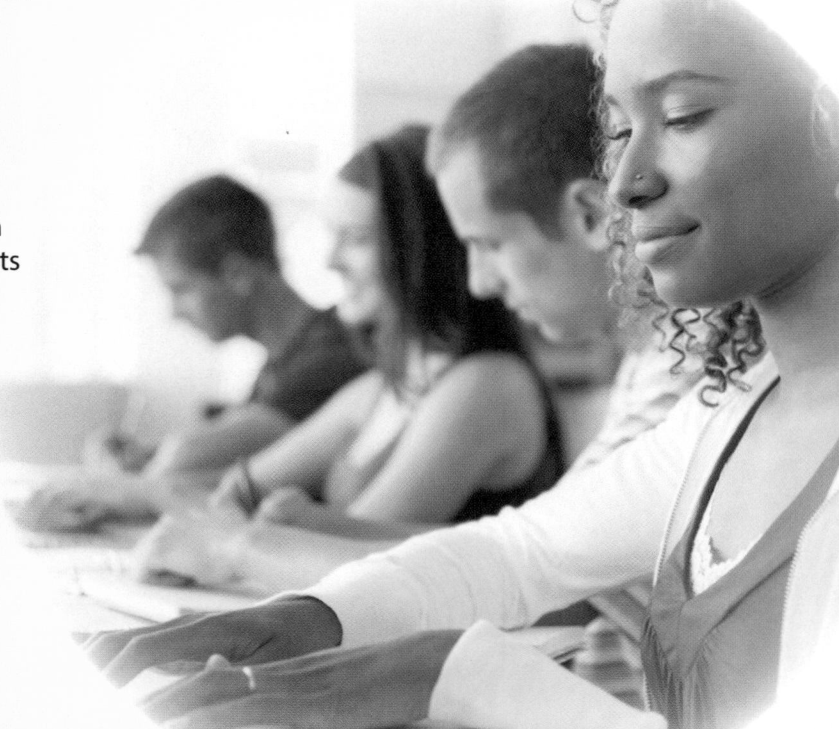

INSTRUCTOR'S EDITION

Vis-à-vis

Beginning French

SIXTH EDITION

Evelyne Amon

Judith A. Muyskens
Nebraska Wesleyan University

Alice C. Omaggio Hadley
Professor Emerita, University of Illinois, Urbana-Champaign

With contributions by:

Viviane Ruellot

Nicole Dicop-Hineline

Amanda LaFleur

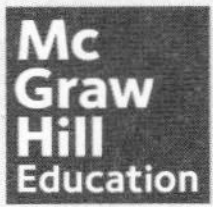

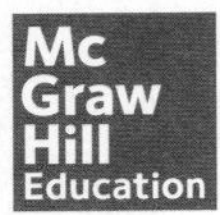

VIS-À-VIS: BEGINNING FRENCH, SIXTH EDITION
Published by McGraw-Hill Education, 2 Penn Plaza, New York, NY 10121.

Some ancillaries, including electronic and print components, may not be available to customers outside the United States.

This book is printed on acid-free paper.

1 2 3 4 5 6 7 8 9 0 DOW/DOW 1 0 9 8 7 6 5 4

ISBN 978–0–07–338647–8
MHID 0–07–338647–2

ISBN 978–1–259–13702–0 (Annotated Instructor's Edition)
MHID 1–259–13702–3

Senior Vice President, Products & Markets: *Kurt L. Strand*
Vice President, General Manager, Products & Markets: *Michael Ryan*
Vice President, Content Production & Technology Services: *Kimberly Meriwether David*
Managing Director: *Katie Stevens*
Senior Brand Manager: *Katherine K. Crouch*
Senior Director of Development: *Scott Tinetti*
Managing Development Editor: *Susan Blatty*
Director of Digital Content: *Janet Banhidi*
Digital Product Analyst: *Sarah Carey*
Digital Development Editor: *Laura Ciporen*
Senior Market Development Manager: *Helen Greenlea*
Executive Marketing Manager: *Craig Gill*
Senior Faculty Development Manager: *Jorge Arbujas*
Editorial Coordinators: *Leslie Briggs / Caitlin Bahrey*
Director, Content Production: *Terri Schiesl*
Content Project Manager: *Kelly A. Heinrichs*
Buyer: *Susan K. Culbertson*
Designer: *Matthew Backhaus*
Cover Image: *Stock Connection Blue/Alamy*
Content Licensing Specialist: *Brenda Rolwes*
Compositor: *Aptara®, Inc.*
Typeface: *10/12 New Aster*
Printer: *R. R. Donnelley*

All credits appearing on page or at the end of the book are considered to be an extension of the copyright page.

Library of Congress Cataloging-in-Publication Data

Amon, Evelyne.
Vis-à-vis: beginning French / Evelyne Amon, Judy Muyskens, Nebraska Wesleyan University; Alice Omaggio Hadley, Professor Emerita, University of Illinois, Urbana-Champaign; Viviane Ruellot, Western Michigan University.—Sixth Edition.
pages cm.
Includes index.
ISBN 978–0–07–338647–8—ISBN 0–07–338647–2 (hard copy : alk. paper)—ISBN 978–1–259–13702–0 (Annotated Instructor's Edition—ISBN 1–259–13702–3 (hard copy: alk. paper) 1. French language—Textbooks for foreign speakers—English. I. Muyskens, Judith A. II. Hadley, Alice Omaggio, 1947– III. Ruellot, Viviane. IV. Title.
PC2129.E5A48 2014
448.2'421–dc23 2013035280

The Internet addresses listed in the text were accurate at the time of publication. The inclusion of a website does not indicate an endorsement by the authors or McGraw-Hill Education, and McGraw-Hill Education does not guarantee the accuracy of the information presented at these sites.

www.mhhe.com

Contents

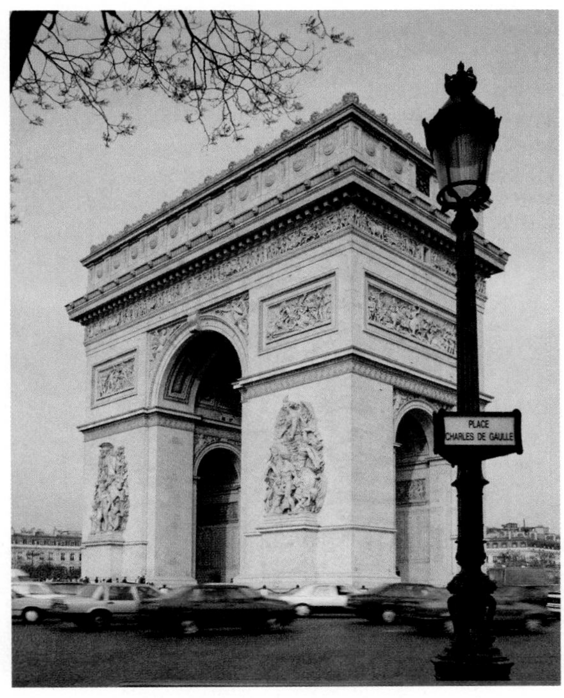

L'Arc de Triomphe, à Paris, en France

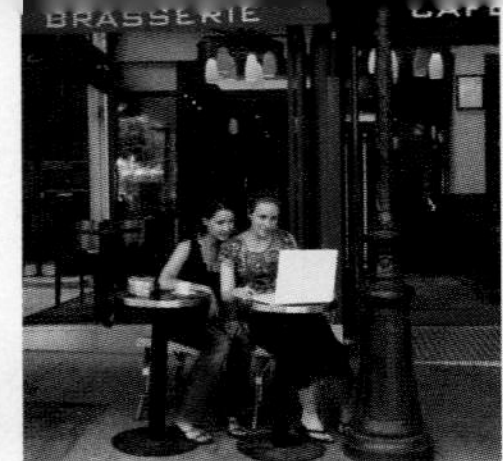
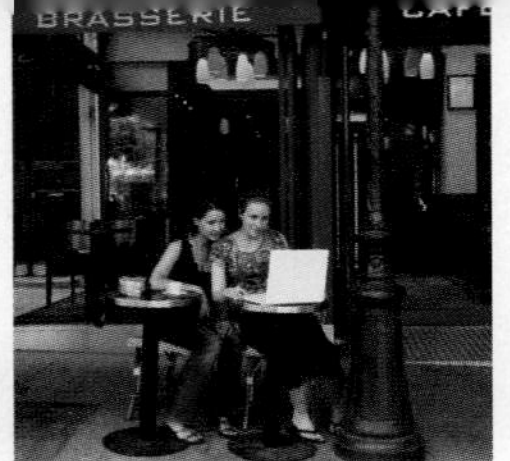

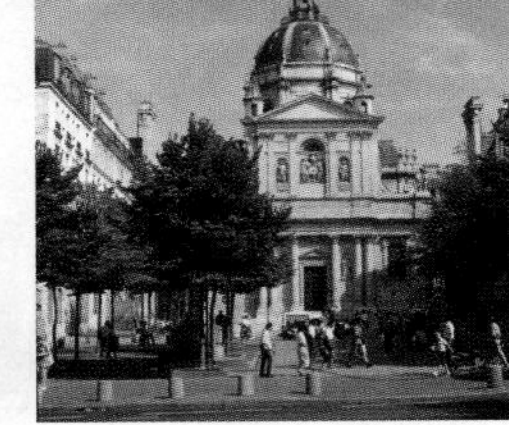

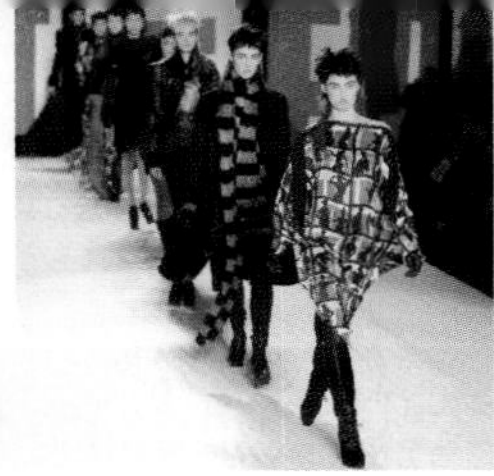

CHAPITRE 3

Elles ont l'air chic! 60

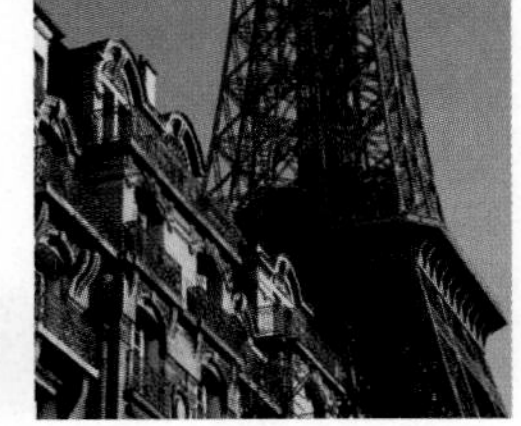

CHAPITRE 4

À la maison 90

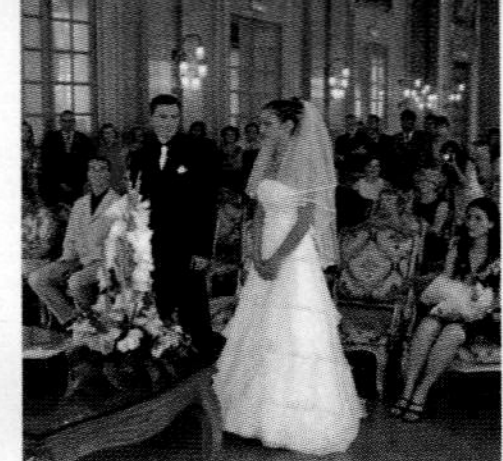

CHAPITRE 5

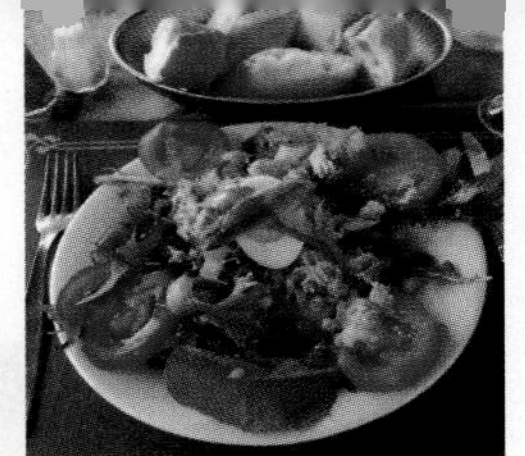

CHAPITRE 6

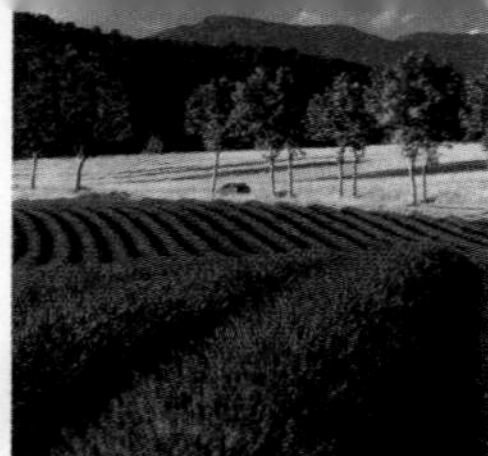

CHAPITRE 9

En route! 232

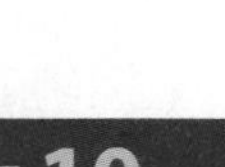

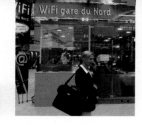

CHAPITRE 10

Comment communiquez-vous? 258

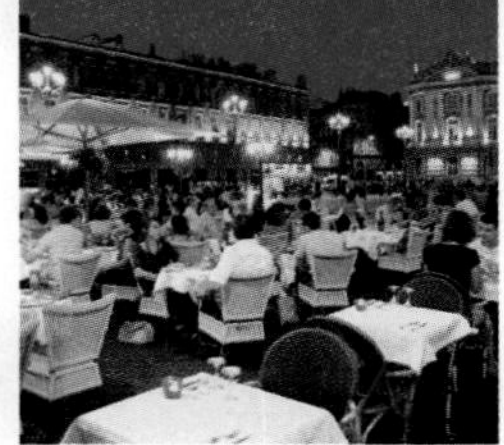

CHAPITRE 11

Vivre en ville 288

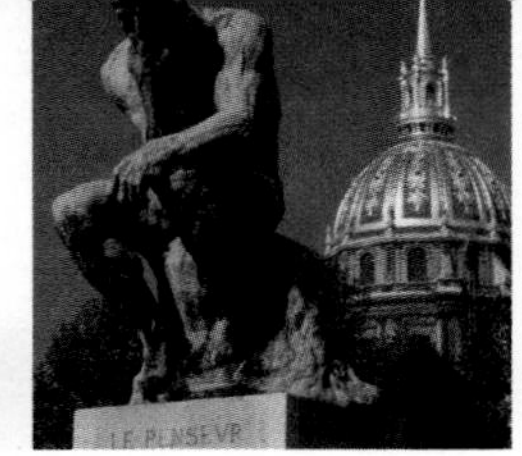

CHAPITRE 12

La passion pour les arts 318

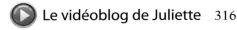

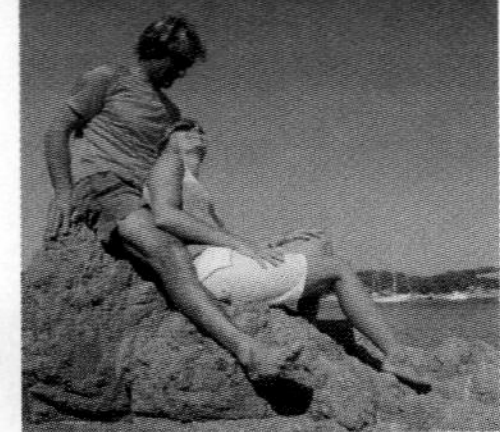

CHAPITRE **13**

La vie quotidienne 352

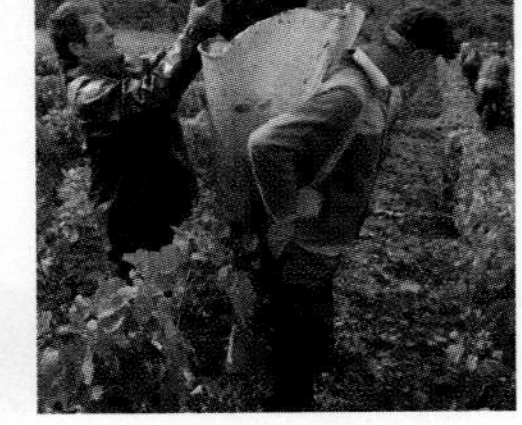

CHAPITRE **14**

Sur le marché du travail 376

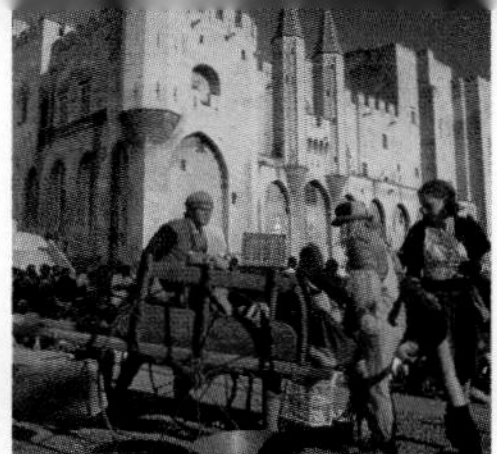

CHAPITRE **15**

Les loisirs 408

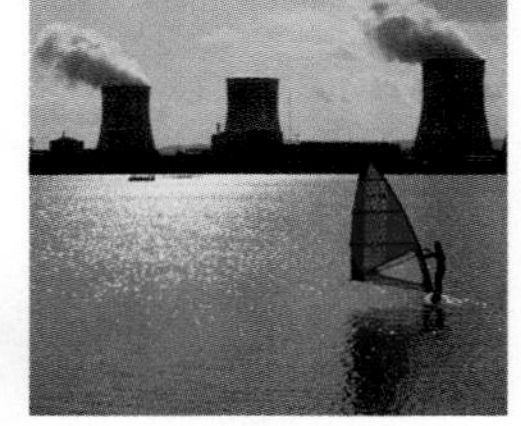

CHAPITRE **16**

Qu'en pensez-vous? 436

APPENDIXES

LEXIQUES

CREDIT

INDEX

About the Authors

Evelyne Amon studied at the Université de Paris-Sorbonne. She holds a DEA in modern literature, a Master in French as a second language, and a CAPES in modern literature. She has taught French language and literature at the secondary and college levels, and for many years has led a training seminar in Switzerland for professors on advances in methodology and pedagogy. She has conducted several training sessions in teaching French as a second language for teachers at the French Institute Alliance Française (FIAF) in New York. As an author, she has written many reference volumes, textbooks, and academic studies for French publishers such as Larousse, Hatier, Magnard, Nathan, and Bordas. She is the author of the McGraw-Hill French reader *C'est la vie!* and has written for successive editions of *Vis-à-vis*.

Judith A. Muyskens, Ph.D., Ohio State University, is Provost and Professor of French at Nebraska Wesleyan University in Lincoln, Nebraska. She continues to visit French-speaking countries and teach French language courses when time allows, especially first- and second-year language classes. For many years, she taught courses in methodology and French language and culture and supervised teaching assistants at the University of Cincinnati. She has contributed to various professional publications, including the *Modern Language Journal*, *Foreign Language Annals*, and the ACTFL Foreign Language Education Series. She is a coauthor of several other French textbooks, including *Rendez-vous: An Invitation to French* and *À vous d'écrire*.

Alice C. Omaggio Hadley, Ph.D., Ohio State University, is a Professor Emerita of French at the University of Illinois at Urbana-Champaign. Before she retired in 2005, she was Director of Basic Language Instruction in French for 25 years, supervising teaching assistants and teaching courses in methodology. She is the author of a language teaching methods text, *Teaching Language in Context*. She has also written articles for various journals and contributed to other professional publications, has been a coauthor of several other French textbooks, and has given numerous workshops for teachers across the country.

Preface

> *"I love the absolutely WONDERFUL* **Vis-à-vis,** *which I still think (after 15 years of teaching) is the best French textbook on the market. In addition to its excellent content, grammar explanations, integration of culture, diverse focus on both France and other Francophone countries (especially Québec, Morocco, Sénégal, Martinique), I love its elegant and useful ORGANIZATION, into chapters with four lessons, and a final review. This makes organizing classes and syllabi so much easier and helpful."*
>
> —Brian Martin, *Williams College*

> *"***Vis-à-vis** *is a fully communicative textbook. It offers a very complete elementary program that fully integrates the four skills, following the ACTFL national standards. It is also strongly attractive for students of all horizons, levels and generations thanks to the digital tools that accompany it."*
>
> —Carole Salmon, *University of Massachusetts, Lowell*

Vis-à-vis engages students with its unique integration of contemporary culture and communicative building blocks, providing the tools they need to build a solid foundation in introductory French. The hallmarks of *Vis-à-vis* are well known:

- an easy-to-navigate chapter structure with four lessons in which vocabulary, grammar, and culture work together as integrated units;
- an abundance of practice activities that range from form-focused to communicative;
- a balanced approach to the four skills;
- diverse coverage of the Francophone world that includes an outstanding video program featuring bloggers and cultural footage from eight different Francophone regions.

These features support the core goals of the introductory French course—communicative and cultural competence—and lay the groundwork for student success.

McGraw-Hill Connect® French and McGraw-Hill LearnSmart®

In its sixth edition, ***Vis-à-vis*** continues to evolve to meet the changing needs of instructors and students by responding to feedback from the users themselves. Employing a wide array of research tools, we identified a number of areas for potential innovation; the new program builds upon the success of the fifth edition with an expanded emphasis on contemporary language, pronunciation, culture, and technology to create a truly communicative, interactive experience. On the digital side, this new edition offers **Connect French** and **LearnSmart,** with their unparalleled adaptive and digital learning resources. These powerful tools, now an integral part of the sixth edition, complement and support the goals of the *Vis-à-vis* program and address the needs of the evolving introductory French course.

Mc Graw Hill Education connect® FRENCH

LEARNSMART®

How do Connect French and LearnSmart Support the Goals of the *Vis-à-vis* Program?

Communicative Competence

One of the major challenges of any introductory language course is to give each student ample exposure to the language and sufficient opportunity for speaking practice to inspire them to communicate with confidence. In **Connect French,** students have full access to the digitally enhanced e-Book, the online *Workbook / Laboratory Manual* activities, **LearnSmart**, and all of the accompanying audio and video resources, giving them the ability to interact with the materials as often as they wish.

Each chapter of the ***Vis-à-vis*** program contains the following exciting enhancements to promote communicative practice and competence:

- **Interactive vocabulary presentations** (**Paroles**) with audio allow students to listen, record, and practice the new vocabulary at home.
- **Interactive textbook and workbook activities for vocabulary and grammar in Connect French,** many of which are auto-graded, give students the opportunity to complete their assignments and come to class better prepared to participate in paired and group activities.
- **Blackboard Instant Messaging** provides the necessary tools for students to work in pairs online or to practice speaking together before coming to class.
- The **Voice Board** feature allows individuals to record their own voice as many times as they wish before they post their recording to which other students may respond.
- New **Prononcez bien!** activities with a recording feature provide students with opportunities for discrete-word and contextualized practice that gives them more confidence in their speaking abilities.

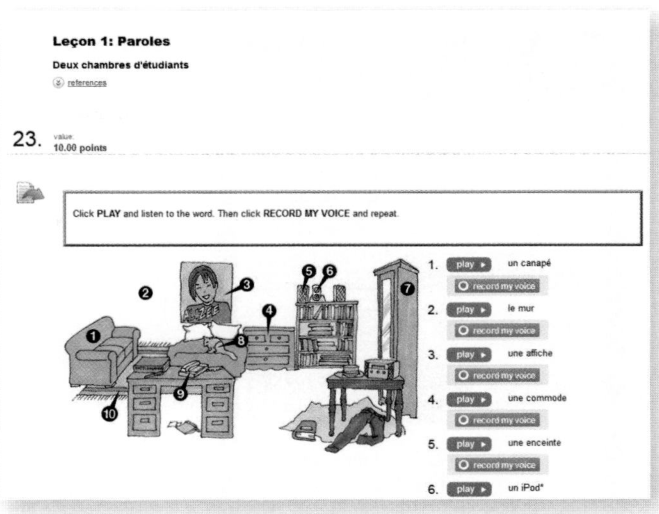

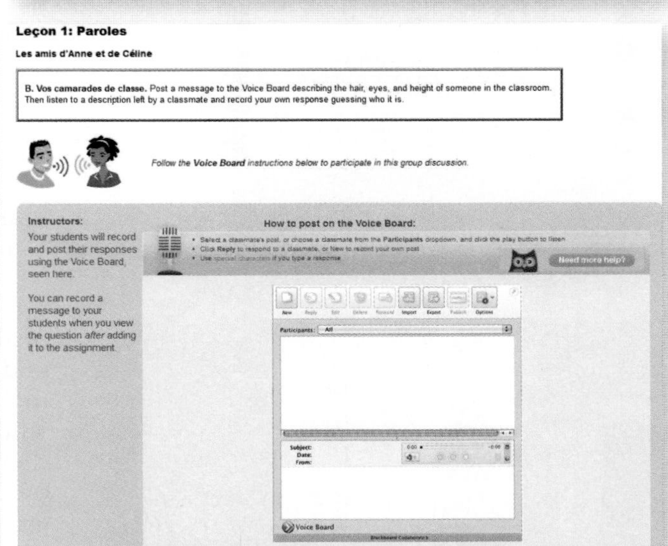

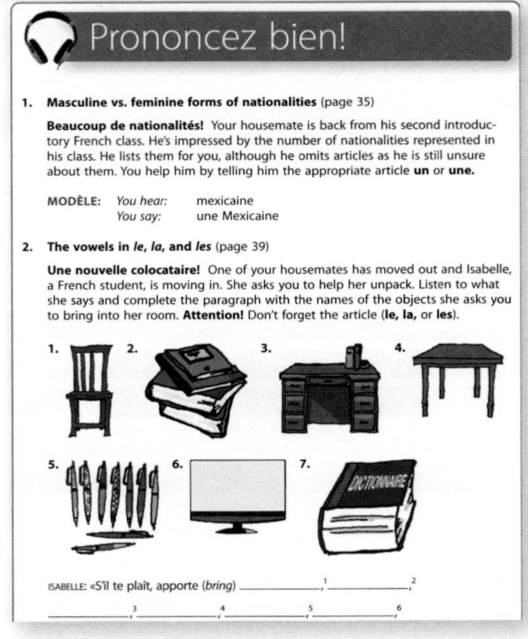

Prononcez bien!

1. **Masculine vs. feminine forms of nationalities** (page 35)

   Beaucoup de nationalités! Your housemate is back from his second introductory French class. He's impressed by the number of nationalities represented in his class. He lists them for you, although he omits articles as he is still unsure about them. You help him by telling him the appropriate article **un** or **une.**

   MODÈLE: *You hear:* mexicaine
   You say: une Mexicaine

2. **The vowels in *le, la,* and *les*** (page 39)

   Une nouvelle colocataire! One of your housemates has moved out and Isabelle, a French student, is moving in. She asks you to help her unpack. Listen to what she says and complete the paragraph with the names of the objects she asks you to bring into her room. **Attention!** Don't forget the article (**le, la,** or **les**).

ISABELLE: «S'il te plaît, apporte (*bring*) ________,[1] ________,[2] ________,[3] ________,[4] ________,[5] ________,[6]

> *I am particularly interested in the inclusion of more pronunciation practice and pronunciation activities. This is what the existing textbooks are usually lacking. The accompanying recording of the explanations and the activities will be very helpful both to students and their instructors.*
>
> —Andrzej Dziedzic, *University of Wisconsin*

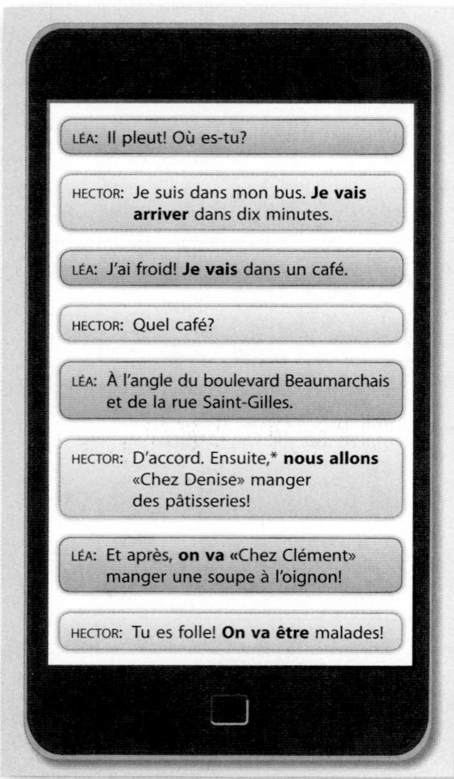
LÉA: Il pleut! Où es-tu?
HECTOR: Je suis dans mon bus. Je vais arriver dans dix minutes.
LÉA: J'ai froid! Je vais dans un café.
HECTOR: Quel café?
LÉA: À l'angle du boulevard Beaumarchais et de la rue Saint-Gilles.
HECTOR: D'accord. Ensuite,* nous allons «Chez Denise» manger des pâtisseries!
LÉA: Et après, on va «Chez Clément» manger une soupe à l'oignon!
HECTOR: Tu es folle! On va être malades!

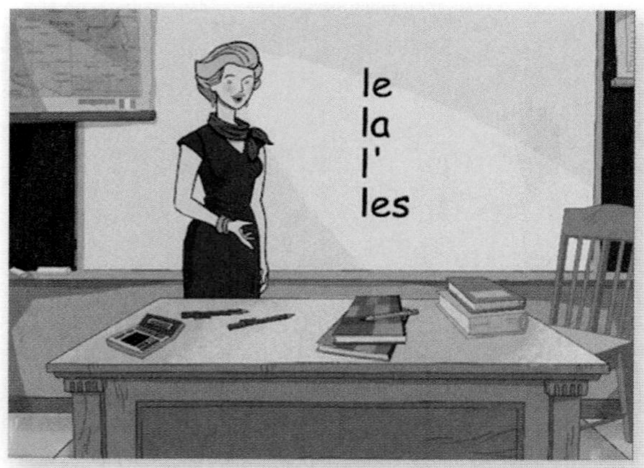
le
la
l'
les

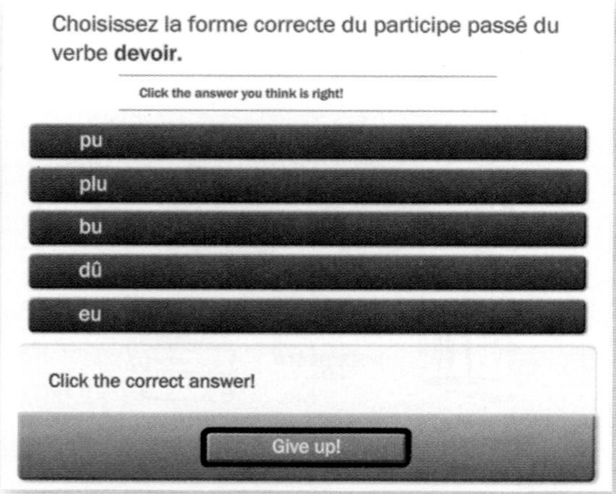
Choisissez la forme correcte du participe passé du verbe devoir.
Click the answer you think is right!
pu
plu
bu
dû
eu
Click the correct answer!
Give up!

> "**Vis-à-vis** *provides a mixed approach that integrates the best of communicative language pedagogy with useful tech tools for technologically enhanced, personalized online language learning. Probably the most up-to-date and refreshing French I out there.*"
>
> —Sarah Gordon, *Utah State University*

- **Four new, lively mini-dialogues** featuring the blog characters have been recorded to provide students with a spirited introduction to the new grammatical structures in context.
- Seventeen **Grammaire interactive** tutorials, each with a brief practice quiz, focus on structures that students typically struggle with, such as the partitive, and the **passé composé** vs. the **imparfait.** These tutorials, accessible only in **Connect French**, give students an alternative means of learning, reviewing, and checking their comprehension of selected grammar points.

In addition to the **Connect French** chapter resources, **LearnSmart** modules for vocabulary and grammar have been developed specifically for ***Vis-à-vis.*** This powerful adaptive system helps students pinpoint their weaknesses and provides them with an individualized study program based on their results. Audio prompts for vocabulary and grammar help students strengthen both their listening and writing skills. All students, no matter their previous language experience, can benefit from using **LearnSmart,** which includes built-in reporting and a competitive scoreboard to increase student engagement. Our research has shown that students using **LearnSmart** have significantly improved their learning and course outcomes.

By using these powerful digital tools, students have myriad opportunities to build their communicative skills. By assigning **Connect French** and **LearnSmart,** instructors save valuable class time for interactive practice.

Cultural Competence

The program's meaningful and extensive exploration of the rich culture of France and the Francophone world is fully supported in **Connect French** through audio and video resources and interactive activities.

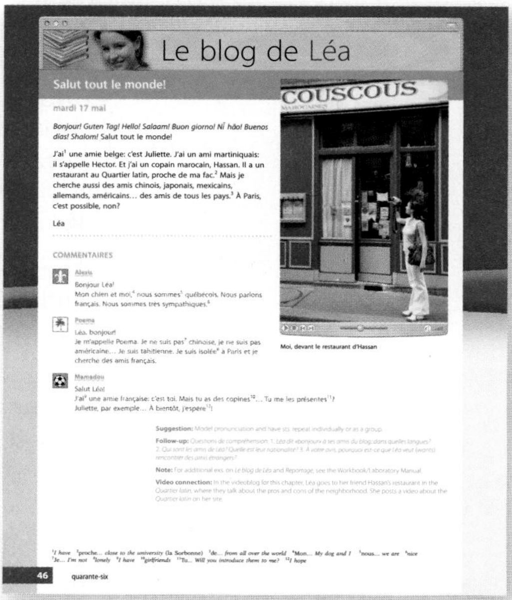

Le blog de Léa

Salut tout le monde!

mardi 17 mai

Bonjour! Guten Tag! Hello! Salaam! Buon giorno! Nǐ hǎo! Buenos dias! Shalom! Salut tout le monde!

J'ai[1] une amie belge: c'est Juliette. J'ai un ami martiniquais: il s'appelle Hector. Et j'ai un copain marocain, Hassan. Il a un restaurant au Quartier latin, proche de ma fac.[2] Mais je cherche aussi des amis chinois, japonais, mexicains, allemands, américains… des amis de tous les pays.[3] À Paris, c'est possible, non?

Léa

COMMENTAIRES

Alexis
Bonjour Léa!
Mon chien et moi,[4] nous sommes[5] québécois. Nous parlons français. Nous sommes très sympathiques.[6]

Poema
Léa, bonjour!
Je m'appelle Poema. Je ne suis pas[7] chinoise, je ne suis pas américaine… Je suis tahitienne. Je suis isolée[8] à Paris et je cherche des amis français.

Mamadou
Salut Léa!
J'ai[9] une amie française: c'est toi. Mais tu as des copines[10]… Tu me les présentes[11]? Juliette, par exemple… À bientôt, j'espère[12]!

Moi, devant le restaurant d'Hassan

Suggestion: Model pronunciation and have sts. repeat individually or as a group.

Follow-up: Questions de compréhension: 1. *Léa dit «bonjour» à ses amis du blog: dans quelles langues?* 2. *Qui sont les amis de Léa? Quelle est leur nationalité?* 3. *À votre avis, pourquoi est-ce que Léa veut (wants) rencontrer des amis étrangers?*

Note: For additional exs. on *Le blog de Léa* and *Reportage*, see the Workbook/Laboratory Manual.

Video connection: In the videoblog for this chapter, Léa goes to her friend Hassan's restaurant in the *Quartier latin*, where they talk about the pros and cons of the neighborhood. She posts a video about the *Quartier latin* on her site.

[1] *I have* [2] **proche…** *close to the university* (**la Sorbonne**) [3] **de…** *from all over the world* [4] **Mon…** *My dog and I* [5] **nous…** *we are* [6] *nice* [7] **Je…** *I'm not* [8] *lonely* [9] *I have* [10] *girlfriends* [11] **Tu…** *Will you introduce them to me?* [12] *I hope*

46 quarante-six

- Every four chapters, ***Vis-à-vis*** introduces a focus on a new French or Francophone character and region. The personal online journal entries in **Le blog de...** , the related **Reportage**, and the **Bienvenue...** readings that precede Chapter 1 and follow Chapters 4, 8, 12, and 16, expose students to contemporary language and the vast diversity of life and culture in France, Belgium, Tunisia, and Martinique. In **Connect French**, instructors may assign the readings and new auto-graded comprehension activities that prepare students for class discussion.

- **Le vidéoblog de...** and the stunning **Bienvenue** video segments give students a window into the sights and sounds of eight different French-speaking regions/countries: France, Belgium, Switzerland, Quebec, Louisiana, Tunisia, Senegal, Martinique, and Tahiti. Each video is accompanied by comprehension and cross-cultural comparison activities that encourage students to make connections between their culture and those of the French-speaking world. The new video activities in **Connect** break the segments into manageable "chunks" that keep students focused on specific information and help improve their listening skills.

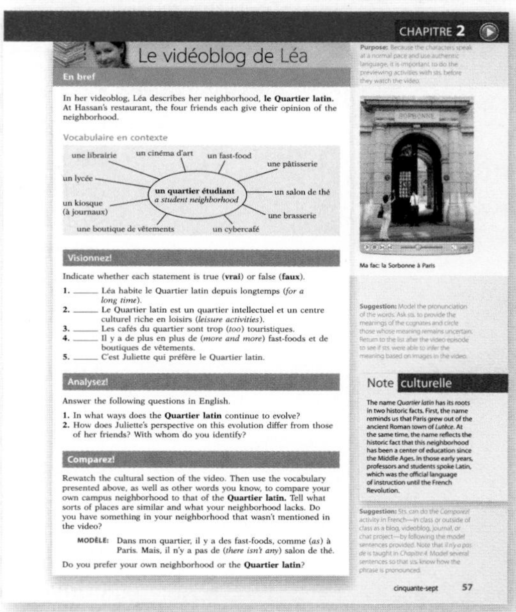

CHAPITRE 2

Le vidéoblog de Léa

En bref

In her videoblog, Léa describes her neighborhood, **le Quartier latin.** At Hassan's restaurant, the four friends each give their opinion of the neighborhood.

Vocabulaire en contexte

Visionnez!

Indicate whether each statement is true (**vrai**) or false (**faux**).

1. ______ Léa habite le Quartier latin depuis longtemps (*for a long time*).
2. ______ Le Quartier latin est un quartier intellectuel et un centre culturel riche en loisirs (*leisure activities*).
3. ______ Les cafés du quartier sont trop (*too*) touristiques.
4. ______ Il y a de plus en plus de (*more and more*) fast-foods et de boutiques de vêtements.
5. ______ C'est Juliette qui préfère le Quartier latin.

Analysez!

Answer the following questions in English.

1. In what ways does the **Quartier latin** continue to evolve?
2. How does Juliette's perspective on this evolution differ from those of her friends? With whom do you identify?

Comparez!

Rewatch the cultural section of the video. Then use the vocabulary presented above, as well as other words you know, to compare your own campus neighborhood to that of the **Quartier latin.** Tell what sorts of places are similar and what your neighborhood lacks. Do you have something in your neighborhood that wasn't mentioned in the video?

MODÈLE: Dans mon quartier, il y a des fast-foods, comme (*as*) à Paris. Mais, il n'y a pas de (*there isn't any*) salon de thé.

Do you prefer your own neighborhood or the **Quartier latin**?

Purpose: Because the characters speak at a normal pace and use authentic language, it is important to do the previewing activities with sts. before they watch the video.

Ma fac: la Sorbonne à Paris

Suggestion: Model the pronunciation of the words. Ask sts. to provide the meanings of the cognates and circle those whose meaning remains uncertain. Return to the list after the video episode to see if sts. were able to infer the meaning based on images in the video.

Note culturelle

The name *Quartier latin* has its roots in two historic facts. First, the name reminds us that Paris grew out of the ancient Roman town of *Lutèce*. At the same time, the name reflects the historic fact that this neighborhood has been a center of education since the Middle Ages. In those early years, professors and students spoke Latin, which was the official language of instruction until the French Revolution.

Suggestion: Sts. can do the *Comparez!* activity in French—in class or outside of class as a blog, videoblog, journal, or chat project—by following the model sentences provided. Note that *il n'y a pas de* is taught in *Chapitre 4*. Model several sentences so that sts. know how the phrase is pronounced.

cinquante-sept 57

- The **Avant de lire** and **Compréhension** activities that accompany the **Lecture** in the **Perspectives** section (**Leçon 4**) of every chapter may now be done online.

The **Connect French** platform gives students the opportunity to interact with the cultural materials as often as they wish and engage them more fully in their language learning.

As we see the modern French classroom changing, we are looking at teaching and learning in a different light. Our research shows that French instructors seek digital tools to extend learning outside of the classroom in more effective ways. The cutting-edge functionality of **Connect French** and **LearnSmart** enables instructors to achieve their course goals using new online presentation activities, improved homework tools, and a better reporting feature. Together, **Connect French and LearnSmart** create a dynamic learning environment that presents communicative practice and rich cultural content as it motivates students to succeed regardless of the delivery platform. We invite you to experience the new ***Vis-à-vis*** program to see how our partnership with today's instructors and students has allowed us to identify and address some of the most common needs in today's French classrooms. Discover the power of ***Vis-à-vis'*** proven approach enhanced by **LearnSmart** and our new digital platform **Connect French.**

> "**Vis-à-vis** *is an exciting, beginning French program that addresses the needs of the 21st century student. There is a rich mixture of language, culture, and technology that will stimulate the reluctant learner.*"
>
> —Dr. Debra Boyd, *North Carolina Central University, Durham*

Program Supplements

Connect French: Used in conjunction with ***Vis-à-vis: Beginning French,*** **Connect French** provides digital solutions for schools with face-to-face, hybrid, or 100% online modes. In addition to the interactive e-Book, complete *Workbook / Laboratory Manual*, grammar tutorials, and audio and video resources described on the preceding pages, some of the key administrative capabilities of **Connect French** include:

- the ability to customize syllabi and assignments to fit the needs of individual programs;
- an integrated gradebook with powerful reporting features;
- the ability to assign **LearnSmart** modules and monitor student progress;
- access to all instructor's resources, including the *Digital Transparencies, Instructor's Manual, Connect French User's Guide*, pre-made exams, and a customizable testing program with audio for the online delivery of assessments;
- access to **Tegrity,** McGraw-Hill's proprietary video capture software that allows instructors to post short videos, tutorials, and lessons for student access outside of class.

MH Campus and Blackboard: Integration of **MH Campus** and **Blackboard** simplifies and streamlines your course administration by integrating with your campus's Learning Management System. With features such as single sign-on for students and instructors, gradebook synchronization, and easy access to all of McGraw-Hill's language content (even from other market-leading titles not currently adopted for your course), teaching an introductory language course has never been simpler.

Annotated Instructor's Edition: The *Instructor's Edition* of the text includes a wide variety of suggestions for presenting each section of the book, ideas for recycling vocabulary, helpful cultural notes, suggested expansion activities, and useful follow-up activities. Answers to the textbook activities are provided in the *Instructor's Manual.*

Workbook / Laboratory Manual: This print supplement provides more conventional, drill-like practice of the **Paroles** and **Structures** sections presented in the textbook using a variety of written and audio activities. In addition, each chapter includes **Le blog de...** and a **Pause-culture** section that expands upon the cultural themes of the chapter. The **Perspectives** section provides additional pronunciation practice, a capstone listening activity (**À l'écoute**), and two writing activities: **Par écrit**, a guided writing activity, and **Journal intime,** a free-writing activity. For students using the print version, the audio files are posted at **Connect French**.

The ***Vis-à-vis*** **Video Program,** which contains **Le vidéoblog de...** and the **Bienvenue...** video segments, is available in **Connect French** and on DVD.

Acknowledgments

The authors wish to acknowledge the team at McGraw-Hill for their continuing support and enthusiasm: Katie Stevens, Scott Tinetti, Janet Banhidi, Katie Crouch, Susan Blatty, Kelly Heinrichs, Brenda Rolwes, Judy Mason, Sue Culbertson, Helen Greenlea, Craig Gill, Jorge Arbujas, Caitlin Bahrey and Leslie Briggs. We would also like to acknowledge our native reader, Nicole Dicop-Hineline, our copyeditor, Peggy Potter, our permissions editor, Veronica Oliva, and our proofreader, Sylvie Waskiewicz. Special thanks as well to the **Connect French** and **LearnSmart** teams for their dedication and creativity in the development of our new digital tools; **Connect French:** Sarah Hill, Laura Ciporen, Jon Fulk, Jason Kooiker, and Justin Swettlen; **LearnSmart:** Bruce Anderson, Abigail Alexander, Géraldine Blattner, Caroline Dequen-McKenzie, Jon Fulk, Lori McMann, Anne-Sabine Nicolas, Françoise Santore, Sandya Shanker, Alicia Soueid, Justin Swettlen, and Valérie Thiers-Thiam.

The authors and the publisher would like to express their gratitude to the following instructors across the country whose valuable suggestions contributed to the preparation of this new edition. The appearance of their names in these lists does not necessarily constitute their endorsement of the text or its methodology.

LearnSmart® Beta Testers

Boston College
Sarah Bilodeau

College of Charleston
Shawn Morrison

Florida Atlantic, Boca Raton
Géraldine Blattner
Robyn Ezersky
Laurine Ferreira
Sophie Ledeme
Rosemary Rahill
Stephanie Sense

Kennesaw State University
Luc Guglielmi

Portland State University
Stéphanie Roulon

Texas State University, San Marcos
Sabrina Hyde
Moira Di Mauro-Jackson, PhD

University of Minnesota, Twin Cities
Adam T. Grant

University of Rhode Island, Kingston
Joann Hammadou Sullivan

Reviewers

Baruch College, CUNY
Ali Nematollahy

Boise State University
Jason Herbeck

Borough of Manhattan Community College, CUNY
Peter Consenstein
Valérie Thiers-Thiam

Broward College
Trent Hoy
Celia M. Roberts
Shirley E. Santry

Cabrillo College
Bette G. Hirsch, PhD
Robyn Marshall

Canisius College
Eileen Angelini

Central Michigan University
Amy J. Ransom
Daniela Teodorescu

City College of New York, CUNY
Maxime Blanchard

Clemson University
Amy Sawyer

College of Charleston
Shawn Morrison, PhD

County College of Morris
Lakshmi Kattepur
Gene Sisti

Dakota College at Bottineau
Linda Grover

Drury University
Catherine Blunk, PhD

Eastern Illinois University
Kathryn M. Bulver, PhD

Eastman School of Music, University of Rochester
Valérie Couderc

Furman University
William Allen

Gordon College
Damon DiMauro

Grand Valley State University
Dan Golembeski

Hostos Community College
Philip Wander

Houston Community College
Maurice Abboud
David Long, PhD

Howard Community College
Heidi Goldenman
Agnès Archambault Honigmann

Illinois Wesleyan University
Lisa Brittingham

Kalamazoo Valley Community College
Jonnie Wilhite

Keene State College
Brian Donovan
Julia Dutton

Kennedy-King College, City Colleges of Chicago
Sonia Elgado-Tall, PhD

Kennesaw State University
Luc D. Guglielmi, PhD

Lee University
James D. Wilkins

Lewis & Clark College
Claudia Nadine

Liberty University
Sharon B. Hähnlen, PhD

Lone Star College–CyFair
Georges Detiveaux

Louisiana College
Cecile Barnhart

Loyola University Chicago
Lisa Erceg

Luther College
Laurie Zaring

Manchester University
Janina Traxler

Mercy College
Alan G. Hartman
Jeanne Marie O'Regan

Mercyhurst University
Douglas Boudreau

Missouri Western State University
Susie Hennessy, PhD

Montana State University
Ada Giusti

Morgan State University
Helen Harrison

Morris College
Catherine Kapi

Mt. San Jacinto College
Jennifer S. Doucet

New Mexico State University
Claude Fouillade

New Paltz, SUNY
Mercedes Rooney

Norco College, Riverside Community College District
Dominique Hitchcock, PhD

North Carolina Central University
Debra Boyd, PhD

North Georgia College & State University
Elizabeth Combier, PhD

North Lake College
Cathy Briggs

Northern Essex Community College
Denise Minnard Campoli

Oakton Community College
Marguerite Solari, PhD

Ohio University
Signe Denbow

Oklahoma State University
Frédérique Knottnerus

Onondaga Community College
Mary-Ellen Faughnan-Kenien, PhD
Elizabeth O'Hara

Pace University
Rosemarie Cristina

Pasadena City College
Michèle Pedrini, PhD
Charlene Potter

Portland State University
Annabelle Dolidon
Jennifer R. Perlmutter
Stéphanie Roulon

Rutgers University
Myriam Alami

Saint Martin's University
Kathleen McKain

Samford University
M. D. Ledgerwood, PhD

San Diego State University
Edith Benkov

San José State University
Jean-Luc Desalvo

Shasta College
Eileen Smith

Southeastern Louisiana University
Aileen Mootoo

Southwestern University
Glenda Warren Carl

St. Catherine University
Jerome Tarmann

St. Cloud State University
María Gloria Melgarejo, PhD

Stephen F. Austin State University
Joyce Carlton Johnston

Stetson University
Richard Ferland

Stony Brook University, SUNY
Madeline Turan

SUNY Fredonia
Kate Douglass
Edward Kolodziej

Texas A&M University
Cheryl Schaile

Union County College
Pamela Mansfield

University of Alabama
Isabelle Drewelow

University of Arkansas
Kathleen Comfort, PhD

University of California, Berkeley
Leslie Martin, PhD

University of California, Riverside
Kelle Truby

University of Cincinnati
Irene Ivantcheva-Merjanska, PhD
Aline Skrzeszewski

University of Denver
Terri Woellners

University of Hawaii at Manoa
Joan Marie Debrah

University of Louisville
Bonnie Fonseca-Greber

University of Maryland
Catherine Savell

University of Massachusetts, Lowell
Carole Salmon

University of Missouri–Saint Louis
Anne-Sophie Blank
Sandra Trapani

University of Nebraska at Omaha
Patrice J. Proulx, PhD

University of New Mexico
Marina Peters-Newell

University of North Carolina, Wilmington
Caroline Hudson

University of North Georgia
Elizabeth Combier, PhD
D. Brian Mann, PhD
Amye Sukapdjo

University of Texas at Arlington
Antoinette Sol, PhD

University of Wisconsin
Andrzej Dziedzic, PhD

Ursinus College
Frances Novack

Utah State University
Sarah Gordon, PhD

Utica College
Marie-Noëlle Little, PhD

Valdosta State University
Ellen Lorraine Friedrich, PhD
Ofélia Nikolova, PhD

Wake Forest University
Elizabeth Barron, PhD

Westminster College
Ingrid Ilinca
Leslie Kealhofer, PhD

Wichita State University
Gail Burkett

William Jewell College
Michael Foster, PhD

Williams College
Brian Martin
Leyla Rouhi

Worcester State University
Judith Jeon-Chapman

Vis-à-vis

Bienvenue à **Vis-à-vis**

Welcome to *Vis-à-vis* and to **la francophonie,** the French-speaking world. In the **blog** sections between **Leçons 2** and **3** in each chapter, you will read the blogs created by four Parisians with different Francophone backgrounds—Léa, Hassan, Juliette, and Hector. You will also have the opportunity to read the commentaries of other French speakers on their blogs and to watch the videoblogs that they have posted on their sites. The *cartes d'identité** and short biographies of these four *blogueurs* are presented below.

RÉPUBLIQUE FRANÇAISE
CARTE NATIONALE D'IDENTITÉ N° : 873099516754
Nationalité française
Nom : BOUCHARD
Prénom(s) : LÉA
Sexe : F
Né(e) le : 22 février 1995
à : PARIS 6ÈME[1]
Taille : 1M65[2]
Signature du titulaire : Léa Bouchard
IDFRABOUCHARD<<<<<<<<<<<<<<<<<<<
8730995167546LÉA<<<<<<<<<9057121G9

Les blogueurs

Chapitres 1–4 feature the blog of Léa Bouchard. **Léa Bouchard,** 19 (dix-neuf) ans,[3] étudiante en 1ère (première) année[4] de Lettres à la faculté de Paris IV Sorbonne. Elle réside avec sa famille, dans un appartement du 6e arrondissement. Sa personnalité: romantique, immature, gracieuse.

Suggestion: You may wish to use the *cartes d'identité* and the descriptions of the characters to point out the number of cognates found in French. Have sts. read the cards and ask them simple questions about the characters. You could also have them create *cartes d'identité* for themselves using these cards as models.

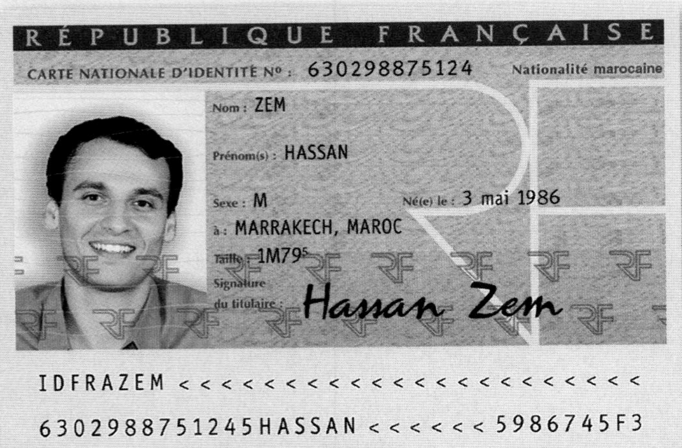
RÉPUBLIQUE FRANÇAISE
CARTE NATIONALE D'IDENTITÉ N° : 630298875124
Nationalité marocaine
Nom : ZEM
Prénom(s) : HASSAN
Sexe : M
Né(e) le : 3 mai 1986
à : MARRAKECH, MAROC
Taille : 1M79[5]
Signature du titulaire : Hassan Zem
IDFRAZEM<<<<<<<<<<<<<<<<<<<<<<<<
6302988751245HASSAN<<<<<<5986745F3

Chapitres 5–8 feature the blog of Hassan Zem. **Hassan Zem,** 28 (vingt-huit) ans, jeune patron[6] d'un restaurant marocain du Quartier latin à Paris. Il occupe un loft du quartier Oberkampf, avec son copain,[7] Abdel. Sa personnalité: charmeur, délicat, généreux.

Suggestion: You may wish to explain that Paris is divided into twenty districts called *arrondissements,* which spiral out clockwise from the center of the city. A map of Paris can be found at the back of this textbook.

[1]sixième (arrondissement) = *6th district of Paris* [2]un mètre soixante-cinq = *5 feet 5 inches* [3]*years old* [4]1ère... = *1st year* [5]un mètre soixante-dix-neuf = *5 feet 10½ inches* [6]*owner* [7]*friend*

---

*The **carte d'identité** is an official national identity card. In addition to the photograph and signature of the cardholder **(titulaire),** it includes such information as date of birth **(né[e] le...),** gender **(sexe),** and height **(taille).** The card is not obligatory for French citizens, but it is free, and is the preferred card for identification purposes.

Chapitres 9–12 feature the blog of Juliette Graf.
Juliette Graf, 22 (vingt-deux) ans, étudiante en Master Multimédia Interactif à l'Université de Paris I Panthéon-Sorbonne. Elle occupe une petite chambre au Quartier latin.
Sa personnalité: raisonnée, méthodique, active.

RÉPUBLIQUE FRANÇAISE
CARTE NATIONALE D'IDENTITÉ N° : 763722399500 Nationalité belge
Nom : GRAF
Prénom(s) : JULIETTE
Sexe : F Né(e) le : 12 août 1992
à : BRUXELLES, BELGIQUE
Taille : 1M70[8]
Signature du titulaire : Juliette Graf
IDFRAGRAF<<<<<<<<<<<<<<<<<<<<<
7637223995004JULIETTE<<<<<3342981A5

Chapitres 13–16 feature the blog of Hector Clément.
Hector Clément, 25 (vingt-cinq) ans, danseur professionnel. Il réside dans un appartement des Halles, avec des camarades.
Sa personnalité: original, susceptible, talentueux.

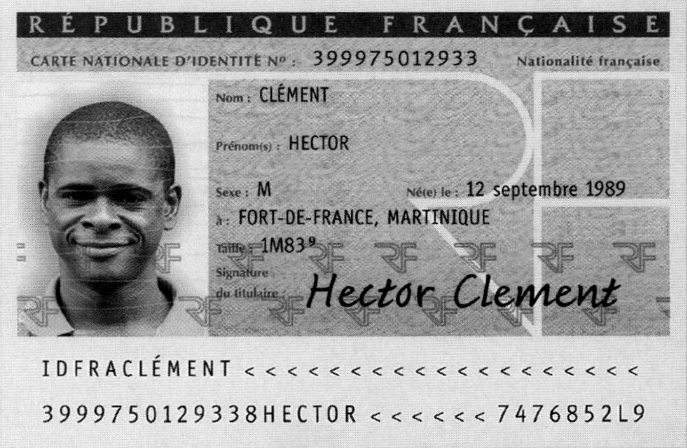

RÉPUBLIQUE FRANÇAISE
CARTE NATIONALE D'IDENTITÉ N° : 399975012933 Nationalité française
Nom : CLÉMENT
Prénom(s) : HECTOR
Sexe : M Né(e) le : 12 septembre 1989
à : FORT-DE-FRANCE, MARTINIQUE
Taille : 1M83[9]
Signature du titulaire : Hector Clement
IDFRACLÉMENT<<<<<<<<<<<<<<<<<<<
3999750129338HECTOR<<<<<<7476852L9

Les commentateurs

The following people offer their commentaries on the blogs.

Alexis Lafontaine, 19 (dix-neuf) ans, étudiant en 1ère année d'économie, de sociologie et de géographie. Il est de Montréal. Il réside à Versailles avec son chien,[10] Trésor.
Sa personnalité: intellectuel, moraliste, solitaire.

Trésor, 3 (trois) ans, chien d'Alexis Lafontaine. Il adore son maître.
Sa personnalité: intelligent, optimiste, indépendant.

Mamadou Bassène, 28 (vingt-huit) ans, journaliste sportif, correspondant du journal[11] sénégalais «Le Soleil». Il est de Dakar. Il réside à Paris, dans le Marais.
Sa personnalité: plein d'humour, relax, charmeur.

Charlotte Cousin, 30 (trente) ans, est traductrice[12] à l'OMS (Organisation Mondiale de la Santé.)[13] Elle réside à Genève. Elle est mariée; elle a[14] un enfant.
Sa personnalité: raisonnable, compliquée, anxieuse.

Poema Dauphin, 22 (vingt-deux) ans, étudiante en maîtrise de Protection de la nature à l'université de Paris XII. Elle est de Tahiti. Elle loge dans une résidence universitaire de Paris, à la Cité internationale du 14e (quatorzième) arrondissement.
Sa personnalité: idéaliste, généreuse, rêveuse.[15]

[8]un mètre soixante-dix = *5 feet 7 inches* [9]un mètre quatre-vingt-trois = *6 feet* [10]*dog* [11]*newspaper* [12]*translator* [13]*OMS... WHO (World Health Organization)* [14]*has* [15]*dreamy*

Les pays francophones

Les... *Francophone countries*

Suggestion: Go over the maps at the back of the book and encourage sts. to refer to them often. Use country names for pronunciation practice. Write country names on the board as sts. say them; then use the list as a basis for group repetition.

More than 220 million people in the world speak French, either as their native language or as a second language used in the workplace. French-speaking regions are found throughout the world.

By following the blogs and videoblogs of Léa, Hassan, Juliette, and Hector in *Vis-à-vis,* you will learn more about the customs, traditions, lifestyles, and everyday routines that define France and many Francophone regions.

Suggestion: Enrich geography knowledge via a quick game of Jeopardy. Divide the class into two or more groups, and have sts. write out (in English) brief definitions of French-speaking areas: A Francophone region of South America. (What is *la Guyane?*) The team with the most correct answers earns a big round of applause!

Note: Bastille Day is the national holiday of France. It is very much like Independence Day in the United States because it is a celebration of the beginning of a new form of government. On July 14, 1789, a large number of French citizens gathered together and stormed the Bastille Prison. Although there were only seven prisoners at the time, the action was a strong symbol of rebellion against the king and marked the beginning of the French Revolution.

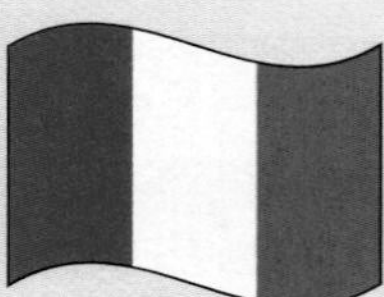

Pays: France (République française)
Nom des habitants: Français
Capitale: Paris
Langue officielle: français
Unité monétaire: euro
Fête nationale: 14 (quatorze) juillet

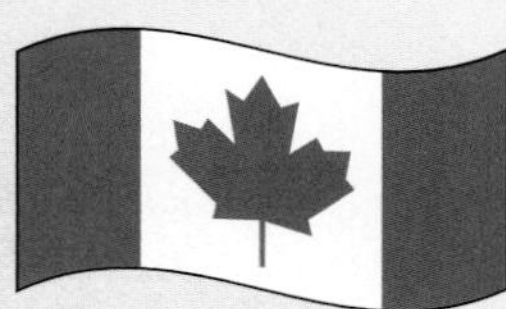

Pays: Canada
Nom des habitants: Canadiens
Capitale: Ottawa
Langues officielles: anglais, français
Unité monétaire: dollar canadien
Fête nationale: 1er (premier) juillet

Note: Canada Day, July 1, is the celebration of the formation of the union of the British North American provinces in a federation.

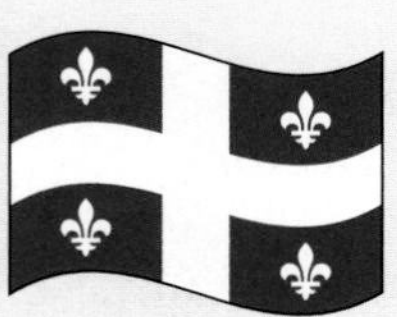

Province (Canada): le Québec
Capitale: Québec
Langue: 80 % (quatre-vingts pour cent) des habitants de la province de Québec parlent (*speak*) français.
Fête nationale: 24 (vingt-quatre) juin

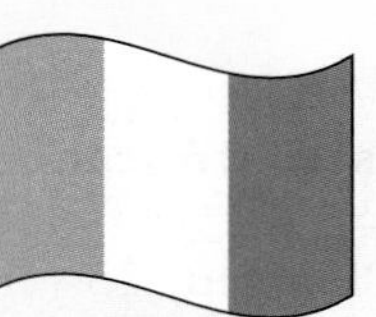

Pays: Côte d'Ivoire (République de Côte d'Ivoire)
Nom des habitants: Ivoiriens
Capitale: Yamoussoukro
Langue officielle: français
Unité monétaire: franc CFA
Fête nationale: 7 (sept) août

Note: Cote d'Ivoire became fully independent from France on August 7, 1960. CFA stands for Communauté Financière Africaine.

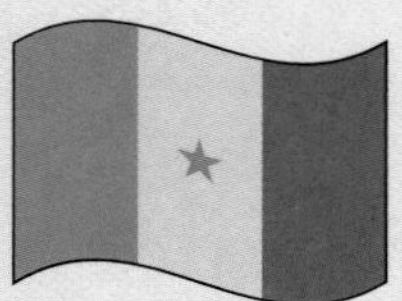

Pays: Sénégal (République du Sénégal)
Nom des habitants: Sénégalais
Capitale: Dakar
Langue officielle: français
Unité monétaire: franc CFA
Fête nationale: 4 (quatre) avril

Note: Senegal celebrates its Independence Day on April 4. It won independence from France on April 4, 1960.

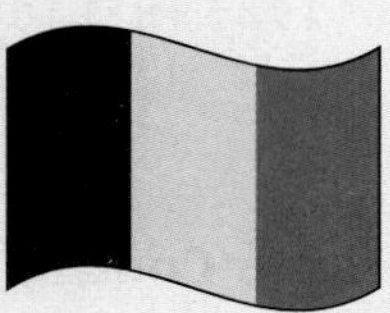

Pays: Belgique (Royaume de Belgique)
Nom des habitants: Belges
Capitale: Bruxelles
Langues officielles: français, allemand (*German*), flamand (*Flemish*)
Unité monétaire: euro
Fête nationale: 21 (vingt et un) juillet

Note: On October 4, 1830, a provisional government in Belgium declared independence from the Netherlands. On July 21, 1831, the first Belgian king, Léopold I, ascended to the throne. The Belgians celebrate this day as their national holiday.

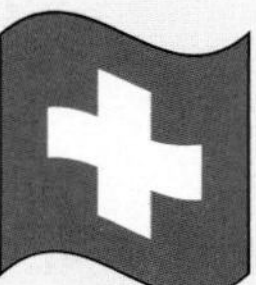

Pays: Suisse (Confédération suisse)
Nom des habitants: Suisses
Capitale: Berne (siège [*seat*] administratif), Lausanne (siège judiciaire)
Langues officielles: allemand, français, italien
Unité monétaire: franc suisse
Fête nationale: 1er (premier) août

Note: The Swiss celebrate their national holiday on August 1 to mark the founding of the Swiss Confederation on August 1, 1291.

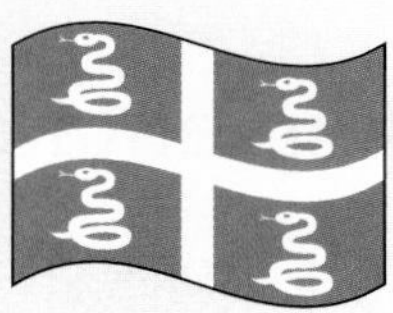

Département d'outre-mer (France): Martinique
Nom des habitants: Martiniquais
Capitale (chef-lieu et préfecture): Fort-de-France
Langue officielle: français
Unité monétaire: euro
Fête nationale: 14 (quatorze) juillet

Note: As an overseas department of France, Martinique celebrates Bastille Day. The flag pictured above is the unofficial flag of Martinique; the French flag is the official flag.

Bienvenue en France

Un coup d'œil° sur Paris, en France

Un... *A glance*

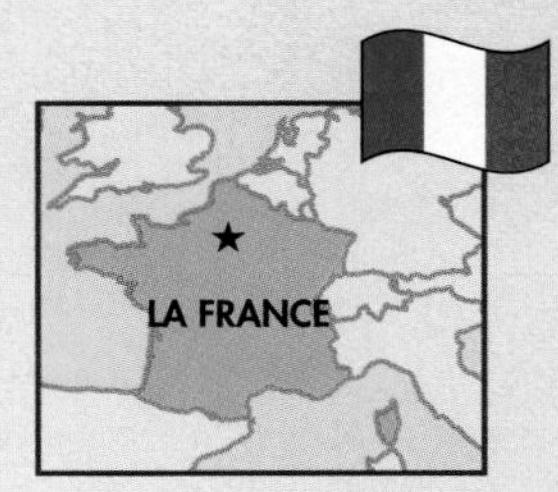

Paris, the City of Light, intrigues, astonishes, provokes, overwhelms . . . and gets under your skin. For centuries, the city has served as a muse, inspiring artists, writers, and musicians alike with its beauty. Paris is the apex of architectural beauty, artistic expression, and culinary delight, and it knows it. As stately as the **Arc de Triomphe,** as disarmingly quaint as the lace-curtained bistros found in each neighborhood, Paris seduces newcomers to enjoy unhurried exploration of its picture-perfect streets.

It is a city of vast, noble perspectives and intimate, medieval streets, of formal **espaces verts** (green open spaces) and quiet squares. This combination of the pompous and the private is one of the secrets of its perennial pull. Another is its size: Paris is relatively small as capitals go, with distances between many of its major sights and museums invariably walkable. Paris is an open history book: a stroll through its streets will take you from the Middle Ages right up to the 21st century.

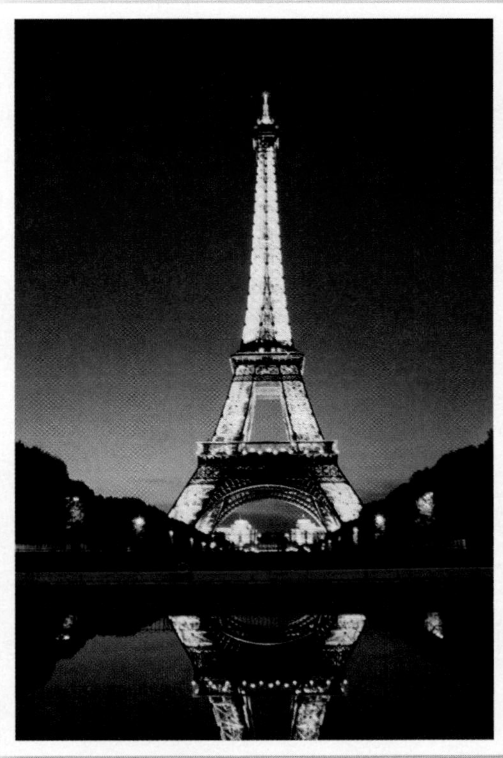

The Eiffel Tower at night

PORTRAIT Astérix

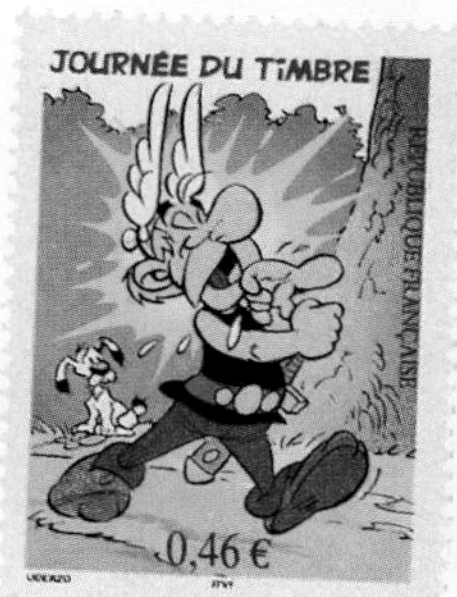

Astérix, the iconic French comic strip character, is a boisterous little Gaul* who lives in a small French village that is holding out against the might of the Roman Empire. Protected by the village druid Panoramix's magic potion, which gives him superhuman strength, Astérix takes the lead in the villagers' perilous attempts to conquer the invading Romans. He is a clever and level-headed warrior who knows when brain is better than brawn. The French see him as a symbol of themselves in his ability to outwit others.

Note: There are cultural video segments that accompany the *Bienvenue* sections before *Chapitre 1* and after *Chapitres 4, 8, 12,* and *16.* The videoscripts for these segments are located in the Instructor's Manual in the Instructor's Resources tab at **Connect French (www.mhconnectfrench.com)**.

Note: The *Bienvenue en France* reading is in English, but the remaining *Bienvenue* pages are in French.

Follow-up: Ask comprehension questions, such as *What are some of the reasons for Paris's popularity as a city over the centuries? Who is Astérix, and why do the French like him?*

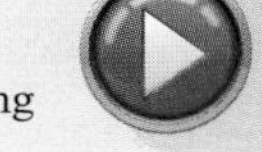

Watch the *Bienvenue en France* video segment to learn more about Paris.

*an inhabitant of the ancient region of Gaul, a province of the Roman Empire including territory corresponding to modern France, Belgium, and northern Italy

CHAPITRE 1

Une nouvelle° aventure

°new

Note: This chapter presents material appropriate to the *Novice Level* of proficiency as described in the *ACTFL Guidelines* and tested in the ACTFL/ETS *Oral Proficiency Interview*. The *Novice Level* is characterized by formulaic expressions, typically involving such subjects as greetings, social amenities, common objects, telling time, counting, and giving dates.

Presentation: Ask sts. to discuss what they see in the photo that tells them this scene is in France and what reminds them of their own country.

Les dossiers de Léa

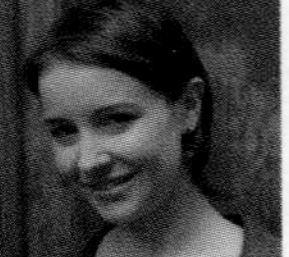

Léa

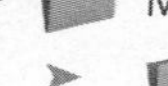

Mes photos

Au café avec Juliette

Vidéo de Juliette pour mon blog

Bonjour ou au revoir?

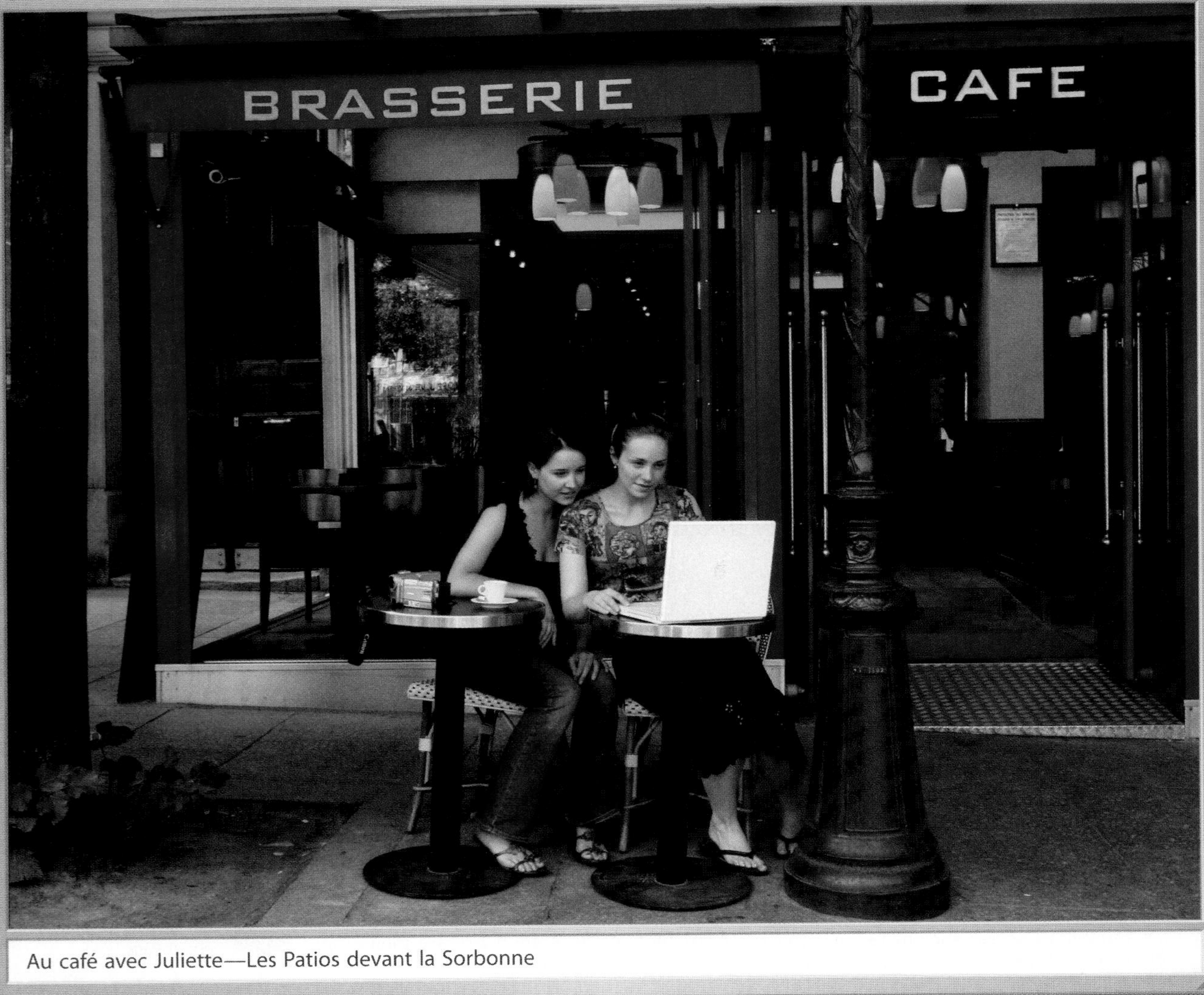

BRASSERIE

CAFE

Au café avec Juliette—Les Patios devant la Sorbonne

Cultural note: *La Sorbonne* is located in the *Quartier latin*, in the 5th *arrondissement* of Paris.

Dans ce chapitre...

OBJECTIFS COMMUNICATIFS

- greeting people
- spelling
- giving numerical information
- introducing yourself
- identifying people, places, and things
- expressing the date
- learning to pronounce the alphabet and selected vowel sounds in French

PAROLES (Leçons 1 et 2)

- Les bonnes manières
- L'alphabet français
- Les accents
- Les mots apparentés
- Les nombres de 0 à 60
- Les jours et les mois

STRUCTURES (Leçon 3)

- Dans la salle de classe
- Les articles indéfinis et le genre des noms

CULTURE

- Le blog de Léa: *Un jour exceptionnel**
- Reportage: *Bisous!*
- Lecture: *Publicité* (Leçon 4)

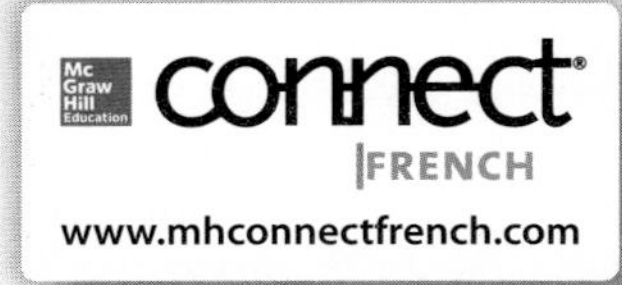

*In **Chapitres 1–4** of *Vis-à-vis*, you will read Léa Bouchard's blog about her life in Paris and the commentaries of other Francophone characters about her blog. See **Bienvenue à *Vis-à-vis*** and **Les pays francophones** (on the preceding pages) for more information on this special feature of *Vis-à-vis*.

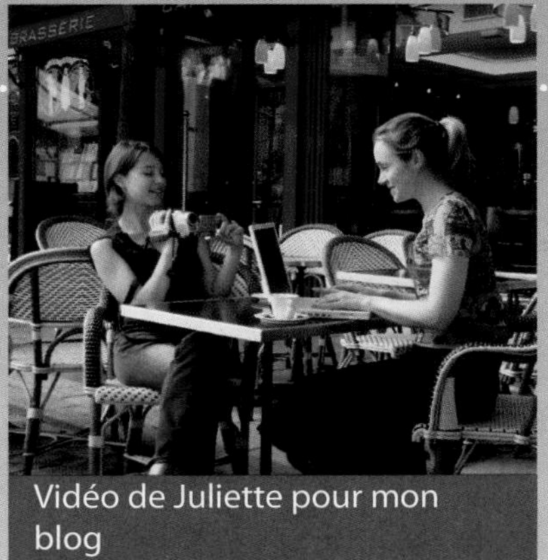

Vidéo de Juliette pour mon blog

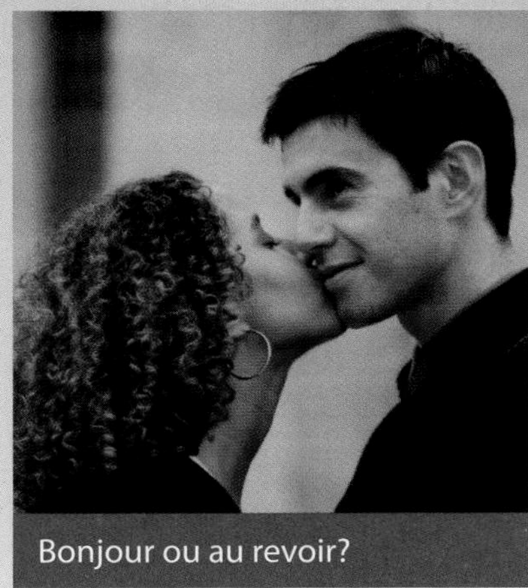

Bonjour ou au revoir?

Purpose: *Vis-à-vis* features a clear and user-friendly organization. The chapter opener presents the communicative objectives and the lexical and grammatical content of the chapter. Each chapter has four *Leçons* with *Le blog de…* and *Reportage* (a two-page cultural spread) separating *Leçons 2* and *3*. The organization of each chapter is as follows: *Leçon 1, Paroles* (vocabulary); *Leçon 2, Structures* (grammar); *Le blog de…* and *Reportage; Leçon 3, Structures* (grammar); *Leçon 4, Perspectives* (reading, writing, listening, and speaking). **Note:** Because *Chapitre 1* focuses more on functional language and basic skills, the first grammar points of the text are introduced in *Leçon 3*.

CHAPITRE 1

Leçon 1

Purpose: In *Chapitre 1,* vocabulary is presented in *Leçons 1, 2,* and part of *Leçon 3.* These *Paroles* sections present words and expressions that will get sts. speaking French. Most terms are illustrated through visual displays. New vocabulary is practiced after each visual presentation and is recycled throughout the chapter and the rest of the book.

PAROLES

Les bonnes manières°

Les... *Good manners*

Suggestion: Although the *tu/vous* distinction is explained in *Chapitre 2,* make sure sts. use informal expressions (*Comment t'appelles-tu?, Et toi?...*) among themselves.

In the French-speaking world, different greetings reflect the differing degrees of familiarity between people. Formality is the general rule; informal expressions are reserved for family, friends of long standing, and close associates and peers (for example, fellow students). All formal greetings are followed by a title: **Bonjour, madame.**

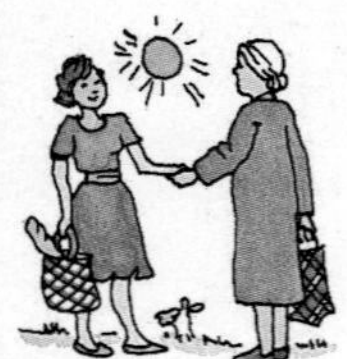

—Bonjour, mademoiselle.
—Bonjour, madame.

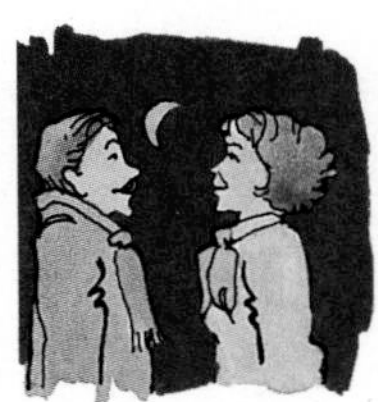

—Bonsoir, monsieur.
—Bonsoir, madame.

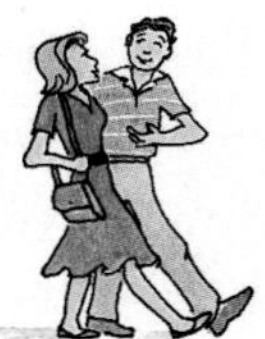

—Je m'appelle Lucas Martin. Et vous, comment vous appelez-vous?
—Je m'appelle Juliette Dupont.

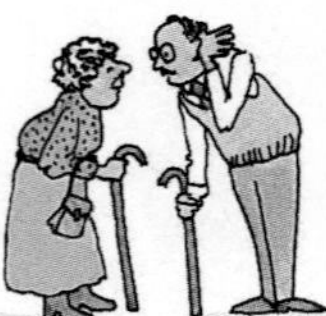

—Comment allez-vous?
—Très bien, merci. Et vous?
—Pas mal, merci.

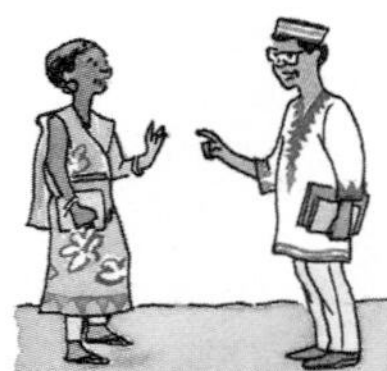

—Salut, ça va?
—Oui, ça va bien. (Ça va mal.) Et toi, comment vas-tu?
—Comme ci comme ça. (Ça peut aller.) (Moyen.)

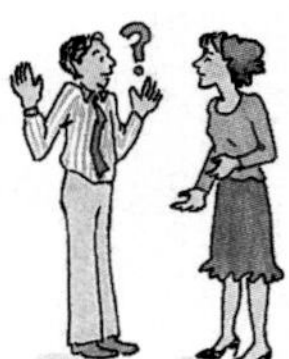

—Comment? Je ne comprends pas. Répétez, s'il vous plaît.
—C'est Lise Bernard.
—Ah oui, je comprends.

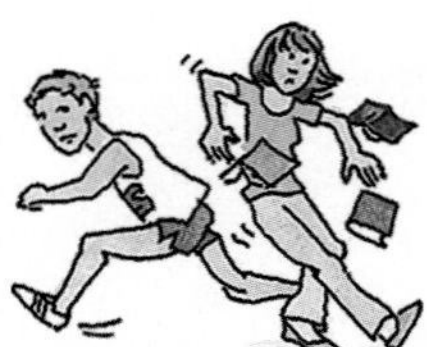

—Oh, pardon! Excusez-moi, mademoiselle.

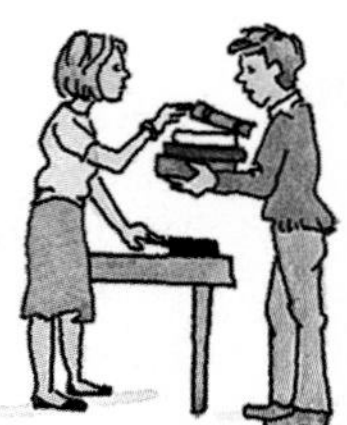

—Merci (beaucoup).
—De rien.

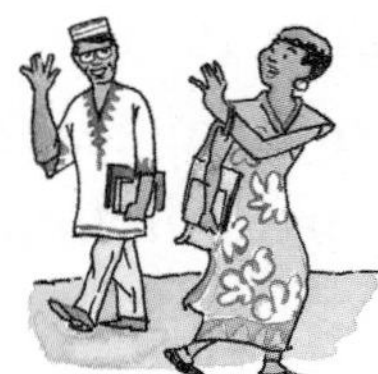

—Au revoir!
—À bientôt!

Suggestions: (1) Use group repetition to reinforce correct pronunciation. (2) Use these expressions in short, complete dialogues with sts. (3) Shake hands with individual sts. whenever appropriate while activating the exchanges.

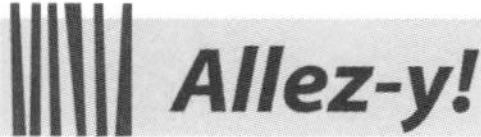

Allez-y!

A. Répondez, s'il vous plaît. Respond in French.

1. Je m'appelle Arthur Lenôtre. Et vous, comment vous appelez-vous? **2.** Bonsoir! **3.** Comment allez-vous? **4.** Merci. **5.** Ça va? **6.** Au revoir! **7.** Bonjour.

B. Soutenu ou familier? (*Formal or informal?*) Decide if each situation shown is formal or informal, then provide an appropriate expression for it.

1.

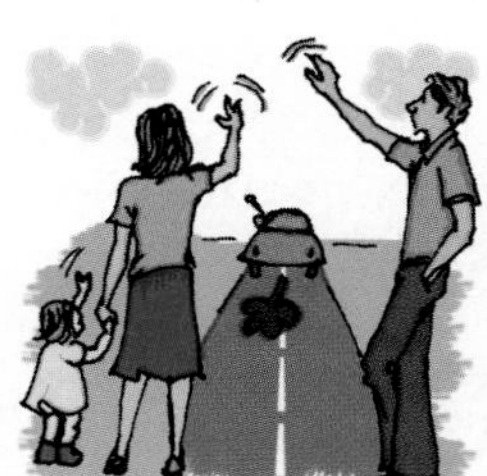

2.

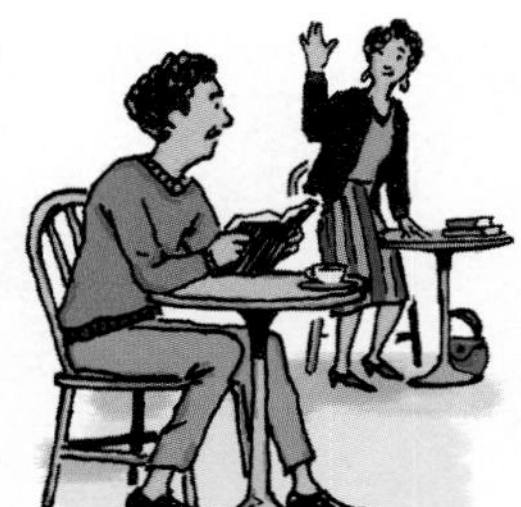

3.

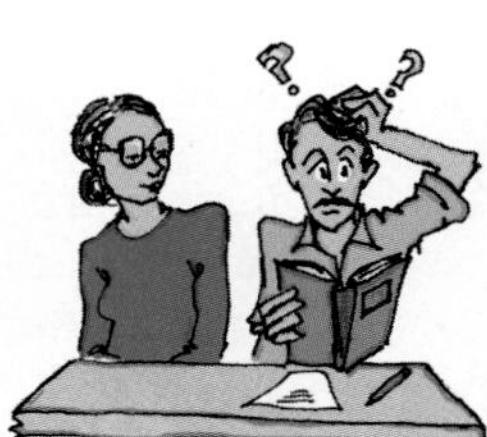

4.

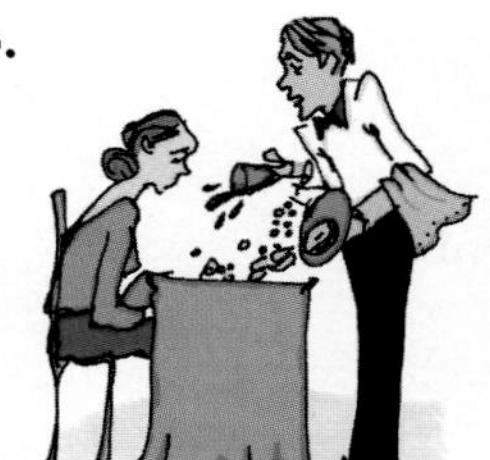

5.

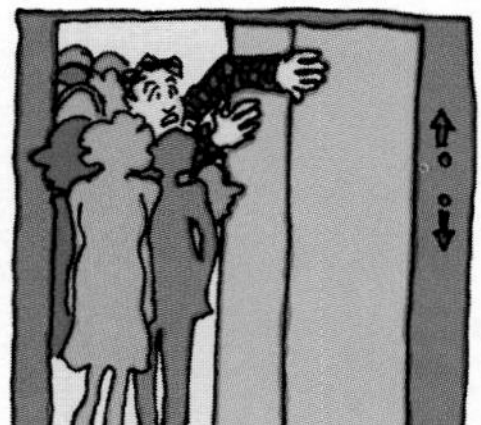

6.

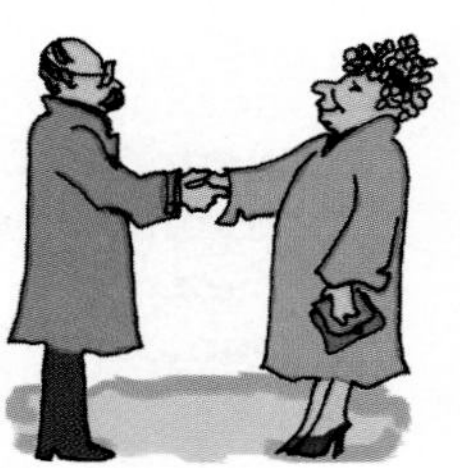

C. Le bon choix. (*The right choice.*) Indicate if the following expressions are used in a formal or informal context. What cues tell you whether it is formal or informal?

1. Comment vous appelez-vous?
2. Et toi?
3. Répète, s'il te plaît.
4. Comment vas-tu?
5. Comment t'appelles-tu?
6. Bonjour, monsieur!
7. Et vous?
8. Salut!
9. Répétez, s'il vous plaît.
10. Comment allez-vous?

Note: Direction lines to exs. are in English through *Chapitre 4*. Starting in *Chapitre 5*, they are in French, glossed where necessary.

Follow-up (A): (1) Sts. work in pairs, practicing handshakes with appropriate dialogue. (2) Sts. take on fictional identities while performing introductions (political figures, musicians, people known on your campus, etc.).

Suggestions (B): (1) Conduct as individual/group response activity. (2) Have sts. write caption first, then give it orally, followed by group repetition.

Le parler jeune

à plus (A+)	à plus tard; à bientôt
ça va super	ça va très bien
c'est la cata	ça va très mal
tchao	au revoir

—Salut! —**À plus!**

—Comment ça va? —**Ça va super!**

Mon mél (*email*) est bloqué: **c'est la cata!**

—Allez **tchao!** —À bientôt!

Presentation (*Le parler jeune*): You may want to point out to sts. that *cata* comes from *catastrophe*.

Purpose: *Le parler jeune* boxes offer contemporary colloquial/slang expressions that correspond to the chapter vocabulary. This vocabulary is presented for student interest and, although generally linked to a conversation activity, is not considered part of the chapter's active vocabulary.

Follow-up (B): How would you greet your English professor at 10:00 AM? at 8:30 PM? your cousin at noon? What would you say if you were standing in an elevator next to someone you didn't know but wanted to meet?

Follow-up (C): Ask sts. to pair informal/formal expressions (*Et toi? / Et vous?*).

L'alphabet français

Suggestion (*L'alphabet*): Make sure the sts. differentiate between sound and letter.

Suggestion: Model pronunciation of the letters. Bring in letters on flash cards. Mix up the letters and have sts. give the letter in French. Spell out places and names and ask sts. to write, guessing the meaning of the words you have spelled.

a	a	**h**	hache	**o**	o	**v**	vé
b	bé	**i**	i	**p**	pé	**w**	double vé
c	cé	**j**	ji	**q**	ku	**x**	iks
d	dé	**k**	ka	**r**	erre	**y**	i grec
e	e	**l**	elle	**s**	esse	**z**	zède
f	effe	**m**	emme	**t**	té		
g	gé	**n**	enne	**u**	u		

L'alphabet phonétique

[a]	**à**, l**a**	[b]	**b**onjour
[ɑ]	p**â**té	[k]	**c**omme, **qu**atre, **k**ilo
[ə]	j**e**, f**e**nêtre	[ʃ]	**ch**aise
[e]	r**é**p**é**t**ez**, all**er**	[d]	**d**imanche
[ɛ]	tr**è**s, mademois**e**lle, fen**ê**tre	[f]	**f**enêtre
[i]	**i**l, st**y**lo	[g]	**g**arçon
[o]	styl**o**, bient**ô**t, bur**eau**	[ɲ]	espa**gn**ol
[ɔ]	p**o**rte	[ʒ]	**j**e, biolo**g**ie
[u]	v**ou**s	[l]	**l**a
[y]	t**u**	[m]	**m**ade**m**oiselle
[ø]	d**eu**x	[n]	**n**euf
[œ]	s**œu**r, n**eu**f	[ŋ]	parki**ng**
[ɑ̃]	comm**en**t, écr**an**	[p]	**p**ardon
[ɛ̃]	bi**en**, c**in**q	[ʀ]	**r**épétez
[ɔ̃]	b**on**jour	[s]	**s**ix, cin**q**, fran**ç**ais, cla**ss**e
[œ̃]	**un**	[t]	**t**able
[j]	b**i**en, mo**y**en, jui**ll**et	[v]	**v**endredi, **w**agon
[ɥ]	h**u**it	[z]	chai**s**e, dou**z**e
[w]*	**ou**i, **w**eek-end		

*The spelling **-oi-** as in "bons**oi**r" is pronounced [wɑ].

Les accents

Suggestion (*Les accents*): Mention that the *circonflexe* is a historical sign for *s* (e.g., forest = *forêt*). You may wish to give examples of how accents distinguish between two words: *ou/où, la/là*.

Accents or diacritical marks sometimes change the pronunciation of a letter and sometimes distinguish between two words otherwise spelled the same. A French word written without its diacritical marks is misspelled.

é e **accent aigu**
à a **accent grave**
ô o **accent circonflexe**
ï i **tréma**
ç c **cédille**

Allez-y!

Follow-up (A): Play hangman, giving a few examples before sts. give their own words.

A. À vous! Spell your name in French. Then spell the name of a city, and see if your classmates can figure out which one it is.

B. Inscription. Several students are signing up to live in the campus international house. Spell their names and cities for the resident assistant.

1. DUPONT Isabelle	Paris	**4.** GUEYE Jérôme	Dakar
2. EL AYYADI Allal	Rabat	**5.** HUBERT Sarah	Lille
3. GOUTAL Ariane	Papeete	**6.** PASTEUR Loïc	Montréal

Suggestion (B): (1) Introduce *majuscule/minuscule.* (2) Have sts. find the cities on the maps at the back of the book.

Les mots apparentés°

°Les… *Cognates*

French and English have many cognates, or **mots apparentés:** words spelled similarly with similar meanings. Their pronunciation often differs dramatically in the two languages.

Here are a few patterns to help you recognize cognates.

FRANÇAIS	ANGLAIS	
-ant	*-ing*	amus**ant** → *amus**ing***
ét-	*st-*	**ét**at → ***st**ate*
-ie, -é	*-y*	cit**é** → *cit**y***
-eux, -euse	*-ous*	séri**eux** → *seri**ous***
-ique	*-ic, -ical*	prat**ique** → *pract**ical***
-iste	*-ist, -istic*	matérial**iste** → *material**istic***
-ment	*-ly*	rapide**ment** → *rapid**ly***
-re	*-er*	ord**re** → *ord**er***

Suggestion: Emphasize the rhythm of the syllables in French.

Be aware that there are also many apparent cognates, called **faux amis** (*false friends*). Here are a few examples along with the correct terms (**mots justes**).

FAUX AMIS		MOTS JUSTES	
collège	*secondary school*	université	*college, university*
librairie	*bookstore*	bibliothèque	*library*
rester	*to stay, remain*	se reposer	*to rest*

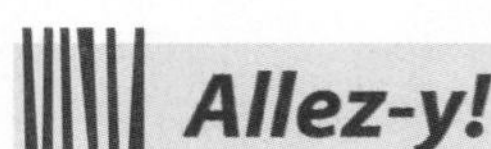

A. Répétez, s'il vous plaît! Pronounce these French cognates as your instructor does.

1. attitude	**4.** bracelet	**7.** injustice	**10.** parfum
2. police	**5.** passion	**8.** hôpital	**11.** magazine
3. balle	**6.** conclusion	**9.** champagne	**12.** présentation

Suggestion (A): You may wish to compare and contrast English and French pronunciation of these cognates.

B. Les mots apparentés. Figure out the English equivalents for the first five words. Then try to figure out the French equivalents for the last five words.

MODÈLES: étranger → *stranger*
generally → généralement

1. logique	**6.** *imperialistic*
2. centre	**7.** *strange*
3. étude	**8.** *tender*
4. liberté	**9.** *logically*
5. courageuse	**10.** *historic*

Suggestion (B): Conduct as group repetition first, then solicit individual responses, if desired.

Leçon 2

PAROLES

Note: Numbers above 60 are presented in *Chapitre 7.*

Presentation: Model pronunciation, followed by group response. Point out the pronunciation of *x* in *deux, six, dix* when the number is used alone, before a vowel, and before a consonant.

Suggestions: For listening comprehension, have sts. write the number they hear: 1, 5, 7, 14, 6, 20, 18, 12, etc., or use flash cards with numbers in random order and have sts. say the number as it appears.

Suggestion: To preview expressing age (*Chapitre 3*), bring in photos of people and ask sts. to guess their ages. Give model: *Il/Elle a… ans.*

Les nombres de 0 à 60°

Les… *Numbers from 0 to 60*

0	zéro	6	six	11	onze	16	seize
1	un	7	sept	12	douze	17	dix-sept
2	deux	8	huit	13	treize	18	dix-huit
3	trois	9	neuf	14	quatorze	19	dix-neuf
4	quatre	10	dix	15	quinze	20	vingt
5	cinq						

21	vingt et un	26	vingt-six	40	quarante
22	vingt-deux	27	vingt-sept	50	cinquante
23	vingt-trois	28	vingt-huit	60	soixante
24	vingt-quatre	29	vingt-neuf		
25	vingt-cinq	30	trente		

Un peu plus…°

Un… *A little more*

Combien de drapeaux y a-t-il?
(How many flags are there?) The French flag has great symbolic value for the nation. It appeared during the French Revolution in 1789 to replace the blue and white flag of the monarchy, the **fleur de lys.** The **tricolore,** as the flag is sometimes called, combines white with blue and red (the colors of Paris). The three colors are often associated with the principles upon which the French republic was founded: **liberté, égalité, fraternité.** The French flag is increasingly displayed alongside the flag of the European Union, blue with a circle of twelve gold stars. The number 12 is a traditional symbol of perfection, completeness, and unity. The circle formation represents solidarity and harmony. What does your national flag symbolize?

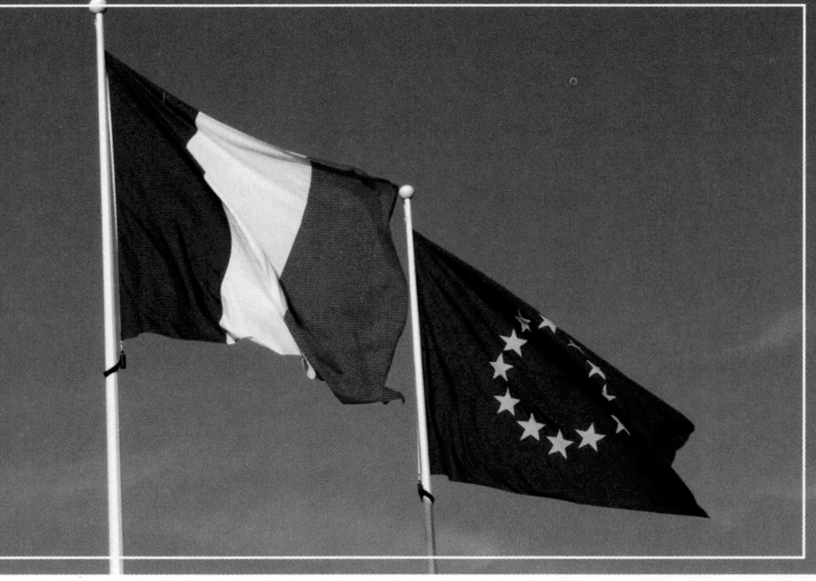

► *Le tricolore et le drapeau de l'Union européenne*

Note: The American flag, sometimes called "The Stars and Stripes", has been changed several times over the history of the United States of America. The colors did not have meaning when the flag was adopted in 1777, but today they are often said to symbolize hardiness and valor (red), purity and innocence (white), and vigilance, perseverence, and justice (blue). In addition, the thirteen stripes (seven red and six white) represent the original thirteen colonies, and the stars represent the fifty states of the Union. In the original Flag Act of 1777, it was resolved that the stars on a blue field represented "a new constellation." The Canadian flag was adopted in 1965. The colors red and white are Canada's official colors (proclaimed in 1921), and the maple leaf is a long-held historical symbol of the land and the people of Canada.

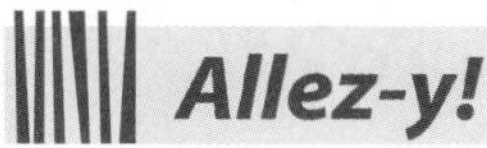

Allez-y!

A. Problèmes de mathématiques. Alternating with a partner, do the following math problems.

VOCABULAIRE UTILE

+ plus, et	− moins	× fois	= font

Combien font 3 plus 10? *How much is 3 + 10?*

MODÈLE: 6 + 2 →
É1*: Combien font six plus (et) deux?
É2: Six plus (et) deux font huit.

1. 8 + 2
2. 5 + 9
3. 4 + 1
4. 3 + 8
5. 43 − 16
6. 60 − 37
7. 56 − 21
8. 49 − 27
9. 2 × 10
10. 3 × 20
11. 6 × 5
12. 7 × 3

B. Les numéros de téléphone. In French, telephone numbers are said in groups of five two-digit numbers. Look at Marine's contact list and, alternating with a partner, read aloud some of her most frequently called numbers.

MODÈLE: É1: Simon Beaujour?
É2: 02.40.29.07.39

MES AMIS

nom	prénom	adresse	tél.
Duclos	Maxime	60, bd. de l'égalité	02.41.48.05.52
Bercegol	Valentine	98, avenue Patton	02.41.46.42.60
de Bailleux	Bénédicte	83, rue des Renardières	02.41.57.13.44
Koehulein	Alice	7, rue de Verneuil	02.41.35.21.08
Beaujour	Simon	12, rue du Temple	02.40.29.07.39

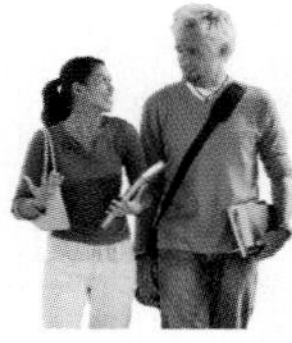

Suggestions (A): (1) Give question *Combien font x et y?* as stimulus for ex. Call on individuals for answers. (2) Do as listening comprehension activity by dictating problems to sts. whose books are closed or to sts. at the board.

Follow-up (A): (1) Write additional problems on flashcards or on the board. Sts. read problems aloud and give answers. (2) Sts. make up additional problems and give them orally. (3) Give a long, continuous problem for fun. For example: 10 + 5 + 4 − 7 − 11 + 6 + 2 + 9 − 1 + 3 = ? (Answer: 20).

Additional activity: *Quel est le plus grand nombre?* 1. *six, seize* 2. *deux, douze* 3. *treize, trois,* etc.

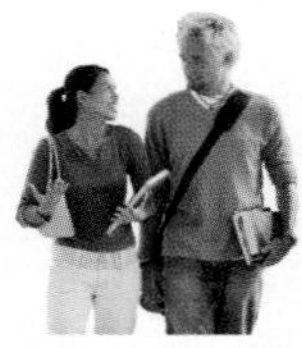

Suggestion (B): To exploit illustration further, model pronunciation of names and have sts. repeat and spell them.

Follow-up (B): Have sts. work in pairs, with one dictating phone numbers to the other, whose book is closed.

*É1 and É2 stand for **Étudiant(e) 1** and **Étudiant(e) 2** (*Student 1* and *Student 2*). These abbreviations are used in partner/pair activities throughout *Vis-à-vis*.

Quel jour sommes-nous?°

Quel... *What day is it?*

La semaine° de Claire

week

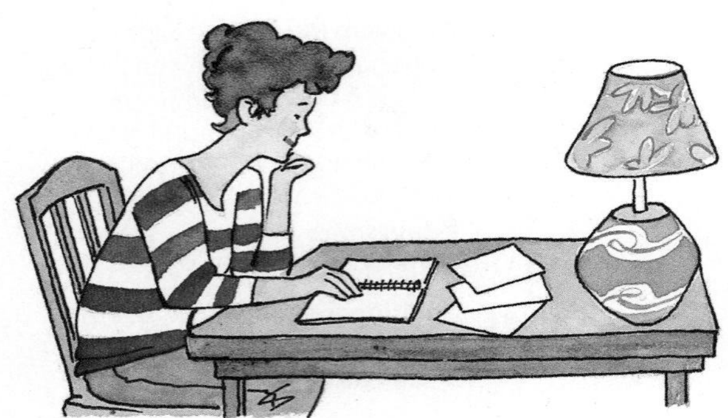

lundi	examen de biologie
mardi	examen de chimie
mercredi	dentiste
jeudi	tennis avec° Augustin
vendredi	laboratoire
samedi	théâtre avec Augustin
dimanche	en famille

°*with*

Presentation: Model pronunciation of days of week and have sts. repeat after your model. Use the following *Allez-y!* with this visual. Practice days of week by asking: *Quel jour sommes-nous? Quels sont les jours du week-end? Quel est votre jour préféré? Quel jour détestez-vous?* In presenting new material, answer questions yourself first, giving your opinion, before asking sts. to answer.

Note: All the days of the week are masculine.

In French, the days of the week are not capitalized. The week begins with Monday.

—Quel jour sommes-nous (aujourd'hui)? / Quel jour est-ce (aujourd'hui)?	*What day is it (today)?*
—Nous sommes mardi. / C'est mardi.	*It's Tuesday.*

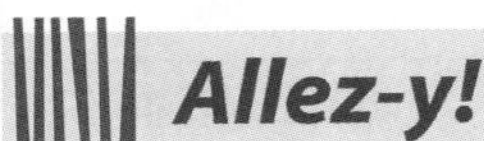

Allez-y!

Suggestion: Present prepositional phrases (*au cours, au laboratoire, chez le dentiste*, etc.) as fixed forms; sts. are not expected to produce them at this point. *Être* appears in *Chapitre 2*, *avoir* in *Chapitre 3*, and *aller* in *Chapitre 5*.

Additional activity: Solicit group response, or call on individuals, with class repeating together. *Quel jour sommes-nous?* MODÈLE: *Easter* → *Nous sommes dimanche.* 1. Thanksgiving 2. Good Friday 3. Labor Day 4. Ash Wednesday 5. Super Bowl

La semaine de Claire. Look over Claire's calendar. Then, alternating with a partner, tell what day of the week it is.

MODÈLE: Claire est au (*is at the*) laboratoire. →
É1: Claire est au laboratoire. Quel jour est-ce? (Quel jour sommes-nous?)
É2: C'est vendredi. (Nous sommes vendredi.)

1. Claire va (*goes*) au théâtre avec Augustin.
2. Claire est chez (*at*) le dentiste.
3. Claire a (*has*) un cours de biologie.
4. Claire est en famille.
5. Claire joue au (*is playing*) tennis avec Augustin.
6. Claire a un examen de chimie.

Quelle est la date d'aujourd'hui?

LES MOIS (*m.*)

décembre	mars	juin	septembre
janvier	avril	juillet	octobre
février	mai	août	novembre

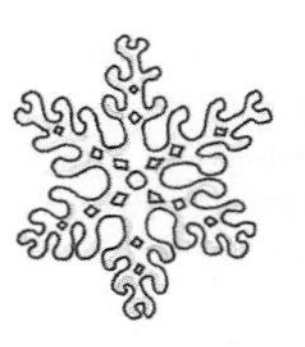
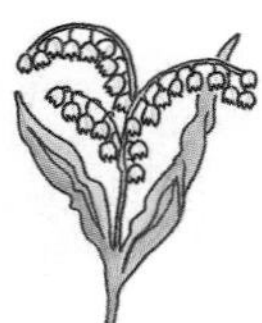
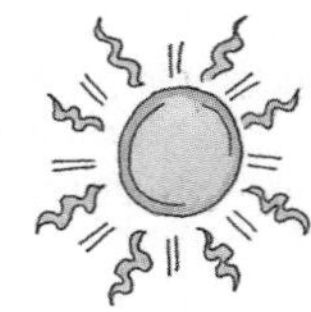
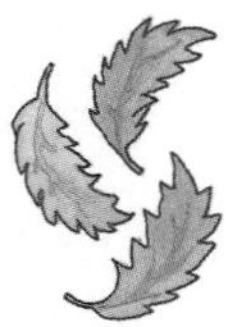

In French, the day is usually followed by the month: **Nous sommes le 21 mars** (abbreviated as 21.3). The word **le** (*the*) usually precedes the day of the month.

Dates in French are expressed with cardinal numbers (**le 21 mars**), with the exception of the first of the month: **le 1er (premier) janvier.**

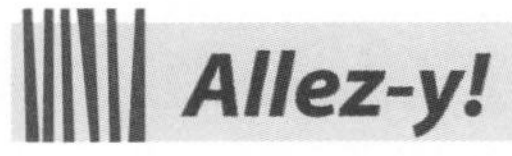

Allez-y!

Continuation (A): Continue with other holidays: *le solstice d'été, Hanoukkah, la fête des rois, le mardi gras,* etc.

A. Fêtes (*Holidays*) **américaines.** What months do you associate with the following holidays?

1. 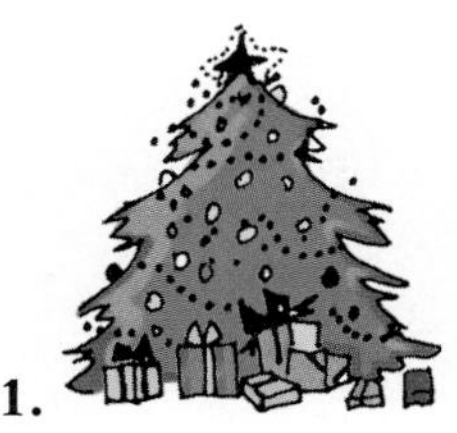
2. 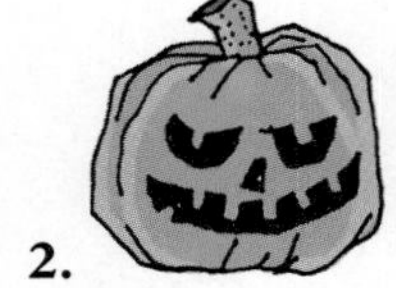
3. 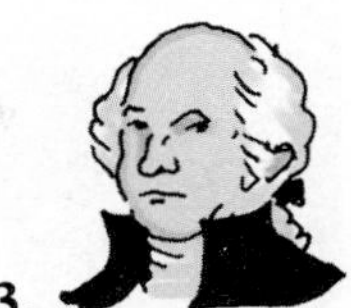
4. 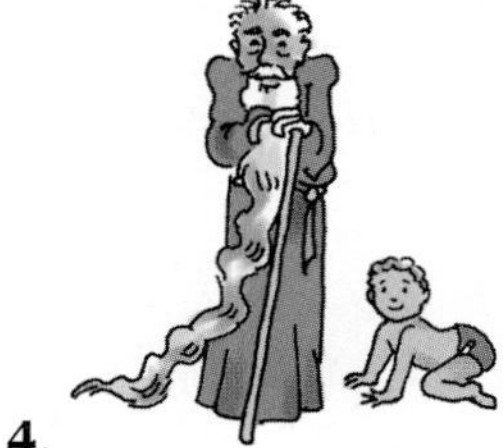
5. 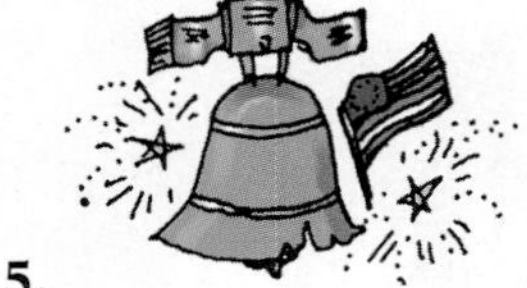
6. 
7. 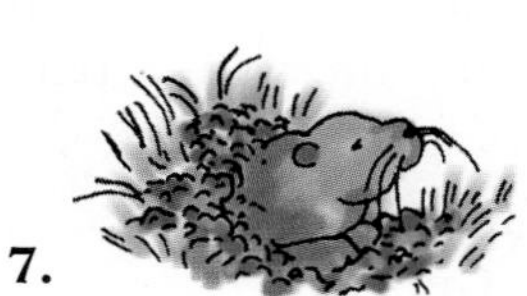
8. 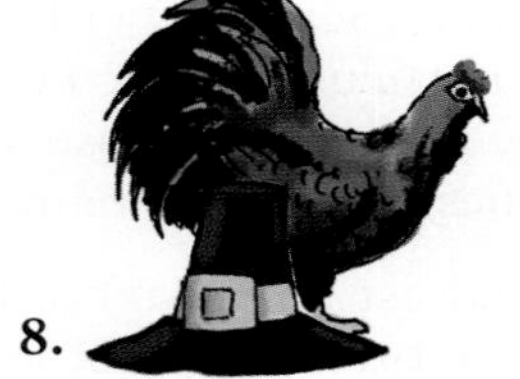

Additional vocabulary: You may want to introduce names of seasons at this time. They are presented in *Chapitre 5*. Years are taught in *Chapitre 8, Leçon 1*.

Suggestion: Teach *Quelle est la date de ton anniversaire?* Ask sts. to find someone in the class with a birthday in each of the 12 months. Sts. write down the names and months; the first to finish wins.

Vocabulary recycling: Quickly review numbers from 1–31. Pick a date, and have sts. call out the date for the previous or the following day. Challenge them to continue in round-robin style for as long as they can.

Additional activity: Have the sts. give the date. You write 22.9, and they say: *le 22 septembre*.

Prononcez bien!

The vowels in *ci, les,* and *mai*

In French, vowels are shorter and pronounced with tenser muscles than they are in English. When you pronounce **ci** [i], **les** [e], and **mai** [ɛ], remember to keep the vowel brief and steady while gradually opening your mouth and relaxing your lips from a smiling position to a neutral shape. Notice the different spellings of each sound.

[i]: **jeudi, souris, stylo**

[e]: **les, et, janvier, répétez**

[ɛ]: **mai, c'est, merci, très, treize, fenêtre**

The vowel sound in **mai** is pronounced with less muscle tension and a mouth open wider than for the vowel sound in **les.**

Purpose: *Prononcez bien!* presents pronunciation tips in order to give sts. practice with difficult sounds and words. As with the *Prononciation* feature in the Workbook/Laboratory Manual, these boxes have been recorded as part of the Audio Program to accompany *Vis-à-vis.*

Pronunciation practice: The *Prononcez bien!* section on page 24 of this chapter contains activities for practicing these sounds.

Note: Realia comes from *Air Canada Magazine.*

Suggestion: If you have sts. from different countries, have them give dates of important national and religious holidays in their country.

Additional activity: *Les fêtes nationales.* Ask sts. to name the national holiday for *Canada (1er juillet); Québec (24 juin); France (14 juillet); Belgique (21 juillet); Suisse (1er août);* etc.

B. Le voyageur bien informé. It can be useful to know the holidays of the countries you visit. Look at the following lists and compare the three countries. Note that the dates of some holidays vary from country to country and from year to year.

SUISSE

1er janv.	Nouvel An
2 janv.	Fête légale
24 mars	Vendredi saint
26 mars	Pâques
27 mars	Lundi de Pâques
4 mai	Ascension
15 mai	Lundi de Pentecôte
1er août	Fête nationale
25 déc.	Noël
26 déc.	Lendemain de Noël

ÉTATS-UNIS

1er janv.	Nouvel An
20 févr.	Anniversaire de Washington
24 mars	Vendredi saint
29 mai	Jour du Souvenir
4 juill.	Fête de l'Indépendance
5 sept.	Fête du Travail
11 nov.	Fête des Anciens Combattants
23 nov.	Action de Grâce
25 déc.	Noël

FRANCE

1er janv.	Nouvel An
27 mars	Lundi de Pâques
1er mai	Fête du Travail
4 mai	Ascension
8 mai	Armistice
15 mai	Lundi de Pentecôte
14 juill.	Fête nationale (Prise de la Bastille)
15 août	Assomption
1er nov.	Toussaint
11 nov.	Jour du Souvenir
25 déc.	Noël

1. Quelles fêtes aux États-Unis ne sont pas célébrées en France? en Suisse? Donnez (*Give*) la date de ces (*these*) fêtes.
2. Y a-t-il plus de (*more*) fêtes religieuses en France et en Suisse qu'aux (*than in the*) États-Unis? Nommez-les (*Name them*) et donnez leur date.
3. Donnez les dates des fêtes nationales dans les trois pays.
4. Quel est votre jour de fête préféré? Pourquoi? (*Why?*)

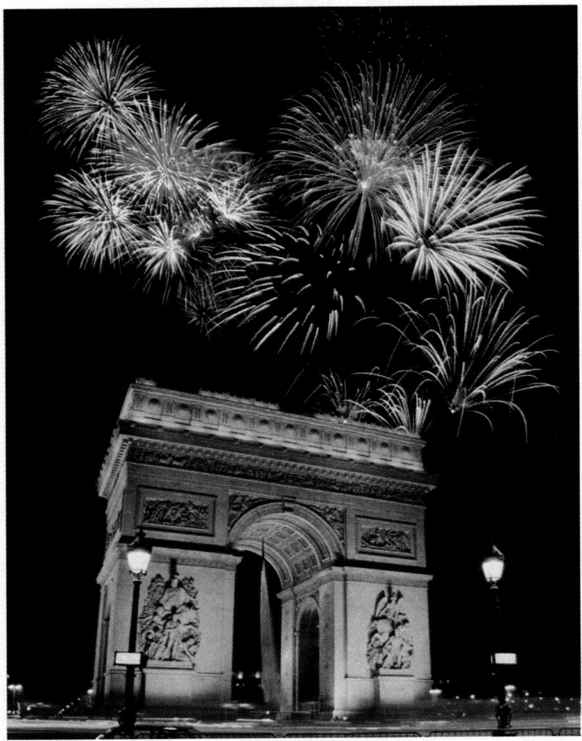

Le 14 juillet, la fête nationale, à Paris

C. La fête des patrons. (*Saint's day.*) In France, each day of the year is associated with a particular saint. Look over the list of names and dates on the following page. Choose six of them and, with a partner, ask and answer questions about name days.

MODÈLE: É1: Quand est (*When is*) la fête de Jules?
É2: Le vingt-trois mai. Et la fête de Gilbert?

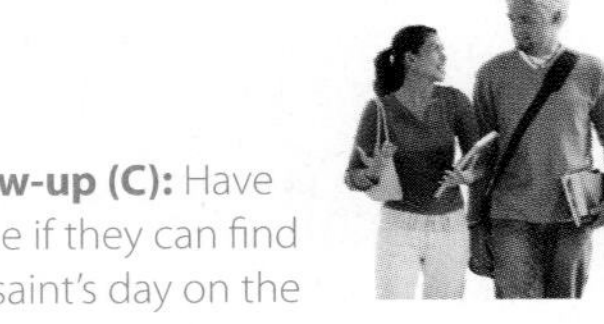

Follow-up (C): Have sts. see if they can find their saint's day on the list.

fêtes à souhaiter°

a

ADOLPHE	30	juin
ADRIEN	8	sept
AGNES	21	janv
AIME	13	sept
AIMEE	20	fév
ALAIN	9	sept
ALBAN	22	juin
ALBERT	15	nov
ALEXANDRE	22	avril
ALEXIS	17	fév
ALFRED	15	août
ALICE	16	déc
ALINE	20	oct
ALPHONSE	1	août
AMAND	6	fév
ANATOLE	3	fév
ANDRE	30	nov
ANGE	5	mai
ANGELE	27	janv
ANNE	26	juil
ANSELME	21	avril
ANTOINE	17	janv
ANTOINETTE	28	fév
ANTONIN	2	mai
ARISTIDE	31	août
ARLETTE	17	juil
ARMAND	8	juin
ARMEL	16	août
ARNAUD	10	fév
ARTHUR	15	nov
AURORE	13	déc

b

BAUDOUIN	17	oct
BEATRICE	13	fév
BENJAMIN	31	mars
BENOIT	11	juil
BERNADETTE	18	fév
BERNARD	20	août
BERTHE	4	juil
BERTRAND	6	sept
BRIGITTE	23	juil

c

CAMILLE	14	juil
CARINE	7	nov
CAROLE	17	juil
CATHERINE	25	nov
CECILE	22	nov
CELINE	21	oct
CHANTAL	12	déc
CHARLES	2	mars
CHRISTEL (LE)	24	juil
CHRISTIAN	12	nov
CHRISTINE	24	juil
CHRISTOPHE	21	août
CLAIRE	11	août
CLAUDE	6	juin
CLEMENCE	21	mars
CLEMENT	23	nov
CLOTILDE	4	juin
COLETTE	6	mars
CORINNE	18	mai
CYRILLE	18	mars

d

DANIEL	11	déc
DAVID	29	déc
DELPHINE	26	nov
DENIS	9	oct
DENISE	15	mai
DIDIER	23	mai
DOMINIQUE	8	août

e

EDITH	13	sept
EDMOND	20	nov
EDOUARD	5	janv
ELIANE	4	juil
ELIE	20	juil
ELISABETH	17	nov
ELISE	17	nov
ELOI	1	déc
EMILE	22	mai
EMILIENNE	5	janv
EMMANUEL	25	déc
ERIC	18	mai
ERNEST	7	nov
ESTELLE	11	mai
ETIENNE	26	déc
EUGENE	13	juil
EVA	6	sept
EVELYNE	27	déc

f

FABIEN	20	janv
FABRICE	22	août
FELIX	12	fév
FERDINAND	30	mai
FERNAND	27	juin
FRANÇOIS	4	oct
FRANÇOISE	12	déc
FREDERIC	18	juil

g

GABRIEL (LE)	29	sept
GAEL	17	déc
GAETAN	7	août
GASTON	6	fév
GAUTIER	9	avril
GENEVIEVE	3	janv
GEOFFROY	8	nov
GEORGES	23	avril
GERALD	5	déc
GERARD	3	oct
GERAUD	13	oct
GERMAIN	31	juil
GERMAINE	15	juin
GERVAIS	19	juin
GHISLAIN	10	oct
GILBERT	7	juin
GILBERTE	11	août
GILLES	1	sept
GINETTE	3	janv
GISELE	7	mai
GODEFROY	8	nov
GONTRAN	28	mars
GREGOIRE	3	sept
GUILLAUME	10	janv
GUSTAVE	7	oct
GUY	12	juin

h

HELENE	18	août
HENRI	13	juil
HERVE	17	juin
HONORE	16	mai
HORTENSE	5	oct
HUBERT	3	nov
HUGUES	1	avril

i

IRENE	5	avril
ISABELLE	22	fév

j

JACINTHE	30	janv
JACQUELINE	8	fév
JACQUES	25	juil
JEAN	24	juin
JEANNE	30	mai
JEROME	30	sept
JOACHIM	26	juil
JOEL	13	juil
JOHANNE	30	mai
JOSEPH	19	mars
JOSETTE	19	mars
JOSSELIN	13	déc
JULES	12	avril
JULIEN	2	août
JULIENNE	16	fév
JULIETTE	30	juil
JUSTE	14	oct

k

KARINE	7	nov

l

LAETITIA	18	août
LAURENT	10	août
LEA	22	mars
LEON	10	nov
LILIANE	4	juil
LINE	20	oct
LIONEL	10	nov
LISE	17	nov
LOIC	25	août
LOUIS	25	août
LOUISE	15	mars
LUC	18	oct
LUCIE	13	déc
LUCIEN	8	janv
LUDOVIC	25	août

m

MADELEINE	22	juil
MARC	25	avril
MARCEL	16	janv
MARCELLE	31	janv
MARIANNE	9	juil
MARIANNICK	15	août
MARIE	15	août
MARIE-THERESE	7	juin
MARTHE	29	juil
MARTIAL	30	juin
MARTINE	30	janv
MARYVONNE	15	août
MATHILDE	14	mars
MATTHIAS	14	mai
MATTHIEU	21	sept
MAURICE	22	sept
MICHEL	29	sept
MICHELINE	19	juin
MIREILLE	15	août
MONIQUE	27	août
MURIEL	15	août

n

NATHALIE	27	juil
NELLY	18	août
NICOLAS	6	déc
NICOLE	6	mars
NOEL	25	déc

o

ODETTE	20	avril
ODILE	14	déc
OLIVIER	12	juil

p

PASCAL	17	mai
PATRICE	17	mars
PAUL	29	juin
PAULE	26	janv
PHILIPPE	3	mai
PIERRE	29	juin
PIERRETTE	31	mai

r

RAOUL	7	juil
RAPHAEL	29	sept
RAYMOND	7	janv
REGINE	7	sept
REGIS	16	juin
REMI	15	janv
RENAUD	17	sept
RENE (E)	19	oct
RICHARD	3	avril
ROBERT	30	avril
RODOLPHE	21	juin
ROGER	30	déc
ROLAND	15	sept
ROLANDE	13	mai
ROMAIN	28	fév
RONALD	17	sept
ROSELINE	17	janv
ROSINE	11	mars

s

SABINE	29	août
SAMUEL	20	août
SANDRINE	2	avril
SEBASTIEN	20	janv
SERGE	7	oct
SIMON	28	oct
SOLANGE	10	mai
SOPHIE	25	mai
STANISLAS	11	avril
STEPHANE	26	déc
SUZANNE	11	août
SYLVAIN	4	mai
SYLVESTRE	31	déc
SYLVIE	5	nov

t

TANGUY	19	nov
THERESE	1	oct
THIBAUT	8	juil
THIERRY	1	juil
THOMAS	3	juil

v

VALENTIN	14	fév
VALENTINE	25	juil
VALERIE	28	avril
VERONIQUE	4	fév
VICTOR	21	juil
VINCENT de Paul	27	sept
VIRGINIE	7	janv
VIVIANE	2	déc

w

WALTER	9	avril
WILFRIED	12	oct

x

XAVIER	3	déc

y

YOLANDE	11	juin
YVES	19	mai
YVETTE	13	janv
YVON	19	mai

°fêtes… *celebrating saints' days*

Suggestion: Use names for pronunciation practice. Comparing pronunciation of cognates illustrates principles of French and English pronunciation clearly.

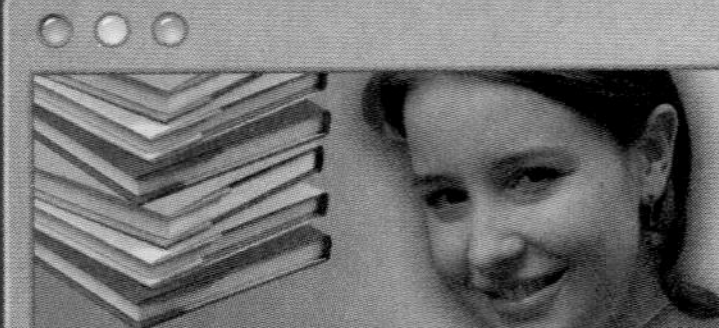

Le blog de Léa

Un jour exceptionnel°

°*jour... special day*

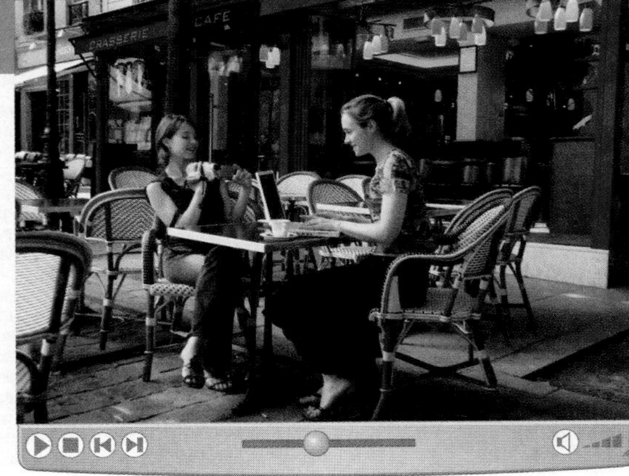

Vidéo de Juliette pour mon blog

vendredi 13 mai

Bonjour! Ça va?

Je m'appelle Léa. Je suis[1] étudiante. Et voilà, je crée un blog avec mes amis[2]! C'est pour communiquer, exprimer[3] des idées, des sentiments, des secrets... Aujourd'hui, c'est le vendredi 13! Un jour exceptionnel. Un jour de chance:[4] Mon blog sera[5] un succès. C'est sûr!

Au revoir, à bientôt
Léa la blogueuse[6]

COMMENTAIRES

Alexis

Léa, le vendredi 13, c'est de la pure superstition!

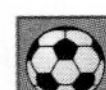

Mamadou

Léa, créer un blog un vendredi 13, c'est risqué! Le vendredi 13, c'est une combinaison fatale. ATTENTION.

Poema

Le vendredi 13: c'est le jour du Super Loto.[7]

Welcome to **Le blog de Léa.** Here, at the center of each chapter of *Vis-à-vis,* you will find:

- The blogs of four Parisians with different Francophone backgrounds. **Chapitres 1–4** feature **Le blog de Léa,** a 19-year-old student at the Sorbonne who lives in the **Quartier latin.** The blogs are followed by commentaries of other Francophone characters.
- The **Reportage** presents up-to-date information related to the chapter theme that depicts life in France, Quebec, North and West Africa, French-speaking Europe, or the Antilles.
- **À vous** offers comprehension questions and personalized questions to accompany the **Reportage.**
- **Parlons-en!** (*Let's talk about it!*) gives students the opportunity to do pair and group work using information from the reading and preceding sections.

[1]Je... *I am* [2]avec... *with my friends* [3]*express* [4]jour... *lucky day* [5]*will be* [6]*person who has a blog* [7]jour... *day of the French lottery drawing with a large cash prize*

Note: For additional activities related to *Le blog de Léa* and *Reportage,* see the Workbook/Laboratory Manual.

Follow-up: You may wish to ask sts. these questions in English and have them answer in French, or you can use this as an opportunity to introduce question words, which are formally presented in *Chapitre 4. Questions de compréhension: 1. Qui est Léa? (Regardez sa carte d'identité, p. 2.) 2. Pourquoi est-ce que Léa crée un blog? 3. Que signifie le vendredi 13 pour Léa? 4. Qui est superstitieux: Alexis? Mamadou? Poema?*

Video connection: In the videoblog for this chapter, Léa and her friends introduce themselves. Léa posts a video on her site about how French speakers typically greet each other and say good-bye.

Purpose: Cultural information appears throughout *Vis-à-vis* but is highlighted in *Le blog de...* and *Reportage. À vous* allows you to expand on the content of the *Reportage* by guiding sts.' conversation with general questions about cultural differences.

REPORTAGE

Bisous!

"Bonjour! Ça va?" With these words, Arielle greets her friend Luc and kisses him on the cheek. This is how French friends typically greet each other.

In France, to say "hello" or "good-bye," you give two, three, or sometimes four kisses, depending on the region in which you find yourself. The **bisou** is a kiss on the cheek. The term **bisou** has an affectionate connotation: You give a **bisou** to children, friends, and family in greeting.

In Belgium, a single kiss suffices, but three are necessary to celebrate joyful occasions.

In Quebec, the custom differs. Maria, who was born in Montreal, explains, "Like Americans, Canadians are warm and charming, but they often maintain a physical distance when greeting newcomers. Close friends and family members, however, share a **bisou.**"

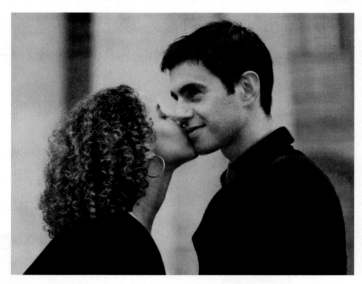

Bonjour ou au revoir? Baiser amical (*friendly kiss*) ou baiser d'amoureux (*lovers'*)? En France, en Belgique, au Canada, au Maroc ou au Sénégal? C'est difficile à dire (*to say*). Que pensez-vous? (*What do you think?*)

In Muslim countries, people typically do not touch but exchange friendly greetings such as **As-salaam'alaykum** (*Peace*) or **Que la paix de Dieu soit avec vous** (*God's peace be with you*).

Remember: You don't give a **bisou** to a person you are meeting for the first time. You politely say **bonjour** and shake his/her hand.

À vous!

1. In your culture, what do you do when you meet someone for the first time? How do you greet friends and family members?
2. What greeting customs from other cultures do you know?

Note: Some of the situations in *Parlons-en!* involve sts. giving one another *la bise*. You may ask sts. to present their situations in front of the class if they feel comfortable doing so.

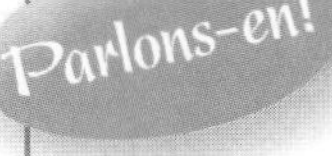

Parlons-en!

Work with a classmate to decide how you would greet the following French speakers in the situations listed below. Be sure to use the appropriate expressions and gestures. Use the information from the **Reportage** and from **Les bonnes manières,** page 8 to guide you.

1. Marie (20 years old) meets her mother at the supermarket in Montreal.
2. Aïcha (15 years old) meets her piano teacher, Madame Clément (40 years old), in the street in Poitiers.
3. Monsieur Kedadou, director of the French department at the Sorbonne, greets Isabelle, a first-year student, in the hall outside of class.
4. Jeanne, who lives in Brussels, greets her best friend, Victoire, who has just arrived to pick her up to go to the movies.

Leçon 3

STRUCTURES

Note: The explanation for the indefinite articles immediately follows *Dans la salle de classe.* Present the article with the noun, giving the translation *a (an)*. Point out that most singular and plural forms of nouns sound alike in French.

Purpose: In *Chapitre 1, Leçon 3* presents more vocabulary and then the first grammar structures—indefinite articles and noun genders and plurals. In this book, each grammar section is introduced by a brief functional dialogue. Contextualized examples recycle the vocabulary of the chapter.

Dans la salle de classe°

Dans... *In the classroom*

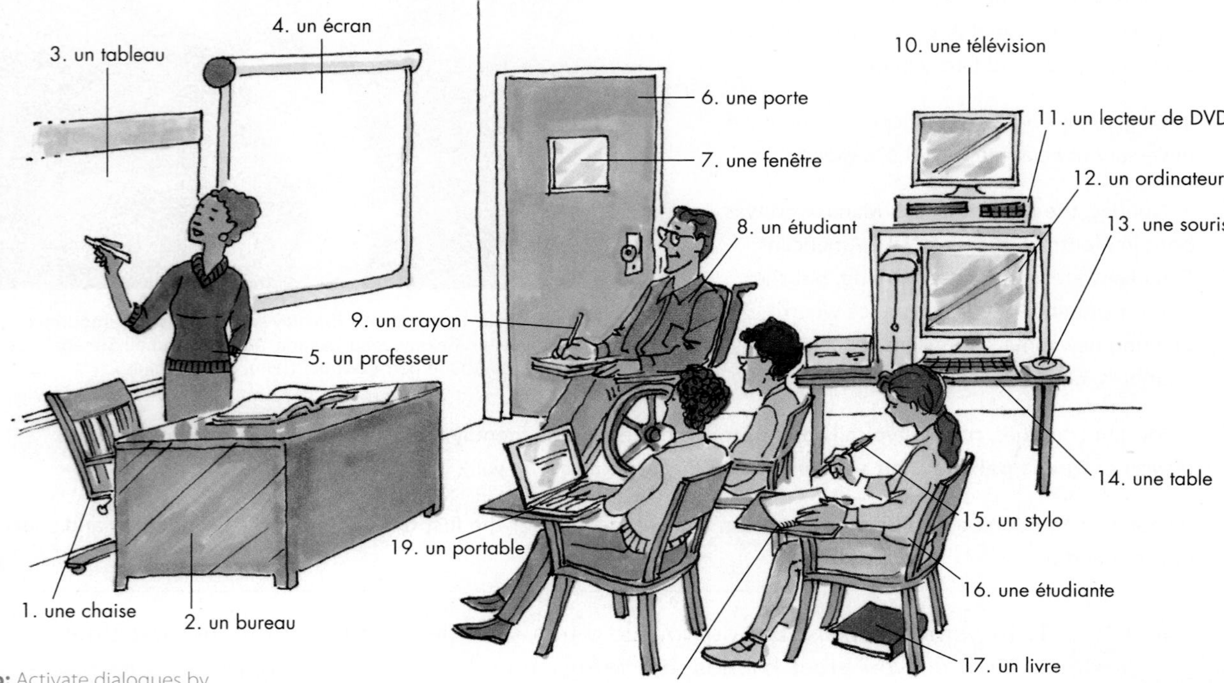

Follow-up: Activate dialogues by pointing to actual classroom objects: *Qu'est-ce que c'est? C'est une porte.*

Additional vocabulary: *une craie, une affiche,* or objects particular to your classroom.

Purpose: *Mots clés* presents lexical items for communication. This feature contains active vocabulary to be used in the activity (activities) it accompanies.

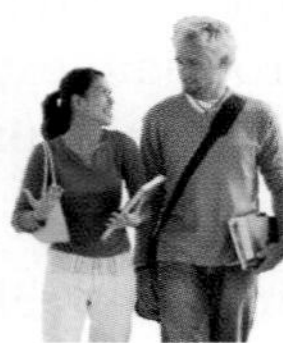

Allez-y!

Note: You may wish to point out to sts. that while *un professeur* is traditionally used for teachers of either gender, *la prof* is becoming more common.

A. Qu'est-ce que c'est? (*What is it?*) **Qui est-ce?** (*Who is it?*) Alternating with a classmate, identify the people and objects in the illustration above.

MODÈLE: É1: Le numéro un, qu'est-ce que c'est?
É2: C'est une (*It's a*) chaise.
É1: Le numéro cinq, qui est-ce?
É2: C'est un professeur.

B. Combien? (*How many?*) Taking turns with a classmate, ask and answer questions about the number of people and objects there are in the illustration. Use the expression **Il y a.**

MODÈLE: étudiants →
É1: Il y a combien d'étudiants?
É2: Il y a quatre étudiants.

Follow-up (B): Use *il y a* to ask about the number of people and objects in your classroom: *étudiant(e)s, professeurs, fenêtres, chaises, tables, télévisions, lecteurs de* DVD, *portes,* etc.

Follow-up (B): For listening comprehension practice, hand out a drawing similar to the one above, and have sts. place a number on an object according to your description: *L'objet numéro 1, c'est une chaise.* Sts. place a *1* on one of the chairs in the sketch.

Mots clés

Using *il y a*

The expression **il y a** (*there is, there are*) is used to state the existence of something or to specify the quantity.

Il y a un cours de français.
There is a French class.

Il y a quatre étudiants dans la classe.
There are four students in the classroom.

Les articles indéfinis et le genre des noms

Identifying People, Places, and Things

Étudier ou communiquer?

Léa contacte Mamadou sur sa page Facebook (Messagerie instantanée).

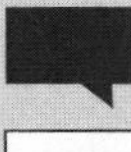

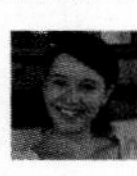

LÉA: Salut Mamadou! J'ai **un** blog et toi, tu as **une** page Facebook!

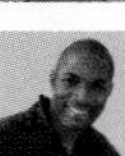

MAMADOU: Oui! J'ai aussi **un** compte Twitter et **un** smartphone. Pour communiquer.

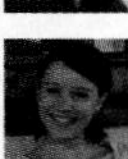

LÉA: Moi, j'ai **une** tablette, **des** cahiers et **des** livres. Pour étudier!

Vrai ou faux?

Léa étudie avec...

1. un blog
2. une page Facebook
3. un compte Twitter
4. un smartphone
5. une tablette
6. des cahiers
7. des livres

Mamadou communique avec...

1. un blog
2. une page Facebook
3. un compte Twitter
4. un smartphone
5. une tablette
6. des cahiers
7. des livres

Pronunciation presentation: Advise sts. to pronounce [y] as they would [i] in *merci*, by closing their mouth and pushing their tongue body to the front of the mouth, but rounding their lips as if to whistle. Model the pronunciation of *tu, salut, étudier.*

Pronunciation practice: The *Prononcez bien!* section on page 24 of this chapter contains activities for practicing these sounds.

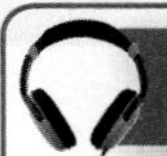

Prononcez bien!

The sounds in *un* and *une*

Note the pronunciation difference between **un** and **une: un** is made of only one sound (the nasal vowel [œ̃]), while **une** has two sounds (the vowel [y] as in **tu,** and the consonant [n]).

Let the air go through both your mouth and your nose when you pronounce **un;** *don't* pronounce the letter *n.*

[œ̃]: **un, lundi, commun**

Let the air go through your mouth only when pronouncing the vowel sound [y] in **une,** and *do* pronounce the *n.*

[y]: **une, lune, brune**

Singular Forms of Indefinite Articles

In French, all nouns (**noms**) are either masculine (**masculin**) or feminine (**féminin**), as are the articles that precede them.

The following chart shows the forms of the singular indefinite article in French, corresponding to *a* (*an*) in English.

MASCULINE		FEMININE	
un ami	*a friend* (*m.*)	**une** amie	*a friend* (*f.*)
un accent	*an accent*	**une** action	*an action*

Un is used for masculine nouns and **une** for feminine nouns. **Un** and **une** can also mean *one,* depending on the context.

Voilà **un** café.	*There's* a *café.*
Il y a **une** étudiante.	*There is* one *student.*

The Gender of Nouns

Note: The concept of number is covered in *Chapitre 2* with the definite articles.

Because the gender (**le genre**) of a noun is not always predictable, it is best to learn it along with the noun; for example, learn **un livre** rather than just **livre.** Here are a few general guidelines to help you determine gender; you will become more familiar with nouns in all of these categories as you work through the chapters of *Vis-à-vis.*

1. Nouns that refer to males are usually masculine; nouns that refer to females are usually feminine.

un homme	*a man*
une femme	*a woman*

2. Sometimes the ending of a noun is a clue to its gender.

MASCULINE		FEMININE	
-eau	un bur**eau**	**-ence**	une différ**ence**
-isme	un pr**isme**	**-ion**	une réact**ion**
-ment	un monu**ment**	**-ie**	une librair**ie**
		-ure	une lect**ure**
		-té	une universi**té**

3. Nouns borrowed from other languages are usually masculine.

   un coca-cola, un couscous, un baklava

4. The names of languages are masculine. They are not capitalized.

   Elle parle un français impeccable! *She speaks perfect French!*

5. Some nouns that refer to people can be changed from masculine to feminine by adding **e** to the noun ending.

un ami	*a friend* (*m.*)	une ami**e**	*a friend* (*f.*)
un étudiant	*a student* (*m.*)	une étudiant**e**	*a student* (*f.*)
un Français	*a French man* (*m.*)	une Français**e**	*a French woman* (*f.*)

Note: Final **t, n, d,** and **s** are silent in the masculine form. When followed by **-e** in the feminine form, they are pronounced.

6. Many nouns that end in **-e** have only one singular form, used to refer to both males and females. Sometimes the gender is indicated by the article.

un touriste	*a tourist* (*male*)
une touriste	*a tourist* (*female*)

Sometimes even the article is the same for both masculine and feminine.

un professeur	*a professor* (*male or female*)
un médecin	*a doctor* (*male or female*)
une personne	*a person* (*male or female*)
une vedette	*a movie star* (*male or female*)

[Allez-y! A]

Note: The information between brackets refers you to an exercise for that grammar point. In this case, **Allez-y!**, Activity A below, will allow you to practice this point.

Plural Forms of Indefinite Articles

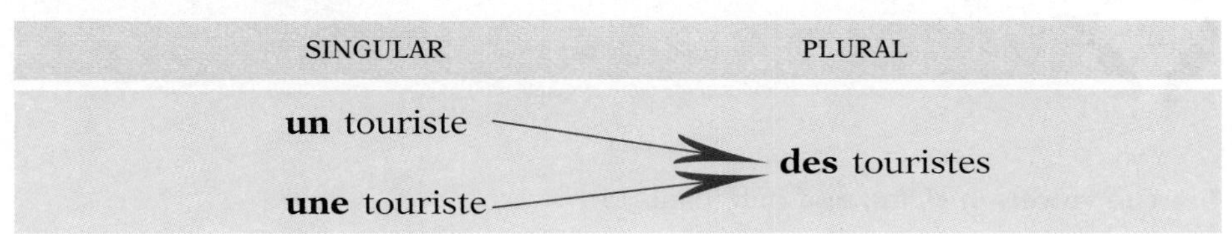

SINGULAR	PLURAL
un touriste	**des** touristes
une touriste	

The plural form (**le pluriel**) of the indefinite articles is always **des.*** Usually, an **s** is added to the noun:

un ami → **des** ami**s**	*a friend; some friends, friends*
une question → **des** question**s**	*a question; some questions, questions*

[Allez-y! B-C]

Grammaire interactive

For more on indefinite articles and the gender and number of nouns, watch the corresponding Grammar Tutorial and take a brief practice quiz at **Connect French.**

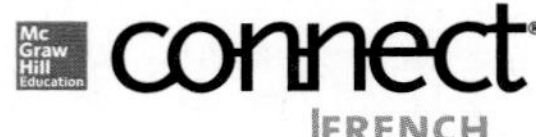

www.mhconnectfrench.com

Suggestion (A, B, C): Emphasize *liaison.*

Allez-y!

A. Qu'est-ce que c'est? (*What is it?*) Working with a partner, identify the following items and people.

MODÈLE: →

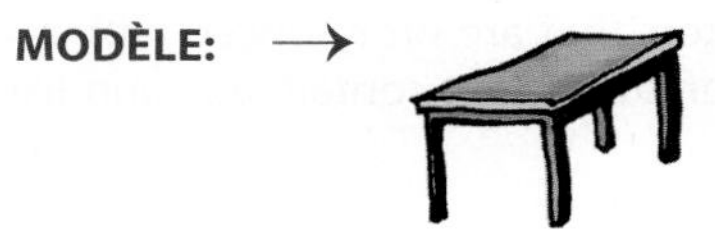

É1: Qu'est-ce que c'est?
É2: C'est une table.

1. 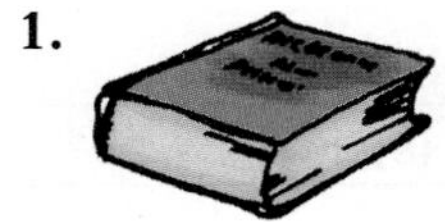

2. 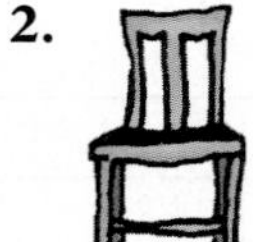

3. 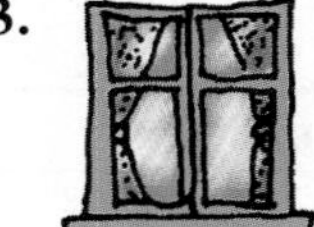

4. 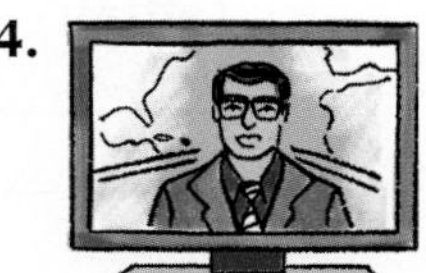

5. 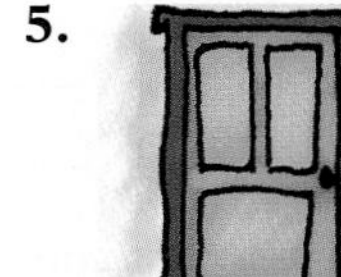

6. 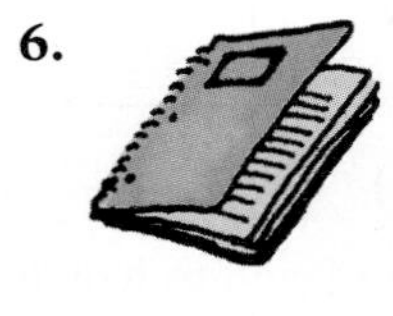

7. 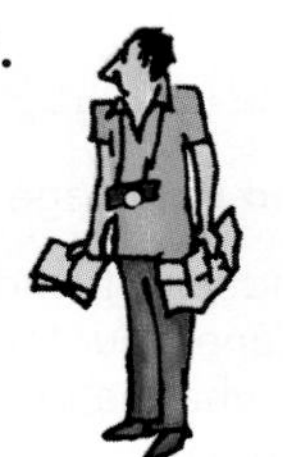

8. 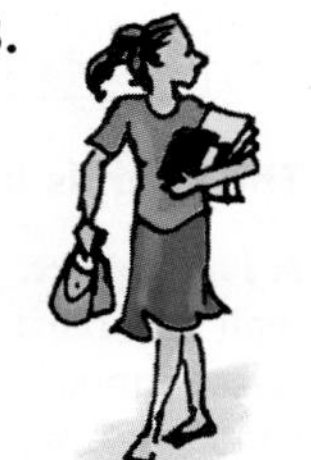

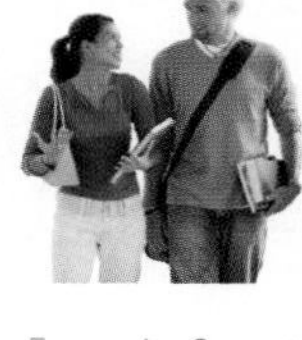

Suggestion: Use this quiz as a preliminary ex. (listening comprehension): Give sts. these words; they respond with *féminin* or *masculin.* 1. *une femme* 2. *une Française* 3. *un touriste* 4. *une comédie* 5. *un étudiant* 6. *une personne* 7. *un stylo* 8. *une fenêtre* 9. *un garçon* 10. *un département*

Follow-up (A): Show pictures of other objects or point to other things in classroom.

B. Dans une salle de classe. Give the plural.

MODÈLE: un stylo → Voilà (*Here are*) des stylos.

1. une table	**3.** une chaise	**5.** une porte
2. un écran	**4.** un ordinateur	**6.** un cahier

---

*In French, the final **s** of the article is usually silent, except when followed by a vowel or vowel sound: **des‿étudiants; des‿hommes.** In these cases, the **s** is pronounced like the letter **z.** This linking is called **liaison.**

C. C'est trop! (*It's too much!*) Give the singular.

MODÈLE: Des jours? ⟶ Non, un jour!

1. Des livres?
2. Des problèmes (*m.*)?
3. Des chaises?
4. Des ordinateurs?
5. Des tables?
6. Des mois?

Prononcez bien!

Script (1A):
*ÉLOÏSE: Bonjour, je m'appe**ll**e Éloïse.*
*ÉRIC: Moi, c'est Ér**i**c. Comment ça va?*
*ÉLOÏSE: Ça peut all**er**.*
(The server brings the bill.)
*LE SERVEUR: Ça fait tr**ei**ze euros, s'il vous plaît.*
*ÉRIC: Voic**i**. À plus tard, Éloïse.*
*ÉLOÏSE: À bientôt, **É**ric.*

Answers (1A): 1. [ɛ] 2. [i] 3. [e] 4. [ɛ] 5. [i] 6. [e]

1. The vowels in *ci*, *les*, and *mai* (page 15)

A. Au café. While waiting to meet your French friends at a Parisian café, you hear the following conversation between a man and a woman sitting at the next table. Listen to their conversation and check the vowel in the right column that corresponds to the bold one in the left column.

	[i]: **ci**	[e]: **les**	[ɛ]: **mai**
1. Bonjour, je m'app**e**lle Éloïse.	☐	☐	☐
2. Moi, c'est Ér**i**c. Comment ça va?	☐	☐	☐
3. Ça peut all**er**.	☐	☐	☐
(*The server brings the bill.*)			
4. Ça fait tr**ei**ze euros, s'il vous plaît.	☐	☐	☐
5. Voic**i**. À plus tard, Éloïse.	☐	☐	☐
6. À bientôt, **É**ric.	☐	☐	☐

Suggestion (1B): This is a whole-class activity. First have sts. pronounce the letters after you. Then have sts. write each one in the appropriate column. Finally, have sts. listen again to check their work.

Answers (1B): [e]: les: p, v, d, g, t, c, b; **[ɛ]: mai:** z, r, s, l, m, f, n

B. L'alphabet français. Your housemate is also an international student who has just started taking French. You help him learn the French alphabet sounds by writing in one column the letters that are pronounced with a sound like the one in **les** and in the other, those that contain a sound like the one in **mai**.

Lettres: z, p, v, r, d, s, g, l, t, c, m, f, b, n

[e]: les	[ɛ]: mai

Script (2A): 1. *une touriste* 2. *un journaliste* 3. *une artiste* 4. *une cycliste* 5. *un dentiste* 6. *un pianiste*

Answers (2A): 1. feminine 2. masculine 3. feminine 4. feminine 5. masculine 6. masculine

2. The sounds in *un* and *une* (page 21)

À l'aéroport. You and your friend are flying to Italy for the weekend. As you wait to board your plane, your friend tries to guess the occupation of the other passengers. Listen to what he says and decide whether he's referring in each case to a man or a woman.

	m.	f.
1.	☐	☐
2.	☐	☐
3.	☐	☐
4.	☐	☐
5.	☐	☐
6.	☐	☐

Leçon 4

Purpose: *Leçon 4: Perspectives* combines and reinforces the vocabulary and grammar structures presented in *Leçons 1–3*, with a special emphasis on skill development.

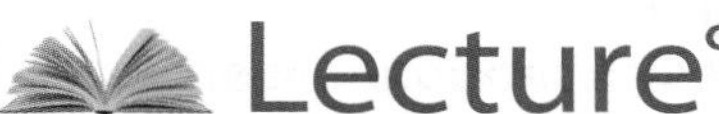

Lecture°

Reading

PERSPECTIVES

Avant de lire°

Avant... *Before reading*

Recognizing cognates. French is a Romance language—that is, it is derived from Latin. English was also heavily influenced by Latin, with the result that the two languages share vocabulary items similar in form and meaning. As you already know (see **Leçon 1**), these words are called cognates (**mots apparentés**). Here are two additional patterns:

FRANÇAIS	ANGLAIS		
-eur	*-or, -er*	vend**eur**	*vendor, seller*
-é	*-ed*	rembours**é**	*reimbursed*

Over the centuries, the French and English languages have borrowed heavily from each other. Although French has absorbed many words from English, some people view these **anglicismes** as threats to the integrity of the language and culture. Words such as **champagne** and **cologne** were borrowed directly from French. Can you think of any others?

The ad on the following page is from the French website **La boutique de l'étudiant.fr.** Just like students everywhere, French students use books or the Internet to make decisions about which school to choose, how to study, or how to prepare for and do well on difficult exams.

Abonnez-vous en ligne means *subscribe online*. What do you think the expression **Profitez d'offres exceptionnelles** means?

Now read the ad through. Then go back and underline all the words you recognize as cognates, and circle the words you don't understand.

Purpose: *Lecture* is the reading selection that appears in every chapter of *Vis-à-vis*. Many of the readings are drawn from authentic contemporary sources; some are author written, and others are literary. Each selection is thematically related to the chapter topic or topics; author-written readings recycle the active vocabulary presented and practiced in the chapter. Unfamiliar words and expressions are glossed in the margin. The reading selections follow a progression through the chapters, from beginning-level texts to increasingly challenging ones, as sts. expand their vocabulary and increase their skills. Each reading selection is followed by a *Compréhension* ex. to verify and expand upon sts.' understanding of the text.

Purpose: *Avant de lire*, which introduces each reading selection in *Vis-à-vis*, presents reading strategies and techniques designed to help sts. approach written texts with greater confidence and efficiency. Each *Avant de lire* presents a specific strategy followed by a brief warm-up ex. These prereading exs. can be done in class or individually by sts. at home.

Cultural note: Historical factors explain some borrowings. In 1066, the French-speaking Normans conquered the British Isles. French was imposed as the official language, and many words entered the English lexicon. Technological innovations have also played a role in borrowings: New technology introduced in one culture may cause a "vocabulary gap" in another; these new words are then borrowed. Prestige is another factor: If a culture is perceived to be prestigious, its vocabulary may be borrowed by another language.

À propos de la lecture...
This ad is taken from a French website for students.

Additional activities: (1) *Le saviez-vous?* Did you know that the following words derive from French? Look for their derivations in a good dictionary.
1. denim → *de Nîmes* 2. jean → *de Gênes* 3. dandelion → *dent de lion.* (2) Point out that associating cognates with the larger context of the text will allow sts. to identify additional non-cognate vocabulary items. Ask them to guess the meaning of the following words from the ad: 1. *librairie* 2. *citations* 3. *livraison* 4. *choisir* 5. *engagements*. At this point, you may wish to remind sts. about the notion of false cognates (*faux amis*), using examples 1 and 5.

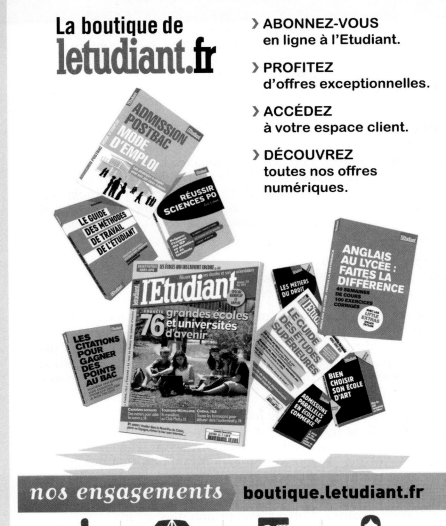

Compréhension

Quel mot? (*Which word?*) Now that you have read the ad, find the word in the text that means:

1. discover
2. studies
3. universities of the future
4. art school
5. to earn points on the «bac» (*French high school exit exam*)
6. guide to higher education
7. make a difference

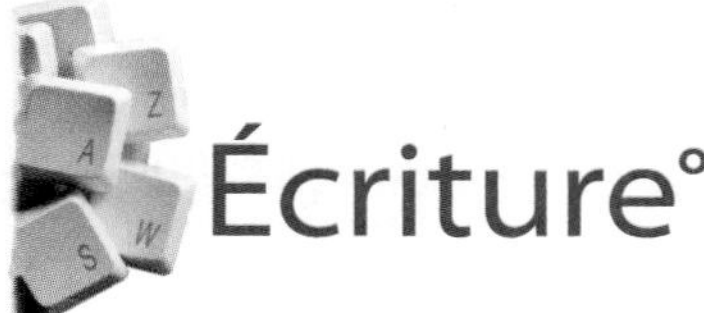

Écriture°

°*Writing*

The writing activities **Par écrit** and **Journal intime** can be found in the Workbook/Laboratory Manual to accompany *Vis-à-vis*.

Purpose: For each chapter in the Workbook/Laboratory Manual, there are two different writing activities that guide sts. through reusing the lexical and grammatical content of the chapter: *Par écrit* emphasizes process-writing and *Journal intime* allows for free-form expression of sts.' own experiences.

Pour s'amuser

Les mots cachés°

°*Les... Word search*

In this grid, find the following words: **avril, bisou, femme, homme, mardi, salut, semaine, soir.**

```
c e d a m a r d i f o d
v s e m a i n e e d i g
b i s o u u s o i r e d
u x a v r i l p o r t i
m a d a m s a l u t m j
f e m m e o h o m m e g
```

La vie en chantant. An activity based on the song "See You Later Alligator" by Louise Attaque can be found in the Instructor's Manual. The song can be purchased at the iTunes store, or sts. can watch the music video on YouTube.

Purpose: Because the characters speak at a normal pace and use authentic language, it is important to do the previewing activities with sts. before they watch the video.

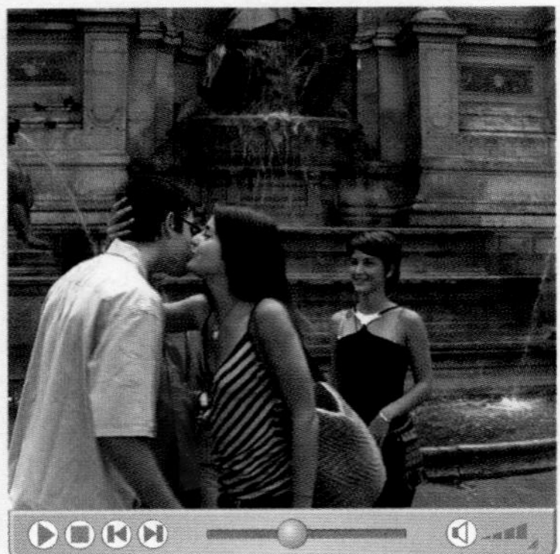

On fait la bise pour dire (*say*) «au revoir».

Suggestion: *Vocabulaire en contexte* presents thematically related words heard in the video episode. Before viewing, model pronunciation as sts. check meanings. Point out the dual meaning of *s'embrasser* and have sts. guess what the *se* before the verb indicates (i.e., reciprocal action).

Suggestion: Introduce questions in *Visionnez!* before watching the video to focus sts.' attention on particular information to listen for and to reinforce the thematically related vocabulary. Return to the questions after viewing to check comprehension.

Suggestion: *Analysez!* and *Comparez!* lead sts. to think more critically about their own culture in relation to what they have just seen in the video. For *Chapitre 1*, analysis can be done as a brief class discussion in English. In later chapters, progressively more French can be used, and the topic can be addressed equally well outside of class as a web-based blog, videoblog, journal, or chat project.

Note culturelle

Juliette is working on her degree, *le Master Multimédia Interactif,* at the *Université Paris I Panthéon-Sorbonne.* This two-year specialization in computer science and multimedia was introduced into the curriculum in 2000. It allows students who have obtained *la licence* after three years of study to further specialize in their chosen field.

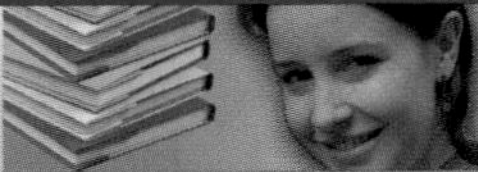

Le vidéoblog de Léa

En bref

In this scene, we first meet Léa and learn about her three friends Hassan, Juliette, and Hector. In her videoblog, Léa describes how French speakers typically greet each other and say good-bye.

Vocabulaire en contexte

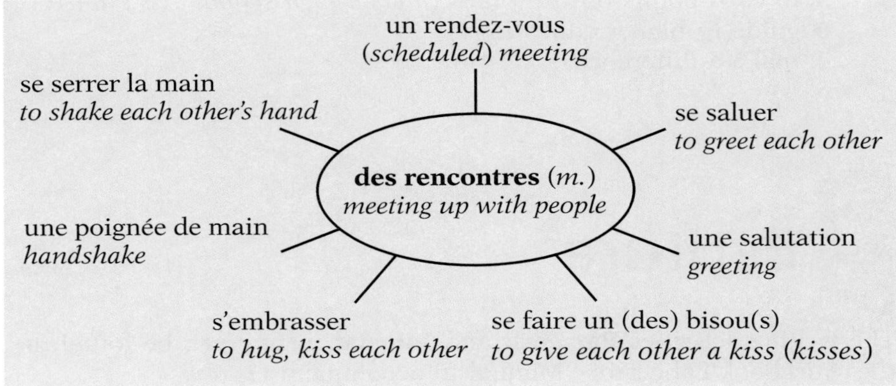

Visionnez!

Choose the correct response.

	Léa	Juliette	Hassan	Hector
1. Qui a (*Who has*) rendez-vous chez le dentiste?	☐	☐	☐	☐
2. Qui étudie le multimédia?	☐	☐	☐	☐
3. Qui a 28 ans?	☐	☐	☐	☐
4. Qui aime (*likes*) la danse?	☐	☐	☐	☐
5. Qui a créé (*created*) un vidéoblog?	☐	☐	☐	☐

Analysez!

Answer the following questions in English.

1. How do greetings differ in France?
2. What do you think the social consequences are of *not* greeting someone in a culturally appropriate way? What impressions can that leave?

Comparez!

Compare appropriate greetings and gestures in your culture to those of a French-speaking culture for the following people: two young female friends, two young male friends, a young male meeting a young female for the first time, a young male or female meeting an older adult male or female for the first time. What conclusions can you draw?

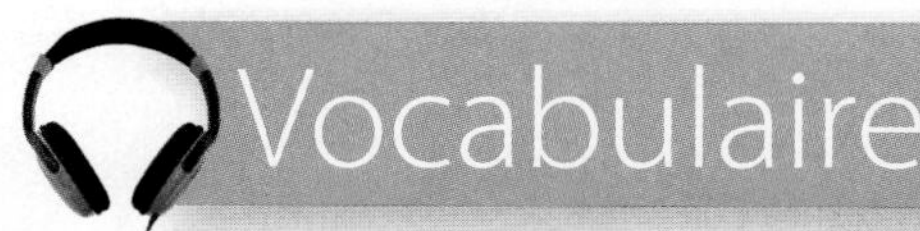

Vocabulaire

Les bonnes manières

À bientôt. See you soon.
Au revoir. Good-bye.
Bonjour. Hello. Good day.
Bonsoir. Good evening.
Ça peut aller. All right. Pretty well.
Ça va? How's it going?
Ça va bien. Fine. (Things are going well.)
Ça va mal. Things are going badly.
Comme ci comme ça. So so.
Comment? What?; How?
Comment allez-vous? / Comment vas-tu? How are you?
Comment vous appelez-vous? / Comment t'appelles-tu? What's your name?
De rien. Not at all. Don't mention it. You're welcome.
Et vous? / Et toi? And you?
Excusez-moi. / Excuse-moi. Excuse me.
Je m'appelle... My name is . . .
Je ne comprends pas. I don't understand.
madame Mrs. (ma'am)
mademoiselle Miss
Merci (beaucoup). Thank you (very much).
monsieur Mr. (sir)
Moyen. All right.
Pardon. Pardon (me).
Pas mal. Not bad(ly).
Répétez. / Répète. Repeat.
Salut! Hi!
S'il vous plaît. / S'il te plaît. Please.
Très bien. Very well (good).

Les nombres de 0 à 60

un, deux, trois, quatre, cinq, six, sept, huit, neuf, dix, onze, douze, treize, quatorze, quinze, seize, dix-sept, dix-huit, dix-neuf, vingt, vingt et un, vingt-deux, etc., **trente, quarante, cinquante, soixante**

Dans la salle de classe

un bureau a desk
un cahier a notebook
une chaise a chair
un crayon a pencil
un écran a screen
un étudiant a (male) student
une étudiante a (female) student
une fenêtre a window
un lecteur de DVD a DVD player
un livre a book
un ordinateur a computer
un portable a laptop
une porte a door
un professeur a professor, instructor (male or female)
une salle de classe a classroom
un smartphone a smartphone
une souris a mouse
un stylo a pen
une table a table
une tablette a tablet computer, an iPad
un tableau a (chalk)board
une télévision a television

Les jours de la semaine

Quel jour sommes-nous / est-ce? What day is it?
Nous sommes / C'est... lundi, mardi, mercredi, jeudi, vendredi, samedi, dimanche. It's . . . Monday, Tuesday, Wednesday, Thursday, Friday, Saturday, Sunday.

Les mois (*m.*)

janvier January
février February
mars March
avril April
mai May
juin June
juillet July
août August
septembre September
octobre October
novembre November
décembre December

Mots et expressions divers

aujourd'hui today
beaucoup very much, a lot
bien well
c'est un/une... it's a (an) . . .
combien de how many
et and
une femme a woman
un homme a man
il y a there is/are
mal badly
non no
oui yes
quel/quelle what; which
Quelle est la date? What is the date?
Qu'est-ce que c'est? What is it?
Qui est-ce? Who is it?

Purpose: *Vocabulaire* contains chapter words and expressions considered *active*. These are the words and expressions sts. are expected to know. Active vocabulary items for each chapter are introduced in the following chapter sections:

- *Leçon 1: Paroles* (In *Chapitre 1*, active vocabulary is also presented in *Leçon 2: Paroles* and in the first part of *Leçon 3*.)
- *Mots clés*
- Grammar paradigms, verb charts, and example sentences from the grammar sections
- Occasionally, from functional brief dialogues that begin grammar sections

The vocabulary list is divided into parts of speech (*Verbes, Substantifs,* etc.), *Mots et expressions divers,* and, occasionally, thematic categories (*Expressions avec* avoir, *Expressions interrogatives,* etc.). Words and expressions within each subgrouping are organized alphabetically.

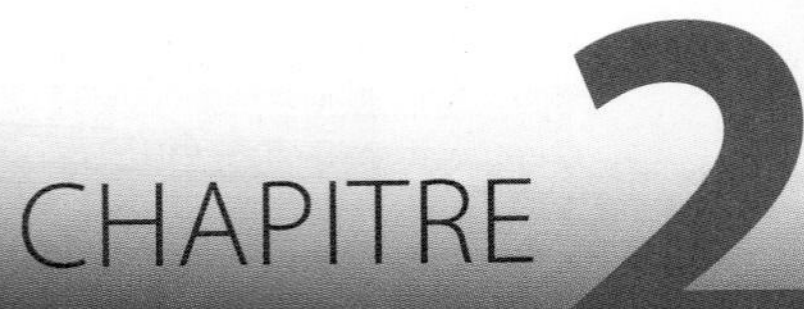

CHAPITRE 2

Nous, les étudiants

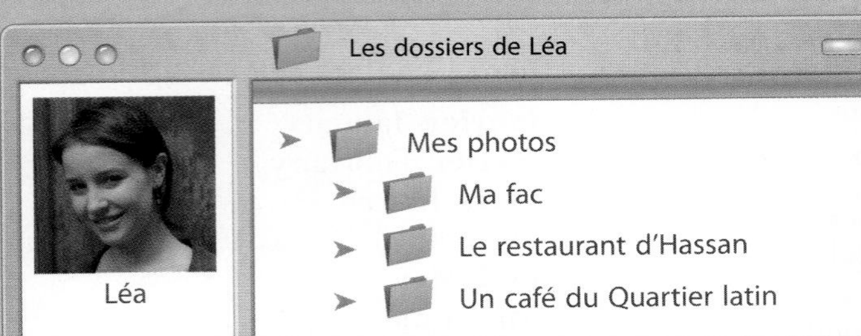

Presentation: Review numbers by counting windows or people or guessing the students' ages. Ask what month it is.

Les dossiers de Léa

Léa

- Mes photos
  - Ma fac
  - Le restaurant d'Hassan
  - Un café du Quartier latin

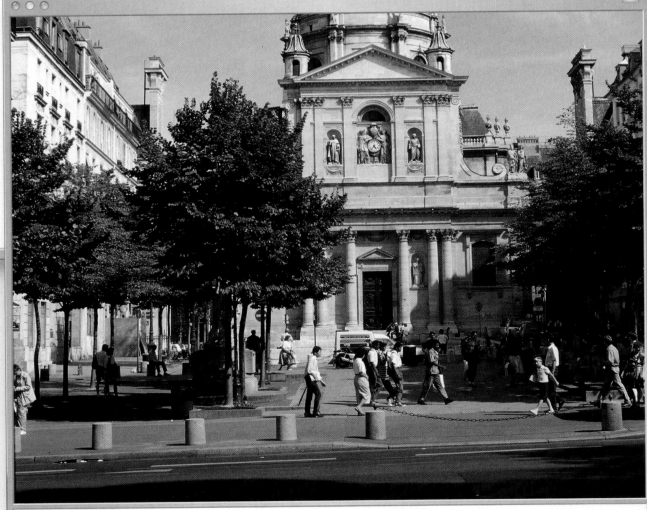

Ma fac: la Sorbonne à Paris

Cultural note: The historical campus of *La Sorbonne* is located in the *Quartier latin*, in the 5th *arrondissement* of Paris.

Dans ce chapitre...

OBJECTIFS COMMUNICATIFS

- identifying people, places, and things
- talking about academic subjects
- talking about nationalities
- expressing actions
- expressing disagreement
- learning to distinguish between and pronounce selected sounds in French

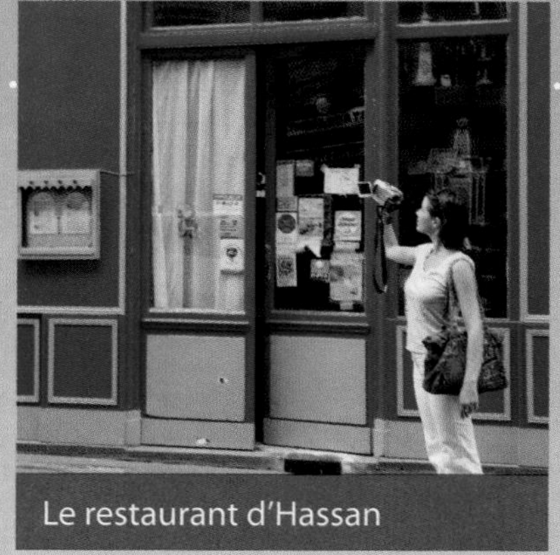

Le restaurant d'Hassan

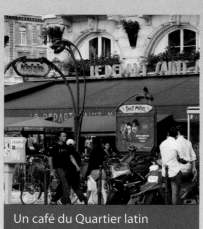

Un café du Quartier latin

PAROLES (Leçon 1)

- Les lieux
- Les matières
- Les pays et les nationalités
- Les distractions

STRUCTURES (Leçons 2 et 3)

- Les articles définis
- Les verbes réguliers en **-er**
- Le verb **être**
- La négation **ne... pas**

CULTURE

- Le blog de Léa: *Salut tout le monde!*
- Reportage: *Quartier latin: le quartier général des étudiants*
- Lecture: *Étudier le français... à Québec, bien sûr!* (Leçon 4)

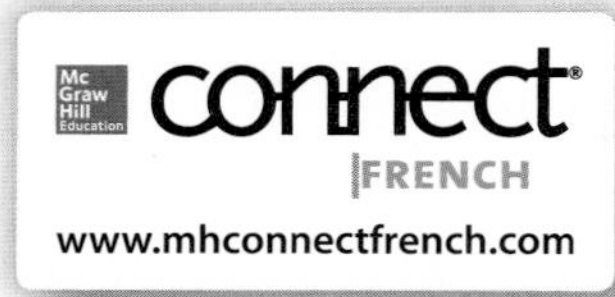

Leçon 1

PAROLES

Purpose: *Leçon 1: Paroles* presents new words and expressions related to the chapter theme. Most new terms are illustrated through visual displays. Additional vocabulary items appear in the *Autres mots utiles* list after the display. New vocabulary terms are practiced after each visual presentation and are recycled throughout the rest of the chapter and in subsequent chapters.

Les lieux°

Les... (*m.*) *Places*

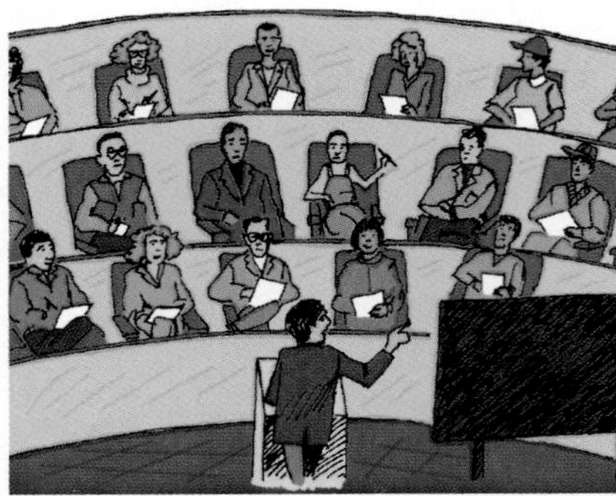

Voici l'amphithéâtre (l'amphi).

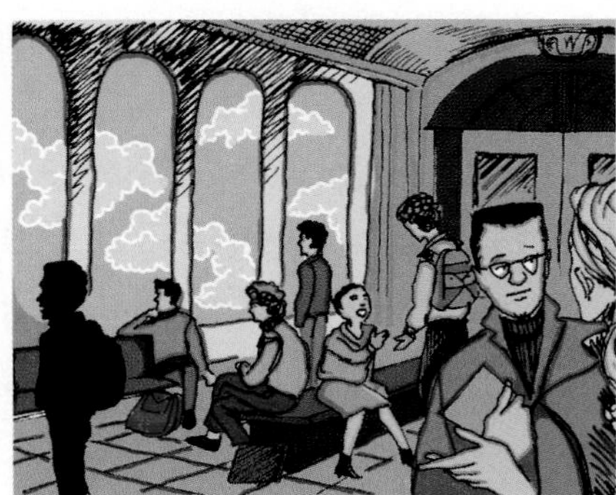

Voici la cité universitaire (la cité-U).

Voici le restaurant universitaire (le resto-U).

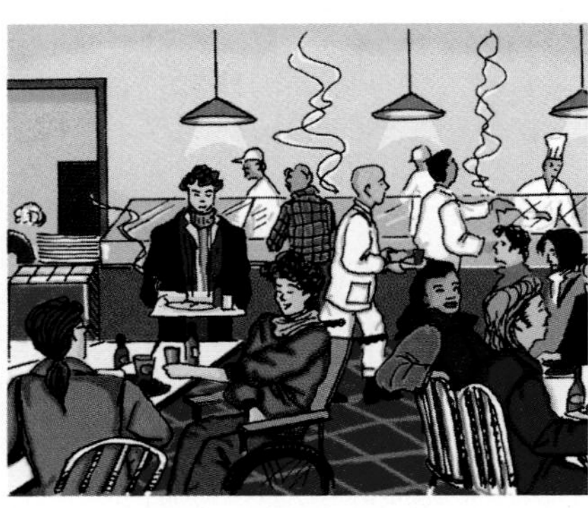

Additional vocabulary: *La cafétéria* and *la cantine* are also used for *school cafeteria.*

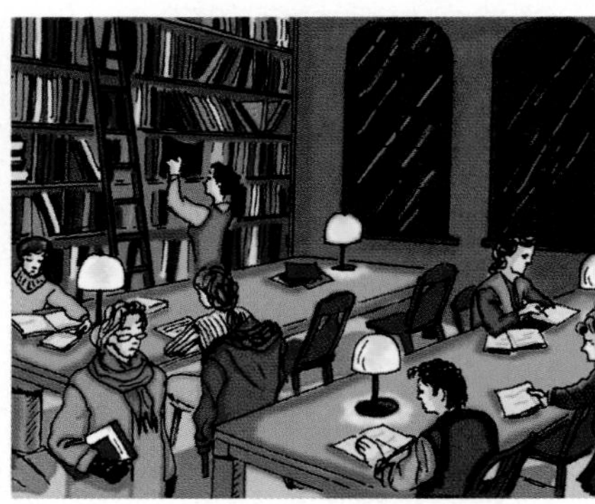

Voici la bibliothèque.

AUTRES MOTS UTILES

le bureau	office
l'école (*f.*)	school
le gymnase	gymnasium
le laboratoire de langues	language lab
la librairie	bookstore
la salle de classe	classroom

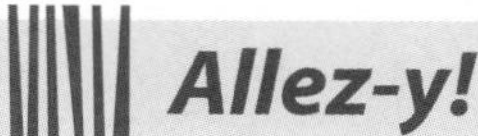

A. Une visite. Associate the following nouns with their location.

MODÈLES: un examen de français → l'amphithéâtre
un coca → le restaurant universitaire

1. un dictionnaire
2. une tablette
3. un casque (*headset*)
4. un livre
5. une télévision
6. un cours de français
7. un sandwich
8. une encyclopédie

B. C'est bizarre? C'est normal? Give your opinion!

MODÈLE: Un match de football dans le restaurant universitaire... → Un match de football dans le restaurant universitaire, c'est bizarre!

1. Un cours de français dans l'amphithéâtre...
2. Une tablette dans la bibliothèque...
3. Un examen dans la cité universitaire...
4. Un café dans l'amphithéâtre...
5. Un dictionnaire dans la bibliothèque...
6. Un magazine dans la librairie...
7. Un smartphone dans la salle de classe

Vocabulary recycling: Continue with terms from *Chapitre 1: un tableau? un stylo? une fenêtre? un professeur? un bureau?* Solicit individual answers, then use group repetition.

Suggestion (A–B): You might want to preview the preposition *à* (*à la, à l', au*) for these exs.

Suggestion (B): Have sts. correct any phrase that is *bizarre*.

Continuation (B): Additional phrases can be given orally: *Un professeur dans le resto-U... ; Une télévision dans la bibliothèque... ; Une étudiante dans l'amphithéâtre... ; Le bureau du professeur dans le restaurant universitaire...*

Follow-up (B): Give sts. a minute to write one or two items to continue this ex. They will read their example for the other sts., who will say: *C'est normal!* or *C'est bizarre!*

Les matières°

Les... (*f.*) *Academic subjects*

À la faculté des lettres et sciences humaines, on étudie (*one studies*)...

la littérature
la linguistique
les langues (*f.*) **étrangères** (*foreign languages*)
- **l'allemand** (*m.*)
- **l'anglais** (*m.*)
- **le chinois**
- **l'espagnol** (*m.*)
- **l'italien** (*m.*)
- **le japonais**

l'histoire (*f.*)
la géographie
la philosophie
la psychologie
la sociologie

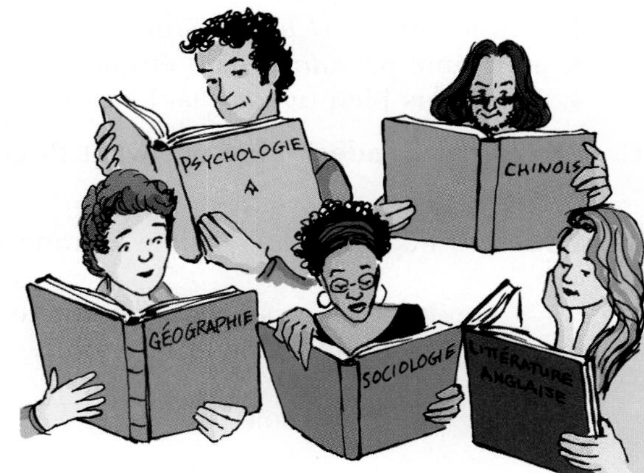

Suggestion: Model pronunciation of the fields of study, having sts. repeat after you. Pay special attention to pronunciation of cognates, especially vowels. Point out that *mathématiques* is always plural in French. Sts. may need additional vocabulary to describe their own studies: *l'archéologie, les relations internationales, l'anthropologie, l'électronique, l'architecture, la médecine, l'art dramatique, la peinture, la danse, les sciences politiques, les sciences économiques, la gestion, la publicité, le marketing, l'administration des affaires*, etc.

Suggestion: Point out the usage of the definite articles *le, la, les* with *les matières* (the general meaning of the definite article is presented in *Leçon* 2).

Additional activity: Ask sts. what they are studying and what *matières* they take.

À la faculté des sciences, on étudie…

les mathématiques (les maths) (*f.*)
l'informatique (*computer science*)
la physique
la chimie (*chemistry*)
les sciences (*f.*) **naturelles**
(la géologie et
la biologie)

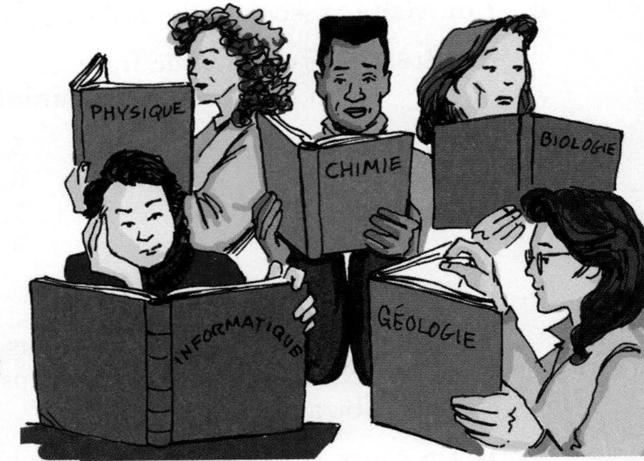

AUTRES MOTS UTILES

le commerce	business
le cours	class
le droit	law
l'économie (*f.*)	economics
le génie	engineering

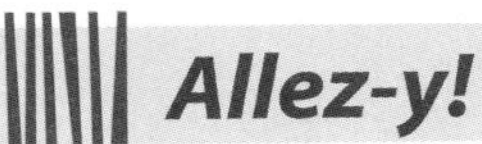

Allez-y!

Suggestion: Bring in photos representative of professions and ask sts. what these people study.

Follow-up: Give the name of a famous person and have sts. indicate what field she or he was in: *Marie Curie, Sigmund Freud, Jean-Paul Sartre, Bill Gates, Jane Austen, Gustave Eiffel,* etc.

A. Les études et les professions. Imagine what subjects are necessary for the following professions.

MODÈLE: un(e) diplomate → On étudie les langues étrangères.

1. un(e) psychologue
2. un(e) chimiste
3. un professeur de physique
4. un professeur d'histoire
5. un(e) ingénieur

B. Mes (*My*) **cours à l'université.** Look back over the lists of **matières,** then tell about yourself by completing the following sentences.

1. J'étudie (*I study*)…
2. J'aime étudier (*I like to study*)…
3. Je n'aime pas (*don't like*) étudier…
4. J'aimerais bien (*would like*) étudier…

Suggestion: Ask one st. to act as recorder and report back other sts.' courses. Encourage sts. to listen carefully and to correct false statements.

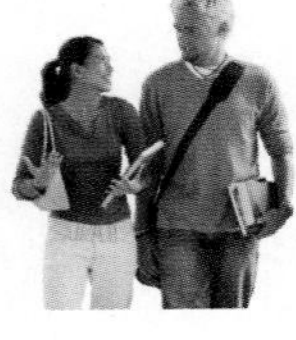

Suggestion: Have various sts. choose someone in class to answer this question. Ask for recall by having them say what each person answered: *Elle étudie…*

C. Et vos camarades? Find out what three classmates are studying this term.

MODÈLE: É1: Moi (*Me*), j'étudie le français, l'histoire et l'informatique. Et toi?
É2: Moi aussi (*too*), j'étudie le français, et j'étudie la philosophie et la chimie.

Presentation: (1) Find these countries on a world map with sts. Point out that the names of countries have gender, though sts. will not be asked to produce the names. (2) Using pictures of famous people, model the pronunciation of the nationalities, using group repetition. (3) Point out differences in pronunciation of masculine and feminine forms. (4) Point out that all languages are masculine, mentioning that they begin with a lowercase letter in French. (5) Possible additions to nationalities are *australien(ne), grec(que), iranien(ne), israélien(ne), norvégien(ne), polonais(e), suédois(e).* Point out that a variety of local languages are spoken in the countries of West Africa. Examples: *wolof* (*Sénégal*), *bantou* (*République Démocratique du Congo*), *baoulé* (*Côte d'Ivoire*).

Note: The definite articles are presented in *Leçon 2.*

Les pays et les nationalités°

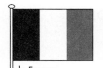

Les... *Countries and nationalities*

la France

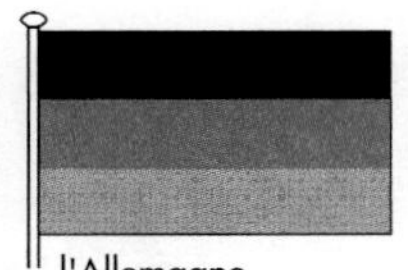
l'Allemagne

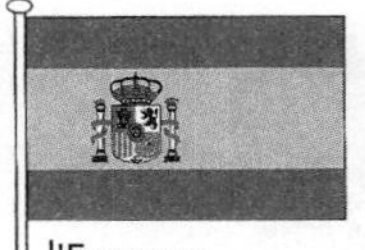
l'Espagne

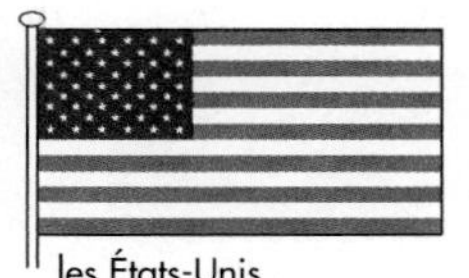
les États-Unis

LES PAYS (*m.*)	LES NATIONALITÉS (*f.*)	
	PERSONNES	ADJECTIFS
l'Algérie	l'Algérien, l'Algérienne	algérien, algérienne
l'Allemagne	l'Allemand, l'Allemande	allemand, allemande
l'Angleterre	l'Anglais, l'Anglaise	anglais, anglaise
la Belgique	le/la Belge	belge
le Canada	le Canadien, la Canadienne	canadien, canadienne
la Chine	le Chinois, la Chinoise	chinois, chinoise
la Côte d'Ivoire	l'Ivoirien, l'Ivoirienne	ivoirien, ivoirienne
l'Espagne	l'Espagnol, l'Espagnole	espagnol, espagnole
les États-Unis	l'Américain, l'Américaine	américain, américaine
la France	le Français, la Française	français, française
l'Italie	l'Italien, l'Italienne	italien, italienne
le Japon	le Japonais, la Japonaise	japonais, japonaise
le Liban	le Libanais, la Libanaise	libanais, libanaise
le Maroc	le Marocain, la Marocaine	marocain, marocaine
le Mexique	le Mexicain, la Mexicaine	mexicain, mexicaine
le Québec*	le Québécois, la Québécoise	québécois, québécoise
la République Démocratique du Congo	le Congolais, la Congolaise	congolais, congolaise
la Russie	le/la Russe	russe
le Sénégal	le Sénégalais, la Sénégalaise	sénégalais, sénégalaise
la Suisse	le/la Suisse	suisse
la Tunisie	le Tunisien, la Tunisienne	tunisien, tunisienne
le Vietnam	le Vietnamien, la Vietnamienne	vietnamien, vietnamienne

The adjective of nationality is identical to the noun except that it is not capitalized. Example: un Anglais; un étudiant anglais.

l'Angleterre

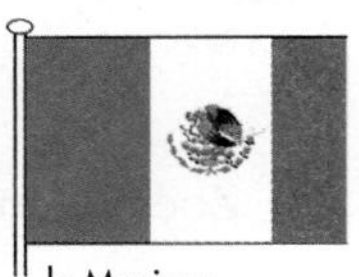
le Mexique

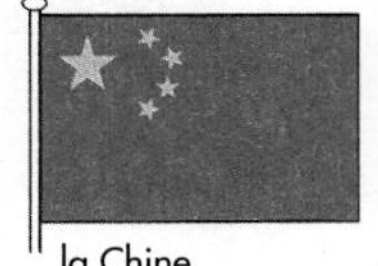
la Chine

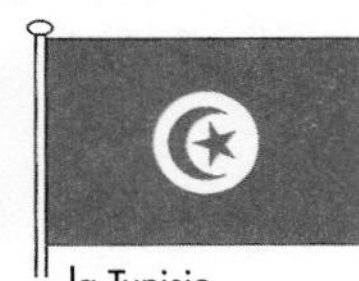
la Tunisie

Pronunciation practice (2): The *Prononcez bien!* section on page 53 of this chapter contains additional activities for practicing these sounds.

Purpose: *Prononcez bien!* presents pronunciation tips in order to give sts. practice with difficult sounds and words. As with the *Prononciation* feature in the Workbook/Laboratory Manual, these boxes have been recorded as part of the Audio Program to accompany *Vis-à-vis.*

*In 2006, the Canadian House of Commons recognized "that the Québécois (*people of Quebec*) form a nation within a united Canada."

Prononcez bien!

Masculine vs. feminine forms of nationalities

Adding **-e** to the masculine forms of most nouns and adjectives of nationality makes them feminine. The final consonant is then pronounced.

allemande, anglaise, chinoise, libanaise

The addition of **-e** to masculine forms ending with the letter *n* denasalizes the vowel [ɛ̃]. It becomes [ɛ], and the *n* is pronounced.

américain [ɛ̃] → **américaine** [ɛn]
marocain → **marocaine**
mexicain → **mexicaine**

Note that when [ɛ̃] is spelled **-ien** in the masculine form, an extra *n* is added in the feminine form.

algérien → **algérienne**
canadien → **canadienne**
tunisien → **tunisienne**

Pronunciation presentation: Explain that the difference in pronunciation between the vowel in *un* [œ̃] and the one in *cinq* [ɛ̃] lies in the shape of the lips: rounded for *un*, stretched for *cinq*. Inform sts. that the contrast in the pronunciation of the two vowels is rarely observed and the vowel [œ̃] is now mostly pronounced like [ɛ̃].

Pronunciation practice (1): Bring cut-outs of a man and a woman (or draw sketches of them on the board). Read the following words aloud to sts. and have them indicate whether they apply to the man or the woman: *ivoirien, marocaine, libanaise, suisse, québécois, vietnamien, sénégalaise, français, japonaise, congolais, belge, Yvonne, François, Simon, Jeanne, Adrienne.*

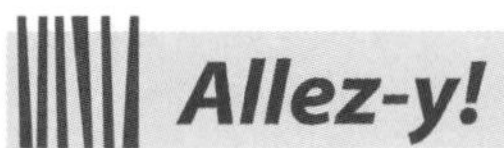

Allez-y!

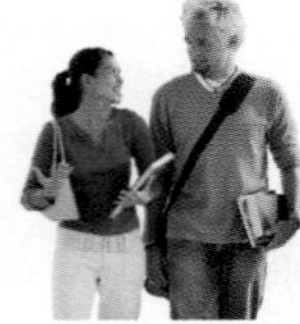

Continuation (A): Have sts. give additional names.

A. Les villes (*Cities*) **et les nationalités.** What nationality are the following people? Ask a classmate to name the nationality.

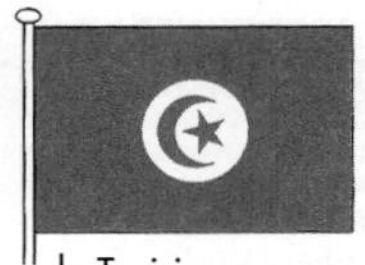

Karim / Tunis

Djamila / Tunis

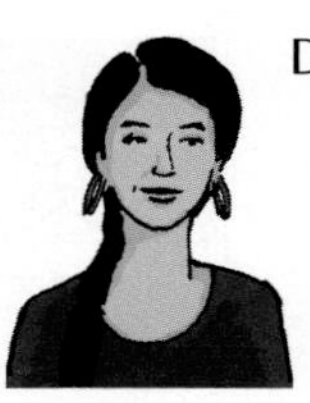

Note: The preposition *à* is practiced further in *Chapitre 3* (contracted forms), and with *aller* in *Chapitre 5;* other prepositions with geographical names are in *Chapitre 8, Leçon 3.*

MODÈLES: É1: Karim habite à (*lives in*) Tunis.
É2: Ah! Il est (*He is*) tunisien, n'est-ce pas?

É1: Djamila habite à Tunis.
É2: Ah! Elle est (*She is*) tunisienne, n'est-ce pas?

Mots clés

The preposition *à* + *ville*

À indicates location or movement. Used before the name of a city, it means you are in the city or going to the city.

J'habite **à** Genève.
I live in Geneva.

Vous allez **à** Montréal.
You are going to Montreal.

Purpose: *Mots clés* presents lexical items for communication. This feature appears twice in each chapter from *Chapitre 2* to *Chapitre 16* and contains active vocabulary to be used in the activity (activities) it accompanies.

Additional activity: Give sts. the nationality of different people and ask them what country they live in. Example: *Hervé est belge. Nommez son pays.*

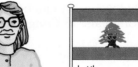

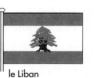

1. Gino / Rome

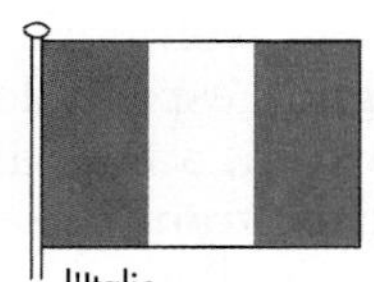

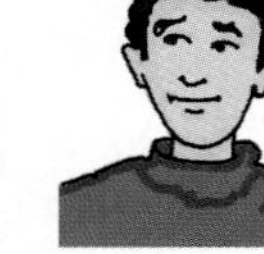

2. Kai / Kyoto

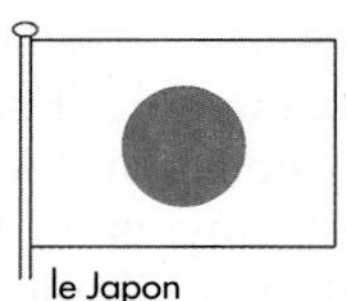

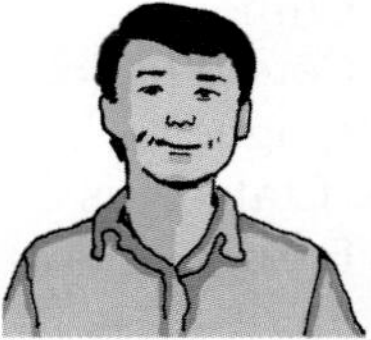

3. Mme Roberge / Montréal

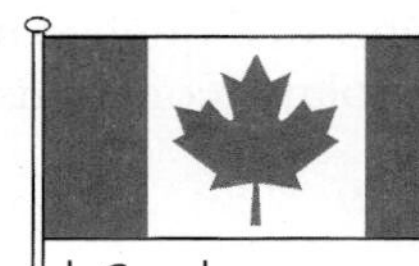

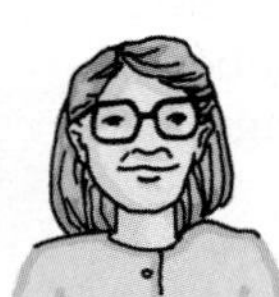

4. Éva / Beyrouth

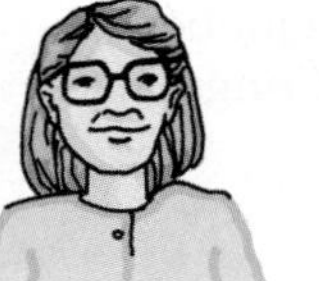

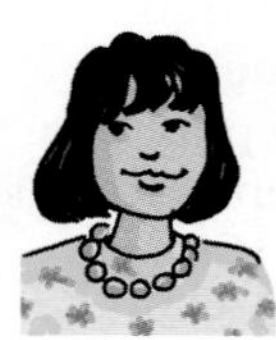

5. Léopold / Dakar

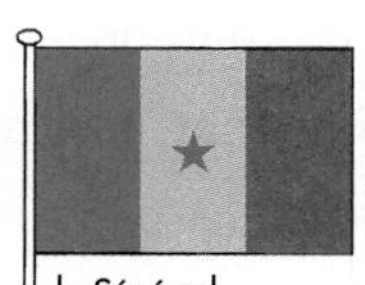

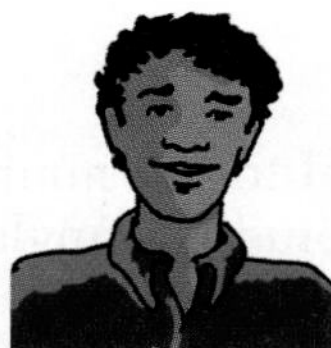

6. Aurélie / Bruxelles

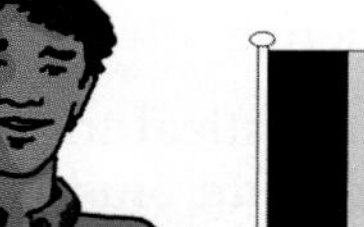

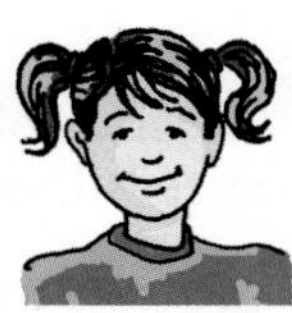

7. Salima / Casablanca

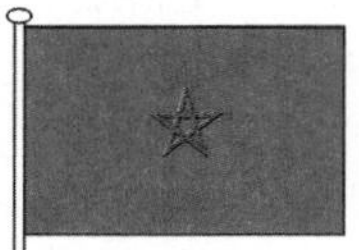

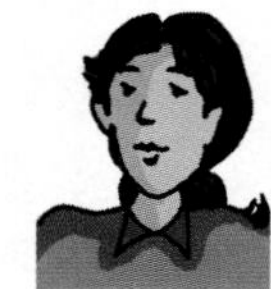

8. Zoé / Genève

la Suisse

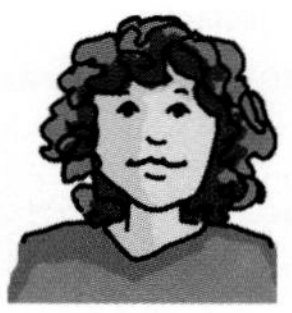

B. Les nationalités et les langues. Working with a partner, give the nationality and probable language(s) of the people from Activity A.

MODÈLES: Karim → É1: Karim?
É2: Karim est tunisien. Il parle (*He speaks*) arabe et français.

Djamila → É2: Djamila?
É1: Djamila est tunisienne. Elle parle (*She speaks*) arabe et français.

Langues: allemand, anglais, arabe, flamand, français, italien, japonais

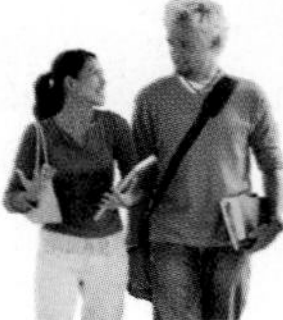

Follow-up: Using a world map, point to important cities and have sts. imagine they live there: *J'habite à Tokyo. Je parle japonais.* Possibilities: *Tokyo, Venise, Seattle, Rio de Janeiro, Québec,* etc.

Les distractions°

°Les... (*f.*) *Entertainment*

Presentation: (1) Model pronunciation; group repetition. (2) Additional cognate vocabulary: *le volley-ball, le ping-pong, le hockey, le golf, les films policiers, les westerns, les comédies musicales, les films documentaires.*

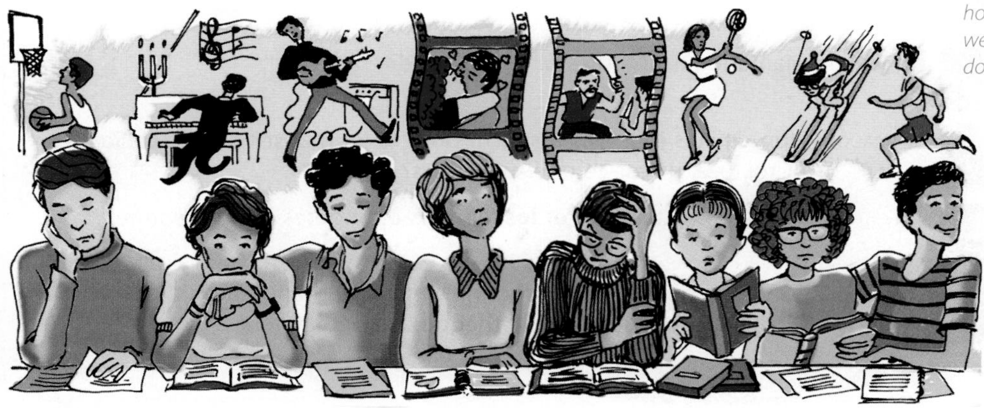

Julien Fatima Rémi Anne-Laure Marc Thu Sophie Allal

LA MUSIQUE	LE SPORT	LE CINÉMA
le jazz	le basket-ball	les films (*m.*) d'amour
la musique classique	le football	les films d'aventures
le rap	le football américain	les films d'horreur
le rock	le jogging	les films de science-fiction
la world music	le ski	
	le tennis	

Suggestion: Practice *les nationalités* with *les distractions: Les Français aiment le football...*

Suggestions: Have sts. circulate for five minutes to exchange information about what they like. For example: *É1* says *Moi, j'aime (je n'aime pas) la musique country. Et toi? É2* replies with his/her own opinion of the same thing—*Moi aussi, j'aime* (*Moi non plus* [neither], *je n'aime pas*) *la musique country.* Pass out a chart on which sts. can jot down findings about 1. *le rap* 2. *le football américain* 3. *les films d'horreur* 4. *le jazz* 5. *les films d'aventures.* Then have them report their findings to the whole class.

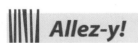

Allez-y!

Préférences. What do these people like?

MODÈLE: Rémi → Rémi aime le rock.

1. Et Thu?
2. Et Sophie?
3. Et Julien?
4. Et Anne-Laure?
5. Et Allal?
6. Et Fatima?
7. Et Marc?
8. Et vous?

Follow-up: Give sts. the name of a famous person in music, sports, or film. They will say *il/elle aime.* For example: *Lady Gaga, Rafa Nadal, Steven Spielberg.*

Leçon 2

Purpose: *Leçons 2* and *3* of *Chapitres 2–16* present the basic structures of the French language. Each grammar point is introduced via a brief functional dialogue. Contextualized examples recycle the vocabulary of the chapter.

Presentation: For ideas on presentation of brief dialogues, see the Instructor's Manual.

STRUCTURES

Les articles définis

Identifying People, Places, and Things

Le journaliste et l'étudiante

Léa contacte Mamadou sur sa page Facebook (Messagerie instantanée).

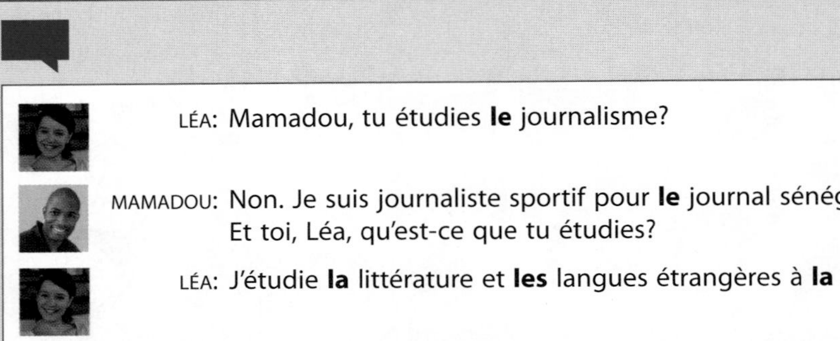

LÉA: Mamadou, tu étudies **le** journalisme?

MAMADOU: Non. Je suis journaliste sportif pour **le** journal sénégalais ***Le** Soleil.* Et toi, Léa, qu'est-ce que tu étudies?

LÉA: J'étudie **la** littérature et **les** langues étrangères à **la** Sorbonne.

MAMADOU: C'est une belle fac, la Sorbonne… il y a **le** grand amphithéâtre Richelieu, **la** superbe bibliothèque… et **la** cafétéria!

Complétez les phrases selon le dialogue.

1. Mamadou est spécialisé dans _____ journalisme sportif.
2. Léa étudie _____ littérature et _____ langues étrangères à _____ fac de _____ Sorbonne.
3. Mamadou apprécie _____ grand amphi Richelieu, _____ bibliothèque et _____ cafétéria de _____ Sorbonne.

Suggestion: Recycle vocab. from *Dans la salle de classe,* p. 20.

Singular Forms of Definite Articles

Here are the forms of the singular definite article (**le singulier de l'article défini**) in French, corresponding to *the* in English.

MASCULINE		FEMININE		MASCULINE OR FEMININE BEGINNING WITH A VOWEL OR MUTE **h***	
le livre	*the book*	**la** femme	*the woman*	**l'**ami	*the friend (m.)*
le cours	*the course*	**la** table	*the table*	**l'**amie	*the friend (f.)*
				l'homme	*the man (m.)*
				l'histoire	*the story (f.)*

*In French, **h** is either *mute* (**muet,** *nonaspirate*) or *aspirate* (**aspiré**). In **l'homme,** the **h** is called *mute,* which simply means that the word **homme** "elides" with a preceding article (**le** + **homme** = **l'homme**). Most **h**'s in French are of this type. However, some **h**'s are aspirate, which means there is no elision; **le héros** (*the hero*) is an example of this. However, in neither case is the **h** pronounced.

1. The definite article in French is used to indicate a specific noun.

   Voici **le** resto-U. — *Here's the university restaurant.*

2. In French, the definite article is also used with nouns employed in a general sense.

   J'aime **le** café. — *I like coffee.*
   C'est **la** vie! — *That's life!*

[Allez-y! A]

Suggestion: To illustrate "specific," preview possession with *de: C'est la lettre de Caroline* as opposed to *C'est une lettre.*

Suggestions: (1) Remind sts. to learn article with noun. (2) Give examples in context of nouns used in a general sense: *J'aime le ski. J'adore la vie. Je déteste le golf.*

Plural Form of Definite Articles

	SINGULAR	PLURAL
Masculine	**le** touriste	**les** touristes
Feminine	**la** touriste	
Before a vowel	**l'**artiste	**les** artistes

1. The plural form (**le pluriel**) of the definite article is always **les.***

   le livre, **les** livres — *the book, the books*
   la femme, **les** femmes — *the woman, the women*
   l'examen, **les** examens — *the exam, the exams*

2. Note that in English, the article is omitted with nouns used in a general sense. In French, the definite articles **le, la, l',** and **les** are used.

   J'aime **le** ski. — *I like skiing.*
   Les Français aiment **le** vin. — *(Generally speaking) French people like wine.*

Prononcez bien!

The vowels in *le, la,* and *les*

Be sure to clearly distinguish between the vowels in **le** (**de, je, fenêtre**), **la** (**ça, madame, ordinateur**), and **les** (**et, cahier, répétez**). Tighten the muscles in your mouth and do the following:

Close your mouth and round your lips for **le.**

[ə]: **le cours**

Open your mouth wide and stretch your lips in a semi-smile for **la.**

[a]: **la table**

Close your mouth and stretch your lips in a wide smile for **les.**

[e]: **les cahiers**

Plural of Nouns

1. Most French nouns are made plural by adding an **s** to the singular, as seen in the preceding examples. Here are some other common patterns.

   - **-s, -x, -z** → no change

   le cour**s** → les cour**s** — *the course, the courses*
   un choi**x** → des choi**x** — *a choice, some choices*
   le ne**z** → les ne**z** — *the nose, the noses*

Pronunciation practice (1): Have sts. indicate whether the following words are (1) *masculin ou féminin: la touriste, la police, le bracelet, la musique, le journaliste, la Russe;* (2) *singulier ou pluriel: la chaise, les écrans, le livre, le stylo, la porte, la télévision, les tables, le bureau, les salles de classe, la radio, le café, les Français, le chimiste.*

Pronunciation practice (2): Write *le, la, les* and the following words on the board and have sts. indicate whether the letter(s) in bold correspond to the sound in *le, la,* or *les: all**er**, je, p**a**rdon, qu**a**torze, **é**cran, mercr**e**di, janvi**er**, **et**, d**a**te, ne**z**.* Remind sts. that the sequence *on* in *m**on**sieur* is pronounced like the vowel in *le* and the *em* in *f**em**me* like the vowel in *la.*

Suggestion: Point out that oral cues to number are often heard only in the article.

Pronunciation practice (3): The *Prononcez bien!* section on page 53 of this chapter contains additional activities for practicing these sounds.

*As with the indefinite article **des,** there is a **liaison** with a vowel or a vowel sound: **les‿étudiants, les‿hommes.**

Suggestion: Point out that one can distinguish the singular or plural of **-al, -ail** nouns orally in both article and noun form.

Suggestion: Have sts. repeat nouns in examples.

- **-eau, -ieu → -eaux, -ieux**

le tabl**eau** → les tabl**eaux**	*the board, the boards*
le bur**eau** → les bur**eaux**	*the desk, the desks*
le **lieu** → les **lieux**	*the place, the places*

- **-al, -ail → -aux**

un hôpit**al** → des hôpit**aux**	*a hospital, hospitals*
le trav**ail** → les trav**aux**	*the work, tasks*

2. Note that the masculine form is used in French to refer to a group that includes at least one male.

un étudian**t** et sept étudian**tes** → des étudian**ts**
un Franç**ais** et une Franç**aise** → des Franç**ais**

[Allez-y! B-C]

Grammaire interactive

For more on definite articles and the gender of nouns, watch the corresponding Grammar Tutorial and take a brief practice quiz at **Connect French.**

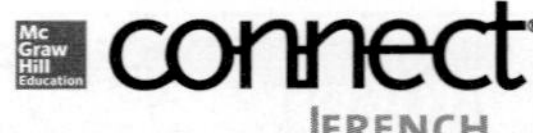

www.mhconnectfrench.com

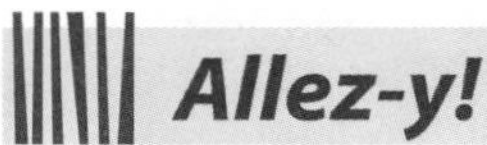

Allez-y!

Suggestion (A): Have sts. give reason for choice of gender by citing the rules presented in *Chapitre 1.*

A. Pensez-y! (*Think about it!*) Figure out the gender of the following words. Then add the definite article.

MODÈLE: femme → féminin; la femme

1. appartement
2. division
3. italien
4. tableau
5. coca-cola
6. biologie
7. université
8. aventure
9. personne
10. tourisme
11. science
12. homme

Follow-up (B): Have sts. continue the tour, giving plural forms of the following nouns: *une table, l'écran, un ordinateur, la cafétéria, une étudiante, le tableau, une chaise.*

Follow-up (B–C): For listening comprehension practice, have sts. indicate whether the following words are *singulier ou pluriel: les dictionnaires, des cours, un examen, les livres, l'amphithéâtre, le bureau, un café, des radios, le film, les étudiants, des amis.*

B. Suivons le guide! (*Let's follow the tour guide!*) Show your guests around campus, using the plural of these expressions.

MODÈLE: la salle de classe → Voilà les salles de classe.

1. la bibliothèque
2. l'amphi(théâtre)
3. le professeur
4. l'étudiant
5. le laboratoire de langues
6. le bureau

C. À l'université. Create sentences using the following words. Then create a different sentence by changing the number and the place.

MODÈLE: étudiante / salle de classe →
Il y a une étudiante dans la salle de classe.
Il y a des étudiantes dans la librairie.
ou Il y a des étudiantes dans les salles d'ordinateurs.

1. tableau / salle de classe
2. une réunion (*meeting*) / amphithéâtre
3. télévision / laboratoire
4. cahier / bureau
5. ordinateur / salle d'ordinateurs
6. Américaine / restaurant
7. dictionnaire / bibliothèque
8. écran / salle de classe

Le parler jeune

la fac	la faculté
une nana	une fille
un mec, un gars	un garçon
potasser	étudier, réviser
un pote	un ami

La **fac** de droit est située rue d'Assas.
Voici Virginie. C'est une **nana** sympa!
Ce **mec,** il travaille chez Virgin.
Allô? Non, pas ce soir, je **potasse** mes maths!
Mon **pote** Jules déteste les maths.

Interaction: Have sts. act out the following situation using the vocabulary and structures from this chapter. *Rendez-vous:* You run into a friend on campus. Greet him or her. Tell him or her about the courses you like and do not like, and then arrange to meet later.

Purpose: *Le parler jeune* boxes offer contemporary colloquial/slang expressions that correspond to the chapter vocabulary. This vocabulary is presented for student interest and, although generally linked to a conversation activity, is not considered part of the chapter's active vocabulary.

Les verbes réguliers en *-er*

Expressing Actions

Note: The minidialogue introduces both subject pronouns and new verb forms (both were previewed in *Leçon 1: Paroles*). You may prefer to focus on subject pronouns alone before introducing the dialogue.

Les étudiants de la Sorbonne

Mamadou téléphone à Léa.

MAMADOU: **Tu aime**s **mieux** la littérature ou les langues étrangères?

LÉA: **J'adore** la littérature et les langues étrangères! Actuellement,* **j'étudie** le russe. Et dans ma classe, nous **commençons** le chinois au deuxième semestre.

MAMADOU: **Vous commencez** le chinois! Bravo! Les étudiants de la Sorbonne sont ambitieux...

LÉA: Et courageux! **Nous travaillons** beaucoup. Mais **nous aimons** aussi les distractions...

*Currently

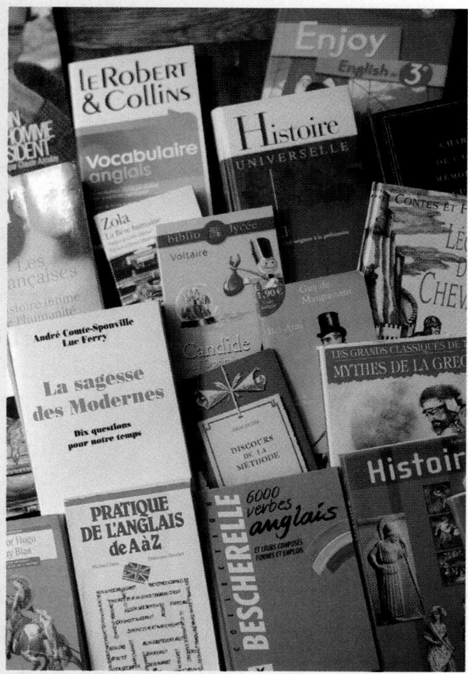

Des livres pour étudier

Trouvez (*Find*) la forme correcte du verbe dans le dialogue.

1. Tu ______ la littérature ou les langues?
2. J' ______ la littérature.
3. J' ______ le russe.
4. Nous ______ le chinois.
5. Vous ______ le chinois!
6. Nous ______ beaucoup.
7. Nous ______ les distractions.

Subject Pronouns and *parler*

Suggestions: A. What pronouns would you use to refer to the following people? 1. yourself 2. yourself and a friend 3. your parents, etc. B. What pronouns refer to the following people? 1. *un professeur* 2. *une femme* 3. *des amis* 4. *maman*, etc.

The subject of a sentence indicates who or what performs the action of the sentence: ***L'étudiant* visite l'université.** A pronoun (**un pronom**) is a word used in place of a noun (**un nom**): ***Il* visite l'université.**

SUBJECT PRONOUNS AND **parler** (*to speak*)					
SINGULAR			PLURAL		
je	parl**e**	*I speak*	nous	parl**ons**	*we speak*
tu	parl**es**	*you speak*	vous	parl**ez**	*you speak*
il	parl**e**	*he, it (m.) speaks*	ils	parl**ent**	*they (m., m. + f.) speak*
elle	parl**e**	*she, it (f.) speaks*	elles	parl**ent**	*they (f.) speak*
on	parl**e**	*one speaks*			

Suggestions: (1) Go over chart on previous page, using forms in complete sentences, such as *je parle français.* Do as group repetition drill. (2) Write all forms of the verb that are pronounced identically on board first; then present *nous, vous* forms to complete paradigm.

1. **Je.** Note that **je** is not capitalized unless it starts a sentence. When a verb begins with a vowel sound, **je** becomes **j'**.

En hiver, **j'aime** faire du ski.	*In winter, I like to go skiing.*

2. **Tu** and **vous.** There are two ways to say *you* in French: **Tu** is used when speaking to a friend, fellow student, relative, child, or pet; **vous** is used when speaking to a person you don't know well or when addressing an older person, someone in authority, or anyone with whom you wish to maintain a certain formality. The plural of both **tu** and **vous** is **vous.** The context will indicate whether **vous** refers to one person or to more than one.

Suggestion: Ask sts. why examples show *vous* or *tu.* This will reinforce previous material.

Note: In English, the *you* form is actually the formal form; the informal form (*thou*) has disappeared in current usage.

Emma, **tu** parles espagnol?	*Emma, do you speak Spanish?*
Madame, où habitez-**vous**?	*Ma'am, where do you live?*
Vous parlez bien français, madame.	*You speak French well, ma'am.*
Pardon, messieurs (mesdames, mesdemoiselles), est-ce que **vous** parlez anglais?	*Excuse me, gentlemen (ladies), do you speak English?*

Suggestion: Point to two women sts. and ask *ils ou elles?* Do the same with two men, and reinforce as needed.

3. **Il** and **elle.** As you know, all nouns—people and objects—have gender in French. **Il** is the pronoun that refers to a masculine person or object, and **elle** refers to a feminine person or object.

Paul travaille. **Il** travaille à la bibliothèque.	*Paul works. He works at the library.*
L'ordinateur est cher, mais **il** est aussi utile.	*The computer is expensive, but it is useful as well.*
Agathe? **Elle** travaille au café.	*Agathe? She works at the café.*
La bibliothèque? **Elle** est ouverte le samedi.	*The library? It is open on Saturdays.*

The plural counterparts **ils** and **elles** are used in the same way as the singular forms. **Ils** corresponds to masculine plural nouns and to a group that includes at least one masculine noun; **elles** corresponds to feminine plural nouns.

Luc et Diane? **Ils** sont toujours ensemble.	*Luc and Diane? They are always together.*

Suggestion: Point out similarity of *on* and English *one,* used for indefinite subjects.

4. **On.** In English, the words *people, we, one,* or *they* are often used to convey the idea of an indefinite subject. In French, the indefinite pronoun **on** is used, always with the third-person singular of the verb.

Ici **on** parle français.	*One speaks French here.* *People (They, We) speak French here.*

On is also used frequently in informal French instead of **nous.**

Nous parlons français. → **On** parle français.

[Allez-y! A]

Present Tense of *-er* Verbs

Most French verbs have infinitives ending in **-er: parler** (*to speak*), **aimer** (*to like; to love*). To form the present tense of these verbs, drop the final **-er** and add the endings shown in the chart.*

PRESENT TENSE OF **aimer** (*to like; to love*)			
j'	aim**e**	nous	aim**ons**
tu	aim**es**	vous	aim**ez**
il/elle/on	aim**e**	ils/elles	aim**ent**

1. Note that the present tense (**le présent**) in French has several equivalents in English.

   Je **parle** français. — *I speak French.* / *I am speaking French.* / *I do speak French.*

2. Other verbs conjugated like **parler** and **aimer** include:

adorer	*to love; to adore*	**fumer**	*to smoke*
aimer mieux	*to prefer* (*to like better*)	**habiter**	*to live*
chercher	*to look for*	**manger**‡	*to eat*
commencer†	*to begin*	**penser**	*to think*
danser	*to dance*	**porter**	*to wear*
demander	*to ask for*	**regarder**	*to watch; to look at*
détester	*to detest; to hate*	**rêver**	*to dream*
donner	*to give*	**skier**	*to ski*
écouter	*to listen to*	**travailler**	*to work*
étudier	*to study*	**trouver**	*to find*
		visiter	*to visit* (*a place*)

   Vous **cherchez** le resto-U? — *Are you looking for the cafeteria?*

   Nous **étudions** l'informatique. — *We're studying computer science.*

3. Some verbs, such as **adorer, aimer (mieux),** and **détester,** can be followed by an infinitive.

   J'**aime écouter** la radio. — *I like listening to the radio.*

   Je **déteste regarder** la télévision. — *I hate watching television.*

[Allez-y! B-C-D-E]

*As you know, final **s** is usually not pronounced in French. Final **z** of the second-person plural and the **-ent** of the third-person plural verb forms are also silent.
†The **nous** form of **commencer** is **commençons.** The **cédille** is added to retain the soft **s** sound.
‡The **nous** form of **manger** is **mangeons.** The **e** is kept to retain the soft **g** sound.

Presentation: You may need to explain what an infinitive is and what conjugating a verb means: An infinitive indicates the action or state, with no reference to who performs it. In English, the infinitive is indicated by *to: to run.* To conjugate a verb means to change the form of the infinitive to correspond to the subject performing the action. In English, this can be illustrated with the verb *to be* (*I am, you are,* etc.).

Note: Point 1 should be emphasized strongly.

Suggestion: After presenting this idea, ask *Comment dit-on? We are visiting Paris, I'm visiting the Sorbonne* (*la Sorbonne*). *She watches the sts. He does love Paris! You* (*Tu*) *hate Paris.*

Suggestion: Point out the use of present-tense questions to indicate near-future action: *Vous travaillez demain?* (Are you going to work tomorrow?)

Suggestion: Model pronunciation of each infinitive several times. Then use the *je* form of each in brief, simple sentences about yourself, repeating several times and pantomiming as appropriate. Transform the base sentence into a simple *vous* question, "coaching" sts. to answer using the *je* form. Example: *danser… J'aime danser. Je danse très bien… Je danse souvent. Et vous, vous aimez danser? Vous dansez souvent?* Emphasize infinitives that include English prepositions in their meaning: *chercher* (to look for), *écouter* (to listen to), *regarder* (to look at). (These are difficult for sts.)

Note: Review use of definite article, if desired. Emphasize use of infinitive after these three verbs.

Grammaire interactive

For more on the present tense of **-er** verbs, watch the corresponding Grammar Tutorial and take a brief practice quiz at **Connect French.**

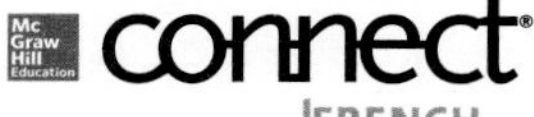

www.mhconnectfrench.com

Allez-y!

Suggestion: Use the following oral rapid response ex. as a preliminary activity. Tell sts. to give the corresponding forms. *je: chercher, écouter, regarder tu: manger, admirer, rêver il/elle: chanter, danser,* etc.

Suggestions: (1) Have sts. write out answers to completion ex. first, then give orally. Reinforce by writing forms on board. (2) Have a few sts. write out answers on board. Use group repetition.

A. Dialogue en classe. Complete the following dialogue with subject pronouns or forms of **parler.**

LE PROFESSEUR: Tout le monde (*Everybody*), _____[1] parlez français?
LA CLASSE: Oui, nous _____[2] français.
LE PROFESSEUR: Ici, en classe, on _____[3] français?
JIM: Oui, ici _____[4] parle français.
GILDAS: Marc et Marie, vous _____[5] chinois?
MARC ET MARIE: Oui, _____[6] parlons chinois.
CHARLOTTE: Jim, tu _____[7] allemand?
JIM: Oui, _____[8] parle allemand.
CÉCILE: Paul parle italien?
JAMEL: Oui, _____[9] parle italien.

Suggestion (B): Ask different sts. to dictate these sentences to others. They may be checked at board or projected using your digital display.

Additional activity: *Qu'est-ce qu'on fait ce soir?* (What are we doing tonight?) *Suivez le modèle.* MODÈLE: *Nous travaillons.* → *On travaille?* 1. *Nous regardons un film.* 2. *Nous étudions l'espagnol.* 3. *Nous visitons le quartier universitaire.* 4. *Nous écoutons la radio.* 5. *Nous donnons une soirée.* 6. *Nous regardons la télévision.* 7. *Nous dansons avec les amis de Pierre.*

B. *Tu* ou *vous*? A student guide is asking questions of various people at the Sorbonne. Complete the questions, using the appropriate pronoun (**tu** or **vous**) and the correct form of the verb in parentheses.

1. Madame, _____ _____ (habiter) près de (*near*) l'université?
2. Romain, _____ _____ (chercher) la faculté des sciences?
3. Paul et Lucie, _____ _____ (visiter) le Quartier latin?
4. Monsieur, _____ _____ (trouver) ce que (*what*) _____ _____ (chercher)?
5. Richard, _____ _____ (demander) des renseignements (*information*) sur la cité universitaire?

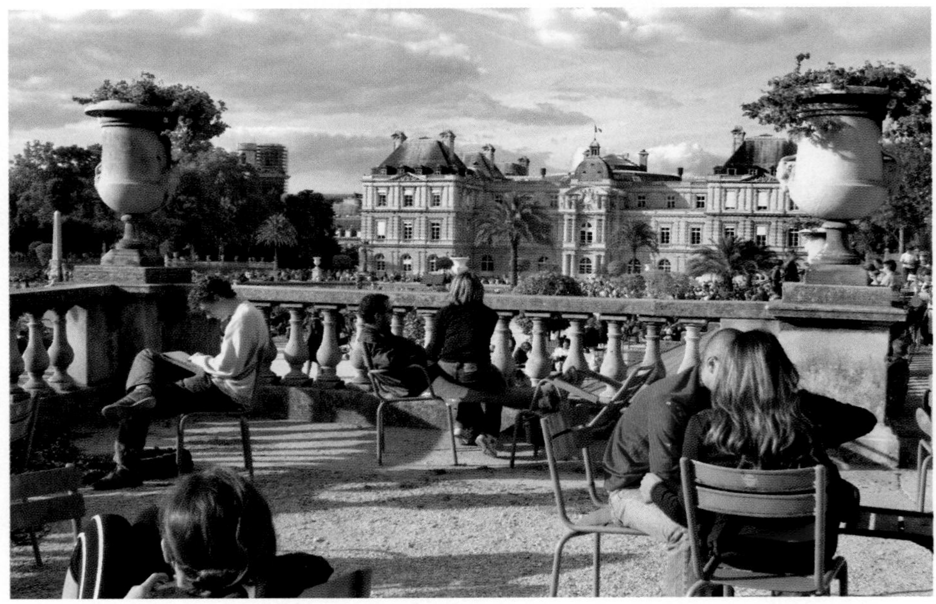

Étudiants au jardin du Luxembourg

C. Portraits. State the preferences of the following people.

MODÈLE: Mon (*My*) cousin... → Mon cousin aime bien le football, mais (*but*) il aime mieux le basket. Il adore le rock et il déteste le travail!

Je...	aimer bien	le tennis
Mon (Ma) camarade...	aimer mieux	le jogging
Mes parents...	adorer	le cinéma
Les étudiants...	détester	la littérature
Le professeur...		les maths
		la physique

Note (C): This is called a "sentence builder." Tell sts. that many sentences can be made using each subject and verb with items from column 3.

D. Une interview. Interview your instructor.

MODÈLE: aimer mieux danser ou (*or*) skier →
Vous aimez mieux danser ou skier?

1. aimer mieux la télévision ou le cinéma
2. aimer ou détester regarder la télévision
3. aimer mieux le rock ou la musique classique
4. aimer mieux la musique ou le sport
5. aimer mieux les livres ou les magazines

Suggestion (D): Sts. recall as many of your responses as possible, stating, for example: *Vous aimez mieux le cinéma, vous…*

Suggestion (Mots clés): Model the pronunciation of these adverbs before sts. use them in sentences. If sts. want to express *not* or *never*, teach *ne… pas* (*jamais*) as lexical items.

E. Curiosité. Find out how your classmate spends his/her free time by asking whether . . .

MODÈLE: il/elle écoute de temps en temps la radio →
É1: Tu écoutes de temps en temps la radio?
É2: Oui, j'écoute quelquefois la radio. Et toi?
É1: Moi, je n'écoute pas la radio.

1. il/elle regarde souvent ou rarement la télévision le week-end
2. il/elle aime le cinéma, en général
3. il/elle mange quelquefois au restaurant
4. il/elle adore ou déteste le sport
5. il/elle skie bien
6. il/elle danse souvent le week-end

Now say which response you find original or strange.

MODÈLE: Sonia déteste le cinéma. C'est bizarre!

Mots clés

To express how often you do something

The following adverbs usually follow the verb.

toujours	*always*
souvent	*often*
quelquefois	*sometimes*
rarement	*rarely*

D'habitude (*Usually*), **en général** (*generally*), and **de temps en temps** (*from time to time*) are adverbs that are most often placed at the beginning of a sentence.

Je regarde **souvent** la télévision.

Annie et moi, nous étudions **quelquefois** à la bibliothèque.

En général, j'étudie le week-end.

Interaction: Have sts. act out the following situation, using the vocabulary and structures from this chapter. *Échange:* Role-play the following situation with a classmate. One of you plays the role of an exchange student from Morocco who speaks French, Arabic, and a Berber dialect but not English. The other plays the role of an interpreter who is giving the exchange student a tour of the campus. Ask the student what subjects he or she likes best. Get to know the student by telling him or her what you enjoy doing. Ask about his or her favorite activities.

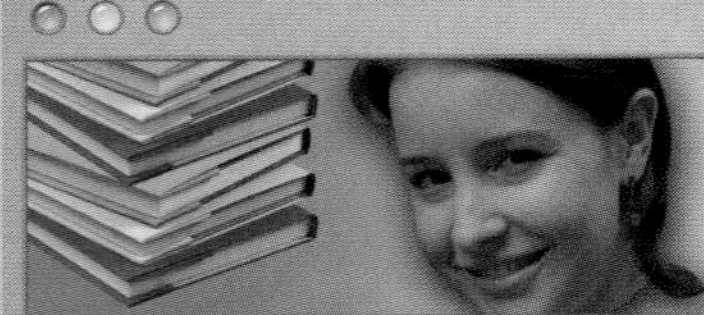

Le blog de Léa

Salut tout le monde!

mardi 17 mai

Bonjour! Guten Tag! Hello! Salaam! Buon giorno! Nǐ hǎo! Buenos días! Shalom! Salut tout le monde!

J'ai[1] une amie belge: c'est Juliette. J'ai un ami martiniquais: il s'appelle Hector. Et j'ai un copain marocain, Hassan. Il a un restaurant au Quartier latin, proche de ma fac.[2] Mais je cherche aussi des amis chinois, japonais, mexicains, allemands, américains… des amis de tous les pays.[3] À Paris, c'est possible, non?

Léa

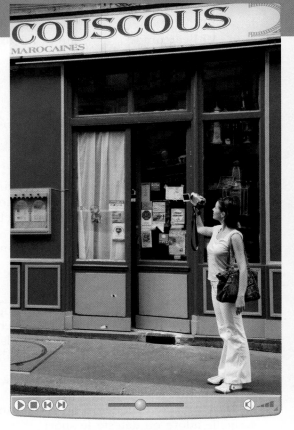

Moi, devant le restaurant d'Hassan

COMMENTAIRES

Alexis

Bonjour Léa!
Mon chien et moi,[4] nous sommes[5] québécois. Nous parlons français. Nous sommes très sympathiques.[6]

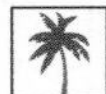

Poema

Léa, bonjour!
Je m'appelle Poema. Je ne suis pas[7] chinoise, je ne suis pas américaine… Je suis tahitienne. Je suis isolée[8] à Paris et je cherche des amis français.

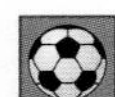

Mamadou

Salut Léa!
J'ai[9] une amie française: c'est toi. Mais tu as des copines[10]… Tu me les présentes[11]?
Juliette, par exemple… À bientôt, j'espère[12]!

Suggestion: Model pronunciation and have sts. repeat individually or as a group.

Follow-up: *Questions de compréhension:* 1. *Léa dit «bonjour» à ses amis du blog: dans quelles langues?* 2. *Qui sont les amis de Léa? Quelle est leur nationalité?* 3. *À votre avis, pourquoi est-ce que Léa veut* (wants) *rencontrer des amis étrangers?*

Note: For additional exs. on *Le blog de Léa* and *Reportage,* see the Workbook/Laboratory Manual.

Video connection: In the videoblog for this chapter, Léa goes to her friend Hassan's restaurant in the *Quartier latin,* where they talk about the pros and cons of the neighborhood. She posts a video about the *Quartier latin* on her site.

[1]*I have* [2]proche… *close to the university* (la Sorbonne) [3]de… *from all over the world* [4]Mon… *My dog and I* [5]nous… *we are* [6]*nice* [7]Je… *I'm not* [8]*lonely* [9]*I have* [10]*girlfriends* [11]Tu… *Will you introduce them to me?* [12]*I hope*

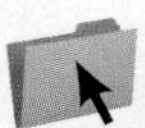

REPORTAGE

Quartier latin: le quartier général des étudiants

À la terrasse du café de la Sorbonne, Éva, d'origine russe, discute avec ses trois amis: Bruno, un étudiant lyonnais, Maren, une jeune Allemande qui étudie le droit social à Paris, et Ahmed, un jeune Marocain en doctorat de cinéma. Cette scène est typique du Quartier latin, zone cosmopolite, sorte de campus international au centre de Paris.

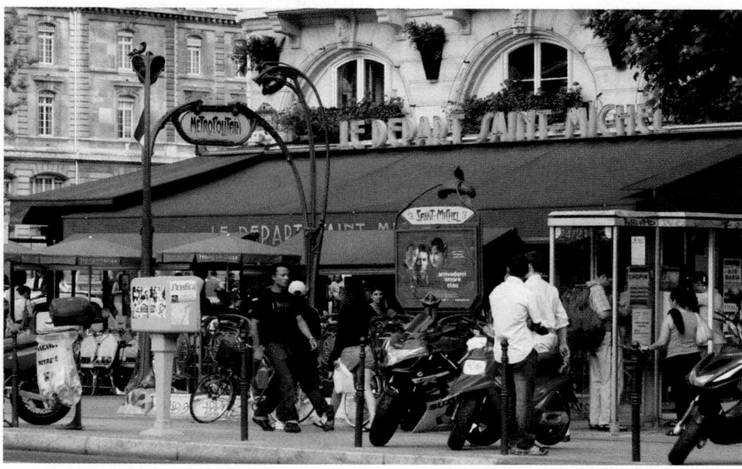

Un café du Quartier latin. Une population jeune, internationale, active et cultivée habite au Quartier latin. C'est le quartier des amitiés éternelles, des idées géniales et des discussions passionnées sur la politique, l'art et la vie. C'est le symbole de la vie étudiante.

Avec ses librairies et ses bibliothèques, le Quartier latin est l'univers de la culture. Les grands lycées (Louis-le-Grand, Henri IV) et les universités comme[1] la célèbre Sorbonne fondée en 1257[2] par Robert de Sorbon continuent à former[3] les élites intellectuelles.

Dans les boutiques du boulevard Saint-Michel, les vêtements[4] remplacent les livres. Mais les petites rues adjacentes ont encore[5] beaucoup de charme: petits restaurants délicieux, cinémas comme le fameux Champollion, boutiques exotiques, bistros et bars animés, cybercafés.

Le jardin du Luxembourg est le parc du quartier. Dans ses allées[6] romantiques, les étudiants discutent, méditent, se relaxent avant ou après un examen. Au Quartier latin, tout est conçu[7] pour le travail et pour le bonheur[8] des étudiants.

[1]*such as* [2]mille deux cent cinquante-sept [3]*educate* [4]*clothes* [5]ont… *still have* [6]*footpaths* [7]*conceived* [8]*happiness*

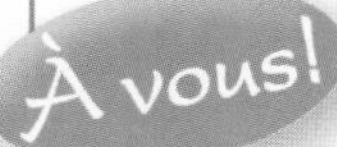

1. Désirez-vous visiter le Quartier latin? Pourquoi? Imaginez votre itinéraire.
2. Le Quartier latin est-il différent d'un campus à l'américaine? Développez votre réponse.
3. Quels détails vous intéressent sur cette photo du Quartier latin?

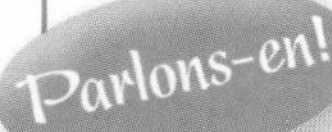

1. Trouvez un plan du Quartier latin sur Internet. Imprimez-le. (*Print it.*)
2. Par groupes de trois étudiants, observez le plan.
3. Situez le boulevard Saint-Michel, la Sorbonne, le lycée Henri IV, le jardin du Luxembourg.
4. À partir du (*Starting from the*) métro Saint-Michel (sur la photo), créez un itinéraire pour visiter le Quartier latin.
5. Présentez votre itinéraire à la classe. Utilisez le verbe *visiter*:

   On visite la Sorbonne, le jardin du Luxembourg…

Leçon 3

Presentation: You may want to teach the minidialogue inductively by having sts. find verb forms and explain how *être* is conjugated.

Le verbe *être*

Identifying People and Things

Les amis de Léa

Appel (Call) *vidéo entre Mamadou et Léa.*

MAMADOU: Salut Léa! Tu parles de tes amis sur ton blog. **Ils sont** sympas?

LÉA: **Mes amis sont** intelligents, amusants et originaux. Juliette et moi, **nous sommes** particulièrement proches.*

MAMADOU: Hector, qui **est-ce?**

LÉA: Hector, **c'est** un danseur professionnel.

MAMADOU: Et Hassan, **c'est** qui?

LÉA: **C'est** un ami adorable!

MAMADOU: Moi aussi, **je suis** adorable! Et toi aussi, **tu es** adorable!

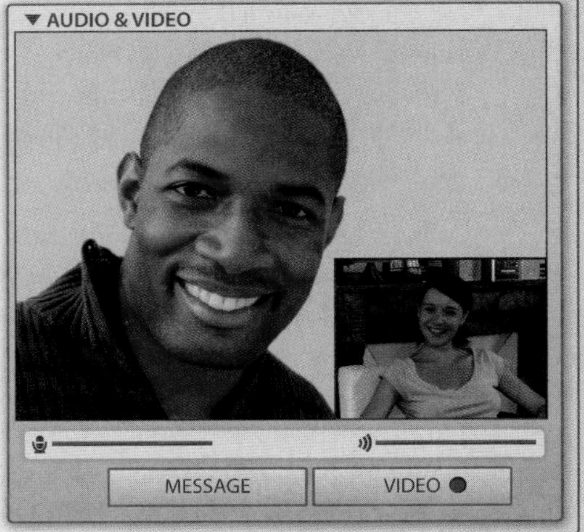

*close

Suggestion: Have sts. correct the false statements.

Vrai ou faux?

1. Les amis de Léa sont amusants.
2. Léa et Juliette sont vraiment (*really*) proches.
3. Hector est l'ami de Mamadou.
4. Hassan est l'ami de Léa.
5. Hassan est danseur.

Suggestion: Model pronunciation. Then have sts. read the roles, in small groups or within whole-class format. See the Instructor's Manual for suggestions on using brief dialogues.

Forms of *être*

PRESENT TENSE OF **être** (*to be*)			
je	**suis**	nous	**sommes**
tu	**es**	vous	**êtes**
il/elle/on	**est**	ils/elles	**sont**

Uses of *être*

1. The uses of **être** closely parallel those of *to be.*

Fabrice **est** intelligent.	*Fabrice is intelligent.*
Est-ce que Clarisse **est** organisée?	*Is Clarisse organized?*
Fabrice et Clarisse **sont** à la bibliothèque.	*Fabrice and Clarisse are at the library.*

2. In identifying someone's nationality, religion, or profession, no article is used following **être.**

Je **suis anglais.**	*I am English.*
Je **suis catholique;** mon ami **est musulman.**	*I'm (a) Catholic; my friend is (a) Muslim.*
—Vous **êtes professeur?**	*Are you a teacher?*
—Non, je **suis étudiant.**	*No, I am a student.*

C'est versus *il/elle est*

1. The indefinite pronoun **ce (c')** is an invariable third-person pronoun. **Ce** has various English equivalents: *this, that, these, those, he, she, they,* and *it.*

2. The expression **c'est** (plural, **ce sont**) is used before modified nouns (always with an article) and proper names; it usually answers the questions **Qui est-ce?** and **Qu'est-ce que c'est?**

—Qui est-ce?	*Who is it?*
—C'est Maxime. C'est un étudiant belge.	*It's Maxime. He is a Belgian student.*
—Ce sont des Français?	*Are they French?*
—Non, ce sont des Italiens.	*No, they're Italian.*
—Qu'est-ce que c'est?	*What is that?*
—C'est un ordinateur.	*That's (It's) a computer.*
—Et ça, qu'est-ce que c'est?	*And that, what is it?*
—Oh ça, c'est une souris.	*Oh, that's a mouse.*

3. **C'est** can also be followed by an adjective, to refer to a general situation or to describe something that is understood in the context of the conversation.

Le français? C'est facile!	*French? It's easy!*
J'adore la France. C'est magnifique!	*I love France. It's great!*

(*continued*)

Suggestion: Explain what an irregular verb is; use *to be* as an English example since it has parallel irregularities. Alternatively, have a st. explain the concept of irregular verbs so you can get insight into sts.' current understanding.

Presentation: Model pronunciation of verb forms, using group repetition. Use complete, simple sentences for modeling: *Je suis intelligent*(e). *Tu es sociable. Il est drôle,* etc. Point out pronunciation of *vous êtes* and *elles sont.* Stress the [z] and [s] sounds.

Suggestion (*Le verbe* être): Compare the structures *Il est français* (adjective) / *C'est un Français* (noun). You may want to explain that what follows *c'est* can be the subject of a sentence (a proper name, a pronoun, or a noun with an article); what follows *il/elle est* cannot stand alone as the subject. Refer to ex. B on page 50.

Suggestion: Ask a st. to explain what "modified" means. Write transformations on board to show equivalence between *Il/Elle est…* (noun) and *C'est un(e)…* (modified noun). Examples: *Il est professeur. C'est un professeur français. Elle est protestante, et elle est sincère. C'est une protestante sincère.* Ask sts. to give alternatives to the following: *C'est un professeur difficile. Il est étudiant, et il est intelligent. Elle est française. C'est une touriste enthousiaste.* Note that sts. rarely learn to produce *c'est* and *il est* correctly in free speech until much later.

Suggestion: Mention the oral structures *C'est qui? C'est quoi?*

Note: The adjective following *c'est* is always masculine singular.

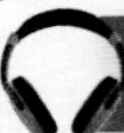

Prononcez bien!

The vowels in *et* and *est*

Be sure to pronounce a single and brief sound in both **et** and **est,** as opposed to the combination of sounds in the English letter *a*. Close your mouth and stretch your lips for [e] in **et** more than for [ɛ] in **est.** The sound [e] is usually found at the end of a syllable or word, whereas [ɛ] tends to appear before a pronounced consonant.*

[e]: **télé, aller, nez, et**

[ɛ]: **matières, être, aime, seize, merci**

*some exceptions: **mai, est, très**

Pronunciation practice (1): Write the following words on the board and have sts. both pronounce them and indicate whether they sound like *et* or *est: adorer, aime, écouter, être, bibliothèque, amphithéâtre, café, cité, librairie, quartier, université, rêve, américain, déteste, française, économie, espagnol, étrangère, après, avec, général, mais.*

Pronunciation practice (2): The *Prononcez bien!* section on page 53 of this chapter contains additional activities for practicing these sounds.

Vocabulary recycling: Use the following as a preliminary ex.: Review classroom vocabulary and practice *être.* Hold up or point to objects, asking *Qu'est-ce que c'est?* Elicit plural forms by holding up two books, three pencils, etc.

Additional activity: *Qui est étudiant? Transformez la phrase selon le modèle.* MODÈLE: *Anne est étudiante. (je, nous, Claire et Hervé, tu, vous, Marc, Jeanne et Catherine, Jacques et Pierre)*

Additional activity: Point to sts. and ask the questions. *MODÈLE: C'est un ami? → Non, ce sont des amis. 1. C'est une étudiante? 2. C'est une touriste? 3. C'est un professeur? 4. C'est une Américaine? 5. C'est un Anglais? 6. C'est une Chinoise?*

Suggestion (B): Can be done orally or in writing.

Note: *ne… pas* is the next point of grammar. Present *ce n'est pas* [snepa] lexically.

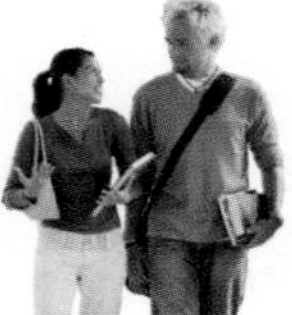

4. **Il/Elle est** (and **Ils/Elles sont**) are generally used to describe someone or something already mentioned in the conversation. They are usually followed by an adjective, a prepositional phrase, and occasionally by an unmodified noun (without an article).

—La librairie?	*The bookstore?*
—Elle est dans la rue Mouffetard.	*It's on Mouffetard Street.*
—Voici Karim. Il est étudiant en biologie.	*Here's Karim. He's a biology student.*
—Il est français?	*Is he French?*
—Oui, il est français, d'origine algérienne.	*Yes, he's French, of Algerian descent.*

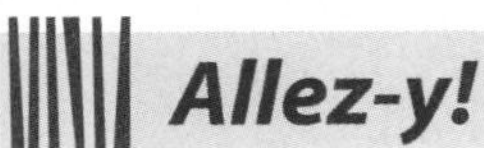

Allez-y!

A. Un examen. Complete the following dialogue between Fabrice and Clarisse using the correct forms of the verb **être.**

FABRICE: Ces livres ______[1] difficiles!
CLARISSE: Pas pour toi, tu ______[2] un génie!
FABRICE: Oui, mais le professeur ______[3] très exigeant (*demanding*).
CLARISSE: Et il dit (*says*) toujours: «Vous ______[4] une étudiante intelligente, mademoiselle.»
FABRICE: Nous ______[5] peut-être (*maybe*) intelligents, mais moi, je ne ______[6] pas prêt pour l'examen!

Qui est-ce? Identify each person described here, based on the dialogue.

1. C'est une personne très exigeante. C'est ______.
2. C'est une étudiante intelligente. C'est ______.
3. Il n'est pas prêt pour l'examen. C'est ______.

B. Deux étudiants africains à Paris. Tell about these young people by completing the descriptions with **c', il,** or **elle.**

Voici Fatima. ______[1] est marocaine. ______[2] est étudiante en philosophie. ______[3] est une personne sociable et dynamique. Son petit ami (*boyfriend*) s'appelle Barthélémy. ______[4] est sénégalais. ______[5] est un jeune homme enthousiaste. ______[6] est aussi un peu timide. ______[7] est un étudiant sérieux.

C. La France et les Français. Taking turns with a classmate, ask and answer questions using **c'est** and **ce n'est pas** (*it's not*).

Suggestion: Point out pronunciation of *lys* [**lis**]. Draw a *fleur de lys* on the board if sts. are not sure what it is.

MODÈLE: le sport préféré des Français: le jogging, le football →
É1: Le sport préféré des Français, c'est le jogging ou le football?
É2: Ce n'est pas le jogging, c'est le football!

1. un symbole de la France: la rose, la fleur de lys
2. un président français: Sartre, Hollande
3. un cadeau (*present*) des Français aux Américains: la Maison-Blanche (*White House*), la Statue de la Liberté
4. une ville avec beaucoup de Français: La Nouvelle-Orléans, St. Louis
5. un génie français: Mme Curie, Albert Einstein
6. parler français: difficile, facile

D. Et vous, comment êtes-vous? Tell a little about yourself.

Je m'appelle ______.
Je suis un(e) ______. (femme / homme)
Je suis ______. (étudiant[e] / professeur)
Je suis ______. (nationalité)
J'habite à ______. (ville)
Je suis l'ami(e) de ______.
J'aime ______.

Now describe one of your classmates using the same guidelines.

Il/Elle s'appelle...

Suggestion: Have sts. write a self-portrait on a 3 × 5 card, deleting their name but adding any details they choose. Collect cards. Then have a st. select a card from deck and read it aloud. Others guess who is being described.

La négation *ne... pas*

Expressing Disagreement

Le Festival du film d'horreur

Juliette téléphone à Léa.

JULIETTE: Allô, Léa, Il y a un festival du film d'horreur au Champollion. Ce soir, c'est *Dracula*.
LÉA: **Je n'aime pas** les films d'horreur.
JULIETTE: **Tu n'aimes pas** les films d'horreur? **Ce n'est pas** possible!
LÉA: C'est possible! Parce que **je n'aime pas** la violence.
JULIETTE: Mais *Dracula*, **ce n'est pas** un film violent! Il y a de l'humour...
LÉA: **Je n'apprécie pas** cette sorte d'humour.
JULIETTE: Qu'est-ce que tu aimes alors?
LÉA: J'adore les films d'amour...
JULIETTE: **Tu n'es pas** originale!

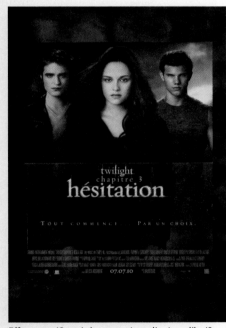

Effrayants (*Scary*), les vampires d'aujourd'hui?

Vrai ou faux?

1. Léa aime les films d'horreur.
2. *Dracula* est un film d'amour.
3. Léa apprécie l'humour du film *Dracula*.
4. Léa n'est pas originale.

1. To make a sentence negative in French, **ne** is placed before a conjugated verb and **pas** after it.

    Je **parle** chinois. → Je **ne parle pas** chinois.
    Elles **regardent** souvent la télévision. → Elles **ne regardent pas** souvent la télévision.

Suggestion: Have sts. correct the false statements.

Grammaire interactive

For more on subject pronouns, the verb **être,** and negation, watch the corresponding Grammar Tutorial and take a brief practice quiz at **Connect French.**

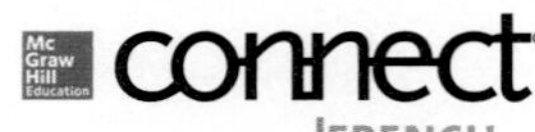

www.mhconnectfrench.com

2. **Ne** becomes **n'** before a vowel or a mute **h.**

   Elle aime les films vampire. → Elle **n'a**ime pas les films vampire.
   Nous habitons ici. → Nous **n'h**abitons pas ici.

3. If a verb is followed by an infinitive, **ne** and **pas** surround the conjugated verb.

   Il aime étudier. → Il **n'aime pas** étudier.

4. In informal conversation, the **e** in **ne** is usually not pronounced; some people do not say the **ne** at all.

   Je **ne** pense **pas** (*I don't think so*).
   Je **n~~e~~** pense **pas.** → J~~e~~ (~~ne~~) pense **pas.**

Presentation: Emphasize that [ʃpɑ̃spa] is an oral phenomenon only.

Note: The structure *pas de* is presented in *Chapitre 4, Leçon 2.*

Allez-y!

A. Portrait de Victor. Here is some information about Victor.

Victor habite à la cité universitaire et, en général, il étudie à la bibliothèque. Après (*After*) les cours, il parle avec ses (*his*) amis au café. Le soir (*In the evening*), il écoute la radio: il aime beaucoup le jazz! Il adore le sport, il skie très bien et le week-end, il regarde les matchs de football à la télévision.

Clarisse is quite different from Victor. Tell what Clarisse doesn't like and doesn't do. Replace **il** with **elle** in the paragraph and make all the verbs negative. **Clarisse…**

Suggestion: Use in whole-class or partner/pair format.

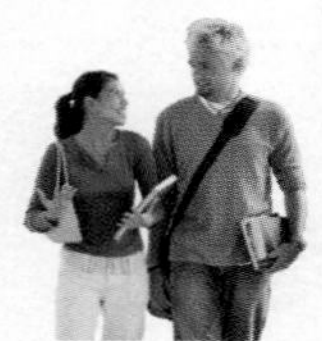

B. Interview à deux. Find out about a classmate by asking about the following activities, habits, and preferences. Answer your partner's questions, too.

MODÈLE: travailler →
É1: Tu travailles?
É2: Non, je ne travaille pas. (Oui, je travaille.) Et toi?

1. parler italien; russe; espagnol; anglais
2. habiter quelle ville; Paris; New York; Abidjan; Cincinnati; la cité-U
3. étudier la psychologie; la littérature; l'informatique; la biologie; le commerce; les langues étrangères
4. aimer les examens; les films de science-fiction; les films d'amour; le rap; la musique country
5. aimer le sport; le football américain; le football; le basket-ball; le hockey
6. détester les maths; l'histoire; la politique; la science; la pyschologie
7. surfer le Web; écouter la radio; parler avec des amis; manger au restaurant; manger au resto-U; skier; danser

Résumez! Now summarize for the class five things you found out about your partner.

Suggestion: Have sts. do orally or in writing, as a whole class or in pairs.

C. Et vous? Tell about yourself by completing the sentences.

1. J'aime ______, mais (*but*) je n'aime pas ______.
2. J'adore ______, mais je déteste ______.
3. J'écoute ______, mais je n'écoute pas ______.
4. J'aime ______, mais j'aime mieux ______.
5. Je n'étudie pas ______. J'étudie ______.

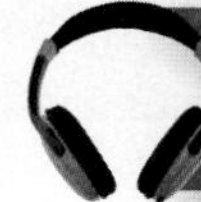

Prononcez bien!

1. **Masculine vs. feminine forms of nationalities** (page 35)

Beaucoup de nationalités! Your housemate is back from his second introductory French class. He's impressed by the number of nationalities represented in his class. He lists them for you, although he omits articles as he is still unsure about them. You help him by telling him the appropriate article **un** or **une.**

MODÈLE: *You hear:* mexicaine
You say: une Mexicaine

Script (1): 1. *canadien* 2. *italienne* 3. *chinoise* 4. *québécois* 5. *vietnamien* 6. *sénégalaise* 7. *allemand* 8. *japonais* 9. *anglaise* 10. *américain*

Answers (1): 1. *un Canadien* 2. *une Italienne* 3. *une Chinoise* 4. *un Québécois* 5. *un Vietnamien* 6. *une Sénégalaise* 7. *un Allemand* 8. *un Japonais* 9. *une Anglaise* 10. *un Américain*

2. **The vowels in *le, la,* and *les*** (page 39)

Une nouvelle colocataire! One of your housemates has moved out and Isabelle, a French student, is moving in. She asks you to help her unpack. Listen to what she says and complete the paragraph with the names of the objects she asks you to bring into her room. **Attention!** Don't forget the article (**le, la,** or **les**).

Script (2): *S'il te plaît, apporte 1. la chaise 2. les livres 3. le bureau 4. la table 5. les stylos 6. la télévision et 7. le dictionnaire. Merci!*

1. 2. 3. 4.

5. 6. 7.

ISABELLE: «S'il te plaît, apporte (*bring*) ____________,[1] ____________,[2] ____________,[3] ____________,[4] ____________,[5] ____________,[6] et ____________.[7] Merci!»

3. **The vowels in *et* and *est*** (page 50)

Où étudier? You are a new student at the university. See what Isabelle has to say about good places to study. Read the following paragraph aloud. Your partner will indicate whether the bold letters correspond to [e] as in **et** or to [ɛ] as in **est**.

Suggestion (3): As sts. work in pairs, circulate in class to monitor their pronuncation.

Answers (3): 1. [e] 2. [e] 3. [ɛ] 4. [e] 5. [e] 6. [ɛ] 7. [e] 8. [e] 9. [ɛ] 10. [ɛ] 11. [ɛ] 12. [ɛ] 13. [ɛ] 14. [e] 15. [ɛ] 16. [e]

En g**é**n**é**ral,[1, 2] j'**ai**me[3] **é**tudi**er**[4, 5] à la biblioth**è**que.[6] Il y a beaucoup de caf**é**s[7] dans le quarti**er**[8] univers**i**t**ai**re,[9, 10] m**ais**[11] pers**o**nn**e**llement,[12, 13] je d**é**t**e**ste[14, 15] y (*there*) **é**tudier[16]: il y a trop de bruit (*too much noise*).

	[e]	[ɛ]		[e]	[ɛ]		[e]	[ɛ]		[e]	[ɛ]
1.	☐	☐	5.	☐	☐	9.	☐	☐	13.	☐	☐
2.	☐	☐	6.	☐	☐	10.	☐	☐	14.	☐	☐
3.	☐	☐	7.	☐	☐	11.	☐	☐	15.	☐	☐
4.	☐	☐	8.	☐	☐	12.	☐	☐	16.	☐	☐

Leçon 4

PERSPECTIVES

Purpose: *Leçon 4: Perspectives* combines and reinforces the vocabulary and grammar structures presented in *Leçons 1–3*, with a special emphasis on skill development.

Purpose: *Avant de lire*, which introduces each reading selection in *Vis-à-vis*, presents reading strategies and techniques designed to help sts. approach written texts with greater confidence and efficiency. Each *Avant de lire* presents a specific strategy followed by a brief warm-up ex. These prereading exs. can be done in class or individually by sts. at home.

Note: In this reading, sts. will practice cognate recognition and contextual guessing. These strategies are intended to sharpen cognitive skills, build confidence in using authentic texts, and discourage overreliance on the dictionary. For this reason, the text has not been pedagogically modified or glossed.

Suggestion: Review presentation of cognates.

Suggestion (3): Lead sts. from the cognate meaning (*plus, formation, bénévolat*) to a related but broader meaning: *more than, training, volunteer.*

Answers (4): The false cognates are *stages* (training, internships), *équipe* (team), *moniteurs* (instructors). Have sts. brainstorm their meaning from cognates. Note that *pratiques* can also be a false cognate, although not in this context.

Purpose: *Lecture* is the reading selection that appears in every chapter of *Vis-à-vis*. Many of the readings are drawn from authentic contemporary sources; some are author written, and others are literary. Each selection is thematically related to the chapter topic or topics; author-written readings recycle the active vocabulary presented and practiced in the chapter. Unfamiliar words and expressions are glossed in the margin. The reading selections follow a progression through the chapters, from beginning-level texts to increasingly challenging ones, as sts. expand their vocabulary and increase their skills. Each reading selection is followed by a *Compréhension* ex. to verify and expand upon sts.' understanding of the text.

Lecture

Avant de lire

Predicting from context. When reading a text in your native language, you constantly—though perhaps unconsciously—make use of contextual information. This information gives you an immediate, overall orientation; it also allows you to figure out the meaning of unfamiliar words. Here are some ways to use contextual information when reading French texts. You will practice these techniques in the reading that follows.

1. Orient yourself using graphic elements: logos, illustrations, headings, and large or heavy type.
   - First, scan the brochure that follows and identify the institution being publicized and its location. Look at the photo. How would you describe the setting? (Is it modern? traditional? cosmopolitan?)
   - Next, quickly read through the first paragraph, underlining the cognates (**mots apparentés**) that you find. How well did your description match the text?

2. Use cognates to help you deduce the meaning of unfamiliar terms.
   - Read the following phrase from the brochure and try to figure out the meaning of the word **logement:**

     logement dans des familles francophones ou dans les résidences universitaires

   Were you able to infer that **logement** means *lodging*?

3. Watch for near cognates.
   - In the following phrases, your developing linguistic intuition should tell you that the words in boldface cannot be translated by the English form that most closely resembles them. Can you find an alternative to them that is close in meaning?

     plus de soixante ans d'expérience
     formation solide des enseignants (*teachers*)
     activités de **bénévolat** en milieu (*setting*) francophone

4. Also be aware of false cognates.
   - What do you think are the false cognates in the following phrases?

     équipe de moniteurs
     stages de travaux pratiques en milieu de travail

5. Now that you have had the chance to refine your ability to recognize cognates, near cognates, and false cognates, scan the bulleted lists beneath each heading in the text and give a suitable English equivalent for them. Although you may not determine the precise meaning of those headings, you should be able to come close.

À propos de la lecture...
This reading is taken from a brochure published by the **Université Laval** in Quebec City. There are many schools and colleges that offer French immersion programs throughout France and the French-speaking world.

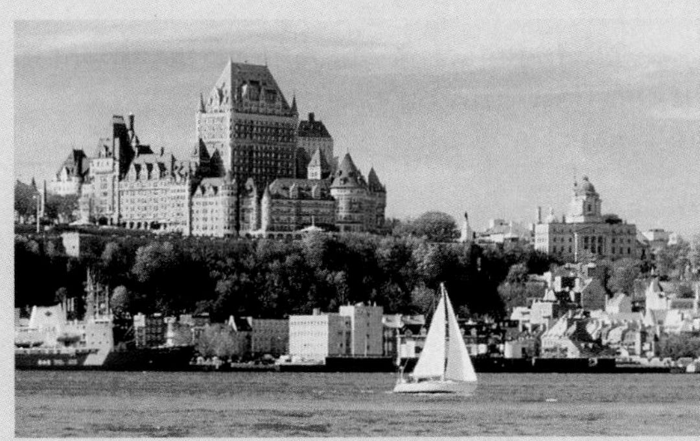

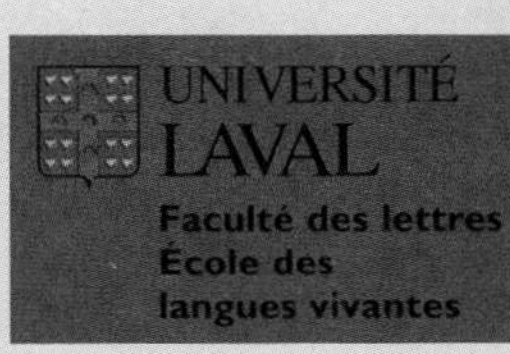

Étudier le français... à QUÉBEC, bien sûr!

Plaque tournante de la francophonie, Québec vous offre le meilleur de deux mondes, le charme européen au cœur de la modernité nord-américaine.

Un séjour linguistique à Québec vous assure une immersion totale dans une ville francophone aux dimensions humaines (632 000 habitants), où vous vous sentirez en toute sécurité.

et à l'Université LAVAL évidemment!

QUALITÉ DES COURS
- plus de soixante-quinze ans d'expérience
- formation solide des enseignants
- matériel pédagogique «sur mesure»

SOUTIEN PÉDAGOGIQUE
- conseillers pédagogiques
- enseignement complémentaire «individualisé» pour les étudiants qui éprouvent des difficultés (trimestres d'automne et d'hiver)
- laboratoires de langues et laboratoires informatiques
- enseignement assisté par ordinateur

ENCADREMENT
- équipe de moniteurs
- activités socio-culturelles et sportives
- excursions
- stages de travaux pratiques en milieu de travail (trimestres d'automne et d'hiver)
- activités de bénévolat en milieu francophone (trimestres d'automne et d'hiver)

Cours à tous les niveaux pendant toute l'année

Programme spécial de français pour non-francophones
Les étudiants peuvent s'inscrire à l'une ou l'autre des sessions suivantes:

ÉTÉ	mai-juin juillet-août	(5 sem. – 7 crédits) (5 sem. – 7 crédits)
AUTOMNE	septembre-décembre	(15 sem. – 16 crédits)
HIVER	janvier-avril	(15 sem. – 16 crédits)

Lors des trimestres d'automne et d'hiver les étudiants du niveau supérieur suivent leurs cours dans le cadre des programmes réguliers de français langue seconde (certificat, diplôme, baccalauréat).

PRIX ABORDABLE
- tous les étudiants de ces programmes de français paient les frais de scolarité des étudiants québécois
- coût de la vie peu élevé
- logement dans des familles francophones ou dans les résidences universitaires

Pour obtenir plus de renseignements sur
- les cours
- l'admission
- le logement
- le visa d'étudiant
- les assurances maladie
- les activités socio-culturelles
- etc.

demandez notre brochure en écrivant à:
École des langues vivantes
Pavillon Charles-De Koninck (2301)
Université Laval
Québec (Québec) G1V 0A6 Canada
Téléphone: (418) 656-2321
Télécopieur: (418) 656-7018
Courriel: elul@elul.ulaval.ca
http://www.elul.ulaval.ca/lecole

Compréhension

À l'Université Laval. Are the following statements true (**vrai**) or false (**faux**)? Underline the words in the brochure on the preceding page that support your answers, and correct any false statements to make them true.

1. V F The **Université Laval** has just begun to offer French courses for foreign students.
2. V F Individualized instruction is offered for those who need help.
3. V F Students may rent apartments in town.
4. V F The university offers both classroom and extracurricular activities.
5. V F Some courses are given in English.

Answers: 1. F (*soixante ans d'expérience*) 2. V (*enseignement individualisé*) 3. F (*logement dans des familles francophones ou dans les résidences universitaires*) 4. V (*les cours, les activités socioculturelles*) 5. F (*immersion totale*)

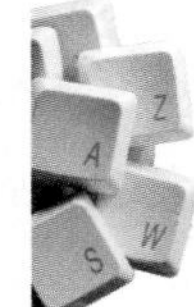

Écriture

The writing activities **Par écrit** and **Journal intime** can be found in the Workbook/Laboratory Manual to accompany *Vis-à-vis*.

Purpose: For each chapter in the Workbook/Laboratory Manual, there are two different kinds of writing activities that guide sts. through reusing the lexical and grammatical content of the chapter: *Par écrit* emphasizes process-writing and *Journal intime* allows for free-form expression of sts.' own experiences.

La vie en chantant. An activity based on the song "Jolie Louise" by Daniel Lanois can be found in the Instructor's Manual. The song can be purchased at the iTunes store, or sts. can watch the music video on YouTube.

Pour s'amuser

Un prof de philo présente un sujet de discussion: «Prouvez que cette chaise n'existe pas.»

Immédiatement, la classe cherche des idées. Les étudiants proposent des arguments, développent des raisonnements compliqués...

Seule Mélanie est silencieuse. Soudain, elle demande: «Quelle chaise?»

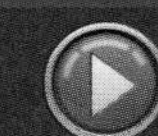

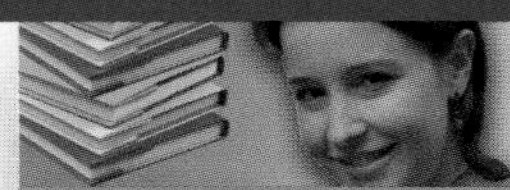

Le vidéoblog de Léa

Purpose: Because the characters speak at a normal pace and use authentic language, it is important to do the previewing activities with sts. before they watch the video.

En bref

In her videoblog, Léa describes her neighborhood, **le Quartier latin.** At Hassan's restaurant, the four friends each give their opinion of the neighborhood.

Vocabulaire en contexte

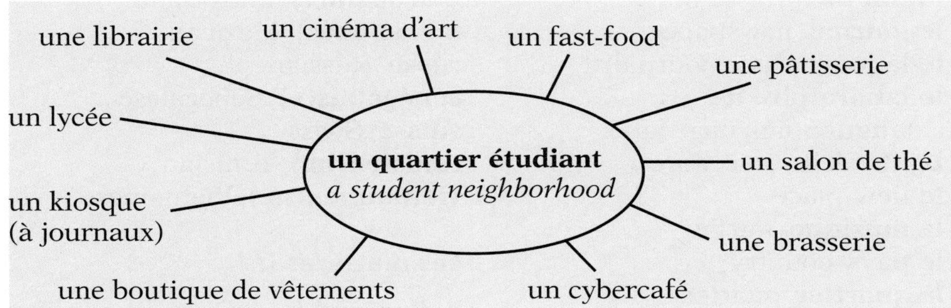

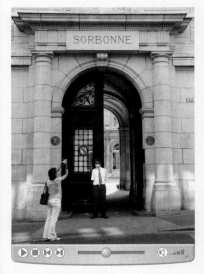

Ma fac: la Sorbonne à Paris

Suggestion: Model the pronunciation of the words. Ask sts. to provide the meanings of the cognates and circle those whose meaning remains uncertain. Return to the list after the video episode to see if sts. were able to infer the meaning based on images in the video.

Visionnez!

Indicate whether each statement is true (**vrai**) or false (**faux**).

1. ______ Léa habite le Quartier latin depuis longtemps (*for a long time*).
2. ______ Le Quartier latin est un quartier intellectuel et un centre culturel riche en loisirs (*leisure activities*).
3. ______ Les cafés du quartier sont trop (*too*) touristiques.
4. ______ Il y a de plus en plus de (*more and more*) fast-foods et de boutiques de vêtements.
5. ______ C'est Juliette qui préfère le Quartier latin.

Analysez!

Answer the following questions in English.

1. In what ways does the **Quartier latin** continue to evolve?
2. How does Juliette's perspective on this evolution differ from those of her friends? With whom do you identify?

Comparez!

Rewatch the cultural section of the video. Then use the vocabulary presented above, as well as other words you know, to compare your own campus neighborhood to that of the **Quartier latin.** Tell what sorts of places are similar and what your neighborhood lacks. Do you have something in your neighborhood that wasn't mentioned in the video?

MODÈLE: Dans mon quartier, il y a des fast-foods, comme (*as*) à Paris. Mais, il n'y a pas de (*there isn't any*) salon de thé.

Do you prefer your own neighborhood or the **Quartier latin**?

Note culturelle

The name *Quartier latin* has its roots in two historic facts. First, the name reminds us that Paris grew out of the ancient Roman town of *Lutèce*. At the same time, the name reflects the historic fact that this neighborhood has been a center of education since the Middle Ages. In those early years, professors and students spoke Latin, which was the official language of instruction until the French Revolution.

Suggestion: Sts. can do the *Comparez!* activity in French—in class or outside of class as a blog, videoblog, journal, or chat project—by following the model sentences provided. Note that *il n'y a pas de* is taught in *Chapitre 4.* Model several sentences so that sts. know how the phrase is pronounced.

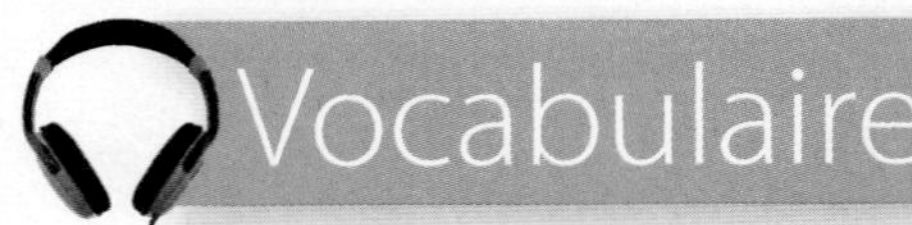

Vocabulaire

Verbes

adorer to love; to adore
aimer to like; to love
aimer mieux to prefer (like better)
chercher to look for
commencer to begin
danser to dance
demander to ask for
détester to detest
donner to give
écouter to listen to
être to be
étudier to study
fumer to smoke
habiter to live
manger to eat
parler to speak
regarder to look at; to watch
rêver to dream
skier to ski
travailler to work
trouver to find
visiter to visit (*a place*)

Substantifs

l'ami(e) (*m., f.*) friend
l'amphithéâtre (*m.*) lecture hall
la bibliothèque library
le bureau office; desk
le café café; cup of coffee
le cinéma movies; movie theater
la cité universitaire (la cité-U) residence halls
le cours course
le dictionnaire dictionary
l'école (*f.*) school
l'examen (*m.*) test, exam
la faculté division (*academic*)
la femme woman
le film film
le gymnase gymnasium
l'homme (*m.*) man
le journal newspaper
le/la journaliste journalist
le laboratoire de langues language lab
la librairie bookstore
le lieu place
la musique music
le pays country
le quartier quarter, neighborhood
la radio radio
le restaurant restaurant
le restaurant universitaire (le resto-U) university cafeteria
le sport sport; sports
le travail work
l'université (*f.*) university
la vie life
la ville city
la visite visit

À REVOIR: **le cahier, l'étudiant(e), le livre, le professeur, la salle de classe**

Les nationalités (*f.*)*

algérien(ne) Algerian
allemand(e) German
américain(e) American
anglais(e) English
belge Belgian
canadien(ne) Canadian
chinois(e) Chinese
espagnol(e) Spanish
français(e) French
italien(ne) Italian
japonais(e) Japanese
libanais(e) Lebanese
marocain(e) Moroccan
mexicain(e) Mexican
russe Russian
sénégalais(e) Senegalese
suisse Swiss
tunisien(ne) Tunisian
vietnamien(ne) Vietnamese

Les matières (*f.*)

l'allemand (*m.*) German
l'anglais (*m.*) English
la biologie biology
la chimie chemistry
le chinois Chinese
le commerce business
le droit law
l'économie (*f.*) economics
l'espagnol (*m.*) Spanish
le flamand Flemish
le génie engineering
la géographie geography
la géologie geology
l'histoire (*f.*) history
l'informatique (*f.*) computer science
l'italien (*m.*) Italian
le japonais Japanese
les langues (*f.*) **étrangères** foreign languages
la linguistique linguistics
la littérature literature
les mathématiques (les maths) (*f.*) mathematics
la philosophie philosophy

Purpose: *Vocabulaire* contains chapter words and expressions considered *active*. These are the words and expressions sts. are expected to know. Active vocabulary items have been introduced in the following chapter sections:

- *Leçon 1: Paroles*
- *Mots clés*
- Grammar paradigms, verb charts, and example sentences from the grammar sections
- Occasionally, from functional brief dialogues that begin grammar sections

The vocabulary list is divided into parts of speech (*Verbes, Substantifs,* etc.), *Mots et expressions divers,* and, occasionally, thematic categories (*Expressions avec* avoir, *Expressions interrogatives,* etc.). Words and expressions within each subgrouping are organized alphabetically.

*These nationalities are capitalized when used as a noun (*e.g.*, **une Algérienne, des Français,** etc.)

la physique physics
la psychologie psychology
les sciences (*f.*) **naturelles** natural sciences
la sociologie sociology

Mots et expressions divers

à at; in
après after
aussi also
avec with
d'accord okay; agreed
dans in
de of, from
de temps en temps from time to time
en in
en général generally
ici here
maintenant now
mais but
moi me
ou or
pour for, in order to
quelquefois sometimes
rarement rarely
souvent often
toujours always
voici here is/are
voilà there is/are

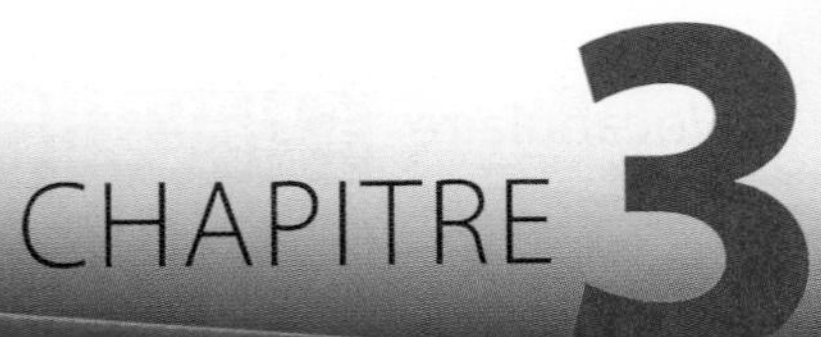

CHAPITRE 3

Elles ont l'air chic!°

Elles... *They look stylish!*

Presentation: Use the photo to review vocabulary from previous chapters by asking: *Il y a combien de femmes? À votre avis, les femmes sont-elles chic? élégantes? bizarres? Quelles sont les nationalités?*

Note: It is becoming more and more common in the press and in contemporary literature to see the invariable adjective *chic* with an *-s* in the plural. The Académie française, however, has not yet made this change official.

Les dossiers de Léa

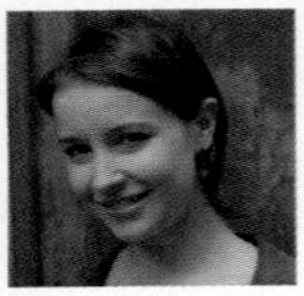

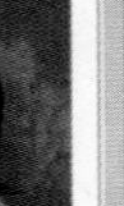

Léa

- Mes photos
  - 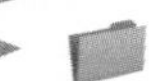 Le nouveau chic parisien
  - 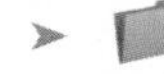 Mes bonnes adresses
  - Le marché aux puces

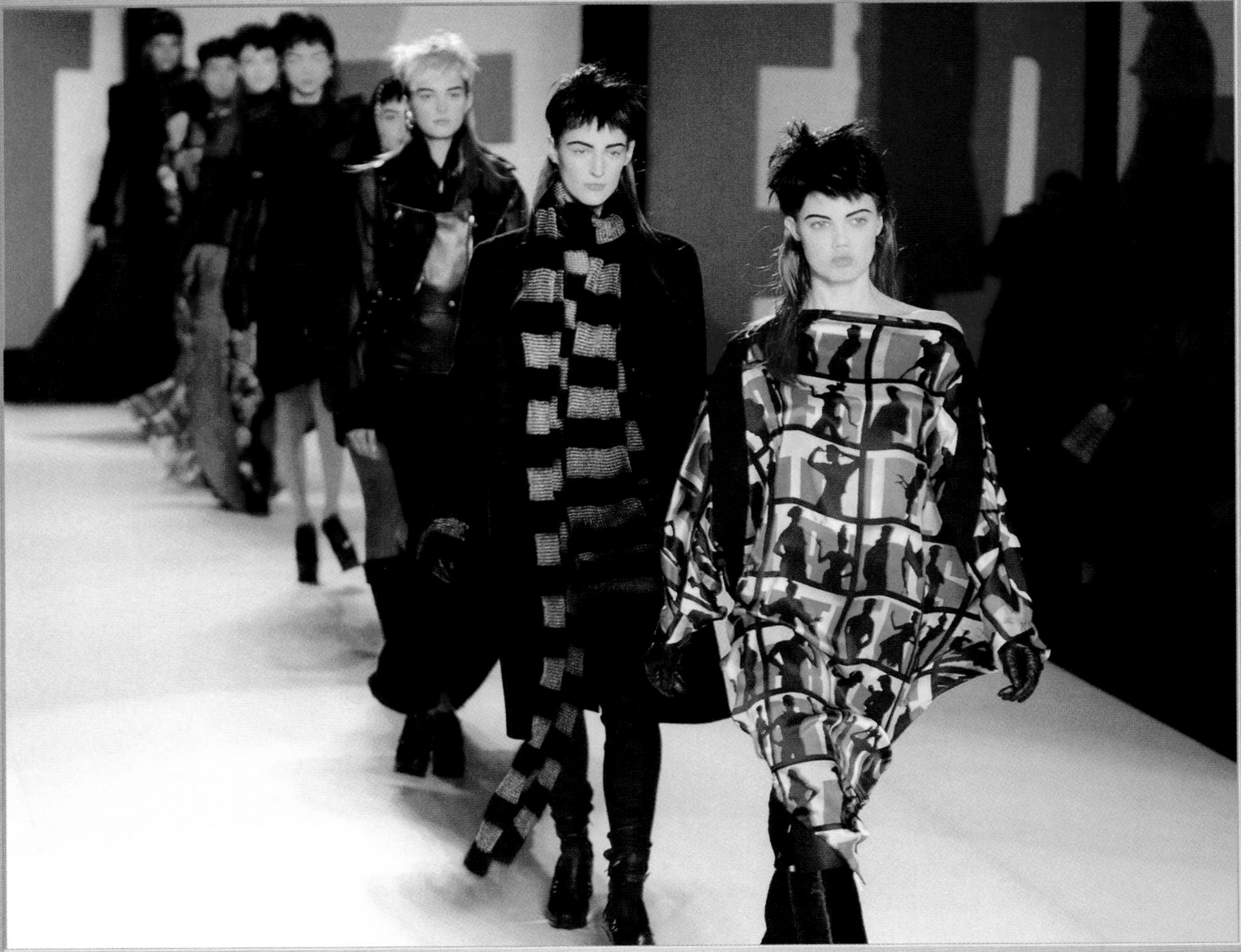

Le nouveau chic parisien

 **Cultural note:** In France, the term *haute couture* is protected by law. Most official *haute couture* houses are located in the 8th *arrondissement* of Paris, in the "Golden Triangle" formed by Avenue Montaigne, Avenue Marceau, and the Champs-Élysées.

Dans ce chapitre...

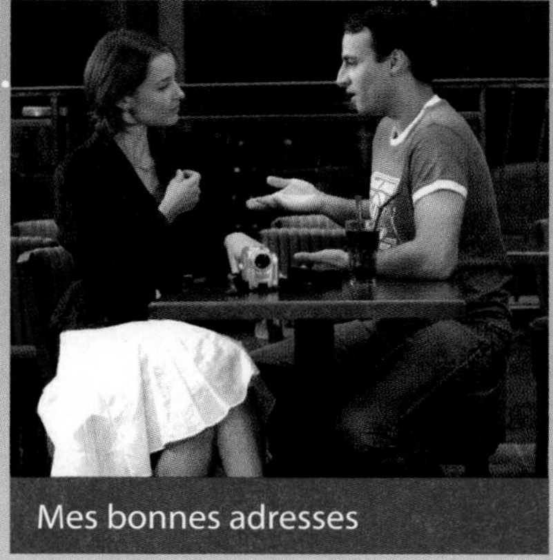
Mes bonnes adresses

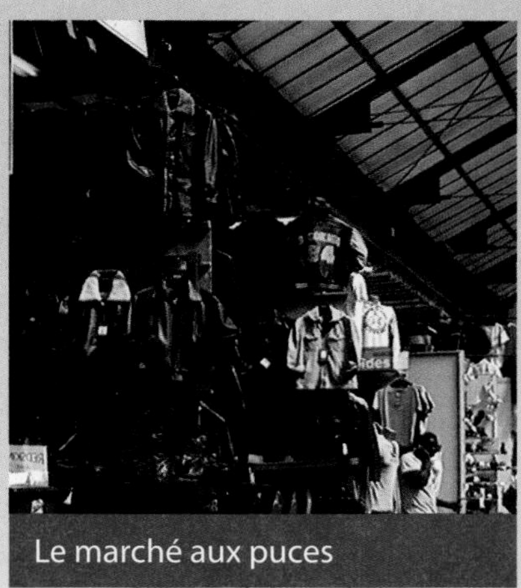
Le marché aux puces

OBJECTIFS COMMUNICATIFS

- describing people, places, and things
- talking about personalities, clothing, and colors
- expressing possession and sensations
- mentioning specific places or people
- getting information
- learning to distinguish between and pronounce selected sounds in French

PAROLES (Leçon 1)

- Les adjectifs de personnalité
- Les vêtements et les couleurs
- Les descriptions physiques et mentales

STRUCTURES (Leçons 2 et 3)

- Le verbe **avoir**
- Les adjectifs qualificatifs
- Les questions à réponse affirmative ou négative
- Les prepositions **à** et **de**

CULTURE

- Le blog de Léa: *En jupe ou en pantalon?*
- Reportage: *Dis-moi où tu t'habilles*
- Lecture: *Paris-Shopping: quelques recommandations* (Leçon 4)

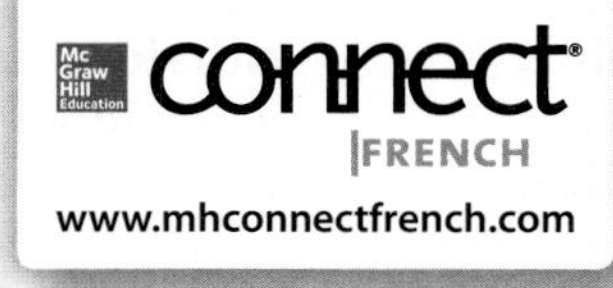

Leçon 1

Quatre personnalités différentes

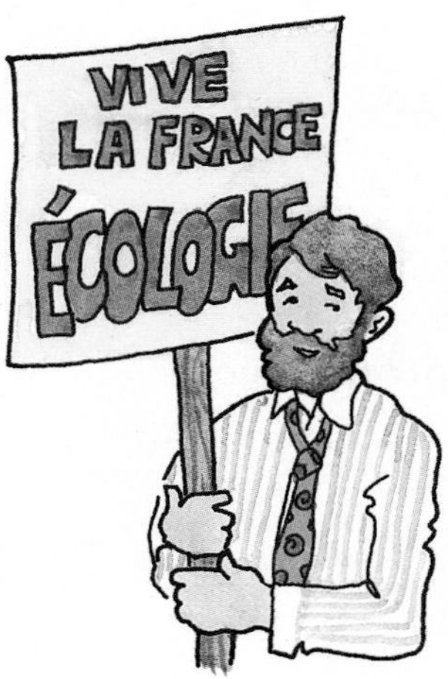

Hadrien est un jeune homme **enthousiaste, idéaliste** et **sincère.** Il est **sensible** (*sensitive*) mais **travailleur** (*hard-working*).

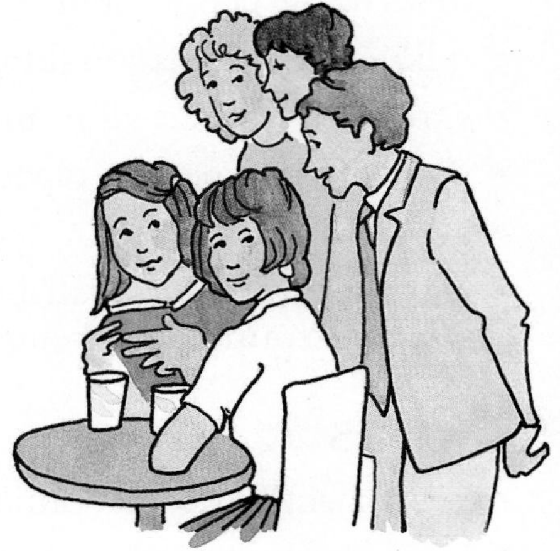

Béatrice est une jeune femme **sociable, sympathique** (*nice, likeable*) et **dynamique.** Elle n'est pas **égoïste** (*selfish*).

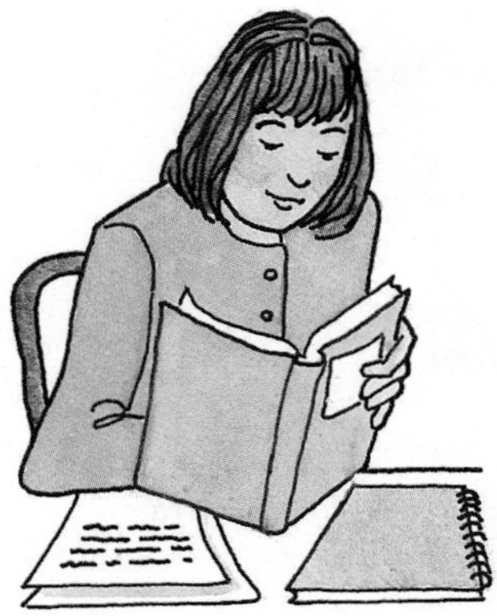

Nathalie est une jeune femme **calme, réaliste** et **raisonnable.** Elle est rarement **triste** (*sad*). Ses études sont assez **difficiles.**

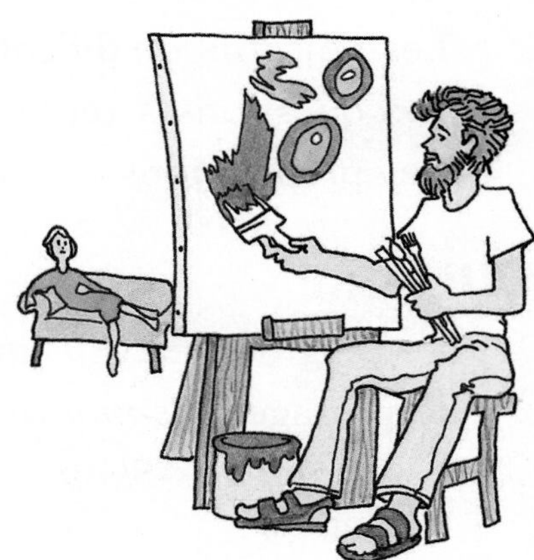

Olivier est un jeune homme **individualiste, excentrique** et **drôle** (*funny*). Il n'est pas **paresseux** (*lazy*).

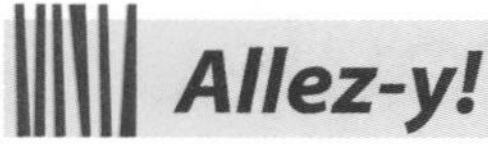

Allez-y!

A. Qualités. Tell about these people by paraphrasing each statement.

MODÈLE: Béatrice aime parler avec des amis. →
C'est une jeune femme sociable.

1. Hadrien parle avec sincérité.
2. Nathalie n'aime pas l'extravagance.
3. Olivier est amusant.
4. Béatrice aime l'action.
5. Hadrien parle avec enthousiasme.
6. Olivier n'est pas conformiste.
7. Nathalie regarde la vie avec réalisme.
8. Olivier aime l'excentricité.
9. Nathalie n'est pas nerveuse.

B. Question de personnalité. What are these different people like? Describe them using at least three adjectives.

Autres adjectifs possibles: antipathique, calme, conformiste, hypocrite, matérialiste, modeste, optimiste, pauvre (*poor*), pessimiste, riche, solitaire

MODÈLE: votre meilleur ami / meilleure amie (*f.*) (*your best friend*) →
Il/Elle est calme, sincère…

1. votre meilleur ami / meilleure amie
2. votre père (*father*)
3. votre mère (*mother*)
4. votre camarade de chambre (*roommate*)
5. votre professeur de français
6. le président américain
7. Lady Gaga
8. LeBron James
9. Bradley Cooper
10. Angelina Jolie

Et vous? Now describe yourself. Begin your sentence with **Je suis… , mais je ne suis pas…**

C. Interview. Ask a classmate the following questions. Use **très, assez, peu,** or **un peu** when appropriate.

MODÈLE: sociable ou solitaire →
É1: Es-tu sociable ou solitaire?
É2: Moi, je suis assez sociable. Et toi?

1. sincère ou hypocrite
2. excentrique ou conformiste
3. triste ou drôle
4. sympathique ou antipathique
5. calme ou dynamique
6. réaliste ou idéaliste
7. raisonnable ou inflexible
8. optimiste ou pessimiste

Now summarize by stating a few characteristics of your classmate, along with their opposites.

Suggestion (A): Do in small groups as an oral or written activity.

Follow-up (A): Personalize activity by changing each statement into a question, using rising intonation. Example: *Vous aimez parler avec des amis? Oui, je suis sociable.* Or name famous people or members of class. Sts. give adjectives they associate with each. Verify correct adjectives by repeating them in complete sentences (*Oui, Steve Carell est drôle.*), making adjectives agree where necessary. **Note:** Sts. will learn agreement of adjectives in *Leçon 2.*

Follow-up (A): Give brief (2–3 sentence) descriptions of famous people. Sts. guess who is being described. Recycle adjectives of nationality.

Mots clés

How to qualify your description

When you first learn a foreign language, you inevitably exaggerate a little because you do not yet have the tools to convey nuances. The following adverbs may be useful.

très	*very*
assez	*somewhat*
peu	*hardly*
un peu	*a little*

Jeanne est **très** calme mais Jacques est **un peu** nerveux.

Mon chien (*dog*) est **peu** intelligent mais il est **assez** drôle.

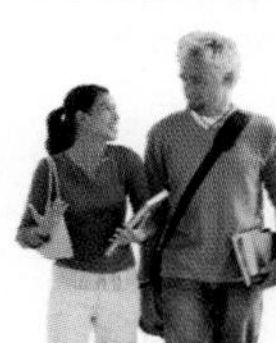

Suggestion (C): Can be done by sts. in pairs or small groups. Sts. describe themselves; partners then give a 3-sentence summary for rest of class.

Presentation: Bring in clothing or pictures of items of clothing.

Additional vocabulary: *une ceinture, des collants, un foulard, des gants, un gilet, un slip, un soutien gorge, un survêtement; à carreaux, à pois, rayé, uni.*

Suggestion: Present clothing with questions and answers involving vocabulary known to sts. Point to relevant items as answers are given. For example: *Qu'est-ce qu'il y a sur l'image? Il y a une chemise? Oui, voici une chemise.*

Presentation: Bring in colored construction paper to present the colors.

Note: The adjectives *orange* and *marron* (chestnut) are invariable.

Les vêtements et les couleurs

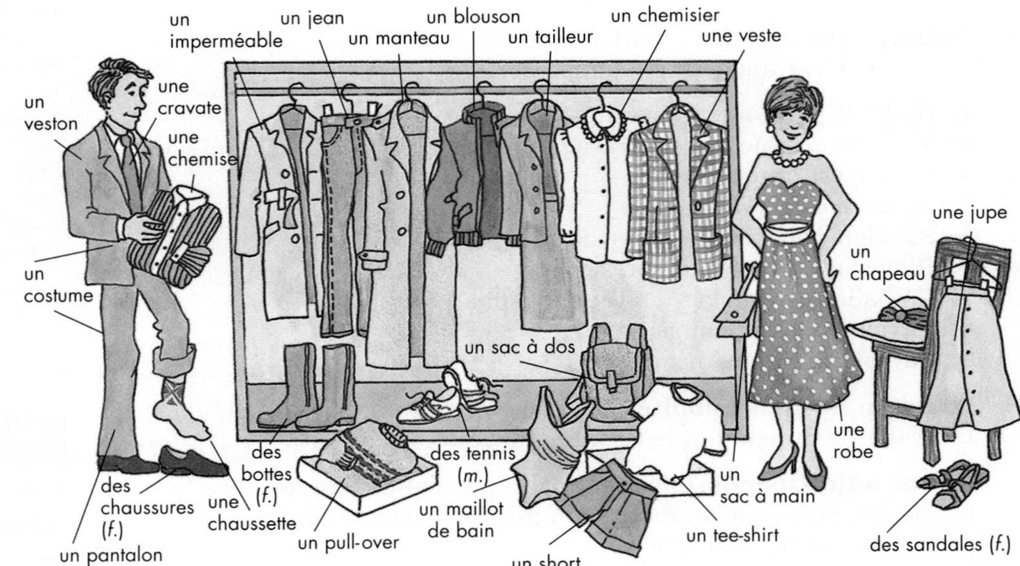

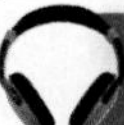

Prononcez bien!

The vowels in *bleu* and *couleur*

For the [ø] in **bleu,** close your mouth as you do for [e] in **et,** but round and purse your lips. Keep your tongue in the front of your mouth.

[ø]: **nerveuse, de, deux, peu**

For the [œ] in **couleur,** open your mouth a bit wider, as you do for [ɛ] in **est,** but round and purse your lips. Position your tongue in the middle of your mouth.

[œ]: **professeur, ordinateur, sœur**

Notice that both vowels are usually spelled **eu,** but [ø] also occurs as **e** in **de, le, me,** and [œ] also occurs as **œ** and **œu.**

Pronunciation practice: The *Prononcez bien!* section on page 83 of this chapter contains activities for practicing these sounds.

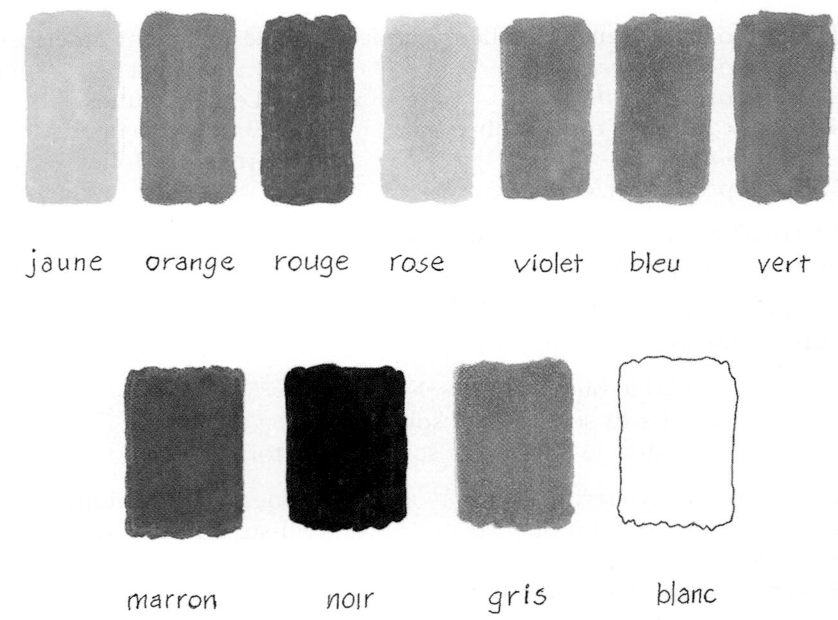

M. Beaujour **porte** (*is wearing*) **un costume gris** et **une cravate orange.**

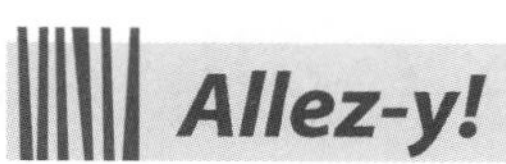

Allez-y!

Additional activity: Sts. describe the clothing of people depicted in photos, magazine ads, slides, etc., taken from Francophone culture, if possible. Ex. can be done orally or in writing. If written, collect descriptions and read in class as you hold up the image described plus two distractors; sts. guess who is described.

A. Qu'est-ce qu'ils portent? Describe what these people are wearing.

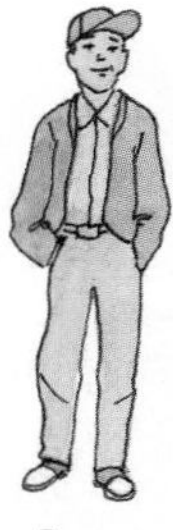
Bruno

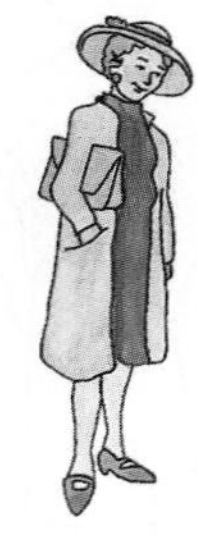
Mme Dupuy

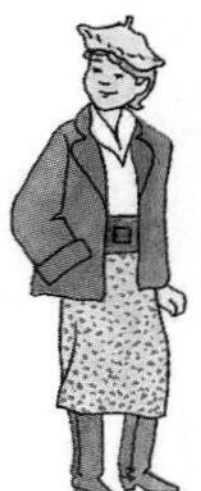
Aurélie

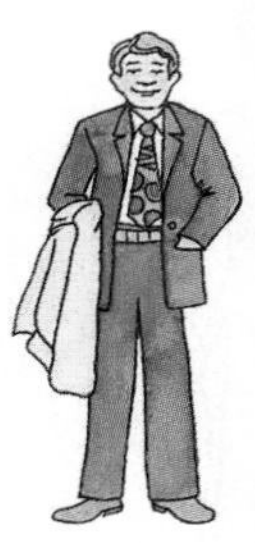
M. Martin

1. Bruno porte une casquette, ______.
2. Mme Dupuy porte ______.
3. Aurélie porte un béret, ______.
4. M. Martin porte ______.

B. Un vêtement pour chaque (*each*) occasion. Describe in as much detail as possible what you wear when you go to these places.

1. à un match de football américain
2. à un concert de rock
3. à une soirée
4. à une interview
5. à l'université
6. à la plage (*beach*)

C. De quelle couleur? Ask a classmate to state the colors of the following things.

MODÈLE: le drapeau (*flag*) américain →
É1: De quelle couleur est le drapeau américain?
É2: Le drapeau américain est rouge, blanc et bleu.

1. le drapeau français
2. le ciel (*sky*)
3. un éléphant
4. le charbon (*coal*)
5. le lait (*milk*)
6. un tigre
7. un zèbre
8. le jade

Le parler jeune

canon	magnifique
classe	chic
déchirer	être original, surprenant, très à la mode
des fringues (*f.*)	des vêtements
un fut	un pantalon
des pompes (*f.*)	des chaussures

Cette fille, elle est **canon**!

Laurent est super **classe** avec son veston noir.

Ton jean rouge, il **déchire.**

Acheter des **fringues,** c'est ma passion.

Est-ce que mon **fut** est trop court?

Je me suis acheté de nouvelles **pompes** pour le mariage de ma sœur.

Follow-up (B): Et ces personnes, qu'est-ce qu'elles portent? *Les rappeurs? Les jeunes* (young people) *chic? Les chanteurs* (singers) *country-western? Les espions* (spies)*? Les goths?*

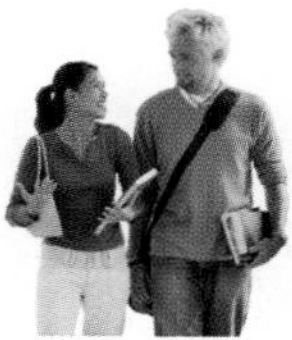

Follow-up (C): Ask sts. to bring in magazine pictures and in small groups describe what people are wearing and the colors of their clothes.

Les amis d'Anne et de Céline

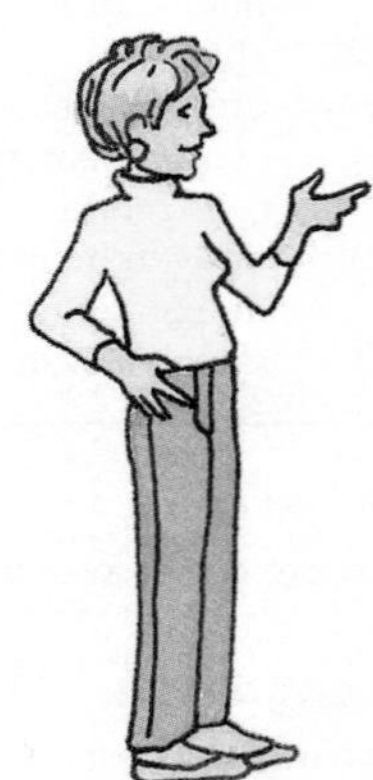

Lise est grande, belle et dynamique. Elle a (*has*) les yeux verts et les cheveux blonds. (Elle est blonde.)

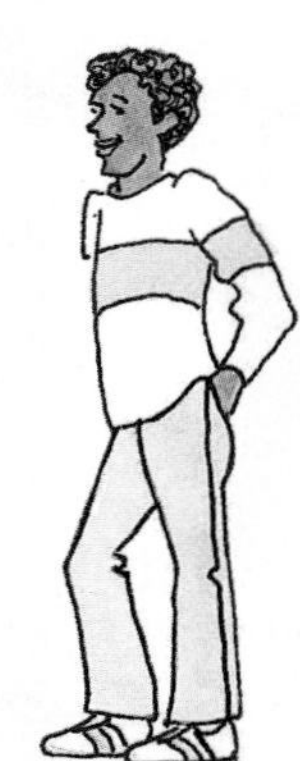

Léo a les cheveux noirs. Il est beau et charmant. Il est de taille moyenne (*medium height*).

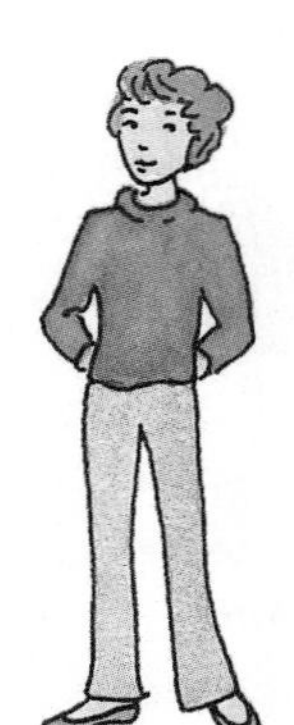

Laure est aussi de taille moyenne. Elle a les yeux marron et les cheveux courts et roux. (Elle est rousse [*redheaded*].)

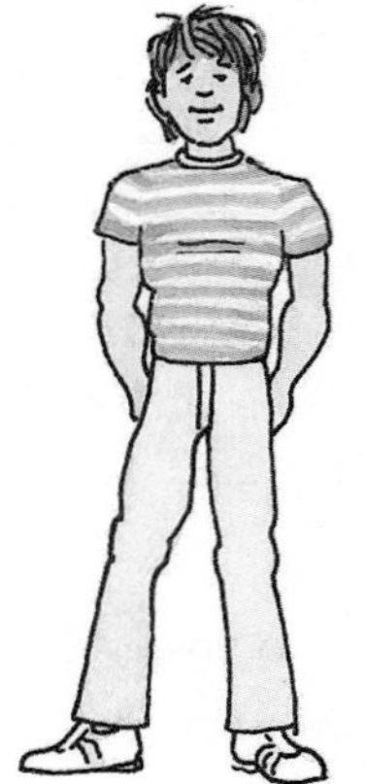

Jacques est très sportif. Il est grand, il a les cheveux longs et châtains* (*light brown*).

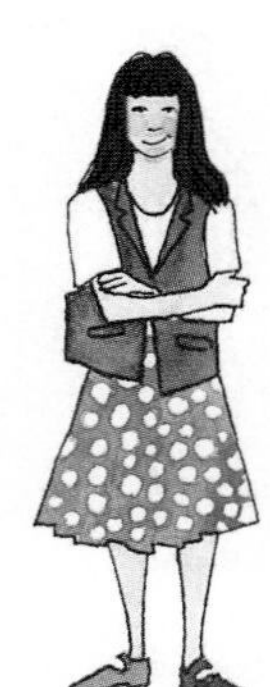

Thu est très petite et intelligente. Elle a les cheveux noirs et raides (*straight*).

Follow-up (Presentation): Display four drawings or pictures of people, giving each a name. Read a brief description using vocabulary words and have sts. indicate whom you are describing.

Continuation (A): Have sts. make up similar short descriptions of people in any visuals you have used in vocabulary presentation.

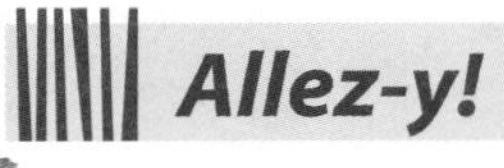

Allez-y!

A. Erreur! Correct any statements that are wrong.

MODÈLE: Léo a les cheveux châtains. → Non, il a les cheveux noirs.

1. Jacques a les cheveux courts. **2.** Laure a les cheveux longs et châtains. **3.** Thu a les cheveux noirs. **4.** Laure a les yeux noirs. **5.** Lise a les cheveux roux. **6.** Léo est très grand. **7.** Lise est de taille moyenne. **8.** Thu est petite. **9.** Léo et Lise sont petits. **10.** Laure est blonde et Lise est rousse.

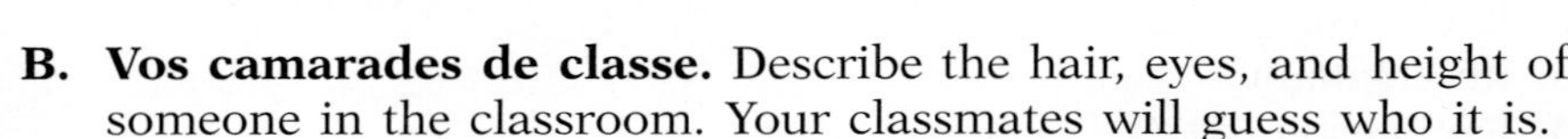

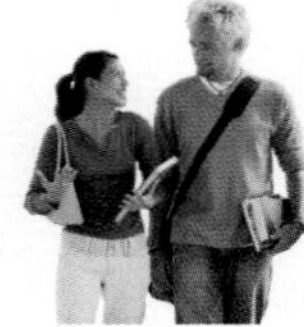

B. Vos camarades de classe. Describe the hair, eyes, and height of someone in the classroom. Your classmates will guess who it is.

MODÈLE: Il/Elle a les cheveux longs et noirs, il/elle a les yeux marron et il/elle est de taille moyenne.

C. Personnalités célèbres. What color hair do the following people have?

MODÈLE: Steve Martin → Steve Martin? Il a les cheveux blancs.

1. Reese Witherspoon
2. Michelle Obama
3. Ron Weasley, l'ami de Harry Potter
4. Brad Pitt

Follow-up (C): Bring in pictures of celebrities or cards with names written on them. Sts. work in groups of two to three to write a brief description. Sts. read description and their classmates guess who is being described.

Follow-up (C): Collect sts.' descriptions and read several, having sts. guess whom you are describing.

*literally, *chestnut;* invariable in gender

Leçon 2

Le verbe *avoir*

Expressing Possession and Sensations

Deux cents amis!

Mamadou contacte Léa sur sa page Facebook (Messagerie instantanée).

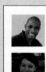

MAMADOU: **Tu as** beaucoup d'amis, Léa!

LÉA: Oui, beacoup. **J'ai de la chance!** Et toi?

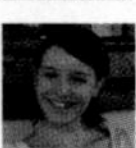
MAMADOU: **J'ai** des amis journalistes. Mais **j'ai envie de** rencontrer d'autres personnes. Toi, par exemple! **Tu as l'air** intéressante. **Ton amie Juliette** aussi **a l'air** sympa.

LÉA: **Tu as** déjà deux cents amis sur ta page Facebook! **Tu n'as pas besoin** de nous!

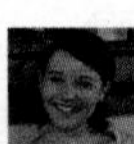
MAMADOU: Oui, mais **j'ai** peu d'amies françaises.

LÉA: Ce soir, **nous avons rendez-vous** au cinéma, Juliette et moi. **Tu as envie** de nous rejoindre?

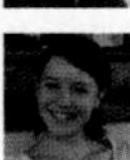
MAMADOU: Oh! **Je n'ai pas de chance*!** Ce soir, c'est impossible parce que **j'ai** du travail.

*Je... *I'm not lucky!*

Suggestion: Have sts. correct the false statements.

Vrai ou faux?

1. Léa a beaucoup d'amis.
2. Mamadou a des amis étudiants.
3. Mamadou a deux cents amis sur sa page Facebook.
4. Mamadou a beaucoup d'amies françaises.
5. Léa a rendez-vous avec Juliette.
6. Mamadou n'a pas de chance.

Forms of *avoir*

The verb **avoir** is irregular in form.

PRESENT TENSE OF **avoir** (*to have*)			
j'	**ai**	nous	**avons**
tu	**as**	vous	**avez**
il/elle/on	**a**	ils/elles	**ont**

Presentation: Model pronunciation. Note the **[z]** sound in *nous avons, vous avez, ils ont,* and *elles ont.* Point out the oral distinction between *ils ont / elles ont* and *ils sont / elles sont.*

Follow-up: For listening comprehension practice, have sts. indicate whether they hear the verb *être* or *avoir* in the following sentences: 1. *Elle est contente.* 2. *Nous avons raison.* 3. *Ils sont américains.* 4. *Ils ont de la chance.* 5. *Elle a l'air contente.* 6. *Tu es française, n'est-ce pas?* 7. *J'ai de la chance aussi.*

Presentation: Bring in other pictures to demonstrate expressions. Interject personalized questions to individual sts. using expressions featured.

—**J'ai** un studio agréable.	*I have a nice studio apartment.*
—**Avez**-vous une camarade de chambre sympathique?	*Do you have a nice roommate?*
—Oui, elle **a** beaucoup de patience.	*Yes, she has lots of patience.*

To ask someone his/her age, use **Quel âge *avez*-vous?** or **Quel âge *as*-tu?**

[Allez-y! A, E]

Expressions with *avoir*

The verb **avoir** is used in many common idioms.

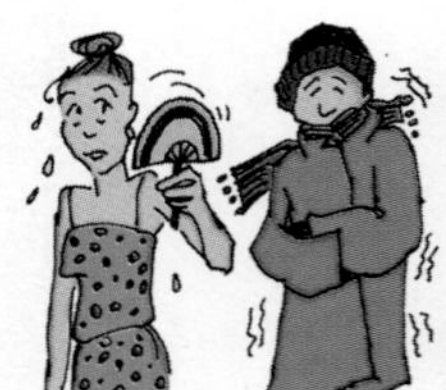

Elle **a chaud.** Il **a froid.**

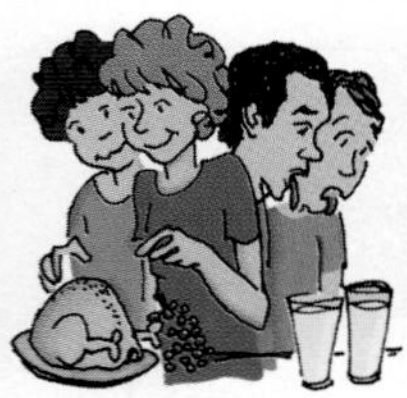

Elles **ont faim.** Ils **ont soif.**

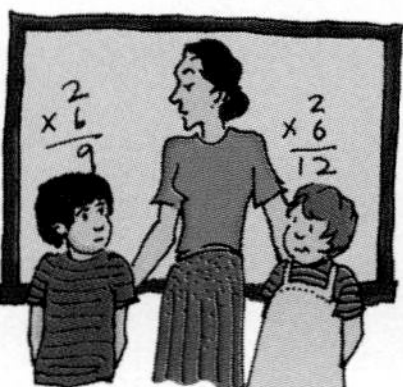

Loïc, tu **as tort.** Magalie, tu **as raison.**

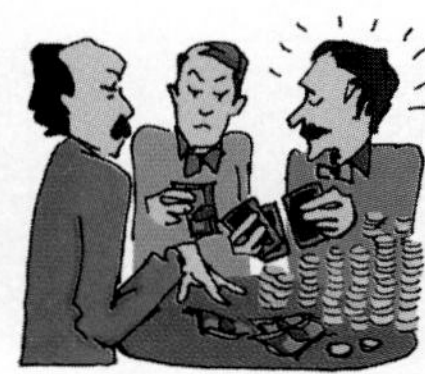

Frédéric **a l'air** content. Il **a de la chance.**

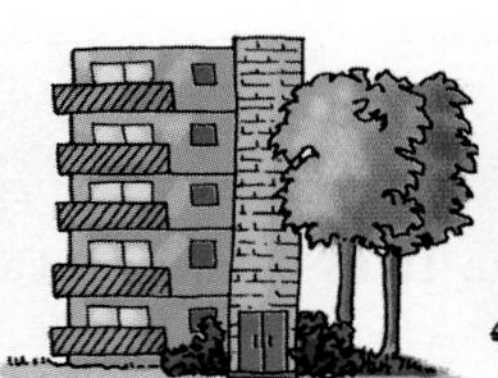

L'immeuble **a l'air** moderne.

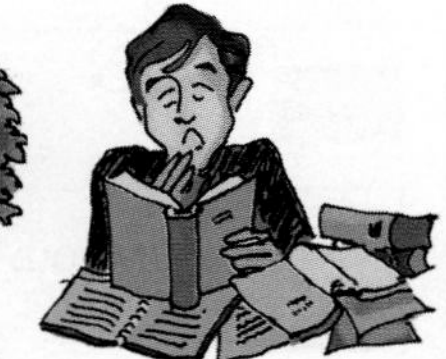

Théo **a sommeil.**

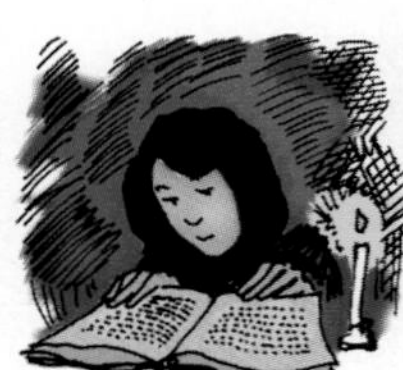

Ingrid **a besoin d'**une lampe.

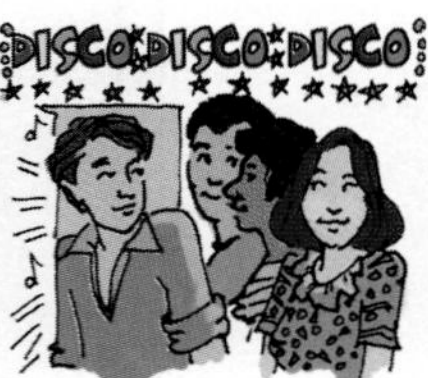

Avez-vous envie de danser?

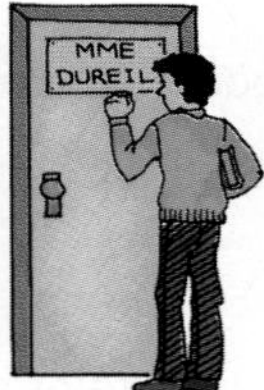

Il **a rendez-vous** avec le professeur.

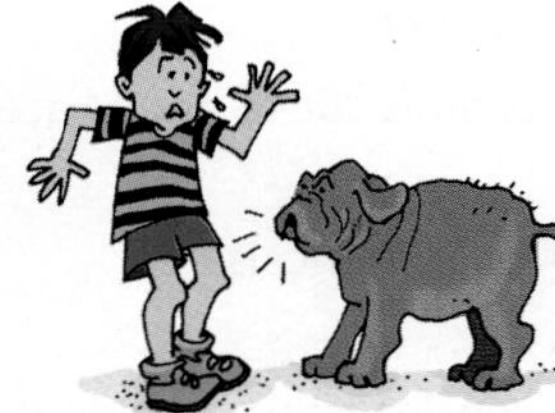

Il **a peur du** chien.

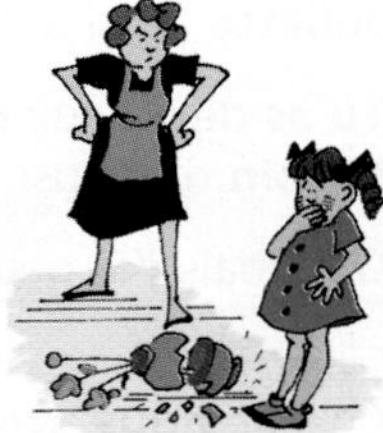

La petite fille **a honte.**

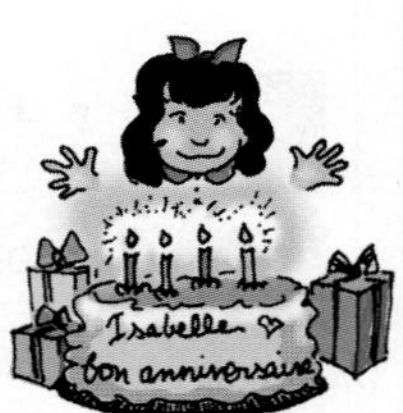

Isabelle **a quatre ans.**

Additional vocabulary: *avoir hâte de* + inf. (*to be looking forward to*)

Note that with **avoir besoin de, avoir envie de,** and **avoir peur de,** the preposition **de** is used before an infinitive or a noun.

[Allez-y! B-C-D]

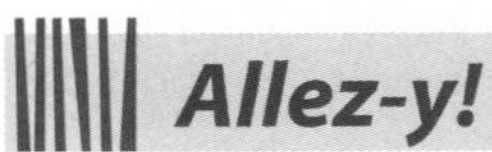

Allez-y!

Additional activity: Ask sts. who in the class has *un iPod / une guitare / une clarinette / un violon / un piano / une flûte*, etc.

A. Vive la musique! You and your friends are planning a musical evening. Say what each person has to contribute to the occasion.

MODÈLE: Isaac / une trompette ⟶ Isaac a une trompette.

1. Yasmine et Marc / un iPod®*
2. vous / une guitare
3. tu / une clarinette
4. je / un violon
5. nous / un piano
6. Isabelle / une flûte

---

*iPod is a registered trademark of Apple Inc.

B. Quel âge ont-ils? Working with a partner, ask and answer questions about the age of the following people. Make educated guesses!

MODÈLE: É1: Quel âge a-t-il?
É2: Il a deux ou trois ans.

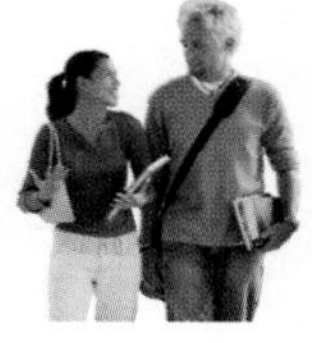

Suggestion: Mention the forms *Ils ont quel âge?* and *Quel âge ils ont?* often used in informal language.

1. 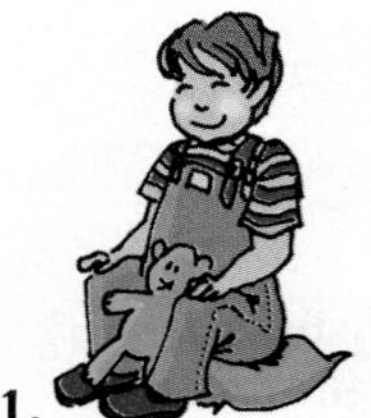
2. 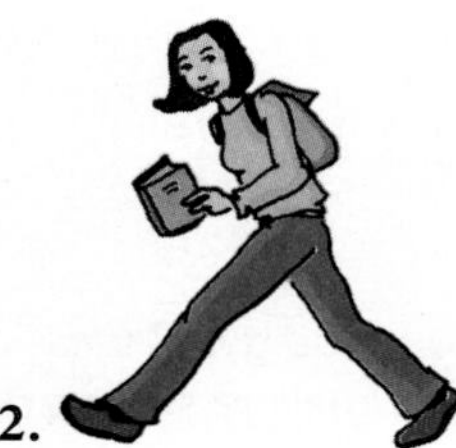
3. 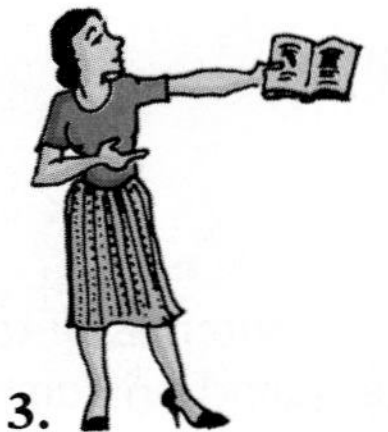
4. 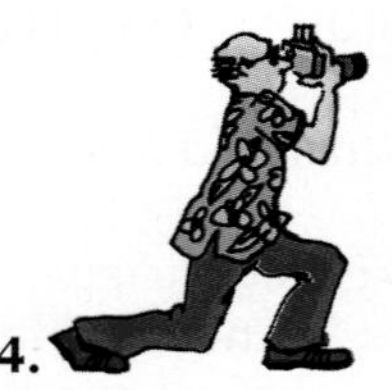

Follow-up: 1. Have sts. estimate ages of others in class. 2. Bring in pictures of people or give names of famous people and have sts. estimate their ages. 3. Teach *environ: Il a environ 40 ans.*

C. Dans quel contexte? For each situation, use an expression with **avoir.**

MODÈLE: Pour moi, un coca-cola, s'il vous plaît. → J'ai soif.

1. Je porte un pull et un manteau.
2. Il est minuit (*midnight*).
3. J'ouvre (*open*) la fenêtre.
4. Je mange une quiche.
5. Paris est la capitale de la France.
6. Des amis français m'invitent (*invite me*) à Paris.

Continuation (C): Provide sts. with more cues to extend the ex. 7. *Je gagne à la roulette.* 8. *Attention, un lion!* 9. *Je casse* (break) *le vase préféré de ma mère.* 10. *Je vais en boîte* (nightclub). 11. *Rome est en Belgique.* 12. *Et une limonade, s'il vous plaît.*

Suggestion: Can be done orally in small groups or in writing. Ask sts. to report some of their answers to the class.

D. Désirs et devoirs (*duties*). What do you and the people you know *want* to do? What do you *have* to do? Use **avoir envie / besoin de** to tell about these people. **Verbes utiles:** danser, écouter, étudier, parler, rêver, skier, travailler, voyager

MODÈLE: je →
J'ai envie de jouer au tennis, mais j'ai besoin d'étudier!

1. je
2. mon meilleur ami / ma meilleure amie
3. mes parents
4. le professeur de français
5. mon/ma camarade de chambre

E. Conversation. Ask a classmate the following questions.

1. Tu as peur de quoi (*what*)?
2. Tu as quoi dans ta chambre?
3. Tu as besoin de quoi pour préparer ton cours de français?
4. Tu as envie de quoi quand tu as faim? quand tu as soif?
5. Tu as envie de quoi maintenant?

Résumez! Now tell the other students the most surprising or unusual fact you learned about your classmate.

MODÈLE: Éric a trois dictionnaires dans sa chambre!

Prononcez bien!

The pronunciation of final consonants

In French, consonant letters ending words are generally not pronounced.*

restauran~~t~~, il~~s~~ dans~~ent~~, cour~~s~~, asse~~z~~, beaucou~~p~~, alleman~~d~~

Final **-c, -r, -f,** and **-l,** however, are pronounced.

avec, bonjour, neuf, mal

Exceptions to this rule include the **c** in blan~~c~~ as well as the **r** in the infinitive of **-er** verbs and in words ending in **-er** and **-ier.**

alle~~r~~, adore~~r~~, quartie~~r~~, cahie~~r~~

*unless they precede a word starting with a vowel (See **Prononcez bien!** on liaison, p. 261)

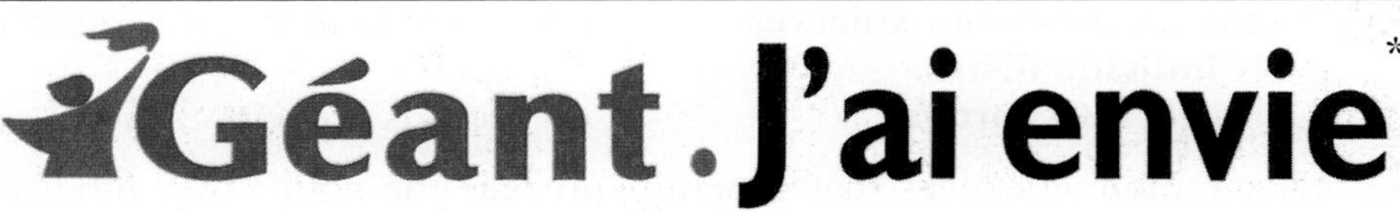

Pronunciation presentation: For more on liaison, please refer to *Leçon 4* in *Chapitre 2* of the Workbook/Laboratory Manual.

Pronunciation practice (1): Write the following expressions on the board and have sts. decide whether the final consonant is pronounced: *ça peut aller, avec l'étudiant, s'il vous plaît, très bien, d'accord, dans l'ordinateur, pour toujours, deux pays, un professeur de chinois, quel jour sommes-nous?*

Pronunciation practice (2): The *Prononcez bien!* section on page 83 of this chapter contains additional activities for practicing these sounds.

*slogan for a French supermarket

Suggestion: Teach how to use two or more adjectives joined by *et*.

Les adjectifs qualificatifs

Describing People, Places, and Things

Des professeurs excellents!

Léa téléphone à Juliette.

LÉA: Salut Juliette! Tu es contente de ton cours de gym? C'est **difficile?**
JULIETTE: Ce n'est pas **facile** quand on commence, mais je suis **persévérante** et la prof est **excellente!**
LÉA: Elle est **patiente?** C'est **important.** La patience, c'est une qualité **essentielle.**
JULIETTE: Elle est toujours **calme.** Elle observe nos mouvements et elle donne des explications très **précises.** Je suis vraiment **contente!** Et toi, ton cours de tennis?
LÉA: On a un **nouveau** prof.
JULIETTE: Il est comment?
LÉA: Il est **grand, beau, charmant...**
JULIETTE: Et **sportif!**

Suggestion: Have two sts. read the dialogue aloud. As they read, write the adjectives on the board in the correct category: *la prof de gym, le prof de tennis, Juliette, les explications.* Ask them what they notice about the forms.

Répondez aux questions.

1. Qui est excellente, patiente et calme?
2. Qui est grand, beau et charmant?
3. Qui est persévérante?
4. La gym, c'est difficile ou c'est facile?
5. Qui donne des explications très précises: le professeur de gym ou le professeur de tennis?

Presentation: Throughout grammar explanation, give or solicit personalized examples. Note that beginning sts. often cannot hear the difference between masculine and feminine forms; they need to learn to recognize the different sounds before they can produce them.

Position of Descriptive Adjectives

Descriptive adjectives (**les adjectifs qualificatifs**) give information about people, places, and things. In French, they usually follow the nouns they modify. They may also follow the verb **être.**

C'est un professeur **intéressant.**	*He's/She's an interesting teacher (professor).*
Le professeur pose des questions **faciles.**	*The teacher (professor) asks easy questions.*
J'aime les personnes **sincères** et **individualistes.**	*I like sincere and individualistic people.*
Gabrielle est **sportive.**	*Gabrielle is athletic.*

A few common adjectives that generally precede the nouns they modify are presented in **Chapitre 4, Leçon 3.**

Agreement of Adjectives

In French, adjectives agree in gender (masculine or feminine) and number (singular or plural) with the nouns they modify. Most adjectives follow the pattern illustrated in the following table.

	MASCULINE	FEMININE
Singular	un étudiant intelligent	une étudiante intelligent**e**
Plural	des étudiants intelligent**s**	des étudiantes intelligent**es**

1. Most feminine adjectives are formed by adding an **e** to the masculine form. Exception: adjectives whose masculine form ends in an unaccented **-e.**

    Hugo est **persévérant.** ⟶ Sylvie est **persévérante.**
    Paul est **triste.** ⟶ Claire est **triste.**

    Remember that final **d, s,** and **t,** usually silent in French, are pronounced when **e** is added.

2. **C'est** can be used to describe a general truth or to refer back to something that has already been mentioned. The adjective that follows **c'est** is always in the masculine singular form.

    Le français? C'est **facile!**
    L'amour (*love*), c'est **essentiel.**

3. Most plural adjectives of either gender are formed by adding an **s** to the singular form. Exception: adjectives whose singular form ends in **-s** or **-x.**

    Elle est **charmante.** ⟶ Elles sont **charmantes.**
    L'étudiant est **sénégalais.** ⟶ Les étudiants sont **sénégalais.**
    Marc est **courageux.** ⟶ Marc et Loïc sont **courageux.**

4. If a plural subject refers to one or more masculine items or people, the plural adjective is masculine.

    Sylvie et Inès sont **françaises.**
    Sylvie et Adam sont **français.**

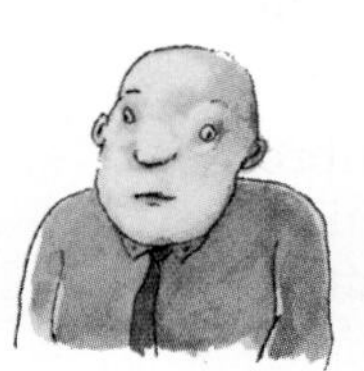
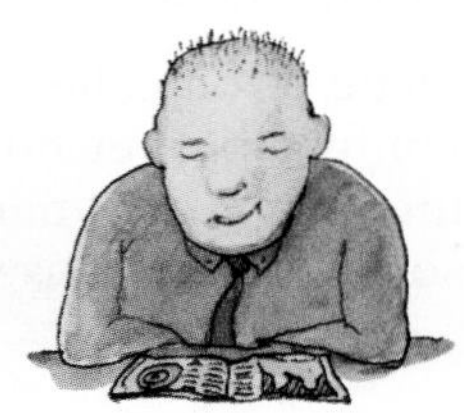
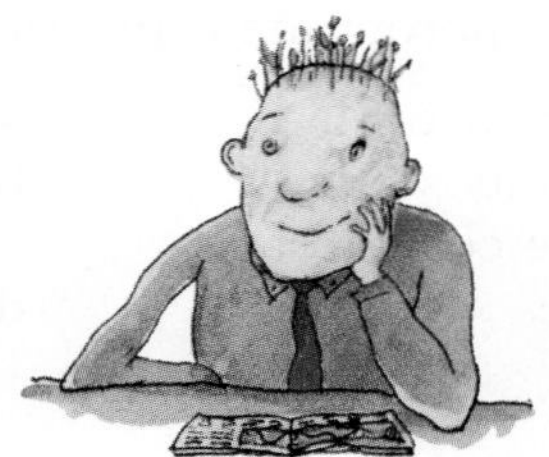
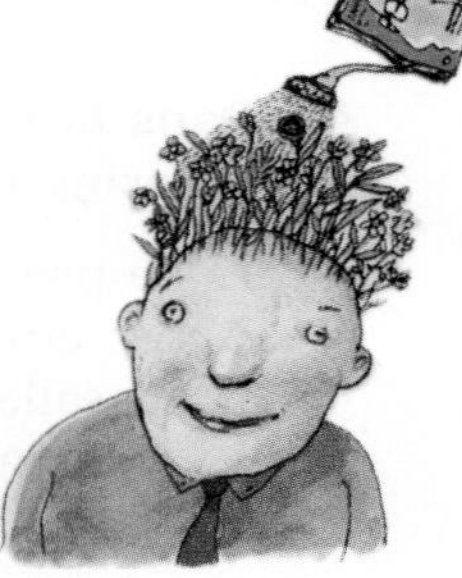

Les magazines.
Accrochants.[1]
Captivants.
Enrichissants.

[1]Catchy.

Suggestion: After presenting the concept of gender agreement, try this listening comprehension ex. (which practices only feminine forms with *-e*). *Masculin ou féminin?* 1. *intelligent* 2. *intelligente* 3. *charmante* 4. *français* 5. *amusant* 6. *amusante* 7. *charmant* 8. *patiente* 9. *américain* 10. *américaine*

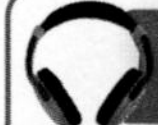

Prononcez bien!

The nasal vowels in *blond, grand,* and *bain*

To pronounce these sounds, let the air coming from your lungs go through both your mouth and nose. Close your mouth and round your lips to say [ɔ̃] as in **blond;** pronounce [ɑ̃] with an open mouth and lips more relaxed in **grand;** for [ɛ̃] in **bain,** your mouth is more open than for [ɔ̃] in **blond,** but less than for [ɑ̃] in **grand,** and your lips are stretched in a smile.

[ɔ̃]: **bonjour, combien**
[ɑ̃]: **comment, quarante, septembre**
[ɛ̃]: **bientôt, vingt, américain, faim**

Pronunciation presentation: For more on nasal vowels, please refer to *Leçon 4* in *Chapitre 3* of the Workbook/Laboratory Manual.

Pronunciation practice (1): Draw or bring in pictures illustrating the following words and ask sts. to name them: *cinq, grand, onze, trente, marron, honte, blond, quarante, blouson, manteau, veston, faim, châtain, crayon, orange, blanc, main, cinquante, imperméable, vingt, restaurant, pantalon, manger, écran, sandales, étudiant, quinze, télévision.*

Pronunciation practice (2): The *Prononcez bien!* section on page 83 of this chapter contains additional activities for practicing these sounds.

Suggestion: Have sts. use the realia for the following activity: *Imaginez une publicité accrochante pour inciter les Américains à acheter* (buy) *des magazines. Utilisez trois ou quatre adjectifs. Est-ce que ce sont les mêmes* (same) *adjectifs que dans la publicité canadienne?*

Descriptive Adjectives with Irregular Forms

PATTERN			SINGULAR		PLURAL	
MASC.		FEM.	MASC.	FEM.	MASC.	FEM.
-eux	} →	**-euse**	heureux (*happy*)	heureuse	heureux	heureuses
-eur			travailleur	travailleuse	travailleurs	travailleuses
-er	→	**-ère**	cher (*expensive*)	chère	chers	chères
-if	→	**-ive**	sportif	sportive	sportifs	sportives
-il	→	**-ille**	gentil (*nice, pleasant*)	gentille	gentils	gentilles
-el		**-elle**	intellectuel	intellectuelle	intellectuels	intellectuelles
-ien	→	**-ienne**	parisien	parisienne	parisiens	parisiennes

Follow-up: For listening comprehension practice, ask sts. to number from 1 to 7 on paper, then indicate whether you are talking about *Michel ou Michèle.* (Write names on board and explain that one is male, the other female.) 1. *Michel est gentil.* 2. *Michel est charmant.* 3. *Michèle est travailleuse.* 4. *Michèle est canadienne.* 5. *Michel est sportif.* 6. *Michel est français.* 7. *Michèle est courageuse.*

Notes: (1) Adjectives ending in *-al* are not treated. You may wish to teach the forms of *idéal, principal, légal,* and *loyal.* Point out the following forms: *idéal, idéaux, idéale, idéales.* Mention the common exception: *finals.* (2) Point out the [j] sound at the end of the feminine form *gentille.*

Additional vocabulary: *ambitieux/euse, impatient(e), généreux/euse, indépendant(e), indiscret/indiscrète.*

Note: For additional exs. on adjectives of color, see Workbook/Laboratory Manual.

Suggestion: Emphasize that the adjective *confortable* is used only with an object (a piece of clothing, furniture, etc.). To express *I am comfortable,* you would use *je suis à l'aise.*

Other adjectives that follow these patterns include **courageux / courageuse, paresseux / paresseuse, sérieux / sérieuse, fier / fière** (*proud*), **naïf / naïve** (*naive*), and **canadien / canadienne.** The feminine forms of **beau** (*handsome, beautiful*) and **nouveau** (*new*) are **belle** and **nouvelle.** The adjective **chic** (*stylish*) is invariable in gender and number.

Adjectives of Color

1. Most adjectives of color have both masculine and feminine forms.

   un chemisier **blanc / bleu / gris / noir / vert / violet**
   une chemise **blanche / bleue / grise / noire / verte / violette**

2. **Jaune, rouge,** and **rose** are invariable in gender.

   un pantalon **jaune** / une robe **jaune**

3. **Marron** and **orange** are invariable in gender and number.

   une robe **marron / orange**   des robes **marron / orange**

Suggestion: Review colors and practice their feminine and plural forms by asking sts. to tell the colors of certain items. MODÈLE: *De quelle couleur est une souris* (mouse)?—*Elle est grise.* 1. *une banane* 2. *une orange* 3. *une rose* 4. *un rubis* 5. *un océan* 6. *un glacier* 7. *une violette* 8. *la neige* (snow) 9. *les plantes* (*f.*) 10. *les fleurs* (*f.*) 11. *les jeans*

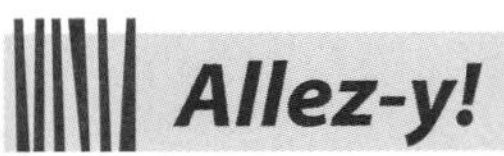

A. Dans la salle de classe. Arthur has a wonderful class. Describe it, choosing the appropriate expressions from the second column.

1. Le professeur est…	**a.** bleue et blanche.
2. Les étudiants sont…	**b.** confortables et nombreuses.
3. La salle de classe est…	**c.** intelligent et dynamique.
4. Les chaises sont…	**d.** sociables et amusants.

B. Des âmes sœurs. (*Soulmates.*) Patrice and Patricia are alike in every respect. Describe them, taking turns with a partner.

MODÈLE: français →
É1: Patrice est français. Et Patricia?
É2: Patricia est française.

1. optimiste
2. intelligent
3. charmant
4. fier
5. sérieux
6. parisien
7. naïf
8. gentil
9. sportif
10. courageux
11. travailleur
12. intellectuel

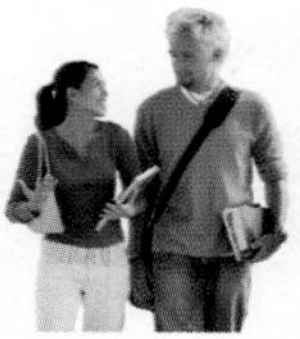

Follow-up (B): Maintenant *Martin parle de Patrice et Patricia. Qu'est-ce qu'il dit?* MODÈLE: *Patrice est français, Patricia aussi est française.* → *Patrice et Patricia sont français.*

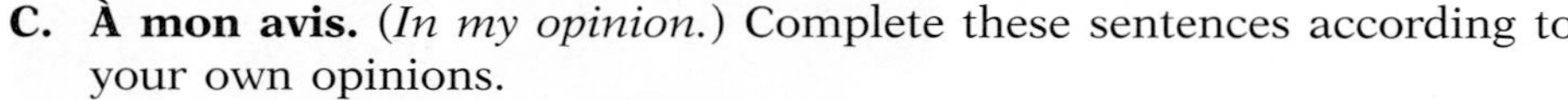

C. À mon avis. (*In my opinion.*) Complete these sentences according to your own opinions.

1. L'homme idéal est ______. Il a une voiture ______ (couleur).
2. La femme idéale est ______. Elle a les yeux ______ (couleur).
3. Le/La camarade de classe idéal(e) est ______.
4. Le professeur idéal est ______.
5. Le chauffeur de taxi idéal est ______.

Continuation (C): Have sts. brainstorm and provide as many completions as possible. This may be done first in groups, or as a whole-class activity. Put sts.' answers on board, or have one st. write on board answers given by classmates. Additional examples: *le/la patron(ne); le/la dentiste; le médecin; le président / la présidente.* Finally, have sts. tell what colors they associate with each person. Tell them to be imaginative.

Follow-up (A–C): Listening Comprehension A. Dictate items: 1. *une chemise noire* 2. *un imperméable gris* 3. *des chaussures blanches* 4. *un pull* (colors of your university) 5. *une chemise noire et blanche* 6. *un tailleur rouge* B. *Qu'est-ce que vous associez avec... ?* (Sts. give items from the *dictée* or their own color associations) 1. *un chanteur (country-western) célèbre* 2. *un prisonnier* 3. *une équipe de base-ball* 4. *un(e) étudiant(e) de votre université* 5. *la femme du président*

D. Un mél. Here is the email that Max dreads receiving from his girlfriend. Transform it into the more positive one that is actually on the way by changing the adjectives and some verbs.

Angers, le 7 janvier

Max,

Je te déteste. Tu es stupide et antipathique. Tous les jours (*Every day*) tu es nerveux, tu ne rêves pas parce que tu es peu idéaliste, et tu es même (*even*) souvent hypocrite. En plus (*Furthermore*) je trouve que tu es paresseux.

Je ne veux pas te revoir. (*I don't want to see you again.*)

Adieu.

Catherine

MODÈLE: Max, je t'adore...

Suggestion: Find photos of people wearing distinctive clothing. Glue them on cards of the same size and cut them in half vertically; you should have one half for each st. Distribute photos; each st. has to find the other half without showing the photo, just by asking yes/no questions about the clothing. Stress that sts. should be careful about the forms of the color adjectives they use.

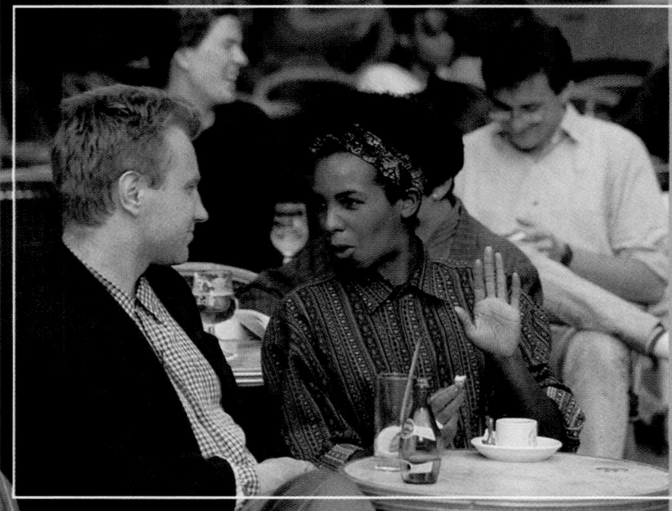

Un peu plus...

Café culture in France.
Cafés in France are important parts of each neighborhood. Many French people go to their favorite café in the morning for a coffee and a croissant, at lunch for a sandwich, or for a drink before dinner, an **apéro (apéritif).** There are **tabacs** in many cafés where one can purchase tobacco, stamps, bus tickets, and other items. Cafés in France are also important places to socialize, where people gather and hold lively conversations. Cafés are also welcoming if you prefer just to sit and relax with a delicious **cappuccino.** Is café culture important in your community? Where do people usually go to socialize?

◄ Qu'est-ce qu'elle dit? (*What is she saying?*)

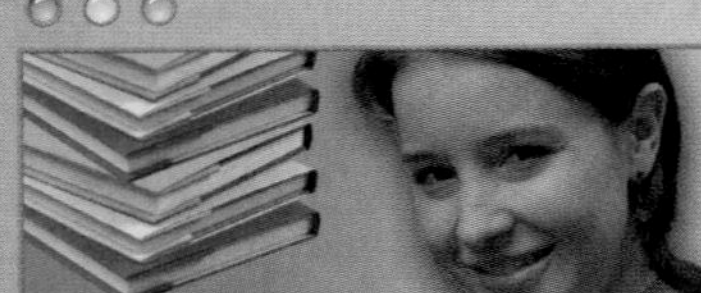

Le blog de Léa

En jupe ou en pantalon?

lundi 23 mai

Samedi soir, il y a une soirée[1] chez mon copain[2] Hector. J'ai envie d'être très belle, très «jeune femme[3]». Mais hélas, j'ai toujours l'air d'avoir 15 ans!

J'ai besoin d'acheter[4] des vêtements originaux et à petit prix.[5] Et aussi des chaussures! Et un sac! La solution, c'est peut-être[6] d'acheter du vintage au marché aux puces[7]?

Je suis petite, brune; j'ai les yeux marron. Vous avez des idées?

Léa

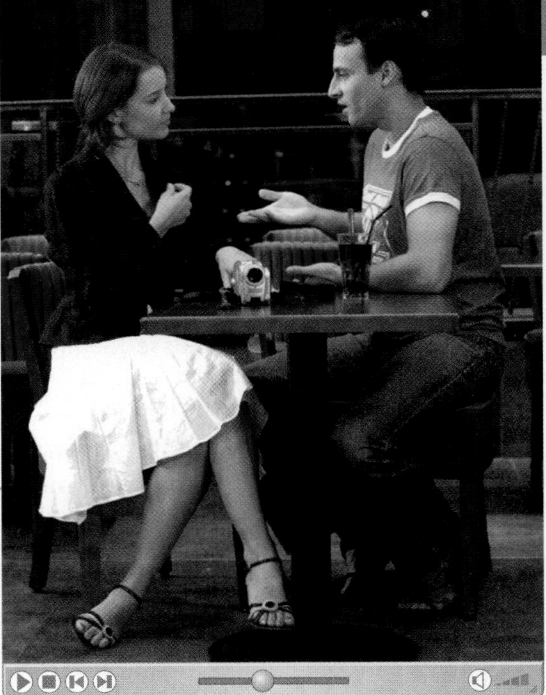

Tu as de bonnes adresses?

COMMENTAIRES

Alexis

Léa,

Pour être[8] originale, tu portes un tee-shirt vert, une veste rose, un jean. Sur le jean, tu mets un short rouge.

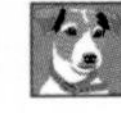

Trésor (chien d'Alexis)

Idiot!

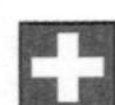

Charlotte

C'est difficile de sélectionner des vêtements pour une soirée. Moi, je suggère une petite robe noire, très courte avec des tennis blanches. Simple, classique, chic.

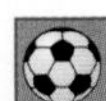

Mamadou

En jupe, en pantalon, en maillot de bain, en short, je suis sûr que tu es charmante!

Suggestion: Model pronunciation and have sts. repeat individually or as a group.

Follow-up: *Questions de compréhension:* 1. *Pourquoi est-il difficile pour Léa d'avoir l'air d'une «jeune femme»?* 2. *Qu'est-ce que Léa doit* (should) *acheter pour la soirée d'Hector?* 3. *Où peut-elle trouver des vêtements originaux et pas chers?* 4. *Que pensez-vous des suggestions d'Alexis et de Charlotte?* 5. *Mamadou est-il sympathique? Pourquoi?*

Note: For additional exs. on *Le blog de Léa* and *Reportage*, see the Workbook/Laboratory Manual.

Video connection: In the videoblog for this chapter, Léa and Hassan discuss where to shop for clothes in Paris and Hassan explains how people dress in Morocco.

[1]*party* [2]*friend* [3]jeune… *young woman* [4]*to buy* [5]à… *cheap* [6]*maybe* [7]marché… *flea market* [8]Pour… *To be*

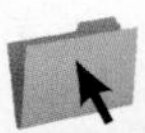

REPORTAGE

Dis-moi où tu t'habilles!°

°*Tell me where you buy your clothes!*

À Paris, est-ce qu'on a besoin d'être riche pour avoir l'air chic? Non! Ce paradoxe a une explication: le fameux chic français n'est pas dans ce qu'[1]on achète mais dans l'art d'assembler les vêtements et les accessoires.

Les étudiants connaissent[2] ce principe essentiel de l'élégance. Et ils font[3] des miracles avec des petits budgets. Mais où trouvent-ils leurs vêtements? D'abord, dans les boutiques pour jeunes comme H&M. Il y a aussi le marché aux puces. Fabien explique: «J'adore la fripe—les vieux vêtements—ils sont originaux.»

Mais que faire si on[4] aime le luxe?

Il y a deux solutions. Anne, par exemple, s'habille dans les «stocks»,[5] magasins où s'accumulent les excès de production de vêtements. Cette semaine, elle a acheté une jupe de la collection Zara pour quinze euros! Gaëlle, qui est BCBG,[6] a une autre solution. Elle va dans un «dépôt-vente» de son quartier où elle achète des vêtements déjà portés mais presque neufs[7]: «Souvent j'ai de la chance, déclare-t-elle. La semaine dernière,[8] pour soixante-neuf euros, j'ai trouvé[9] un foulard[10] Hermès!»

[1]ce... *what* [2]*understand* [3]*create* [4]que... *what do you do if you* [5]*outlet stores* [6]*preppy* [7]presque... *almost new* [8]*last* [9]ai... *found* [10]*scarf*

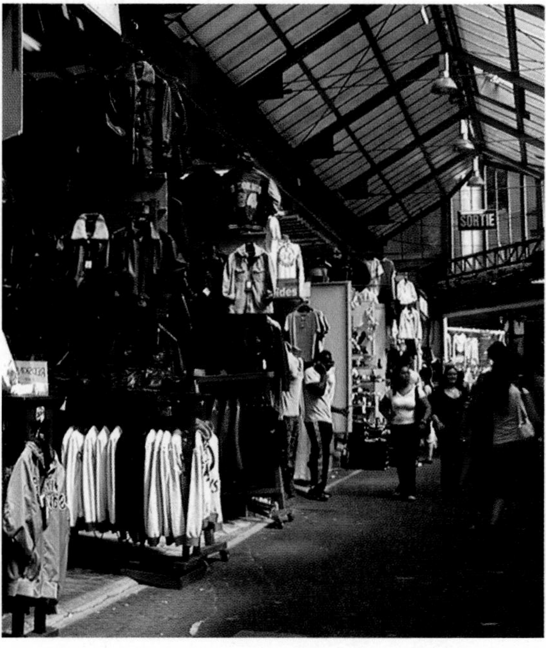

Le marché aux puces de la Porte de Clignancourt. C'est une véritable caverne d'Ali-Baba: les amateurs visitent le marché de préférence le samedi matin. Ils cherchent, ils explorent, ils achètent. Ils ont raison! Avec un peu de chance et beaucoup d'efforts, ils trouvent des trésors parmi (*among*) des montagnes de vêtements.

À vous! Dans quels magasins trouvez-vous vos vêtements? Êtes-vous plutôt comme Fabien, comme Anne ou comme Gaëlle? Expliquez vos préférences.

Parlons-en! Cet été, vous participez à un programme universitaire d'été, à Nice, sur la Côte d'Azur. Vous achetez des vêtements pour ce voyage. Vous avez un budget de $300.

1. Travaillez en groupes de trois ou quatre. Préparez deux listes: une pour les filles (*girls*), une pour les garçons (*boys*).
2. Dans chaque liste, proposez les vêtements nécessaires: tee-shirt, short, chemise, chemisier, pantalon, jupe, etc. Précisez le nom des magasins (*stores*) où vous achetez ces vêtements et donnez les prix.
3. Comparez la liste de votre groupe aux listes des autres. Quel groupe a la liste la plus (*the most*) adaptée à un programme universitaire d'été? la plus économique? la plus classique? la plus extravagante?
4. Quelle est la liste idéale? Votez!

Leçon 3

STRUCTURES

Cultural note: Point out that the French are more animated in discussions than people in the U.S. usually are, often raising their voices and gesticulating vigorously.

Les questions à réponse affirmative ou négative

Getting Information

Une robe noire ou une robe grise?

Appel vidéo entre Juliette et Léa.

JULIETTE: Finalement, **est-ce que tu portes** une jupe pour la soirée d'Hector?
LÉA: Non, je porte un jean avec un chemisier blanc. **Est-ce** assez chic?
JULIETTE: Oui! Un chemisier blanc, c'est très chic! Mais le jean… **tu ne penses pas que** c'est un peu commun?
LÉA: Commun? Certainement pas! C'est simple et élégant. Et toi, **tu portes** une robe?
JULIETTE: Oui, mais j'hésite entre une robe noire et une robe grise. C'est un choix impossible! (Elle rit.*)

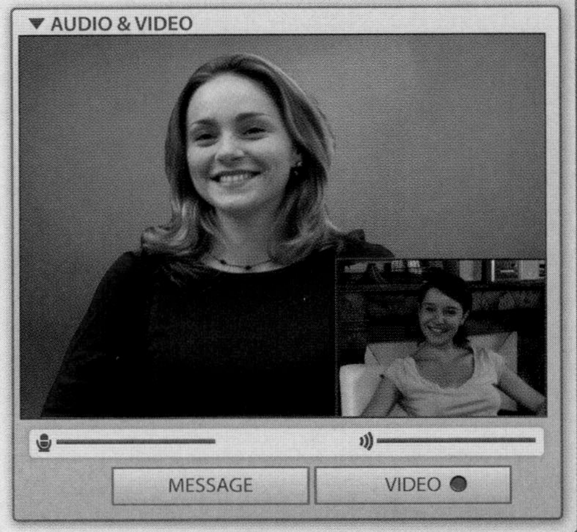

*Elle… *She laughs*

Voici les réponses. Trouvez les questions dans le dialogue.

1. Non, je porte un jean avec un chemisier blanc.
2. Oui! Un chemisier blanc, c'est très chic!
3. Oui, mais j'hésite entre une robe noire et une robe grise.

Note: Make sure sts. understand the difference between yes/no questions and information questions.

Suggestion: Model pronunciation of questions in examples, having sts. repeat after your model.

Suggestion: Practice *si* by asking obvious questions: *Vous n'êtes pas américain/canadien? Vous n'aimez pas la musique?* etc.

In French, there are several ways to ask a question requiring a *yes* or *no* answer.

Questions Without Change in Word Order

1. You can raise the pitch of your voice at the end of a sentence.

—Vous ne parlez pas anglais?	*You don't speak English?*
—Si, un peu.*	*Yes, a little.*

*Note that **si,** not **oui,** is used to answer *yes* to a negative question.

2. When confirmation is expected, add the tag **n'est-ce pas** to the end of the sentence.

Il aime la musique, **n'est-ce pas?**	*He likes music, doesn't he?*
Nous ne mangeons pas au resto-U, **n'est-ce pas?**	*We don't eat at the cafeteria, do we?*

3. Another way is to precede a statement with **Est-ce que (Est-ce qu'** before a vowel sound).

Est-ce que Nathan étudie l'espagnol?	*Does Nathan study Spanish?*
Est-ce qu'elles écoutent la radio?	*Are they listening to the radio?*

[Allez-y! A-B with **Mots clés**]

Note: Point out variety of English tags: *Isn't that so? Right? Don't you think? . . . doesn't she? . . . isn't he? . . . haven't they?* etc.

Suggestion: Mention that although *est-ce que* is one of the easiest ways to form questions, it is not used as much in writing as it is orally.

Questions with Change in Word Order

Questions can also be formed by inverting the subject and the verb. This question formation is more common in written French.

1. When a pronoun is the subject of the sentence, the pronoun and verb are inverted and hyphenated.

PRONOUN SUBJECT	
Statement:	Il est touriste.
Question:	**Est-il** touriste?

Es-tu étudiante en philosophie?	*Are you studying philosophy?*
Aiment-ils les discussions animées?	*Do they like animated discussions?*

The final **t** of third-person plural verb forms is pronounced when followed by **ils** or **elles: aiment-elles.** When third-person singular verbs end with a vowel, **-t-** is inserted between the verb and the pronoun.

Elle aim**e** les jupes. →	**Aime-t-elle** les jupes?
Il port**e** un veston. →	**Porte-t-il** un veston?

Je is seldom inverted. **Est-ce-que** is used instead: **Est-ce que je suis élégant?**

2. When a noun is the subject of the sentence, the noun subject is retained; the third-person pronoun corresponding to the subject follows the verb and is attached to it by a hyphen.

NOUN SUBJECT	
Statement:	Paul est touriste.
Question:	**Paul est-il** touriste?

Marc est-il étudiant?	*Is Marc a student?*
Delphine travaille-t-elle beaucoup?	*Does Delphine work a lot?*
Les amis arrivent-ils ce soir?	*Are our friends arriving tonight?*

[Allez-y! C-D]

Note: You might want to teach inversion with noun subjects for passive recognition only at this point, reentering this type of question formation later in the year for active practice.

Suggestion: Point out that the inserted *t* does not mean anything; it is used to avoid the juxtaposition of two vowels.

Note: At this level, you might want to emphasize intonation and *est-ce que* for yes/no questions. Simple inversion is also presented in *Vis-à -vis,* because we represent the current usage. Sts. are already familiar with some inversion structures (*Comment vas-tu?*). We avoid inversion with 3rd pers. (*A-t-il peur?; Paul a-t-il faim?*) and will never use inversion with *je,* because it is almost never used in day-to-day language.

Suggestion: In all exs. in this section, encourage sts. to think of other ways to ask the same questions. Stress especially the easiest ways: rising intonation, tag questions, and *est-ce que*, with inversion using nouns for recognition only at this point.

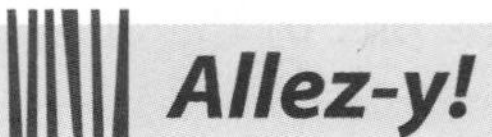

Allez-y!

A. C'est difficile à croire! You find it hard to believe what Manon is telling you. Express your surprise by turning each statement into a question. (Your intonation should express your disbelief!)

MODÈLE: Jade est de Paris. → Jade est de Paris?

1. Pascal est aussi de Paris.
2. Jade et Pascal sont belges.
3. Louis est le camarade de Pascal.
4. C'est un garçon drôle.
5. Il n'habite pas à Paris.
6. Sandra est canadienne.

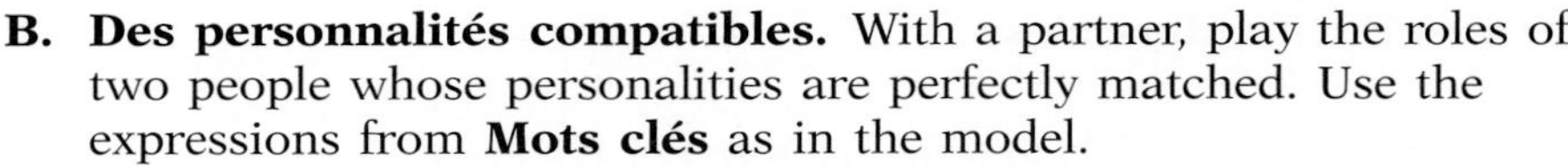

B. Des personnalités compatibles. With a partner, play the roles of two people whose personalities are perfectly matched. Use the expressions from **Mots clés** as in the model.

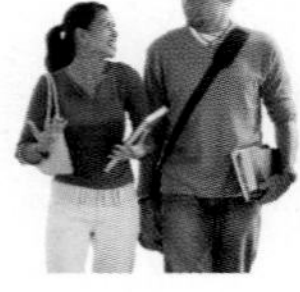

MODÈLE: calme →
É1: Est-ce que tu es calme?
É2: Oui, je suis calme. Et toi? *or* Non, je ne suis pas calme. Et toi?
↓ ↓
É1: Moi aussi, je suis calme. *or* Moi non plus, je ne suis pas calme.

1. sympathique
2. sportif / sportive
3. curieux / curieuse
4. sérieux / sérieuse
5. patient(e)
6. travailleur / travailleuse

Mots clés

The expressions *moi aussi, moi non plus*

If you agree with someone's comment, your answer will be either **moi aussi** (*me too*) or **moi non plus** (*me neither*).

—Je suis fatigué!
—Moi aussi!

—Mais je n'ai pas faim!
—Moi non plus!

C. Étudiants à la Sorbonne. You are writing an article on student life in Paris. Verify the information you have jotted down by expressing your statements as questions.

MODÈLE: Stéphane étudie à la Sorbonne.→
Est-ce que Stéphane étudie à la Sorbonne?

1. Il est belge.
2. Vous admirez Stéphane.
3. Stéphane et Carole sont étudiants en philosophie.
4. Ils sont sympathiques.
5. Carole habite à la cité-U.

Note (C): You might want to do this ex. using inversion.

Interaction: Have sts. act out the following situation, using the vocabulary and structures from this chapter. *Journaliste:* You are a reporter for the school newspaper; a classmate plays the role of a visiting celebrity. Find out everything you can about this person: likes and dislikes, whether he or she likes to go certain places, some personality characteristics.

D. Portrait d'un professeur. Ask your instructor about his or her personality, tastes, and clothing. Use inversion in your questions. **Verbes suggérés:** aimer, danser, écouter, être, parler, regarder, skier

MODÈLES: Êtes-vous pessimiste?
Aimez-vous les cravates orange?

Now see if your classmates were listening. Ask a classmate three questions about your instructor.

MODÈLE: Est-ce que le professeur est pessimiste?

Les prépositions *à* et *de*

Mentioning Specific Places or People

Tennis, poker ou restaurant?

Léa contacte Hector sur sa page Facebook (Messagerie instantanée).

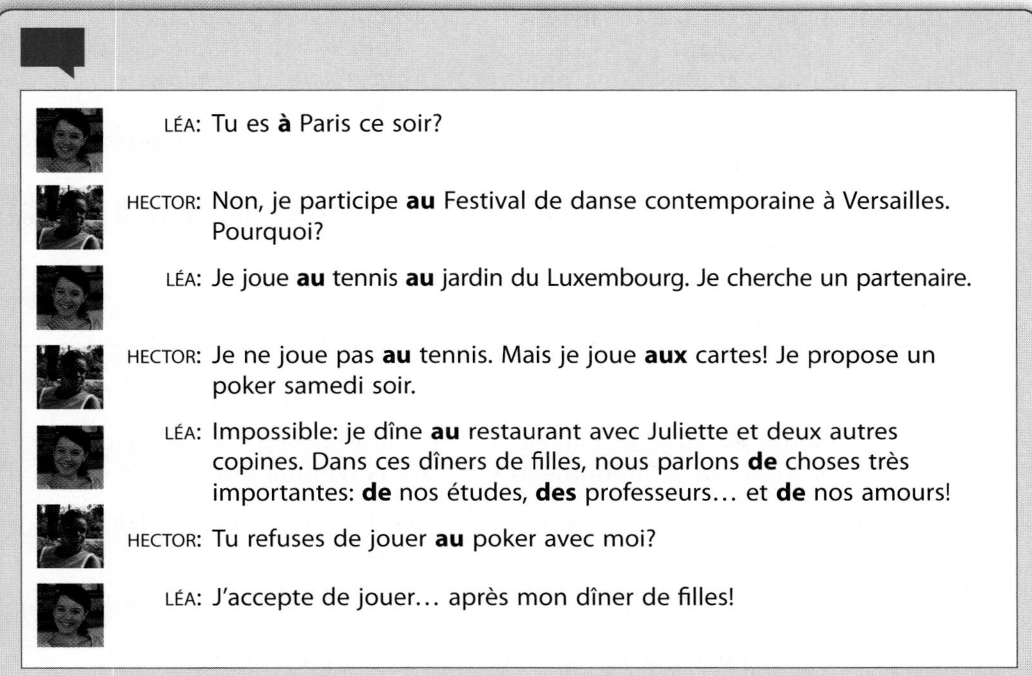

LÉA: Tu es **à** Paris ce soir?

HECTOR: Non, je participe **au** Festival de danse contemporaine à Versailles. Pourquoi?

LÉA: Je joue **au** tennis **au** jardin du Luxembourg. Je cherche un partenaire.

HECTOR: Je ne joue pas **au** tennis. Mais je joue **aux** cartes! Je propose un poker samedi soir.

LÉA: Impossible: je dîne **au** restaurant avec Juliette et deux autres copines. Dans ces dîners de filles, nous parlons **de** choses très importantes: **de** nos études, **des** professeurs… et **de** nos amours!

HECTOR: Tu refuses de jouer **au** poker avec moi?

LÉA: J'accepte de jouer… après mon dîner de filles!

Complétez les phrases.

Hector

1. Hector est ______ Versailles.
2. Il participe ______ Festival de danse.
3. Il ne joue pas ______ tennis.
4. Il joue ______ cartes.
5. Il joue ______ poker.

Léa

6. Léa est ______ Paris.
7. Elle joue ______ jardin du Luxembourg.
8. Elle dîne ______ restaurant avec des copines.
9. Elles parlent ______ choses importantes.

Prepositions (**les prépositions**) give information about the relationship between two words. Examples in English are *at, before, for, in, of, to, under, without.* In French, the prepositions **à** and **de** sometimes contract with articles.

Note: Articles are not used before names of most cities. Exceptions are *La Nouvelle-Orléans, Le Havre,* and *Le Caire.*

Suggestion: Urge sts. to learn these verbs that take indirect objects. You may need to explain in more detail what an indirect object is. Using the example *I gave the ball to Cathy,* ask sts. to identify the direct and indirect objects. Point out that *à + name of person* is the sign for the indirect object in French.

The Preposition *à*

1. À indicates location or destination. It has several English equivalents.

Arnaud habite **à** Paris.	*Arnaud lives in Paris.*
Il étudie **à** la bibliothèque.	*He studies at (in) the library.*
Il arrive **à** Bruxelles demain.	*He's coming to Brussels tomorrow.*

2. With verbs such as **donner, montrer, parler,** and **téléphoner, à** introduces the indirect object (usually a person) even when *to* is not used in English.

Arnaud **donne** un livre **à** son copain.	*Arnaud gives his friend a book.*
Arnaud **montre** une photo **à** Delphine.	*Arnaud shows Delphine a photo.*
Il **parle à** un professeur.	*He's speaking to a professor.*
Il **téléphone à** un ami.	*He's calling a friend.*

The preposition *to* is not always used in English, but **à** must be used in French with these verbs.

The Preposition *de*

1. De indicates where something or someone comes from.

Medhi est **de** Casablanca.	*Medhi is from Casablanca.*
Il arrive **de** la bibliothèque.	*He is coming from the library.*

2. De also indicates possession (expressed by *'s* or *of* in English) and the concept of belonging to, being a part of.

Voici la librairie **de** Madame Vernier.	*Here is Madame Vernier's bookstore.*
J'aime mieux la librairie **de** l'université.	*I prefer the university bookstore (the bookstore of the university).*

3. When used with **parler, de** means *about.*

Nous parlons **de** la littérature contemporaine.	*We're talking about contemporary literature.*

Note: Point out the pronunciation of *aux* before a consonant and before a vowel (*aux courts de tennis / aux amis*).

The Prepositions *à* and *de* with the Definite Articles *le* and *les*

à + le = au	Arnaud arrive **au** cinéma.
à + les = aux	Arnaud arrive **aux** cours.
à + la = à la	Arnaud arrive **à la** librairie.
à + l' = à l'	Arnaud arrive **à l'**université.
de + le = du	Arnaud arrive **du** cinéma.
de + les = des	Arnaud arrive **des** cours.
de + la = de la	Arnaud arrive **de la** librairie.
de + l' = de l'	Arnaud arrive **de l'**université.

The Verb *jouer* with the Prepositions *à* and *de*

When **jouer** is followed by the preposition **à,** it means to play a team sport or a game. When it is followed by **de,** it means to play a musical instrument.

Follow-up: With sts., make a list of team sports and musical instruments; always give the gender.

Note: The structure *faire de* (+ individual sports) is presented in *Chapitre 5, Leçon 3.*

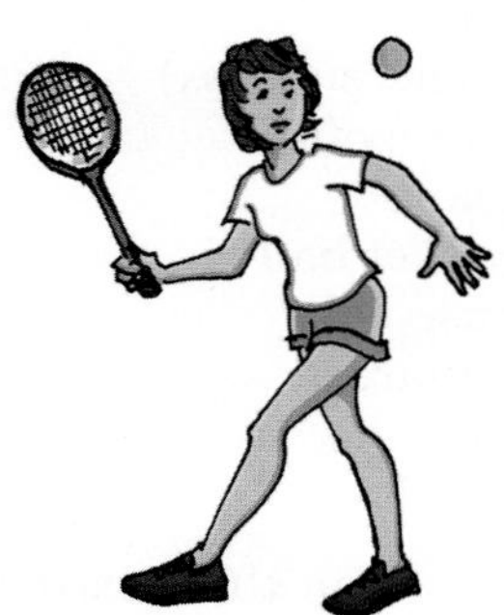

Naïma
joue au tennis.

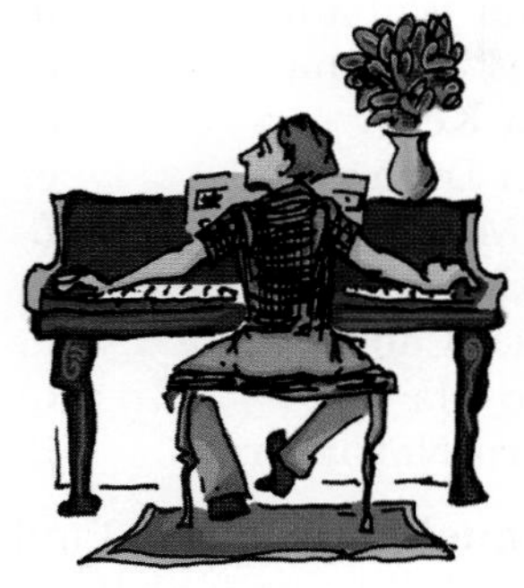

Philippe
joue du piano.

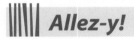

Allez-y!

A. Où est-ce qu'on va? (*Where do we go?*) Answer, taking turns with a partner. **Suggestions:** l'Alliance (*Institute*) française, l'amphithéâtre, la bibliothèque, le café, le cinéma, le concert, les courts de tennis, le Quartier latin, le restaurant universitaire, la salle de sport

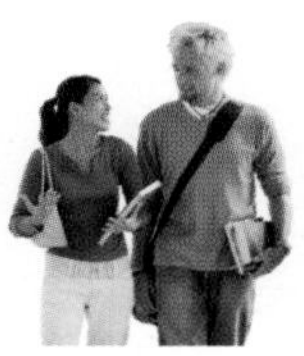

MODÈLE: pour écouter une symphonie →
É1: Où est-ce qu'on va pour écouter une symphonie?
É2: On va au concert.

1. pour regarder un film **2.** pour jouer au tennis **3.** pour jouer au volley-ball **4.** pour écouter le professeur **5.** pour apprendre (*learn*) le français **6.** pour étudier **7.** pour manger **8.** pour visiter la Sorbonne **9.** pour parler avec des amis

B. Camille, une personne très active. Adapt the following sentences, using the words in parentheses.

Suggestion: Do as rapid response drill. Alternatively, dictate sentences to sts. at board (with other sts. writing at their seats) and have them do transformations in writing, with group repetition as needed.

1. Camille téléphone *à Sophie.* (le professeur / les amies / Gabriel / le restaurant)
2. Elle parle *de la littérature africaine.* (le rap / la politique française / les livres de Marguerite Duras / le cours de japonais)
3. Camille arrive *de la librairie.* (le resto-U / New York / la bibliothèque / les courts de tennis)
4. Elle aime jouer *au football.* (le piano / les cartes / le basket-ball / la guitare)

C. Les passe-temps. Complete the following sentences with **jouer à** or **de.** Match the players with the sports or instruments they play.

MODÈLE: Aaron Rodgers → Aaron Rodgers joue au football américain.

Answers (C): 1. d 2. j 3. h 4. e 5. f 6. b 7. i 8. g 9. a 10. c.

1. Wynton Marsalis	**a.** le violoncelle
2. Serena Williams	**b.** le golf
3. Carlos Santana	**c.** les échecs (*chess*)
4. Alicia Keys	**d.** la trompette
5. Kevin Durant	**e.** le piano
6. Phil Mickelson	**f.** le basket-ball
7. David Beckham	**g.** le base-ball
8. Miguel Cabrera	**h.** la guitare
9. Yo-Yo Ma	**i.** le foot
10. Hikaru Nakamura	**j.** le tennis

Suggestion (D): See who can find the most names in the shortest time. Show sts. how to prepare a form with activities listed vertically on the left, with plenty of room for names next to each.

D. Trouvez quelqu'un qui... Find someone in the classroom who does each of the following activities. On a separate piece of paper, note down his/her name next to the activity. See who can complete the list the fastest.

MODÈLE: Est-ce que tu joues au tennis?
Oui, je joue au tennis. (*ou* Non, je ne joue pas au tennis.)

aimer le laboratoire de langues	jouer au volley
aimer les films français	jouer aux cartes
jouer au base-ball	jouer de la clarinette
jouer au bridge	jouer de la guitare
jouer au poker	manger à la cafétéria aujourd'hui
jouer au tennis	?

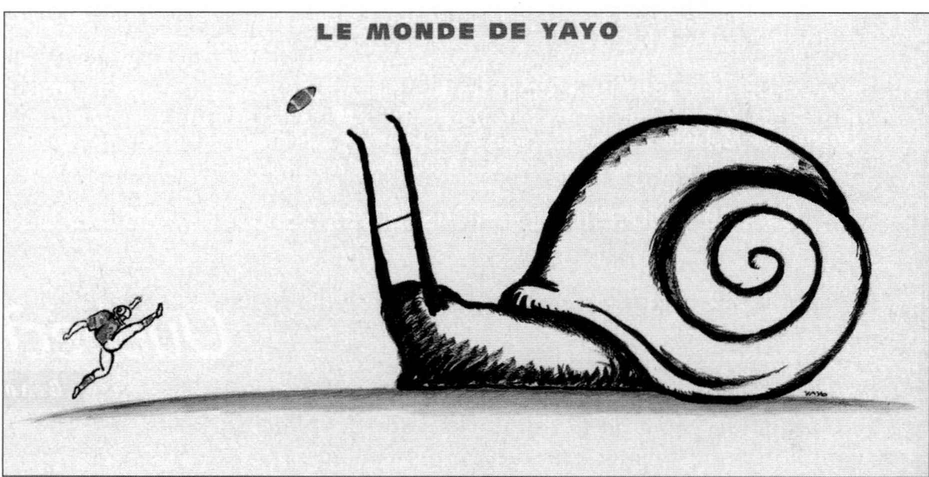

Qu'est-ce que vous pensez de cette illustration?

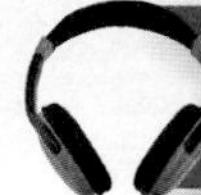

Prononcez bien!

1. **The vowels in *bleu* and *couleur*** (page 64)

   A. **Nathalie et Olivier.** Isabelle talks about two of your mutual friends. Listen to her and indicate whether she's referring to Nathalie or to Olivier.

   B. **Trouvez l'intrus.** You and Isabelle are playing *Odd Man Out*. Read each series of words aloud and your partner will say the word that doesn't belong.

      1. deux, peu, fleur, bleu, cheveux
      2. sœur, deux, couleur, œuf, peur
      3. yeux, jeudi, danseuse, peu, jeune

2. **The pronunciation of final consonants** (page 69)

   Stéphane. Isabelle is talking about Stéphane. You know you've met him but you can't remember much about him. First, read her description of Stéphane and indicate whether the final consonants in bold are pronounced or not. Then, read the paragraph aloud.

   Rappelle-toi (*Remember*)! Stéphane est étudian**t** en alleman**d**. Il est gran**d**, sporti**f** et intellectue**l**. Il travaille dans un restauran**t** du quartie**r** le vendredi soi**r**. Il porte souven**t** un pantalo**n** gri**s**, un tee-shirt ver**t** et un sa**c** blan**c**. D'accor**d**? Tu vois (*see*) maintenan**t**?

3. **The nasal vowels in *blond, grand,* and *bain*** (page 71)

   A. **Le jeu des voyelles nasales.** Your French instructor has invented a game to help you practice the French nasal vowels. You will hear three sets of seven words, each containing one of the three sounds listed below. Write the words you hear from each set in the correct category.

      1. [ɔ̃] as in **blond**
      2. [ɑ̃] as in **grand**
      3. [ɛ̃] as in **bain**

   B. **Les soldes.** You and your housemates took advantage of the department store sales to update your wardrobes. With your partner, take turns reading the list of what you all bought, making sure to distinguish between the sounds [ɔ̃] as in **blond,** [ɑ̃] as **grand,** and [ɛ̃] as in **bain.**

   Nous av**on**s acheté c**in**q blous**on**s bl**an**cs, qu**in**ze p**an**tal**on**s marr**on**, trois m**an**teaux or**an**ge, v**in**gt s**an**dales et deux gr**an**ds sacs à m**ain**!

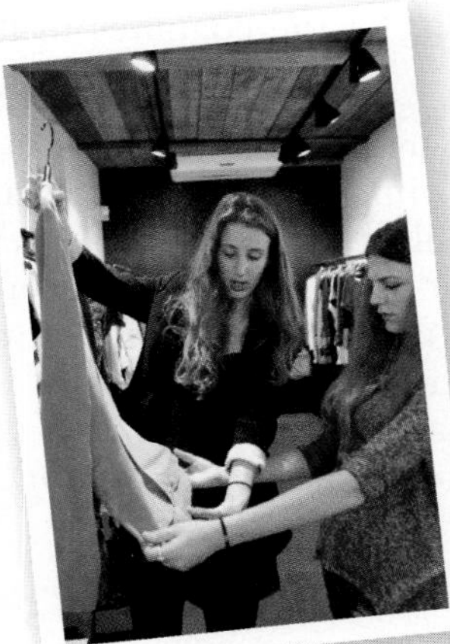

Est-ce que la jeune femme va acheter ce chemisier?

Suggestion (1A): Have students write *N* or *O* on a sheet of paper as you say each adjective.

Script (1A): 1. *paresseux* 2. *nerveuse* 3. *travailleuse* 4. *chauffeur* 5. *danseuse*

Answers (1A): 1. *Olivier* 2. *Nathalie* 3. *Nathalie* 4. *Olivier* 5. *Nathalie*

Answers (1B): 1. *fleur* 2. *deux* 3. *jeune*

Answers (2): Pronounced: *sportif, intellectuel, soir, sac;* Not pronounced: *étudiant, allemand, grand, restaurant, quartier, souvent, pantalon, gris, vert, blanc, D'accord, maintenant*

Suggestion (3): Write the sounds on the board and remind students how to articulate the vowels by reviewing the explanation in the *Prononcez bien!* box on p. 71.

Script (3A): Set 1: *bien, bonsoir, bientôt, bonjour, comment, vendredi, pardon* Set 2: *juin, janvier, américain, raison, danser, science, besoin* Set 3: *dimanche, sympathique, envie, long, sincère, souvent, combien*

Answers (3A): 1. blond: *bonsoir, bonjour, pardon* 2. grand: *janvier, danser, science* 3. bain: *sympathique, sincère, combien*

Leçon 4

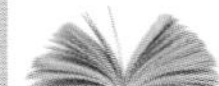

Lecture

Avant de lire

Gaining confidence in your reading skills. You have already practiced two strategies that facilitate comprehension of a written text: recognizing cognates (**Chapitre 1**) and predicting the content using the context (**Chapitre 2**). These strategies *do* work. The more you practice them, the more confidence you will gain, enabling you to read texts in French with greater ease and enjoyment. Here is some additional advice:

- *Read and reread.* Read the text once to get the general sense. Then read it a second time, using the techniques you already know to fill in the gaps.
- *Don't fret over every word.* Break the habit of reading for word-for-word translation. Concentrate on getting the meaning of larger "chunks" of text—phrases and entire sentences.
- *Use the dictionary as a last resort.* After using all of your reading strategies, try to decide whether the meaning of an unfamiliar word is truly crucial for your comprehension of the general meaning. If it is, consult a dictionary. The dictionary is an important tool, but it should be used with moderation.

Parlons de la mode. Paris is one of the great centers of the fashion industry, and French fashion terms have been incorporated extensively into English. For this reason, in fashion advertising in English, it is not unusual to see French words used unaltered. Do you know the meanings of the following words?

parfum	boutique	haute couture
couturier	mode	prêt-à-porter

Des mots apparentés! The following sentences are excerpted from the reading selection. Guess the meaning of the cognates in italics.

1. Mais c'est dans le Marais que les jeunes *créateurs* sont rassemblés. Dans des boutiques très *originales*, ils *proposent* des vêtements et des *accessoires innovants*, parfois vraiment *excentriques*. Les garçons et les filles (*boys and girls*) *adorent!*
2. Pour les étrangers (*foreigners*) *en visite* à Paris, acheter des vêtements et des chaussures est une *expérience intéressante* et même une *aventure*! Mais attention: la *politesse* avant tout!
3. *Bravo!* Vous êtes *éduqué*(*e*), aimable, *respectueux/respectueuse*: dans un magasin, vous êtes *sûr*(*e*) d'obtenir (*to obtain*) une *assistance immédiate*.

Paris-shopping: quelques recommandations

> **À propos de la lecture...**
> This reading was written by one of the authors of *Vis-à-vis*.

Paris est la ville des jolies boutiques de mode. Pour les filles, pour les garçons, pour les jeunes, pour les adultes, pour les seniors, il y a le choix. On trouve tout, à tous les prix.[1]

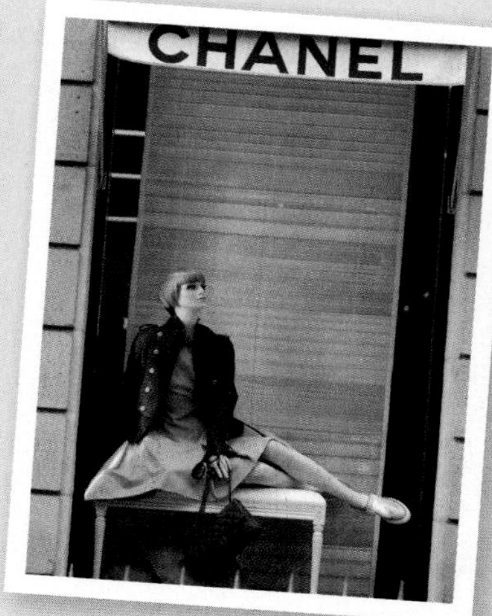

Le prêt-à-porter de luxe

Les Champs-Élysées et le Marais

Les beaux quartiers privilégient les marques[2] prestigieuses (et chères!): Louis Vuitton, Christian Dior, Hermès ou Chanel. Sur les Champs-Élysées, rue François 1er, rue Montaigne et rue Saint-Honoré, les magasins chic exposent les trésors fabuleux du prêt-à-porter de luxe: foulards, sacs, chemises, cravates et costumes.

Mais c'est dans le Marais que les jeunes créateurs sont rassemblés. Dans des boutiques très originales, ils proposent des vêtements et des accessoires innovants, parfois vraiment excentriques. Les garçons et les filles adorent, par exemple, les sacs de la boutique Matières à réflexion fabriqués avec du vieux cuir[3] recyclé.

Expédition shopping

Pour les étrangers en visite à Paris, acheter des vêtements et des chaussures est une expérience intéressante et même une aventure! Mais attention: la politesse avant tout! Voici donc quelques recommandations pour vos expéditions-shopping:

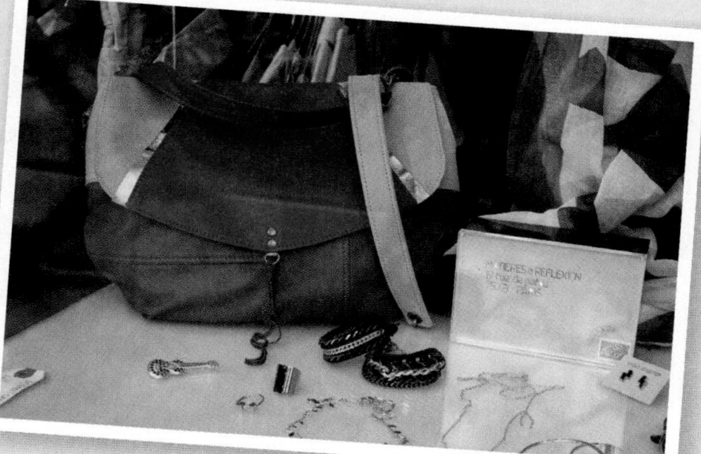
Des créations originales

- Pour être bien reçu(e)[4] dans les boutiques de mode, respectez les bonnes manières: Un «bonjour» est indispensable quand vous poussez la porte!
- Puis quand on vous demande: «Est-ce que je peux vous aider?[5]», vous répondez: «Non, merci; je regarde». Ou bien vous posez une question: «S'il vous plaît, quel est le prix des chaussures noires exposées dans la vitrine?[6]»
- Enfin, quand la vendeuse vous présente les fameuses chaussures, surtout n'oubliez pas de dire «merci»!

Bravo! Vous êtes éduqué(e), aimable, respectueux/respectueuse: dans un magasin, vous êtes sûr(e) d'obtenir une assistance immédiate! Et un sourire![7]

[1]à... *at all (different) prices* [2]*brands* [3]*leather* [4]*received, welcomed* [5]Est-ce que... *May I help you?* [6]*shop window* [7]*smile*

Suggestion: If you wish to treat this topic in more depth, print out the dialogue between the salespeople and the clients and the list of useful expressions from the Instructor's Manual and distribute them to the class. This will allow students to see the expressions used in context before they create their own scenarios.

Compréhension

1. Où est-ce qu'on trouve les magasins et boutiques de luxe à Paris? Quelles sortes de vêtements est-ce qu'on y trouve?
2. Dans quel quartier est-ce qu'on trouve des vêtements et des accessoires originaux appréciés des jeunes?
3. À votre avis, quelle est l'expression la plus utile à connaître pour une expédition shopping agréable à Paris?

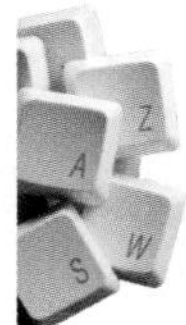

Écriture

The writing activities **Par écrit** and **Journal intime** can be found in the Workbook/Laboratory Manual to accompany *Vis*-à-*vis*.

Pour s'amuser

Mots en désordre°

Mots... *Word scramble*

The letters of these words have been scrambled. Find the original words. (Hint: They all have to do with clothing and colors.)

o r e s

n a j e

l a n b c

p e u j

l e i l a t u r

n a l p o n t a

m e c h e s i

Answers: rose, jean, blanc, jupe, tailleur, pantalon, chemise

La vie en chantant. An activity based on the song "Couleur café" by Serge Gainsbourg can be found in the Instructor's Manual. The song can be purchased at the iTunes store, or sts. can watch the music video on YouTube.

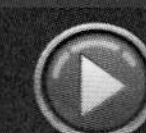

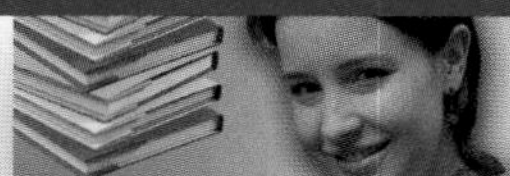

Le vidéoblog de Léa

En bref

In this episode, Léa and Hassan meet at a café, where they talk about clothing. In her videoblog, Léa describes the various places one can buy clothing in Paris; Hassan talks about how people dress in Morocco.

Vocabulaire en contexte

la mode *fashion*

- une bonne adresse *good/favorite place to shop*
- dépenser de l'argent *to spend money*
- être en solde *to be on sale*
- le luxe *luxury*
- le marché aux puces *flea market*
- la haute couture *high fashion, designer clothing*
- un (petit, gros) budget vêtements *(small, large) clothing budget*

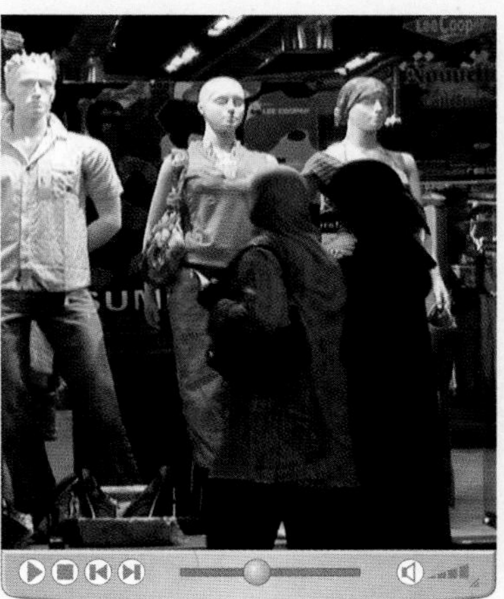

On fait (*does*) du shopping au Maroc.

Visionnez!

	Léa	Hassan	Les deux
1. Qui ne dépense pas beaucoup d'argent pour ses vêtements?	☐	☐	☐
2. Qui a une liste de bonnes adresses?	☐	☐	☐
3. Qui porte presque (*almost*) toujours un jean?	☐	☐	☐
4. Qui est quelquefois sportif, quelquefois élégant?	☐	☐	☐
5. Qui aime les vêtements chic?	☐	☐	☐

Suggestion: Ask sts. yes/no questions based on the vocabulary to aid their comprehension of the video episode: *Tu as un petit ou un gros budget vêtements? Tu aimes acheter des vêtements en solde? Y a-t-il un marché aux puces en ville?* etc.

Suggestion: Before watching the video, ask sts. the *Visionnez!* questions about their classmates, then return to the questions after the video for a quick comprehension check.

Note: Beginning in this chapter, the *Analysez!* questions can be done in French using the model sentences provided.

Analysez!

Voici une liste de vêtements marocains traditionnels mentionnés par Hassan: **des babouches, une djellaba, un fez / un tarbouch, un foulard** (*scarf*). Qui porte chaque (*each*) vêtement—un homme, une femme ou les deux? Ces vêtements ont-ils des équivalents occidentaux (*Western*)?

MODÈLE: Un homme porte un fez. Un fez est une sorte de chapeau.

Comparez!

Make a list of the **bonnes adresses** in your area. Which stores are good for a small clothing budget, which are good for a large one, and which articles of clothing in particular are these stores known for? How do these stores compare to those described in the video?

MODÈLE: Si vous avez un petit budget vêtements, le magasin Marshall's est super: on y trouve (*finds there*)…

Note culturelle

French families are spending a much smaller percentage of their income on clothing than they used to (5.6% today compared to 11% in 1960). Clothing is now less of a social symbol. It is a way of expressing one's identity. France is still known as the land of luxury products, however, and the new tendencies determined by *haute couture* collections are still carefully dissected on news broadcasts every season. Some of the most famous *couturiers* are Dior, Chanel, Givenchy, Ungaro, Gaultier, Lacroix, to name only a few.

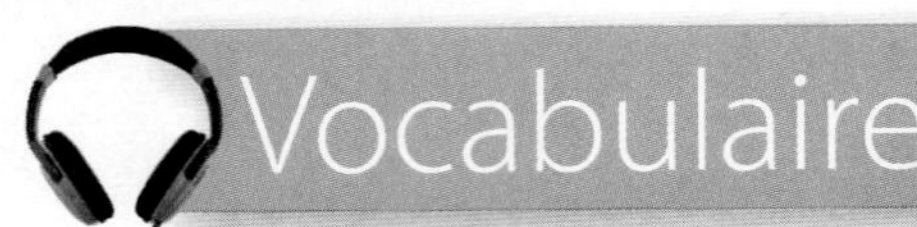

Vocabulaire

Verbes

arriver to arrive
avoir to have
jouer to play
  jouer à to play (*a sport or game*)
  jouer de to play (*a musical instrument*)
montrer to show
porter to wear; to carry
téléphoner à to telephone

À REVOIR: **regarder, travailler**

Expressions avec *avoir*

avoir (20) ans to be (20) years old
avoir besoin de to need (to)
avoir chaud to be warm
avoir de la chance to be lucky
avoir envie de to want (to), feel like (*doing s.th.*)
avoir faim to be hungry
avoir froid to be cold
avoir honte to be ashamed
avoir l'air (+ *adj.*); **avoir l'air de** (+ *inf.*) (+ *noun*) to seem, look, appear
avoir peur (de) to be afraid (of, to)
avoir raison to be right
avoir rendez-vous avec to have a meeting (date) with
avoir soif to be thirsty
avoir sommeil to be sleepy
avoir tort to be wrong

Substantifs

le/la camarade de chambre roommate
les cartes (*f.*) cards
les cheveux (*m. pl.*) hair
les échecs (*m. pl.*) chess
la fille girl
le garcon boy
la jeune femme young woman
le jeune homme young man
le magasin store
la personne person
la soirée party
les yeux (*m.*) eyes

À REVOIR: **l'ami(e), la bibliothèque, l'université**

Adjectifs

antipathique unpleasant
beau / belle beautiful
blond(e) blond
châtain (*inv. in gender*) chestnut brown
cher / chère expensive
chic (*inv.*) stylish
court(e) short
drôle funny, odd
égoïste selfish
facile easy
fatigué(e) tired
fier / fière proud
gentil(le) nice, pleasant
grand(e) tall, big
heureux / heureuse happy; fortunate
hypocrite hypocritical
nouveau / nouvelle new
paresseux / paresseuse lazy
pauvre poor
petit(e) small, short
prêt(e) ready
raide straight
roux / rousse redheaded
sensible sensitive
sportif / sportive *describes someone who likes physical exercise and sports*
sympa(thique) nice, likeable
travailleur / travailleuse hardworking
triste sad

À REVOIR: **espagnol(e), français(e), italien(ne)**

Adjectifs apparentés

amusant(e), blond(e), calme, charmant(e), conformiste, content(e), courageux / courageuse, curieux / curieuse, (dés)agréable, différent(e), difficile, dynamique, élégant(e), enthousiaste, essentiel(le), excellent(e), excentrique, extraordinaire, idéal(e), idéaliste, (im)patient(e), important(e), individualiste, inflexible, intellectuel(le), intelligent(e), intéressant(e), long(ue), modeste, naïf / naïve, nerveux / nerveuse, optimiste, ordinaire, parisien(ne), patient(e), persévérant(e), pessimiste, précis(e), raisonnable, réaliste, riche, sérieux / sérieuse, sincère, snob, sociable, solitaire

Les vêtements

le béret beret
le blouson windbreaker
les bottes (*f.*) boots
la casquette baseball cap
le chapeau hat
les chaussettes (*f.*) socks
les chaussures (*f.*) shoes
la chemise shirt
le chemisier blouse
le costume (*man's*) suit
la cravate tie
l'imperméable (*m.*) raincoat
le jean jeans
la jupe skirt
le maillot de bain swimsuit

le manteau coat
le pantalon pants
le pull-over sweater
la robe dress
le sac à dos backpack
le sac à main handbag
les sandales (*f.*) sandals
le short shorts
le tailleur woman's suit
le tee-shirt T-shirt
les tennis (*m.*) tennis shoes
la veste sports coat, blazer
le veston suit jacket

Les couleurs

blanc / blanche white
bleu(e) blue
gris(e) gray
jaune yellow
marron (*inv.*) brown
noir(e) black
orange (*inv.*) orange
rose pink
rouge red
vert(e) green
violet(te) violet

Mots et expressions divers

assez somewhat
de taille moyenne of medium height
moi aussi me too
moi non plus me neither
n'est-ce pas? isn't it so?
peu not very; hardly
un peu a little
Quel âge avez-vous (as-tu)? How old are you?

CHAPITRE 4

À la maison°

À... *At home*

Presentation: Have sts. look at the photo. Ask *Qu'est-ce que c'est?* pointing to the building, the Eiffel Tower, the windows, etc. Use this also as an opportunity to introduce *Chapitre 4* vocabulary, prepositions of location, and question words. You can also recycle adjectives such as *grand, élégant, beau,* and color words.

Les dossiers de Léa

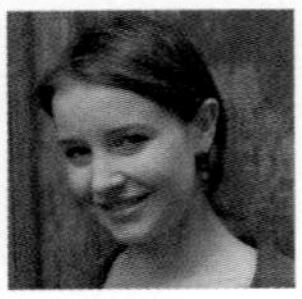

Léa

- Mes photos
  - Des appartements de luxe
  - Un petit «chez moi»
  - De vieilles maisons à Montréal

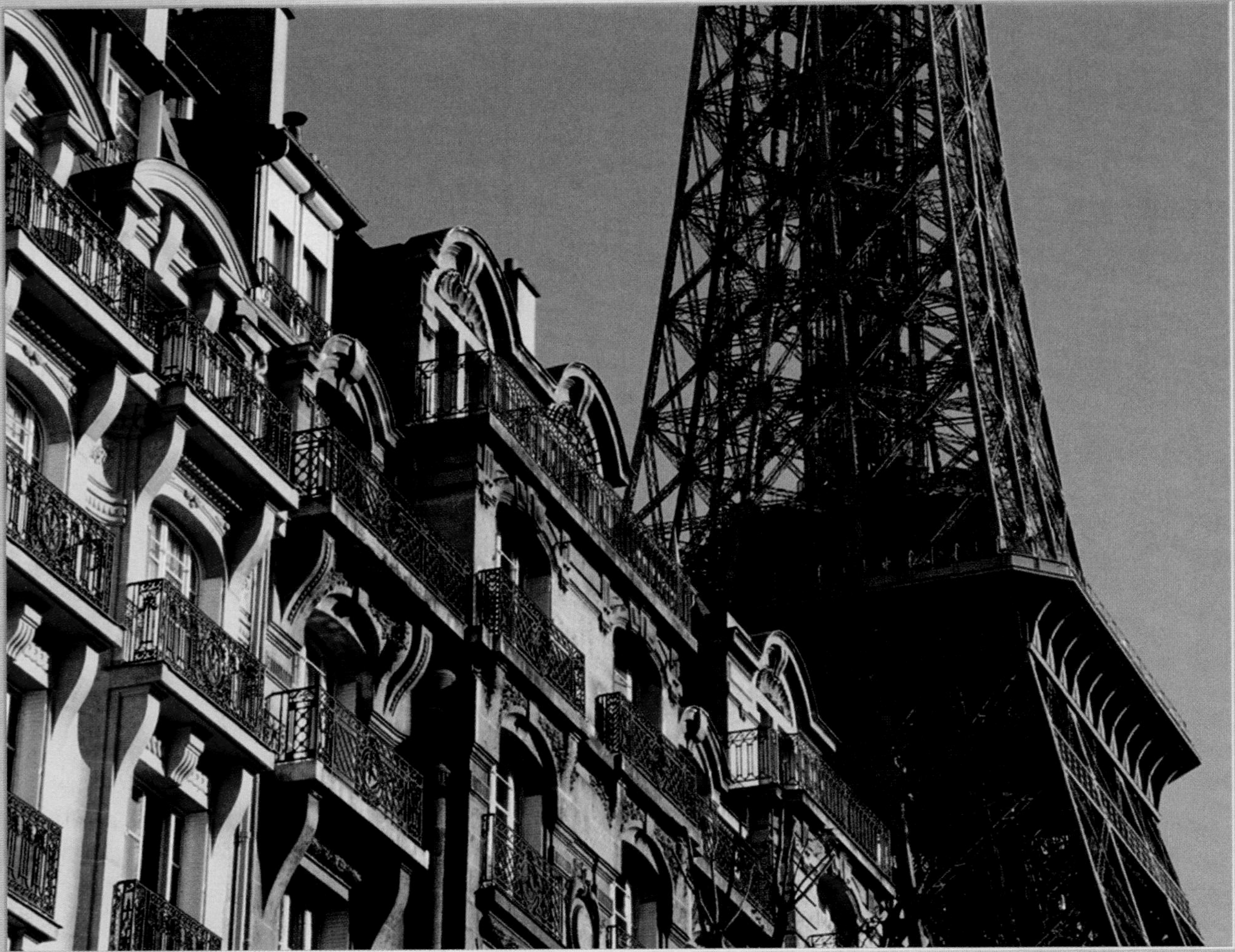

Des appartements de luxe dans le septième arrondissement

 **Cultural note:** The Eiffel Tower was built for the *Exposition Universelle* in 1889. It is located on the *Champ-de-Mars* in the 7th *arrondissement* of Paris.

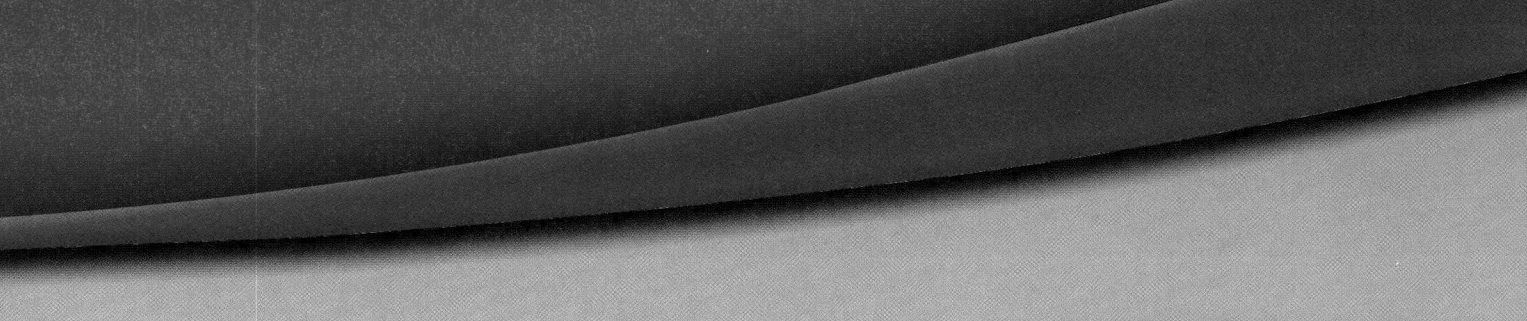

Dans ce chapitre...

OBJECTIFS COMMUNICATIFS

- locating people and objects
- expressing the absence of something
- getting information
- expressing actions
- describing people, places, and things
- learning to distinguish between and pronounce selected sounds in French

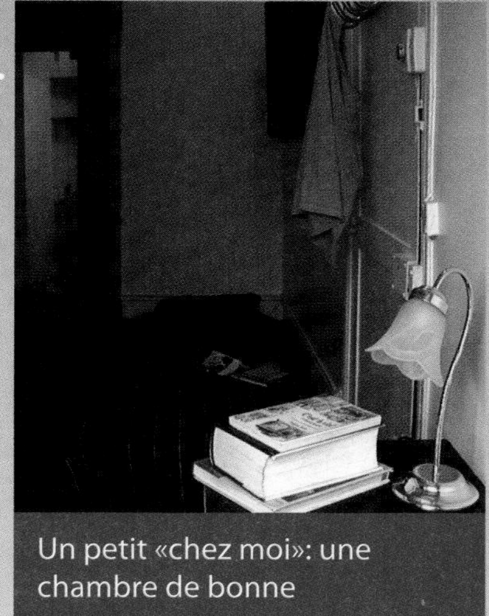

Un petit «chez moi»: une chambre de bonne

PAROLES (Leçon 1)

- Les prépositions de lieu
- L'ameublement

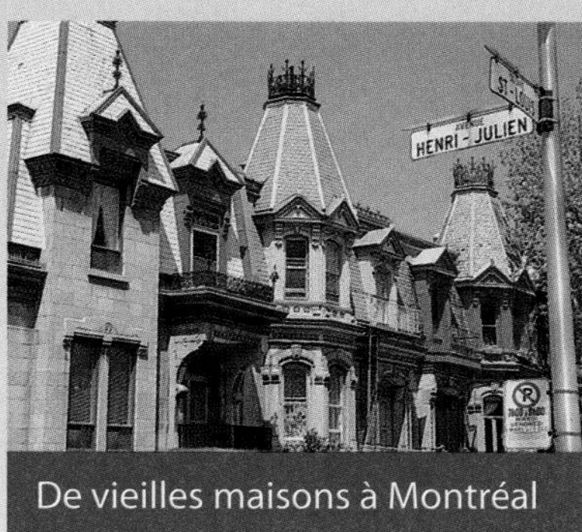

De vieilles maisons à Montréal

STRUCTURES (Leçons 2 et 3)

- Les articles indéfinis après **ne... pas**
- Les mots interrogatifs
- Les verbes en **-ir**
- La place de l'adjectif qualificatif

CULTURE

- Le blog de Léa: *Chez moi*
- Reportage: *Montréal: vivre en français*
- Lecture: *La colocation* (Leçon 4)

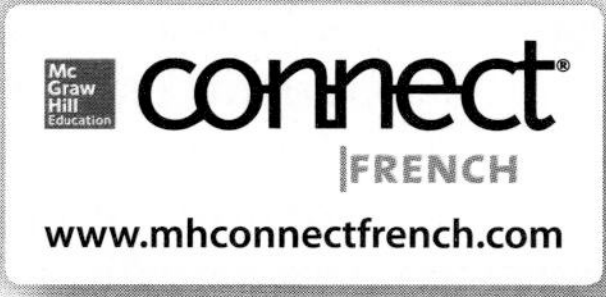

Leçon 1

Suggestion: Read sentences and have sts. match them to drawings, covering captions.

PAROLES

Clarisse, Justin et la voiture°

°*car*

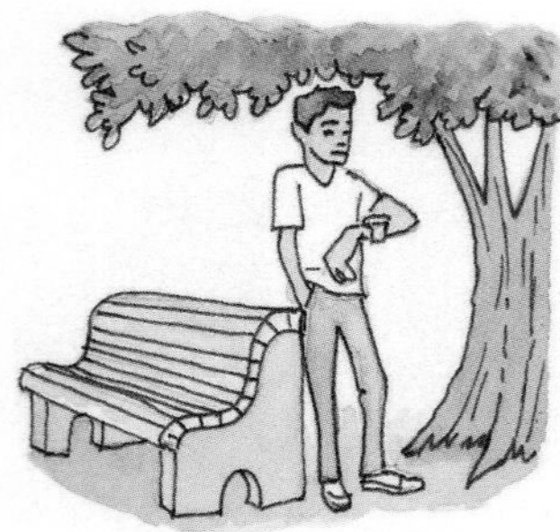

Justin est **dans** le parc, **entre** le banc (*bench*) et l'arbre (*tree*).

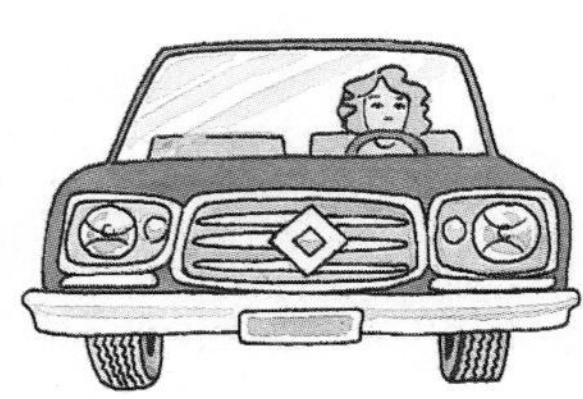

Clarisse est **dans** sa voiture, **loin du** parc.

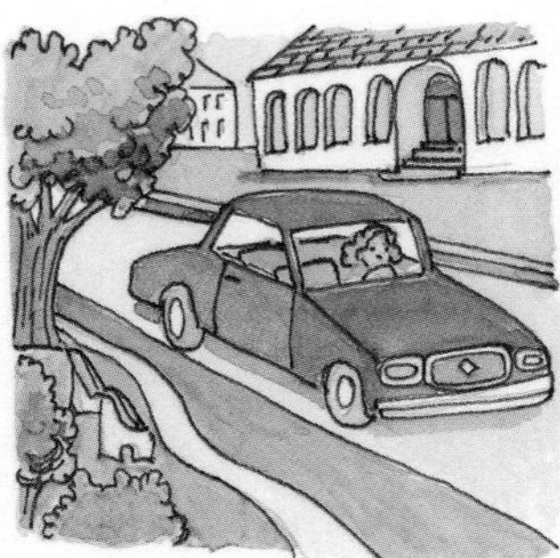

Maintenant, elle est **en face de** l'université, **près du** parc.

Suggestion: Point out the contractions with *de*.

Suggestion: Using your classroom layout, ask: *Où est* (name/object)*?* Have sts. answer: *Il/Elle est à côté de… , près de… ,* etc.

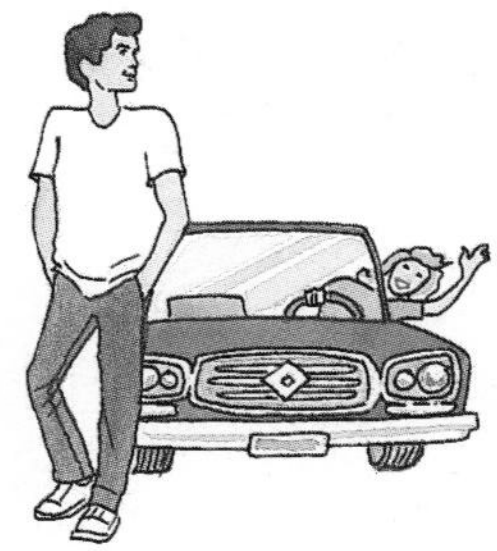

Justin est **devant** la voiture.

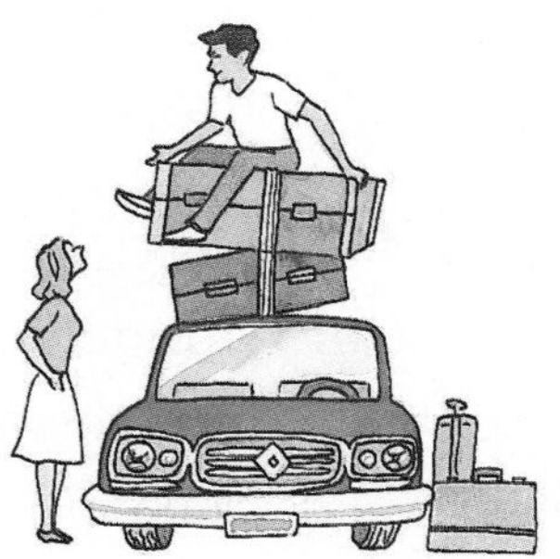

Clarisse est **à côté de** la voiture. Justin est **sur** la voiture.

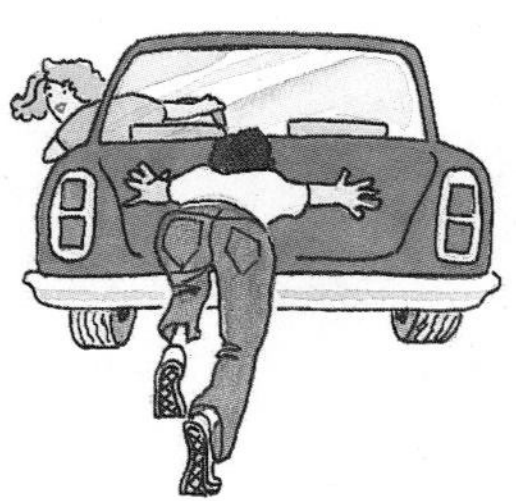

Justin pousse la voiture. Il est **derrière** la voiture.

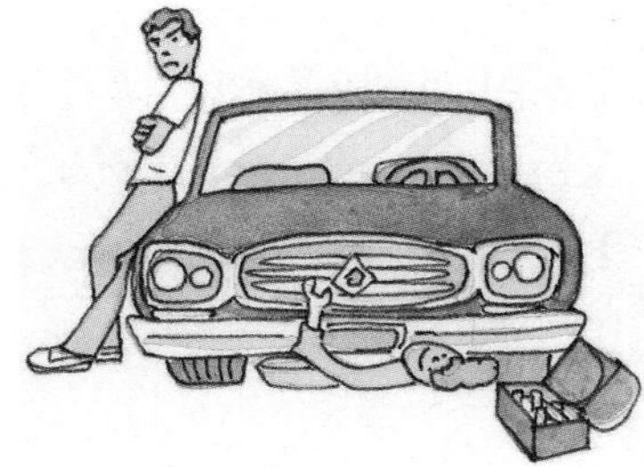

Clarisse est **sous** la voiture. Justin est **à gauche de** la voiture. Les outils (*tools*) sont **par terre, à droite de** la voiture.

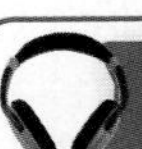

Prononcez bien!

The vowels in *sous* and *sur*

The difference between these two vowels lies in tongue position: in the back of your mouth for [u] in **sous,** and all the way to the front, pressing against your lower teeth, with tensely rounded and protruding lips, for [y] in **sur.**

[u]: **joue, court, blouson**

[y]: **jupe, cure, salut**

To help you produce the sound [y], pronounce the sound [i] in **dit,** and progressively round your lips, making sure your tongue does not shift to the back of your mouth: **du.**

dit → du

vie → vue

lit → lu

Pronunciation practice (1): Write the words *sous* and *sur* on the board, and have sts. decide whether the following words sound like the former or the latter: *université, roux, curieux, blouson, costume, jupe, pull-over, rouge, trouver, bureau, musique, plus, étudier, voiture, salut.*

Pronunciation practice (2): The *Prononcez bien!* section on page 110 of this chapter contains additional activities for practicing these sounds.

LES PRÉPOSITIONS DE LIEU	
dans	*in*
entre	*between*
chez	*at the home of; at the office of*
à côté de	*next to, beside*
en face de	*across from, opposite*
devant ≠ derrière	*in front of ≠ behind*
sur ≠ sous	*on ≠ under*
à gauche de ≠ à droite de	*to the left of ≠ to the right of*
près de ≠ loin de	*near ≠ far from*
par	*by; through*
par terre	*on the ground*

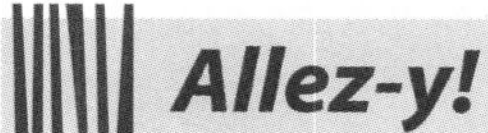

Allez-y!

A. Vrai ou faux? The following statements correspond (by number) to the drawings on the previous page. Correct any statements that are wrong.

1. Justin est assis (*seated*) sur le banc.
2. Clarisse est à côté du parc.
3. Elle est près de l'université.
4. Justin est derrière la voiture.
5. Clarisse est à gauche de la voiture.
6. Justin est en face de la voiture.
7. Clarisse est sur la voiture.

B. Désordre. Justin has a problem with clutter! Describe his room, using **les prépositions de lieu.**

MODÈLE: Il y a deux livres sous la chaise.

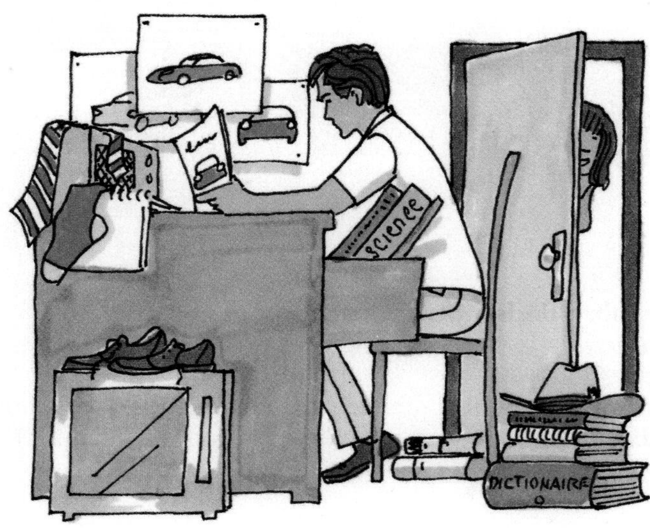

Follow-up: Place classroom objects on desk as in drawing. Ask sts. to describe scene. Move objects around several times to elicit different descriptions.

Additional activity: For listening comprehension practice, describe a simple scene and ask sts. to draw a sketch according to the description. Example: *Il y a une table. Derrière la table, il y a deux chaises. À côté de la table, il y a une étudiante. Sur la table, il y a des livres. Sous la table, il y a un chat,* etc.

Additional activity: Make copies of a simple drawing of a typical room. Sts. work in pairs: one st. describes the drawing, and the other st. reproduces it. As a follow-up, show the drawings in class and ask sts. to describe each (because they will vary).

Suggestions: (1) Model pronunciation, reinforcing with group and individual work. (2) Have sts. name object(s) that (a) can be held in the hand; (b) make noise; (c) one can sit on; (d) are for studying; (e) are decorative. (3) *Devinettes:* Indicate objects by describing their location: *Il est sur la table.* Sts. identify: *C'est le magazine.* Note that clothing vocabulary can be reentered here. (4) Hold up images of various objects and have sts. identify them.

Deux chambres d'étudiants

La chambre de Céline est en désordre. Elle loue un appartement dans un immeuble moderne.

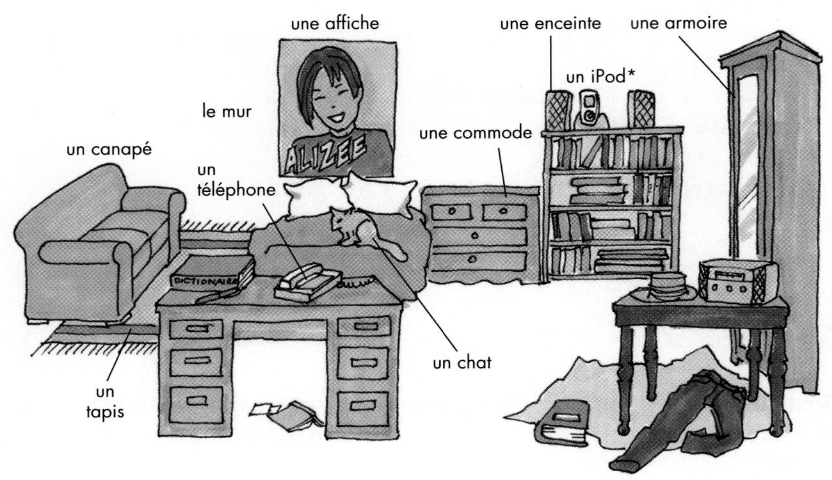

La chambre d'Anne est en ordre. Elle habite dans une maison.

Note: Cellphones and laptops are both called *portables.*

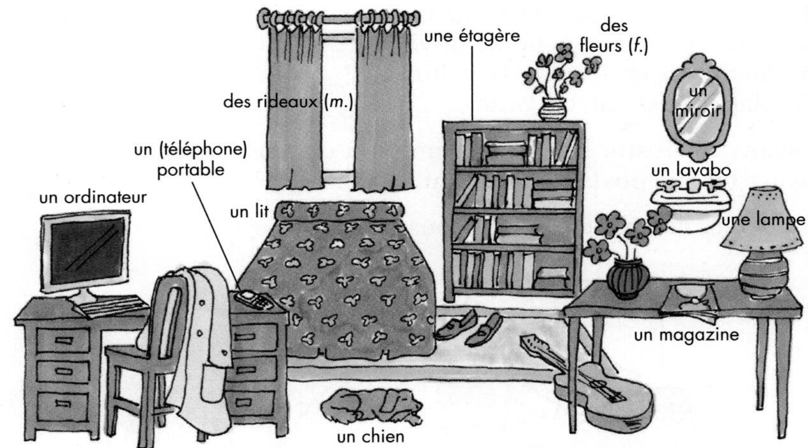

Note: *Chambres de bonne* are former maid's quarters on the top floor of 19th-century buildings. They are now often converted into lodgings and rented out to sts. as *studettes.*

AUTRES MOTS UTILES

une chambre de bonne	a maid's room; a garret
un meuble	a piece of furniture
un réveil	an alarm clock
une station d'accueil	a docking station (iPod, cellphone)
un studio	a studio (one-room apartment)

*iPod is a trademark of Apple, Inc.

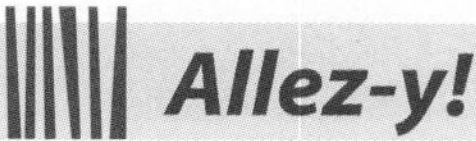

Allez-y!

A. Deux chambres. Taking turns with a partner, ask and answer questions about the two rooms. Start with **Qu'est-ce qu'il y a...** (*What is there . . .*).

MODÈLE: derrière l'étagère d'Anne? ⟶
É1: Qu'est-ce qu'il y a derrière l'étagère d'Anne?
É2: Il y a un mur.

1. sur le bureau de Céline? d'Anne?
2. à côté du lit de Céline? d'Anne?
3. sous la table de Céline? d'Anne?
4. sur le lit de Céline?
5. sur l'étagère de Céline? d'Anne?
6. devant le lit d'Anne?
7. à côté du téléphone de Céline?
8. sur le mur de Céline? d'Anne?
9. par terre dans la chambre de Céline? d'Anne?
10. sur la table d'Anne?
11. à côté de l'étagère d'Anne?
12. sur le tapis de Céline? d'Anne?

B. L'intrus. Three items are similar and one is different in each of the following series. Find the items that are out of place.

1. lit / commode / armoire / fleur
2. iPod / affiche / guitare / enceintes
3. lavabo / livre / magazine / étagère
4. miroir / affiche / rideaux / magazine

C. Préférences. What might you find in the room of a person with the following interests?

MODÈLE: les arts ⟶
Sur le mur, il y a des affiches; il y a des livres d'art dans l'étagère et à côté du lit,...

1. étudier
2. écouter de la musique
3. parler à des amis
4. le sport
5. la mode
6. le cinéma

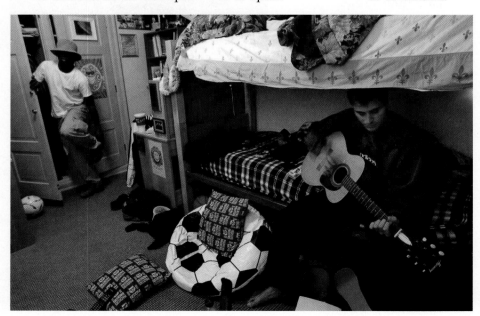

Décrivez (*Describe*) cette chambre d'étudiant à la cité-U.

Follow-up: Have sts. create a *devinette* as described in the previous marginal note.

Additional activity: *Quels objets dans les chambres d'Anne et de Céline associez-vous avec les mots suivants?* 1. *Taylor Swift* 2. *Paris-Match* 3. *la fenêtre* 4. *les livres* 5. *la rose* 6. *les murs* 7. *une définition* 8. *Calvin Klein*

Note (A): Make sure sts. use the indefinite article with the structure *Il y a*. Compare: *Il y a un mur derrière l'étagère* with *Le mur est derrière l'étagère.*

Follow-up (B): Have sts. add another word to each category. They can explain their choices in English. Possibilities: 1. *étagère* 2. *radio* 3. *dictionnaire* 4. *téléphone*

Suggestion (C): Do as a listening activity, with sts. writing down as many different items as they can.

Suggestions (C): (1) Ask several sts. to give a different answer for each question until possibilities are exhausted. (2) Could be done in pairs or small groups.

Leçon 2

Les articles indéfinis après *ne... pas*

Expressing the Absence of Something

Un logement pour une copine

Léa téléphone à Juliette.

LÉA: Salut Juliette! Est-ce que tu as un canapé dans ton nouveau studio?

JULIETTE: Léa**, je n'ai pas de** studio, mais simplement une chambre de bonne! Et **je n'ai pas de** canapé: c'est minuscule, chez moi! J'ai un lit, une chaise, une commode et un bureau. C'est tout!

LÉA: Ah… c'est ennuyeux… C'est pour une copine italienne. Elle est à Paris pour deux jours et **elle n'a pas de** logement.

JULIETTE: Elle a certainement de l'argent pour un petit hôtel au Quartier latin… Elle a de la famille… des amis…

LÉA: Non. **Elle n'a pas d**'argent… **pas de** famille à Paris… et **pas d**'amis, excepté moi.

JULIETTE: Et moi, **je n'ai pas de** place.

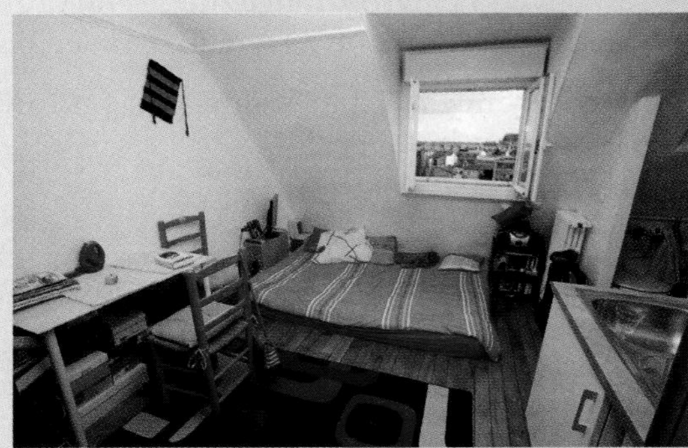

Une chambre de bonne sous les toits (*rooftops*)

Complétez les phrases selon le dialogue.

1. Juliette n'a pas… (*trois choses*)
2. L'amie italienne n'a pas… (*quatre choses*)

Presentation: Using simple drawings demonstrating sentences or using sts. as examples may make presentations more interesting. For example: *Maria (une étudiante) a un stylo, mais pas de papier,* etc.

Note: Point out that *pas de* is used as a negative expression of quantity to state the absence of something.

Presentation: Model pronunciation of sentences so sts. can hear the difference between *des* and *de.*

1. In negative sentences, the indefinite article (**un, une, des**) becomes **de (d')** after **pas.**

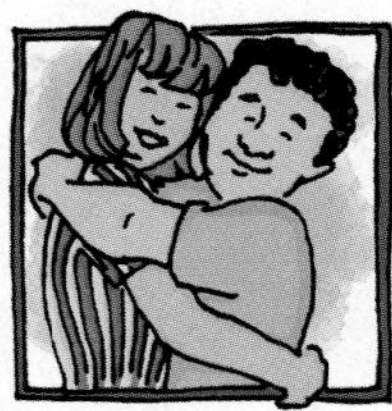

Il a une amie.

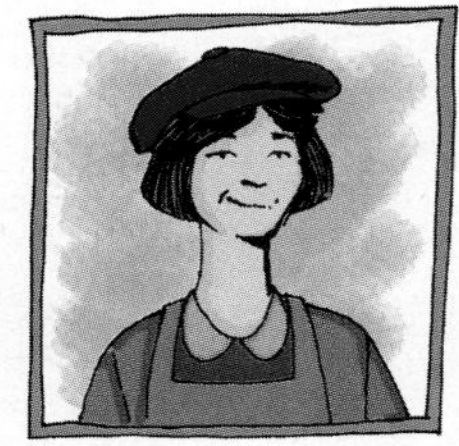

Elle porte une casquette.

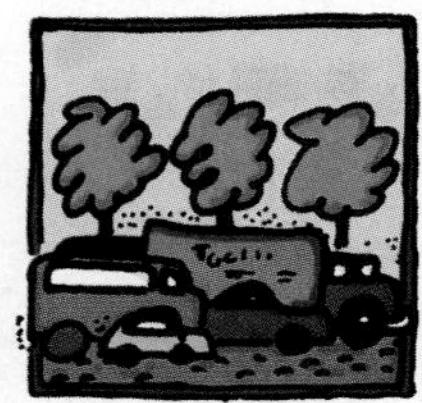

Il y a des voitures dans la rue.

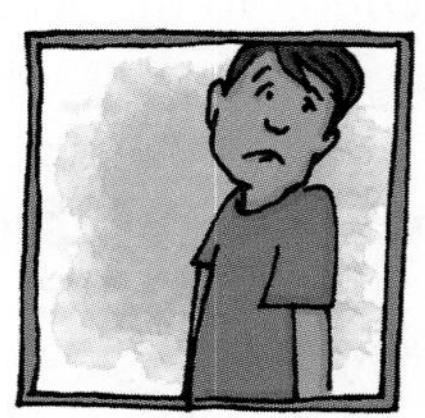

Il n'a pas d'amie.

Elle ne porte pas de casquette.

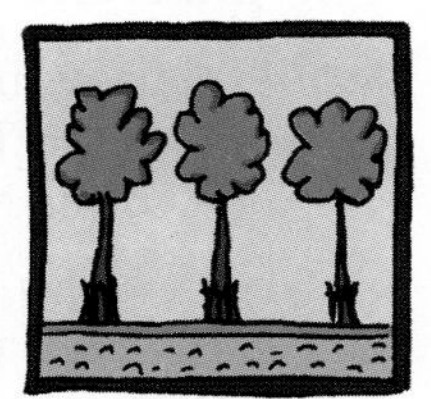

Il n'y a pas de voitures dans la rue.

Suggestion: To reinforce placement of *ne… pas de,* draw a picture of a hamburger on board or transparency, labeling the bun *ne,* the burger *the conjugated verb,* and the bottom bun *pas de.* This shows that the conjugated verb is "sandwiched" between *ne* and *pas de.* Note that this image can be recycled later when teaching direct and indirect objects, the *passé composé,* etc.

—Est-ce qu'il y a **un livre** sur la table?	*Is there a book on the table?*
—Non, il n'y a **pas de livre** sur la table.	*No, there is no book on the table.*
—Est-ce qu'il y a **des fleurs** sur la table?	*Are there any flowers on the table?*
—Non, il n'y a **pas de fleurs** sur la table.	*No, there aren't any flowers on the table.*

Suggestion: To help sts. memorize this structure, ask *Des problèmes / Des questions?* Have them answer *Pas de problème / Pas de question!* frequently.

Note: The negation *pas de* can be followed by a singular noun or a plural with no change in meaning: *pas de livre* and *pas de livres* both mean *no books.*

[Allez-y! A]

2. In negative sentences with **être,** however, the indefinite article does not change.

   —C'est un livre?
   —Non, ce n'est pas un livre.

3. The definite article **(le, la, les)** does not change in a negative sentence.

   —Elle a **la** voiture aujourd'hui?
   —Non, elle n'a pas **la** voiture.

[Allez-y! B]

Grammaire interactive

For more on the verb **avoir** and negation, watch the corresponding Grammar Tutorial and take a brief practice quiz at **Connect French.**

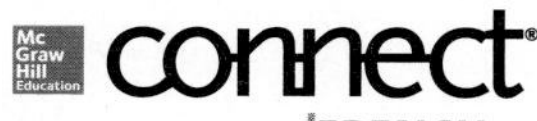

www.mhconnectfrench.com

Allez-y!

A. **Chambre à louer.** (*Room for rent.*) The room Jacob is inquiring about is very sparsely furnished. Play the roles of Jacob and his prospective landlord or landlady, following the example.

MODÈLE: une télé →
É1: Est-ce qu'il y a une télé dans la chambre?
É2: Non, il n'y a pas de télé.

1. un lavabo
2. une armoire
3. des tapis
4. des étagères
5. une commode
6. un lit

Additional activities: Ask the following questions pertaining to the classroom: *Est-ce qu'il y a une lampe dans la salle de classe? un lavabo? des étagères? des tapis? un miroir? un lit? une télévision?*

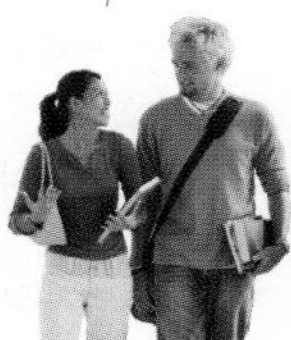

Vocabulary recycling: Review classroom items from *Chapitre 1, Leçon 3* along with prepositions from *Leçon 1* of this chapter. Have sts. write out 2–3 questions of their own, and encourage them to come up with bizarre possibilities: *Est-ce qu'il y a un professeur sous la table? Est-ce qu'il y a une étudiante sur le bureau?*

Follow-up: Dictate the following paragraph and then have sts. make each sentence negative. *Nous avons des CD. Ce sont des CD français. Il y a un CD de Carla Bruni ici. Tu as des CD intéressants.*

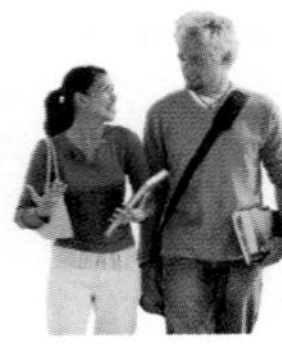

B. Une interview. Interview a classmate. Pay close attention to the articles.

MODÈLES: avoir un ordinateur →
É1: Tu as un ordinateur?
É2: Non, je n'ai pas d'ordinateur. *or* Oui, j'ai un ordinateur.

aimer les ordinateurs →
É1: Tu aimes les ordinateurs?
É2: Non, je n'aime pas les ordinateurs. *or* Oui, j'aime les ordinateurs.

1. étudier le russe (l'italien, l'allemand)
2. avoir une chambre (un appartement, une maison)
3. travailler le soir (*in the evening*) (le samedi, le dimanche)
4. avoir des albums de Beyoncé (des albums de musique classique, des albums de jazz)
5. aimer les chats (les chiens)
6. ?

Résumez! Now summarize what you have learned about your classmate for the rest of the class: **Il/Elle a… , mais il/elle n'a pas de (d')…**

Presentation: Model pronunciation. Have half the class take the role of Hassan and the other half the role of Léa.

Les mots interrogatifs

Getting Information

Studio à louer

Appel vidéo entre Hassan et Léa.

HASSAN: **Comment** vas-tu, Léa?
LÉA: Très bien… Je révise. J'ai un examen de littérature.
HASSAN: **Quand?** Demain?
LÉA: Non, jeudi. **Pourquoi**[1]**?**
HASSAN: Parce que[2] je visite un appartement tout à l'heure. Tu m'accompagnes?
LÉA: Mais, c'est nouveau! Tu déménages? **Où?** Dans **combien de** temps?
HASSAN: Dans quelques[3] jours, peut-être. Il y a un studio à louer, juste en face de mon restaurant. C'est une opportunité!
LÉA: **Qui** est le propriétaire?
HASSAN: C'est un client! Un jeune homme charmant…
LÉA: Vraiment? Alors, j'arrive!

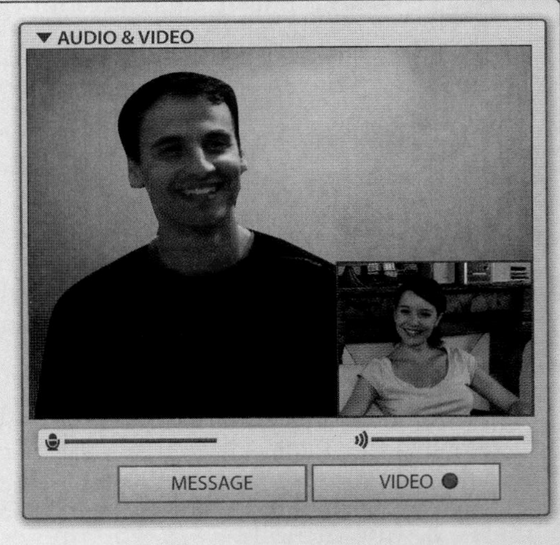

[1]*Why?* [2]*Parce... Because* [3]*several*

Trouvez les mots interrogatifs qui correspondent aux réponses ci-dessous.

1. Très bien.
2. Jeudi.
3. Parce que je visite un appartement.
4. En face de mon restaurant.
5. Dans quelques jours, peut-être.
6. Un client.

Information Questions with Interrogative Words

Information questions ask for new information or facts. They often begin with interrogative expressions. Here are some of the most common interrogative adverbs in French.

où	*where*	**pourquoi**	*why*
quand	*when*	**combien de**	*how much, how many*
comment	*how*		

Information questions can be formed with **est-ce que** or with a change in word order. (You may wish to review the presentation of yes/no questions in **Chapitre 3, Leçon 3.**) The interrogative word is usually placed at the beginning of the question.

1. These are information questions with **est-ce que.**

   Où / **Quand** / **Comment** / **Pourquoi** } **est-ce que** Samuel joue du banjo?

   Combien de fois par semaine (*times a week*) **est-ce que** Samuel joue?

2. These are information questions with a change in word order.

PRONOUN SUBJECT	NOUN SUBJECT
Où / **Quand** / **Comment** / **Pourquoi** } étudie-t-il la musique?	**Où** / **Quand** / **Comment** / **Pourquoi** } Samuel étudie-t-il la musique?
Combien d'instruments a-t-il?	**Combien d'**instruments Samuel a-t-il?

3. These are information questions consisting of a noun subject and verb only. With **où, quand, comment,** and **combien de,** it is possible to ask information questions using only a noun subject and the verb, with no pronoun.

   Où / **Quand** / **Comment** } étudie Samuel?

   Combien d'instruments a Samuel?

   However, the pronoun is almost always required with **pourquoi.**

   Pourquoi Samuel étudie-t-**il?**

[Allez-y! A-B-F]

Note: It is important that sts. understand the distinction between information questions and yes/no questions.

Suggestion: Remind sts. that *je* is almost never inverted with the verb; *est-ce que* is used instead.

Note: Questions with intonation are more familiar (*Où tu vas? Tu vas où?*). Questions with *est-ce que* are part of everyday language. Inversion is considered more formal in certain circumstances; it is used in writing and is preferred in formal conversation.

Note: You may wish to use this opportunity to introduce the interrogative expression *D'où* (From where)—*D'où viens-tu?* (Where are you from?).

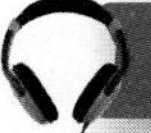

Prononcez bien!

The pronunciation of *quand*

Unlike English, in which *qu* is often pronounced [kw], in French, **qu** is generally pronounced [k], as in **que.**

[k]: **que, quand, quatre, Québec, physique**

Only when **qu** precedes **oi** is it pronounced [kw]: **pourquoi.**

In liaison, the **d** of **quand** is pronounced [t].

[t]: **quand est-ce que, quand on parle**

Information Questions with Interrogative Pronouns

Some of the most common French interrogative pronouns (**les pronoms interrogatifs**) are **qui, qu'est-ce que,** and **que. Que** becomes **qu'** before a vowel or mute **h. Qui** is invariable.

Suggestion: Point out that *qui* can be a subject, a direct object, or the object of a preposition.

Suggestion: Point out that when a verb is used with a preposition (remind sts. of *téléphoner à*, *montrer à*, *donner à* from *Chapitre 3*), the preposition will precede *qui* in a question.

Suggestion: Ask sts. to listen to the following paragraph for *who, what, when, where,* and *why* information. Afterward, they will ask each other those questions about the passage. *Marina habite à la cité universitaire. Elle a une chambre agréable mais petite. Le matin, elle est à l'université parce qu'elle a des cours. Elle est très contente parce qu'elle aime la vie universitaire.*

1. **Qui** (*who, whom*) is used to ask about a person or people.

Qui étudie le français?	*Who studies French?*
Qui regardez-vous? **Qui** est-ce que vous regardez?	*Whom are you looking at?*
À qui Samuel parle-t-il? **À qui** est-ce que Samuel parle?	*Whom is Samuel speaking to?*

2. **Qu'est-ce que** and **que** (*what*) refer to things or ideas. **Que** requires inversion.

Qu'est-ce que vous étudiez? **Qu'**étudiez-vous?	*What are you studying?*
Que pense-t-il de la chambre?	*What does he think of the room?*

[Allez-y! C-D-E-F]

Allez-y!

Suggestion: Use the following as preliminary exs.: A. *Transformez en questions:* 1. *Michel travaille.* (*où, quand, comment, pourquoi*) 2. *Marie achète des affiches.* (*qui, qu'est-ce que, combien de*) B. *Posez la question qui convient en utilisant qui ou qui est-ce que.* 1. *Richard a une nouvelle radio.* 2. *Les Boucher habitent près d'ici.* 3. *Marie cherche son amie Annick sur le campus.* C. *Maintenant posez des questions avec que ou qu'est-ce que.* 1. *Il y a de belles lampes ici.* 2. *Nous regardons les tables et les chaises.* 3. *Jacques cherche une nouvelle chambre.*

A. De l'argent. Monsieur Harpagon is sometimes stingy. Respond to these statements as he would, using **pourquoi.**

MODÈLE: J'ai besoin d'un manteau. →
Pourquoi avez-vous besoin d'un manteau?

1. Nous avons besoin d'une étagère.
2. Ariane a besoin d'un dictionnaire d'anglais.
3. Paul a besoin d'une voiture.
4. J'ai besoin d'un nouveau tapis.

B. Une chambre d'étudiant. Complete the conversation with the appropriate interrogative expressions. **Suggestions:** comment, où, pourquoi, quand, combien de...

MODÈLE: SABINE: Comment est la chambre?
JULIEN: La chambre est *très agréable.*

SABINE: ______?
JULIEN: La chambre est *sur la rue Napoléon.*
SABINE: ______?
JULIEN: J'emménage (*I move in*) *jeudi.*
SABINE: ______?
JULIEN: La chambre est *petite mais confortable.*

Additional activity: *Votre camarade joue le rôle d'un francophone qui passe une année à votre université. Vous demandez:* 1. where he/she is from 2. where he/she is living and with whom 3. how many courses he/she is taking 4. whether he/she is working and where 5. his/her feelings about the university or town.

SABINE: ______?
JULIEN: Il y a *deux* chaises et *une* table.
SABINE: ______?
JULIEN: La lampe est *à côté de la station d'accueil.*
SABINE: ______?
JULIEN: J'ai un iPod *parce que j'adore la musique.*
SABINE: ______?
JULIEN: J'écoute de la musique *quand j'étudie.*

C. Une visite chez Camille et Lola. Ask a question in response to each statement about Camille and Lola's new apartment. Use **qu'est-ce que** or **que.**

MODÈLE: Nous visitons le logement de Camille et Lola. →
Qu'est-ce que vous visitez? (*ou* Que visitez-vous?)

1. Nous admirons l'ordre de la chambre de Camille.
2. Il y a un miroir sur le mur.
3. Je regarde les affiches de Camille.
4. Je trouve des magazines intéressants.
5. Habib n'aime pas les rideaux à fleurs.
6. Nous aimons bien la vue et le balcon.
7. Ah non, la porte est ouverte! Tout le monde cherche le chat de Camille.

D. Les étudiants et le logement. With a little help from her friends, Brigitte finds a new room. Create a question, using **qui** or **à qui,** that corresponds to each item of information.

MODÈLE: *Brigitte* cherche un logement. →
Qui cherche un logement?

1. *Mme Boucher* a une petite chambre à louer dans une maison.
2. Vanessa et Richard parlent de Mme Boucher à *Brigitte.*
3. Brigitte téléphone à *Mme Boucher.* **4.** Mme Boucher montre la chambre à *Brigitte.* **5.** *Brigitte* loue la chambre de Mme Boucher.

E. Voici les réponses. Invent questions for these answers.

MODÈLE: Dans la chambre de Claire. →
Où est-ce qu'il y a des affiches de cinéma?
Où sont les livres de Cécile?

1. C'est un magazine français.
2. À l'université.
3. Parce que je n'ai pas envie d'étudier.
4. Vingt-quatre étudiants.
5. À Laure.
6. Djamila.
7. Très bien.
8. Parce que j'ai faim.
9. Maintenant.

F. Êtes-vous curieux/curieuse? Why is it always the instructor who asks questions? It's your turn to question him/her. Be formal; use inversion.

MODÈLES: D'où êtes-vous?
Pourquoi aimez-vous le français?

Mots clés

Giving reasons

To answer the question **pourquoi?,** use **parce que** (**parce qu'** before a vowel sound).

Je travaille **parce que** j'ai besoin d'argent.

Note (Mots clés): The structure *à cause de* (*because of*) is used before a noun.

Additional activity: *Une interview.* Interview a classmate. Answer using *il(s), elle(s),* and *c'est* when needed. 1. *D'où es-tu? Comment est la ville?* 2. *Où habites-tu, dans une maison, un appartement ou une résidence universitaire? Avec qui? Comment est ta chambre?* 3. *Est-ce que tu aimes l'université? Pourquoi? Combien de cours as-tu ce semestre? Comment sont tes cours?* 4. *Comment est ton/ta camarade de chambre?* 5. *Est-ce que tu parles avec tes amis après les cours? Où?*

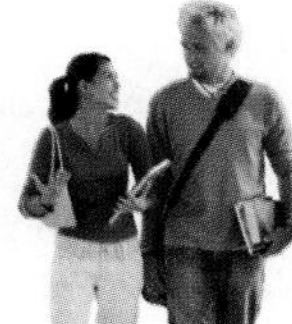

Suggestion: Give sts. a minute to think of questions to ask you. Or have sts. write their questions on cards to be handed in to you.

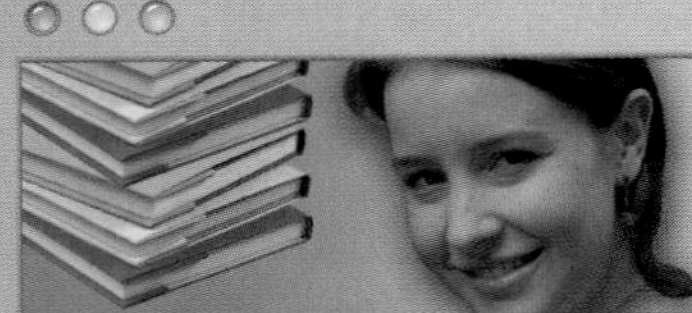

Le blog de Léa

Chez moi

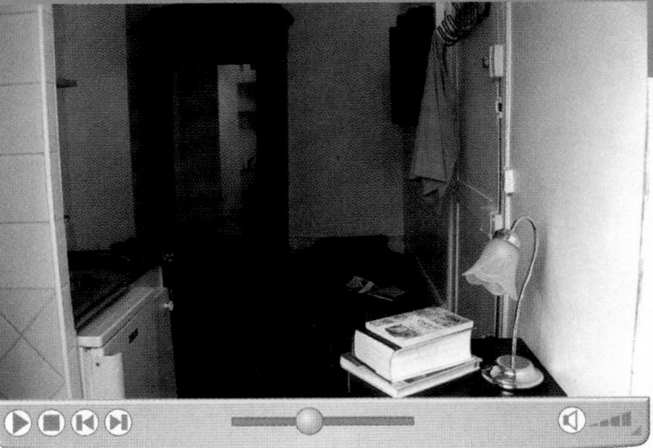

Un petit «chez moi»: une chambre de bonne

mercredi 25 mai

Chers amis du blog, j'ai un problème.

J'ai 19 ans et j'habite encore avec maman et papa. Ils trouvent ça normal. Pas moi.

Habiter un petit «chez moi», c'est mon rêve.[1] Juste un studio ou une simple chambre de bonne avec un lit, une armoire et une douche. Comme Juliette.

Voilà mon idéal: une petite chambre sous les toits,[2] à côté de la fac.

Mais ce n'est pas facile de trouver un logement à Paris, spécialement au Quartier latin. Je cherche, je regarde les petites annonces[3]... Rien.[4]

Quand est-ce que je vais trouver?

Hassan me conseille la colocation[5]: il a peut-être raison...

Léa

COMMENTAIRES

Alexis

Salut Léa!

Au Québec, comme aux États-Unis, les étudiants n'habitent pas chez leurs parents. Ils ont une chambre à l'université. Déménage[6]! Tu es une adulte, après tout.

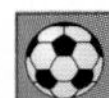

Mamadou

Moi aussi, Léa, pour étudier en France, j'ai déménagé à Paris. Ma famille habite toujours au Sénégal.

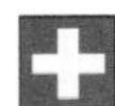

Charlotte

Pourquoi déménager? On est bien chez ses parents...

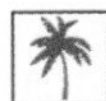

Poema

Ton copain[7] Hassan n'a pas tort: la colocation, c'est une solution intéressante. Propose à tes parents! D'ailleurs,[8] à côté de chez moi, il y a une chambre à louer. Elle a l'air pas mal. C'est une colocation. Regarde l'annonce sur Internet: «Étudiante d'origine québécoise cherche colocataire. Propose jolie chambre de 12 m^2 [9] dans bel appartement. Immeuble avec concierge. Au 5e étage[10] sans ascenseur.[11] 500 euros/mois, charges comprises.[12]»

Suggestion: Model pronunciation and have sts. repeat individually or as a group.

Follow-up: *Questions de compréhension: 1. Quel est le problème de Léa? 2. Expliquez la situation des étudiants québécois et sénégalais. Est-ce qu'ils habitent chez leurs parents? 3. Comment Léa imagine-t-elle son futur logement? 4. Expliquez les différentes solutions proposées par chaque commentateur. Quelle solution préférez-vous personnellement? 5. Que pensez-vous de l'annonce d'Internet? De la photo du «petit chez moi» de Léa?*

Video connection: In the videoblog for this chapter, Léa films her visit to the apartment offered by the student from Quebec and posts a video about Montreal on her site.

[1]*dream* [2]sous... *on the top floor* (lit. *under the roof*) [3]petites... *classified advertisements* [4]*Nothing* [5]me... *is advising me to get a roommate* [6]*Move out!* [7]*buddy* [8]*Moreover* [9]12 mètres carrés = *12 square meters = approx. 129 sq. ft.* [10]cinquième... = *6th floor* (of an American building) [11]sans... *without elevator* [12]*included*

REPORTAGE

Montréal: vivre en français

Parler français, dans une ambiance française, mais sur le continent américain, est-ce que c'est possible? Bien sûr!

Il y a près de chez vous un territoire francophone. C'est la province de Québec, au Canada. Dans cette région, le français est la langue officielle des administrations, du travail, du commerce et des communications.

Combien de membres représente cette communauté? Huit millions de personnes. Très actives et passionnément francophiles, elles désirent protéger leur héritage culturel francophone.

Étudiante américaine, Deborah étudie le français à l'université de Montréal pour devenir professeur. Tous les jours, elle lit[1] *Le journal de Montréal* ou *La presse.* À la télévision, elle regarde des programmes français proposés par le Réseau de l'Information[2] (RDI).

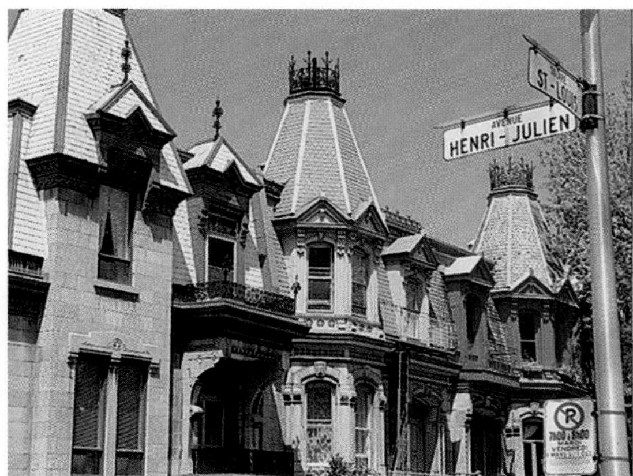

Montréal est la ville des contrastes: Les demeures (*residences*) anciennes du Vieux-Montréal et d'autres quartiers montréalais s'opposent aux grands immeubles ultra modernes d'autres secteurs de la ville.

Elle aime se promener[3] dans les rues tranquilles de la vieille ville. «J'ai l'impression d'être en Europe», dit-elle. On comprend[4] pourquoi: Montréal a été fondé[5] par les Français en 1642.[6] Ses origines sont évidentes dans son architecture, dans les noms des rues, dans le Vieux-Port. Mais surtout,[7] à Montréal, on attache une importance essentielle à la beauté de l'environnement et à la qualité de vie. Exactement comme à Paris, à Rome ou à Madrid.

[1]*reads* [2]Réseau... *Information Network* [3]se... *to walk* [4]*understands* [5]a... *was founded* [6]mille six cent quarante-deux [7]*especially*

À vous!

1. Regardez la carte à la fin du livre. Où est la province de Québec? la ville de Montréal?
2. Pourquoi est-ce qu'on parle français à Montréal?
3. Pourquoi Deborah aime-t-elle particulièrement Montréal?
4. Sur la photo, quels détails suggèrent que Montréal est une ville francophone?

Parlons-en!

Travaillez à deux. Répondez, tour à tour, à ces deux questions que vous pose votre camarade:

Comment s'appelle la ville où tu es né(e) (*born*)? Où est-elle située? Utilisez les prépositions de lieu données dans votre manuel (page 93). Suivez le modèle.

MODÈLE: Je suis né(e) à La Nouvelle-Orléans. La ville est située sur le Mississippi. La Nouvelle-Orléans n'est pas loin du Golfe du Mexique.

Additional activity: Have sts. work in pairs. Display or print out a map of Quebec. Each person chooses a city or town with a French name. Have them take turns asking and answering the following questions: *Comment s'appelle la ville? Où est-elle située?*

Leçon 3

STRUCTURES

Les verbes en *-ir*

Expressing Actions

Du camping à Londres?

Léa et Juliette discutent au café.

JULIETTE: **Tu réfléchis à** nos vacances?
LÉA: Oui! J'ai envie de faire du ski d'été dans les Alpes. Ou bien de visiter Londres. **Tu choisis!**
JULIETTE: Léa, **on finit** toujours par aller où tu désires! Alors, tu décides!
LÉA: Bon: c'est Londres!
JULIETTE: Ça va. J'aime bien l'Angleterre. Si **nous réussissons** à trouver un petit hôtel pas cher, c'est d'accord.
LÉA: Non. L'hôtel, c'est impersonnel. **Je réfléchis à** une autre solution de logement.
JULIETTE: Le camping, par exemple? (Elle rit.)

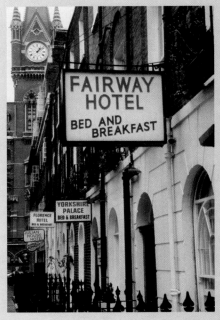

Londres, une des destinations préférées des jeunes français

Complétez les phrases par les verbes en **-ir** qui figurent dans le dialogue.

1. Tu ______ à nos vacances?
2. Tu ______ les Alpes ou Londres?
3. Comme toujours, on ______ par aller où tu désires!
4. Nous ______ à trouver un petit hôtel.
5. Je ______ à une solution.

Vocabulary recycling: Quickly review forms of regular *-er* verbs (*parler, visiter, danser*) before beginning regular *-ir* verbs. Have sts. lead classmates in rapid-response drills using their own original examples. Model pronunciation of verb forms. Compare the pronunciation of *ss* [s] to *s* [z] between vowels.

Note: Many *-ir* verbs are derived from descriptive adjectives (*vieil* → *vieillir*; *blanc* → *blanchir*; *grand* → *grandir*, etc.). For extra conjugation practice, use "color" verbs: *bleuir, brunir, jaunir, noircir, rougir, verdir.*

Although the infinitives of the largest group of French verbs end in **-er,** those of a second group end in **-ir.** To form the present tense of these verbs, drop the final **-ir** and add the endings shown in the chart.

PRESENT TENSE OF **finir** (*to finish*)			
je	fin**is**	nous	fin**issons**
tu	fin**is**	vous	fin**issez**
il/elle/on	fin**it**	ils/elles	fin**issent**

The **-is** and **-it** endings of the singular forms have silent final consonants. The double **s** of the plural forms is pronounced.

1. Other verbs conjugated like **finir** include:

agir	*to act*
choisir	*to choose*
réfléchir (à)	*to reflect (upon), to consider*
réussir (à)	*to succeed (in)*

J'**agis** toujours avec logique. — *I always act logically.*
Nous **choisissons** des affiches. — *We're choosing some posters.*

2. The verb **réfléchir** requires the preposition **à** before a noun when it is used in the sense of *to consider, to think about,* or *to reflect upon something.*

Elles **réfléchissent aux** questions de Paul. — *They are thinking about Paul's questions.*

3. The verb **réussir** requires the preposition **à** before an infinitive or before the noun* in the expression **réussir à un examen** (*to pass an exam*).†

Je **réussis** souvent **à** trouver les réponses. — *I often succeed in finding the answers.*
Marc **réussit** toujours **à** l'examen d'histoire. — *Marc always passes the history exam.*

4. The verb **finir** requires the preposition **de** before an infinitive. When **finir** is followed by **par** + infinitive, it means *to end up* (*doing*).

En général, je **finis d'**étudier à 8 h 30. — *I usually finish studying at 8:30.*
On **finit** souvent **par** regarder la télé. — *We often end up watching TV.*

Additional vocabulary: *-ir* verbs: *grandir, grossir, maigrir, obéir (à), pâlir, punir, réagir*

Note: Stress the use of the preposition *à* after *réfléchir* and *réussir*, and *de* or *par* when *finir* is followed by an infinitive.

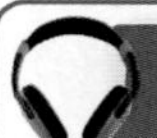

Prononcez bien!

The consonant *s*

When the letter **s** begins a word and when it occurs between a vowel and a consonant, pronounce it as [s].

[s]: **réponse**

When it is surrounded by two vowels, pronounce it as [z].

[z]: **choisir**

To make an [s] sound between two vowels, the spelling is usually **ss.** Remember to write **ss** in conjugations that require it.

[s]: **finissez, réussissons**

Notice that the sound [s] can also be produced by other letters.

[s]: **merci, ça, nation, soixante**

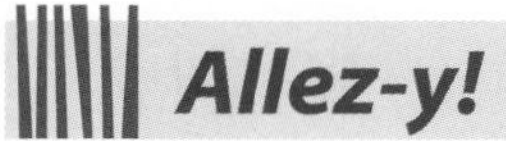

Allez-y!

Suggestion (A): Can be done orally or in writing. You may want to let sts. work through ex. in writing first and then give answers orally.

A. À la bibliothèque. Read the following description of Céline's visit to the library. Then imagine that Céline and Anne are there together and restate the account using **nous.**

Je choisis un livre de référence sur la Révolution française. Je réfléchis au sujet. Je réussis à trouver une revue intéressante sur la Révolution. Je finis très tard.

B. En cours de littérature. Complete the sentences with appropriate forms of **agir, choisir, finir, réfléchir,** or **réussir.**

1. Le professeur _____ des textes intéressants.
2. Les étudiants _____ avant de répondre aux questions du professeur.
3. Pierre et Anne _____ toujours leur travail très vite (*fast*).
4. Nous _____ toujours aux examens.
5. Toi, tu _____ souvent sans (*without*) réfléchir.

Pronunciation practice (1): Pronounce the following words and have sts. decide whether they are spelled with one *s* or two: *bonsoir, six, professeur, mademoiselle, finissons, pessimiste, chaise, monsieur, réfléchissez, philosophie, intéressant, blouson, salut, besoin, rousse, amusant.*

Pronunciation practice (2): The *Prononcez bien!* section on page 110 of this chapter contains additional activities for practicing these sounds.

Additional activity (A): *En français, s'il vous plaît.* 1. Marie-Josée always chooses difficult courses. 2. She thinks about university studies and succeeds in finding dynamic professors. 3. She never acts without thinking (*sans réfléchir*). 4. She finishes studying at the library.

*Note the exception: **réussir sa vie** (*to make a success of one's life*) does not require the preposition **à.**
†**Passer un examen** means *to take an exam,* not *to pass* one.

C. Choisissez! What might these people pick out for their new rooms? **Suggestions:** une armoire, des enceintes, des étagères, un iPod, un miroir, un ordinateur

MODÈLE: Karim. Il aime la musique. → Il choisit un iPod.

1. Ako. Elle étudie l'informatique. **2.** Fatima et Julie. Elles ont beaucoup de livres. **3.** Luc. Il est vaniteux (*vain*). **4.** Antoine et Romain. Ils ont beaucoup de vêtements. **5.** Chantal. Elle aime écouter la musique très fort (*loud*).

Follow-up: Ask the class the same questions using *Qui…* (*Qui dans la classe agit sans réfléchir?*). Solicit responses that require sts. to talk about their partners.

D. Une conversation. Use the following cues as a springboard for discussion with a classmate.

MODÈLE: réussir / aux examens →
É1: Est-ce que tu réussis toujours aux examens?
É2: Oui, bien sûr, je réussis toujours aux examens!
É1: Ah, tu es intelligent(e)! Moi, je ne réussis pas toujours aux examens.

1. agir / souvent / sans réfléchir
2. finir / exercices / français
3. choisir / cours (difficiles, faciles,…)
4. réfléchir / problèmes (politiques, des étudiants,…)
5. choisir / camarade de chambre (patient, intellectuel, calme,…)

La place de l'adjectif qualificatif

Describing People, Places, and Things

Cinquante euros la nuit

Léa téléphone à Juliette.

LÉA: Juliette, je suis sur le site Booking.com. Voici une proposition **intéressante:** «Loue **beau** studio dans **joli petit** immeuble **ancien. Bon** quartier de Londres.»
JULIETTE: Tu as des photos?
LÉA: Oui, deux photos. Je regarde… Ah! La vue est horrible: un parking!
JULIETTE: Comment est la salle de bains?
LÉA: Il y a une **petite** douche avec un **vieux** rideau. Les murs sont jaunes!
JULIETTE: Stop! C'est non! Je déteste le jaune!
LÉA: Mais Juliette, ce n'est pas cher! 50 euros la nuit!

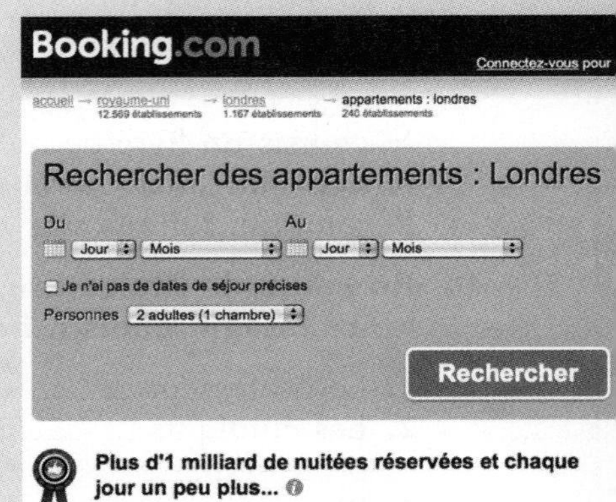

Le boom des réservations sur Internet

Quelles sont les caractéristiques du studio, de l'immeuble et du quartier? Utilisez les adjectifs du dialogue.

1. C'est un _____ studio.
2. C'est un _____ _____ immeuble ancien.
3. C'est un _____ quartier.
4. C'est une _____ douche.
5. C'est un _____ rideau.

Adjectives That Usually Precede the Noun

Presentation: Use the mnemonic device BAGS (beauty, age, goodness, size) to help sts. remember the short adjectives that precede. Show pictures of famous people, and describe them using these adjectives (*C'est un bon acteur; C'est un petit homme;* etc.).

1. Certain short and commonly used adjectives usually precede the nouns they modify.

REGULAR	IRREGULAR	IDENTICAL IN MASCULINE AND FEMININE
grand(e)* *big, tall; great*	**ancien / ancienne*** *old; former*	**autre** *other*
joli(e) *pretty*	**beau / belle** *beautiful, handsome*	**chaque** *each, every*
mauvais(e) *bad*	**bon(ne)** *good*	**jeune** *young*
petit(e) *small, little*	**cher / chère*** *dear; expensive*	**pauvre*** *poor; unfortunate*
vrai(e) *true*	**dernier / dernière** *last*	
	faux / fausse *false*	
	gentil(le) *nice, kind*	
	gros(se) *large; fat, thick*	
	long(ue) *long*	
	nouveau / nouvelle *new*	
	premier / première *first*	
	vieux / vieille *old*	

Marise habite une **petite** chambre en cité-U. — *Marise lives in a small room at the university dormitory.*
Les **jeunes** étudiants aiment bien le cinéma. — *Young students like to go to the movies.*
C'est une **bonne** idée! — *It's a good idea!*

2. The adjectives **beau, nouveau,** and **vieux** are irregular. They have two masculine forms in the singular.

SINGULAR		
MASCULINE	MASCULINE BEFORE VOWEL OR MUTE **h**	FEMININE
un **beau** livre	un **bel** appartement	une **belle** voiture
un **nouveau** livre	un **nouvel** appartement	une **nouvelle** voiture
un vieux livre	un **vieil** appartement	une **vieille** voiture
PLURAL		
MASCULINE		FEMININE
de **beaux** appartements		de **belles** voitures
de **nouveaux** appartements		de **nouvelles** voitures
de **vieux** appartements		de **vieilles** voitures

[Allez-y! A]

*More information about **grand, ancien, cher,** and **pauvre** can be found on the next page.

Grammaire interactive

For more on the gender, number, and position of adjectives, watch the corresponding Grammar Tutorial and take a brief practice quiz at **Connect French.**

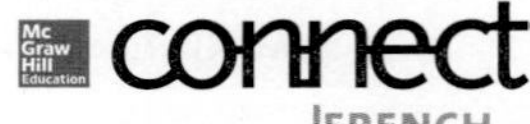

www.mhconnectfrench.com

Adjectives Preceding Plural Nouns

When an adjective precedes a noun in the plural form, the plural indefinite article **des** generally becomes **de.***

J'ai **des** livres de français. ⟶ J'ai **de** nouveaux livres de français.
Il y a **des** films à la télé. ⟶ Il y a **de** vieux films à la télé.

[Allez-y! B-C]

Adjectives That Can Precede or Follow Nouns They Modify

The adjectives **ancien / ancienne** (*old; former*), **cher / chère** (*dear; expensive*), **grand(e),** and **pauvre** can either precede or follow a noun, but their meaning depends on their position. Generally, the adjective in question has a literal meaning when it follows the noun and a figurative meaning when it precedes the noun.

LITERAL SENSE	FIGURATIVE SENSE
Il a des chaises **anciennes.** *He has antique chairs.*	M. Sellier est l'**ancien** propriétaire. *Mr. Sellier is the former landlord.*
C'est un lecteur de DVD très **cher.** *That's a very expensive DVD player.*	Ma **chère** amie… *My dear friend . . .*
C'est un homme très **grand.**† *He's a very tall man.*	C'est un très **grand** homme. *He's a great man.*
Les étudiants **pauvres** reçoivent une bourse de l'État. *Poor (not rich) students* receive a scholarship from the state.	**Pauvres** étudiants! Il y a un examen demain! *The poor (unfortunate) students! There is an exam tomorrow!*

Placement of More Than One Adjective

When more than one adjective modifies a noun, each adjective precedes or follows the noun as if it were used alone.

C'est une **petite** femme **blonde.**
J'ai de **bons** livres **français.**
C'est un **vieil** immeuble **agréable.**

---

*In informal speech, **des** is often retained before the plural adjective: **Elle a toujours *des belles* plantes.**

†The adjective **grand(e)** is placed *after* the noun to mean *big* or *tall* only in descriptions of people. In descriptions of things and places, **grand(e)** is placed *before* the noun to mean *big, large,* or *tall:* **les grandes fenêtres, un grand appartement, une grande table.**

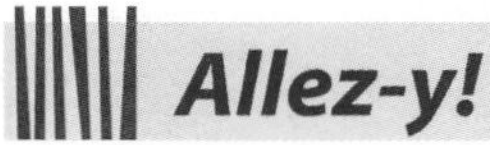

Allez-y!

A. Vous déménagez? You are moving out of the apartment you share with a friend. Specify which items you are taking with you.

MODÈLE: la table / vieux → J'emporte la vieille table.

1. le lit / petit
2. les tapis / grand
3. l'ordinateur / nouveau
4. le lecteur de DVD / vieux
5. la commode / grand
6. les chaises / beau

B. David emménage! David has moved into his new apartment, and he's explaining where everything goes. Give the plural form of the nouns, and make the appropriate agreements.

MODÈLE: Je place un beau vase sur l'étagère. →
Je place de beaux vases sur l'étagère.

Pour décorer, je mets une vieille affiche[1] sur le mur. Près du lit, il y a une petite lampe[2]. J'ai une nouvelle chaise[3] pour la table de cuisine. À la fenêtre, j'installe un long rideau.[4] Pour me détendre (*relax*), je passe (*play*) un bon album.[5] Pour finir, j'invite un vieux copain[6] (*buddy*).

C. L'amie de David. David's friend Julie has joined him to go shopping for things for his new apartment. For each sentence, provide the proper form and placement for the adjectives within parentheses.

MODÈLE: David regrette les _______ excursions _______. (ennuyeux, long) →
David regrette les longues excursions ennuyeuses.

1. Il cherche une _______ commode _______. (ancien, autre)
2. Julie est une _______ femme _______. (petit, sympathique)
3. Elle porte une _______ robe _______. (beau, blanc)
4. Le petit ami de Julie est un _______ homme _______. (dynamique, jeune)
5. Il aime les _______ voitures _______. (américain, vieux)

D. Jeu de logique. Complete the following thoughts logically using **les mots de liaison** found in the **Mots clés.**

1. J'habite dans un beau quartier, _______ c'est un peu cher.
2. Je vais déménager (*I'm going to move*) _______ je trouve un nouvel appartement.
3. J'ai envie d'habiter dans le vieux quartier de la ville _______ en banlieue (*in the suburbs*).
4. Pour le moment, mon amie Jeanne n'a pas d'argent, _______ elle habite chez ses (*her*) parents.
5. C'est une femme calme _______ organisée.
6. Elle commence un nouvel emploi (*job*) le mois prochain (*next*), _______ elle pense emménager avec moi.

E. Chez moi. Ask a classmate to describe his/her room. Use questions to get information on placement, color, size, and so on. As he/she gives you the details, draw a plan of the room. Then repeat the exercise, answering his/her questions about your room.

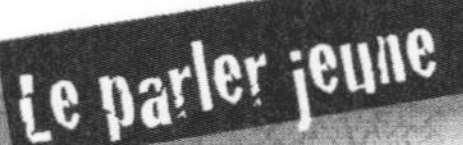

Le parler jeune

un appart	un appartement
un coloc	un colocataire
une piaule	une chambre
un pieu / un plumard	un lit
un proprio	un propriétaire

Mon **appart** est joli mais trop petit!

Ton **coloc** est un ami?

Max loue une **piaule** au Quartier latin.

Le matin, impossible de sortir de mon **pieu**!

Ton **proprio,** il est sympa?

Mots clés

Using conjunctions

To make more complex and interesting sentences, use the following words:

et	*and*
alors	*so*
ou	*or*
mais	*but*
si	*if*
donc	*therefore*

Geneviève est riche **et (mais)** généreuse.

J'habite près de l'université **donc (alors)** j'étudie souvent à la bibliothèque.

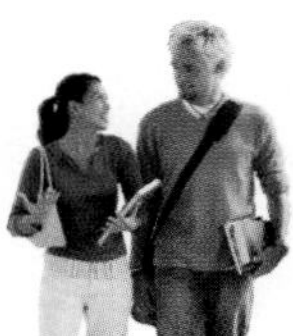

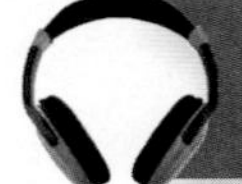

Prononcez bien!

Script (1A): *Rappelle-toi! Elle était rousse, aux cheveux courts, avec une jupe, un pull-over et des chaussures rouges; étudiante à l'université, en musique; intelligente et curieuse.*

Answers (1B): 1. *court/cours* 2. *joue/joues/jouent* 3. *du* 4. *vous* 5. *tu* 6. *nous* 7. *pour*

1. **The vowels in *sous* and *sur*** (page 92)

A. Questions pour un champion! You and your roommate Hugo are watching your favorite game show on TV. Hugo is talking about Justine, one of the contestants from the day before. You don't remember her, so Hugo describes her. Listen and complete the paragraph with the words you hear. Each one contains the sound [u] as in **sous** or [y] as in **sur**.

HUGO: Rappelle-toi! Elle était (*was*) __________,[1] aux cheveux __________,[2] avec une __________,[3] un __________[4] et des __________[5] __________;[6] __________[7] à l' __________,[8] en __________;[9] intelligente et __________.[10]

B. Le jeu de l'autre mot. The show starts with a game in which the host says a word containing either [u] as in **sous** or [y] as in **sur** and asks contestants to come up with a similar-sounding word containing the other vowel. Your partner will play the **présentateur/présentatrice** (*host*) and read the following words while you play one of the **candidats** (*contestants*) and give the answers.

MODÈLE: PRÉSENTATEUR/PRÉSENTATRICE: rousse
CANDIDAT(E): russe

1. cure **2.** jus (*juice*) **3.** doux (*soft*) **4.** vue (*view*) **5.** tout (*all*) **6.** nu (*naked*) **7.** pur(e)

Script (2A): *Bonsoir! Je m'appelle Sébastien. Je suis professeur de philosophie à l'université de la Sorbonne. Mes étudiants aiment bien mes cours. Ils disent qu'ils sont difficiles, mais intéressants et, parfois, amusants. Quand les étudiants font des efforts et qu'ils réfléchissent beaucoup, ils réussissent bien au cours.*

Script: (2B): 1. *rose, danser, télévision, gymnase, visiter* 2. *classe, université, russe, travailleuse, chaussette*

Answers (2B): 1. *danser* 2. *travailleuse*

2. **The consonant *s*** (page 105)

A. Un nouveau joueur. One of the contestants was eliminated and replaced by a new one, who is now introducing himself. Listen and complete the sentences.

__________[1]! Je m'appelle __________.[2] Je suis __________[3] de __________[4] à l' __________[5] de la Sorbonne. Mes étudiants aiment bien mes cours. Ils __________[6] qu'ils sont __________,[7] mais __________[8] et, parfois, __________.[9] Quand les étudiants font des efforts et qu'ils __________[10] beaucoup, ils __________[11] bien au cours.

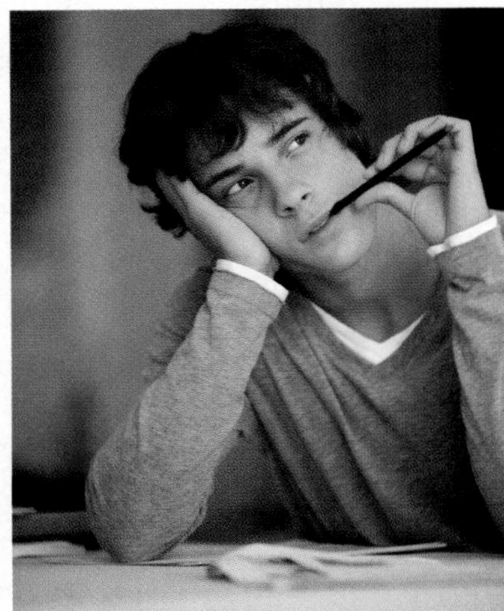

B. Trouvez l'intrus. After the contestants' introduction, the show resumes with two *Odd Man Out* games. The presenter will read two lists of five words that contain the letter s. Say the word that doesn't belong, based on its sound.

Leçon 4

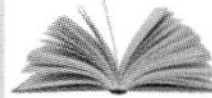

Lecture

Avant de lire

Predicting content from titles. The title of a reading selection often helps you anticipate content by activating your background knowledge about a topic. Brainstorming topics based on a title before you read will make reading easier, because you will already have information in mind that can aid your comprehension.

The text you will read in this section is called "La colocation." What do you already know about renting a room or a house with another person? Make a short list of the advantages and disadvantages. Use the following questionnaire as a guide. Then, as you read, see how many of the items you mentioned appear in the text.

Acceptable ou inacceptable? Which of the following situations would you consider acceptable or unacceptable behavior from a housemate?

	ACCEPTABLE	INACCEPTABLE
1. Votre colocataire (*housemate*) organise une soirée; vous n'êtes pas invité(e).	☐	☐
2. Les amis de votre colocataire arrivent à l'improviste (*unexpectedly*).	☐	☐
3. Le petit ami / La petite amie de votre colocataire emménage chez vous.	☐	☐
4. Votre colocataire mange vos provisions, mais il/elle aime cuisiner (*to cook*) pour vous.	☐	☐
5. Votre colocataire déménage sans donner de préavis (*without notice*).	☐	☐

Additional activities: A. Ask sts. about their own living situations; use the following questions and vocabulary: *Habitez-vous seul(e) ou avec un(e) colocataire? Quels sont les avantages et les désavantages de votre situation? Vocabulaire utile: aimer la vie privée / la compagnie des autres; c'est pratique / économique / cher; le loyer* (rent) / *l'hypothèque* (mortgage); *coûter cher / peu; préférer le calme / le confort.* MODÈLE: *J'habite seul(e) parce que je préfère le calme.* B. *Comparez-vous à votre camarade de chambre, votre colocataire ou un bon ami / une bonne amie. Utilisez les expressions suivantes ou d'autres que vous connaissez.* (The conjugation of *faire* is introduced in *Chapitre 5;* encourage sts. to follow the model and use the infinitive form after conjugated verbs such as *aimer, détester,* and *préférer.*) *Vocabulaire: l'ordre, le désordre, les factures* (bills), *le téléphone; ordonné(e), désordonné(e), organisé(e), désorganisé(e); nettoyer, ranger, payer, partager, aimer / détester faire le ménage* (to do housework), *faire la vaisselle* (to do the dishes), *faire des tâches ménagères* (to do chores); *tout le temps, souvent, quelquefois, ne… jamais,* etc.

La colocation

En France: un phénomène nouveau et populaire

Vous êtes jeune, avec un petit budget, et vous cherchez un logement? Bonne chance! Trouver un logement indépendant à Paris et dans les grandes villes est presque[1] impossible! Pourquoi? Parce que les chambres de bonne sous les toits, les studettes[2] et les studios pour étudiants sont rares et chers. Et les candidats très nombreux. Mais il y a une solution: partager[3] un appartement avec des amis.

[1]*almost* [2]*maids' rooms, typically with shared bathrooms and showers* [3]*share*

À propos de la lecture…
This reading was adapted from *Quo* magazine.

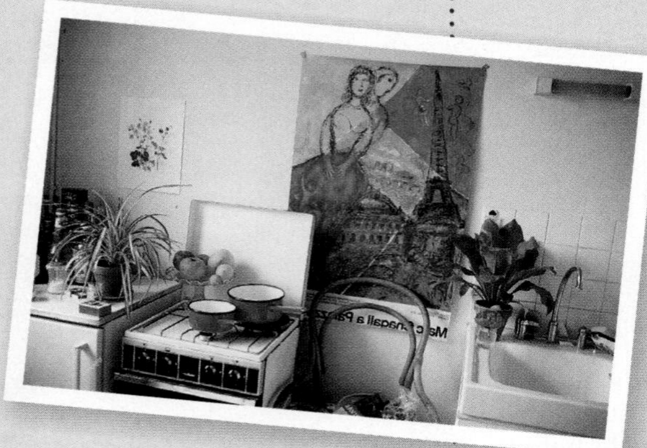

Voici un petit appartement à partager. Est-ce que vous aimez le décor? Pourquoi / Pourquoi pas?

Une expérience unique

Vivre ensemble dans un appartement, étudier, partager la même salle de bains, faire les courses, préparer à dîner, c'est amusant, mais ce n'est pas facile. Pour les Français qui sont très indépendants, la colocation, ce phénomène nouveau, demande des efforts et de la patience. Mais quelle expérience enrichissante! Voilà une occasion unique d'apprendre la tolérance et d'établir des amitiés éternelles.

Bien vivre en colocation

Pour une colocation réussie, voici quelques règles de vie commune.

- **Les amis.** N'encouragez pas vos amis à venir à l'improviste, surtout juste avant un examen. Présentez vos amis à votre colocataire.
- **Les soirées.** Écrivez les dates de vos soirées sur un calendrier commun pour éviter[4] de mauvaises surprises. Invitez votre colocataire à vos soirées de temps en temps.
- **Le petit ami / La petite amie.** Si le contrat stipule deux personnes, la colocation n'est pas pour trois ou quatre personnes!
- **La nourriture.[5]** Achetez la nourriture séparément et ne mangez pas les provisions de l'autre.
- **Le ménage.[6]** Il y a des degrés variables de tolérance au désordre. Il est nécessaire de parler de ce sujet avec votre colocataire et de partager le travail.

Et n'oubliez pas[7]: le dialogue et l'humour sont essentiels quand on partage un appartement!

[4]*avoid* [5]*Food* [6]*Housework* [7]*n'... don't forget*

Compréhension

A. Pourquoi? Expliquez pourquoi...

1. les étudiants choisissent la colocation plus souvent que les autres groupes.
2. il est difficile pour les Français de vivre en colocation.
3. la colocation est une expérience enrichissante.

B. Oui ou non? Indiquez si l'auteur du texte conseille (*recommends*) ou déconseille les comportements suivants.

1. Si le petit ami / la petite amie de votre colocataire emménage chez vous, accueillez-le/la (*welcome him/her*).
2. Désignez une personne pour faire le ménage, une autre pour faire la cuisine.
3. Parlez des problèmes immédiatement.
4. N'invitez pas votre colocataire à vos soirées.
5. La nourriture dans le frigo appartient à (*belongs to*) tout le monde.

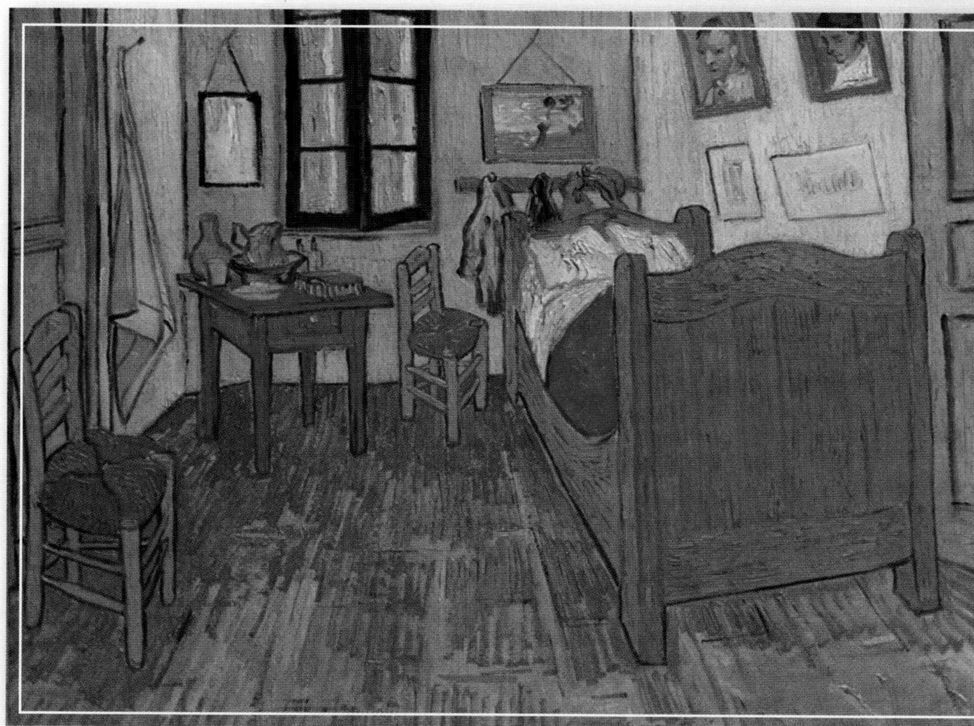

Un peu plus...

Vincent Van Gogh.
Van Gogh (1853–1890) was born in the Netherlands but lived and worked most of his life in France. Early in his career, he lived in Paris among a community of artists in Montmartre, a neighborhood in the northern part of the city. He later left Paris for the south of France, where he was particularly inspired by the vivid colors of nature. The colors and bright sunlight of Provence are captured in some of his more well-known paintings of sunflowers, gardens, and his bedroom in Arles. Art critics speak of the intensity of emotion associated with this painting, *Chambre d'Arles.* What makes this work so intense?

◀ Vincent Van Gogh: *Chambre d'Arles,* 1888. (Musée d'Orsay, Paris)

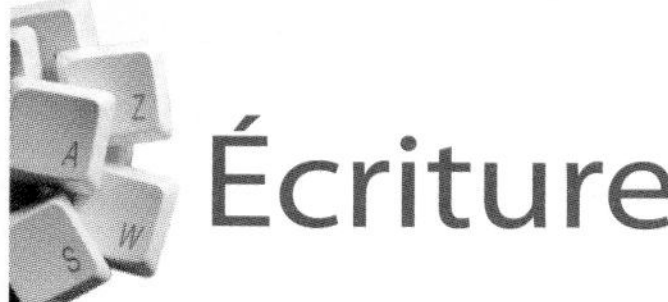

Écriture

The writing activities **Par écrit** and **Journal intime** can be found in the Workbook/Laboratory Manual to accompany *Vis-à-vis*.

La vie en chantant. An activity based on the song "Le vieux château" by Georges Brassens can be found in the Instructor's Manual. The song can be purchased at the iTunes store, or sts. can watch the music video on YouTube.

Pour s'amuser

Le rébus

Work with a partner and use the lexique to solve the puzzle.

\+ + + + 2 +

Answer: Je déménage demain (jeu + dés + mai + nage + deux + main).

Suggestion: To aid comprehension of the video episode, ask: *As-tu un(e) colocataire? Aimes-tu ton appartement ou préfères-tu déménager? Aimes-tu les autres locataires dans ton immeuble?*

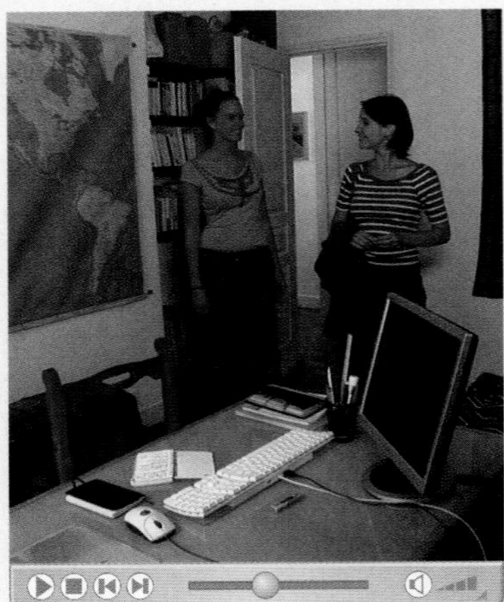

Léa visite l'appartement de Sonia

Suggestion (*Visionnez!*): Have sts. read the statements aloud and guess which will be the right adjective before they watch the video. Return to this activity after watching the video for a quick comprehension check.

Suggestion (*Analysez!*): Using the video images, go over additional vocabulary from the cultural segment on Montreal before sts. answer the questions: *un gratte-ciel, le quartier branché, leurs escaliers exterieurs, leurs balcons et leurs terrasses, les rues bordées d'arbres, un grand fleuve*. For the first question, contrast *ancien* and *moderne* and challenge the association that many North Americans make between European style as "old" and North American style as "modern."

Note culturelle

In France, campus housing is managed by **CNOUS (Centre national des œuvres universitaires et scolaires).** Regional centers (**CROUS**) exist to help students find lodging in the **cité-U.** Priority is given to students who study far from home and whose parents are of modest means. The monthly rent (**le loyer mensuel**) for a traditional room in Paris is about 180 euros and between 330 and 550 euros for a more comfortable **studette** or **studio,** including electricity, heating, and water.

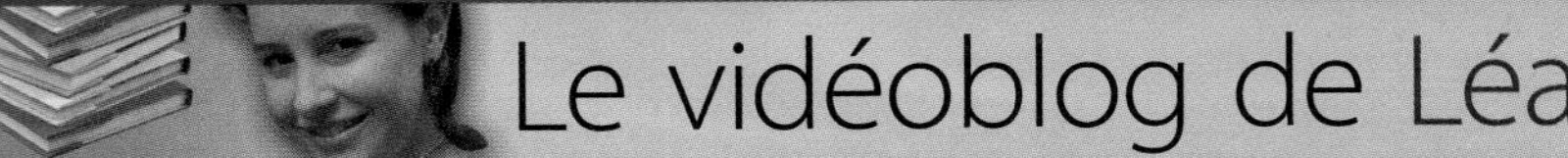

Le vidéoblog de Léa

En bref

In this episode, Léa meets Sonia, a young woman originally from Montreal who lives in Paris and is looking for a roommate to share her apartment. After being shown around the apartment, Léa asks Sonia to describe the architectural landscape of Montreal for her videoblog.

Vocabulaire en contexte

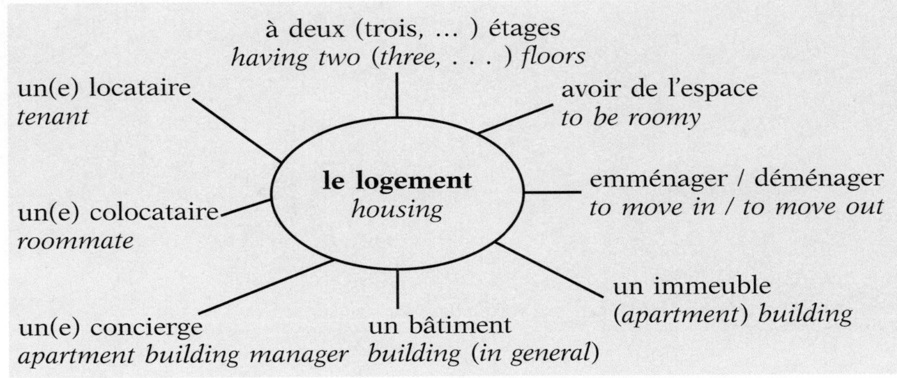

Visionnez!

For each statement, choose the adjective that best describes Sonia's apartment and neighborhood.

1. Léa trouve que l'appartement de Sonia est petit / grand.
2. Elle pense que le séjour (*living room*) est très sombre / clair.
3. La chambre de Sonia est simple / en désordre.
4. La chambre à louer (*for rent*) est petite / grande.
5. L'appartement est dans un quartier super / désagréable.
6. Les locataires sont vraiment cool / désagréables.

Analysez!

1. Sonia dit (*says*) que Montréal est une ville «où l'architecture du passé et du présent coexistent». Donnez des exemples.
2. Sonia dit aussi que Montréal est une ville «ouverte». Expliquez.

Comparez!

Watch Léa's visit to Sonia's apartment again. Is Sonia's apartment similar to student apartments near your campus? Using the vocabulary presented above, as well as other words you know, describe the housing possibilities for students in your area.

MODÈLE: Il y a de petits appartements dans des immeubles à deux étages, et il y a aussi…

Follow-up: After sts. have talked about the housing possibilities in their campus neighborhood, you may wish to have them discuss the architecture in the area and compare it to what they saw of Montreal in the video.

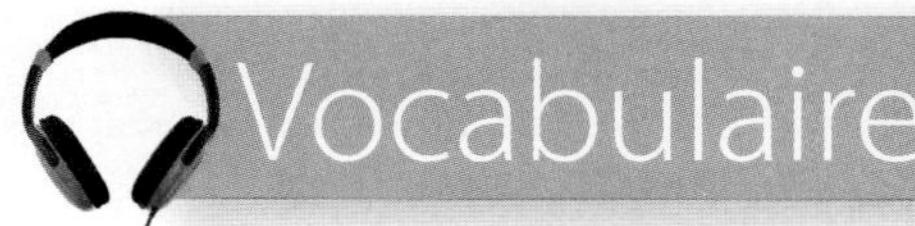

Vocabulaire

Verbes

agir to act
bavarder to chat
choisir to choose
déménager to move out
emménager to move in
finir (de + *inf.*) to finish (*doing s.th.*)
  finir par + *inf.* to end up (*doing s.th.*)
louer to rent
passer un examen to take an exam
réfléchir (à) to think (about)
réussir (à) to succeed (in); to pass (*a test*)

Substantifs

l'affiche (*f.*) poster
l'appartement (*m.*) apartment
l'armoire (*f.*) wardrobe, closet
le (baladeur) iPod iPod (player)
le canapé sofa
la chambre bedroom
  chambre de bonne maid's room; garret
le chat cat
le chien dog
la commode chest of drawers
le couloir hallway
la douche shower
l'enceinte (*f.*) speaker
l'étagère (*f.*) shelf
la fleur flower
la guitare guitar
l'immeuble (*m.*) apartment building
la lampe lamp
le lavabo bathroom sink
le lit bed
la location rent
le logement lodging, place of residence
le magazine magazine
la maison house
le meuble piece of furniture
le miroir mirror
le mur wall
le réveil alarm clock
le rideau curtain
la rue street
la station d'accueil docking station (iPod, cell phone)
la studette small studio (apartment) with shared bathroom
le studio studio (apartment)
le tapis rug
le téléphone telephone
le (téléphone) portable cell phone
les toilettes (*f. pl.*) **(les W.-C.)** restroom
la voiture car

À REVOIR: **le bureau, la chaise, l'ordinateur, la table, la télé(vision)**

Adjectifs

ancien(ne) old, antique; former
autre other
bon(ne) good
chaque each
dernier / dernière last
faux / fausse false
gros(se) large; fat; thick
jeune young
joli(e) pretty
mauvais(e) bad
premier / première first
vieux / vieil / vieille old
vrai(e) true

À REVOIR: **beau / bel / belle, cher / chère, facile, gentil(le), grand(e), long(ue), nouveau / nouvel / nouvelle, pauvre, petit(e)**

Prépositions de lieu

à côté de beside
à droite de on the right of
à gauche de on the left of
chez at the home of; at the office of
derrière behind
devant in front of
en face de across from
entre between
loin de far from
par by
  par terre on the ground
près de near
sous under
sur on

Mots interrogatifs

combien (de) how many, how much
comment how, what
où where
pourquoi why
qu'est-ce que, que what
quand when
qui who, whom

Mots et expressions divers

alors so; then
donc then; therefore
en désordre disorderly
en ordre orderly
parce que because
si if

Bienvenue...

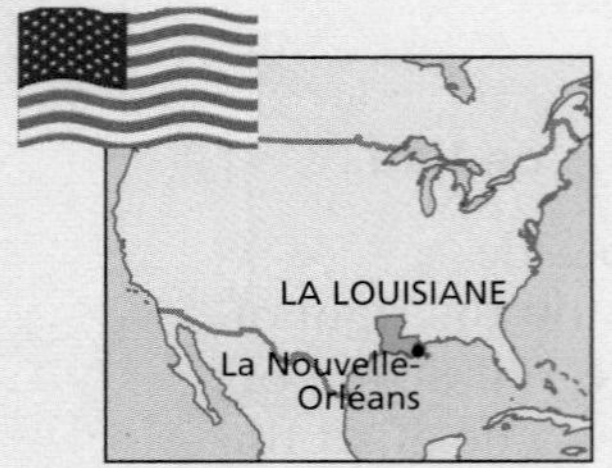

Un coup d'œil sur La Nouvelle-Orléans et le pays des Cadiens,° en Louisiane

° Cajuns

Quand on parle de la Louisiane, on pense souvent à La Nouvelle Orléans et au Mardi Gras. Et c'est vrai, il y a des traces françaises dans l'architecture, la cuisine, les noms et les traditions de La Nouvelle Orléans. Mais à l'extérieur de cette grande ville, il y a toute une autre culture francophone à découvrir—le pays des Cadiens. Au sud-ouest de la ville, vous pouvez[1] explorer les bayous et parler français avec les habitants des communautés de nom français, comme LaRose et Belle Rivière. Si vous continuez plus vers le nord-ouest, vous allez traverser le Bassin de l'Atchafalaya, un grand marais[2] entre Bâton Rouge et Lafayette. Si vous avez le temps, allez à Henderson pour faire une visite guidée de l'Atchafalaya en bateau—vous allez peut-être y voir des cocodrils[3]! Si vous avez faim, goûtez du boudin* ou des écrevisses.[4] On mange bien en Louisiane!

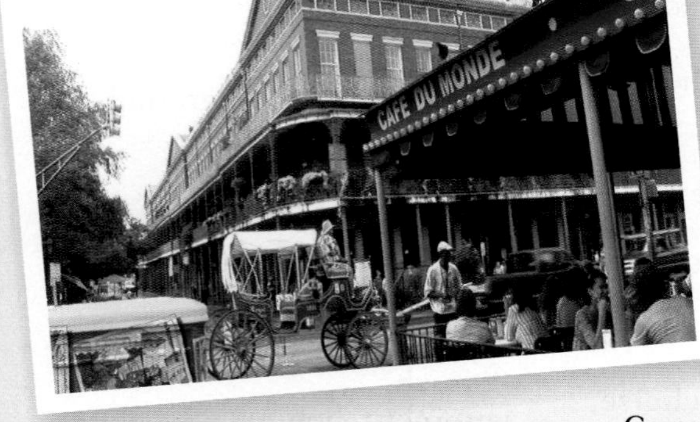

Le célèbre Café du Monde à La Nouvelle-Orléans

Qui sont les Cadiens? Ce sont les descendants des Acadiens, un peuple d'origine française, exilés du Canada par les Anglais en 1755. Alors, beaucoup d'Acadiens s'installent en Louisiane, qui est un territoire francophone. Ce qu'on appelle «cadien» aujourd'hui est vraiment un mélange[5] de cultures. La musique, la cuisine et même la langue cadiennes sont influencées par les Créoles, les Espagnols, les Amérindiens[6] et d'autres groupes ethniques en Louisiane. La Louisiane française, c'est un véritable gombo!

[1]*can* [2]*swamp* [3]*alligators (Cajun)* [4]*crawfish* [5]*mixture* [6]*Native Americans*

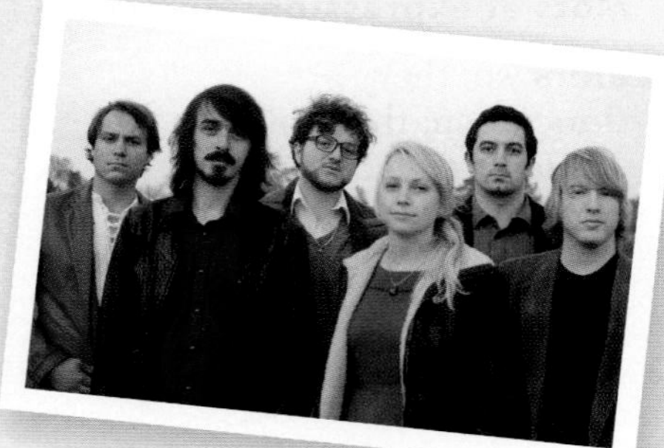

Feufollet: un groupe de jeunes musiciens de Louisiane

PORTRAIT Feufollet†

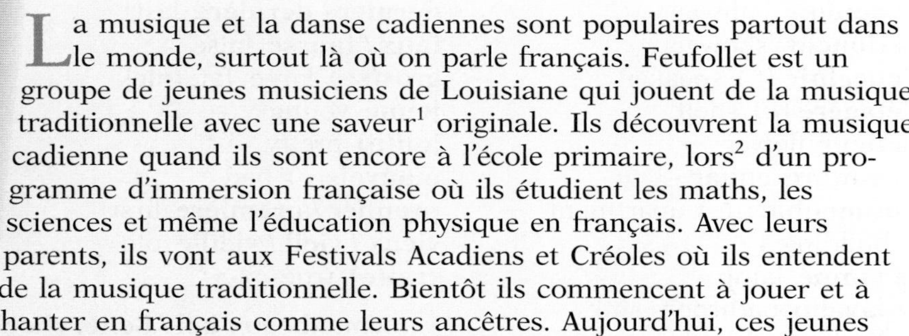

La musique et la danse cadiennes sont populaires partout dans le monde, surtout là où on parle français. Feufollet est un groupe de jeunes musiciens de Louisiane qui jouent de la musique traditionnelle avec une saveur[1] originale. Ils découvrent la musique cadienne quand ils sont encore à l'école primaire, lors[2] d'un programme d'immersion française où ils étudient les maths, les sciences et même l'éducation physique en français. Avec leurs parents, ils vont aux Festivals Acadiens et Créoles où ils entendent de la musique traditionnelle. Bientôt ils commencent à jouer et à chanter en français comme leurs ancêtres. Aujourd'hui, ces jeunes adultes jouent leur musique en Louisiane, en France, au Canada—et aux Festivals Acadiens et Créoles! Les musiciens de Feufollet trouvent qu'il est important de comprendre et de parler la langue qu'ils chantent. Ils s'amusent, ils gagnent de l'argent et ils préservent leur héritage.

[1]*flavor* [2]*during*

***Boudin** is a spicy sausage made of rice, ground pork, onions, and other seasonings. It is sold widely in local grocery stores as a quick snack or meal. The traditional blood sausage that the French call **boudin** also exists in Louisiana, where it is known as **boudin rouge.**

†In southwestern Louisiana, the **feu follet** refers to a shining light seen over the swamps at night. Folk tales came up with many different meanings for these lights, such as the souls of babies who had died without being baptized.

en Amérique du Nord

Un coup d'œil sur Québec, au Canada

Est-ce que vous aimez faire du ski[1]? Avez-vous envie de faire du magasinage,[2] ou est-ce que vous préférez visiter les musées? Venez voir la ville de Québec, la capitale de la province de Québec, et l'une des seules[3] villes fortifiées en Amérique du Nord. Les Québécois sont toujours très fiers de leur héritage francophone et, pour environ[4] 80 % des Québécois, le français est leur langue maternelle.

Dans le Vieux-Québec, il y a beaucoup de magasins chic et de bons restaurants. Visitez le musée de la Civilisation, qui propose des expositions sur l'histoire et la culture contemporaine du Québec. Sur la terrasse Dufferin, derrière le château Frontenac, vous pouvez écouter des musiciens québécois pendant l'été[5] ou faire des glissades[6] pendant l'hiver.[7] Chaque février pendant le carnaval de Québec, on célèbre les plaisirs de l'hiver avec des feux d'artifice,[8] de la musique et une grande compétition de sculptures sur neige[9]!

[1]faire... *go skiing* [2]faire... *go shopping* (*Quebec expression*)
[3]*only* [4]*approximately* [5]pendant... *during the summer*
[6]faire... *go tobogganing* [7]*winter* [8]feux... *fireworks*
[9]sculptures... *snow sculptures*

L'hiver dans le Vieux-Québec

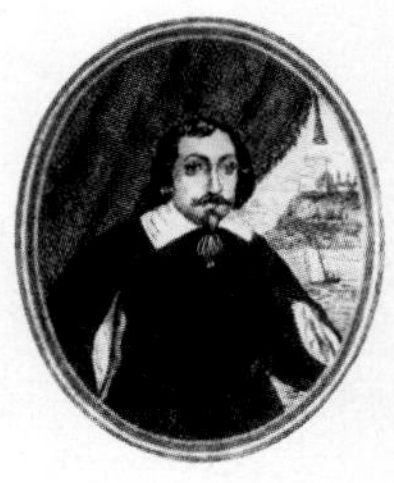

PORTRAIT Samuel de Champlain (c. 1567[1]–1635[2])

Grand géographe et explorateur français, Samuel de Champlain explore, entre 1603[3] et 1633,[4] les régions du fleuve[5] Saint-Laurent, l'Acadie (appelée[6] aujourd'hui la Nouvelle-Écosse et le Nouveau-Brunswick) et le Québec. Champlain devient[7] l'ami des Amérindiens Hurons et des Algonquins, qui lui font découvrir[8] leur pays. Il fonde la ville de Québec en 1608.[9]

[1]mille cinq cent soixante-sept [2]mille six cent trente-cinq [3]mille six cent trois [4]mille six cent trente-trois
[5]*river* [6]*called* [7]*becomes* [8]qui... *who help him discover* [9]mille six cent huit

Note: See the Instructor's Manual for follow-up questions about this *Bienvenue* section.

Watch the *Bienvenue en Amérique du Nord* video segments to learn more about Cajun Country and Quebec.

CHAPITRE 5

De génération en génération

Les dossiers d'Hassan

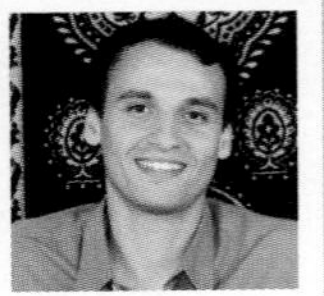

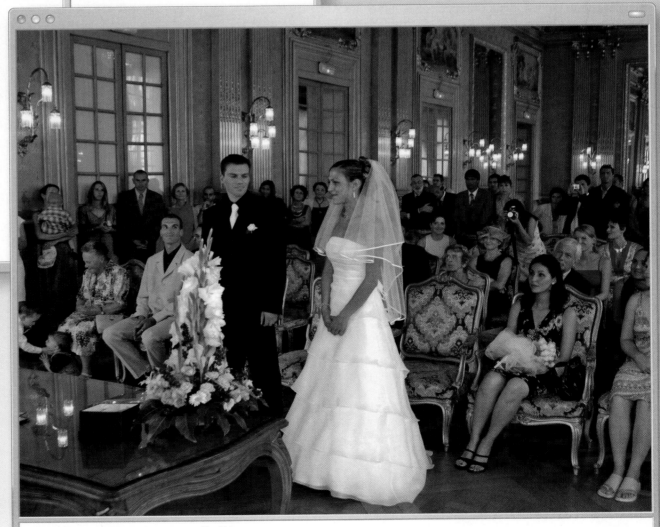

Hassan

- Mes photos
  - Un mariage à Rennes
  - Abdel, Carole et moi
  - Une famille marocaine

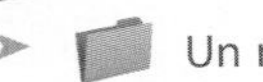

Presentation: Have sts. describe the clothing of the bride and groom and several of the guests using colors and other adjectives. Also ask them to imagine the personalities and ages of some of the people in the photo.

Un mariage à Rennes dans une salle élégante

Culture note: Rennes is located in northwest France. It is the *chef-lieu* of the *Ille-et-Vilaine* department and the largest city in *La Bretagne*.

Dans ce chapitre...

OBJECTIFS COMMUNICATIFS

- talking about family and relatives
- identifying rooms in a house
- talking about weather
- expressing possession
- talking about plans and destinations
- expressing what you are doing and making
- expressing actions
- learning to distinguish between and pronounce selected sounds in French

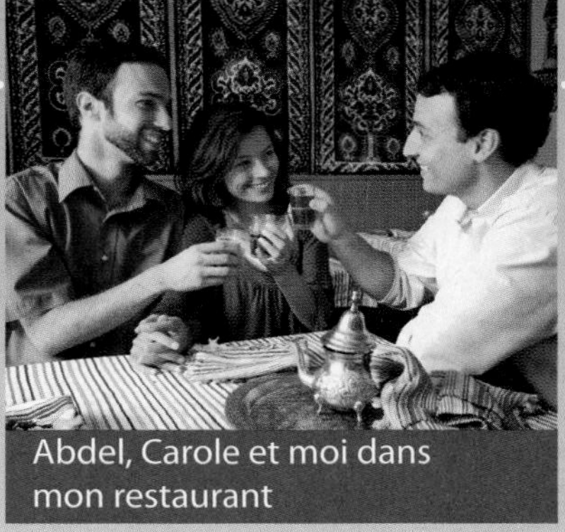

Abdel, Carole et moi dans mon restaurant

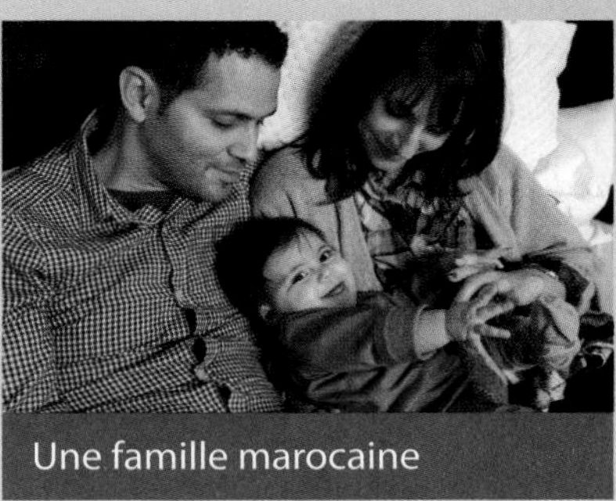

Une famille marocaine

PAROLES (Leçon 1)

- La famille
- La maison
- Les saisons et le temps

STRUCTURES (Leçons 2 et 3)

- Les adjectifs possessifs
- Le verbe **aller** et le futur proche
- Le verbe **faire**
- Les verbes en **-re**

CULTURE

- Le blog d'Hassan: *Un mariage franco-marocain**
- Reportage: *La famille au Maroc: une valeur sûre*
- Lecture: *Giverny: le petit paradis de Monet* (Leçon 4)

Note: Starting in *Chapitre 5*, all ex. instructions are in French, with glosses as needed.

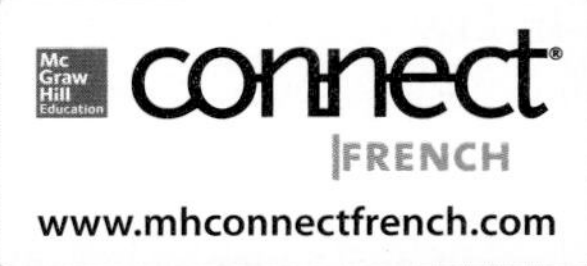

*In **Chapitres 5–8**, you will read Hassan Zem's blog. He will write about Moroccan wedding customs, food, and vacation options. Other characters will offer commentaries on his blog.

CHAPITRE 5

Leçon 1

PAROLES

Trois générations d'une famille

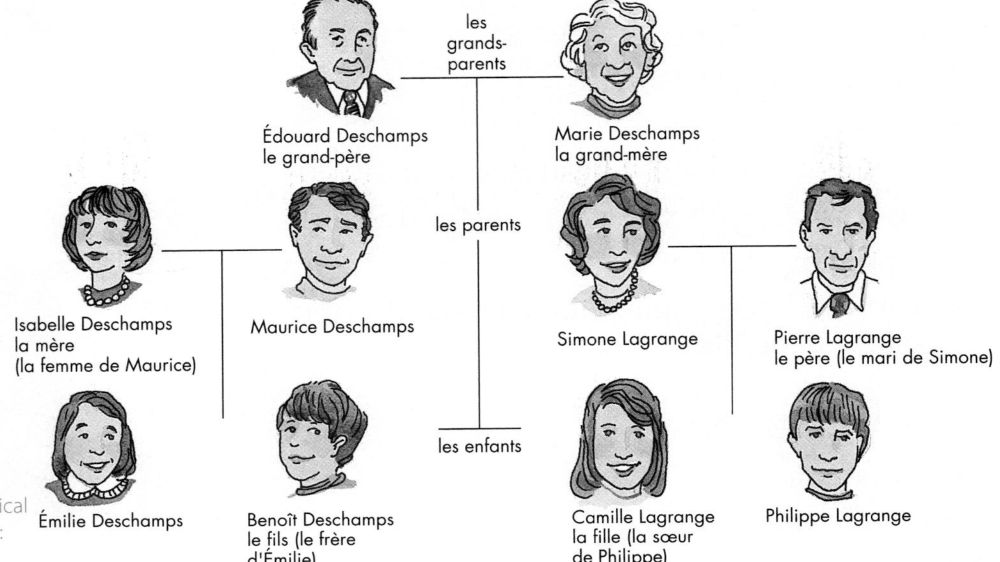

Presentation: Bring in pictures of famous families (Obamas, Bushes) to reinforce vocabulary. Once sts. have mastered the new nouns, make illogical statements and have sts. correct you: *Barack Obama est le père de Michelle.*

Suggestion: Point out the difference in pronunciation of *fils* [fis] and *fille* [fij].

Note: When *demi* is placed before a noun, it is linked to the noun by a hyphen and remains invariable: *des demi-frères.* When *grand* is part of a compound noun, it also is linked to the noun by a hyphen. However, *grand* agrees in number with the noun: *un grand-père, des grands-pères.* Note however, that *grand* does not agree in gender in *grand-mère.*

Additional vocabulary: *filleul(e)* (godson, goddaughter), *parrain* (godfather), *marraine* (godmother).

AUTRES MOTS UTILES

le petit-enfant grandchild
la petite-fille granddaughter
le petit-fils grandson

le cousin, la cousine cousin
le neveu nephew
la nièce niece
l'oncle (*m.*) uncle
la tante aunt

le parent parent (*or* relative)
les arrière-grands-parents (*m. pl.*) great-grandparents

célibataire single
divorcé(e) divorced
marié(e) married
pacsé(e) joined legally by a PACS*

le beau-frère brother-in-law
la belle-sœur sister-in-law
le demi-frère half brother (*or* stepbrother)
la demi-sœur half sister (*or* stepsister)
le beau-père father-in-law (*or* stepfather)
la belle-mère mother-in-law (*or* stepmother)
le gendre son-in-law
la bru daughter-in-law

---

*The **Pacte civil de solidarité** is a type of civil union voted into French law in 1999 by the National Assembly. Two adults (same sex or not) may enter into a **PACS** by registering with the court clerk. Same sex marriage became legal in France on May 18, 2013.

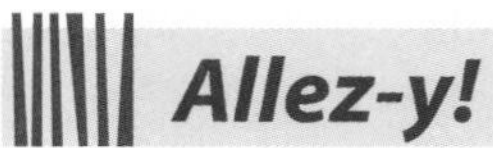

Allez-y!

Suggestion (A): Can be done in pairs. Spot check some of the answers afterward.

A. La famille Deschamps. Étudiez l'arbre généalogique (*family tree*) de la famille Deschamps et répondez aux questions.

1. Comment s'appelle la femme d'Édouard?
2. Comment s'appelle le mari d'Isabelle?
3. Comment s'appelle la tante d'Émilie et de Benoît? Et l'oncle?
4. Combien d'enfants ont les Lagrange? Combien de filles et de fils?
5. Comment s'appelle le frère d'Émilie?
6. Combien de cousins ont Émilie et Benoît? Combien de cousines?
7. Comment s'appelle la grand-mère de Philippe? Et le grand-père?
8. Combien de petits-enfants ont Édouard et Marie? Combien de petites-filles? Combien de petits-fils?
9. Comment s'appelle la sœur de Philippe?
10. Comment s'appellent les parents de Maurice et de Simone?

B. Qui sont-ils? Complétez les définitions suivantes.

1. Le frère de mon père est mon ______.
2. La fille de ma tante est ma ______.
3. Le père de ma mère est mon ______.
4. La femme de mon grand-père est ma ______.

Maintenant définissez les personnes suivantes .

5. une nièce
6. des arrière-grands-parents
7. une tante
8. un grand-père
9. une belle-sœur
10. un demi-frère

Suggestion (B): Before doing this ex., present the poss. adj. *mon* and *ma* lexically.

Suggestion (B): Can be done in pairs or groups of three. Sts. should take notes and report answers.

C. Une famille américaine. Posez (*Ask*) les questions suivantes à votre camarade.

1. As-tu des frères, des sœurs, des demi-frères ou des demi-sœurs? Combien? Comment s'appellent-ils/elles? (Ils/Elles s'appellent...)
2. As-tu des grands-parents? Combien? Habitent-ils chez toi, dans une maison ou dans un appartement?
3. As-tu des cousins ou des cousines? Combien? Habitent-ils/elles près ou loin de la famille?
4. Combien d'enfants (de fils ou de filles) désires-tu avoir? Combien d'enfants est-ce qu'il y a dans une famille idéale?

D. Une famille française. Avec un(e) camarade, décrivez la famille sur la photo. Donnez le nombre de personnes, et devinez (*guess*) qui sont les personnes et quel âge elles ont. Puis imaginez leur (*their*) profession, leurs goûts (*tastes*), leur personnalité. Donnez le plus de détails (*as many details as*) possibles.

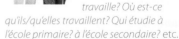

Follow-up: Ask 3–4 sts. to give a short description of the family of one of the other sts. interviewed, while the whole class takes notes. The class then asks you questions about information shared. Divide class members into two teams for this activity. When a team "stumps" you, it gets a point. The team with most questions missed by you wins.

Mots clés

La préposition *chez*

Chez, which generally refers to someone's residence, means **à la maison de.** It can also refer to a place of business (doctor's office, butcher shop, etc.).

On travaille **chez** toi ou **chez** moi?
Are we working at your place or my place?

J'habite **chez** Éric.
I live at Éric's place.

Tu as rendez-vous **chez** le dentiste?
Do you have a dentist appointment?

Note: *Chez* can also be used before the name of a store if it is a proper name; e.g., *chez McDonald's.* It can also be used before a nationality, in which case it means *dans le pays de*, e.g., *Chez les Français, on aime bien le vin.*

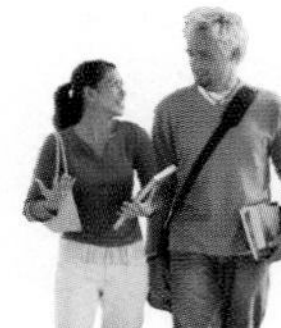

Additional activities: A. Focus on one family member and review his/her relationship to others in family: *Comment s'appelle la mère de Simone? Qui est la belle-sœur de Simone?* B. Sts. invent details about members of the Deschamps family as you ask questions, using *-er* verbs. *Qui travaille? Où est-ce qu'ils/qu'elles travaillent? Qui étudie à l'école primaire? à l'école secondaire?* etc.

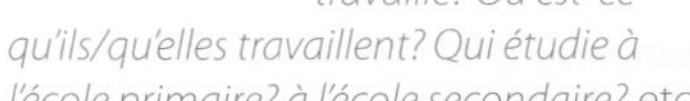

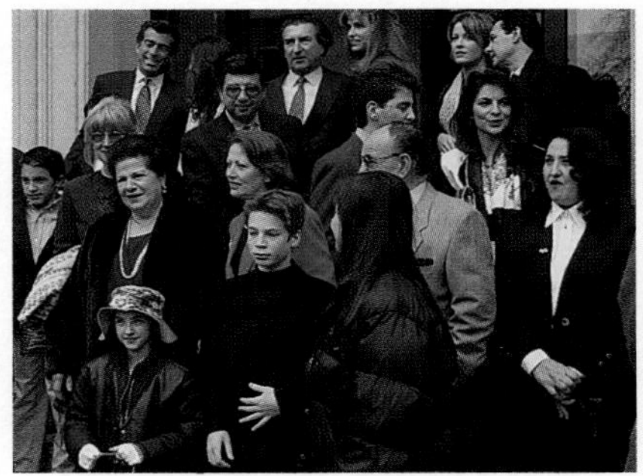

C'est une affaire de famille. Qui voyez-vous?

Note: You may wish to point out that in French, no plural is formed in the family name when it is preceded by *les.*

Chez les Chabrier

Presentation: Use magazine pictures in class for identification of rooms and furniture.

MAISON À LOUER: 3 pièces (*f.*) + cuisine, salle de bains

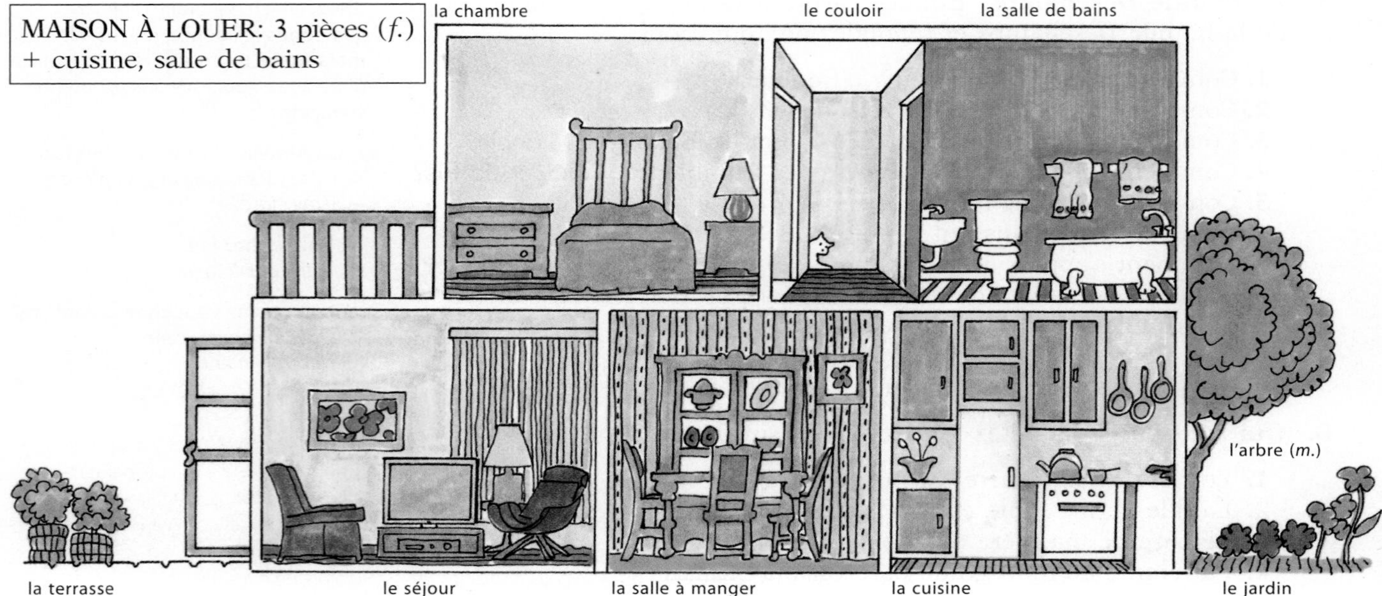

Additional vocabulary: *la cuisinière, le frigo, le vaisselier, la table de chevet, la baignoire.*

Note: Sts. often have trouble with the difference between *premier étage* and *first floor.* A drawing on the board may help.

Vocabulary recycling: *Le plan de la maison. Décrivez la maison des Chabrier.* MODÈLE: *sous / salle de bains → La cuisine est sous la salle de bains. 1. à côté de / séjour 2. à côté de / salle de bains 3. à côté de / salle à manger 4. sous / chambre 5. à côté de / maison*

Follow-up: Ask sts. to describe their ideal apartment.

Additional activity: Sts. think of as many words as they can (in French) that they associate with their own lodgings.

Continuation (B): Ask questions such as the following: *Où est-ce qu'on joue aux cartes? Où est-ce qu'on parle avec des ami(e)s? Où est-ce qu'on dîne?*

AUTRES MOTS UTILES

le bureau	study, office
la clé	key
l'escalier (*m.*)	stairway
le rez-de-chaussée	ground floor
le premier (deuxième) étage	second (third) floor (*in North America*)
le sous-sol	basement

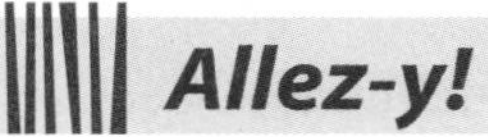

Allez-y!

A. Les pièces de la maison. Trouvez les pièces d'après (*according to*) les définitions suivantes.

MODÈLE: C'est un lieu qui donne sur (*that overlooks*) la terrasse. → C'est le balcon.

1. la pièce où il y a une table pour manger **2.** la pièce où il y a une télévision **3.** la pièce où il y a un lavabo **4.** la pièce où on prépare le dîner **5.** un lieu de passage **6.** la pièce où il y a un lit

B. Dans quelle pièce? Regardez encore une fois la maison des Chabrier. Où est-ce qu'on fait (*does*) les choses suivantes? Commencez vos phrases avec **On...**

1. regarder la télé: sur le balcon / dans le séjour
2. planter des fleurs: dans le jardin / dans la chambre
3. jouer avec le chat: dans la salle de bains / dans le couloir
4. manger: dans le couloir / dans la salle à manger
5. préparer un café: dans la cuisine / sur le balcon

Quel temps fait-il? Les saisons et le temps°

°Quel... *How's the weather? Seasons and weather*

Presentation: Have sts. repeat seasons and weather expressions after your model. Using images from the Internet, PowerPoint slides, or flashcards with pictures like these, review seasons and weather expressions in random order.

Suggestion: Point out that all seasons are masculine; explain the uses of *au* (before consonant) and *en* (before vowel).

Suggestion: Point out *il impersonnel;* compare to *il y a.*

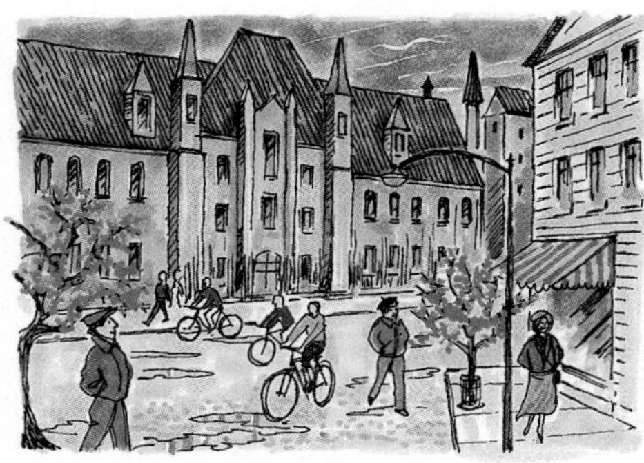

Au **printemps,** chez les Belges...
Le temps est nuageux.
Il fait frais.

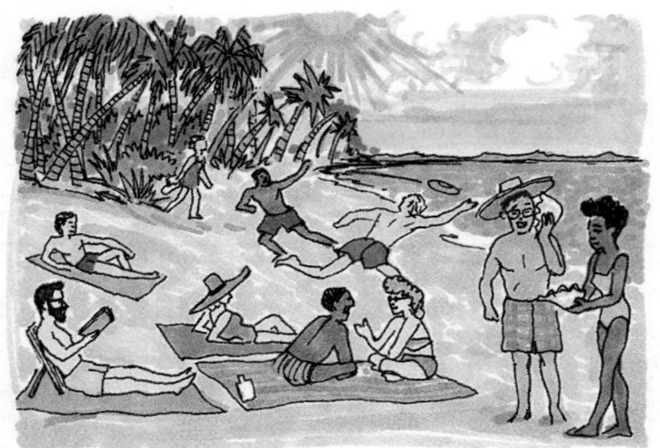

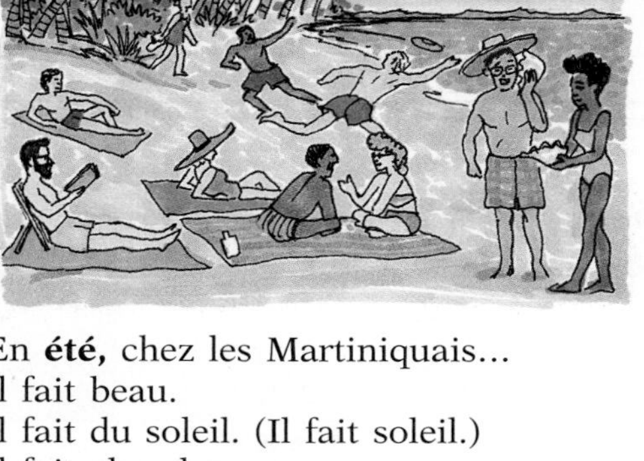

En **été,** chez les Martiniquais...
Il fait beau.
Il fait du soleil. (Il fait soleil.)
Il fait chaud.

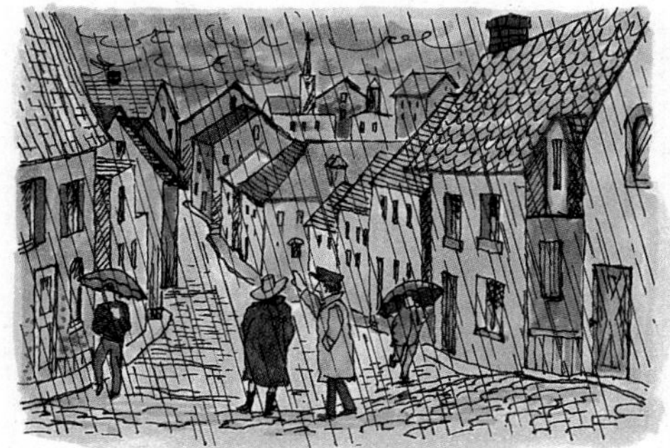

En **automne,** chez les Bretons...
Il pleut.
Il fait mauvais.
Le temps est orageux.

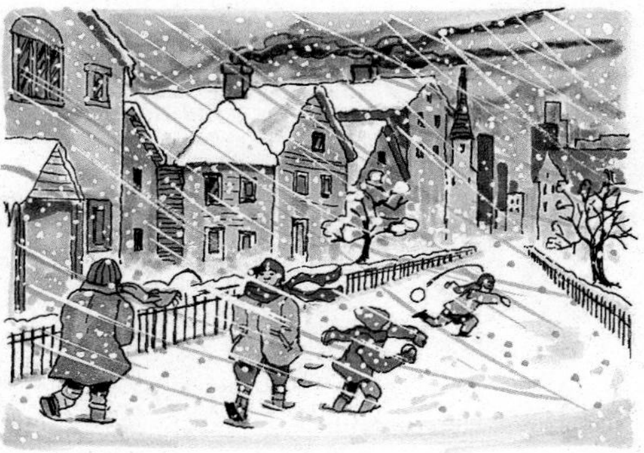

En **hiver,** chez les Québécois...
Il neige.
Il fait froid.
Il fait du vent. (Il y a du vent.)

- To ask about the weather:

  Quel temps fait-il?

- To tell about the season:

  Nous sommes au printemps (en été, en automne, en hiver).

Pronunciation presentation: Remind sts. of (1) the liaison [n] between *en* and *été, automne,* and *hiver;* (2) the silent *m, p,* and *s* in *temps.*

Pronunciation practice (1): Ask sts. to produce, in association with the following words, the appropriate version of (1) *premier: Le* ______ *étudiant, ordinateur, cahier, août, chapeau, octobre, bureau, hiver, tapis;* (2) *dernier: Le* ______ *ami, camarade, examen, café, manteau, appartement, chat, immeuble, oncle.*

Pronunciation practice (2): The *Prononcez bien!* section on page 138 of this chapter contains additional activities for practicing these sounds.

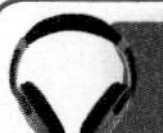

Prononcez bien!

The pronunciation of *premier*

The **-er** in **premier** and **dernier** (*last*) has two different pronunciations: [e], as in **et,** when it ends a sentence or is followed by a word starting with a consonant, and [ɛʀ], as in **mère,** when it precedes a word beginning with a vowel sound.

[e]: **le premier jour, le dernier mois**

[ɛʀ]: **le premier étage, le dernier été, le premier homme**

Note (B): See the Instructor's Manual for ideas about using authentic materials in class.

Follow-up (B): Ask sts. to work in small groups to prepare *la météo* of the United States or of the provinces in Canada, using a weather map from the newspaper or the Internet. They can pick a *météorologiste* from their group to present the weather to the class.

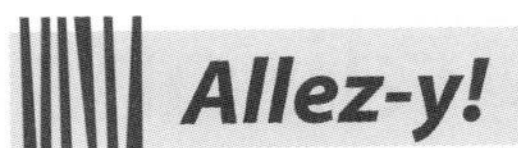

Continuation (A): Ask sts. to describe the weather on Martin Luther King Day, Valentine's Day, American Independence Day, and Labor Day.

A. Parlons du temps. Répondez aux questions suivantes.

1. En quelle saison est Pâques (*Easter*)?
2. Quel temps fait-il en hiver en Alaska?
3. Est-ce qu'il fait beau l'hiver à Seattle?
4. En quelle saison est le Jour d'action de grâce (*Thanksgiving Day*)?
5. C'est le mois de mai. Quel temps fait-il chez vous?

MÉTÉO

MATIN — NUAGEUX

Rhin & Moselle ASSURANCES

Groupe Allianz Via Assurances

APRES-MIDI — NUAGEUX

SITUATION:
Après le passage de la zone orageuse sur l'Alsace, nous allons retrouver pour ce milieu de semaine des températures beaucoup plus supportables.

PLAINE D'ALSACE:
Matinée encore nuageuse et brumeuse. Dans la journée retour de belles périodes ensoleillées. Humidité de l'air revenant à 60 pour 100. Températures moins élevées que ces jours derniers.

VOSGES ET FORÊT-NOIRE:
Déclin des pluies d'orages, temps d'abord nuageux puis en amélioration grâce au retour d'éclaircies. Baisse importante des températures.

POUR LES TROIS JOURS SUIVANTS:
De jeudi à vendredi beau temps à nouveau plus chaud ce qui pourrait nous ramener des orages pour le prochain week-end.

Jean Breton

SAVERNE +19°/+23°
STRASBOURG +20°/+25°
VENT 15KmH
COLMAR +21°/+26°
GUEBWILLER +20°/+25°
MULHOUSE +20°/+24°

STOCKHOLM 18°/22°
LONDRES 17°/23°
BERLIN 23°/26°
BONN 22°/25°
VARSOVIE 22°/29°
PARIS 18°/25°
VIENNE 22°/31°
BORDEAUX 21°/27°
NICE 24°/28°
ROME 26°/32°
MADRID 25°/33°
ATHENES 26°/30°
ALGER 28°/37°

Infographie DNA Studio

B. Les prévisions de la météo. (*Weather forecast.*) Regardez le temps prévu pour l'Alsace et l'Europe et répondez aux questions suivantes.

1. Quel temps fait-il en Alsace?
   a. Il neige.
   b. Le temps est nuageux.
   c. Il pleut.
2. Quel temps fait-il à Berlin?
   a. Il fait (du) soleil.
   b. Le temps est orageux.
   c. Il fait beau.
3. Quel temps fait-il à Alger?
   a. Il fait mauvais.
   b. Il fait froid.
   c. Il fait (du) soleil.

C. Le temps et les goûts. Qu'est-ce que vous aimez porter quand… ?

1. il fait très chaud
2. il fait froid et qu'il neige
3. il fait beau et frais
4. il pleut

Additional activity: In groups, sts. prepare descriptions of a particular state or city, identifying it as one or the other. They mention characteristic weather and appropriate clothing, as well as a few telling characteristics. Each group reads its description to the class, and the others guess the place described. If sts. cannot guess immediately, which is probable, allow them to ask five yes/no questions to get more information.

Leçon 2

Les adjectifs possessifs

Expressing Possession

Vacances d'été

Mamadou contacte Léa sur sa page Facebook (Messagerie instantanée).

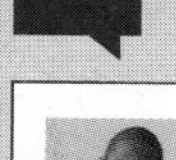

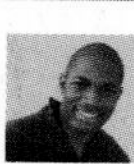

MAMADOU: Léa, quels sont **tes** projets pour l'été?

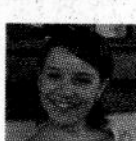

LÉA: **Mon** programme de juillet est très agréable: un petit voyage à Londres avec **mon** amie Juliette, et deux semaines à la montagne avec **ma** sœur et **son** mari, **mes** parents, **leur** chien… et **mon** chat!

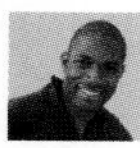

MAMADOU: Il a de la chance, **ton** chat! Et en août?

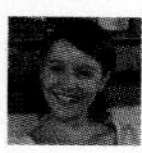

LÉA: **Ma** sœur, **mes** cousins, **mon** chat et moi sommes chez **nos** grands-parents dans **notre** maison de famille en Normandie. C'est une tradition.

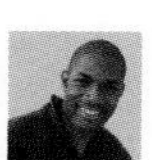

MAMADOU: Quand est-ce que **vos** vacances finissent?

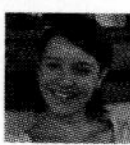

LÉA: Le 31 août. Nous retournons tous à Paris!

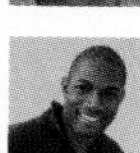

MAMADOU: Avec **ton** chat?

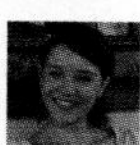

LÉA: Avec **mon** chat!

Vrai ou faux?

1. Léa voyage en juillet avec son amie Juliette.
2. Juliette va (*is going*) à la montagne avec sa sœur, ses parents et leur chien.
3. En août, Léa et sa sœur vont (*are going*) chez leurs grands-parents.
4. Leurs cousins aussi vont être chez leurs grands-parents.
5. Léa retourne à Paris sans (*without*) son chat.

One way to indicate possession in French is to use the preposition **de: la maison *de* Claudine.** Another way is to use the possessive adjectives presented on the next page.

	SINGULAR		PLURAL
	MASCULINE	FEMININE	MASCULINE AND FEMININE
my	**mon** père	**ma** mère	**mes** parents
your (informal)	**ton** père	**ta** mère	**tes** parents
his, her, its, one's	**son** père	**sa** mère	**ses** parents
our	**notre** père	**notre** mère	**nos** parents
your (formal and plural)	**votre** père	**votre** mère	**vos** parents
their	**leur** père	**leur** mère	**leurs** parents

Presentation: Model pronunciation, using a short sentence: *Mon père est sympathique. Ma mère est agréable,* etc.

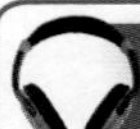

Prononcez bien!

The vowels in *notre* and *nos*

Clearly distinguish between the vowel [ɔ] in the singular form **notre/votre** and the vowel [o] in the plural form **nos/vos** of the possessive adjective.

Open your mouth and keep your tongue in a central position for **notre/votre;** close your mouth further, shift your tongue to the front of your mouth, and let your lips protrude for **nos/vos.**

The sound [ɔ] is generally spelled **o: divorcé, sol, alors.**

The sound [o] is also often spelled **o** when it is the last pronounced sound in the syllable: **lavabo, joli.**

Other spellings for the sound [o] include **bientôt, chaud,** and **beau.**

Pronunciation practice: The *Prononcez bien!* section on page 138 of this chapter contains activities for practicing these sounds.

1. In French, possessive adjectives agree in gender and number with the nouns they modify.

Mon frère et **ma sœur** aiment le sport.	*My brother and my sister like sports.*
Voilà **notre maison.**	*There's our house.*
Habitez-vous avec **votre sœur** et **vos parents?**	*Do you live with your sister and your parents?*
Ils skient avec **leurs cousins** et **leur oncle.**	*They're skiing with their cousins and their uncle.*

2. The forms **mon, ton,** and **son** are also used before feminine nouns that begin with a vowel or mute **h.**

   affiche (*f.*) ⟶ **mon affiche**
   amie (*f.*) ⟶ **ton amie**
   histoire (*f.*) ⟶ **son histoire**

3. Pay particular attention to the use of **son, sa, ses** (*his, her*). Whereas English has two possessives, corresponding to the gender of the possessor (*his, her*), French has three, corresponding to the gender and number of the noun possessed (**son, sa, ses**).

SINGULAR NOUNS:

Masculine	Il / Elle } aime **son** chien.
Feminine	Il / Elle } aime **sa** maison.
PLURAL NOUNS:	Il / Elle } aime **ses** oncles et **ses** tantes.

Note: Mention that *Elle aime sa maison* can also mean *She likes his house,* but that the French often say *sa maison à elle / à lui* for clarity. The stressed pronouns are presented in *Chapitre 12.*

Suggestion: Use the following as a preliminary ex.: *Comment dit-on… en français?* 1. *Anne is looking at her mother.* 2. *Anne is looking at her father.* 3. *Anne is looking at her parents.* 4. *Marc is listening to his father.* 5. *Marc is listening to his mother.* 6. *Marc is listening to his brothers and sisters.*

In the preceding examples, **son, sa,** and **ses** can all mean *his* or *her*. Usually, their meaning will be clear in context. Look at the following examples.

Carine habite une grande maison. **Son** jardin est magnifique.	*Carine lives in a big house. Her garden is magnificent.*
Pierre a deux enfants: **sa** fille a 5 ans et **son** fils a 3 ans. **Ses** enfants sont jeunes.	*Pierre has two children: His daughter is 5 years old and his son is 3 years old. His children are young.*

Grammaire interactive

For more on possessive adjectives, watch the corresponding Grammar Tutorial and take a brief practice quiz at **Connect French.**

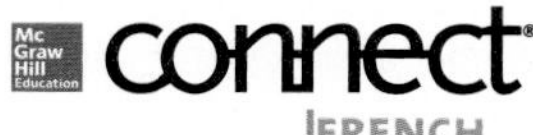

www.mhconnectfrench.com

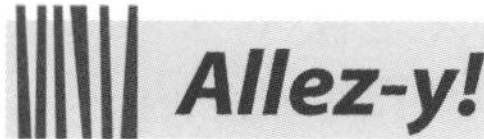

A. Le vide-grenier. (*Garage sale.*) À la fin du semestre, les étudiants organisent un vide-grenier. Formulez des questions et répondez.

MODÈLES: la lampe de Nicolas? (oui) ⟶
É1: Est-ce que c'est la lampe de Nicolas?
É2: Oui, c'est sa lampe.

les lampes de Nicolas (non) ⟶
É1: Est-ce que ce sont les lampes de Nicolas?
É2: Non, ce ne sont pas ses lampes.

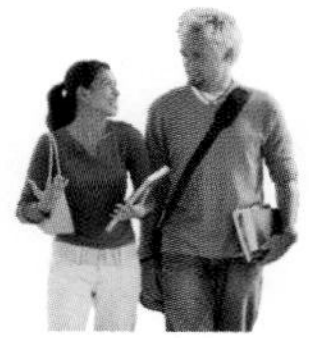

1. la chaise de Pierre? (oui)
2. la commode de Léa? (non)
3. les affiches de Jean? (non)
4. le piano de Pierre et de Sophie? (oui)
5. les meubles d'Annick? (non)
6. les bureaux des parents? (oui)
7. l'ordinateur de Fatima? (oui)
8. l'étagère de Fabrice? (non)

B. Casse-tête familial. (*Family puzzle.*) Posez rapidement les questions suivantes à un(e) camarade.

MODÈLE: Qui est le fils de ton oncle? ⟶ C'est mon cousin.

1. Qui est la mère de ton père?
2. Qui est la fille de ta tante?
3. Qui est la femme de ton oncle?
4. Qui est le père de ton père?
5. Qui est le frère de ta mère?
6. Qui est la sœur de ta mère?
7. Qui sont les femmes de tes frères?
8. Qui sont les enfants de tes sœurs?

Follow-up (B): Sts. invent questions of their own, trying to stump other sts. For example: *Qui est le frère de mon père?*

Le parler jeune

un copain/mec	un petit ami
une copine/meuf	une petite amie
sortir avec	avoir comme copain ou copine
un(e) frangin(e)	un frère / une sœur
un(e) gosse	un(e) enfant

J'ai un nouveau **copain.**

Il parle des heures au téléphone avec sa **meuf.**

Mathilde **sort** avec le frère de sa meilleure amie.

J'ai une **frangine** et deux **frangins.**

Dans ma famille, on était trois **gosses.**

Presentation: You may want to point out to sts. that *meuf* is the *verlan* (backward) slang term for *femme*.

Additional activity: *À la maison. Faites les substitutions et les changements nécessaires. 1. Avec qui habitez-vous? → J'habite avec mon* <u>*père*</u>*. (sœurs, grand-mère, oncle, amis) 2. Qu'est-ce que tu aimes dans ma chambre? → J'aime ton* <u>*chat*</u>*. (affiches, lampe, livres, armoire) 3. À qui téléphone ma cousine Claire? → Elle téléphone à votre* <u>*père*</u>*. (parents, tante, cousin) 4. Avec qui habitent-ils? → Ils habitent avec leurs* <u>*parents*</u>*. (frère, amis, mère, grands-parents)*

C. La fête des voisins. Les gens du quartier organisent un barbecue à l'occasion de la fête des voisins. Complétez les dialogues suivants avec les adjectifs possessifs. Étudiez bien le contexte avant de (*before*) choisir l'adjectif.

1. É1: Paul et Florence adorent les animaux.
   É2: Oui, ils ont un chien et deux chats: ______ chien s'appelle Marius et ______ chats Minou et Félix.
2. É1: Tiens, voilà Pierre. Avec qui est-il?
   É2: Il est avec ______ parents et ______ amie Laure.
   É1: Et ______ sœur n'est pas là?
   É2: Non, elle est en vacances au Maroc.
3. É1: Salut, Alain!
   É2: Salut, Pierre. Dis, la jolie fille aux cheveux blonds, c'est ______ cousine belge?
   É1: Oui. Viens. (*Come.*) Alain, je te présente ______ cousine Sylvie.
   É2: Enchanté, mademoiselle.
4. É1: Pardon, vous êtes Monsieur et Madame Legrand, n'est-ce pas?
   É2: Oui.
   É1: Je suis Monsieur Smith, le professeur d'anglais de ______ enfants.
   É2: Oh, mais ce ne sont pas ______ enfants, ce sont les fils de mon frère Laurent. Voici ______ fils.
5. É1: Tu as de la chance, tu as une famille super! ______ parents sont très sympas! Est-ce que ______ grand-père habite avec vous?
   É2: Non, mais il est souvent à la maison.
   É1: ______ grand-père, malheureusement (*unfortunately*), habite très loin.

Follow-up (D): Have sts. write a short description of their partner's relative and hand it in at end of interview activity. Use this st. material for dictations or listening passages the next class day.

D. Interview. Posez les questions suivantes à un(e) camarade de classe.

1. Quel membre de ta famille (un cousin, une cousine, un neveu, et cetera) est-ce que tu admires particulièrement? Pourquoi?
2. Comment s'appelle-t-il/elle?
3. Où est-ce qu'il/elle habite? Avec qui? Comment est sa maison?
4. Quel est son sport préféré? sa musique favorite?

Maintenant faites le portrait du parent proche (*close relative*) préféré de votre camarade.

Le verbe *aller* et le futur proche

Talking About Plans and Destinations

Un bon programme

Léa et Hector échangent des textos (SMS).

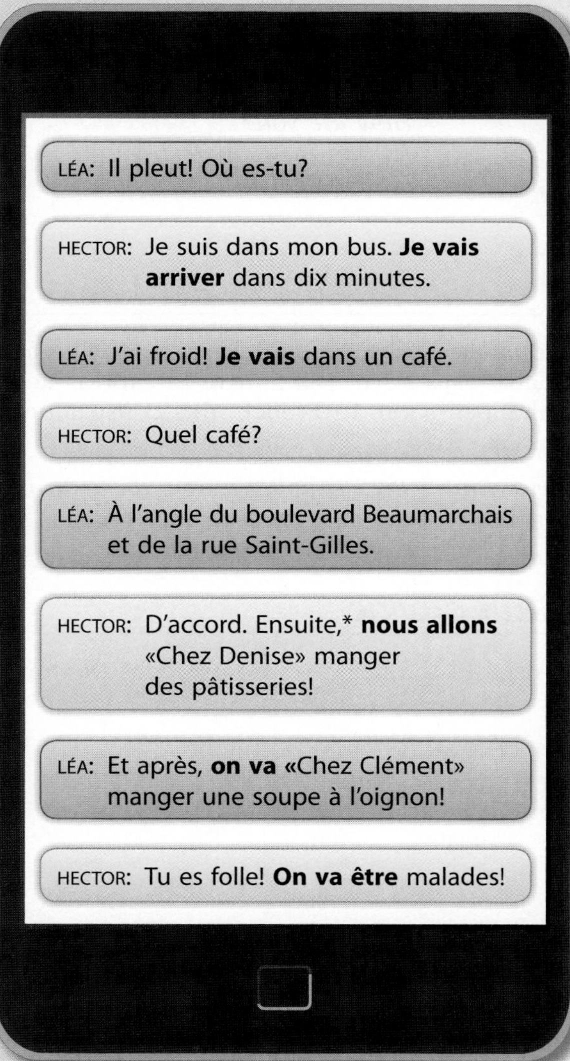

LÉA: Il pleut! Où es-tu?
HECTOR: Je suis dans mon bus. **Je vais arriver** dans dix minutes.
LÉA: J'ai froid! **Je vais** dans un café.
HECTOR: Quel café?
LÉA: À l'angle du boulevard Beaumarchais et de la rue Saint-Gilles.
HECTOR: D'accord. Ensuite,* **nous allons** «Chez Denise» manger des pâtisseries!
LÉA: Et après, **on va** «Chez Clément» manger une soupe à l'oignon!
HECTOR: Tu es folle! **On va être** malades!

*Then

Vrai ou faux?

1. Hector va arriver dans dix minutes.
2. Léa va dans un café.
3. Hector et Léa vont «Chez Denise» pour manger une soupe à l'oignon.
4. Hector et Léa vont «Chez Clément» pour manger des pâtisseries.
5. Hector et Léa vont être malades.

Forms of *aller*

The verb **aller** is irregular in form.

Suggestion: Emphasize the pronunciation of *je vais* [ʒvɛ].

PRESENT TENSE OF **aller** (*to go*)			
je	**vais**	nous	**allons**
tu	**vas**	vous	**allez**
il/elle/on	**va**	ils/elles	**vont**

Note: Point out that when using the verb *aller* with a destination, you must use a preposition, e.g., *à*, *dans*, *chez*.

Allez-vous à Grenoble pour vos vacances? — *Are you going to Grenoble for your vacation?*
Comment est-ce qu'**on va à** Grenoble? — *How do you go to (get to) Grenoble?*

You have already used **aller** in several expressions.

Comment **allez-vous**? — *How are you?*
Salut, ça **va**? — *Hi, how's it going?*
Ça **va** bien / mal. — *Fine. / Badly.*

[Allez-y! A]

Aller + Infinitive

In French, **aller** + infinitive is used to express an event that will occur in the near future. English also uses *to go* + infinitive to express actions or events that are going to happen soon. In French, this construction is called **le futur proche.**

Paul **va louer** un appartement. — *Paul is going to rent an apartment.*
Allez-vous **visiter** la France cet été? — *Are you going to visit France this summer?*

Mots clés

Exprimer le futur proche

tout à l'heure	*in a while*
tout de suite	*immediately*
bientôt	*soon*
demain	*tomorrow*
la semaine prochaine	*next week*
l'année prochaine	*next year*
dans quatre jours	*in four days*
ce week-end	*this weekend*
ce matin	*this morning*
cet après-midi	*this afternoon*
ce soir	*this evening*

Ne… pas and the *futur proche*

When the **futur proche** is used in the negative, **ne** precedes the form of **aller,** and **pas** follows.

Sylvie **ne** va **pas** étudier ce week-end. — *Sylvie is not going to study this weekend.*

[Allez-y! B-C-D]

Note: The *futur simple* (presented in *Chapitre 14*) is usually preferred in the negative form.

Grammaire interactive

For more on the verb **aller,** the **futur proche,** and the preposition **à** and its contractions, watch the corresponding Grammar Tutorial and take a brief practice quiz at **Connect French.**

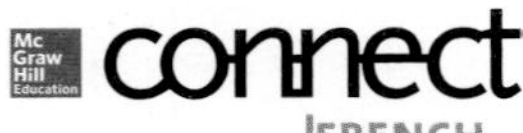

www.mhconnectfrench.com

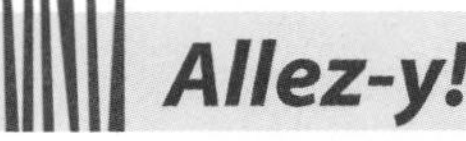

A. Où est-ce qu'on va? La solution est simple!

MODÈLE: J'ai envie de regarder un film. → Alors, je vais au cinéma!

1. Nous avons faim.
2. Il a envie de parler français.
3. Elles ont besoin d'étudier.
4. J'ai soif.
5. Tu as sommeil.
6. Vous avez envie de regarder la télévision.

dans le séjour
à la bibliothèque
dans la cuisine
à Paris
dans la salle à manger
dans la chambre
au cinéma

Suggestion (A): Can be done as a paired writing activity. Several sts. can share their answers with the class at the end.

B. Des projets. (*Plans.*) Qu'est-ce qu'on va faire (*to do*)?

MODÈLE: tu / regarder / émission (*show*) préférée / soir →
Tu vas regarder ton émission préférée ce soir.

1. je / finir / travail / semaine prochaine
2. nous / écouter / du jazz
3. vous / jouer / guitare
4. Frédéric / trouver / livre de français / bientôt
5. je / choisir / film préféré
6. les garçons / aller au cinéma / voiture / après-midi
7. tu / aller / concert / avec / amis

C. À vous la parole! Répondez aux questions suivantes.

1. Avec qui allez-vous prendre le petit déjeuner (*eat breakfast*) demain?
2. Qu'est-ce que vous allez faire demain après-midi?
3. Est-ce que vous allez faire du sport ce soir?
4. Quand allez-vous retourner à la maison ce soir?
5. Quand est-ce que vous allez passer votre prochain test de français?
6. La semaine prochaine, allez-vous aller au cinéma?
7. L'année prochaine, allez-vous continuer à étudier le français?

D. Quels sont vos projets pour le week-end? Interviewez un(e) camarade de classe. Rapportez à la classe les projets de votre camarade. Utilisez **peut-être** (*maybe*) si vous n'êtes pas certain(e).

Suggestions: rester (*stay*) à la maison, écouter la radio (de la musique), préparer un dîner (des leçons), regarder un film (la télévision), travailler à la bibliothèque (dans le jardin), aller au restaurant (au cinéma), parler avec des amis, finir un livre intéressant, et cetera.

MODÈLE: aller au cinéma →
É1: Vas-tu aller au cinéma?
É2: Oui, je vais peut-être aller au cinéma. (*ou* Non, je ne vais pas aller au cinéma.) Et toi?

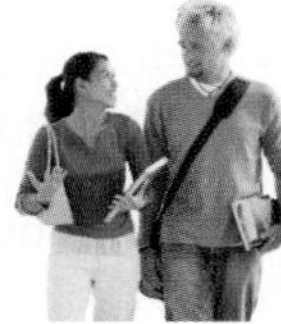

Follow-up: Have sts. report a few answers to class, or write a short composition on their partner's responses. Sts. can count the affirmative sentences to see who is the most active person in class.

Follow-up: Ask sts. to give their *projets pour demain* to a small group. They can choose responses from those presented or add other ideas.

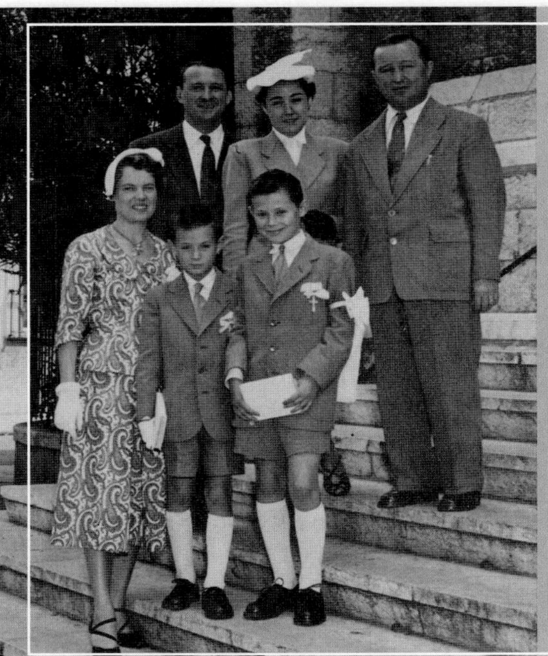

Un peu plus...

La famille.
La photo date des années 50 (*the 1950s*): à cette époque (*at that time*), on se marie et ensuite, on a des enfants. Aujourd'hui, le mariage n'est plus le seul moyen (*only means*) acceptable de former une famille. En France, 56,6 % des enfants sont nés (*born*) de parents non-mariés.
Et chez vous?

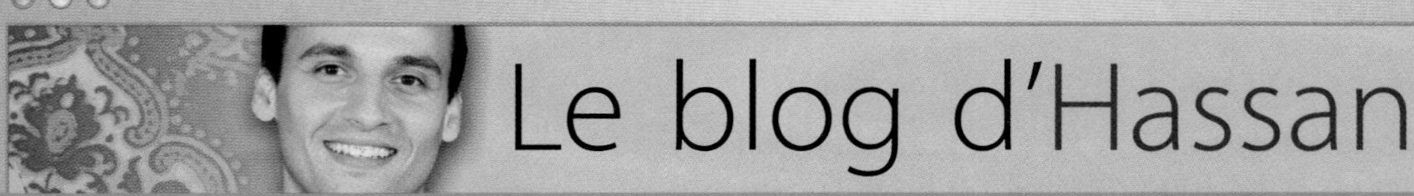

Le blog d'Hassan

Un mariage franco-marocain

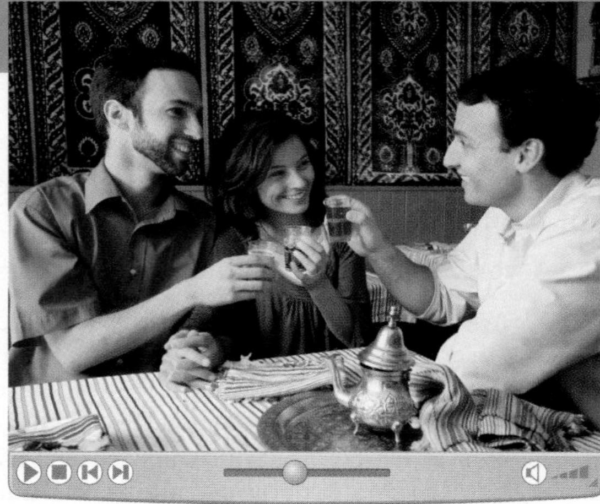

Abdel, Carole et moi dans mon restaurant

jeudi 2 juin

Salut! Vous entrez dans le blog d'Hassan. Pour le moment j'écris,[1] mais bientôt je vais aussi faire des films vidéos comme un vrai pro des nouvelles technologies!

J'ai une grande nouvelle[2]: Mon copain Abdel va se marier.[3] Il est amoureux! Sa chérie s'appelle Carole. Elle est française.

Ça va être un mariage franco-marocain, un mariage interculturel.

Mais va-t-il être célébré en France ou au Maroc? Je ne sais pas: les fiancés n'ont pas encore pris leur décision.[4]

En tout cas, on va bien manger, c'est sûr! Et pourtant,[5] ce n'est pas moi qui vais préparer le repas de noces[6]...

On prévoit[7] au moins 110 invitations pour les parents, les grands-parents, les oncles et les tantes, les cousins et les cousines des deux côtés.[8] Et aussi les amis!

Hassan

Suggestion: Model pronunciation and have sts. repeat individually or as a group.

Follow-up: 1. *Que savez-vous* (What do you know) *d'Hassan? (Regardez sa carte d'identité,* p. 2). 2. *Qu'est-ce qu'un mariage interculturel?* 3. *Où va se passer* (take place) *le mariage d'Abdel? Qui va être invité?* 4. *Le mariage et la famille: quelle est l'opinion des commentateurs? Quels pays et quelles cultures représentent-ils?* 5. *Que pensez-vous personnellement du mariage et de la famille?*

Video connection: In the videoblog for this chapter, Hassan, Abdel, and Carole explore possible wedding sites: a barge on the Seine, l'Institut du monde arabe, la Tour Montparnasse in Paris, or a beautiful *ryad* in Morocco.

COMMENTAIRES

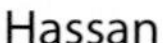

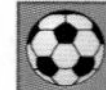

Mamadou

Salut, Hassan
Chez nous, en Afrique, la famille c'est synonyme de bonheur et de puissance.[9]
Si Abdel est comme un frère pour toi, tu vas bientôt avoir de nouveaux neveux et nouvelles nièces! Tu vas devenir tonton[10] adoptif! Tu es content?

Alexis

Tu es célibataire, Hassan? Veinard[11]! Le mariage, c'est une horrible invention humaine!

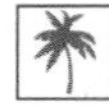

Poema

Tu es cynique, Alexis! Moi, je veux me marier,[12] je veux un mari et des enfants.
En Polynésie, la famille c'est une bénédiction.

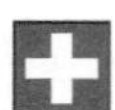

Charlotte

Tu as raison, Poema. Le mariage, c'est l'équilibre! Ici, à Genève, j'ai une petite fille adorable et un mari très présent, et je suis heureuse.

[1]*I am writing* [2]grande... *big news* [3]va... *is getting married* [4]n'ont... *have not yet decided* [5]*however* [6]repas... *wedding meal* [7]On... *We are planning* [8]*sides* [9]bonheur... *happiness and strength* [10]*uncle* (fam.) [11]*Lucky you!* [12]veux... *want to get married*

REPORTAGE

La famille au Maroc: une valeur sûre

Le Maroc change: en 2003, le Roi[1] Mohammed VI modernise le code de la famille. Le nouveau code introduit un principe révolutionnaire dans une société traditionnelle: l'égalité entre l'homme et la femme. Comme la Tunisie et le Liban, deux autres pays francophones, le Maroc choisit donc le progrès.

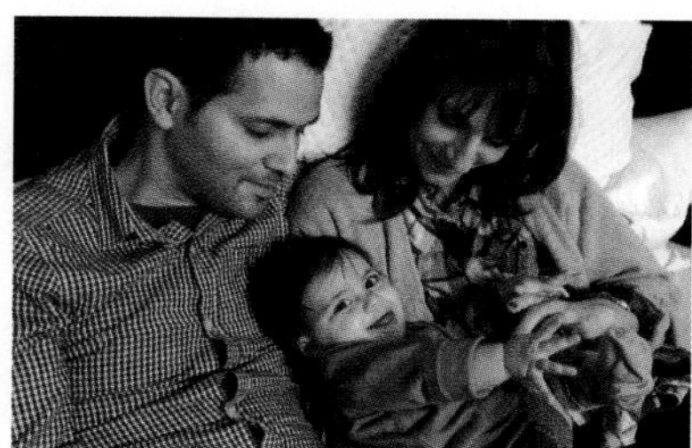
Une famille marocaine

Dans le couple d'aujourd'hui, l'homme et la femme ont des droits[2] et des obligations réciproques. Dans la société marocaine traditionnelle, au contraire, la femme devait[3] obéir à son mari et la polygamie était autorisée. Maintenant aussi, la femme a le droit de demander le divorce et, dans ce cas, elle a, en priorité, la garde[4] des enfants.

«C'est à travers une multitude de petits faits significatifs que l'on peut apprécier l'évolution de la société marocaine, explique Dounia, jeune mère et femme active. L'âge légal du mariage pour les femmes est de 18 ans au lieu de[5] 15 ans. La politique s'ouvre[6] aux femmes: le Maroc a des ambassadrices, et le Roi accepte d'avoir des conseillères. Dans les entreprises, les femmes ont accès à des postes de responsables.» Et Dounia ajoute: «Nous avons maintenant l'élection d'une Miss Maroc! Tout cela était inconcevable pour nos parents.»

Elle continue: «Mais attention! Le modèle européen n'est pas applicable chez nous. Le Maroc a des traditions qui fondent sa culture. Nous ne voulons pas y renoncer.[7] Par exemple, pour une Française ou une Américaine, servir son mari, c'est de la soumission. Pour une femme marocaine, c'est un moyen[8] d'établir son influence.»

Le mariage est toujours fortement valorisé[9] au Maroc. Plus de 90[10] pour cent des Marocains pensent qu'il est préférable aux hommes et aux femmes de se marier et d'avoir des enfants. Et la solidarité familiale reste fondamentale: pour les Marocains, les parents âgés doivent être pris en charge[11] par les enfants et non pas par l'État.

[1]*King* [2]*rights* [3]*had to* [4]*care* [5]au... *instead of* [6]*is opening up* [7]y... *reject them* [8]*means* [9]fortement... *highly valued* [10]quatre-vingt-dix [11]doivent... *should be cared for*

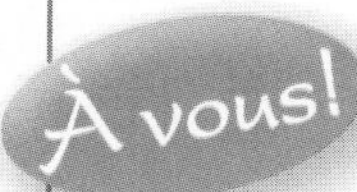

1. Que fait le Roi du Maroc en 2003 pour améliorer (*to improve*) la condition et le statut (*status*) de la femme marocaine?
2. Quels sont les nouveaux droits de la femme marocaine?
3. Expliquez: «Le modèle européen n'est pas applicable chez nous. Le Maroc a des traditions qui fondent sa culture.»
4. Comment s'exprime (*is expressed*) la solidarité familiale au Maroc? Et dans votre culture? Comment les Marocains traitent-ils leurs parents âgés? Et les Américains?

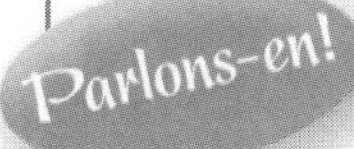

1. Dans quels domaines l'égalité entre les hommes et les femmes est-elle effective dans la société américaine? Parlez des études, du travail, du couple, du ménage et de la cuisine.
2. Comparez les droits de la femme marocaine et de la femme américaine. Qui est la plus émancipée—la femme marocaine ou la femme américaine? Expliquez. Qui valorise le plus le mariage? les enfants? les responsabilités professionnelles?

Leçon 3

STRUCTURES

Le verbe *faire*

Expressing What You Are Doing or Making

Je fais tout!

Hector téléphone à Hassan.

HECTOR: Salut Hassan: ton restaurant, ça va?
HASSAN: Non. C'est terrible! Mon chef de cuisine est absent. **Je fais** tout!
HECTOR: **Tu fais** le service?
HASSAN: **Je fais** les courses, **je fais** la cuisine, **je fais** le service.
HECTOR: Moi aussi, **je fais** beaucoup de choses!
HASSAN: Toi, **tu fais** de la danse: c'est différent, c'est de l'art…
HECTOR: Mais avec mes colocataires, nous aussi, **nous faisons** tout à la maison: **nous faisons** le marché, la lessive, le ménage… Et ça, ce n'est pas de l'art!

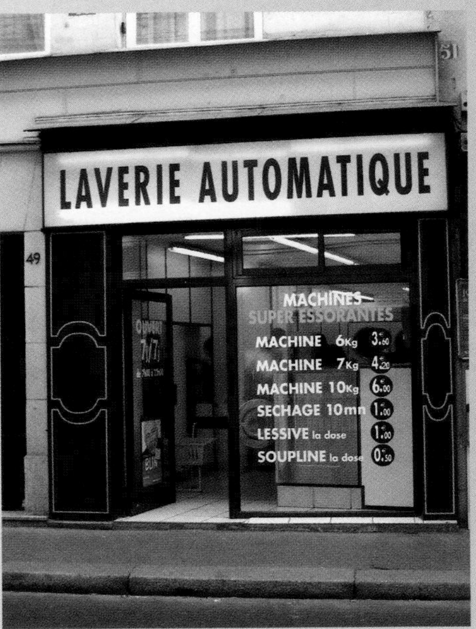

Faire la lessive à la laverie automatique, ça, ce n'est pas de l'art!

Répondez aux questions.

1. Qu'est-ce qu'Hassan fait au restaurant?
2. Qui fait de la danse?
3. Qu'est-ce qu'Hector et ses colocataires font dans la maison?

Forms of *faire*

The verb **faire** is irregular in form.

Presentation: Model the pronunciation of verb forms in short sentences, taken from the dialogue. Examples: *Tu fais le service? Je fais les courses. Nous faisons le ménage.*

Suggestion: Mention the pronunciation of *je fais* [ʃfɛ] and *nous faisons* [fəzɔ̃].

PRESENT TENSE OF **faire** (*to do; to make*)			
je	**fais**	nous	**faisons**
tu	**fais**	vous	**faites**
il/elle/on	**fait**	ils/elles	**font**

Note the difference in pronunciation of **fais / fait, faites,** and **faisons.**

Je fais mon lit. — *I make my bed.*
Nous faisons le café. — *We're making coffee.*
Faites la vaisselle. — *Do the dishes.*

Expressions with *faire*

The verb **faire** is used in many idiomatic expressions.

faire attention (à)	*to pay attention (to); to watch out (for)*
faire la connaissance (de)	*to meet (for the first time), make the acquaintance (of)*
faire les courses	*to do errands*
faire la cuisine	*to cook*
faire ses devoirs	*to do one's homework*
faire la lessive	*to do the laundry*
faire le marché	*to do the shopping; to go to the market*
faire le ménage	*to do the housework*
faire une promenade	*to take a walk*
faire la queue	*to stand in line*
faire un tour (en voiture)	*to take a walk (a ride)*
faire la vaisselle	*to do the dishes*
faire un voyage	*to take a trip*

Le matin je **fais le marché,** et le soir je **fais mes devoirs.** — *In the morning I do the shopping, and in the evening I do my homework.*

1. **Faire** is also used to talk about individual sports: **faire du sport, faire du jogging, de la voile** (*sailing*), **du ski, de l'aérobic.**
2. As seen in **Leçon 1, il fait** is also used to describe the weather.

Il fait tellement beau! — *It's so nice outside!*

Presentation: Model pronunciation of *faire* expressions. You may want to use expressions in short personalized questions as you present them: *Aimez-vous faire la cuisine? Où faites-vous vos devoirs?* If possible, display images from the Internet depicting these actions. You may need to explain what an idiomatic expression is: An idiom (*une expression idiomatique*) is a group of words that has meaning to the speakers of a language but that does not necessarily appear to make sense when examined word by word. Idiomatic expressions are often different from one language to another. For example, in English, *to pull Mary's leg* usually means to tease her, not to grab her leg and pull it.

Additional vocabulary: *faire la fête* (*to party*), *faire du shopping* (*to shop;* note: in Quebec, *magasiner*).

Note: All martial arts are used with *faire* and *golf* is used with *jouer à*.

Allez-y!

A. Faisons connaissance! À une petite soirée à l'université, les gens se rencontrent (*meet each other*). Suivez le modèle.

MODÈLE: je / le professeur d'italien ⟶
Je fais la connaissance du professeur d'italien.

1. tu / la sœur de Louise
2. nous / un cousin
3. Élodie / une étudiante sympathique
4. les Levêque / les parents de Clara
5. je / la femme du professeur
6. vous / la nièce de M. de La Tour

B. Activités du week-end. Qui fait les activités suivantes? Faites des phrases logiques avec les éléments des deux colonnes.

1. Tu...	**a.** faisons du jogging dans le parc.
2. Pierre...	**b.** ne fais pas le ménage.
3. Anne et Laure...	**c.** faites vos devoirs de français.
4. Mon frère et moi, nous...	**d.** fais la cuisine pour tes amis.
5. Benoît et toi, vous...	**e.** font des courses en ville.
6. Non, moi le dimanche, je...	**f.** fait du sport avec ses copains.

Suggestion: Encourage sts. to use other idiomatic expressions with *faire*.

Suggestion: Bring in magazine pictures of people doing activities that require *faire* expressions and have sts. describe pictures.

Note (C): Emphasize that the use of the definite article in this context means a repetitive or habitual action.

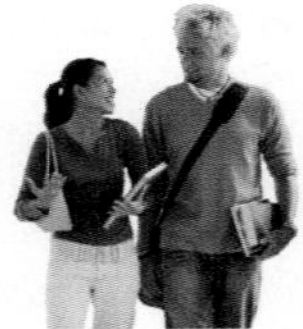

C. D'habitude, qu'est-ce que vous faites? Avec un(e) camarade de classe, faites une liste de vos activités habituelles. Utilisez les expressions suivantes: **le matin, le midi, le soir; le lundi (matin), le mardi,** et cetera; **le week-end, une fois par semaine** (*once a week*), **tous les jours** (*every day*).

MODÈLE: É1: D'habitude, qu'est-ce que tu fais le soir?
É2: Je fais du jogging tous les soirs.

D. Mimes. Formez deux groupes. Choisissez une expression avec **faire** en le tirant par hasard d'un chapeau. Faites deviner cette expression par les membres de votre groupe. Si votre équipe (*team*) devine la réponse, elle a un point. L'équipe qui a le plus de points gagne (*wins*).

Vocabulary recycling: Before presenting *-re* verbs, quickly review *-er*, *-ir*, and a handful of irregular verbs. Have sts. write out brief, original examples and lead classmates in rapid-response drills: *Je cherche mes cahiers* (*Bruno, les étudiantes, tu, nous*); *Ils choisissent leurs cours* (*je, Mireille, vous, tu*); *Nous allons au cinéma* (*Marc, tu, vous, je*), etc.

Les verbes en *-re*

Expressing Actions

J'arrive!

Juliette téléphone à Léa.

JULIETTE: Allô, allô! **Tu entends?**
LÉA: **J'entends** mal; je suis dans le métro, à Opéra.
JULIETTE: **Tu descends** à quelle station?
LÉA: **Je descends** à Bastille.
JULIETTE: Je suis avec Hector. **Nous attendons** devant le cinéma UGC. Nous faisons la queue. Le film commence à 20 h.
LÉA: J'arrive! **Vous m'attendez,** hein!

Vrai ou faux?

1. Juliette demande à Léa si elle entend.
2. Léa entend mal.
3. Léa descend à Opéra.
4. Juliette et Hector attendent Léa au café.
5. Léa demande à ses amis d'attendre.

Note: Point out that all three singular forms of *-re* verbs sound alike.

Suggestion: For listening-comprehension practice, have sts. indicate whether they hear a singular or plural verb in the following sentences: 1. *Elles attendent le dessert.* (Solicit two reasons for plural: *liaison* and *d* sound.) 2. *Il rend le poulet au chef.* 3. *Elles perdent leur appétit.* 4. *Il entend le chien.* 5. *Il répond à la question de son ami.*

Note: Provide lots of examples with *attendre*, which poses problems because the English equivalent requires a preposition. *Rendre visite à* and *répondre à* also pose problems because of comparison with English.

Suggestion: Point out the phonetic opposition between *attendre* [atɑ̃dʀ] and *entendre* [ɑ̃tɑ̃dʀ].

A third group of French verbs has infinitives that end in **-re.**

PRESENT TENSE OF **vendre** (*to sell*)			
je	vend**s**	nous	vend**ons**
tu	vend**s**	vous	vend**ez**
il/elle/on	vend	ils/elles	vend**ent**

1. Other verbs conjugated like **vendre** include the following.

attendre	*to wait (for)*	**rendre**	*to give back, return*
descendre	*to go down; to get off*	**rendre visite à**	*to visit (someone)*
entendre	*to hear*		
perdre	*to lose; to waste*	**répondre à**	*to answer*

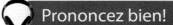

Elle attend le dessert.	*She's waiting for dessert.*
Nous descendons de l'autobus.	*We're getting off the bus.*
Le commerçant rend la monnaie à la cliente.	*The storekeeper gives change back to the customer.*
Je réponds à sa question.	*I'm answering his/her question.*

2. The expression **rendre visite à** means to visit a *person* or *people.* The verb **visiter** is used only with places or things.

   Je rends visite à mon ami.
   Les touristes visitent les monuments de Paris.

Additional activity (A): *Qu'est-ce qu'on fait maintenant? Changez du singulier au pluriel ou vice versa.* MODÈLE: *Je vends ma guitare. → Nous vendons notre guitare.* 1. *Tu rends visite à ton amie Paulette.* 2. *Vous rendez un livre à la bibliothèque.* 3. *J'entends la voiture qui arrive.* 4. *Nous descendons de la voiture.* 5. *Elles perdent du temps au café.* 6. *Il répond aux questions de sa sœur.*

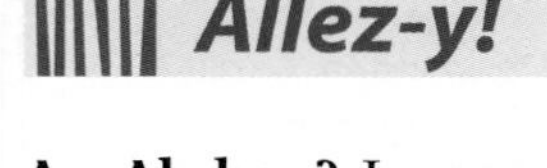

Allez-y!

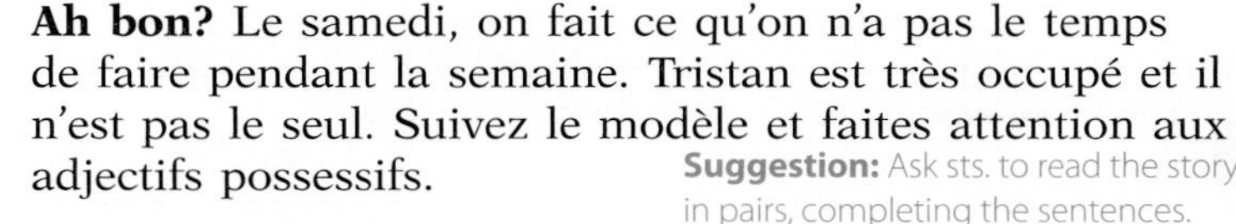

A. Ah bon? Le samedi, on fait ce qu'on n'a pas le temps de faire pendant la semaine. Tristan est très occupé et il n'est pas le seul. Suivez le modèle et faites attention aux adjectifs possessifs.

Suggestion: Ask sts. to read the story in pairs, completing the sentences.

MODÈLE: vendre des DVD sur eBay (moi) →
É1: Tristan vend des DVD sur eBay.
É2: Ah bon? Moi aussi je vends des DVD sur eBay!

1. rendre ses livres à la bibliothèque (nous)
2. attendre le bus pour aller faire des courses (mon frère)
3. descendre au sous-sol (vous)
4. perdre trop de temps à lire ses méls (toi)
5. entendre à la radio une publicité pour un concert (mes copains)
6. répondre à beaucoup de coups de téléphone (*phone calls*) (moi)

B. Un week-end à Paris. Complétez l'histoire avec les verbes à droite.

Alain et Marie-Lise habitent à Bruxelles. Aujourd'hui ils _____[1] à Paris en train. Ils vont _____[2] visite à leur cousine Pauline. Les trois cousins ont toujours beaucoup de projets et ne _____[3] pas une minute quand ils sont ensemble (*together*). Alain et Marie-Lise aiment beaucoup Pauline parce qu'elle _____[4] toujours à leurs méls. Pauline aime aussi ses cousins, et elle _____[5] leur arrivée avec impatience. Elle _____[6] enfin la sonnette (*doorbell*)!

attendre
descendre
entendre
perdre
rendre
répondre

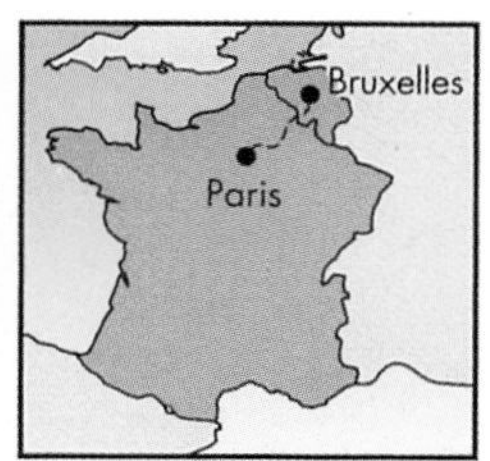

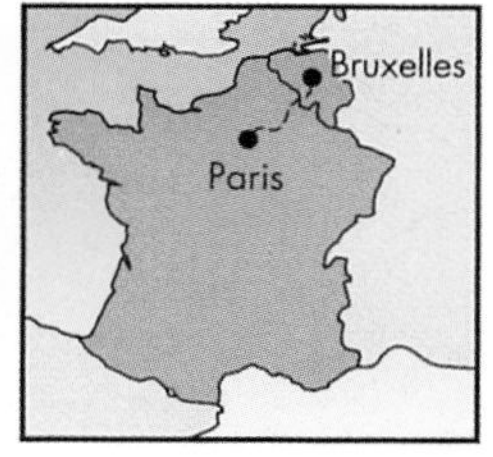

C. Perdez-vous souvent patience? Interviewez un(e) camarade de classe. Il/Elle utilise **souvent, pas souvent** ou **toujours** dans sa réponse.

MODÈLE: É1: Tu attends l'autobus, mais il n'arrive pas. Est-ce que tu perds patience?
É2: Oui, je perds souvent patience.

1. Tu attends un coup de téléphone. La personne ne téléphone pas. **2.** Un ami / Une amie ne répond pas à tes textos. **3.** Tu perds les clés de ta voiture ou de ton appartement. **4.** Tu as rendez-vous avec un ami / une amie. Tu attends longtemps (*for a long time*), mais il/elle n'arrive pas.

Follow-up: (1) Take tally of results of interviews. *Qui est patient? Qui est normal? Qui n'est pas du tout patient?* (2) Expand answers by asking sts. to say what they do in each situation. Example of expansion with model sentence: *Je prends un taxi.*

Interaction: Have sts. act out the following situation, using the vocabulary and structures they've learned. *Conversation:* You are left alone in a room with a friend's parents (two classmates) while your friend prepares to go out with you. Make polite conversation with them. Talk about your family, your home, where you and your friend will go, and what you will do together this evening.

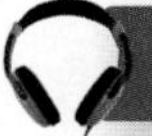

Prononcez bien!

The consonant *r*

When you pronounce a French **r,** the back of your tongue almost touches the back of your palate. Force air out, as when you pronounce an **h,** and maintain that very narrow passage between the back of your tongue and the back of your palate. You will get that rattling sound characteristic of the French **r.**

[ʀ]: **parent, pour, arriver, rhume**

The **r** occurring at the end of a word is usually pronounced, with the exception of the following:

- infinitive verbs ending in **-er: aller, donner, parler**
- professions ending in **-er: boucher, plombier**

Pronunciation presentation: To help sts. become aware of the narrow passage between the back of their tongue and the back of their palate, invite them to reflect on the position of their articulators when they gargle after brushing their teeth, and when they clear their throat to spit out.

Pronunciation practice (1): Using the family tree at the beginning of the chapter, elicit sts.' pronunciation of the following words: *père, mère, frère, sœur, mari, parent, grands-parents.*

Pronunciation practice (2): Using the drawing of the house in this chapter, elicit sts.' pronunciation of the following words: *bureau, chambre, jardin, rez-de-chaussée, séjour, terrasse.*

Pronunciation practice (3): Additional activities to practice these sounds can be found on page 138.

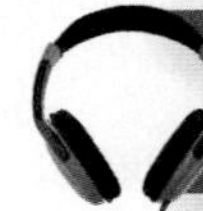

Prononcez bien!

1. The pronunciation of *premier* (page 123)

Journal intime. Vous rangez (*clean*) votre chambre et retrouvez le journal intime que vous avez commencé à votre arrivée en France. Avec un(e) camarade, lisez les phrases suivantes à voix haute (*aloud*) en faisant attention à la prononciation de «premier».

Cher journal,

1. Aujourd'hui, c'est le ***premier*** août.
2. Je suis très content(e) parce que j'emménage dans mon ***premier*** appartement avec Hugo.
3. Hugo, c'est mon ***premier*** ami français!
4. Je vais avoir mon ***premier*** bureau.
5. Je vais acheter mon ***premier*** ordinateur.
6. Et je vais avoir mon ***premier*** lit aussi. C'est super!

2. The vowels in *notre* and *nos* (page 126)

Week-end chez les parents d'Hugo. Vous passez le week-end avec Hugo chez ses parents. Sa mère pose des questions sur votre vie aux États-Unis. Complétez les phrases avec **notre, nos** ou **votre, vos.** Ensuite, jouez la scène avec un(e) camarade de classe.

Answers (2): 1. *votre* 2. *votre* 3. *notre* 4. *vos* 5. *nos*

LA MÈRE: Comment est ______[1] maison aux États-Unis? Est-ce que ______[2] cuisine est grande, comme celle-ci (*like this one*)?
VOUS: ______[3] maison est grande et jolie, mais la cuisine est plus petite.
LA MÈRE: Est-ce que vous habitez chez ______[4] parents?
VOUS: Oui, et nous avons deux chiens aussi. Ils adorent jouer dans le jardin de ______[5] voisins!

3. The consonant *r* (page 137)

A. La famille d'Hugo. Vous continuez votre conversation avec la mère d'Hugo. Jouez le rôle de la mère et lisez sa description de la famille à voix haute. Faites attention à la prononciation du *r*.

Les grands-parents paternels d'Hugo sont morts (*dead*). Moi, j'ai encore (*still*) mon père, Gérard—il a 80 ans!—et ma mère, Catherine. J'ai aussi quatre frères et trois sœurs. En tout (*Altogether*), Hugo a quatorze cousins et cousines! J'ai invité (*invited*) Christophe et Karine, les cousins les plus proches (*closest*) d'Hugo, à manger avec nous ce soir.

B. Devinettes. En attendant l'arrivée des cousins d'Hugo, vous jouez aux devinettes (*riddles*) avec lui (*him*). Trouvez les pièces de la maison qui correspondent aux définitions que lit Hugo (votre camarade de classe).

MODÈLE: É1: C'est la pièce où il y a un ordinateur et des livres pour travailler.
É2: C'est le bureau!

1. C'est la pièce où il y a un lit.
2. C'est la pièce où il y a un canapé, des fauteuils et une télévision.
3. C'est la partie de la maison où il y a le séjour, la salle à manger et la cuisine.
4. C'est l'espace (*area*) où il y a des arbres et des roses.
5. C'est l'espace où il y a des chaises longues et où on prend le petit déjeuner (*breakfast*) en été.

Answers (3B): 1. *la chambre* 2. *le séjour / la salle de séjour* 3. *le rez-de-chaussée* 4. *le jardin* 5. *la terrasse*

 Lecture

Avant de lire

Identifying a pronoun's referent. As you know, a pronoun may "stand in" for a noun. By using a pronoun to replace a noun, an author can avoid repeating the noun, which would result in unnatural sounding language. To illustrate this, reformulate the following sentence from the text by replacing the pronoun **il** with the noun it refers to:

> C'est en 1883[1] que l'artiste s'installe avec sa famille à Giverny, en Normandie, à 75[2] kilomètres de Paris. Il va y habiter pendant 43 ans. Il adore Giverny. Il transforme sa propriété en un jardin riche en symétries, en perspectives et en couleurs.

Without the pronoun, the text sounds repetitive and awkward.

A pronoun may also refer to a person or group that can be identified by context. For example, this text begins:

> Nous sommes à Giverny, chez le peintre Claude Monet...

You can infer that the subject **nous** includes the reader as well as the author; the use of this inclusive **nous** creates a bond between the reader and the author, inviting the reader to "come along for the ride."

Recall too that French does not have a single pronoun that corresponds to "it"; a third-person pronoun such as **il, elle,** or **ce** plays this role. In the sentence below, which **il** refers to Monet and which is an impersonal pronoun?

> Monet aime observer la nature quand il fait beau, quand il pleut, quand il fait du vent, et analyser la lumière du matin, de l'après-midi, du soir. C'est à Giverny qu'il trouve son inspiration et qu'il définit son art.

As you read the text, be sure that you are able to identify the referent for each pronoun to ensure accurate comprehension.

[1]mille huit cent quatre-vingt-trois [2]soixante-quinze

À propos de la lecture...
Les auteurs de *Vis-à-vis* ont écrit ce texte.

«Mon cœur[1] est à Giverny, toujours et toujours... »
Claude Monet

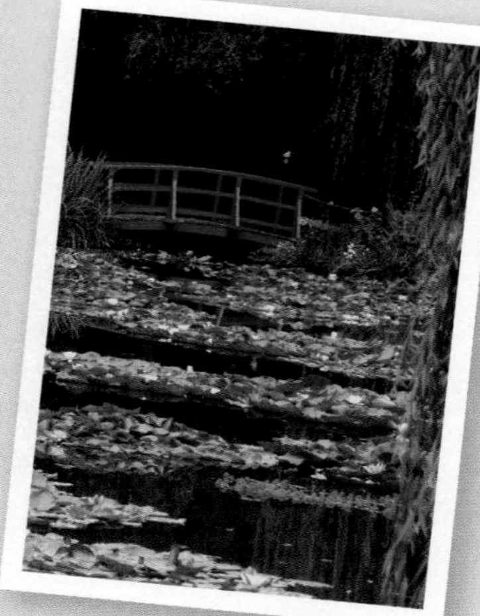

Le pont japonais à Giverny

Giverny: le petit paradis de Monet

Une destination touristique

Nous sommes à Giverny, chez le peintre Claude Monet (1840[2]–1926[3]). Chaque année, 500 000[4] visiteurs découvrent avec émotion ce petit paradis. Dans la maison, toutes les pièces semblent encore habitées: la salle à manger, les salons et les chambres. Devant la maison rose qui a aussi charmé les amis de Monet (les peintres Cézanne, Renoir et Matisse, et l'écrivain Zola), les visiteurs découvrent le Clos normand,[5] un immense jardin symétrique planté de fleurs et d'arbres et, plus loin, le Jardin d'eau[6] avec son célèbre[7] pont japonais.

Une inspiration pour le père de l'impressionnisme

C'est en 1883[8] que l'artiste s'installe[9] avec sa famille à Giverny, en Normandie, à 75[10] kilomètres de Paris. Il va y habiter pendant 43 ans. Il adore Giverny. Il transforme sa propriété en un jardin riche en symétries, en perspectives et en couleurs, et arrange les fleurs dans un désordre apparent. Le résultat est une véritable œuvre d'art.[11]

Monet aime observer la nature quand il fait beau, quand il pleut, quand il fait du vent, et analyser la lumière[12] du matin, de l'après-midi, du soir. C'est à Giverny qu'il trouve son inspiration et qu'il définit son art. Cet endroit magnifique inspire à l'artiste des œuvres célèbres comme *Le Champ d'iris jaunes à Giverny* (1887[13]), le *Printemps, Giverny* (1890[14]) et les *Nymphéas*, une série de 250[15] tableaux qui évoquent les nénuphars[16] du bassin.

«Je veux réussir à traduire ce que je ressens[17]» explique-t-il. Ses peintures ne reproduisent pas les objets mais une impression ou une émotion. C'est un nouveau mouvement de peinture. Monet est bien le père de l'impressionnisme.

[1]*heart* [2]mille huit cent quarante [3]mille neuf cent vingt-six [4]cinq cent mille [5]Clos... *field in the Norman style* [6]*water* [7]*famous* [8]mille huit cent quatre-vingt-trois [9]*settles* [10]soixante-quinze [11]œuvre... *work of art* [12]*light* [13]mille huit cent quatre-vingt-sept [14]mille huit cent quatre-vingt-dix [15]deux cent cinquante [16]*water lilies* [17]réussir... *to succeed in translating what I feel*

Compréhension

Une brochure publicitaire. Create a travel brochure for Monet's garden in Giverny by filling in the blanks with the appropriate expressions from the text.

Un petit paradis terrestre? Ça existe à quelques ______[1] de Paris! Découvrez Giverny où le peintre ______[2] a trouvé son inspiration. Son œuvre ne reproduit pas les objets, mais ______[3] ou ______[4] —c'est le principe de l'impressionnisme.

La maison a l'air toujours ______,[5] marquée par la présence des amis illustres de Monet, parmi eux (*among them*), l'écrivain ______.[6]

Devant la maison de Monet, on trouve un immense jardin symétrique qui s'appelle «______».[7] En traversant le célèbre Pont japonais, on arrive au fameux ______[8] qui a donné naissance à une série de 250 ______[9] appelés «______».[10]

Giverny, c'est la nature, la lumière, les couleurs, les nuances. Venez découvrir ce lieu privilégié!

Answers: 1. *kilomètres* 2. *Monet* 3. *une impression* 4. *une émotion* 5. *habitée* 6. *Zola* 7. *le Clos normand* 8. *Jardin d'eau* 9. *tableaux* 10. *Nymphéas*

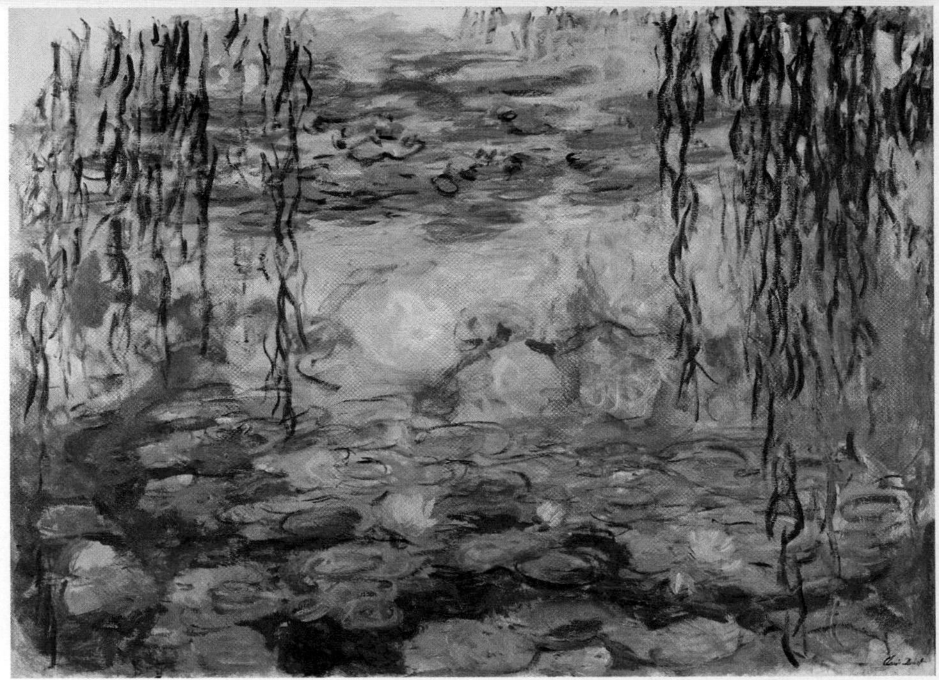

Claude Monet: *Nymphéas,* 1916–1919. (Musée Marmottan Monet, Paris)

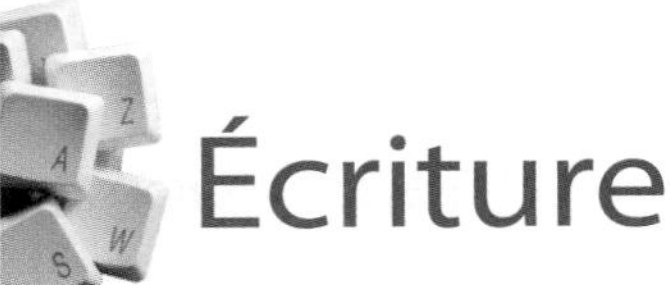

Écriture

The writing activities **Par écrit** and **Journal intime** can be found in the Workbook/Laboratory Manual to accompany *Vis-à-vis*.

Pour s'amuser

Un homme raconte ses vacances à son collègue.

—La première semaine, on a eu (*we had*) mauvais temps: la pluie, la neige, le vent, le froid...
—Et la deuxième semaine? ...
—Une catastrophe!
—Vraiment? Pourquoi?
—Mes beaux-parents sont arrivés...

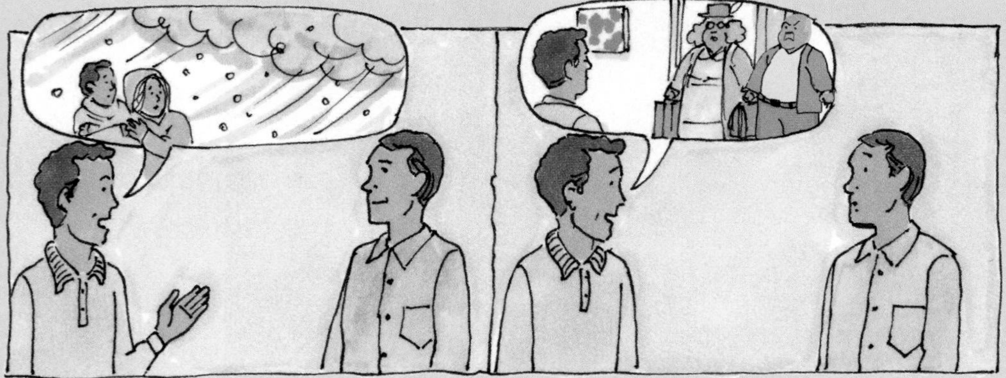

La vie en chantant. An activity based on the song "Je suis une enfant" by Carla Bruni can be found in the Instructor's Manual. The song can be purchased at the iTunes store, or sts. can watch the music video on YouTube.

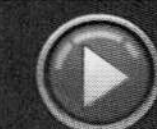

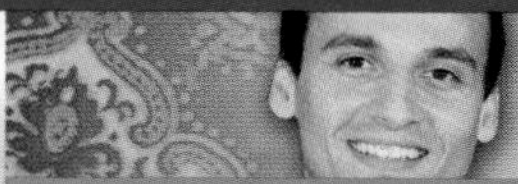

Le vidéoblog d'Hassan

En bref

Dans cet épisode, Hassan est dans son restaurant avec son copain Abdel et Carole, la fiancée d'Abdel. Abdel et Carole mentionnent des endroits (lieux) possibles pour leur cérémonie et leur réception de mariage.

Vocabulaire en contexte

Indiquez vos préférences pour une cérémonie et une réception idéale de mariage.

Les invités

- ☐ **seulement** (*only*) moi et mon fiancé / ma fiancée
- ☐ seulement les deux familles
- ☐ seulement de très bons amis
- ☐ les deux familles et de bons amis
- ☐ **tout le monde** (*everyone*)!

Les lieux

- ☐ sur une **péniche** (*river barge*)
- ☐ au **56e** étage d'une **tour** (*tower*)
- ☐ sur la terrasse d'un musée ou d'un institut
- ☐ dans un hôtel de grand **luxe** (*luxury*)
- ☐ dans une église (*church*), une mosquée, une synagogue

Visionnez!

Choisissez la bonne réponse.

1. Pour Carole, le détail le plus (*most*) important est ______.
   a. le nombre d'invités **b.** le lieu **c.** le mois de l'année
2. Pour Carole, une réception de mariage sur une péniche ______.
   a. **coûte** (*costs*) trop cher **b.** est très romantique **c.** est une mauvaise idée
3. La tour Montparnasse et l'Institut du **monde** (*world*) arabe offrent de belles vues ______.
   a. quand il fait beau **b.** seulement le soir **c.** seulement en été
4. On fête un mariage au Maroc ______.
   a. à la plage (*beach*) **b.** chez les parents du marié **c.** dans un **ryad** (*Moroccan villa*)

Analysez!

Répondez aux questions.

1. De quels lieux à Paris parlent-ils dans la vidéo? Quel est l'avantage et/ou l'inconvénient de chaque (*each*) lieu? Quel lieu préférez-vous?
2. Abdel et Carole forment-ils un couple «traditionnel»? Pourquoi?

Comparez!

Faites la description d'une cérémonie ou d'une réception de mariage typique dans votre culture. Regardez encore une fois (*once more*) la partie culturelle de la vidéo: les lieux de mariage en France ressemblent-ils aux lieux de mariage aux États-Unis? Expliquez.

Suggestion: In *Chapitres 5–8*, certain vocabulary relevant to the video segment is presented in the form of checklists, from which sts. select their preferences. After you model the pronunciation and review the meanings of the words in boldface (which are words actually contained in the video transcript), have sts. select their preference(s) in each column. Afterward, a comparison and "tally" of preferences can be done in groups or as a whole-class activity.

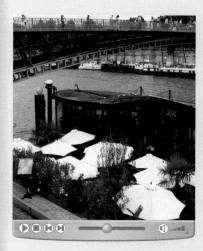

Une péniche pour la réception de mariage

Additional vocabulary: Other vocabulary you may wish to present before viewing includes *compter, il faut d'abord décider, je veux quelque chose d'exceptionnel, prix, quelque chose.*

Suggestion: Use *Visionnez!* to introduce additional vocabulary and concepts and to check comprehension after viewing. Ask sts. to read the questions before they watch the video. Review the meanings of the words in boldface. Return to these questions afterward for a quick comprehension check.

Note culturelle

Un ryad (ou riad) est une belle maison bourgeoise, d'architecture traditionnelle mauresque[1] construite autour d'un patio, généralement avec une fontaine. Les ryads, qui servent souvent aujourd'hui de Maisons d'hôtes,[2] sont souvent luxueux, avec plusieurs salons et chambres, et un décor typiquement marocain.

[1]*Moorish* [2]Maisons… *small hotels*

CHAPITRE **5**

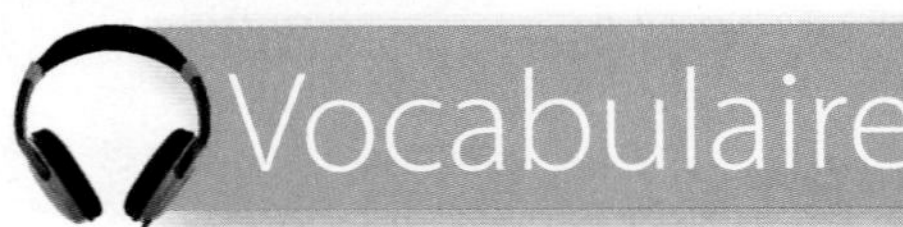

Vocabulaire

Verbes

aller to go
aller + *inf.* to be going (to do something)
aller mal to feel bad (ill)
attendre to wait (for)
descendre to go down; to get off
entendre to hear
faire to do; to make
perdre to lose; to waste
préparer to prepare
rendre to give back; to return; to hand in
rendre visite à to visit (*someone*)
répondre à to answer
rester to stay, remain
vendre to sell

À REVOIR: **étudier, habiter, jouer (à) (de), manger**

Substantifs

l'arbre (*m.*) tree
l'autobus (*m.*) (city) bus
le bruit noise
la clé key
la famille family
la météo weather forecast
les projets (*m. pl.*) plans
le temps time; weather
les vacances (*f. pl.*) vacation

À REVOIR: **l'affiche** (*f.*), **le chien, la commode, le couloir, le lavabo, le lit, le logement**

Adjectifs

célibataire single (*person*)
divorcé(e) divorced
marié(e) married
pacsé(e) joined legally by a **PACS**
préféré(e) favorite, preferred

La famille

les arrière-grands-parents great-grandparents
le beau-frère brother-in-law
le beau-père father-in-law; stepfather
la belle-mère mother-in-law; stepmother
la belle-sœur sister-in-law
la bru daughter-in-law
le cousin cousin (*male*)
la cousine cousin (*female*)
le demi-frère half brother; stepbrother
la demi-sœur half sister; stepsister
l'enfant (*m., f.*) child
la femme wife
la fille daughter
le fils son
le frère brother
le gendre son-in-law
la grand-mère grandmother
le grand-parent (les grands-parents) grandparent(s)
le grand-père grandfather
le mari husband
la mère mother
le neveu nephew
la nièce niece
l'oncle (*m.*) uncle
le parent parent; relative
le père father
la petite-fille granddaughter
le petit-enfant grandchild
le petit-fils grandson
la sœur sister
la tante aunt

La maison

le balcon balcony
le bureau office
la chambre bedroom
la cuisine kitchen
l'escalier (*m.*) stairway
le jardin garden
la pièce room
le premier/deuxième étage second/third floor
le rez-de-chaussée ground (first) floor
la salle à manger dining room
la salle de bains bathroom
le séjour living room
le sous-sol basement
la terrasse terrace

Expressions avec *faire*

faire attention (à) to pay attention (to); to watch out (for)
faire la connaissance (de) to meet (*for the first time*), make the acquaintance (of)
faire les courses to do errands
faire la cuisine to cook
faire ses devoirs to do one's homework
faire la lessive to do the laundry
faire le marché to do the shopping, go to the market
faire le ménage to do the housework
faire une promenade to take a walk
faire la queue to stand in line
faire du sport to play/do sports
faire de l'aérobic to do aerobics; **... du jogging** to run, jog; **... du ski** to ski; **... du vélo** to go cycling; **... de la voile** to go sailing
faire un tour (en voiture) to take a walk (ride)
faire la vaisselle to do the dishes
faire un voyage to take a trip

Le temps

Quel temps fait-il? How's the weather?
Il fait beau. It's nice (out).
Il fait chaud. It's hot.
Il fait (du) soleil. It's sunny.
Il fait du vent. (Il y a du vent.) It's windy.
Il fait frais. It's cool.
Il fait froid. It's cold.
Il fait mauvais. It's bad (out).
Il neige. It's snowing.
Il pleut. It's raining.
Le temps est nuageux. It's cloudy.
Le temps est orageux. It's stormy.

Les saisons

Au printemps (*m.*)... In spring . . .
En automne (*m.*)... In fall . . .
En été (*m.*)... In summer . . .
En hiver (*m.*)... In winter . . .

Mots et expressions divers

l'année prochaine next year
après after; afterward
bientôt soon
ce week-end this weekend
cet après-midi / ce matin / ce soir this afternoon / morning / evening
chez at the home (establishment) of
dans quatre jours in four days (from now)
demain tomorrow
d'habitude usually
une fois par semaine once a week
le lundi / le vendredi soir on Mondays / on Friday evenings
peut-être maybe
la semaine prochaine next week
tous les jours every day
tout à l'heure in a while
tout de suite immediately
le week-end on weekends

CHAPITRE 6

À table!°

À... *Let's eat!*

Les dossiers d'Hassan

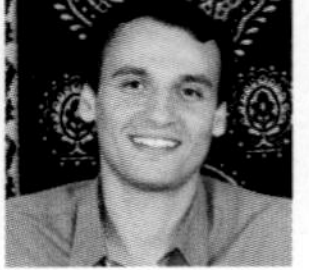
Hassan

- Mes photos
  - Une belle salade niçoise
  - Leçon 1—une salade marocaine
  - Mangez, bougez!°

Presentation: Ask sts. to describe what they see in the photo. Review colors by asking questions such as *Est-ce que la salade niçoise est un plat coloré? Quelles couleurs voyez-vous* (do you see)? *De quels ingrédients a-t-on besoin pour faire cette salade?*

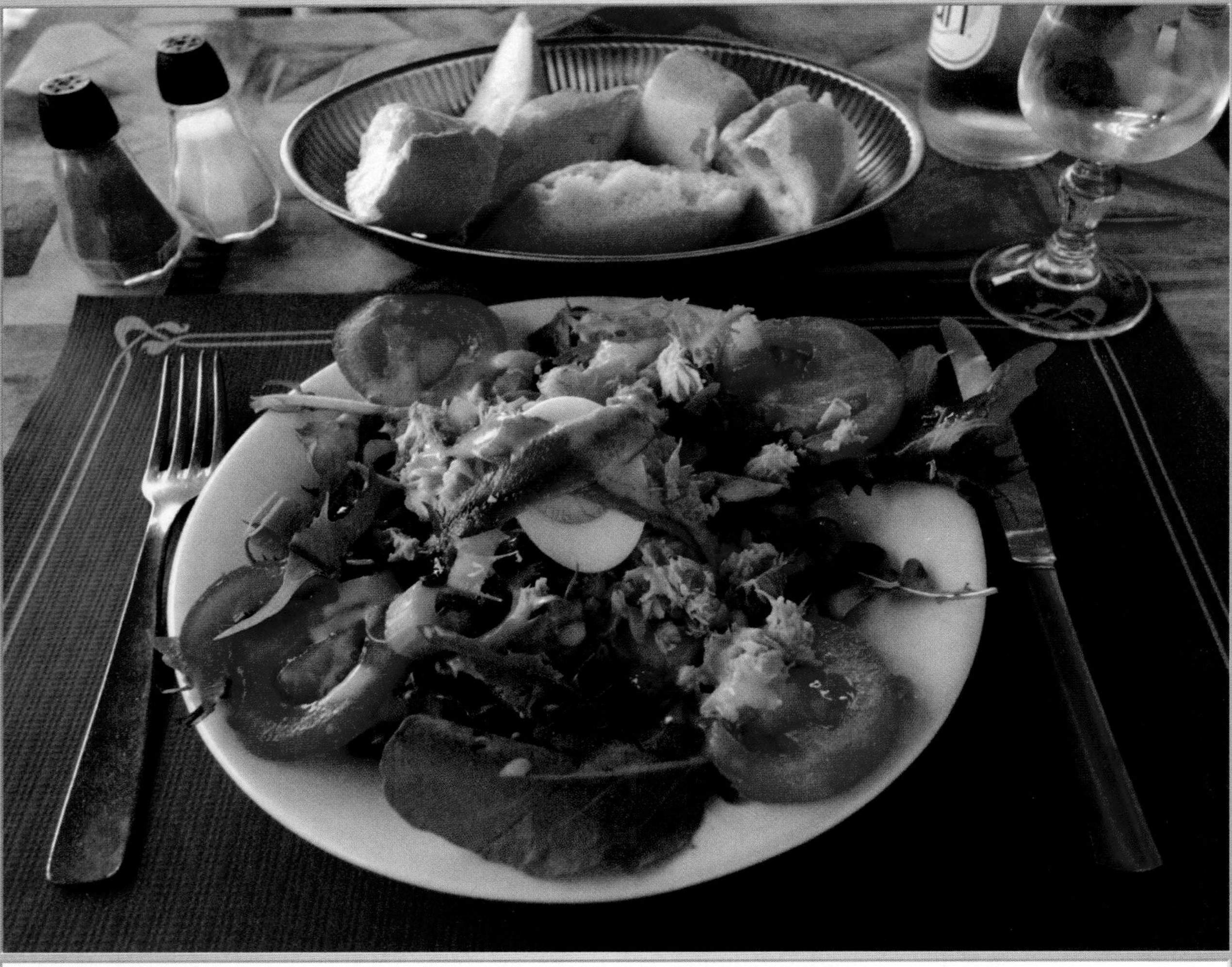

Mangez... *Eat, move!*

Une belle salade niçoise avec de la laitue, du thon, des olives noires, des œufs durs, des tomates et des anchois

Cultural note: *Salade niçoise* is a classic example of the cuisine of *Provence* and the *Côte d'Azur* in southeastern France. Other specialities of this region include *aïoli*, *bouillabaisse*, and *ratatouille*.

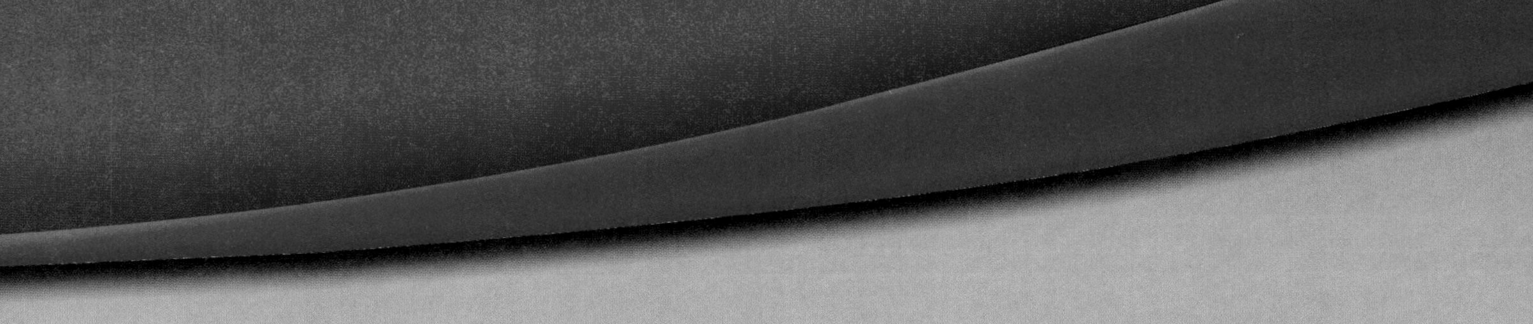

Dans ce chapitre...

OBJECTIFS COMMUNICATIFS

- talking about food and drink
- expressing quantity
- giving commands
- telling time
- learning to distinguish between and pronounce selected sounds in French

PAROLES (Leçon 1)

- Les repas, la nourriture et les boissons
- Le verbe **préférer**
- Le couvert à table

STRUCTURES (Leçons 2 et 3)

- Les verbes **prendre** et **boire**
- Les articles partitifs
- L'impératif
- L'heure

CULTURE

- Le blog d'Hassan: *Miam-miam!*
- Reportage: *Mangez, bougez!*
- Lecture: *Saveurs du monde francophone* (Leçon 4)

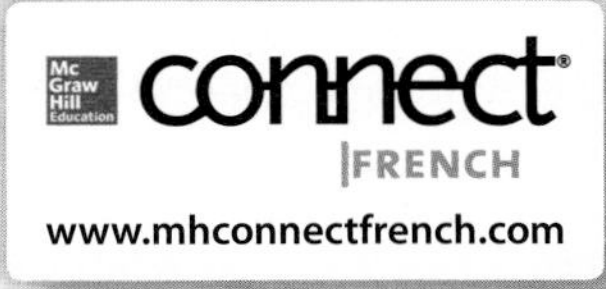

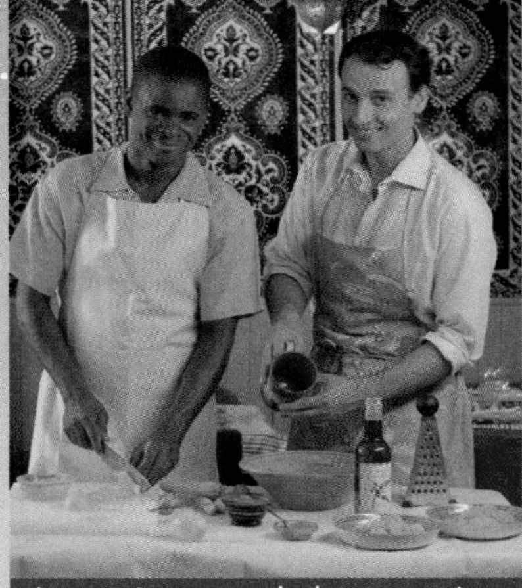

Leçon 1—une salade marocaine de carottes râpées à l'orange

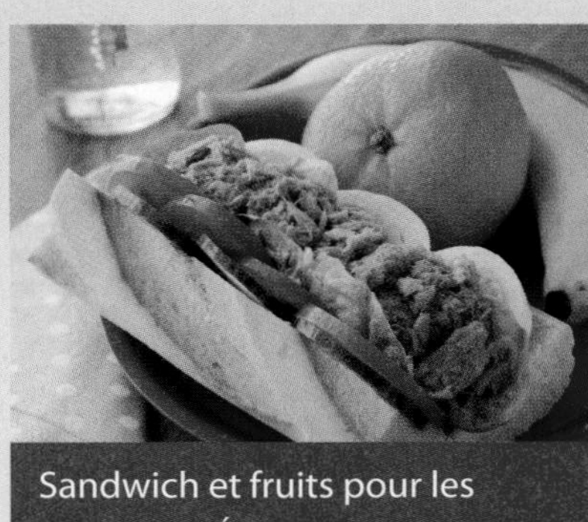

Sandwich et fruits pour les gens pressés

Leçon 1

PAROLES

Note: In familiar language, *le petit déj'* [p(ə)tidɛʒ] is often used.

Cultural note: *Le déjeuner, le dîner,* and *le souper* are the original names for meals; they are still used in some areas (Quebec, Belgium).

Suggestion: Point out that *déjeuner, dîner,* and *souper* can also be used as verbs.

Suggestion: Emphasize the pronunciation of *un œuf* [œ̃nœf] and *des œufs* [dezø].

Suggestion: Present the partitive articles lexically; *du* (*m.*), *de la* (*f.*), and *de l'* (before a vowel) are introduced in *Leçon 2*.

Suggestion: Show photos of French meals and ask sts. to guess which meal it is.

Presentation: Bring in pictures or real examples of the various foods portrayed.

Les repas de la journée*

Voilà des aliments (*m.*) populaires en France.

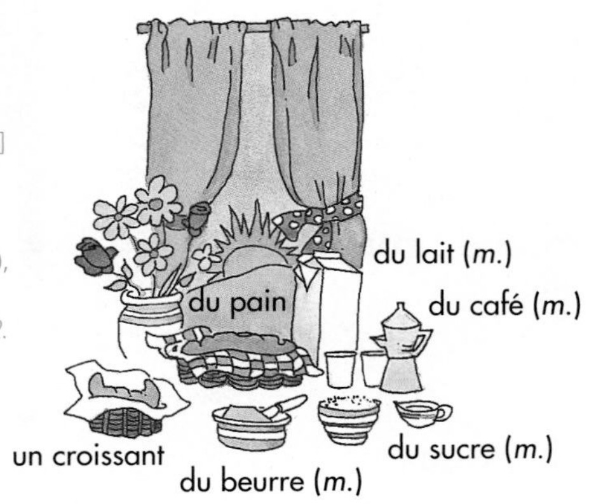

Le matin: le petit déjeuner

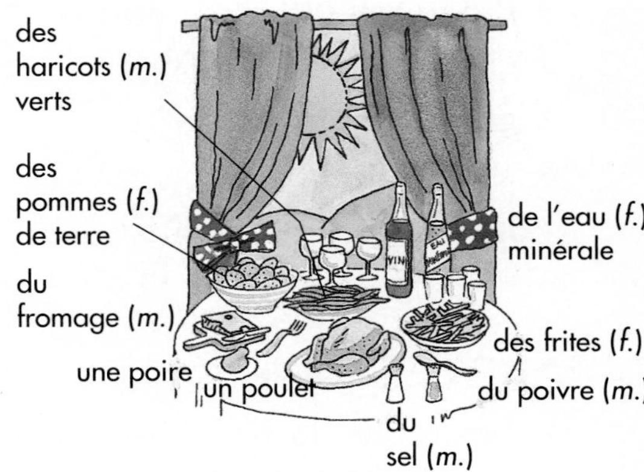

Le midi: le déjeuner

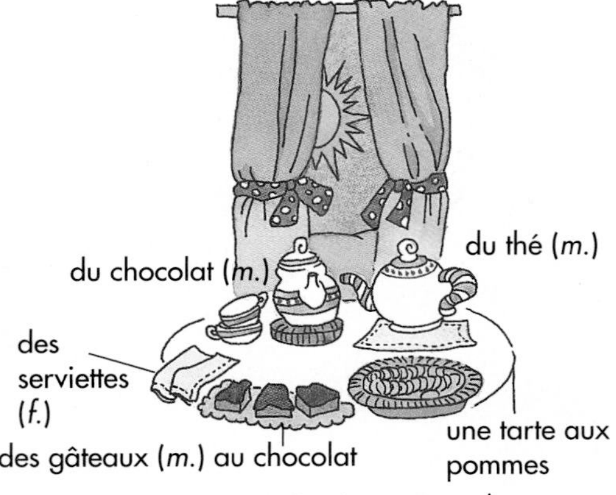

L'après-midi: le goûter†

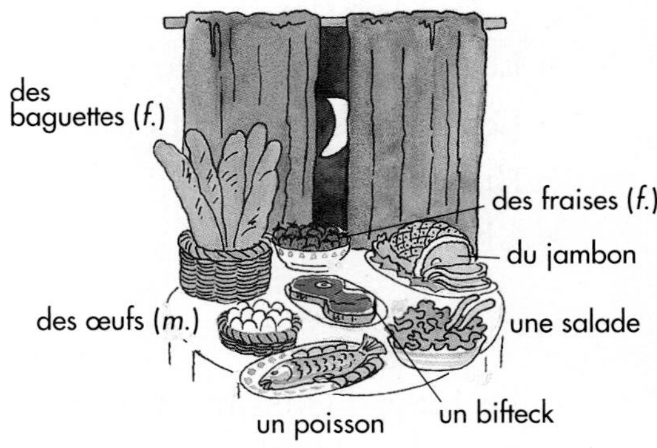

Le soir: le dîner

Cultural note: Talk about the custom of bringing a small gift when one is invited for a meal. Talk about the tradition of serving wines with special meals, as well as an *apéritif* and sometimes a *digestif.*

Additional vocabulary: *les boissons: un café au lait, un citron pressé, un coca, une infusion* (herb tea), *une limonade, un Orangina, un Perrier, un thé au citron, un thé au lait,* etc.

---

*__La journée__ (*The day*) is used instead of **le jour** to emphasize the notion of an entire day, as in the expression **Quelle journée!** (*What a day!*) or **Bonne journée!** (*Have a nice day!*).

†**Le goûter** is an afternoon snack: **des petits pains au chocolat pour les enfants; du thé ou du café et des gâteaux pour les adultes.**

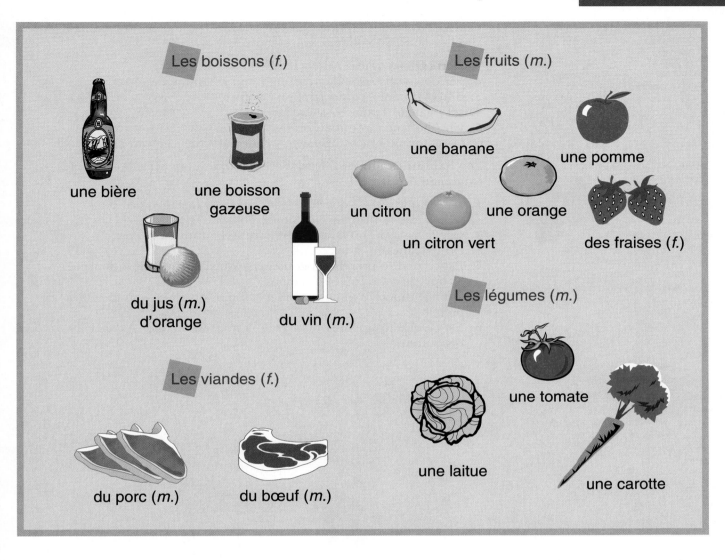

Les boissons (*f.*)

une bière

une boisson gazeuse

du jus (*m.*) d'orange

du vin (*m.*)

Les fruits (*m.*)

une banane

une pomme

un citron

une orange

un citron vert

des fraises (*f.*)

Les légumes (*m.*)

une tomate

une laitue

une carotte

Les viandes (*f.*)

du porc (*m.*)

du bœuf (*m.*)

AUTRES MOTS UTILES

les brocolis (*m.*)	broccoli	**le poivron**	bell pepper
le champagne	champagne	**le plat**	dish (of food)
le champignon	mushroom	**les produits** (*m.*) **frais**	fresh products
la crème	cream		
le dessert	dessert	**déjeuner**	to eat lunch
l'oignon (*m.*)	onion	**dîner**	to eat dinner

Suggestion: Emphasize the use of *déjeuner* and *dîner* to express "to eat lunch" and "to eat dinner." Sts. tend to translate literally using *manger.*

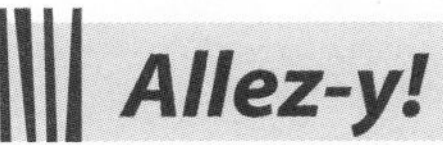

A. Catégories. Ajoutez (*Add*) d'autres aliments dans les catégories mentionnées.

MODÈLE: La mousse au chocolat est *un dessert.*→
Le gâteau, la tarte aux pommes et les fraises sont aussi des desserts.

1. La bière est *une boisson.*
2. La pomme de terre est *un légume.*
3. Le porc est *une viande.*
4. La banane est *un fruit.*

Additional activity: *Définitions. Suivez le modèle.* MODÈLE: *Le goûter → Le goûter est le repas de l'après-midi.* 1. *le petit déjeuner* 2. *le dîner* 3. *le déjeuner*

Suggestion (B): Do as a listening activity, with sts. writing down the *intrus* as they hear each list.

Follow-up (B): Have sts. add another word to category that *does* belong.

B. L'intrus. Dans les groupes suivants, trouvez le mot qui ne va pas avec les autres. Expliquez votre choix.

1. café / fraise / bière / thé / lait
2. haricots verts / salade / carotte / œuf / pomme de terre
3. bifteck / porc / pain / jambon / poulet
4. sel / gâteau / poivre / sucre / beurre
5. vin / banane / pomme / orange / melon
6. tarte aux pommes / fromage / chocolat / thé / gâteau au chocolat

Additional activities: A. *Plats. Faites une liste des ingrédients nécessaires à chaque plat.* MODÈLE: *une mousse au chocolat* → *le chocolat, le beurre, les œufs* 1. *une soupe* 2. *un café au lait* 3. *une omelette* 4. *une salade de fruits* 5. *un sandwich* 6. *une fondue* B. *Associations. Quels mots est-ce que vous associez avec… ?* 1. *un petit déjeuner américain* 2. *une salade césar* 3. *un régime* (diet) 4. *un bon repas marocain* 5. *un pique-nique*

C. Les habitudes alimentaires. Posez les questions suivantes à un(e) camarade de classe.

1. D'habitude, est-ce que tu prends un petit déjeuner? Si oui, qu'est-ce que tu manges? Sinon, pourquoi pas?
2. Quelle boisson préfères-tu prendre le matin?
3. Où déjeunes-tu et avec qui?
4. Est-ce que tu prends un goûter quelquefois pendant la journée? Si oui, qu'est-ce que tu manges?
5. Pour le dîner, tu aimes cuisiner? Si oui, qu'est-ce que tu aimes préparer?
6. Est-ce que tu préfères manger à la maison ou aller manger au restaurant?

Cultural note: Tell students that if they want to find the best chocolate shops in France, Switzerland, or Belgium, they can use a French search engine to look for the *Portail du chocolat* or a similar website.

Le verbe *préférer*

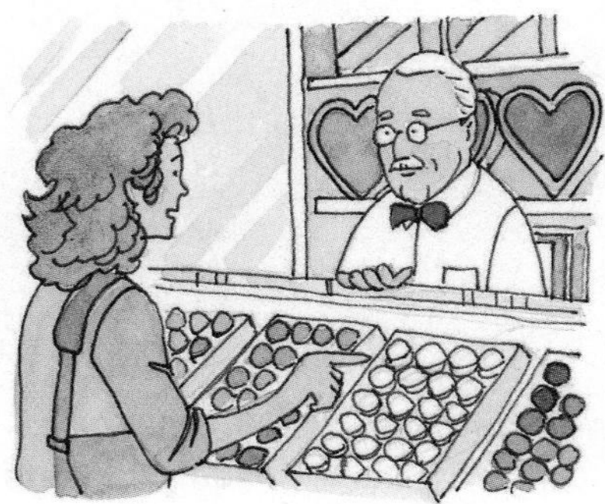

Elle préfère le chocolat blanc.

Presentation: You may wish to point out that *préférer* and similar verbs, along with other stem-changing verbs such as *acheter* (*Chapitre 8*), *appeler* (*Chapitre 10*), and *envoyer* (*Chapitre 10*), are sometimes called "boot" or "shoe" verbs, because if you circle the forms that have stem changes in the conjugation table, the resulting shape looks like a boot or shoe. See the verb charts in Appendix B for the complete conjugations of *-er* verbs with spelling changes.

PRESENT TENSE OF **préférer** (*to prefer*)			
je	**préfère**	nous	préférons
tu	**préfères**	vous	préférez
il/elle/on	**préfère**	ils/elles	**préfèrent**

Although the endings are regular, the verb **préférer** is irregular. For the forms of **je, tu, il/elle/on,** and **ils/elles,** the second **é** from the stem (**préfér-**) changes to **è (je préfère).** The **nous** and **vous** forms are regular. Verbs conjugated like **préférer** include **répéter, espérer** (*to hope*), **célébrer,** and **considérer.**

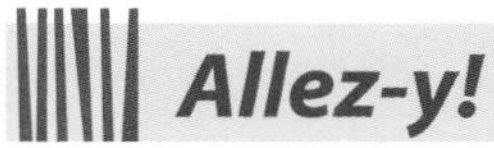

Allez-y!

A. **Fiche** (*Form*) **gastronomique.** Demandez à un(e) camarade de classe quelles sont ses préférences, et complétez la fiche. Utilisez **quel** (*m.*) ou **quelle** (*f.*) et le verbe **préférer.**

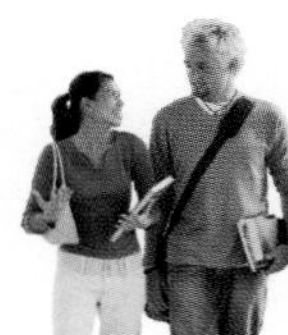

Suggestion: Could be done as a poll where sts. circulate and interview several class members.

MODÈLE: É1: Quelle boisson préfères-tu?
É2: Je préfère le/la…

boisson: ______________________

viande: ______________________

légume: ______________________

fruit: ______________________

dessert: ______________________

repas: ______________________

plat: ______________________

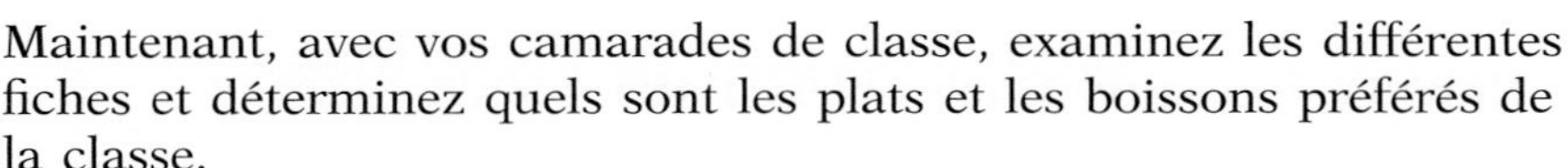

Maintenant, avec vos camarades de classe, examinez les différentes fiches et déterminez quels sont les plats et les boissons préférés de la classe.

B. **Question de préférence.** Avec un(e) camarade, répondez aux questions suivantes.

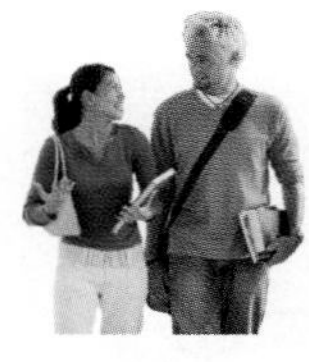

1. Quel repas est-ce que tu préfères? Pourquoi?
2. Est-ce que, selon toi (*in your opinion*), tu es bon cuisinier / bonne cuisinière (*cook*)?
3. Dans quel restaurant est-ce que tu espères aller prochainement (*next*)?
4. Chez toi, quelles fêtes est-ce qu'on célèbre? Qu'est-ce que vous préparez pour célébrer cette/ces (*this/those*) fête(s)?

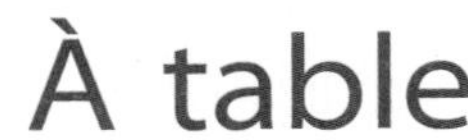

À table

Presentation: Distinguish between *l'assiette creuse* and *l'assiette plate*. Distinguish between the use of *plat* and *assiette* for *dish*.

Suggestions: (1) Bring in items to set table. Demonstrate different setting and style of eating in France. (2) Have sts. comment in English about differences in table settings in France and the U.S.

Additional vocabulary: *la corbeille à pain, le rond de serviette*

Suggestion: Make the distinction between *verre à vin* (the glass itself) and *verre de vin* (glass and its contents).

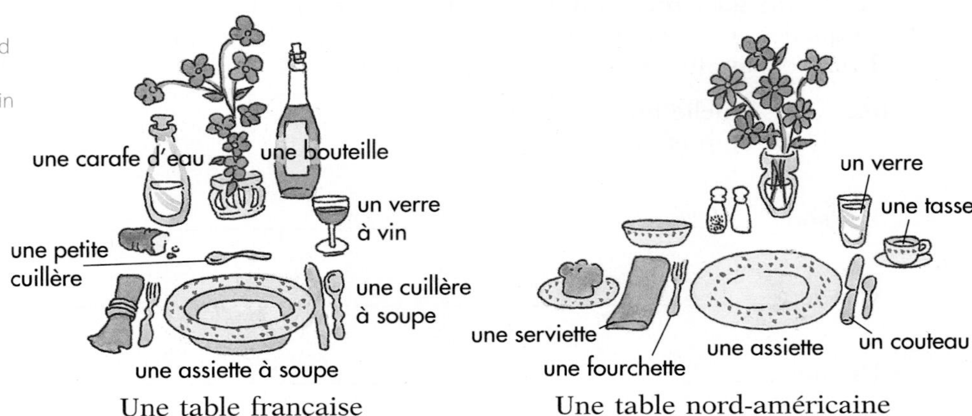

AUTRES MOTS UTILES

un bol	bowl-shaped cup (*for* **café au lait**)
une nappe	tablecloth
la soupe	soup

Allez-y!

Suggestion (A): Do as rapid-response activity, individual response with occasional group repetition. Solicit a variety of answers (*assiette, couteau*, etc.)

Continuation (A): *le beurre, la tarte aux pommes, le lait, le fromage*

A. L'objet nécessaire. Quels objets utilisez-vous?

MODÈLE: le café au lait →
J'utilise un bol pour le café au lait.

1. le vin
2. la viande
3. la soupe
4. la salade
5. le thé
6. la mousse au chocolat
7. l'eau
8. le café express

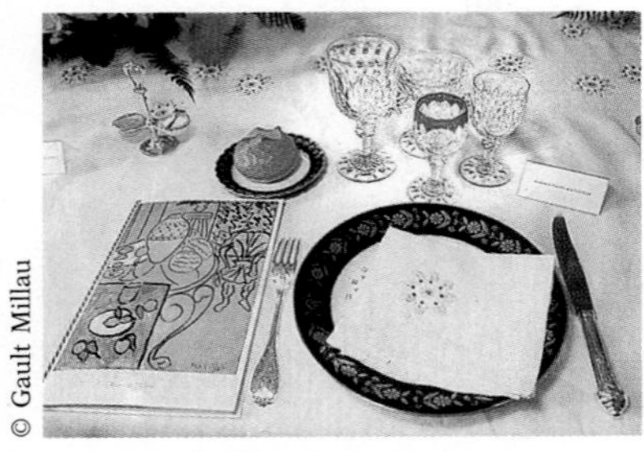

© Gault Millau

Une table élégante

B. L'art de la table. Mettre le couvert (*Setting the table*) est souvent un art. Regardez la photo tirée du magazine *Gault Millau* et répondez aux questions.

1. Décrivez ce qu'il y a sur la table. Est-ce une table pour un repas simple ou élégant? Quel est l'objet en papier à gauche?
2. À votre avis, pourquoi est-ce qu'il y a quatre verres?
3. Et chez vous, qu'est-ce qu'on place sur la table au petit déjeuner, au déjeuner, au dîner, pour un repas spécial?

Follow-up (B): Use the Rose technique to practice vocabulary, speaking, and listening: Ask one st. to draw a place setting; she or he will describe it to a partner who will draw without looking at the picture. At the end, sts. confirm comprehension by looking at the first st.'s picture.

Presentation: Have pairs of sts. take turns reading the dialogue aloud.

Les verbes *prendre* et *boire*

Talking About Food and Drink

Petit déjeuner entre amis

Hassan et Abdel échangent des textos (SMS).

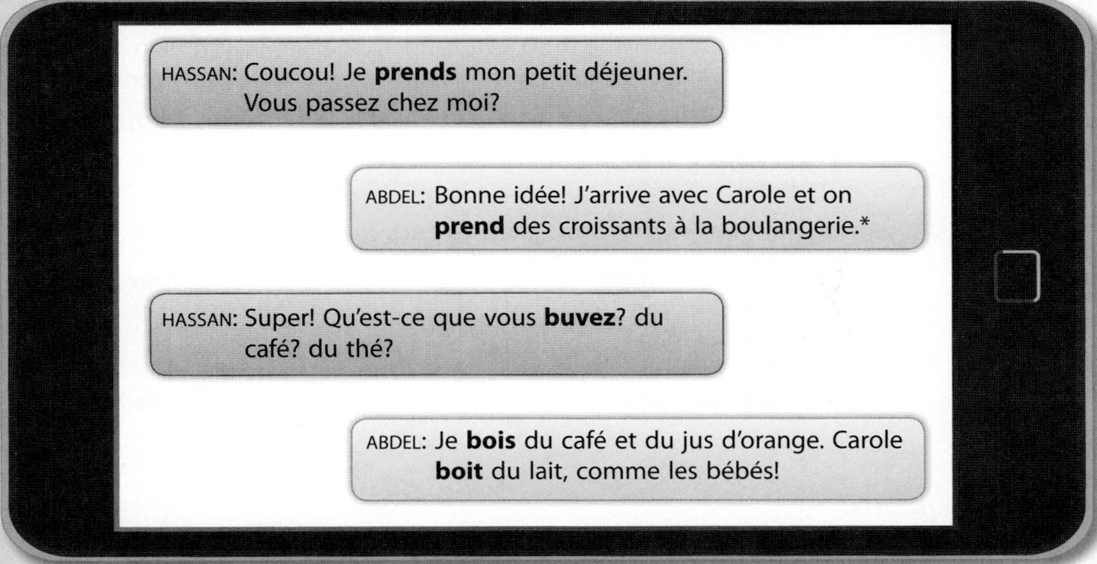
HASSAN: Coucou! Je **prends** mon petit déjeuner. Vous passez chez moi?
ABDEL: Bonne idée! J'arrive avec Carole et on **prend** des croissants à la boulangerie.*
HASSAN: Super! Qu'est-ce que vous **buvez**? du café? du thé?
ABDEL: Je **bois** du café et du jus d'orange. Carole **boit** du lait, comme les bébés!

**bakery*

Répondez aux questions.

1. Quel repas prend Hassan?
2. Qu'est-ce qu'Abdel et Carole prennent à la boulangerie?
3. Qu'est-ce qu'Abdel boit?
4. Pourquoi est-ce qu'Abdel compare Carole à un bébé?
5. Qu'est-ce que vous buvez le matin?

Prendre and Similar Verbs

The verb **prendre** is irregular in its plural forms.

PRESENT TENSE OF **prendre** (*to take*)			
je	**prends**	nous	**prenons**
tu	**prends**	vous	**prenez**
il/elle/on	**prend**	ils/elles	**prennent**

Presentation: Use whole sentences to model pronunciation, such as *Je prends du poulet, Tu prends du poisson,* etc. Emphasize the use of *prendre* (not *avoir*) with meals (*prendre le petit déjeuner*) and certain dishes (*prendre le* [*du*] *porc*) and drinks (*prendre du vin*).

1. Verbs conjugated like **prendre** include **apprendre** (*to learn*) and **comprendre** (*to understand; to include*).

—Qu'est-ce que vous **prenez?** —Je **prends** la salade verte.	*What are you having?* *I'm having the green salad.*
Il **apprend** l'espagnol.	*He's learning (how to speak) Spanish.*
Est-ce que tu **comprends** l'allemand?	*Do you understand German?*
Le menu à 20 euros **comprend** une entrée, un plat et un dessert.	*The meal for 20 euros includes an appetizer, the main course, and a dessert.*

2. When an infinitive follows **apprendre,** the preposition **à** must be used.

Apprenez-vous **à** skier?	*Are you learning (how) to ski?*

Apprendre can also mean *to teach.* In this case, the person taught is preceded by **à.** If the thing taught is a verb, it is also preceded by **à.**

J'apprends le russe à Lola.	*I'm teaching Lola Russian.*
J'apprends à Lola à parler russe.	*I'm teaching Lola to speak Russian.*

Suggestion: For listening comprehension practice, have sts. say whether verbs are singular or plural. You may want to do this as a *dictée. Il prend le poulet à la crème. Elles prennent un sandwich au fromage. Ils prennent de la bière. Elle prend une pizza. Ils comprennent le menu. Elle apprend le français. Ils apprennent à choisir le vin. Ça prend du temps.*

3. Some common expressions with **prendre** include:

prendre du temps	*to take (a long) time*
prendre son temps	*to take one's time*
prendre un repas	*to eat a meal*
prendre le petit déjeuner	*to have breakfast*
prendre un verre	*to have a drink (usually alcoholic)*

Suggestion: Ask sts. to make up sentences using these expressions.

Boire

The verb **boire** is also irregular in form.

Note: Stress pronunciation of [y] in *buvons.*

PRESENT TENSE OF **boire** (*to drink*)			
je	**bois**	nous	**buvons**
tu	**bois**	vous	**buvez**
il/elle/on	**boit**	ils/elles	**boivent**

Tu **bois** de l'eau minérale.	*You're drinking mineral water.*
Nous **buvons** de la bière.	*We're drinking beer.*

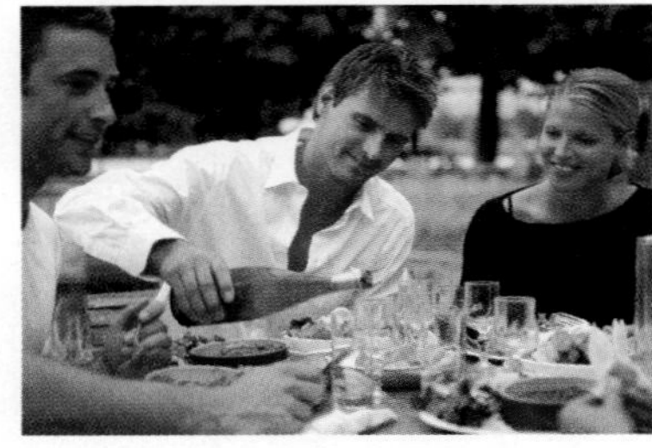

Offrir un verre aux amis, c'est sympa! Qu'est-ce qu'on boit ici? Qu'est-ce qu'on mange?

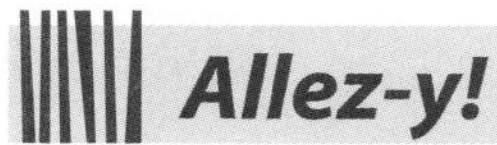

Allez-y!

A. Des étudiants modèles? Lisez les phrases, puis faites les substitutions suivantes: (1) tu, (2) mon meilleur ami / ma meilleure amie, (3) mon/ma camarade et moi, (4) je, (5) mes copains.

1. Vous apprenez le français. **2.** Vous comprenez presque (*almost*) toujours le professeur. **3.** Pour préparer les examens, vous prenez des livres à la bibliothèque. **4.** Pour faire votre travail, vous prenez votre temps. **5.** Mais malheureusement (*unfortunately*), vous buvez trop de (*too much*) café.

Suggestion (A): Sts. do as dictation at board, transforming sentences after writing the first cue.

B. Qu'est-ce qu'on boit? Choisissez la boisson qui convient à chaque situation.

Boissons: de la bière, du café, du champagne, de l'eau, du jus d'orange, du jus de pomme, du lait chaud, de la limonade, du thé, du vin

MODÈLE: Nous sommes le 31 décembre. (Loïc) →
Il boit du champagne.

1. Il fait très chaud. (vous) **2.** Il fait froid. (Christian) **3.** Il est minuit (*midnight*). (tu) **4.** Il est huit heures du matin (*8 AM*). (je) **5.** Nous sommes au café. (nous) **6.** Emma et Inès sont au restaurant. (elles)

C. Conversations au café. Vous êtes au café. Qu'est-ce que les gens disent? Complétez les conversations avec les verbes **prendre, apprendre** et **comprendre.**

1. FANNY: Est-ce que tu ______ un café?
AZIZ: Non, je ______ une bouteille d'eau minérale.
2. LÉA: Est-ce que tu ______ l'anglais?
FRANCO: Oui, et j' ______ aussi l'anglais à mes enfants. Et vous deux, qu'est-ce que vous ______ comme (*as*) langue étrangère?
CLÉMENT: Nous, nous ______ le japonais.
3. CLAUDE: Est-ce que vous ______ toujours le professeur de philosophie?
DAVID: Non, mais les autres (*others*) ______ tout!

Suggestion (C): Have sts. write out answers first and then solicit individual responses from class.

Suggestion (C): Have sts. first complete the dialogues with a partner. Have one group read each minidialogue aloud. Then each group picks a dialogue to expand into a more lengthy dialogue. Have several groups read their newly constructed dialogue to the class. Ask comprehension questions as a follow-up.

D. Mission impossible? Posez une question avec **Est-ce que tu...** pour trouver un(e) camarade de classe qui (*who*)...

1. ne prend pas de petit déjeuner **2.** prend en général des crêpes (*pancakes*) au petit déjeuner **3.** boit cinq tasses de café ou plus par jour **4.** boit un verre de lait à chaque repas **5.** apprend un nouveau sport ce semestre **6.** comprend le sens de la vie (*meaning of life*)

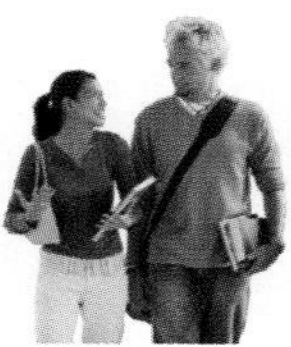

Continuation (D): Add a few more personalized questions that will interest/amuse your class.

Suggestion: You may wish to teach the concept inductively using a chocolate bar, asking *Aimez-vous le chocolat? Voulez-vous du chocolat? Je prends du chocolat.*

Les articles partitifs

Expressing Quantity

Pas de gâteau pour le dessert!

Suggestion: Emphasize that an article is always needed in French.

Suggestion: After sts. read the grammar section, have them reread the mini-dialogue and find other types of articles. Ask them to explain, based on what they have just learned, why they think those are not partitive articles.

Hassan téléphone à Carole.

HASSAN: Salut, Carole! Alors, le dîner que tu prépares pour les parents d'Abdel, il est prêt[1]?

CAROLE: Non... mais mon menu est prêt: **du** poulet avec des pommes de terre. **De la** salade verte. Et pour finir, **du** fromage et des fruits. J'adore les repas simples!

HASSAN: C'est un menu quotidien[2] trop banal pour une grande occasion. Pourquoi pas une belle salade niçoise avec **de la** laitue, des œufs, **du** thon,[3] des oignons? Et ensuite,[4] un bœuf aux carottes avec **de l'**huile[5] d'olive? Ce n'est pas compliqué...

CAROLE: Et pour le dessert, un gâteau?

HASSAN: **Pas de** gâteau: **De la** mousse au chocolat! Avec **du** citron: c'est original, et... très très facile!

Délicieuse, la mousse au chocolat!

[1]*ready* [2]*daily* [3]*tuna* [4]*next* [5]*oil*

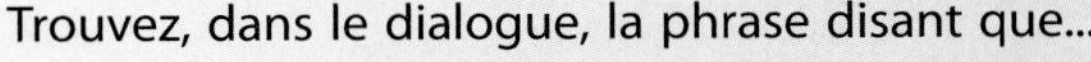

Trouvez, dans le dialogue, la phrase disant que...

1. Carole compose un menu avec de la viande, des légumes et des fruits.
2. Carole n'aime pas les repas compliqués.
3. Dans la salade niçoise, il y a plusieurs (*several*) ingrédients.
4. Hassan n'est pas favorable au gâteau pour le dessert.
5. La mousse au chocolat, c'est facile à préparer.

Suggestion: Point out how each noun in the examples refers to divisible or measurable quantities rather than nondivisible, countable nouns. Some grammarians consider that true partitives are used only in singular.

Forms of Partitive Articles

In addition to the definite and indefinite articles, there is a third article in French, called the partitive (**le partitif**). It has three forms: **du** (*m.*), **de la** (*f.*), and **de l'** (before a vowel or mute **h**). It agrees in gender and number with the noun it precedes.

Prenez-vous **du** jambon?	*Are you having (some) ham?*
de la salade?	*(some) salad?*
de l'eau minérale?	*(some) mineral water?*

Follow-up: Dictate sentences and have sts. explain why partitive or indefinite article is used: *Il y a une assiette (un couteau, une tasse, du beurre, des croissants, du café, etc.)*

Partitive versus Indefinite Articles

1. The partitive article is used to indicate part of a quantity that is measurable but not countable. This idea is sometimes expressed in English by *some* or *any;* usually, however, *some* is only implied.

Examples of noncountable nouns (also called *mass nouns*) include **beurre, chocolat, eau, glace, lait, pain, sucre, viande, vin, argent,** and **temps.**

Avez-vous **du** thé?	*Do you have tea?*
Je voudrais **du** sucre.	*I would like (some) sugar.*
Mangez-vous **du** poisson?	*Do you eat fish?*

2. When something is countable or is considered as a whole, the indefinite article is used instead.

Après le dîner, je prends **un** thé.	*After dinner, I have (a cup of) tea.*
Je voudrais **un** sucre dans mon café.	*I would like one (cube of) sugar in my coffee.*
Je mange **un** poisson par semaine.	*I eat a (whole) fish every week.*

Partitive versus Definite Articles

1. The partitive article is used with verbs such as **acheter,* boire, manger,** and **prendre,** because they usually involve consuming or buying a *portion* of something. However, after verbs of preference such as **adorer, aimer, aimer mieux, détester,** and **préférer,** the definite article is used, because these verbs generally express a reaction to an entire category.

Beaucoup de Français mangent **du** fromage à la fin du repas, mais moi, je déteste **le** fromage.	*Many French people eat cheese at the end of the meal, but I hate cheese.*

2. The partitive is also used with abstract qualities attributed to people, whereas the definite article is used to talk about these qualities in general.

Elle a **du** courage.	*She has (some) courage.*
Elle déteste **l'**hypocrisie.	*She hates hypocrisy.*

Partitives in Negative Sentences

1. In negative sentences, partitive articles become **de** (**d'**), except after **être.** This is also true with the plural indefinite article **des.**

Je bois **du** lait.	→	Je ne bois **pas de** lait.
Elle mange **de la** soupe.	→	Elle ne mange **pas de** soupe.
Tu prends **de l'**eau.	→	Tu ne prends **pas d'**eau.
BUT: C'est **du** vin espagnol.	→	Ce n'est pas **du** vin espagnol.
Vous mangez **des** carottes.	→	Vous ne mangez **pas de** carottes.
BUT: Ce sont **des** poires.	→	Ce ne sont **pas des** poires.

***Acheter** means *to buy.* It will be presented in *Chapitre 8*. Meanwhile, see Appendix B for the conjugation of **acheter.**

Mots clés

Exprimer un désir

Je voudrais means *I would like.* It is used to make a polite request and can be followed by a noun or an infinitive.

Je voudrais un café, s'il vous plaît.
I would like a cup of coffee, please.

Je voudrais prendre le menu du jour.
I would like to have the special of the day.

Note: *Vis-à-vis* presents the comparison between the partitive and definite articles as soon as possible after explaining the partitive because many sts. grasp the concept of partitive only when they see this contrast. At this early stage, it may be helpful to emphasize the somewhat simplified rule of thumb given: *aimer, détester, préférer* take the definite article; *boire, manger, prendre, acheter* usually take the partitive article.

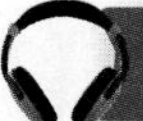

Prononcez bien!

The vowels in *du* and *de*

Be sure to clearly distinguish between the vowels in **du** [dy] and **de** [də]. For **du,** round your lips and close your mouth, push the body of your tongue forward, pressing the tip against your lower teeth, and make your lips protrude. For **de,** open your mouth slightly more than for **du,** shift your tongue to the center of your mouth, and round your lips without having them protrude.

[y]: Il y a **du** poulet.

[ə]: Il n'y a pas **de** poulet.

Pronunciation practice: The *Prononcez bien!* section on page 168 of this chapter contains activities for practicing these sounds.

Grammaire interactive

For more on the verbs **boire** and **prendre,** the expression **je voudrais,** and the partitive articles, watch the corresponding Grammar Tutorial and take a brief practice quiz at **Connect French.**

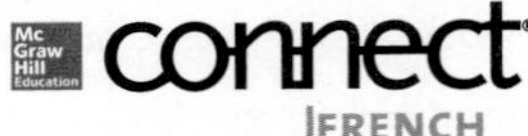

www.mhconnectfrench.com

2. The expression **ne... plus** (*no more, no longer, not any more*) surrounds the conjugated verb, like **ne... pas.**

Nils et Zoé? Ils **ne** mangent **plus** de viande.	*Nils and Zoé? They don't eat meat anymore.*
Je suis désolé, mais nous **n'**avons **plus** de vin.	*I'm sorry, but we have no more wine.*

[Allez-y! A]

Partitives with Expressions of Quantity

Partitive articles also become **de** (**d'**) after expressions of quantity.

Suggestion: Go over picture captions orally, then change *vin* to *bière.*

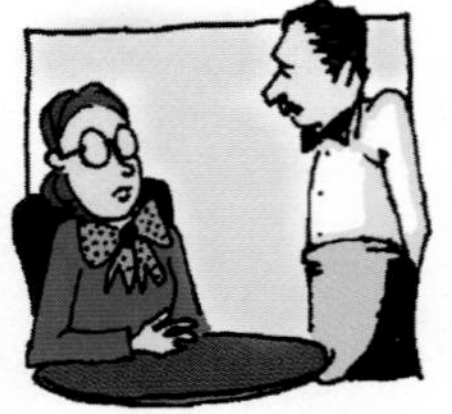

Elle commande **du vin.**

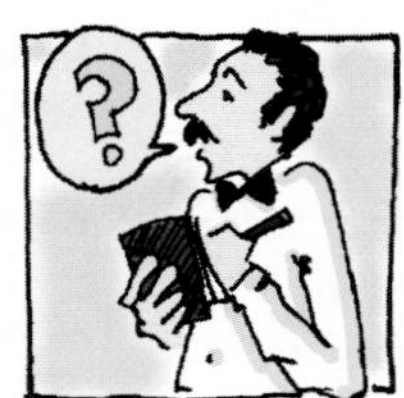

Combien de verres est-ce qu'elle commande?

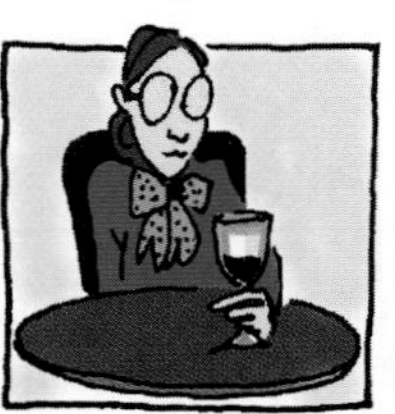

Elle commande **un peu de vin.**

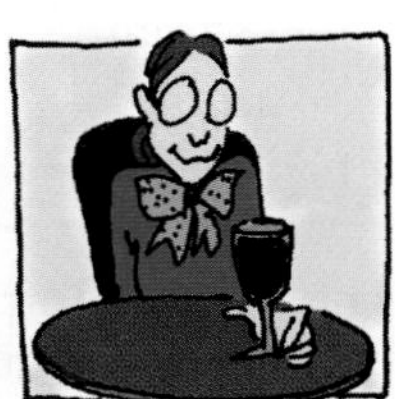

Elle commande **beaucoup de vin.**

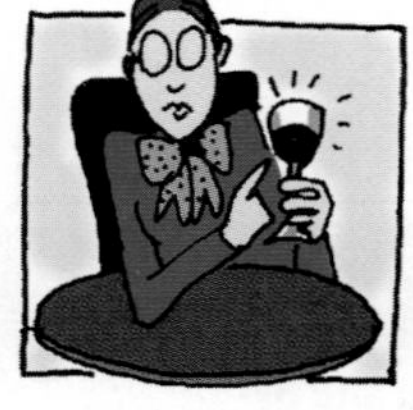

Elle commande **un verre de vin.**

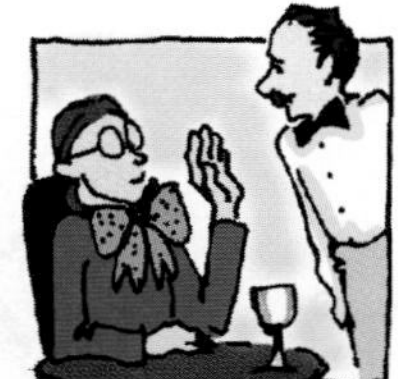

Elle a **assez de vin.**

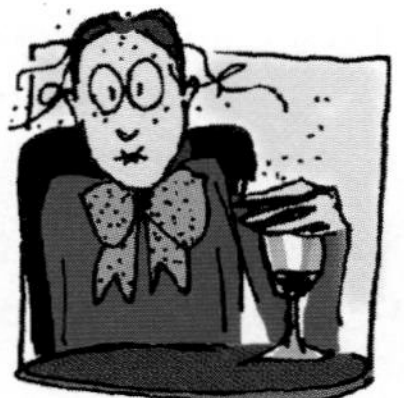

Elle boit **trop de vin.**

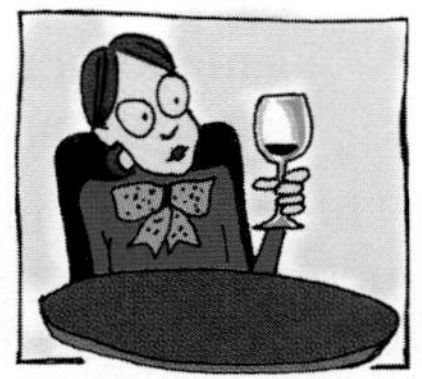

Dans son verre, il y a **peu de vin.**

Suggestion: You might want to present expressions such as *une boite de, un bol de, une bouteille de, un morceau de, une tranche de.*

Suggestion: Point out the difference between *peu de* (little, not many/much) and *un peu de* (a little of).

Suggestion (A): Can be done first in small groups or in writing and then reviewed orally with the whole class.

Continuation (A): Hold up food items or pictures of food items from magazines to continue the activity.

[Allez-y! B-C]

Additional activities: A. *À table! Qu'est-ce qu'on mange?* MODÈLE: *le poulet → On mange du poulet.* 1. *la salade* 2. *les pommes de terre* 3. *le poisson* 4. *la viande* 5. *le pain* 6. *les fruits* 7. *le melon* 8. *les œufs* 9. *la soupe* 10. *l'omelette* 11. *la tarte aux pommes* 12. *les sandwichs* B. *Au restaurant. Faites des phrases complètes pour décrire la scène.* 1. *Thibaut / demander / bifteck* 2. *nous / demander / lait* 3. *vous / commander / bière* 4. *Jules et Manon / manger / sandwichs* 5. *le serveur (waiter) / avoir / patience / avec nous*

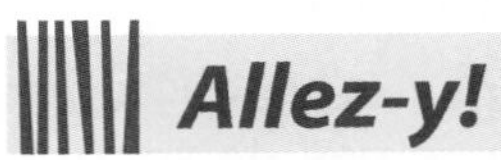

A. À table! Qu'est-ce que vous prenez, en général, à chaque repas? Qu'est-ce que vous ne prenez pas? Pensez-y!

Possibilités: du bacon, un bifteck, du café au lait, des croissants, des frites, du fromage, un fruit, un hamburger, de la pizza, du poulet, des spaghettis...

MODÈLE: Au petit déjeuner... →
Au petit déjeuner, je prends du jus d'orange, mais je ne prends pas de café au lait.

1. Au petit déjeuner... 2. Au déjeuner... 3. Au dîner...

B. Dîner d'anniversaire (*birthday*). Avec un(e) camarade, vous préparez un dîner surprise pour fêter l'anniversaire d'un ami / d'une amie. Mais avez-vous tous (*all*) les ingrédients nécessaires?

MODÈLE: carottes (assez) / (ne... pas) tomates ⟶
É1: Est-ce que tu as des carottes?
É2: Oui, j'ai assez de carottes, mais je n'ai pas de tomates.

1. eau minérale (3 bouteilles) / (ne... plus) jus d'orange
2. café (un peu) / (ne... plus) thé
3. fraises (beaucoup) / (ne... pas) melon
4. chocolat (trop) / (ne... pas) œufs
5. viande (assez) / (ne... pas) légumes
6. sucre (un bol) / (ne... plus) sel

C. La réponse est simple! Trouvez des solutions aux problèmes suivants. Utilisez les verbes **boire, apprendre, comprendre** et **prendre** et des expressions avec **prendre.**

MODÈLE: Je désire parler avec un ami. ⟶ Je prends un verre au café avec un ami.

1. J'ai faim. **2.** J'ai soif. **3.** Je désire bien parler français.
4. Je désire étudier les mathématiques. **5.** Je n'aime pas le vin.
6. Je ne suis pas pressé(e) (*in a hurry*).

D. Dis-moi ce que tu manges! Regardez les résultats d'une enquête sur les habitudes alimentaires des Français et répondez aux questions suivantes.

1. Est-ce que les Français dépensent (*spend*) plus pour acheter des boissons alcoolisées ou non alcoolisées (sans compter le lait)?
2. Nommez deux catégories de produits frais que les Français aiment consommer.
3. Quels sont les produits que les Français végétariens ne consomment pas?
4. Dans la liste, nommez deux catégories de produits que l'on (*that one*) achète généralement au marché en plein air (*open-air*).
5. À votre avis, quelles sont les différences entre les habitudes alimentaires des Français et des Nord-Américains?

Additional activity (D): Ask sts. to organize the categories according to their own eating habits. Use the words *souvent, quelquefois,* and *rarement*; e.g., *Je mange souvent du fromage.*

Additional activity: *Conversation et interview.* 1. *Est-ce que vous mangez beaucoup de viande? de poisson? de légumes? de fruits?* 2. *Qu'est-ce que vous aimez manger? Qu'est-ce que vous n'aimez pas manger?* 3. *Qu'est-ce que vous prenez au petit déjeuner? Est-ce que vous prenez des œufs, des céréales, du pain et du beurre? Qu'est-ce que vous buvez au petit déjeuner? Qu'est-ce que vous prenez pour votre déjeuner? pour votre dîner? Qu'est-ce que vous buvez?* 4. *Qu'est-ce que vous aimez manger comme dessert?* 5. *Est-ce que vous faites souvent la cuisine? Qu'est-ce que vous aimez préparer?* 6. *Imaginez que vous allez faire un pique-nique avec des amis. Qu'est-ce que vous allez apporter?*

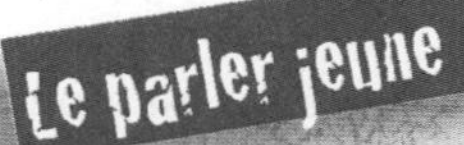

la bouffe	la nourriture, le repas
un casse-dalle	un sandwich
un kawa	un café
une patate	une pomme de terre
le pinard	le vin

Ce soir, on a décidé de faire une petite **bouffe** à la maison.

À midi, je mange un **casse-dalle** au café du coin.

Un petit **kawa** après le dessert?

Un steak avec des **patates** frites: c'est le bonheur!

Je te sers un peu de **pinard**?

Ce que les Français consomment (en % du total des dépenses alimentaires)

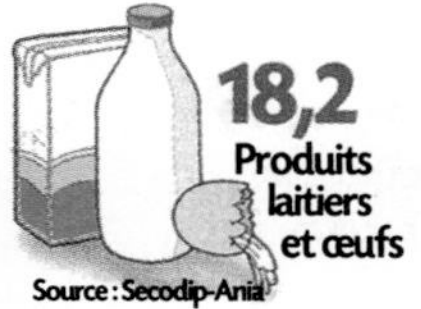
18,2
Produits laitiers et œufs
Source : Secodip-Ania

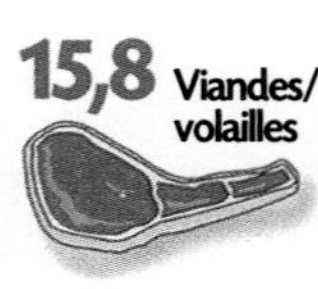
15,8 Viandes/volailles

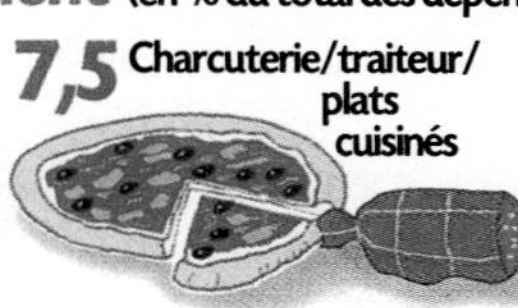
7,5 Charcuterie/traiteur/plats cuisinés

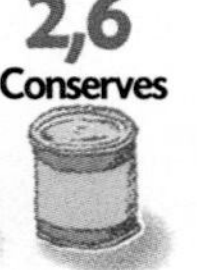
2,6 Conserves

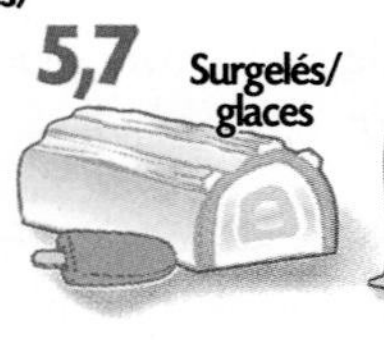

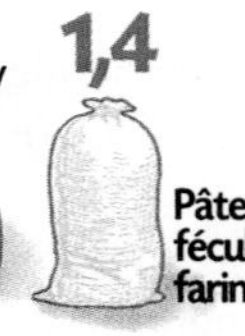
1,4 Pâtes/féculents/farines

Pain 0,7

Produits de la mer (poissons, crustacés...) 3,5

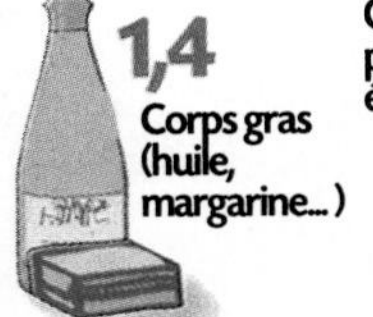
1,4 Corps gras (huile, margarine...)

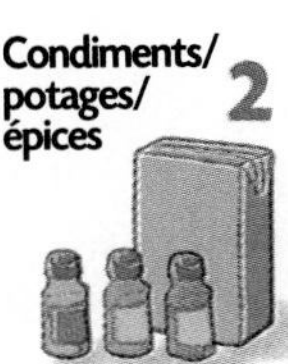
Condiments/potages/épices 2

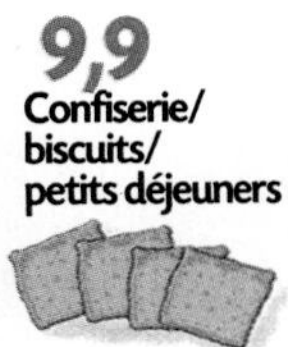
9,9 Confiserie/biscuits/petits déjeuners

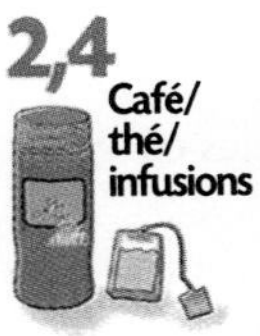
2,4 Café/thé/infusions

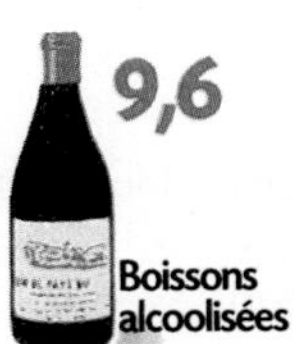
9,6 Boissons alcoolisées

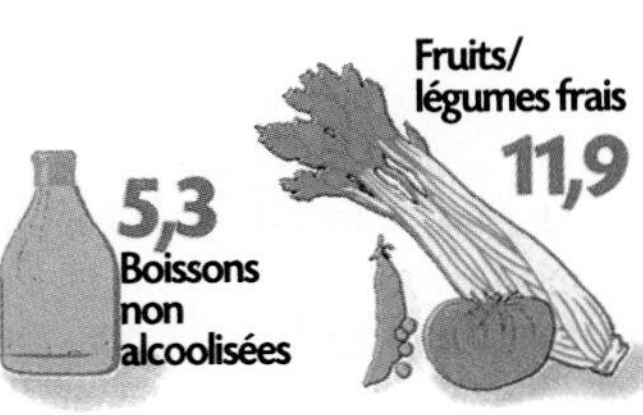

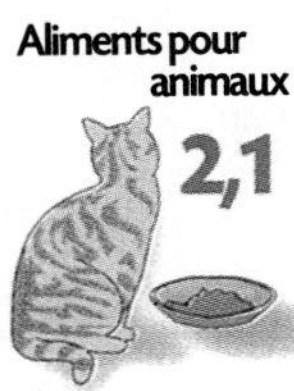
Aliments pour animaux 2,1

Presentation: You may want to point out to sts. that *la bouffe* comes from the verb *bouffer*, which is usually translated as *to eat,* but literally means *to puff.*

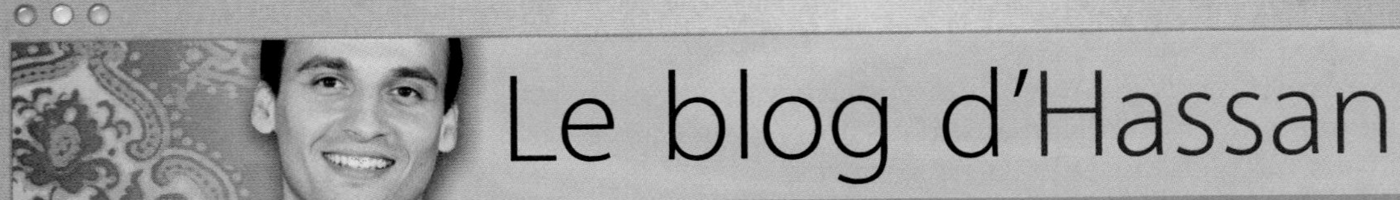

Miam-miam!°

°Miam... *Yum yum!*

vendredi 5 juin

Suggestion: Model pronunciation and have sts. repeat individually or as a group.

Salut les ennemis de la cuisine!

Vous adorez les bons petits plats mais vous détestez cuisiner? C'est parfait! Je vais créer un blog culinaire pour vous: un blog avec plein de recettes[1] délicieuses à accomplir en 10 minutes maximum. Les explications vont être simples, avec des photos et des petits films vidéo.

Je vais proposer des recettes marocaines diététiques, réalisées[2] avec des produits du marché: du poisson, du poulet, de la viande de bœuf, des légumes, des fruits. Dans ces plats, je vais utiliser des épices pour donner du goût[3]: du cumin, du safran, de l'harissa.[4]

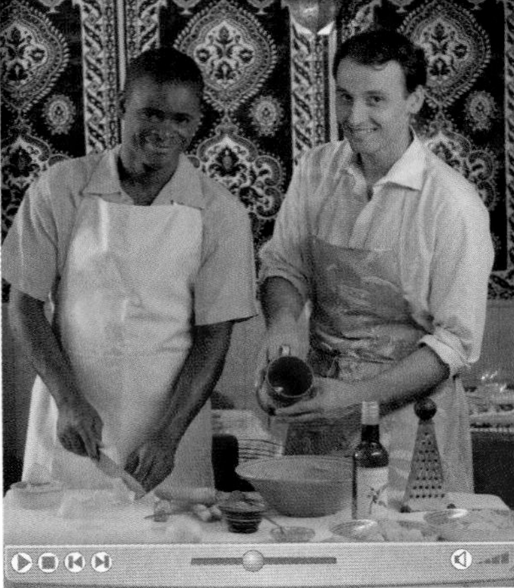

Leçon 1—une salade marocaine de carottes râpées à l'orange

Mon copain Hector est mon premier «client»! Il est danseur et il doit absolument avoir une alimentation équilibrée.[5] Je vais lui apprendre à cuisiner. Regardez la vidéo: c'est notre première leçon. Hector prépare une salade marocaine de carottes râpées[6] à l'orange! C'est un étudiant très sérieux. Je suis content de lui.

Bon appétit les amis,
Hassan

Follow-up: 1. *Que projette Hassan? Quels sont les aspects originaux de son concept?* 2. *Que pensez-vous personnellement de son idée?* 3. *Qu'ont en commun les cuisines marocaine et sénégalaise? Quels produits donnent du goût aux cuisines marocaine et sénégalaise?* 4. *Pourquoi Poema attend-elle avec impatience les recettes d'Hassan?* 5. *Commentez les réactions d'Alexis et de Trésor. Qui est enthousiaste? Pourquoi? Qui n'est pas enthousiaste? Pourquoi?*

Video connection: In the videoblog for this chapter, Hassan and Hector prepare *une salade marocaine de carottes râpées à l'orange* as part of Hassan's cooking blog. The recipe for this dish is in the *Lecture* for this chapter.

COMMENTAIRES

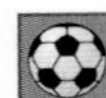

Mamadou

Dans la cuisine africaine, on utilise beaucoup d'épices. C'est le secret du goût.

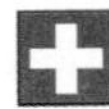

Charlotte

Hassan, j'attends ton blog! La cuisine, ça prend trop de temps. Préparer un bon dîner en 10 minutes, c'est le top[7]!

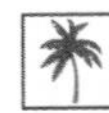

Poema

Personnellement, je suis au régime.[8] Bravo pour les recettes diététiques marocaines! Je vais craquer[9] pour ton blog!

Alexis

Tu vas nous faire mourir[10] avec tes recettes minceur[11]! Moi, je mange et je bois de tout: «Bonne cuisine et bon vin, c'est le paradis sur terre[12]». C'est une parole du roi[13] Henri IV...

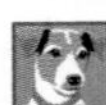

Trésor

Tu vas aussi inventer des recettes pour les chiens? Moi, j'adore les os[14] avec de la sauce!

[1]plein... *lots of recipes* [2]*prepared, made* [3]épices... *spices to give flavor* [4]*North African spice made from ground or pureed peppers* [5]alimentation... *well-balanced diet* [6]*grated* [7]*best* [8]au... *on a diet* [9]Je... *I'll be unable to resist* [10]nous... *kill us* [11]*slimming* [12]*earth* [13]parole... *saying of King* [14]*bones*

REPORTAGE

Mangez, bougez!

«Encore un peu de fromage avec un bon petit verre de vin pour finir le repas? Et pour le dessert, du gâteau au chocolat?»

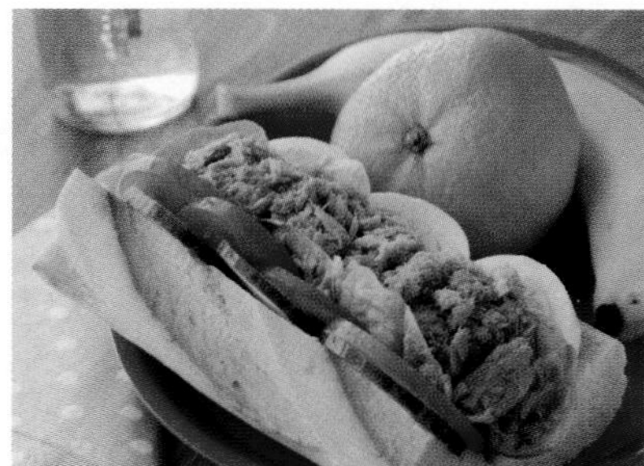

Sandwich et fruits pour les gens pressés

En France, la nourriture est une cause nationale; manger est un plaisir,[1] et même une passion. Un anniversaire, une promotion, une fête,[2] tout est prétexte à faire un bon repas en famille ou avec des amis.

Mais bien manger signifie souvent trop manger. Et ce n'est pas bon pour la santé[3]! Alors, comment faire? Avec son programme officiel «Manger-Bouger», l'Institut national de prévention et d'éducation pour la santé propose une solution: manger oui, mais à condition de consommer des produits frais, d'équilibrer[4] ses repas et d'avoir des activités physiques.

Les Français sont d'accord, comme Zoé, une étudiante en médecine qui nous parle de ses habitudes alimentaires[5]: «Pour le petit déjeuner, je prends des céréales, je mange beaucoup de pain avec du beurre et de la confiture, je bois du jus d'orange. Pour le déjeuner, je n'ai pas beaucoup de temps, alors, une pomme ou une banane me suffisent. Dans la journée, je bois du thé et je mange du chocolat... trop de chocolat! Le soir, je prépare un vrai dîner: je mange des pâtes ou du riz, parce que c'est facile à préparer, des légumes et des fruits parce que c'est bon pour la santé. Je cuisine peu de viande et de poisson parce que c'est cher! Je précise aussi que je suis très sportive: je marche[6] beaucoup; je fais de la gym et du tennis une fois par semaine. Je sais[7] que mes repas ne sont pas toujours équilibrés, mais j'apprends à manger correctement… C'est important!»

Luc, étudiant en Droit, est très sérieux: il boit du lait le matin et de l'eau à tous les repas; il adore les légumes; il achète du poisson deux fois par semaine, de la viande tous les lundis et il fait du sport chaque jour. «Vous pensez que je suis trop raisonnable? Mais non! Quand je suis avec mes copains, mon menu change: je bois de la bière—jamais[8] trop de bière—et je mange des frites, mon plat préféré! Et le lendemain,[9] je fais un footing[10]… ».

Vous voyez, les habitudes alimentaires des Français ne sont pas encore parfaites. Mais le programme «Manger-Bouger» fait réfléchir et progresser. Même[11] les enfants apprennent à sélectionner leurs aliments et à cuisiner. Et pour l'activité physique, pas de problème: ils sont toujours en mouvement… parce que ce sont sont des enfants!

[1]*pleasure* [2]*holiday* [3]*health* [4]*balance* [5]habitudes… *eating habits* [6]*walk* [7]*know* [8]*never* [9]*the next day* [10]fais… *go for a run* [11]*Even*

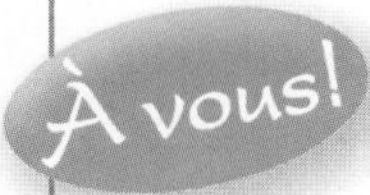

1. Les Français aiment bien manger. Et les Américains? Expliquez.
2. Que mange Zoé?
3. Que mange Luc? Est-il raisonnable quand il mange avec ses copains? Commentez son attitude.
4. Et vous, quels sont vos plats préférés?
5. Présentez le programme «Manger-Bouger». Selon vous, est-ce qu'il est difficile à appliquer? Expliquez.

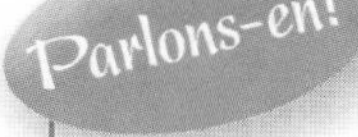

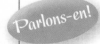

1. Travaillez en groupes de trois. Composez un petit déjeuner, un déjeuner ou un dîner équilibré pour le programme «Manger-Bouger». Associez des activités physiques à vos menus.
2. Présentez votre menu et votre programme d'activités physiques à la classe. Répondez aux commentaires et aux suggestions de vos camarades. Qui a le programme le plus réussi (*successful*)? Votez!

Suggestion: Once sts. have prepared their own menus, have them compare their choices with those listed for the same meal on the *Manger-Bouger* website. Ask them to comment on the similarities and/or differences.

Leçon 3

STRUCTURES

L'impératif

Giving Commands

Deux baguettes et du sel!

Abdel et Carole échangent des textos (SMS).

CAROLE: **Sois**[1] gentil, **apporte**[2] deux baguettes pour ce soir.

ABDEL: Je prends un gâteau pour le dessert?

CAROLE: Non. **Achète**[3] du sel.

ABDEL: Du sel pour le dessert?

CAROLE: Idiot! Du sel pour mon bœuf aux carottes. **Ne perds pas** de temps. Tes parents arrivent dans 20 minutes!

ABDEL: **Fais** attention: mes parents sont toujours en avance…

CAROLE: **Dépêche-toi,**[4] **dépêche-toi!**

Trouvez la phrase où…

1. Carole demande gentiment (*politely*) à Abdel d'apporter deux baguettes.
2. Carole demande à Abdel d'acheter du sel.
3. Abdel explique que ses parents vont bientôt arriver.
4. Carole ordonne à Abdel de se dépêcher.

[1]*Be* [2]*bring* [3]*Buy* [4]*Hurry up*

The imperative is the command form of a verb. It is used to express an order, a piece of advice, or a suggestion. There are three forms in French. As in English, subject pronouns are not used with the imperative.

(tu)	**Arrête** de parler!	*Stop talking!*
(nous)	**Allons** au restaurant!	*Let's go to the restaurant!*
(vous)	**Passez** une bonne journée!	*Have a nice day!*

1. Verbs ending in **-er:** The imperatives are the same as the corresponding present-tense forms, except that the **tu** form does not end in **-s.**

INFINITIVE	tu	nous	vous
regarder	**Regarde!**	**Regardons!**	**Regardez!**
entrer	**Entre!**	**Entrons!**	**Entrez!**

Écoute!	*Listen!*
Regardez! Un restaurant russe.	*Look! A Russian restaurant.*
Entrons!	*Let's go in!*

The imperative forms of the irregular verb **aller** follow the pattern of regular **-er** imperatives: **va, allons, allez.**

2. Verbs ending in **-re** and **-ir:** The imperative forms are identical to their corresponding present-tense forms. This is true even of most irregular **-re** and **-ir** verbs.

INFINITIVE	tu	nous	vous
attendre	**Attends!**	**Attendons!**	**Attendez!**
finir	**Finis!**	**Finissons!**	**Finissez!**
faire	**Fais... !**	**Faisons... !**	**Faites... !**

Attends! Finis ton verre!	*Wait! Finish your drink!*
Faites attention!	*Pay attention!* (*Watch out!*)

3. The verbs **avoir** and **être** have irregular command forms.

INFINITIVE	tu	nous	vous
avoir	**Aie... !**	**Ayons... !**	**Ayez... !**
être	**Sois... !**	**Soyons... !**	**Soyez... !**

Sois gentil, Michel.	*Be nice, Michel.*
Ayez de la patience.	*Have patience.*

4. In negative commands, **ne** comes before the verb and **pas** follows it.

Ne prends pas de sucre!	*Don't have any sugar!*
Ne buvons pas trop de café.	*Let's not drink too much coffee.*
N'attendez pas le dessert.	*Don't wait for dessert.*

Follow-up: Have sts. decide whether the following commands should be in the affirmative or negative: 1. *faire ses devoirs après le dîner* 2. *jeter* (throw) *sa serviette par terre* 3. *manger vite* 4. *être poli(e).*

(*continued*)

5. When using these command forms, you should be aware that they are not the most polite way of expressing your wishes. Later on you will learn about indirect commands or requests with the conditional, which are much more polite. With the imperative, the use of **s'il vous plaît** and **s'il te plaît** will make your requests more polite.

Aie de la patience, **s'il te plaît.**	*Please have patience.*
Ne fumez pas, s'il vous plaît.	*Please don't smoke.*

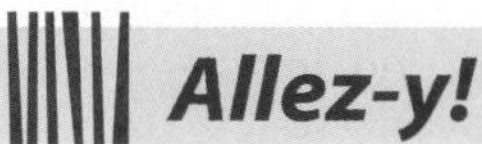

Additional activity: *Préparatifs.* MODÈLE: *Vous faites le marché.* → *Faites le marché.* 1. *Vous allez vite au marché.* 2. *Nous attendons l'autobus.* 3. *Tu descends de l'autobus.* 4. *Vous achetez du pain frais* (fresh). 5. *Nous choisissons un camembert.* 6. *Tu commandes un poulet chaud.* 7. *Tu prends ta fourchette. Maintenant, mettez les phrases précédentes à la forme négative de l'impératif.*

Follow-up (A-B): Play *Jacques a dit* (Simon Says). For example: *Jacques a dit: Prenez votre livre de français. Prenez votre stylo. Jacques a dit: Regardez le mur. Dites bonjour à votre camarade de classe.*

A. **Les bonnes manières.** Vous êtes à table avec un enfant. Dites-lui ce qu'il faut (= il est nécessaire de) faire ou ne pas faire.

MODÈLE: ne pas jouer avec ton couteau →
Ne joue pas avec ton couteau!

1. attendre ton frère **2.** prendre ta serviette **3.** finir ta soupe **4.** manger tes carottes **5.** regarder ton assiette **6.** être sage (*good* [*lit., wise*]) **7.** ne pas manger de sucre **8.** boire ton verre de lait **9.** ne pas demander de dessert

B. **Un job d'été.** Vous travaillez comme serveur/serveuse dans un café. Voici les recommandations de la patronne (*owner*).

MODÈLE: faire attention aux clients → Faites attention aux clients.

1. être aimable **2.** avoir de la patience **3.** écouter les clients **4.** répondre aux questions **5.** ne pas perdre de temps **6.** rendre correctement la monnaie (*change*)

Maintenant vous parlez avec un autre serveur / une autre serveuse de ce qu'il faut faire au travail. Répétez les recommandations de la patronne.

MODÈLE: faire attention aux clients → Faisons attention aux clients!

Suggestions (C): (1) Give sts. a few minutes to develop responses. Then solicit individual responses orally, or send 3–4 sts. to board to write their answers. Compare sts.' results. (2) You may want to do a set of orders first to show sts. how to create a chain of actions. Have various sts. play the robot.

C. **Le robot.** Vous avez un robot qui travaille pour vous. La classe choisit un étudiant / une étudiante pour jouer le rôle du robot. Donnez cinq ordres en français au robot. Il/Elle est obligé(e) d'obéir. Utilisez «s'il te plaît».

MODÈLE: Va au tableau, s'il te plaît!

L'heure

Telling Time

Suggestion: Point out the difference between *heure* (clock time), *temps* (time to do something; weather), *fois* (occasion; arithmetic operation); give examples.

Note: Digital watches have made the use of 24-hour system (formal time) more frequent.

Quelle heure est-il?

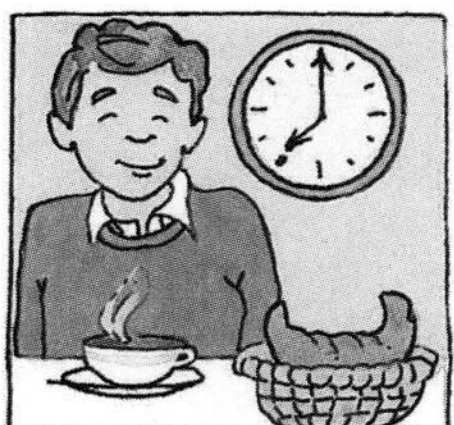

Il est **sept heures.** Quel repas est-ce que Vincent prend?

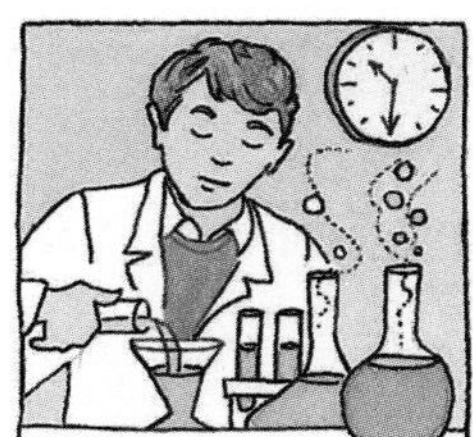

Il est **dix heures et demie.*** Où est Vincent?

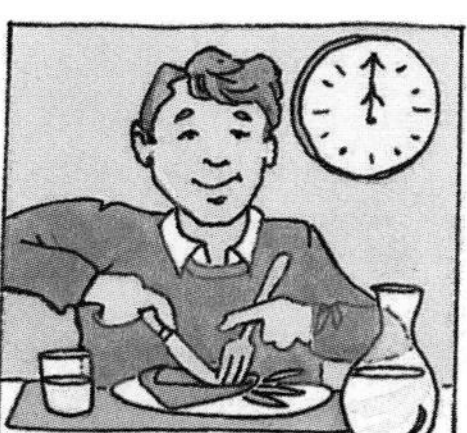

Il est **midi.** Quel repas est-ce qu'il prend?

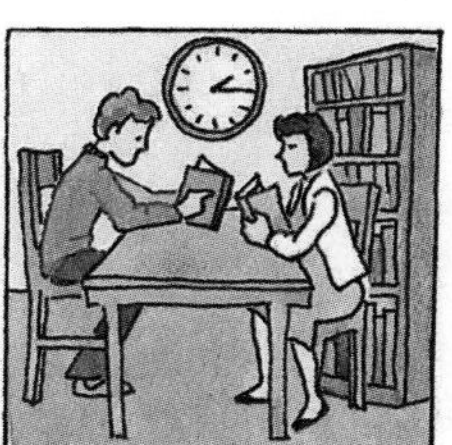

Il est **deux heures et quart.** Où est Vincent?

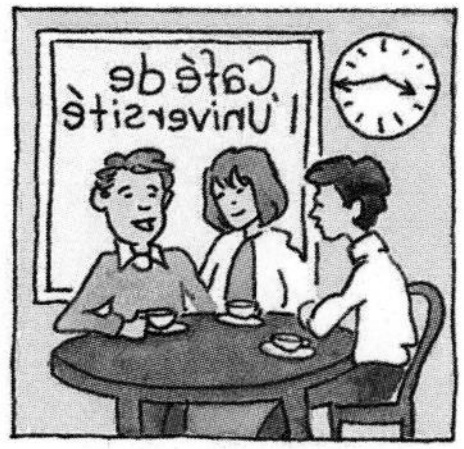

Il est **quatre heures moins le quart.** Qu'est-ce qu'il fait?

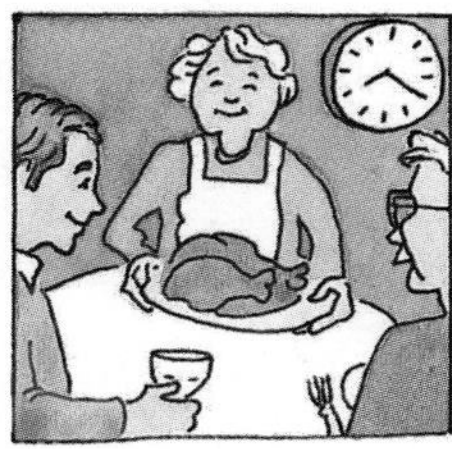

Il est **huit heures vingt.** Il dîne en famille?

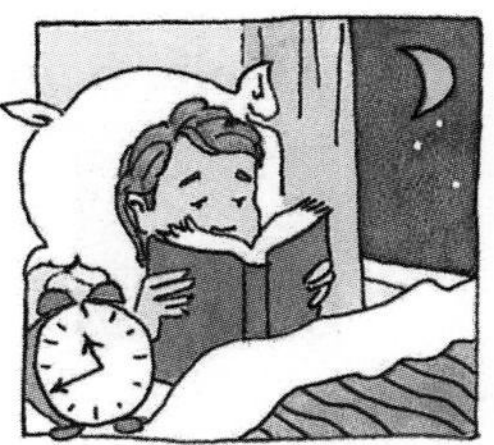

Il est **minuit moins vingt.** Est-ce qu'il étudie encore?

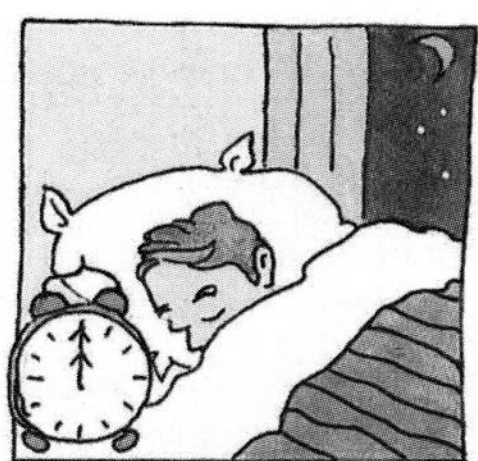

Il est **minuit,** et Vincent dort (*is sleeping*).

Presentation: Model pronunciation of captions with group repetition. Use cardboard clock to show times as they are repeated and to illustrate principles of telling time.

Additional vocabulary: *Il arrive vers* (around) *2 h. Il est environ* (about) *2 h. Arrivez à 2 h pile* (sharp).

1. To ask the time:

Excusez-moi, quelle heure est-il?	*Excuse me, what time is it?*

2. To ask at what time something happens:

—**À quelle heure** commence le film?	*At what time does the movie start?*
—**À** deux heures et demie.	*At 2:30.*

3. To tell the time:

Il est une **heure.**	*It is 1:00.*
Il est deux **heures.**	*It is 2:00.*
Il est presque **midi / minuit.**	*It's almost noon / midnight.*

4. To make a distinction between A.M. and P.M.:

Il est neuf heures **du matin.**	*It's 9 A.M. (in the morning).*
Il est quatre heures **de l'après-midi.**	*It's 4 P.M. (in the afternoon).*
Il est onze heures **du soir.**	*It's 11 P.M. (in the evening, at night).*

Prononcez bien!

Liaison with *heures*

Note the pronunciation of the last letter in the following numbers when they are followed by the word **heures.**

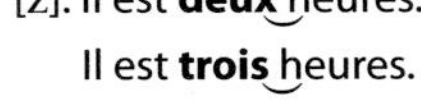

[z]: Il est **deux** heures.
Il est **trois** heures.
Il est **six** heures.
Il est **dix** heures.
[v]: Il est **neuf** heures.

Pronunciation practice: The *Prononcez bien!* section on page 168 of this chapter contains activities for practicing these sounds.

---

*To tell the time on the half hour, **et demie** is used after the feminine noun **heure(s)** and **et demi** is used after the masculine nouns **midi** and **minuit.**

Il est trois heures **et demie.**	*It's 3:30 (half past three).*
Il est midi **et demi.**	*It's 12:30 (half past noon).*

Suggestion: Use the following as preliminary listening exs. A. Hold up clock face, arrange hands to show various times and simultaneously say them, correctly or incorrectly. Sts. respond *oui* or *non*. B. Give the following times and ask sts. to draw the corresponding clock face. Then put the correct answers on the board for immediate feedback. *Il est…* 1. *9 h* 2. *10 h 30* 3. *11 h 45* (*midi moins le quart*) 4. *2 h 15* 5. *24 h*, etc.

Mots clés

Exprimer le temps de façon générale

Il est **tard.**
It's late.

Il est **tôt.**
It's early.

Jamal prend son repas **de bonne heure.**
Jamal eats early.

Gabriel est **en retard** aujourd'hui.
Gabriel is late today.

D'habitude, il est **en avance.**
Usually, he's early.

Camille est toujours **à l'heure.**
Camille is always on time.

Interaction: Have sts. act out the following situation, using the vocabulary and structures from this chapter. *Conseils:* A French exchange st. has recently arrived at your university and wants to know the hours when the campus dining places are open (= *ouvert*) and the kinds of foods they serve. Give him/her some information and simple advice about what and where to eat.

The 24-hour clock is used for official announcements (e.g., TV or transportation schedules), to make appointments, and to avoid ambiguity. For time expressed in figures, **h** (**heures**) is used (without a colon).

	OFFICIAL 24-HOUR	12-HOUR
9 h 15	neuf heures quinze	neuf heures **et quart** (du matin)
15 h 30	quinze heures trente	trois heures **et demie** (de l'après-midi)
18 h 45	dix-huit heures quarante-cinq	sept heures **moins le quart** (du soir)
20 h 50	vingt heures cinquante	neuf heures **moins dix** (du soir)

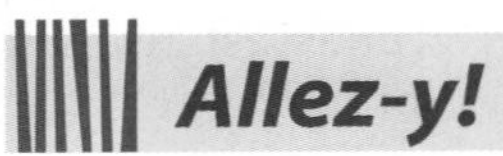

Vocabulary recycling: Ask sts. at what time they typically eat breakfast, lunch, snack, and dinner, and what each meal typically consists of.

Suggestion: Do as whole-class response activity, or in pairs, after modeling first few items for whole group.

A. Quelle heure est-il? Donnez l'heure selon les deux systèmes.

1. 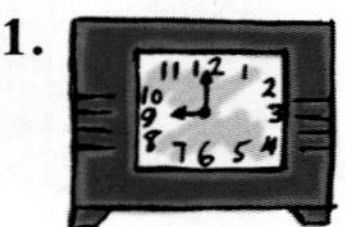
2. 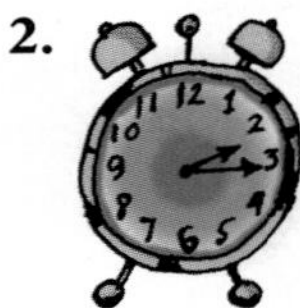
3. 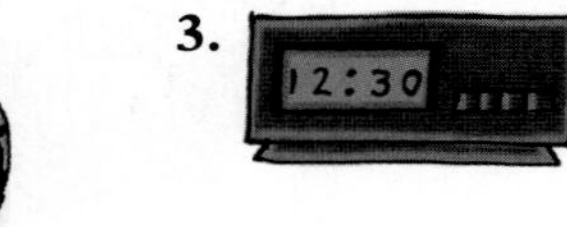

4. 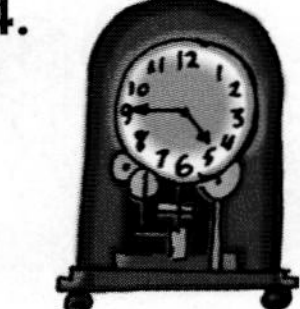
5. 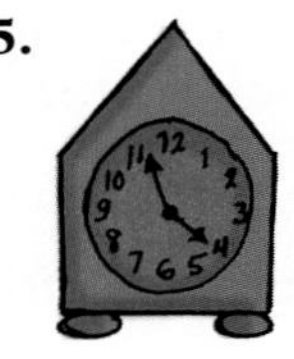
6. 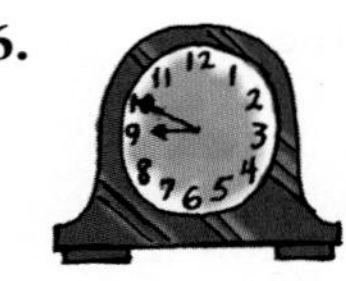
7. 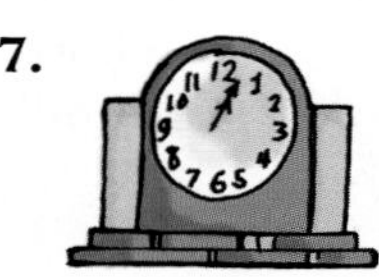
8. 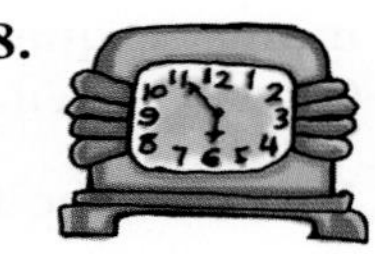
9. 
10. 
11. 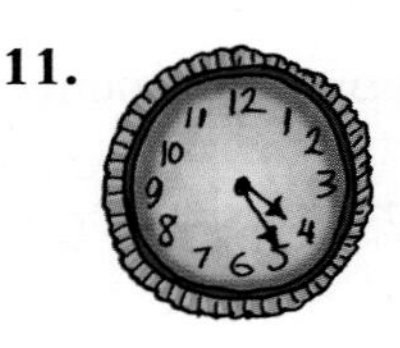
12. 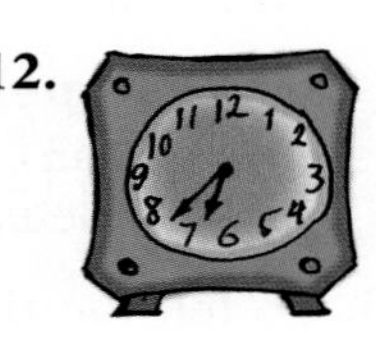

B. Quelle heure est-il pour vous? Qu'est-ce que vous faites?

1. 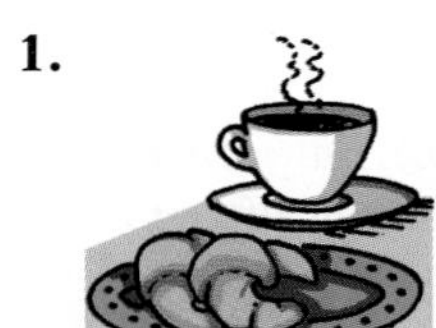
2. 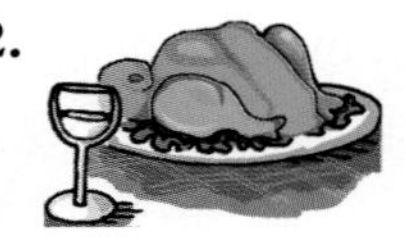
3. 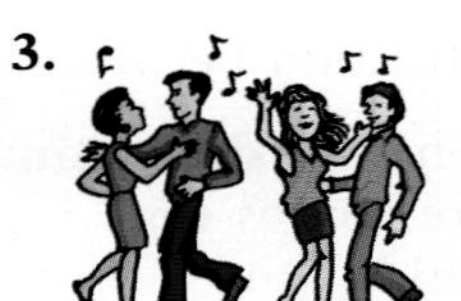
4. 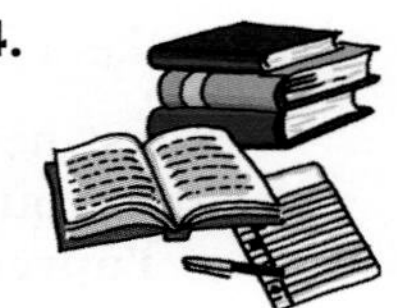

C. Les bars et restaurants de Carcassonne. Imaginez que vous êtes à Carcassonne et que vous consultez la liste des restaurants et cafés de la ville. Voici des informations sur quatre établissements et leurs horaires (*schedules*).

1. À quelle heure préférez-vous prendre votre petit déjeuner? Où pouvez-vous (*can you*) aller? Est-il possible de prendre votre repas à sept heures et demie dans ce restaurant? à huit heures et demie?
2. Samedi, vous voulez (*want*) surfer sur Internet pendant votre déjeuner à midi. Est-ce que le QC est ouvert (*open*)? À quelle heure décidez-vous d'aller au QG?
3. Où allez-vous pour manger une spécialité méditerranéenne? À quelle heure s'arrête le service du déjeuner? À quelle heure commence le service du dîner?
4. Est-il possible de dîner à l'Auberge des Chênes le lundi? Pourquoi? Est-il possible de déjeuner dans ce restaurant le lundi? À quelle heure?
5. Quel restaurant reste ouvert après minuit? Jusqu'à (*Until*) quelle heure?

LES BARS ET RESTAURANTS de CARCASSONNE

L'Auberge des Chênes
Formule midi 15€ en semaine - Menus 22€ à 42€ - Carte
Fermé° lundi soir et samedi midi
1 Rte de Limoux - Tél. 04 68 25 40 11

Closed

L'ESCALIER
Pizzas - TEX-MEX
Spécialités méditerranéennes
De 12h à 14h et de 19h à minuit.
La pizzeria qui fait disjoncter
le Guide du Routard
22, bd Omer Sarraut 11000 CARCASSONNE
Tél. 04 68 25 65 66

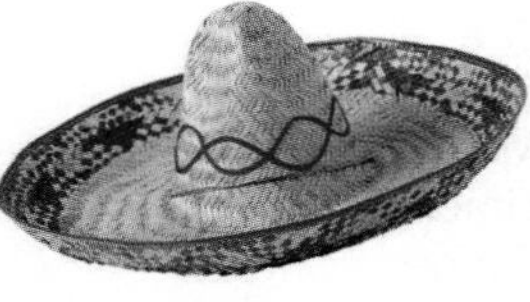

Cyber Café le QG

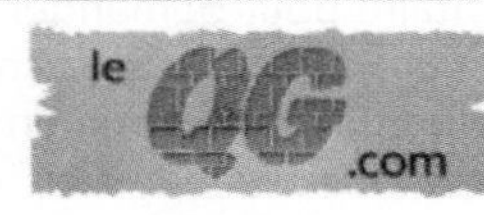

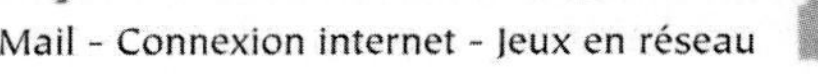
Mail - Connexion internet - Jeux en réseau
Restauration rapide à toutes heures - Boissons chaudes/froides
Ouvert° du lundi au vendredi 8h-19h - Samedi 13h-19h fermé le dimanche
80 allée d'Iéna - Tél. 0811 094 015

Open

Le Colonial Lounge
Restaurant - Bar d'ambiance
Vous invite à l'évasion tous les jours de 11h à 16h
et de 19h à 2h du mat' - Formule à partir de 10€50 et sa carte
Au bord du canal, face à la gare - 3, avenue Maréchal Foch
Tél. 04 68 72 48 43 - mail.lecoloniallounge@aol.com

Follow-up: A. Have sts. give times in both official and conversational ways. B. Ask sts. to role-play a situation in which two friends go to the *Cyber Café le QG* for lunch, but when they arrive they find it is closed because it is Sunday. They consult the advertisements and discuss where else they could go and at what time, or whether they should wait until the next day to return to *le QG*.

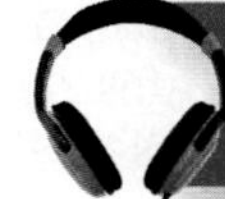

Prononcez bien!

Script (1A): 1. *du lait* 2. *du thé* 3. *du chocolat* 4. *de sucre* 5. *du jambon* 6. *de poisson*

Answers (1A): 1. a 2. a 3. a 4. b 5. a 6. b

Answers (1B): *Il n'y a pas de beurre, pas de café, pas de céleri, pas de fromage. Il y a du poivre. Il n'y a pas de poulet, pas de raisin. Il y a du sel et du thon. Il n'y a pas de vin.*

1. La voyelle dans *du* et *de* (page 157)

A. Au supermarché. Vous êtes au supermarché, mais vous n'avez pas votre liste avec vous. Vous téléphonez à votre colocataire. Elle vous dit (*tells you*) les choses que vous avez et que vous n'avez pas. La communication est mauvaise et vous avez des difficultés à entendre si elle dit « il y a **du** ____ » ou « il n'y a pas **de** ____ »? Faites attention à la prononciation des voyelles **u** et **e** dans les articles pour choisir la bonne réponse.

1. a. Il y a du lait.	**b.** Il n'y a pas de lait.
2. a. Il y a du thé.	**b.** Il n'y a pas de thé.
3. a. Il y a du chocolat.	**b.** Il n'y a pas de chocolat.
4. a. Il y a du sucre.	**b.** Il n'y a pas de sucre.
5. a. Il y a du jambon.	**b.** Il n'y a pas de jambon.
6. a. Il y a du poisson.	**b.** Il n'y a pas de poisson.

B. Au restaurant. Vous êtes au restaurant avec votre ami(e) et un serveur passe avec un plat qui a l'air délicieux (la photo de ce plat est à la page 146). Votre ami(e) vous demande s'il y a les ingrédients suivants dans ce plat: **beurre, café, céleri, fromage, pain, poivre, poulet, raisin, sel, tomates, thon, vin.**

MODÈLE: É1: Est-ce qu'il y a du café?
É2: Non, il n'y a pas de café.

Suggestion (2A): Before sts. begin the activity, be sure they understand the meaning of *pendant*.

Script (2A): *Christophe va voyager pendant deux heures et Zoé pendant treize heures. Le voyage d'Éric et Isabelle va durer six heures; le voyage de Marc trois heures. Simon, lui, va voyager pendant seize heures et Carine pendant douze heures.*

Answers (2A) 1. a 2. b 3. a 4. a 5. b 6. b

Suggestion (2B): Review the times with the sts. before they begin, then circulate in class and monitor their pronunciation as they do the activity.

Answers (2B): 1. Elle arrive à neuf‿heures (v) cinquante-cinq. 2. Il arrive à deux‿heures (z) cinq. 3. Elle arrive à deux‿heures (z) dix. 4. Il arrive à trois‿heures (z) vingt-neuf. 5. Il arrive à six‿heures (z) trente. 6. Elle arrrive à six‿heures (z) quarante-cinq.

2. Liaison with *heures* (page 165)

A. Un week-end entre amis! Les amis de votre colocataire, qui n'habitent pas tous en France, viennent (*are coming*) passer le week-end avec vous. Votre colocataire parle de la durée de voyage de ses amis. Cochez les temps mentionnés.

1. Christophe	**a.** 2 h	**b.** 12 h
2. Zoé	**a.** 3 h	**b.** 13 h
3. Éric et Isabelle	**a.** 6 h	**b.** 16 h
4. Marc	**a.** 3 h	**b.** 13 h
5. Simon	**a.** 6 h	**b.** 16 h
6. Carine	**a.** 2 h	**b.** 12 h

B. Horaires des arrivées. Les amis de votre colocataire (votre camarade de classe) vont arriver en train à des heures différentes. Vous téléphonez à votre colocataire pour demander leurs heures d'arrivée. Posez les questions 1 à 3 à votre colocataire selon le modèle. Ensuite, changez de rôle pour les questions 4 à 6. Faites bien attention à la liaison avec le mot **heures.**

MODÈLE: Christophe (8 h 45)
É1: À quelle heure arrive Christophe?
É2: Il arrive à 8 h 45.

1. Zoé (9 h 55)	**3.** Isabelle (2 h 10)	**5.** Simon (6 h 30)
2. Éric (2 h 05)	**4.** Marc (3 h 29)	**6.** Carine (6 h 45)

Leçon 4

Lecture

Avant de lire

Scanning (Part 1). You are planning a dinner party featuring dishes from a number of French-speaking countries. One of your guests doesn't eat fish; another is allergic to dairy products. As you look for recipes, you rapidly *scan* the list of ingredients, rejecting those that contain salmon and/or cream, for example. Scanning allows you to read more efficiently. Instead of reading line by line, you can skip much of a text and still find the information you need.

Scan the recipes in this section. Would you be able to prepare both of them for the guests described here?

Le vocabulaire culinaire. In recipes, instructions are often given in the infinitive form, which can be translated by an imperative in English.

Râper finement les carottes.	*Finely grate the carrots.*
Couper en morceaux un kilo de poissons.	*Cut up a kilo of fish into pieces.*

In addition, many cooking instructions include the verbs **faire** and **laisser.** Read the following examples carefully.

Faire bouillir...	*Boil . . .*
Laisser mijoter...	*Let simmer . . .*

Can you guess the meaning of the expression **laisser cuire**? (Note that the verb **cuire** is related to the noun **cuisine**).

Voyons voir... Parcourez rapidement (*Scan*) les recettes à la page suivante et décidez si les affirmations sont vraies ou fausses.

1. V F La salade marocaine est sucrée.
2. V F On sert la soupe avec du riz.
3. V F La soupe se cuit (*cooks*) assez rapidement.
4. V F Il y a du jus d'orange dans la salade.
5. V F La soupe contient beaucoup de matières grasses (*fat*).

À propos de la lecture...
Ces recettes sont tirées et adaptées de deux sites Web.

Note: Tell sts. that *eau de fleur d'oranger* is a flavoring used in Moroccan dishes.

Saveurs du monde francophone

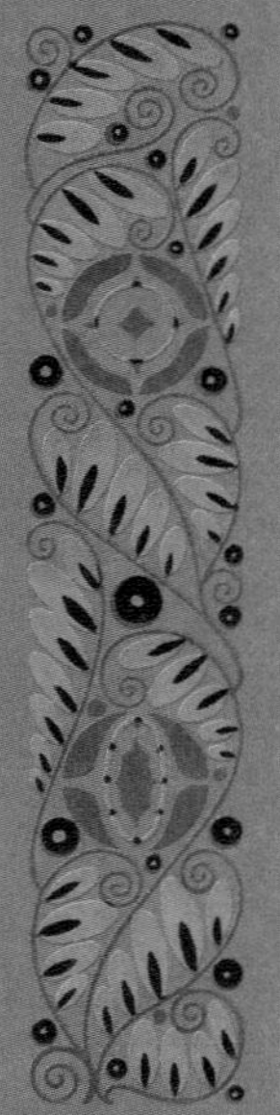

Salade marocaine de carottes râpées à l'orange

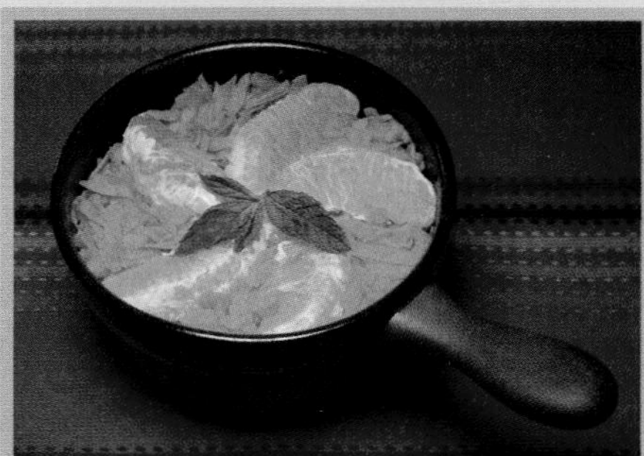

Ingrédients

500 g de carottes
1 pincée de cannelle[1]
1 cuillerée à soupe de sucre en poudre
1 cuillerée à soupe d'eau de fleur d'oranger
1 verre de jus d'orange
le jus d'un citron
2 oranges

Préparation

Râper finement les carottes. Les arroser du mélange cannelle, jus de citron, sucre, eau de fleur d'oranger, jus d'orange. Mélanger. Disposer sur assiettes et décorer de tranches[2] d'oranges pelées à vif.[3]

Servir frais.

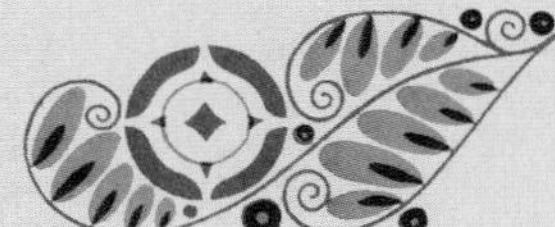

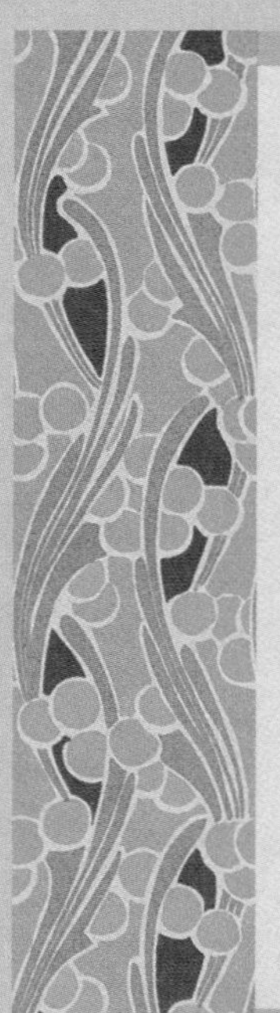

Blaff de poissons martiniquais°

Blaff... *Fish poached in broth, Fish soup*

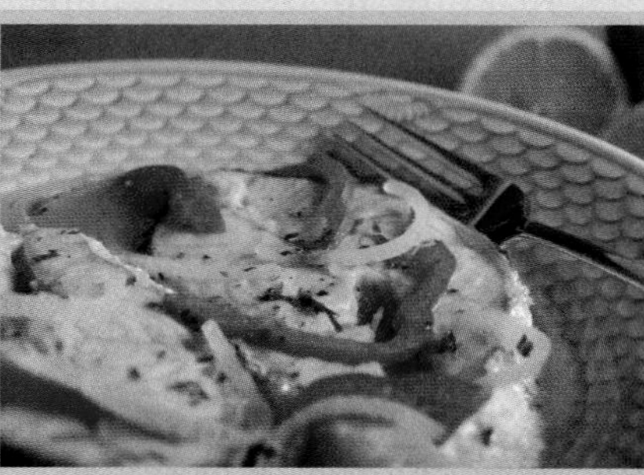

Ingrédients

1 kilo de poissons variés
1 citron vert
1 citron
2 oignons
1 gousse d'ail[4]
1 clou de girofle[5]
1 pincée de thym
2 cuillerées à soupe de persil finement haché[6]
3 cives[7] hachées
un morceau de piment[8]
du sel et du poivre

Préparation

Préparer le court-bouillon: Faire bouillir longuement dans une casserole[9] d'eau le girofle, le thym, le persil, et les oignons préalablement[10] coupés en rondelles,[11] les cives hachées, le sel, le poivre, et le piment. Couper en morceaux[12] un kilo de poissons, les frotter[13] de citron vert et les plonger dans le court-bouillon.

Laisser cuire de 10 à 15 minutes. Ajouter[14] le jus d'un citron et la gousse d'ail écrasée.[15] Laissez mijoter pendant quelques minutes.

Servir les poissons dans ce bouillon très parfumé.[16]

[1]pincée... *pinch of cinnamon* [2]*slices* [3]pelées... *peeled with the zest removed* [4]gousse... *clove of garlic* [5]*clove* [6]*chopped* [7]*chives* [8]*hot pepper* [9]*pot* [10]*ahead of time* [11]*round slices* [12]*pieces* [13]*rub* [14]*Add* [15]*crushed* [16]*flavorful*

Compréhension

Quel verbe, quel ingrédient? Choisissez l'ingrédient de la colonne de droite qui suit logiquement le verbe dans la colonne de gauche. **Attention:** Parfois il y a plus d'une réponse possible.

1. Écraser _______.	**a.** l'eau
2. Hacher _______.	**b.** les oranges
3. Faire bouillir _______.	**c.** les carottes
4. Peler _______.	**d.** les oignons
5. Râper _______.	**e.** la gousse d'ail
6. Couper _______.	**f.** les cives

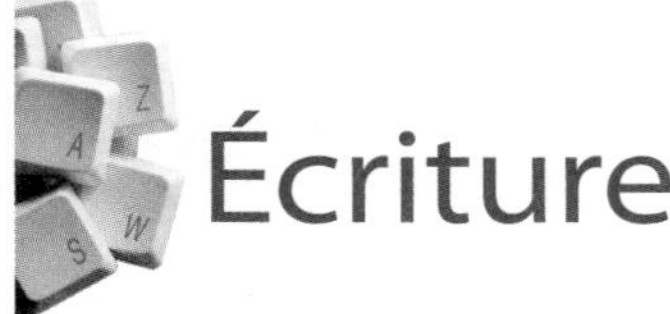

Écriture

The writing activities **Par écrit** and **Journal intime** can be found in the Workbook/Laboratory Manual to accompany *Vis-à-vis*.

Additional activity/Follow-up: *Goûts et préférences. Regardez de nouveau la liste des ingrédients de ces deux plats: est-ce qu'il y a des ingrédients que vous adorez? que vous n'aimez pas du tout? Est-ce que vous avez envie d'essayer les deux recettes, ou préférez-vous l'une des deux? Expliquez.*

Additional vocabulary: *appétissant* (appetizing), *avoir l'air épicé / piquant* (spicy), *fade* (bland), *le goût* (taste), *salé* (savory, "salty"), *la saveur* (flavor, taste), *sucré* (sweet).

Pour s'amuser

«Le vin est la partie intellectuelle d'un repas. Les viandes et les légumes n'en sont que la partie matérielle.»

—Alexandre Dumas

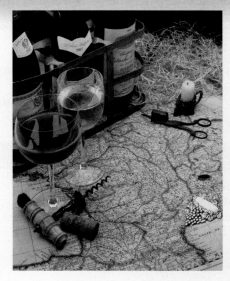

Selon vous, est-ce que le vin est une boisson «intellectuelle»? Expliquez.

La vie en chantant. An activity based on the song "Sénégal fast food" by Amadou et Miriam can be found in the Instructor's Manual. The song can be purchased at the iTunes store, or sts. can watch the music video on YouTube.

Le vidéoblog d'Hassan

En bref

Dans cet épisode, Léa et Juliette regardent le vidéoblog d'Hassan. Le jeune homme donne une petite leçon de cuisine à Hector. Les deux amis préparent une salade marocaine traditionnelle: des carottes râpées à l'orange. Ensuite, Hector parle de la cuisine martiniquaise.

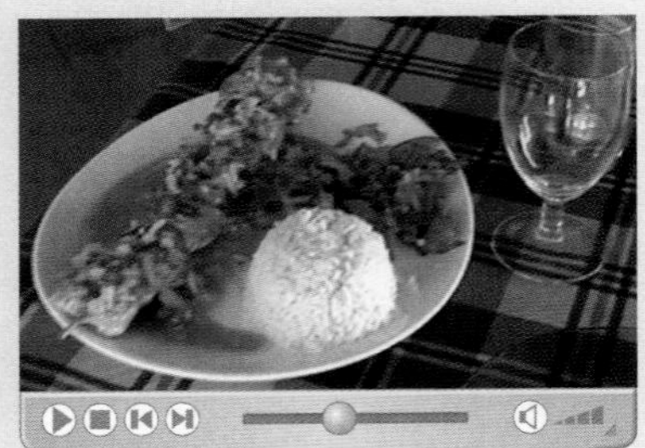

Une brochette de poisson à la martiniquaise

Vocabulaire en contexte

Mesurez *votre* talent en cuisine et décrivez *votre* repas typique.

Votre talent en cuisine

- ☐ Moi, je suis un excellent cuisinier / une excellente cuisinère!
- ☐ **Je sais** (*I know how*) préparer de bons **plats.**
- ☐ Il y a un ou deux plats que je sais préparer.
- ☐ Je suis incapable de faire un sandwich!

Votre repas typique

- ☐ un repas **diététique** composé de produits frais
- ☐ un repas équilibré traditionnel
- ☐ un repas lourd et gras (*heavy and greasy*)
- ☐ un repas fast-food

Suggestion: After you model the pronunciation and review the meanings of the words in boldface (which are words actually contained in the video transcript), have sts. select their preference(s) in each column. Afterward, a comparison and "tally" of preferences can be done in groups or as a whole-class activity.

Additional vocabulary: Other vocabulary you may wish to present before viewing includes *Est-ce que tu peux, marrant, parfumer.*

Suggestion: The *Visionnez!* activity has two uses: to introduce additional vocabulary and concepts and then as a postviewing comprehension check. Ask sts. to read the activity before they watch the video. Model the pronunciation of the words in boldface. You may wish to explain before viewing that *l'eau de fleur d'oranger* is a flavoring. After viewing, return to these questions for a quick whole-class comprehension check.

Visionnez!

Regardez la vidéo et trouvez l'équivalent des mots en caractères gras.

1. ______ Hassan **râpe** les carottes.
2. ______ Hector **coupe** les oranges en tranches fines (*thin slices*).
3. ______ Hector **verse** le jus de citron sur les carottes.
4. ______ Hassan **ajoute** du sucre et de l'eau de fleur d'oranger.
5. ______ Hassan **met** un peu de cannelle sur la salade.
6. ______ Hassan **mélange** les ingrédients.

a. *cuts*
b. *adds*
c. *pours*
d. *grates*
e. *mixes*
f. *puts*

Analysez!

Répondez aux questions.

1. Le climat a une influence sur la cuisine d'un pays. Existe-t-il d'autres influences? Donnez des exemples.
2. Trouvez-vous la cuisine martiniquaise appétissante? Pourquoi (pas)?

Comparez!

Qu'est-ce qui influence la cuisine de votre région? Quels sont les plats et les ingrédients typiques? Regardez encore une fois la partie culturelle de la vidéo: préférez-vous la cuisine de votre région ou la cuisine martiniquaise? Expliquez.

Note culturelle

Au Maroc, pays à l'hospitalité légendaire, le thé à la menthe[1] vous est proposé à toute heure. Préparé dans une théière[2] de métal, on vous le présente bien chaud et très sucré. On le verse[3] très haut[4] dans un petit verre. Refuser un thé à la menthe est impoli. C'est parfois[5] considéré comme une offense.

[1]*mint* [2]*teapot* [3]*pours* [4]*high* [5]*sometimes*

Note: Other influences might include religion (prohibitions against certain foods), population (space available for growing food), and daily life (amount of time one can spend preparing and eating food).

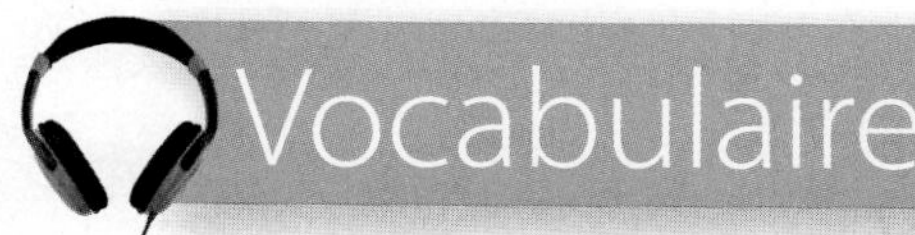

Vocabulaire

Verbes

apporter *to bring*
apprendre to learn
boire to drink
célébrer to celebrate
commander to order (*in a restaurant*)
comprendre to understand; to include
considérer to consider
déjeuner to eat lunch
dîner to dine, eat dinner
espérer to hope
passer to pass, spend (*time*)
préférer to prefer
prendre to take; to have (to eat; to order)
  prendre le petit déjeuner to have breakfast
  prendre du temps to take (a long) time
  prendre son temps to take one's time
  prendre un repas to eat a meal
  prendre un verre to have a drink (*usually alcoholic*)

À REVOIR: **aimer mieux, préparer**

Substantifs

l'après-midi (*m.*) afternoon
la cuisine cooking; kitchen
le déjeuner lunch
le dîner dinner
le goûter afternoon snack
la journée (whole) day
le matin morning
le midi noon
le plat dish (*of food*)
le petit déjeuner breakfast
le produit product
le repas meal
le soir evening

Les provisions

l'aliment (*m.*) food
le beurre butter
la bière beer
le bifteck steak
le bœuf beef
la boisson gazeuse soft drink
le champignon mushroom
le citron lemon
le citron vert lime
la crème cream
l'eau (*f.*) **(minérale)** (mineral) water
la fraise strawberry
les frites (*f. pl.*) French fries
le fromage cheese
le gâteau cake
les haricots* (*m. pl.*) **verts** green beans
le jambon ham
le jus (d'orange) (orange) juice
le lait milk
le légume vegetable
la nourriture food
l'œuf (*m.*) egg
l'oignon (*m.*) onion
le pain bread
la poire pear
le poisson fish
le poivre pepper
le poivron bell pepper
la pomme de terre potato
le poulet chicken
les produits (*m.*) **frais** fresh products
le sel salt
le sucre sugar
la tarte pie
le thé tea
la viande meat
le vin wine

À table

l'assiette (*f.*) plate
le bol wide cup
la bouteille bottle
le couteau knife
la cuillère (à soupe) (soup) spoon
la fourchette fork
la glace ice cream
la nappe tablecloth
la serviette napkin
la tasse cup
le verre glass

Substantifs apparentés

la baguette, la banane, les brocolis (*m. pl.*), **la carafe, la carotte, le champagne, le chocolat, le croissant, le dessert, le fruit, la laitue, l'orange** (*f. pl.*), **le porc, la salade, la soupe, la tomate**

Adjectif

frais/fraîche fresh

L'heure

Quelle heure est-il? What time is it?
Il est... heure(s). It is . . . o'clock.
  ... et demi(e) half past (the hour)
  ... et quart quarter past (the hour)
  ... moins le quart quarter to (the hour)
  ... du matin in the morning
  ... de l'après-midi in the afternoon
  ... du soir in the evening, at night
Il est midi. It's noon.
Il est minuit. It's midnight.
À quelle heure... ? At what time . . . ?

Les expressions de quantité

assez de enough of
beaucoup de a lot of
peu de little of
trop de too much of, too many of
un peu de a little of

Mots et expressions divers

à l'heure on time
de bonne heure early
Dépêche-toi! *Hurry up!*
en avance early
en retard late
je voudrais I would like
ne... plus no more, no longer, not any more
plusieurs several
presque almost
Sois gentil! *Be nice!*
tard late
tôt early
vers around, about (*with time expressions*)

*The initial **h** is aspirate here, which means there is no elision with the article **les**.

CHAPITRE 7

Les plaisirs de la cuisine

Les dossiers d'Hassan

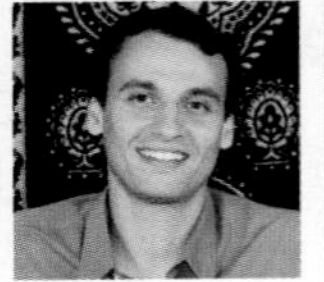

Hassan

- Mes photos
  - Un beau marché en plein air
  - Faire le marché
  - Un tajine marocain

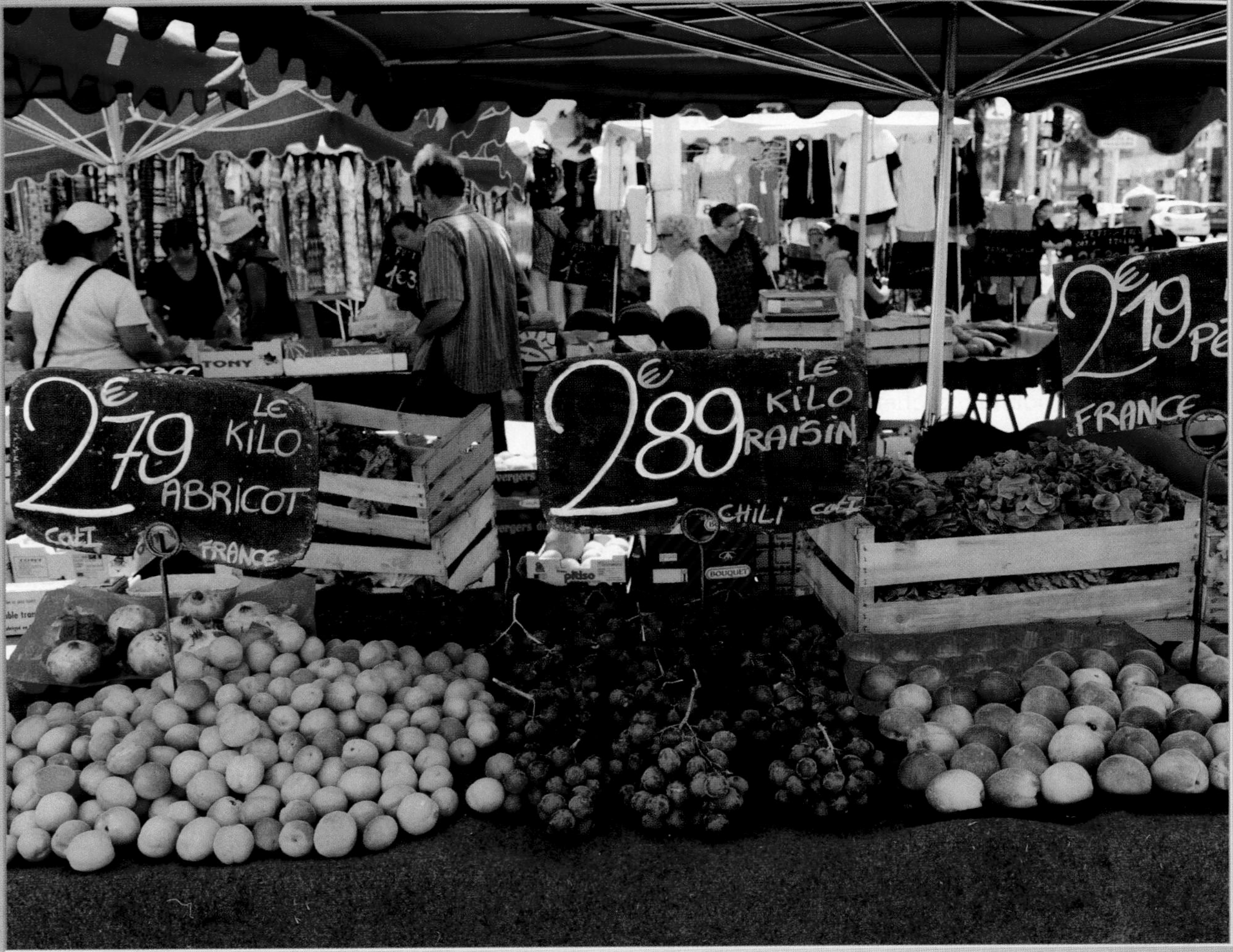

Presentation: Ask sts. to describe what they see. Review food vocabulary by asking sts. to name what other products might be sold in this market. Numbers above 60 are presented in this chapter. You can use the signs in the photo to introduce them.

Un beau marché en plein air

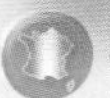 **Cultural note:** Every French city and town has an open-air market on designated days of the week. In addition to food, there are often booths selling clothes, kitchen utensils and gadgets, wine, and local artisanal products, such as pottery, salad bowls, table linens, fabric, etc.

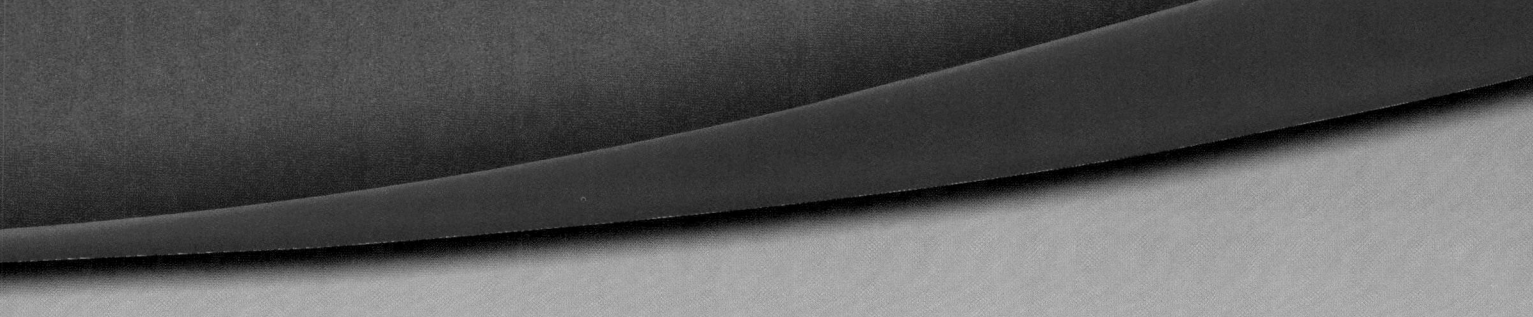

Dans ce chapitre...

OBJECTIFS COMMUNICATIFS

- asking about choices
- pointing out people and things
- expressing desire, ability, necessity, and obligation
- talking about past events
- learning to distinguish between and pronounce selected sounds in French

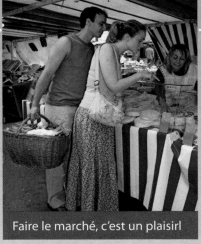
Faire le marché, c'est un plaisirl

PAROLES (Leçon 1)

- Les magasins d'alimentation
- Au restaurant
- Les nombres supérieurs à 60

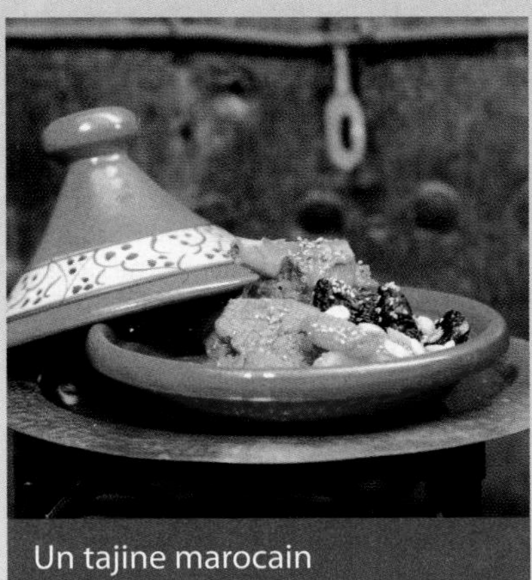
Un tajine marocain

STRUCTURES (Leçons 2 et 3)

- L'adjectif interrogatif **quel**
- Les adjectifs démonstratifs
- Les verbes **vouloir, pouvoir** et **devoir**
- Le passé composé avec l'auxiliaire **avoir**

CULTURE

- Le blog d'Hassan: *Marché ou cybermarché?*
- Reportage: *Comment voyager dans son assiette?*
- Lecture: *Les grandes occasions* (Leçon 4)

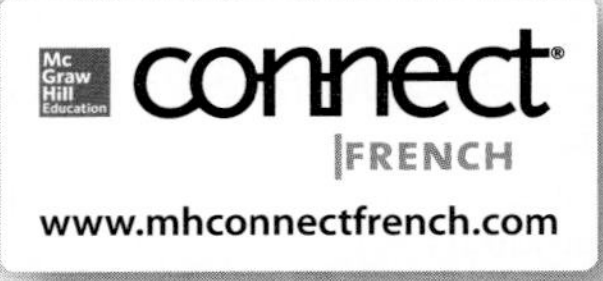

CHAPITRE 7

Leçon 1

PAROLES

Presentation: (1) Model pronunciation. (2) Have sts. name foods that are: *sucré, salé, des légumes, des fruits, des produits laitiers, du porc, du bœuf, des poissons, des fruits de mer, des pâtisseries,* etc. Mention that the French do not mix *sucré* and *salé* in the same dish. (3) If available, show images of French markets of various types, including open-air, supermarkets, and specialty shops. Have sts. name foods and stores seen in the presentation.

Les magasins (*m.*) d'alimentation

Mme Barbet va d'abord (*first*) à la boulangerie, puis (*then*) à la poissonnerie, et ensuite (*then*) à la boucherie.

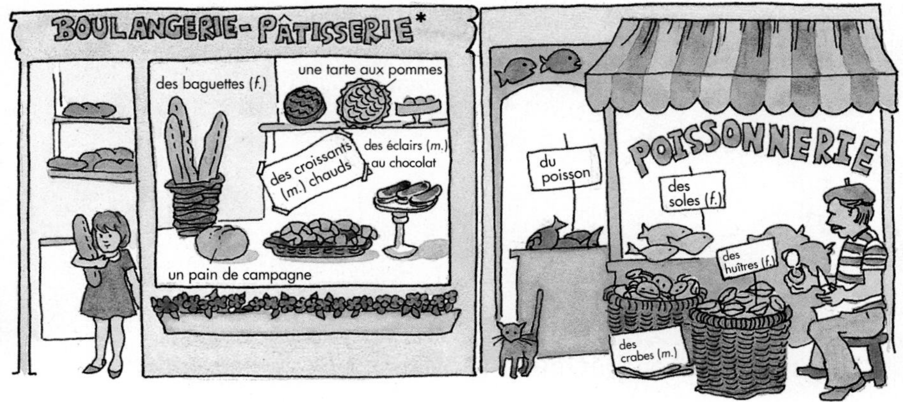

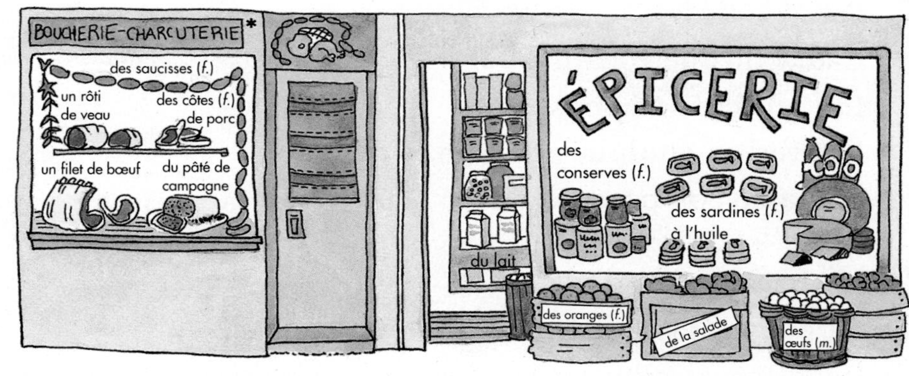

Additional vocabulary: *de l'agneau, un pain au chocolat, de la pizza, des pommes frites, du riz,* etc.

Prononcez bien!

The semivowel in *ail*

Pronounce the semivowel [j] the same way you pronounce the first letter of the English word *you*, with the sides of your tongue pressing against the sides of your palate. Below are the most common spellings of the sound [j].

[j]: **bien, yeux, maillot***

The **-il** at the end of a word is also pronounced [j].

[j]: **ail, travail, sommeil, vieil**

One exception to this rule is **gentil,** where the **-il** is pronounced [i].

***mille, ville, villa, village, tranquille** are exceptions to this rule and the **-ill** is pronounced [il].

AUTRES MOTS UTILES

de l'ail (*m.*)	garlic	**de l'huile** (*f.*)	oil
une boîte (de conserve)	a can (of food)	**des pâtes**	pasta
		un saucisson	a salami
des crevettes (*f.*)	shrimp	**du saumon**	salmon
un homard†	a lobster		

Cultural note: In Quebec, a convenience store is called *un dépanneur;* it is essentially a small *épicerie.* For *pain au chocolat,* the word *chocolatine* is used.

Note: Point out that one says *à la boucherie* but *chez le boucher,* etc.

Pronunciation practice (1): Show sts. pictures of the following items and ask them to name them: *cuillère, serviette, famille, chien, réveil, télévision, yeux, chemisier, maillot de bain, tailleur, violet, cahier.*

Pronunciation practice (2): The *Prononcez bien!* section on page 195 of this chapter contains additional activities for practicing these sounds.

*There are also separate stores; **la boulangerie,** where one buys bread, **la pâtisserie,** where one buys pastries, **la boucherie,** where one buys beef and poultry, and **la charcuterie** where one buys pork products.

†The **h** in **homard** is aspirate, which means that there is no "elision" with the article **le** (i.e., **le homard**). Note how this is different from **l'huître,** which has a mute **h.** In both cases, the **h** is silent.

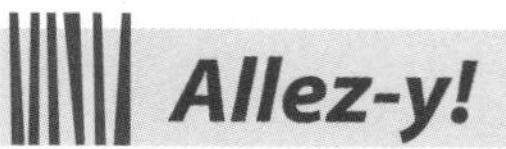

Follow-up: One st. chooses a store and names one product that can be bought there. Another repeats the product and names a new one, and so on. Do this for several stores. *MODÈLE: —À la boulangerie-pâtisserie, j'achète un éclair au chocolat. —J'achète un éclair au chocolat et une baguette. —J'achète un éclair au chocolat, une baguette et…*

Les magasins du quartier. Où est-ce qu'on va pour acheter les produits suivants?

MODÈLE: des éclairs au chocolat →
Pour acheter des éclairs au chocolat, on va à la boulangerie-pâtisserie.

1. des saucisses et un rôti de veau
2. des huîtres et des crabes
3. des sardines à l'huile
4. des côtes de porc
5. de la sole et du saumon
6. du pâté de campagne et du filet de bœuf
7. de l'ail et des boîtes de conserve
8. un pain de campagne

Suggestion (Au restaurant): Bring in menus from French restaurants. Use some of the following questions: *Quel est le nom du restaurant? Lisez le nom de chaque catégorie de plats. Est-ce que «l'entrée» veut dire* plat principal *ou* premier plat? *Que signifient «nos formules» probablement? «nos fromages»? «les desserts»? «les plats»?*

Au restaurant

Restaurant La Guirlande de Julie

Ouvert de 12 h 00 à 14 h 30 et de 19 h 00 à 22 h 30.
Fermé le lundi.

Pour commencer

Kir[1]	*9 euros*
Coupe[2] *de champagne*	*15 euros*
Américano	*8 euros*

Nos formules[3]

(excepté le soir, le samedi, le dimanche et les jours fériés)

Plat du marché	*14 euros*
Entrée, plat du marché	*18 euros*
ou	
Plat du marché, dessert	*18 euros*
Entrée, plat du marché, dessert	*20 euros*

Les entrées

Fromage de chèvre au basilic et à l'huile d'olive	*7 euros*
Escargots de Bourgogne	*9 euros*
Terrine de gibier,[4] *petite salade «selon saison»*	*9 euros*
Foie gras de canard[5] *maison*	*15 euros*

Les plats

Notre spécialité «Pot-au-feu[6] *royal»*	*16 euros*
Confit de canard, pommes bûcheronnes, champignons	*17 euros*
Rognons de veau[7] *bordelais et petits oignons*	*15 euros*
Saumon braisé en croûte d'herbes, tagliatelle de légumes	*18 euros*

Nos fromages

Petit chèvre frais mariné à l'huile vierge	*7 euros*
Assiette de fromages	*7 euros*

Les desserts

Tarte aux pommes, glace à la cannelle	*8 euros*
Crème brûlée à la vanille de Bourbon	*8 euros*
Glaces et sorbets, parfums au choix	*8 euros*

Prix nets, service compris

[1]*White wine with blackcurrant liqueur* [2]*Goblet* [3]*Special of the day generally including* un plat *and* une entrée *or* un dessert. [4]Terrine… *Game paté* [5]*duck* [6]*Stew* [7]Rognons… *Veal kidneys*

Note: The *menu à prix fixe* (*fixed-price menu*) is a feature of many French restaurants. Customers ordering from it select their courses from a list of choices that is somewhat smaller than the regular menu, *la carte*. The beverage is often included (*boisson comprise*) in the cost of the *menu à prix fixe*. When service is included (*service compris*), tipping is not expected.

AUTRES MOTS UTILES

l'addition (*f.*)	check
l'argent (*m.*)	money
autre chose	something else
la carte	menu
compris(e)	included
l'entrée (*f.*)	first course
les escargots (*m.*)	snails
goûter	to taste
le menu	fixed-price meal (*usually including* **une entrée, un plat,** *and* **du fromage** *or* **un dessert**)
la mousse au chocolat	chocolate mousse
le plat	course (*of a meal*); dish (*type of food*)
le plat principal	main course
le pourboire	tip
le prix	price
quelque chose	something
le serveur / la serveuse	waiter / waitress

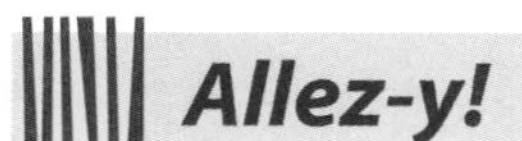

Note: *Vis-à -vis* avoids use of *garçon* for *serveur;* the former is now considered demeaning by many French-speaking people.

A. La Guirlande de Julie. Mettez le dialogue dans le bon ordre. Numérotez les phrases de 1 à 10.

LE SERVEUR

_______ Vous désirez quelque chose à boire?
_______ (*plus tard*) Vous désirez autre chose?
_______ Une eau minérale. Vous désirez une entrée?
_______ Bonjour, madame. Avez-vous choisi? (*Have you decided?*)
_______ Très bien, madame. (*plus tard*) Prenez-vous du fromage, un dessert?

LA CLIENTE

_______ Une eau minérale, s'il vous plaît.
_______ Oui, j'ai fait mon choix (*choice*).
_______ Oui, comme entrée, je vais prendre le foie gras de canard, et ensuite, le pot-au-feu.
_______ Euh, je vais prendre une crème brûlée à la vanille, s'il vous plaît.
_______ Non, merci. Apportez-moi (*Bring me*) l'addition, s'il vous plaît.

Additional activity: *Qui est-ce? Est-ce que c'est un client, une cliente, un serveur ou une serveuse?* 1. *Il a faim.* 2. *Elle arrive avec la carte.* 3. *Elle prend le menu à 20 euros.* 4. *Il commande un repas.* 5. *Il prend la commande.* 6. *Il apporte les entrées.* 7. *Elle boit son vin.* 8. *Elle apporte l'addition.* 9. *Il paie l'addition et laisse un pourboire.* 10. *Elle prend le pourboire.*

B. Au restaurant. Avec un(e) camarade, regardez la carte de La Guirlande de Julie. Jouez les rôles du serveur / de la serveuse et du client / de la cliente. Notez ce que le client / la cliente commande.

MODÈLE: LE SERVEUR / LA SERVEUSE: Qu'est-ce que vous prenez comme entrée? (plat principal, boisson…)
LE CLIENT / LA CLIENTE: Je prends le/la*…

Vocabulary recycling: *Préférez-vous _______?* 1. *le café ou le thé?* 2. *le porc, le bœuf, le veau ou le poulet?* 3. *la viande ou le poisson?* 4. *le gâteau ou les fruits?* 5. *le pain ou les croissants?* 6. *la tarte aux pommes ou la tarte à la crème?*

Follow-up (B): After group work, have several sts. describe each meal. Ask class *Qui a le repas le plus* (the most) *intéressant?*

*The definite article, rather than the partitive, is often used when one orders a dish from a menu.

Les nombres supérieurs à 60

Presentation: If possible, bring in coins and banknotes from French-speaking countries.

60	soixante	72	soixante-douze	90	quatre-vingt-dix
61	soixante **et** un	73	soixante-treize	91	quatre-vingt-onze
62	soixante-deux	80	quatre-vingt**s**	92	quatre-vingt-douze
63	soixante-trois	81	quatre-vingt-un	93	quatre-vingt-treize
70	soixante-dix	82	quatre-vingt-deux	100	cent
71	soixante **et** onze	83	quatre-vingt-trois		

- Note that **quatre-vingts** takes an **-s,** but that numbers based on it do not: **quatre-vingt-un,** and so on.

101	cent un	600	six cents
102	cent deux	700	sept cents
200	deux cents	800	huit cents
201	deux cent un	900	neuf cents
300	trois cents	999	neuf cent quatre-vingt-dix-neuf
400	quatre cents	1 000	mille
500	cinq cents	999 999	?

- Note that the **-s** of **cents** is dropped if it is followed by any other number: **deux cent un, sept cent trente-cinq.**
- Like **cent, mille** (*one thousand*) is expressed without an article. **Mille** is invariable and thus never ends in **-s: mille quatre, sept mille, neuf mille neuf cent quatre-vingt-dix-neuf.**

Préférez-vous les légumes, les fruits de mer ou la viande?

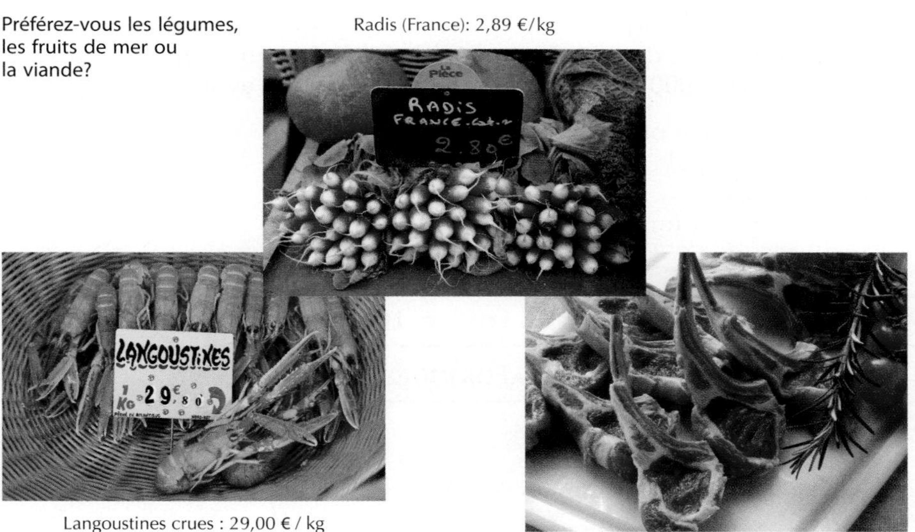

Radis (France): 2,89 €/kg

Langoustines crues : 29,00 € / kg

Côtes d'agneau : 19,06 € / kg

Vocabulary recycling: Quickly review numbers from 1 to 60, presented in *Chapitre 1, Leçon 2.* A. Sts. stand and count by one's, two's, three's, etc., round-robin style. B. Sts. write out four math problems (addition, multiplication, subtraction, division), then circulate, putting their questions to several classmates. C. Sts. circulate and find out the birthdays of four classmates (also useful for reviewing dates, presented in *Chapitre 1, Leçon 2*).

Presentation: Model pronunciation of numbers 60 to 100. Ask sts. to (1) count from 60 to 100 by two's, three's, or five's; (2) say the numbers on flashcards held up for them, prepared before class and presented in random order; (3) guess number of pennies (candies, other small objects) in a jar by suggesting numbers from 60 to 100. St. guessing right number gets the "prize." Then present numbers 100 to 999 by explaining system briefly.

Note: Point out that the French count by tens from 1 to 60 but by twenties from 61 to 100: 61-79, 80-99. Note that *et* is used with the numbers 61 and 71 (as with 21, etc.) but not with 81 and 91. There is no *liaison* in *quatre-vingt-un* [katrəvɛ̃œ̃], *quatre-vingt-huit* [katrəvɛ̃ɥit], and *quatre-vingt-onze* [katrəvɛ̃ɔ̃z]. Note also the use in French of a blank space where English uses a comma to indicate thousand(s); a period (*un point*) is sometimes also used. *Deux mille deux cent cinquante* is written either 2 250 or 2.250. The French use the comma (*la virgule*), not a period, in decimal numbers: 3,25 (three and 25/100) is said as *trois virgule vingt-cinq.*

Cultural note: *Septante* (70), *octante / huitante* (80), and *nonante* (90) are often used in Belgium and Switzerland.

Additional activity: *Les nombres à la chaîne.* This can be done with 2- or 3-digit numbers. You choose a number, e.g.: 54. The first st. must say a number starting with the last digit of that number: 48. The next st. then says a number starting with 8, etc.

Suggestion: Check for the current rate of the *euro.* At printing, 1,00 euro = 1.30 USD = 1.32 CAD.

- French currency is **l'euro** (*m.*)(€); it is divided into **centimes.** The most common way of writing prices in **euros** is: 48,50 €, **(quarante-huit euros cinquante).**
- The nouns **million** and **milliard** (*billion*) take **-s** in the plural. When introducing a noun, they are followed by **de (d').**

Ce château a coûté sept **millions d'**euros.	*This chateau cost seven million euros.*

Suggestion (A): Have sts. do this ex. in pairs. Use as listening comprehension as follows: Dictate the problem by saying *Combien font… ?* Sts. write down problem and volunteer answer by a show of hands. Problems and answers can be done at board by a few sts. during this ex.

Cultural note: *Le menu* refers to a full meal including *un hors-d'œuvre* (a cold light snack before the meal), *une entrée* (a hot or cold meal starter that precedes the main dish), *un plat principal,* and *du fromage* or *un dessert.* The price is fixed and the tip is included. Many restaurants have at least two *menus:* an inexpensive one and a more expensive one. The word *formule* is also used to describe *un menu* with *un plat* and *une entrée* or *un dessert.* If you want to order a single dish, you can order *à la carte.* Wines and desserts are usually listed in sections called *la carte des vins* and *la carte des desserts.*

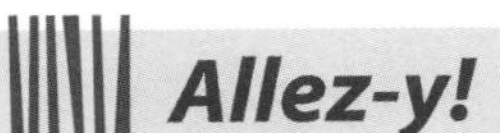

Allez-y!

A. Problèmes de mathématiques. Inventez six problèmes, puis demandez à un(e) camarade de les résoudre (*solve them*).

Vocabulaire utile: + (plus, et), − (moins), × (fois), ÷ (divisé par), = (font, égalent)

MODÈLES: 37 + 42 →
É1: Trente-sept plus (et) quarante-deux?
É2: Trente-sept plus (et) quarante-deux font (égalent) soixante-dix-neuf.

10 × 10 000 →
É1: Dix fois dix mille?
É2: Dix fois dix mille font (égalent) cent mille.

B. La cuisine diététique. Votre partenaire et vous avez un restaurant français qui sert de la cuisine diététique. Créez un menu à moins de (*fewer than*) 1 000 calories. Le menu doit (*must*) avoir…

un hors-d'œuvre ou une entrée
un plat principal
des légumes
un fromage ou un dessert

VALEUR CALORIQUE DE QUELQUES ALIMENTS (pour 100 grammes)							
TRÈS CALORIQUES		CALORIQUES		PEU CALORIQUES		TRÈS PEU CALORIQUES	
Saucisson	559	Brie	271	Banane	97	Poire	61
Chocolat	500	Pain	259	Crevettes	96	Pomme	61
Pâté de foie gras	454	Côte d'agneau	256	Pommes de terre	89	Carotte	43
Biscuits secs	410	Filet de porc	172	Lait	67	Fraise	40
Macaronis, pâtes	351	Œufs	162	Artichaut	64	Orange	40
Riz	340	Poulet	147			Champignons	31
Camembert	312	Canard	135			Tomates	22

C. Les promotions du mois. Ce soir, vous faites des courses. Vous allez dans un magasin spécialisé en produits surgelés (*frozen*). Vous achetez un plat principal, des légumes et un dessert. Qu'est-ce que vous allez choisir?

Follow-up: Have sts. role-play shopping with a friend and choosing the items for their meal. They can use the expressions *plus cher, moins cher, de bonne qualité.*

CHEZ PICARD SURGELÉS

Côtes d'agneau
(pièces de 60 g environ)
le sac de 1 kg 15,80

Gigot d'agneau prêt à découper
(pièce de 1,4 à 1,8 kg) le kg 12,60

4 steaks hachés
(100 g) Picard, *le kg 9,45 €*,
la boîte de 400 g 5,90

10 steaks hachés
(100 g) Picard,
la boîte de 1 kg 10,20

Crevettes crues
(10-20 au kg) élevées à Madagascar, *le kg 37,50 €*,
l'étui de 800 g 32,00

Magret de canard
(pièce de 300-400 g)
le kg 18,40

2 cuisses de poulet rôties
avec partie de dos,
le kg 11,40 €, le sac de 400 g 6,60

Poulet à la mexicaine
hauts de cuisses marinés,
cuits (5 pièces) *le kg 13,62 €*,
le sac de 400 g 6,95

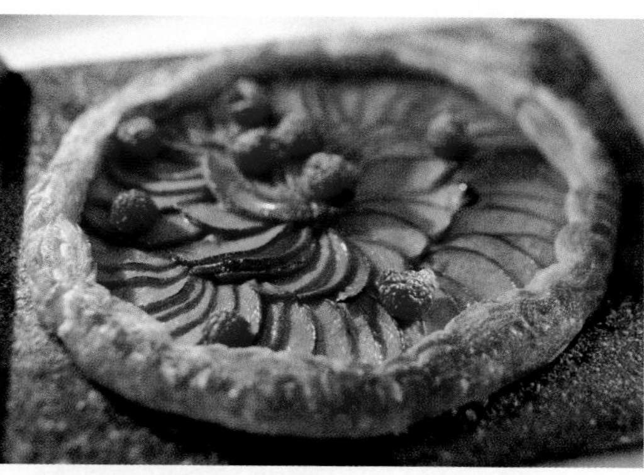

Tarte aux pommes : *le kg 7.84 €*, 5,20 € la piece de 680 g

Petits pois doux extra-fins et jeunes carottes
le kg 2,84 €, le sac de 450 g........ 4,30

Petits pois doux à la française
(avec laitue en tablettes et petits oignons blancs)
le sac de 1 kg........ 5,70

Carottes jeunes entières extra-fines
le sac de 1 kg........ 5,10

Carottes en rondelles
le sac de 1 kg........ 4,90

20 crêpes au jambon-fromage
la boîte de 1 kg 7,20

2 crêpes savoyardes
reblochon, pommes de terre, lardons, oignons,
le kg 13,36 €, la boîte de 250 g........ 4,40

4 crêpes campagnardes
champignons, jambon, lard fumé, *le kg 10,56 €*,
la boîte de 460 g........ 5,90

Framboises brisées
Chili, le sac de 1 kg 8,20

Framboises entières
Chili, le sac de 1 kg 6,90

2 mousses au chocolat
Picard, *le kg 15,70 €*,
la boîte de 170 g 5,10

2 Petits Plaisirs au chocolat
recette Lenôtre, Brossard,
le kg 33,38 €, la boîte de 130 g 5,50

2 Tiramisù
crème au mascarpone, génoise imbibée de café, saupoudrage cacao, Picard,
le kg 19,25 €, la boîte de 200 g 4,80

Composez votre menu.

Maintenant calculez le prix de ce que vous allez acheter.

	PRIX
Plat principal	______
Légumes	______
Dessert	______
Total	______

Enfin, donnez votre menu et les résultats de vos calculs à la classe. Qui compose le menu le plus cher (*most expensive*), le plus original?

Additional activity: *Dans votre porte-monnaie. Comptez vos pièces de monnaie selon les modèles.* MODÈLES: *5 € + 50 c* → cinq euros cinquante; *10 c + 5 c + 1 c* → seize centimes. 1. *50 c + 20 c + 10 c + 5 c + 1 c* 2. *50 c + 20 c + 20 c + 5 c + 1 c* 3. *50 c + 10 c + 1 c* 4. *5 € + 1 € + 50 c + 20 c + 5 c* 5. *5 € + 1 € + 1 € + 50 c + 10 c* 6. *2 € + 1 € + 10 c + 10 c + 5 c + 1 c* 7. *10 € + 1 € + 20 c + 5 c* 8. *10 € + 5 € + 2 € + 20 c + 5 c*

CHAPITRE 7

Leçon 2

STRUCTURES

L'adjectif interrogatif *quel*

Asking About Choices

Tout le monde° au restaurant!

°*Everybody*

Hector téléphone à Hassan.

HECTOR: Allô, Hassan? J'organise une petite fête.[1]
HASSAN: Super! **Quel** jour? Pour **quelle** occasion?
HECTOR: Pour le 14 juillet: la fête[2] nationale! On dîne et ensuite, on va danser avec des amis.
HASSAN: **Quels** amis?
HECTOR: J'invite Juliette... Léa... son copain Mamadou... Abdel et sa fiancée...
HASSAN: Tu cuisines?
HECTOR: Non. J'invite tout le monde au restaurant!
HASSAN: C'est une bonne idée. Dans **quel** restaurant?
HECTOR: Dans TON restaurant!

[1]*party, celebration* [2]*holiday*

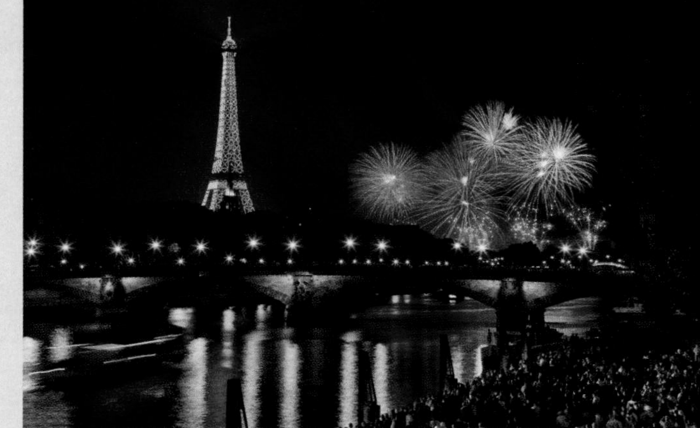
Paris en fête

Trouvez dans le dialogue, la question qui correspond à ces réponses en utilisant la forme correcte de **quel.** Faites des phrases complètes.

1. *Pour le 14 juillet*, Hector organise une petite fête.
2. *Pour la fête nationale,* Hector propose de dîner et ensuite d'aller danser avec des amis.
3. Hector invite *Juliette, Léa, son copain Mamadou, Abdel et sa fiancée.*
4. Hector invite tout le monde *dans le restaurant d'Hassan.*

Presentation: Remind sts. that different interrogative forms reflect differences in the questioner's expectations about information he or she will receive in response. Questions with inversion and *est-ce que* indicate that the questioner seeks a yes/no answer. Questions with *qu'est-ce que* imply that the questioner is seeking new information. In questions with *quand, pourquoi,* and *où,* the questioner seeks information about specific circumstances. In questions with interrogative adjective *quel(le)(s),* the questioner seeks more precise information.

Forms of *quel*

Quel (quelle, quels, quelles) means *which* or *what.* It agrees in gender and number with the noun it modifies. You are already familiar with **quel** in expressions such as **Quelle heure est-il?** and **Quel temps fait-il?** It is used to obtain more precise information about a noun already mentioned or implied. Questions with **quel** can be formed either with inversion or with **est-ce que.**

Quel fromage voulez-vous goûter?	*Which* (*What*) *cheese would you like to try?*
À **quelle** heure est-ce que vous dînez?	(*At*) *what time do you eat dinner?*

Dans **quels** restaurants aimez-vous manger?	*In what (which) restaurants do you like to eat?*
Quelles boissons préférez-vous?	*What (Which) beverages do you prefer?*

Quel is also used in exclamations.

Quel plat exemplaire!	*What an exemplary dish!*
Quelle horreur!	*How awful!*

[Allez-y! A-B]

Suggestion: Ask sts. to give other exclamations. Contexts: in French class, with a young child, in a food store, buying a car, etc.

Additional activity (A): *Préparatifs. Vous organisez une soirée avec un(e) camarade. Formez des questions complètes en utilisant un adjectif interrogatif.* MODÈLE: *quel / boisson / apporter / tu?* → *Quelle boisson apportes-tu?* 1. *quel / viande / préparer / tu?* 2. *quel / légumes / préférer / tu?* 3. *quel / plat / apporter / tu?* 4. *quel / salade / préparer / tu?* 5. *quel / fromage / acheter / tu?* 6. *quel / fruits / avoir / tu?* 7. *quel / dessert / choisir / tu?* 8. *quel / amies / inviter / tu?*

Quel with *être*

Quel can also stand alone before **être** followed by the noun it modifies.

Quel est le prix de ce champagne?	*What's the price of this champagne?*
Quelle est la différence entre le Perrier et l'Évian?	*What's the difference between Perrier and Évian?*

Allez-y!

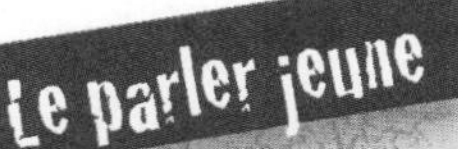

avoir la dalle	avoir faim
le resto	le restaurant
se taper la cloche	faire un bon repas
le troquet	le café; le bar

J'ai pas mangé depuis ce matin: **j'ai la dalle**!

On va dîner au **resto**, après le cinéma?

Dimanche, on s'est **tapé la cloche** en famille.

On prend un café au **troquet** du coin?

A. Qui vient dîner? Mme Guilloux veut organiser un dîner demain soir. Son mari l'interroge (*asks her questions*). Complétez leur dialogue avec **qu'est-ce que, quel(le)** ou **qui.**

M. GUILLOUX: ______[1] vas-tu inviter?
MME GUILLOUX: Maxime, Isabelle et Laurence.
M. GUILLOUX: Et ______[2] tu vas préparer?
MME GUILLOUX: Un rôti de bœuf avec des pommes de terre sautées.
M. GUILLOUX: Oh là là, ______[3] chance (*luck*)! Mais ______[4] va faire les courses?
MME GUILLOUX: Toi, bien sûr.
M. GUILLOUX: Bien voyons! ______[5] vin est-ce que je dois acheter?
MME GUILLOUX: Je ne sais pas. ______[6] tu préfères?
M. GUILLOUX: Un vin rouge. Un bordeaux, par exemple.
MME GUILLOUX: Très bien. ______[7] heure est-il?
M. GUILLOUX: 18 h 30.
MME GUILLOUX: Déjà! ______[8] tu attends? Dépêche-toi (*Hurry up*), les magasins vont bientôt fermer.

B. Une conversation à table. Parlez avec vos camarades de leurs goûts. Utilisez l'adjectif interrogatif **quel** et variez la forme de vos questions.

MODÈLE: sport → Quel sport est-ce que tu préfères? *ou* Quel sport préfères-tu?

1. boisson
2. légume
3. viande
4. repas
5. distractions
6. chansons (*f.*)
7. boîte (*f.*) de nuit (*nightclub*)
8. émission (*f.*) de télévision (*TV program*)
9. livres
10. magazines
11. couleur
12. matières
13. vêtements
14. films

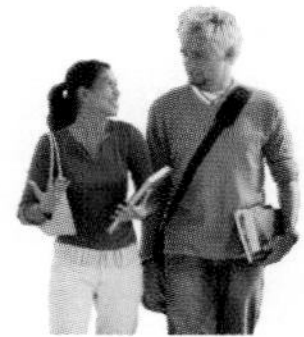

Suggestion: Have sts. do this in small groups as if they are at a dinner party, or dictate questions to sts., with some at board and others at their seats, after which they write a response. Compare responses at board and among members of class.

Les adjectifs démonstratifs

Pointing Out People and Things

À table!

Hassan, Hector, Juliette, Léa, Mamadou, Abdel discutent au restaurant d'Hassan.

LÉA: **Cette** salade marocaine, c'est un délice!
JULIETTE: Et **ces** brochettes grillées! Une merveille!
MAMADOU: Parlons aussi de **ce** filet de bœuf: il est exquis!
ABDEL: Moi, c'est **ce** gâteau au caramel que je trouve super. Donne-nous la recette,* Hassan!
HECTOR: Nous sommes tous d'accord: **ce** dîner est exceptionnel!
HASSAN: Quel triomphe, mes amis! Mais **ces** compliments sont un peu exagérés…
HECTOR: Pas du tout! Ne sois pas modeste!
LÉA: Hassan, tu vas avoir un bon pourboire! (*Elle rit.*)

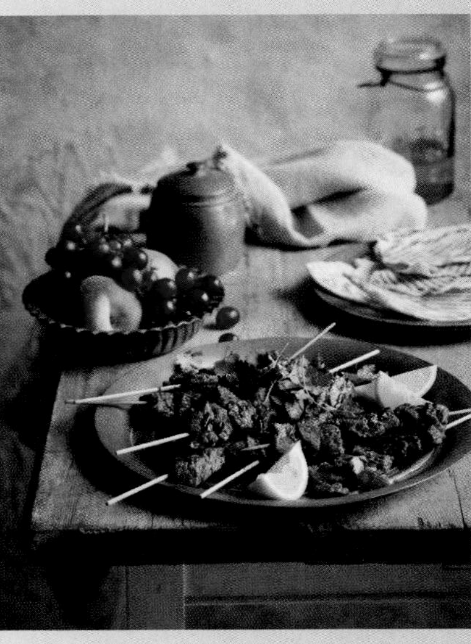

Bon appétit!

Qu'est-ce qu'ils disent? Trouvez les phrases du dialogue qui répondent aux questions suivantes.

*Donne… *Give us the recipe*

Qu'est-ce qui est…

1. un délice?
2. une merveille?
3. exquis?
4. super?
5. exceptionnel?
6. exagéré?

Presentation: (1) Review rules (*Chapitre 1*) for determining gender of nouns. (2) Use pictures to present the demonstrative adjectives inductively: *Je préfère cette voiture-ci. Et vous, préférez-vous cette voiture-ci ou cette voiture-là? Je préfère cet acteur-là . Et vous?*, etc.

Forms of Demonstrative Adjectives

Demonstrative adjectives (*this / that, these / those*) are used to specify a particular person, object, or idea. They agree in gender and number with the nouns they modify.

	SINGULAR	PLURAL
Masculine	**ce** magasin	**ces** magasins
	cet escargot	**ces** escargots
	cet homme	**ces** hommes
Feminine	**cette** épicerie	**ces** épiceries

Note that **ce** becomes **cet** before masculine nouns beginning with a vowel or mute **h.**

[Allez-y! A-B]

Use of *-ci* and *-là*

In English, *this / these* and *that / those* indicate the relative distance to the speaker. In French, the suffix **-ci** is added to indicate closeness, and **-là** , to indicate greater distance.

—Prenez-vous **ce** gâteau**-ci?**	*Are you having this cake* (*here*)?
—Non, je préfère **cet** éclair**-là.**	*No, I prefer that éclair* (*over there*).

[Allez-y! C]

Note: These suffixes are not always needed, because one can say *ce gâteau* and point to it.

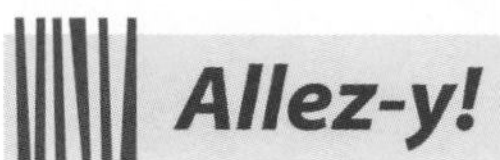

A. Au supermarché. Qu'est-ce que vous achetez?

MODÈLE: une bouteille d'huile → J'achète cette bouteille d'huile.

1. une boîte de sardines **2.** un camembert **3.** des tomates **4.** une bouteille de vin **5.** quatre poires **6.** une bouteille d'eau minérale **7.** des pommes de terre **8.** un éclair au café **9.** un artichaut

Suggestion (A): Have sts. do this in pairs, or use sentences for board work.

Suggestion (A): You might want to present the irregular *-er* verb *acheter* (*Chapitre 8*).

B. Exercice de contradiction. Vous allez faire un pique-nique. Vous faites des courses avec un(e) camarade, mais vous n'êtes pas d'accord! Jouez les rôles.

MODÈLE: pain / baguette →
É1: On prend ce pain?
É2: Non, je préfère cette baguette.

1. saucisson / tranche (*f.*) (*slice*) de jambon
2. pâté / poulet froid
3. filet de bœuf / rôti de veau
4. haricots verts / oignons
5. pizza (*f.*) / sandwich
6. pommes / bananes
7. tarte / éclair
8. gâteau / glace
9. jus de fruits / bouteille de vin
10. boîte de sardines / morceau (*m.*) (*piece*) de fromage

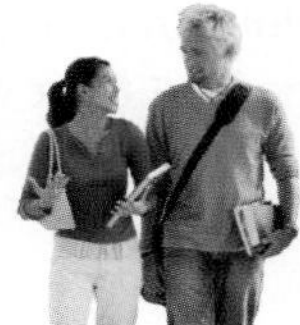

Suggestion (B): Do this activity in pairs. Have whole class go over a few responses to check small-group work.

C. Chez le traiteur. (*At the delicatessen.*) Jouez les rôles du client / de la cliente et du traiteur.

MODÈLE: poulet →
LE CLIENT / LA CLIENTE: Donnez-moi un poulet, s'il vous plaît.
LE TRAITEUR: Quel poulet? Ce poulet-ci ou ce poulet-là?
LE CLIENT / LA CLIENTE: Ce poulet-ci. Et donnez-moi aussi un peu de ce fromage.
LE TRAITEUR: Tout de suite, monsieur / madame.

1. salade
2. rôti
3. légumes
4. pâté
5. pizza
6. saucisses

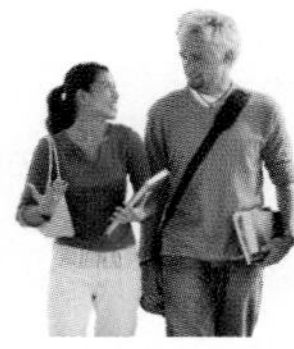

Additional activity: *À la boulangerie-pâtisserie. Qu'est-ce que vous allez prendre?* (Bring in photos and allow sts. to choose items.) MODÈLE: *tartes → Je vais prendre ces tartes.* 1. *éclair* 2. *gâteau* 3. *tarte aux pommes* 4. *baguette* 5. *pain* 6. *croissants chauds*

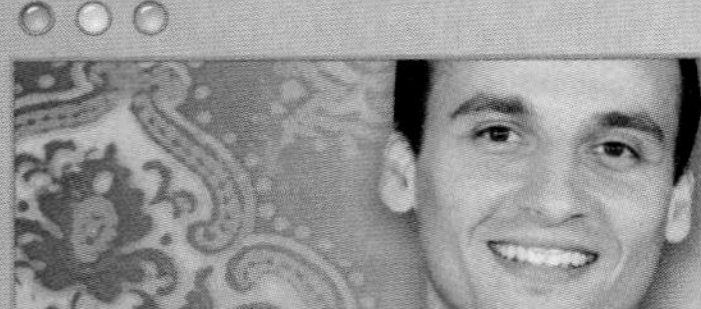

Le blog d'Hassan

Marché ou cybermarché?

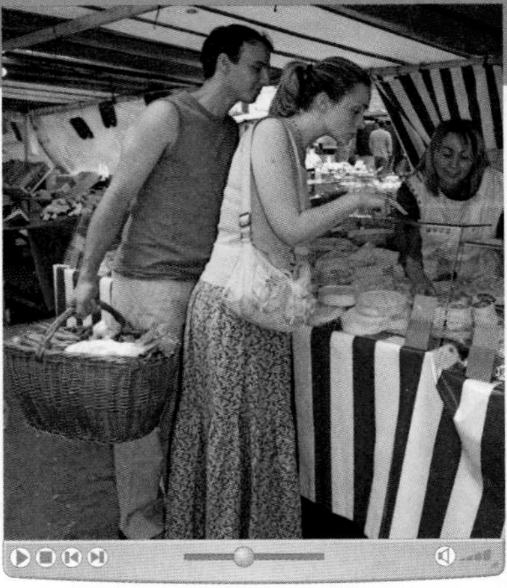

Faire le marché, c'est un plaisirl

dimanche 7 juin

Suggestion: Model pronunciation and have sts. repeat individually or as a group.

Salut tout le monde!

Dimanche prochain, Juliette et moi on va faire les courses au marché de la place Monge. Ensuite, avec nos potes,[1] on va préparer le déjeuner chez moi. Hector et Léa vont acheter une tarte pour le dessert, Juliette va préparer les légumes et moi le poisson! Ça va être marrant[2]!

Juliette aime bien le marché, mais elle préfère les cybermarchés. Un seul clic et tout apparaît[3] sur l'écran: la charcuterie, l'épicerie, la poissonnerie et la pâtisserie. La livraison[4] est souvent gratuite.[5]
Je dois dire que c'est pas mal…

Mais moi, je préfère le marché: c'est animé; je peux sentir[6] l'odeur des produits frais; je peux toucher, peser,[7] sélectionner et quelquefois goûter! C'est vraiment agréable!

Et vous? Vous faites vos courses en ligne ou au marché?

Hassan

Video connection: The *marché de la place Monge* in the *5ᵉ arrondissement* is one of Paris's upscale markets. Sts. will see this market in the videoblog for this chapter as Hassan and Juliette shop for food for a party.

COMMENTAIRES

Alexis

Moi aussi, je commande sur Internet, c'est tellement[8] facile! Tu cliques sur un rôti de bœuf, et il est dans ton assiette!

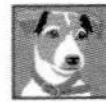

Trésor

Alexis, je déteste le cybermarché: la bouffe, ce n'est pas virtuel! C'est réel!

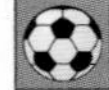

Mamadou

Chez moi, au Sénégal, tous les matins, ma mère fait son marché. Le marché africain, c'est l'odeur du poivre et des épices associé au parfum des mangues et des poissons frais.

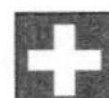

Charlotte

Tu sais Hassan, pour une mère de famille, le supermarché c'est la solution idéale. À Genève, je fais les courses le samedi matin et je suis tranquille pour huit jours. Et il y a toujours des promotions!

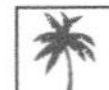

Poema

Les marchés de Papeete sentent le tiare—c'est la fleur emblème de Tahiti—l'ananas[9] et la vanille.

Cultural note: Online grocery shopping is a growing trend in France. Telemarket.fr and Houra.fr are the most popular cybermarkets. Some large supermarket chains such as Auchan and Carrefour also offer this service. More and more people are grocery shopping online, but traditional markets are still preferred by the French. For links to these online markets, go to **Connect French (www.mhconnectfrench.com).**

Follow-up: 1. *Comment est organisé le déjeuner programmé chez Hassan? Pourquoi est-ce que «ça va être marrant»?* 2. *Quels aspects du cybermarché Juliette apprécie-t-elle? Pourquoi Hassan préfère-t-il le marché?* 3. *Que pensez-vous de la réflexion de Trésor? Êtes-vous d'accord avec lui?* 4. *Quelles sont les particularités du marché africain? du marché tahitien?* 5. *Décrivez les marchés de votre ville.*

[1]*buddies* [2]*lots of fun* [3]*appears* [4]*delivery* [5]*free* [6]je… *I can smell* [7]*weigh* [8]*so* [9]*pineapple*

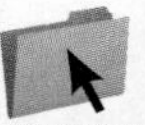

REPORTAGE

Comment voyager dans son assiette?

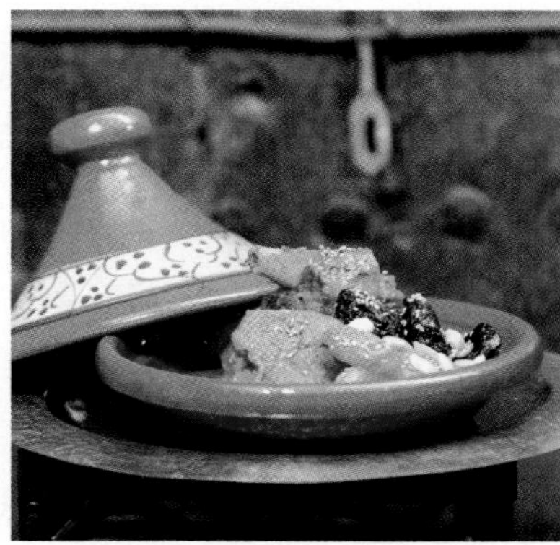
Un tajine marocain

Chaque nation dans le monde a une spécialité culinaire. Le plat national, c'est un peu le drapeau d'un pays, sa culture, son âme.[1]

Pour connaître les saveurs[2] des tables francophones, faisons un voyage culinaire…

Nous voilà d'abord en Suisse. Quel est le plat national ici? La fondue! Arrêtons-nous maintenant en Belgique. Que mange-t-on dans les petits restaurants populaires de Bruxelles? Des moules-frites[3]! Faisons une petite excursion en France. C'est étrange: au pays de la gastronomie, le plat du jour idéal, c'est tout simplement un steak-frites accompagné d'un petit vin rouge!

Maintenant, nous voyageons au Québec. Ici «la poutine» est sur tous les menus de restaurants. Inventé dans les années 1950, ce plat est préparé avec des frites, du fromage et de la sauce brune.[4] C'est parfait pour un pays froid!

Enfin, nous visitons l'Afrique. Au Cameroun, on adore le «n'dolé», une préparation d'épinards,[5] de crevettes, de poisson ou de viande mélangés à des arachides.[6] En Algérie, le couscous, à base de semoule,[7] est sur toutes les tables. On peut le préparer de mille et une façons.[8] C'est la même chose pour «le tajine», le plat national du Maroc. Ce ragoût[9] de viande, de volaille,[10] de poisson et de légumes est délicieux pour la bouche et beau pour les yeux. Regardez la photo!

Tous ces plats traditionnels des pays francophones vous invitent au voyage. Partez! L'aventure commence dans votre assiette.

[1]*soul* [2]*flavors* [3]*mussels with French fries* [4]sauce… *gravy* [5]*spinach* [6]*peanuts* [7]*semolina* [8]*ways* [9]*stew* [10]*poultry*

À vous!

1. Qu'est-ce qu'un «plat national»?
2. Quel est le plat national de chaque pays francophone mentionné dans ce reportage? Quels autres plats de ces pays connaissez-vous? Si possible, citez aussi les plats nationaux d'autres pays francophones.
3. Quand vous voyagez, aimez-vous goûter des aliments ou des plats nouveaux? Racontez une de vos découvertes culinaires dans un pays étranger ou dans un restaurant étranger de votre ville.
4. Quel est le plat national de votre pays? Comment est-il préparé?
5. Quels ingrédients y a-t-il dans le tajine sur la photo? Avez-vous envie de le goûter? Expliquez.

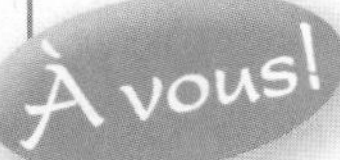

Parlons-en!

Travaillez en petits groupes et répondez aux questions suivantes. Qui est le plus aventurier / la plus aventurière du groupe?

1. En France, on mange des grenouilles, des escargots, du lapin (*rabbit*) et du cheval. Vous acceptez de manger ces plats? Pourquoi?
2. Combien d'étudiants dans votre groupe accepte cette aventure culinaire? Comptez!
3. Quels plats français les étudiants moins aventuriers aimeraient-ils essayer (*to try*)? Pour quelle raison?
4. Quels plats extraordinaires avez-vous déjà essayés? C'était bon?

Suggestion: Have each group present their results to find out who the most adventurous eater in the class is.

Leçon 3

Les verbes *vouloir, pouvoir* et *devoir*

Expressing Desire, Ability, and Obligation

Les vins de Napa Valley

Hector et Hassan échangent des textos (SMS).

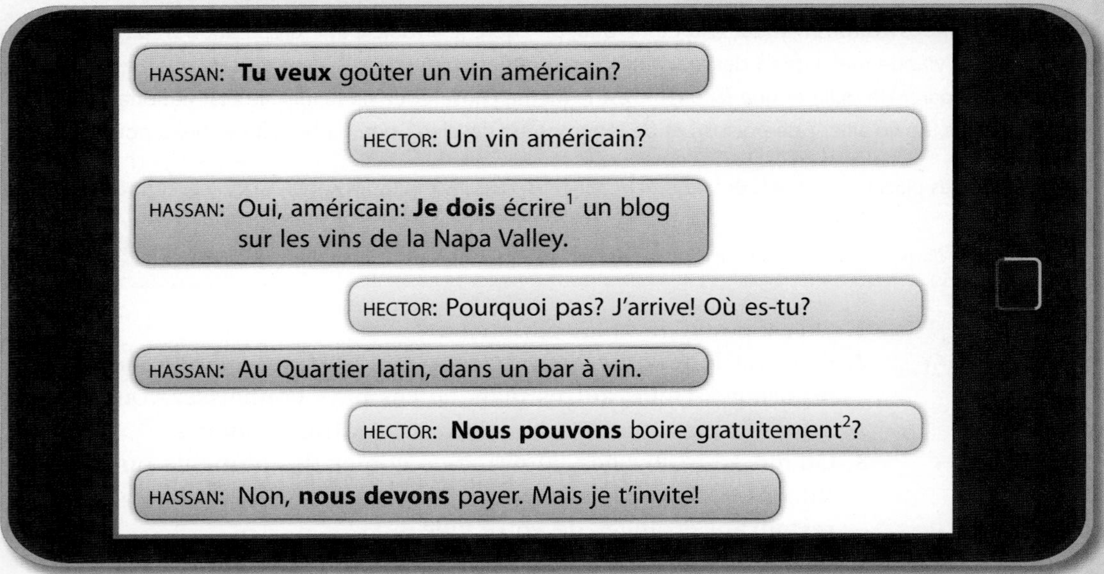
HASSAN: **Tu veux** goûter un vin américain?
HECTOR: Un vin américain?
HASSAN: Oui, américain: **Je dois** écrire[1] un blog sur les vins de la Napa Valley.
HECTOR: Pourquoi pas? J'arrive! Où es-tu?
HASSAN: Au Quartier latin, dans un bar à vin.
HECTOR: **Nous pouvons** boire gratuitement[2]?
HASSAN: Non, **nous devons** payer. Mais je t'invite!

[1]*to write* [2]*for free*

Vrai ou faux? Corrigez les phrases fausses.

1. Hassan propose à Hector de goûter des vins français.
2. Il doit écrire un blog sur les vins de la Napa Valley.
3. Hector accepte de goûter ces vins avec Hassan.
4. Ils doivent payer pour boire.
5. Hassan veut inviter Hector.

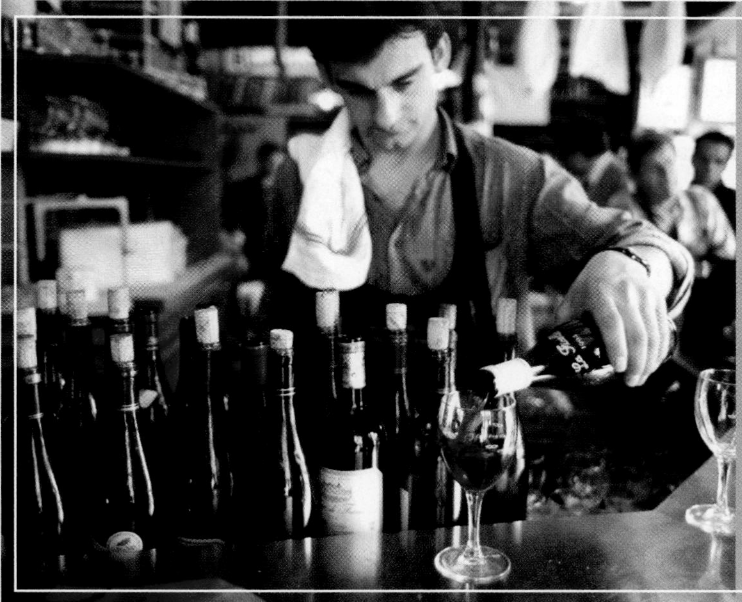

Un peu plus…

Le Jugement de Paris.
Les vins français ont depuis longtemps une réputation mondiale. Tous les amateurs de vin connaissent les vins rouges de Bordeaux, comme le Château Mouton-Rothschild, ou les blancs de Bourgogne, comme le Beaune Clos des Mouches de la Maison Joseph Drouhin. En 1976, on a organisé un concours de vin pour comparer les vins français et les vins californiens de la Napa Valley. Cet événement, appelé le Jugement de Paris, a eu lieu le 24 mai à Paris. Il y avait 11 juges et personne ne pensait que les vins californiens avaient une chance de gagner. La dégustation (*tasting*) s'est faite à l'aveugle (*was done blind*). Ce sont deux vins américains qui ont gagné: le chardonnay 1973 de Chateau Montelena et le cabernet sauvignon 1973 de Stag's Leap Wine Cellars. La réputation de la Napa Valley était faite!

◄ *Un bar à vin à Paris: Quels vins voulez-vous déguster?*

Forms of *vouloir, pouvoir,* and *devoir*

The verbs **vouloir** (*to want*), **pouvoir** (*to be able to*), and **devoir** (*to have to; to be obliged to; to owe*) are all irregular in form.

vouloir		pouvoir		devoir	
je	**veux**	je	**peux**	je	**dois**
tu	**veux**	tu	**peux**	tu	**dois**
il/elle/on	**veut**	il/elle/on	**peut**	il/elle/on	**doit**
nous	**voulons**	nous	**pouvons**	nous	**devons**
vous	**voulez**	vous	**pouvez**	vous	**devez**
ils/elles	**veulent**	ils/elles	**peuvent**	ils/elles	**doivent**

Uses of *vouloir, devoir,* and *pouvoir*

1. **Vouloir** can be followed by a noun or an infinitive.

   Je **veux** un café. — *I want a cup of coffee.*
   Je **veux** commander un café. — *I want to order a cup of coffee.*

   Vouloir bien means *to be willing to, be glad* (*to do something*). **Vouloir dire** expresses *to mean.*

   Il **veut bien** goûter les escargots. — *He's willing to taste the snails.*
   Qu'est-ce que ce mot **veut dire**? — *What does this word mean?*

2. **Devoir,** followed by an infinitive, expresses necessity, obligation, or probability.

   Je suis désolé, mais nous **devons** partir. — *I'm sorry, but we must leave.*
   Marc est absent; il **doit** être malade. — *Marc is absent; he must be sick.*

Pronunciation practice (1): Have sts. indicate whether the subject of the following verbal phrases is *singulier* or *pluriel*: *peut visiter la maison, veulent lire un livre, veut louer l'appartement, peuvent voter, veulent vendre la maison, peut vendre la télévision, veut laisser son numéro de téléphone.*

Pronunciation practice (2): The *Prononcez bien!* section on page 195 of this chapter contains additional activities for practicing these sounds.

Note: You could mention the use of *veuillez* + infinitive to express polite requests in writing and the use of *puis-je* orally. Remind sts. also that they have already learned *je voudrais* + infinitive or noun to politely express something they want to do or have.

Suggestion: Ask sts. questions: *Qu'est-ce que vous voulez faire ce soir? Qu'est-ce que vous devez faire ce soir?* Demonstrate the difference between one's desires (*vouloir*) and one's obligations (*devoir*).

Prononcez bien!

The vowels in *veux* and *veulent*

Make sure to distinguish between the two vowel sounds [ø] and [œ] as you pronounce the singular and plural forms of **vouloir** and **pouvoir.** Remember to round your lips for both sounds.

For the [ø] in **veux, veut, peux,** and **peut,** close your mouth and keep your tongue in the front of your mouth.

[ø]: **Je veux** du fromage.

For the [œ] in **veulent** and **peuvent,** open your mouth a bit wider and slightly shift your tongue to the middle of your mouth.

[œ]: Ils **peuvent** dormir.

Pronunciation presentation: You may want to point out that *je peux* can become [ʃpø] orally.

When not followed by an infinitive, **devoir** means *to owe.*

—Combien d'argent est-ce que tu **dois** à tes amis?	*How much money do you owe to your friends?*
—Je **dois** 10 euros à Jacques et 20 euros à François.	*I owe Jacques 10 euros and François 20 euros.*

3. **Pouvoir** is usually followed by an infinitive.

Vous **pouvez** arriver à 15 h?	*Can you arrive at 3:00 P.M.?*

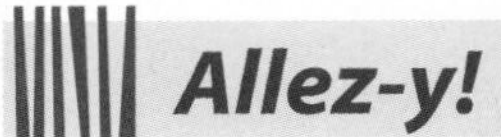

Suggestion: Ask sts. to write individually and then to read resulting dialogue in pairs.

A. Une soirée compliquée. Composez un dialogue entre Noémie et Simon.

NOÉMIE: je / avoir / faim / et / je / vouloir / manger / maintenant
SIMON: tu / vouloir / faire / cuisine?
NOÉMIE: non… / est-ce que / nous / pouvoir / aller / restaurant?
SIMON: oui, je / vouloir / bien
NOÉMIE: où / est-ce que / nous / pouvoir / aller?
SIMON: on / pouvoir / manger / couscous / Chez Bébert
NOÉMIE: nous / devoir / inviter / Carole
SIMON: tu / pouvoir / inviter / Jean-Pierre / aussi
NOÉMIE: ce / soir / ils / devoir / être / cité universitaire?
SIMON: oui, ils / devoir / préparer / un / examen
nous / pouvoir / parler / de / ce / examen / restaurant

B. Le Ritz. Pour fêter son anniversaire (*To celebrate his birthday*), Stéphane invite ses amis américains Ben et Jessica au restaurant «le Ritz». Complétez leur dialogue avec les verbes **pouvoir, devoir** et **vouloir** à la forme appropriée. Quelquefois plusieurs réponses sont possibles.

BEN: Qu'est-ce qu'on ______[1] prendre?
STÉPHANE: Comme entrée, vous ______[2] prendre le pâté de lapin, il est excellent. Et comme plat de résistance…
JESSICA: Pardon, que ______[3] dire «plat de résistance»?
STÉPHANE: Bon, c'est le plat principal du repas. Vous ______[4] absolument essayer (*try*) la truite (*trout*) aux amandes, c'est la spécialité de la maison. Comme dessert si vous ______[5], vous ______[6] prendre une charlotte aux framboises.
JESSICA: Ça ______[7] être très nourrissant (*rich, fattening*) tout ça, non?
STÉPHANE: Un peu, mais ce n'est pas tous les jours mon anniversaire. Tu ______[8] oublier ton régime pour aujourd'hui.

C. Vos impressions. Complétez les phrases suivantes à la forme affirmative ou à la forme négative, selon votre opinion personnelle. Utilisez **devoir, pouvoir** ou **vouloir** + infinitif dans chaque phrase.

MODÈLE: Les étudiants ______. → Les étudiants ne doivent pas étudier jusqu'à (*until*) minuit tous les soirs.

1. Le professeur ______. **2.** Les parents ______. **3.** Mes camarades ______. **4.** Les hommes ______. **5.** Les femmes ______. **6.** Je ______.

Suggestions (C): (1) Dictate incomplete sentences, with as many sts. as possible at board and others at seats. Compare completions provided by a variety of sts. (2) Can be done in small groups.

Additional activity: *Au restaurant. Faites les substitutions indiquées. 1. Qu'est-ce que vous voulez prendre? (nous, les étudiantes, Paul et vous) 2. Tu dois commander maintenant. (ils, nous, elle, je) 3. Elle veut bien essayer les huîtres. (je, tu, Marc et Pierre) 4. Vous pouvez apporter le plat. (nous, les étudiants, tu) 5. Combien est-ce que je dois? (vous, tu, nous, ils, Fernand) 6. Qu'est-ce que tu veux dire? (Patrick et Jeanne, vous, elles, la serveuse) 7. Elle doit payer cent euros. (je, les étudiants)*

Additional activity: *Des projets. Racontez les histoires suivantes. Utilisez les verbes* vouloir, devoir *et* ne pas pouvoir, *selon le modèle.* MODÈLE: *Jacques / être riche / travailler / aller souvent au cinéma → Jacques veut être riche. Il doit beaucoup travailler. Il ne peut pas aller souvent au cinéma. 1. les étudiants / réussir aux examens / écouter le professeur / parler en cours 2. Claudine / préparer une mousse au chocolat / utiliser du sucre, du chocolat et de la crème / utiliser des huîtres 3. l'épicier / avoir beaucoup de clients / être agréable / être désagréable 4. Pierre / être serveur / prendre correctement les commandes / boire au restaurant où il travaille*

Mots clés

Demander poliment et remercier

Je voudrais (presented in **Chapitre 6**) and **je pourrais** (*I could*) are conditional forms of **vouloir** and **pouvoir,** respectively. They are used to make a request sound more polite.

Je veux l'addition.
I want the check.

Je **voudrais** l'addition.
I would like the check.

Est-ce que je peux avoir de l'eau?
Can I have some water?

Est-ce que je **pourrais** avoir de l'eau?
Could I have some water?

Don't forget to add **s'il vous plaît** to your request and to say **merci.**

The appropriate answers for **merci** are:

De rien. (*more familiar*)
Il n'y a pas de quoi.
Je vous en prie, madame.* (*formal*)

*In polite conversation in French, **monsieur, madame,** and **mademoiselle** are used much more often than *ma'am* or *sir* in English.

D. Soyons polis! Avec un(e) partenaire, demandez et remerciez selon le modèle.

MODÈLE: vouloir / tasse / café
É1: Je voudrais une tasse de café, s'il vous plaît.
É2: Voilà, madame / monsieur.
É1: Merci, monsieur / madame.
É2: Il n'y a pas de quoi.

1. pouvoir avoir / carafe / eau?
2. vouloir / morceau / fromage
3. pouvoir avoir / bouteille / vin?
4. vouloir / kilo / poulet

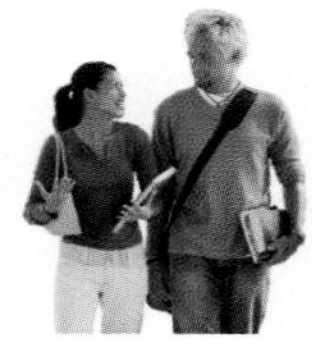

Suggestion: Have sts. read the *Mots clés* box on page 190 before they begin Activity D.

Le passé composé avec l'auxiliaire *avoir*

Talking About the Past

Le vin: un sujet très sérieux!

Hector contacte Léa sur la page Facebook d'Hector (Messagerie instantanée).

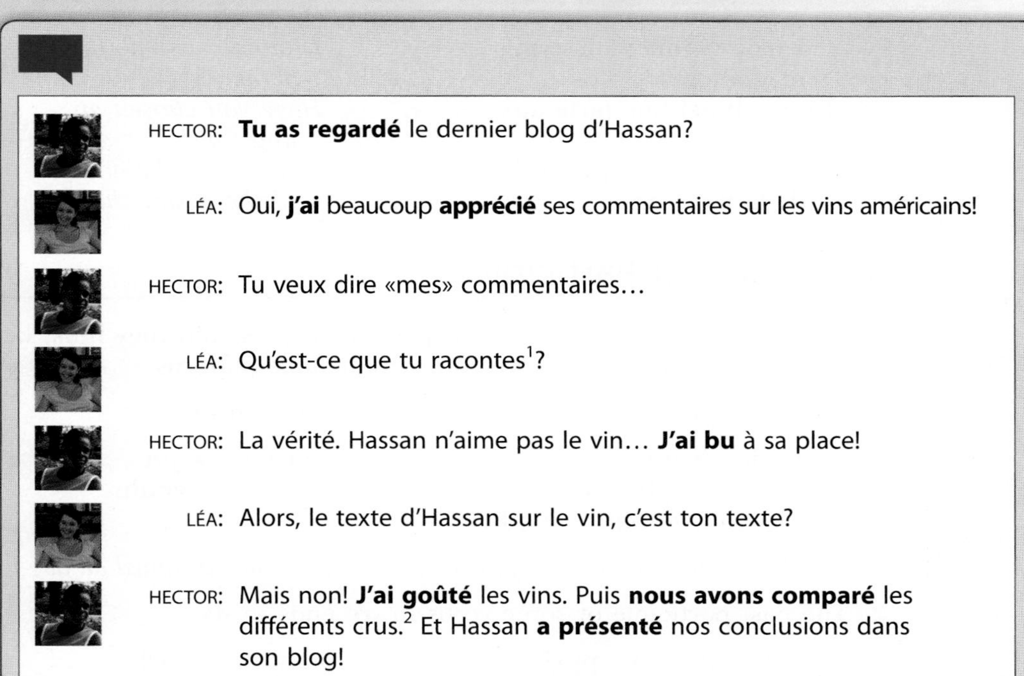

HECTOR: **Tu as regardé** le dernier blog d'Hassan?

LÉA: Oui, **j'ai** beaucoup **apprécié** ses commentaires sur les vins américains!

HECTOR: Tu veux dire «mes» commentaires…

LÉA: Qu'est-ce que tu racontes[1]?

HECTOR: La vérité. Hassan n'aime pas le vin… **J'ai bu** à sa place!

LÉA: Alors, le texte d'Hassan sur le vin, c'est ton texte?

HECTOR: Mais non! **J'ai goûté** les vins. Puis **nous avons comparé** les différents crus.[2] Et Hassan **a présenté** nos conclusions dans son blog!

[1]Qu'est-ce que... *What are you talking about?* [2]*vintages*

Répondez aux questions. Faites des phrases complètes.

1. Qui a regardé le blog d'Hassan?
2. Qui a apprécié ses commentaires?
3. Qui a goûté les vins?
4. Qui a présenté les conclusions dans son blog?

Suggestion: Review the conjugation of *avoir* before presenting *passé composé* with *avoir.* You may wish to point out that the *passé composé* is the past tense form used most frequently in conversation.

Note: The expression *prendre le dîner* is also used to mean *to eat dinner.* The *passé composé* of that expression is *J'ai pris le dîner* (see Point 2 below).

The **passé composé** is a compound past tense. It relates events that began and ended at some point in the past. The **passé composé** of most verbs consists of the present tense of the auxiliary verb (**le verbe auxiliaire**) **avoir** plus the past participle (**le participe passé**) of the verb in question.

PASSÉ COMPOSÉ OF **dîner** (*to dine, eat dinner*)			
j'	**ai dîné**	nous	**avons dîné**
tu	**as dîné**	vous	**avez dîné**
il/elle/on	**a dîné**	ils/elles	**ont dîné**

The **passé composé** has several equivalents in English. For example, **j'ai dîné** can mean *I dined* (*ate dinner*), *I have dined* (*have eaten dinner*), *I did dine* (*did eat dinner*), according to the context.

Presentation: Model pronunciation of past participles.

Regular Past Participles

The following chart illustrates the formation of regular past participles.

Verbs ending in **-er:**	**-er** → **-é**	trouv**er** → trouv**é**
Verbs ending in **-ir:**	**-ir** → **-i**	chois**ir** → chois**i**
Verbs ending in **-re:**	**-re** → **-u**	perd**re** → perd**u**

J'**ai trouvé** une pâtisserie magnifique. — *I found a wonderful pastry shop.*
Tu **as choisi** une tarte aux pommes? — *Have you chosen an apple pie?*
Non, nous **avons perdu** l'adresse de la pâtisserie. — *No, we lost the address of the pastry shop.*

Irregular Past Participles

Note: In *dû,* the circumflex is not a historical sign; it simply differentiates the past participle from the contraction *du.*

Note: *Devoir* expresses probability (*Il a dû arriver en retard.* [He must have arrived late.]) and obligation (*Il a dû partir sans elle.* [He had to leave without her.]).

Most irregular verbs have irregular past participles, and they must be memorized. However, there are some predictable patterns.

1. The past participle of many verbs in **-oir** ends in **-u.**

avoir → **eu**
devoir → **dû**
pleuvoir (*to rain*) → **plu**
pouvoir → **pu**
vouloir → **voulu**

Hier, il **a plu** toute la journée. — *Yesterday, it rained all day long.*

2. The past participle of some verbs in **-re** ends in **-is.**

apprendre → **appris**
comprendre → **compris**
prendre → **pris**

J'**ai pris** l'autobus à la boulangerie. — *I took the bus to the bakery.*

Suggestion: (After the presentation and for listening comprehension): Read the following sentences. Sts. indicate whether they hear *passé composé* or *présent:* 1. *Il a plu hier.* 2. *Martine a porté un imperméable.* 3. *Georges a perdu un livre.* 4. *Il boit un café.* 5. *Nous avons vu Jeanne au cinéma.* 6. *Tu as vu Jeanne aussi?* 7. *Je fais une promenade.*

3. Other important irregular past participles include:

boire → **bu**
être → **été**
faire → **fait**

Elle **a fait** le marché. — *She did the shopping.*

[Allez-y! A-B]

Negative and Interrogative Sentences in the *passé composé*

1. In negative sentences, **ne... pas** surrounds the auxiliary verb (**avoir**).

Nous **n'avons pas** préparé les hors-d'œuvre.	*We have not prepared the hors-d'œuvres.*
Vous **n'avez pas** pris de dessert?	*Didn't you have a dessert?*

2. In questions with inversion, only the auxiliary verb and the subject are inverted.

As-tu oublié le dessert?	*Did you forget dessert?*

[Allez-y! C-D]

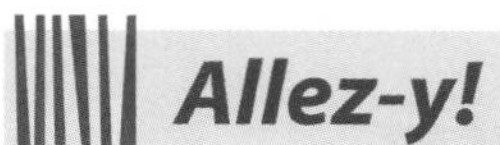

Allez-y!

A. Un voyage. Qu'est-ce que ces personnes ont fait dans le sud de la France? Faites des phrases complètes au passé composé.

MODÈLE: nous / choisir / huîtres
Nous avons choisi des huîtres.

1. vous / goûter / crevettes
2. Sylvie / finir / bouteille de vin
3. toi et moi, nous / boire / coca-cola / café
4. Thibaut / perdre / porte-monnaie (*wallet*)
5. Julie et Martin / visiter / pâtisserie magnifique
6. Morgane et toi, vous / apprendre / à parler avec l'accent marseillais
7. je / faire / de la planche à voile (*windsurfing*)

Additional activity: *Au marché. Faites les substitutions et les changements nécessaires. 1. Vous allez faire les courses? —Oui, nous avons trouvé un excellent supermarché.* (*je, Marc, ils, elle*) *2. Avez-vous choisi un plat principal? —J'ai choisi le pot-au-feu.* (*nos cousins, nous, Michel et Paul*) *3. Que cherchez-vous? —Marie a perdu la liste des achats* (shopping list). (*nous, je, vous, Marc et Michel*)

B. Une carte postale. Complétez la carte postale de Marie. Choisissez le verbe approprié et conjuguez-le au passé composé.

commencer	**être**	**passer**	**rendre**
décider	**faire**	**préparer**	**visiter**

Chère Eva,

J' ______[1] mes vacances d'hiver une semaine avant Noël avec Yasmine. Nous ______[2] deux semaines à la montagne en Suisse.

Nous ______[3] de rester à Zermatt. Nous ______[4] du ski et du shopping. Nous ______[5] une fondue délicieuse. Au retour, nous ______[6] visite à des amis à Genève et nous ______[7] le Palais des Nations de l'ONU. Notre séjour et les repas en Suisse ______[8] inoubliables. Je t'embrasse,

Marie

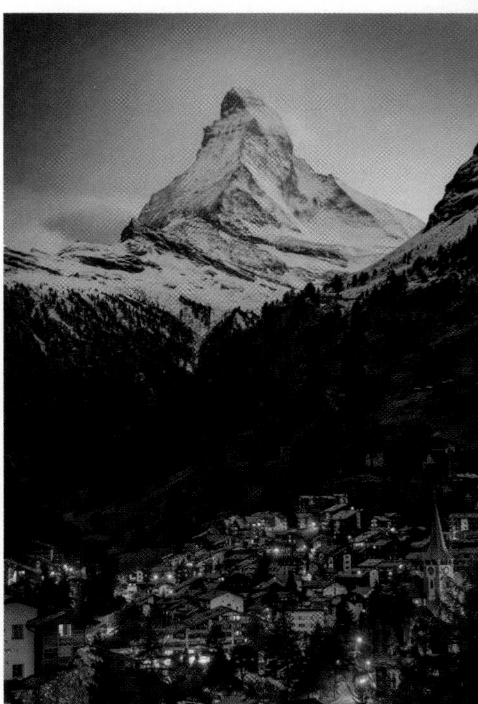

Le Mont Cervin et le village de Zermatt, en Suisse

Suggestion (C): Do in groups of three; one st. asks questions and other two alternate answering.

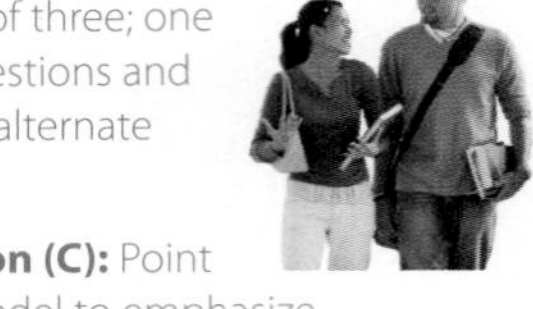

Suggestion (C): Point out the model to emphasize transformation of the indefinite article to *pas de* (C. 2, 6, 7).

Mots clés

Exprimer le passé

avant-hier
the day before yesterday

hier, hier matin, hier soir
yesterday, yesterday morning, last night

le mois / l'hiver **dernier (passé)**
last month, last winter

la semaine / l'année **dernière (passée)**
last week, last year

toute la matinée / la journée / la soirée* / la nuit
all morning, all day, all evening, all night

*Use **matinée, journée,** and **soirée** rather than **matin, jour,** and **soir** if you wish to express a duration. They are often used with **toute.**

Suggestion (*Mots clés*): Model pronunciation of these words, and encourage sts. to use them in subsequent activities.

C. À Orange. Tristan pose des questions à ses cousins Zoé et Thibaud, qui (*who*) ont visité la ville historique d'Orange, près d'Avignon. Jouez les rôles avec deux camarades.

MODÈLE: trouver un restaurant pas cher à Orange →
TRISTAN: Avez-vous trouvé un restaurant pas cher à Orange?
THIBAUD: Non, nous n'avons pas trouvé de restaurant pas cher à Orange.

1. prendre le petit déjeuner près de l'amphithéâtre romain
2. faire une promenade dans la vieille ville
3. contempler la vieille fontaine
4. étudier les inscriptions romaines
5. apprendre l'histoire de France
6. chercher des fruits à l'épicerie
7. envoyer (*to send*) une description de la ville à vos parents

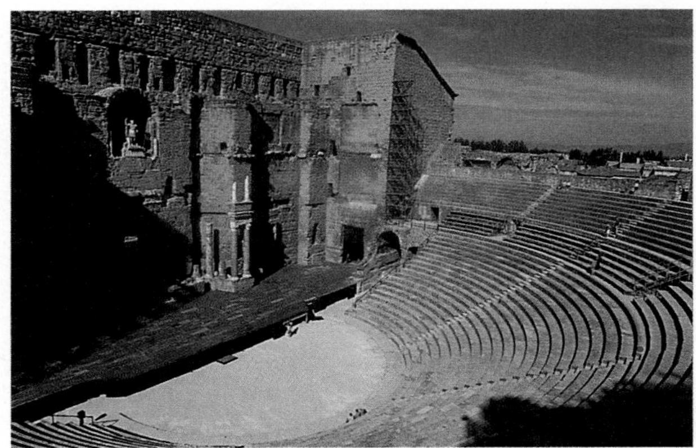

L'amphithéâtre à Orange, près d'Avignon, en France. Combien de personnes peuvent s'y asseoir (*sit there*)?

Suggestion (D): Have sts. do in pairs and report one thing their partners did.

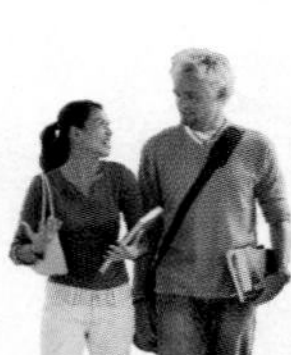

D. Interview. Posez des questions à un(e) camarade sur ses activités passées. Essayez d'utiliser les expressions des **Mots clés.** Voici des suggestions:

Le matin: boire du café, faire du sport, faire le marché, prendre le petit déjeuner, regarder la télévision, …

L'après-midi / Le soir: étudier une leçon, inviter des amis, jouer aux cartes, pique-niquer, skier, …

La semaine / L'année dernière: dîner au restaurant, finir une dissertation, rendre visite à des amis, travailler dans un magasin, voyager en Europe, …

MODÈLE: É1: Est-ce que tu as fait du sport hier matin?
É2: Oui, j'ai fait du jogging jusqu'à onze heures. (Non, je n'ai pas fait…) Et toi?

Puis racontez à la classe ce que votre camarade a fait.

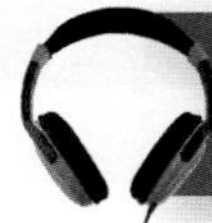

Prononcez bien!

1. The semivowel in *ail* (page 176)

A. Dîner d'anniversaire. Hugo et son ami Yann discutent du dîner d'anniversaire de leur ami Rémi. Avec votre camarade, lisez leur conversation à voix haute en faisant bien attention à la prononciation des mots français *en italique.*

HUGO: Je suis arrivé en *premier* et j'ai garé (*parked*) ma voiture devant celle (*the one*) de Rémi.
YANN: Moi, je suis arrivé en *dernier* et j'ai garé ma moto *derrière* sa voiture!
HUGO: Au dîner, j'ai mangé à côté d'une *fille* qui s'appelle *Camille*.
YANN: Ah oui, elle a de beaux *yeux* bleus.

B. Dîner d'anniversaire (suite). Hugo et Yann parlent de leur repas. Avec votre camarade, lisez leur conversation à voix haute et complétez les phrases à l'aide des images.

HUGO: Qu'est-ce que tu as pris: du poisson ou de la __________[1] ?
YANN: Du poisson, avec une demi- __________[2] de vin blanc. Et toi, qu'est-ce que tu as bu?
HUGO: Oh, juste une __________[3] .
YANN: C'est tout?! Tu n'es pas dans ton __________[4] (*aren't feeling well*) ce matin?
HUGO: Si, mais j'ai encore sommeil.

Answers (1B): 1. *viande* 2. *bouteille* 3. *bière* 4. *assiette*

2. The vowels in *veux* and *veulent* (page 189)

A. Un nouveau joueur. La famille d'Hugo va bientôt déménager. Écoutez les phrases et décidez si Hugo parle de ses parents ou de son petit frère.

	Les parents	Le petit frère
1. vendre la maison	☐	☐
2. habiter dans un grand appartement en ville	☐	☐
3. vendre le lit et l'armoire de la chambre d'amis	☐	☐
4. visiter des appartements dès (*as early as*) le week-end prochain	☐	☐
5. une grande chambre	☐	☐

Script (2A): 1. *Ils veulent vendre la maison.* 2. *Il veut habiter dans un grand appartement en ville.* 3. *Il peut vendre le lit et l'armoire de la chambre d'amis.* 4. *Ils peuvent visiter des appartements dès le week-end prochain.* 5. *Il veut une grande chambre.*

Answers (2A): 1. *les parents* 2. *le petit frère* 3. *le petit frère* 4. *les parents* 5. *le petit frère*

B. Un dîner. Vos colocataires et vous organisez un dîner chez vous. Chaque invité va apporter quelque chose (*something*). Avec votre camarade, lisez les phrases à voix haute et complétez-les avec la forme appropriée du verbe entre parenthèses.

1. Annette __________ (vouloir) apporter l'entrée.
2. Éric et Christine __________ (pouvoir) se charger (*be in charge of*) du plat principal.
3. Isabelle, tu __________ (pouvoir) faire le dessert?
4. Christophe et Karine __________ (vouloir) apporter du pain.
5. Moi, je __________ (pouvoir) m'occuper (*take care of*) de la salade.

Answers (2B): 1. *veut* 2. *peuvent* 3. *peux* 4. *veulent* 5. *peux*

Leçon 4

Lecture

Avant de lire

Using titles and visuals. You have already used a number of strategies to help you guess the content of a text before you start reading. In many cases, visuals such as photos, graphs, and diagrams also allow you to anticipate the major themes of the text. Look at the title, the photos, and the photo captions in the following reading selection: What kinds of information do you think you might find in this passage? After you have read through the text, decide whether the title describes the content adequately. If not, suggest a title that is more descriptive. How well do the photos correspond to the text? What other ideas in the text would you like to see illustrated?

Ça se fête! Quelles sont les plus grandes occasions de l'année pour vous: votre anniversaire, Noël, le nouvel an? Comment célébrez-vous ces occasions? Faites une liste des plats que vous mangez.

Suggestion: Once sts. have read the reading, have them compare their lists to the list of dishes that the French prepare for the same holidays. Ask them to explain the similarities and differences.

À propos de la lecture...
Les auteurs de *Vis-à-vis* ont écrit ce texte.

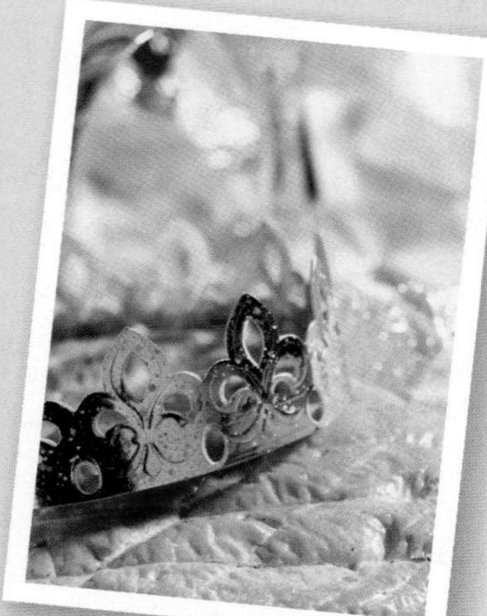

Une galette des Rois

Les grandes occasions

En France, les jours de fête sont l'occasion de se réunir[1] en famille ou entre amis. À chaque fête, on mange des plats typiques qui varient parfois[2] selon les régions. Voici les fêtes les plus gourmandes[3] du calendrier français.

*La fête des Rois**

Pour la fête des Rois, le 6 janvier, on achète chez le pâtissier une galette. C'est un gâteau qui contient une fève.[4] La personne qui trouve la fève dans son morceau de gâteau est le roi (ou la reine),[5] et cette personne choisit sa reine (ou son roi). La famille ou les amis boivent à leur santé.[6]

Pâques[7]

Pâques est, bien sûr, la fête du chocolat. C'est aussi un jour où l'on se retrouve ensemble, en famille à l'église et à table. On

[1]se... *get together* [2]*sometimes* [3]les plus... où l'on mange bien [4]*bean* [5]roi... *king* (*or queen*) [6]*health* [7]*Easter*

*This Christian holiday, Epiphany, also called Twelfth Night, commemorates Christ's appearance to the Gentiles (represented by the Three Kings).

fait un grand repas, et au dessert, grands et petits mangent des œufs, des cloches,[8] des poules ou des poissons en chocolat remplis[9] de bonbons.

Noël

Noël est peut-être la fête des fêtes. Le Réveillon[10] de Noël est un grand dîner que l'on prend le plus souvent après la messe[11] de minuit. Au menu: huîtres, foie gras, dinde aux marrons[12] et beaucoup de champagne! Au dessert, on mange une bûche[13] de Noël, un gâteau roulé au chocolat en forme de bûche. Les enfants, bien sûr, attendent avec impatience l'arrivée du Père Noël.

[8]*bells* [9]*filled* [10]Le... *Midnight supper* [11]cérémonie catholique [12]dinde... *turkey with chestnuts* [13]*log*

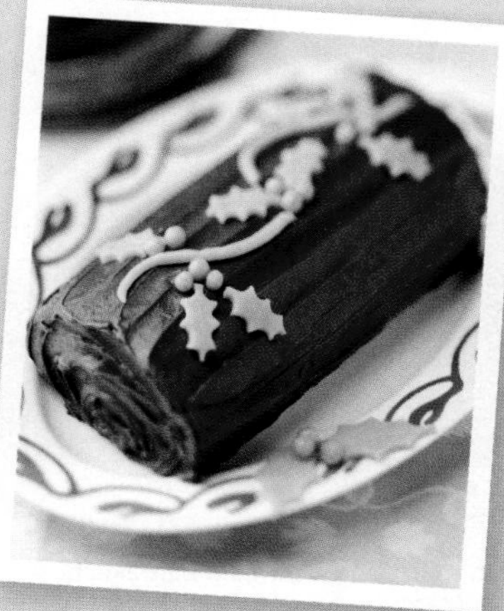
Une bûche de Noël pour le Réveillon

Compréhension

Match the following quotations with the relevant paragraphs in "Les grandes occasions."

1. «C'est ma fête préférée parce que j'adore les œufs en chocolat.»
2. «Je suis le roi!»
3. «Nous attendons toujours avec impatience l'arrivée de la bûche.»

Additional activity: Have sts. create a word association chain about two holidays in North America. Then use these as a basis for comparison of traditions and customs in the two countries.

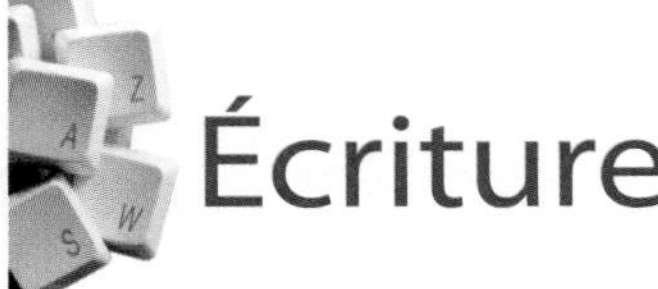

Écriture

The writing activities **Par écrit** and **Journal intime** can be found in the Workbook/Laboratory Manual to accompany *Vis-à-vis.*

La vie en chantant. An activity based on the song "Aïcha" by Khaled can be found in the Instructor's Manual. The song can be purchased at the iTunes store, or sts. can watch the music video on YouTube.

Pour s'amuser

Un monsieur très avare dit à ses enfants:

—Si vous êtes gentils ce soir, je vous montrerai la photo de quelqu'un qui mange une glace.

Le vidéoblog d'Hassan

En bref

Dans cet épisode, Juliette et Hassan sont au marché. Ils cherchent des ingrédients pour le dîner qu'ils vont préparer pour Léa et Hector. Dans son vidéoblog, Hassan décrit ses marchés préférés à Paris et au Maroc et Hector décrit les marchés à la Martinique.

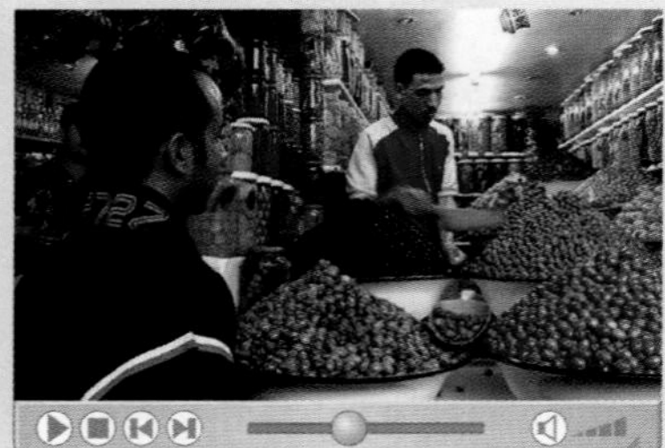

Un marchand d'olives à Marrakech, au Maroc

Additional vocabulary: Other vocabulary you may wish to present before viewing includes: *tu sais, il faut acheter, on arrête, on rentre.*

Vocabulaire en contexte

Imaginez que vous faites votre marché en France. Quels produits dans la liste désirez-vous avoir pour votre propre (*own*) dîner ce soir?

Provisions possibles

- ☐ des **fruits de mer** (*seafood*)
- ☐ du saumon frais
- ☐ des **huîtres** (*oysters*)
- ☐ des fruits/légumes bio (*organic*)
- ☐ du fromage **de chèvre** (*goat*)
- ☐ du pain **de campagne**
- ☐ des **épices/piments** (*spices/ hot peppers*)
- ☐ des fleurs
- ☐ tout (*everything*)

Visionnez!

Qu'est-ce que les quatre amis vont manger ce soir? Écoutez bien et faites le menu.

Entrée	**Pain**	**Dessert**
________	________	________
Plat principal	**Fromages**	**Boisson**
________	________	________
________	________	
________	________	

Analysez!

Répondez aux questions.

1. Quelles différences y a-t-il entre les marchés de France et les marchés d'autres pays francophones?
2. Qu'est-ce qu'un marché offre à sa clientèle qu'un *supermarché* n'offre pas?

Comparez!

Où allez-vous normalement «faire votre marché»? Y a-t-il un marché semblable (*similar*) aux marchés parisiens dans votre région? Regardez encore une fois la partie culturelle de la vidéo: où préférez-vous faire votre marché? Expliquez.

Note culturelle

Le souk[1] est un élément fondamental de la vie marocaine. Il joue un rôle social et économique: 40 000 artisans et 5 000 commerçants travaillent dans les souks de Marrakech et aussi des milliers[2] de porteurs, guides, marchands ambulants, et cetera. Vous pouvez tout acheter: du téléphone portable aux babouches faites main.[3] Noter qu'en français, le mot «souk» désigne aussi un lieu en désordre («C'est un vrai souk, ici!»).

[1]marché marocain [2]*thousands*
[3]babouches… *handmade slippers*

Suggestion: Ask sts. to describe a typical dinner they might prepare with friends and ask them to compare their meal to the one in the video.

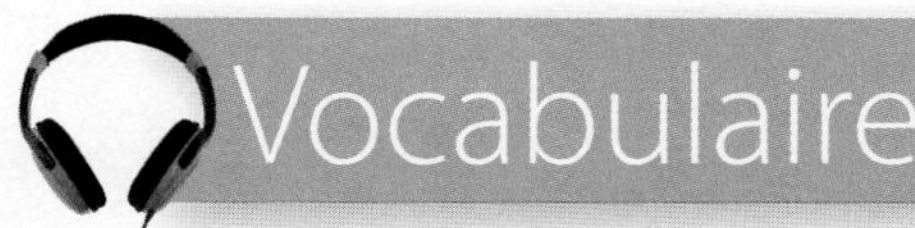

Vocabulaire

Verbes

apporter to bring; to carry
coûter to cost
devoir to have to, be obliged to; to owe
goûter to taste
laisser to leave (behind)
pleuvoir to rain
pouvoir to be able to, can
vouloir to want
vouloir bien to be willing; to agree
vouloir dire to mean

À REVOIR: **apprendre, avoir, boire, choisir, commander, comprendre, dîner, être, faire, perdre, prendre, préparer, trouver, vendre**

Substantifs

l'addition (*f.*) bill, check (*in a restaurant*)
l'ail (*m.*) garlic
l'argent (*m.*) money
la boîte (de conserve) can (*of food*)
la carte menu
le centime 1/100th of a euro
les conserves (*f. pl.*) canned goods
le copain/la copine (boy)friend/(girl)friend
la côte chop
la chose thing
les crevettes (*f.*) shrimp
l'éclair (*m.*) eclair (*pastry*)
l'entrée (*f.*) first course
l'escargot (*m.*) snail
l'euro (*m.*) euro (*European Union currency*)
la fête holiday; party; celebration
le filet fillet (*beef, fish, etc.*)
le homard lobster
l'huile (*f.*) **(d'olive)** (olive) oil
l'huître (*f.*) oyster
le kilo(gramme) kilo(gram)
le magasin store, shop
la matinée morning
le menu fixed (price) menu
le morceau piece
la mousse au chocolat chocolate mousse
la nuit night
le pain de campagne country-style wheat bread
le pâté de campagne (country-style) pâté
les pâtes (*f.*) pasta
le plat course (*meal*)
plat principal main dish
le pourboire tip
le prix price
le régime diet
le rôti roast
les sardines (à l'huile) (*f.*) sardines (in oil)
la saucisse sausage
le saucisson salami
le saumon salmon
le serveur / la serveuse waiter / waitress
la soirée evening
la sole sole (*fish*)
la tranche slice
le veau veal

À REVOIR: **l'assiette** (*f.*), **le bœuf, la boisson, le crabe, la cuisine, le déjeuner, le dîner, le fromage, la glace, le gâteau, les haricots verts, le matin, le pain, le petit déjeuner, la pomme, la pomme de terre, le porc, le soir, la viande, le vin**

Les magasins

la boucherie butcher shop
la boulangerie bakery
la charcuterie pork butcher's shop (delicatessen)
l'épicerie (*f.*) grocery store
la pâtisserie pastry shop; pastry
la poissonnerie fish store

Expressions temporelles

avant-hier the day before yesterday
dernier / dernière last
hier yesterday
hier soir last night
passé(e) last
toute la matinée / la journée / la soirée / la nuit all morning / day / evening / night

Mots et expressions divers

autre chose something else
ça this, that
ce (cet, cette) / ces this, that / these, those
compris(e) included
d'abord first
ensuite next, then
Il n'y a pas de quoi. You're welcome.
je pourrais I could
Je vous en prie. You're welcome. (*formal*)
(et) puis (and) then, next
quel(le)(s) which, what
tout le monde everybody

À REVOIR: **je voudrais, de rien**

CHAPITRE 8

Vive les vacances!

Les dossiers d'Hassan

Hassan

- Mes photos
  - Les Contamines dans les Alpes
  - À La Nouvelle-Orléans
  - En vacances à Cannes

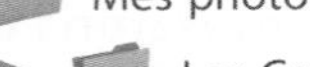

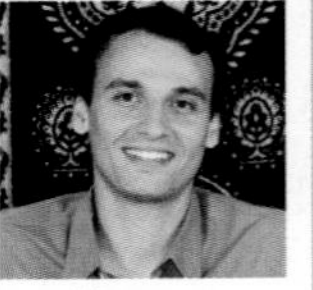

Note: À l'origine, *vive* est la forme exclamative du verbe *vivre* au subjonctif (*qu'il vive*). Par ce terme, on souhaite une vie longue, heureuse et prospère à une personne importante. Exemple: *Vive le roi!* Par extension, on utilise aussi cette exclamation pour célébrer une chose agréable à laquelle on attache une valeur particulière. Exemple: *Vive les vacances!*

Presentation: Review weather expressions and leisure activities by asking questions such as *Quel temps fait-il? Aimez-vous faire du ski? Aimez-vous la neige? Où faites-vous du ski?*

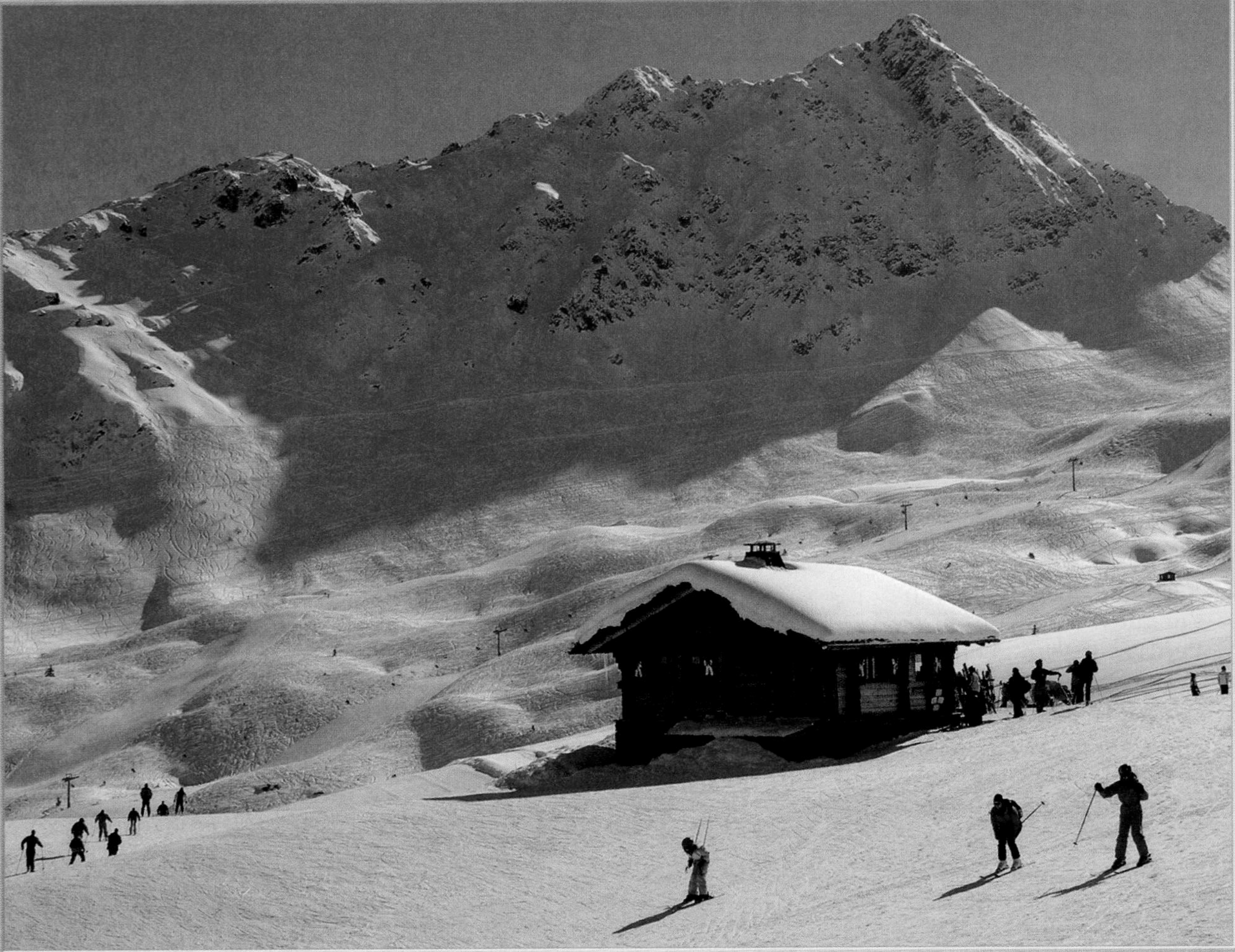

Un beau jour aux Contamines près de Chamonix dans les Alpes françaises

Cultural note: Les Contamines-Montjoie is located near *Mont Blanc* in the *Haute-Savoie* department of the *Rhône-Alpes* region.

Dans ce chapitre...

OBJECTIFS COMMUNICATIFS

- talking about vacation, recreational equipment
- expressing dates and actions
- talking about the past
- expressing how long ago something happened
- expressing location
- learning to distinguish between and pronounce selected sounds in French

PAROLES (Leçon 1)

- Les régions de la France et les loisirs
- Le verbe **acheter**
- L'équipement de sport et de voyage
- L'année

STRUCTURES (Leçons 2 et 3)

- Quelques verbes irréguliers en **-ir**
- Le passé composé avec l'auxiliaire **être**
- L'expression impersonnelle **il faut**
- Les prépositions devant les noms de lieu

CULTURE

- Le blog d'Hassan: *Partir!*
- Reportage: *France: le pays des grandes vacances*
- Lecture: *Des vacances au Maroc* (Leçon 4)

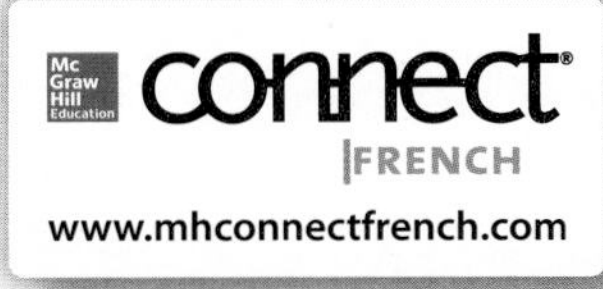

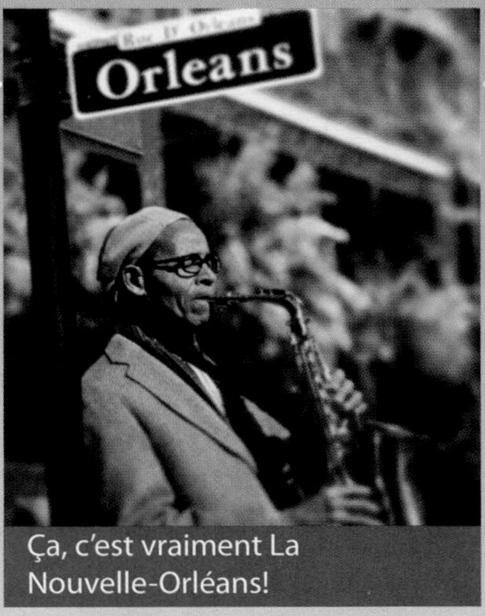

Ça, c'est vraiment La Nouvelle-Orléans!

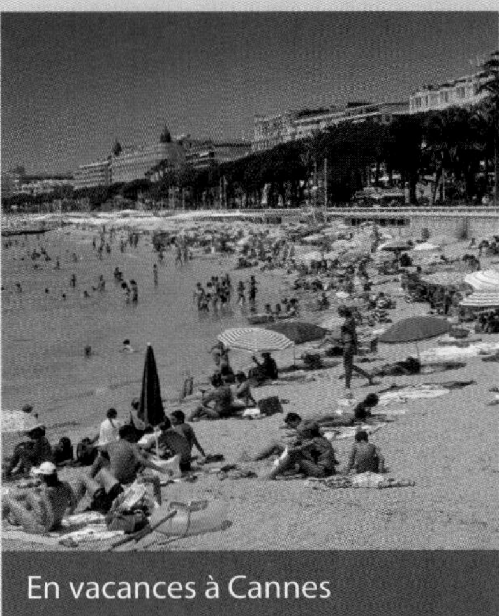
En vacances à Cannes

CHAPITRE **8**

Leçon 1

PAROLES

En vacances

Pronunciation presentation: Model pronunciation of the following words: *Charlemagne, oignon, champagne, ignorer, campagne, union, espagnol.*

Pronunciation practice: The *Prononcez bien!* section on page 224 of this chapter contains activities for practicing these sounds.

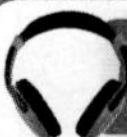

Prononcez bien!

The pronunciation of *montagne*

To pronounce the sequence **gn** as [ɲ], blend the sounds [n] and [j] as you do in the English words *onion* and *union*. This sound is most often spelled **gn,** and sometimes **ni.**

[ɲ]: **magnifique, champignon, dernier**

For words ending in **-gne,** make sure you don't pronounce the final **-e.**

[ɲ]: **montagne, campagne**

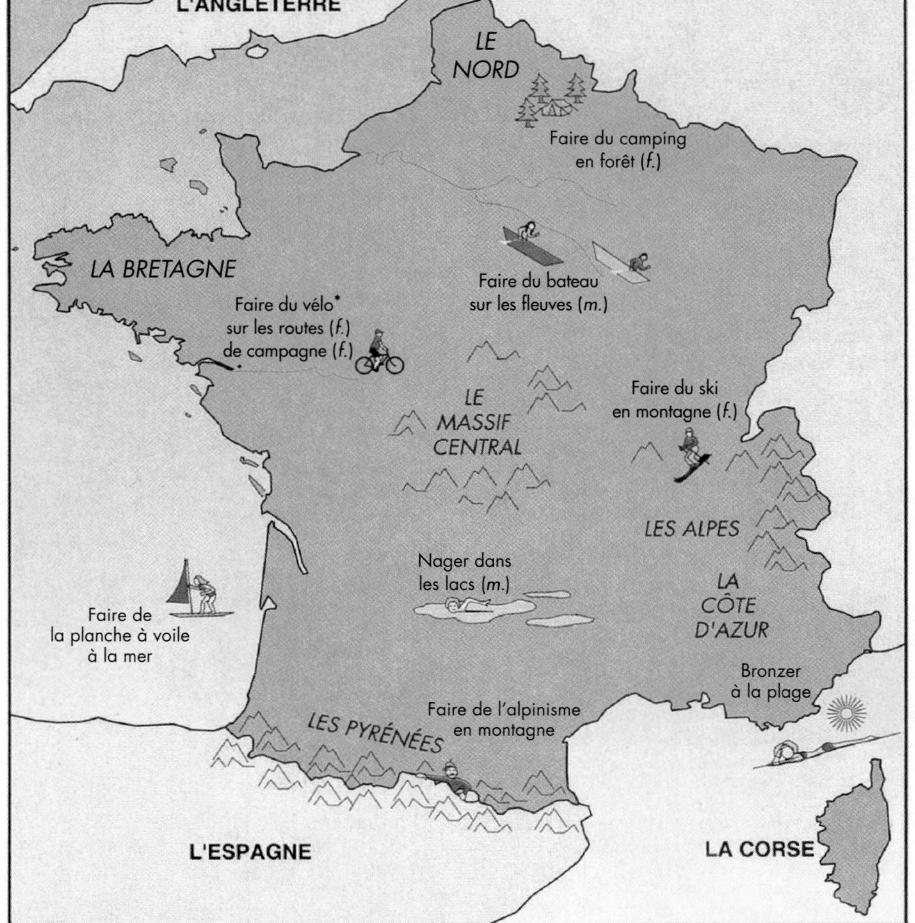

Additional vocabulary: *aller à la chasse, faire du jogging, faire du patinage, faire du roller, faire du snowboard, faire du vélo de montagne (du VTT), faire de la voile, jouer au golf, jouer au tennis,* etc.

Suggestion: Provide sts. with other expressions, depending on how they spend their vacations.

Suggestion: Review *faire de, jouer à.*

AUTRES MOTS UTILES

faire... du cheval, de l'équitation	to go . . . horseback riding
de la plongée libre	snorkeling
de la plongée sous-marine	scuba diving
du ski nautique	waterskiing
du ski alpin	downhill skiing
du ski de fond	cross-country skiing
une randonnée	for a hike
aller à la pêche	to go fishing
patiner	to skate
prendre des vacances	to take a vacation
un endroit	a place

*__Faire du vélo__ is synonymous with **faire de la bicyclette.**

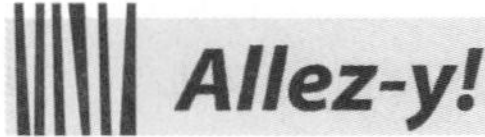

Allez-y!

A. Où passer les vacances? Quels sont les avantages touristiques des endroits suivants?

1. Qu'est-ce qu'on peut faire en montagne?
2. Au bord d'un lac?
3. À la plage?
4. Sur une route de campagne?
5. Sur un fleuve?
6. En forêt?
7. À la mer?

Maintenant expliquez où vous voulez passer vos prochaines vacances et quelles activités on peut faire à cet endroit.

B. Activités de vacances. Qu'est-ce qu'ils font?

1. Que fait un nageur / une nageuse? Où est-ce qu'on trouve beaucoup de nageurs?
2. Que fait un campeur / une campeuse? Où est-ce qu'on fait du camping en France? aux États-Unis?
3. Que fait un skieur / une skieuse? Où est-ce qu'on fait du ski en France? aux États-Unis?
4. Que fait un(e) cycliste? Où est-ce qu'on fait du vélo en France? aux États-Unis?
5. Combien de nageurs, de campeurs, de skieurs, de cyclistes est-ce qu'il y a dans la classe? D'habitude, où est-ce qu'ils passent leurs vacances?

Suggestion: Have sts. make list in groups and share responses with class.

Additional activity: *Vos vacances. 1. Préférez-vous passer les vacances d'été à la mer, en montagne, à la campagne? 2. Qu'est-ce que vous aimez faire en vacances? 3. Où allez-vous aller l'été prochain?*

Additional activity: Start at the front of the classroom and have each st. answer the following question: *Qu'est-ce que tu aimes faire pendant tes vacances?* Each st. must repeat the preceding responses and then add their own. Ask sts. to give original answers each time.

Additional activity: *Qu'est-ce qu'ils vont faire? 1. Maurice cherche ses skis. 2. Claire apporte sa tente. 3. Dominique achète une bicyclette. 4. Serge loue un bateau. 5. Sylvie prend des leçons de natation. 6. Les Vasseur achètent de la crème solaire* (suntan lotion).

Le verbe *acheter*

The verb **acheter** (*to buy*) is irregular. The **e** from the stem (**achet-**) becomes **è** for the forms of **je, tu, il/elle/on,** and **ils/elles.** The forms of **nous** and **vous** are regular. Note that all the endings are regular.

PRESENT TENSE OF **acheter**			
j'	**achète**	nous	achetons
tu	**achètes**	vous	achetez
il/elle/on	**achète**	ils/elles	**achètent**

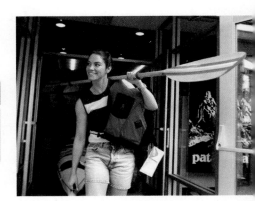

Faire du shopping en vue des vacances. Va-t-elle faire du bateau ou du vélo en vacances? Qu'est-ce qu'elle achète? Qu'est-ce qu'elle porte?

Additional vocabulary: *un kayak, une rame* (paddle, oar)

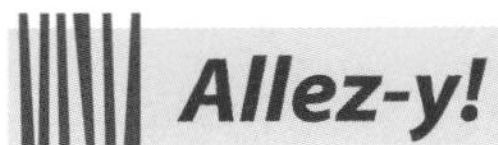

Les besoins sont différents. Ces personnes préparent leurs vacances. Complétez les phrases avec la forme appropriée du verbe **acheter.**

1. Caroline veut aller à la plage. Elle ______ un maillot de bain.
2. Nous voulons passer les vacances de Noël à la Martinique. Nous ______ des shorts et des tee-shirts.
3. Tu veux bien aller à la montagne. Tu ______ un sac à dos.
4. Rock et Marine organisent un voyage à Londres. Ils ______ des imperméables.
5. L'été prochain, vous voulez rendre visite à des amis à Paris. Vous ______ une jupe noire et un pull rouge.

Presentation: Bring in pictures or examples of these clothing items to teach vocab.

Additional vocabulary: *un bikini, des espadrilles.*

Au magasin de sports

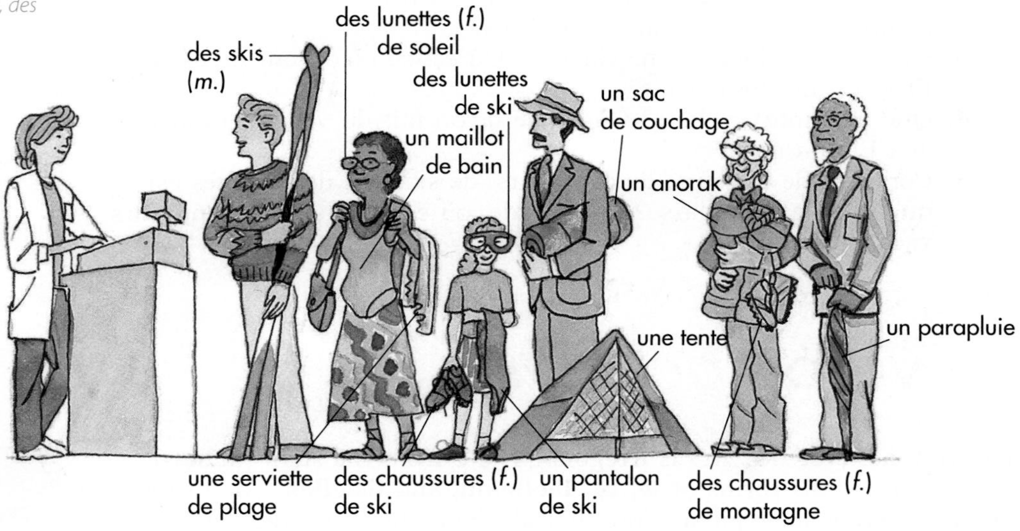

AUTRES MOTS UTILES

un casque	helmet	**des gants** (*m.*)	gloves
une crème solaire	suntan lotion	**un sac à dos**	backpack
un écran solaire	sunblock	**une valise**	suitcase

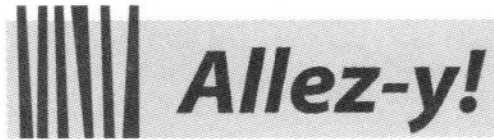

Allez-y!

A. Achats. (*Purchases.*) Complétez les phrases en vous basant sur le dessin à la page 204.

1. Le jeune homme va acheter des ______. Il va passer ses vacances à Grenoble où il veut ______.
2. La jeune femme veut acheter un ______, une ______ et des ______. Elle va descendre sur la Côte d'Azur (*French Riviera*) où elle va ______ et ______.
3. La jeune fille a envie d'acheter des ______ de ski, des chaussures de ______ et un ______ de ski. Sa famille va passer les vacances dans les Alpes où elle va ______.
4. L'homme va acheter un ______ et une ______. Il va ______ dans le nord de la France ce week-end.

Suggestion (A): Could be done for listening comprehension by changing completed items into questions. Ask sts. to look at pictures. Read items and have sts. identify pictures.

Continuation (A): 5. *La vieille dame est très sportive. Elle va acheter un ______ et des ______ Ce week-end, elle va ______ avec son mari dans les Pyrénées.* 6. *Le vieux monsieur a l'air patient. Il veut acheter un ______.*

B. L'intrus. Dans les groupes suivants, trouvez le mot qui ne va pas avec les autres. Expliquez votre choix.

1. le maillot de bain / les lunettes de soleil / la crème solaire / l'anorak
2. la tente / le maillot de bain / le sac de couchage / le sac à dos
3. les gants de ski / la serviette de plage / les skis / l'anorak
4. les lunettes de soleil / les chaussures de ski / le short / le maillot de bain

Suggestions (B): (1) Could be done for listening comprehension with books closed. (2) After sts. have found odd word, have them try to think of one more word that is related in some way to other words.

C. Choix de vêtements. Qu'est-ce qu'on porte pour faire les activités suivantes?

MODÈLE: pour aller à la pêche →
Pour aller à la pêche, on porte un chapeau…

1. pour faire du ski nautique **2.** pour aller à la montagne **3.** pour faire une promenade dans la forêt **4.** pour faire du vélo **5.** pour faire du bateau **6.** pour faire du ski de fond

Et vous? Décrivez les vêtements que vous portez quand vous faites votre sport favori.

Vocabulary recycling: Refer sts. to previous clothing vocab. from *Chapitre 3* for review.

Continuation (C): (1) *Pour aller au cinéma; pour aller aux offices religieux; pour aller danser.* (2) Ask sts. to name one thing they would *not* wear during these activities.

Follow-up (C): Bring in a clothing size chart from France to show how sizes are different. Teach *la taille, la pointure,* and *Je chausse du…* (*My shoe size is…*).

D. Conseils pratiques. Vous préparez un voyage en Tunisie. Voici les vêtements qu'on vous recommande.

> ***Les vêtements***
> *En hiver : quelques pulls, un imperméable et des vêtements de demi-saison.*[1]
> *En été : des vêtements légers*[2] *en fibres naturelles, maillot de bain, lunettes de soleil, chapeau, chaussures aérées,*[3] *tenues*[4] *pratiques pour les excursions. Sans oublier un léger pull pour les soirées et les hôtels climatisés.*[5]

[1]*spring or autumn* [2]*lightweight* [3]*well-ventilated* [4]*outfits, clothes* [5]*air-conditioned*

1. Selon (*According to*) la brochure, quels vêtements sont recommandés pour un voyage en hiver, en été? Donnez des exemples.
2. À votre avis, quel temps fait-il en Tunisie en hiver, en été?

Imaginez maintenant que vous travaillez dans une agence de voyages. Quels vêtements allez-vous conseiller (*to suggest*) à des touristes qui vont en Alaska, au Mexique ou dans le Grand Canyon? Quels autres achats conseillez-vous?

Suggestion (D): Encourage sts. to tell what they know about Tunisia.

Suggestion (D): Take this opportunity to discuss other African francophone countries: *l'Algérie, le Bénin, le Burkina Faso, le Burundi, le Cameroun, le Congo, la Côte d'Ivoire, le Gabon, la Guinée, le Mali, le Maroc, la Mauritanie, le Niger, la République Centrafricaine, le Rwanda, le Sénégal, le Tchad, le Togo.* Have sts. locate these countries on the map of Africa at the back of the book.

Follow-up (D): Have sts. play the roles of *agent de voyages* and *voyageur / voyageuse.*

Presentation: You may introduce *Quand êtes-vous né(e)?* and *Je suis né(e) en…* as lexical items to have sts. practice saying years. Reenter dates and seasons by having sts. guess each other's birthdays. Suggested question sequence: *Est-ce que ton anniversaire est… en automne? au printemps?* etc. *au mois de novembre?* etc. *le 13? le 14?*

Des années importantes

La machine à calculer inventée par Blaise Pascal en **1642** (mille six cent quarante-deux).

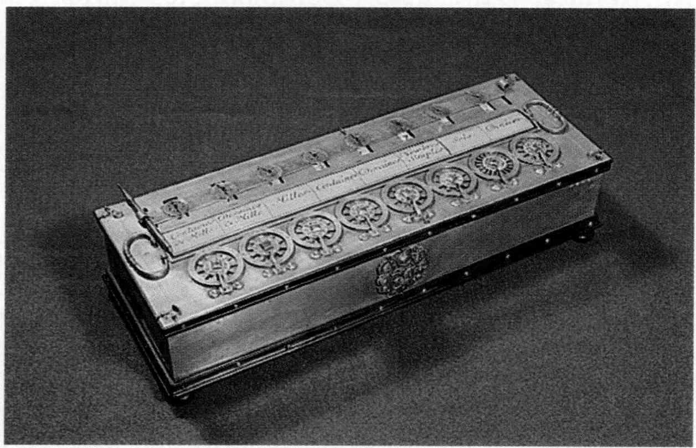

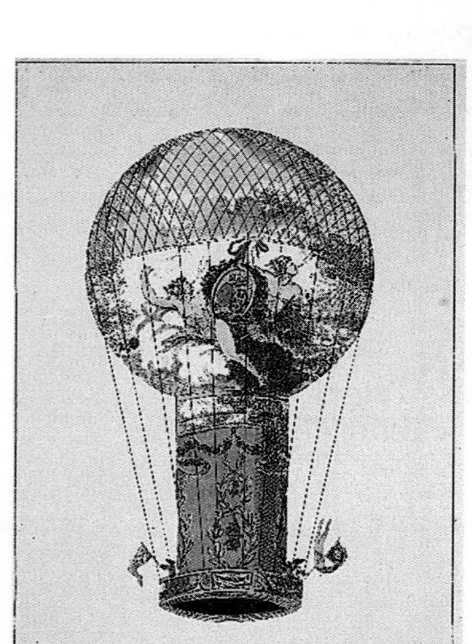

Le ballon à air chaud inventé par les frères Montgolfier en **1783** (mille sept cent quatre-vingt-trois).

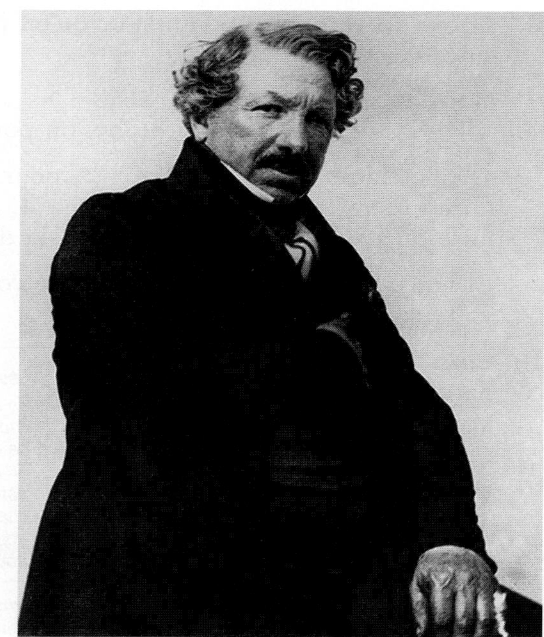

Les procédés de développement des images photographiques inventés par Jacques Daguerre en **1835** (mille huit cent trente-cinq).

- In French, years are expressed with a multiple of **mille** or with **cent.**

  mille neuf cents (*or* dix-neuf cents) *1900*
  mille neuf cent quatre-vingt-dix-neuf *1999*
  (*or* dix-neuf cent quatre-vingt-dix-neuf)
  deux mille quatorze *2014*

- The preposition **en** is used to express *in* with a year.

  en mille neuf cent vingt-trois *in 1923*

- Note the expression **les années 50** (*the* [*nineteen*] *fifties*): **les années cinquante.**

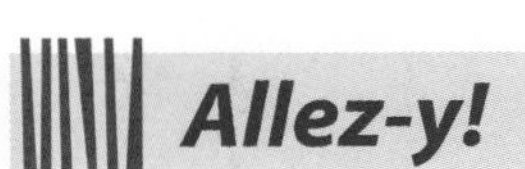

Continuation (A): *Maintenant, chaque étudiant(e) nomme un événement historique. Les autres donnent la date de l'événement en question. Qui est l'historien(ne) de la classe? Suggestions: le voyage autour du monde de Magellan; l'arrivée de Christophe Colomb en Amérique; la rédaction de la Constitution américaine; la vente de la Louisiane aux États-Unis par Napoléon*

A. Un peu d'histoire. Êtes-vous bon(ne) en histoire? Avec un(e) camarade, trouvez la date qui correspond à chaque événement historique. Les événements sont présentés par ordre chronologique!

1. Charlemagne est couronné (*crowned*) empereur d'Occident.	**a.** 1944
2. Guillaume, duc de Normandie, conquiert (*conquers*) l'Angleterre	**b.** 1804
3. Jeanne d'Arc bat (*beats*) les Anglais à Orléans.	**c.** 1889
4. Prise de la Bastille.	**d.** 1066
5. Napoléon est couronné empereur des Français.	**e.** 1429
6. Gustave Eiffel construit la tour Eiffel.	**f.** 1789
7. Débarquement (*Landing*) anglo-américain en France.	**g.** l'an 800

B. L'avenir. (*The future.*) Quels sont vos projets d'avenir? Posez les questions suivantes à un(e) camarade. Ensuite, présentez à la classe une observation sur l'avenir de votre camarade.

1. En quelle année vas-tu obtenir (*to obtain*) ton diplôme universitaire?
2. En quelle année vas-tu passer des vacances en France?
3. En quelle année vas-tu avoir 65 ans?

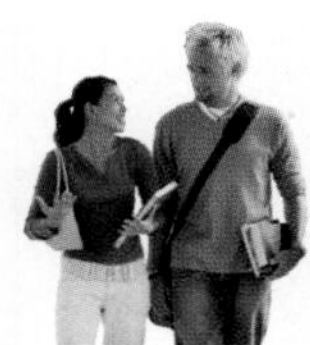

Continuation (B): 4. *En quelle année vas-tu aller à Paris? à Montréal? en Europe? en Afrique? en Asie?* 5. *En quelle année tes enfants vont-ils commencer leurs études universitaires?*

Follow-up (B): Ask sts. to guess year of birth of their partner based on information they have received.

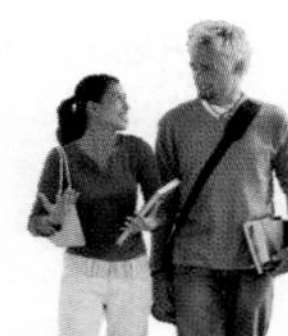

Answers (A): 1. g 2. d 3. e 4. f 5. b 6. c 7. a

Follow-up (A): For listening comprehension practice, give sts. years orally and have them choose an event during that year.

Cultural note (A): Held by many in the Anglo-Saxon world to be one of history's chief villains, *Guillaume, Duc de Normandie,* and his conquest of England (1066) are depicted in the Bayeux Tapestry, displayed at the *Bibliothèque de Bayeux* in northwest France. The Norman conquest had immense consequences for the language and culture of England: the gallicizing of the local Germanic tongue and the birth of middle English; the development of common law, the feudal system, and a centralized state; ecclesiastical reform; and the start of the centuries-long dominance of French mores and letters across *la Manche.*

Leçon 2

Quelques verbes irréguliers en *-ir*

Expressing Actions

Vacances à Versailles

Alexis contacte Poema sur sa page Facebook (Messagerie instantanée).

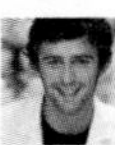

ALEXIS: Poema, **tu pars** cet été?

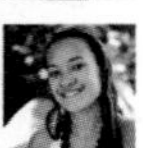

POEMA: **Je pars** à la Guadeloupe au mois d'août. Et toi?

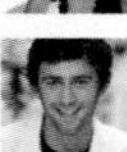

ALEXIS: Moi, **je reviens** juste de Montréal. Je suis fatigué. **Je dors** toute la journée!

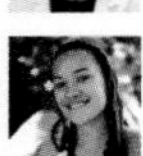

POEMA: **Tu dors**! Tu ne travailles pas?

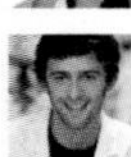

ALEXIS: Non. Je suis en vacances!

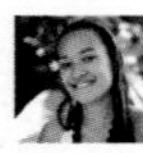

POEMA: **Tu viens** à la Guadeloupe avec moi?

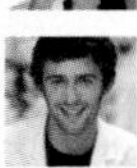

ALEXIS: Merci pour l'invitation, mais Trésor et moi nous restons à Versailles.

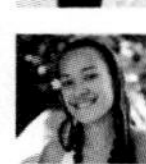

POEMA: À Versailles? Mais qu'est-ce qu'on fait à Versailles en été?

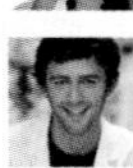

ALEXIS: **On dort** le matin, on fait du vélo dans le parc du château l'après-midi, **on sort** le soir.

Vrai ou faux? Corrigez les phrases fausses.

1. Poema part au Canada cet été.
2. Alexis revient de Montréal.
3. Poema est fatiguée. Elle dort toute la journée.
4. Poema demande à Alexis de venir à la Guadeloupe avec elle.
5. Alexis dit: «On sort le matin, on dort le soir».

Dormir and Similar Verbs

The verb **dormir** (*to sleep*) has an irregular conjugation.

PRESENT TENSE OF **dormir**			
je	**dors**	nous	**dormons**
tu	**dors**	vous	**dormez**
il/elle/on	**dort**	ils/elles	**dorment**

Presentation: Point out that the consonant sound of the verb stem is heard in third-person plural but not in singular, which helps the listener distinguish singular from plural.

Je **dors** très bien. — *I sleep very well.*
Dormez-vous à la belle étoile? — *Do you sleep in the open air?*
Nous **dormons** jusqu'à 7 h 30. — *We sleep until 7:30.*

Verbs conjugated like **dormir** include:

partir *to leave, depart*
sentir *to feel; to sense; to smell*
servir *to serve*
sortir *to leave; to go out*

Je **pars** en vacances. — *I'm leaving on vacation.*
Ce plat **sent** bon/mauvais. — *This dish smells good/bad.*
Nous **servons** le petit déjeuner à 8 h. — *We serve breakfast at 8:00.*
À quelle heure allez-vous **sortir** ce soir? — *What time are you going out tonight?*

Suggestion: Use the following as a listening discrimination ex. Sts. write *S* or *P* next to each number. *Singulier ou pluriel?* 1. *Ils servent le dîner.* 2. *Elle sent le pain chaud.* 3. *Ils sentent les fleurs sur la table.* 4. *Elle dort après le dîner.* 5. *Ils dorment devant la télé.* 6. *Elles sortent ce soir.* Go over ex., asking sts. to explain their answers.

Suggestion: You might want to teach *je me sens bien* (I feel good) as a lexical item to avoid confusion with *je sens bon* (I smell good).

Partir and *sortir*

Partir and **sortir** mean *to leave,* but they are used differently.

1. **Partir** is the opposite of **arriver.** It can be used alone or followed by a preposition.

   Je **pars** demain. — *I'm leaving (departing) tomorrow.*
   Elle **part** de/pour Cannes. — *She's leaving from/for Cannes.*

2. **Sortir** is the opposite of **entrer** (*to enter*). It can also be used alone or followed by a preposition.

   Ils **sortent** du théâtre. — *They're leaving the theater.*
   Elle **sort** de la caravane. — *She's getting out of the camper.*
   Sortons de l'eau! — *Let's get out of the water!*

Sortir can also mean that one is going out for the evening, or seeing another person regularly.

Tu **sors** ce soir? — *Are you going out tonight?*
Iris et Édouard **sortent** ensemble. — *Iris and Édouard are going out together.*

Note: **Quitter** (a regular **-er** verb) means *to leave* (*go away from*) *something or someone.* It always requires a direct object, either a place or a person.

Je **quitte** Paris. — *I'm leaving Paris.*
Elle **quitte** son ami. — *She's leaving her boyfriend.*

[Allez-y! A-D]

Grammaire interactive

For more on regular **-re** and **-ir** verbs and verbs like **sortir,** watch the corresponding Grammar Tutorial and take a brief practice quiz at **Connect French.**

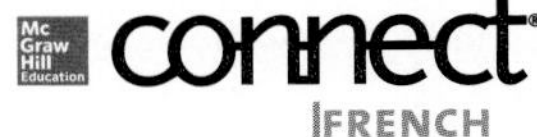

www.mhconnectfrench.com

Note: To express *I quit* (*my job*), one can say *j'ai quitté mon emploi,* but not *j'ai quitté* by itself.

Presentation: Write forms of *venir* on board as you model them, with the three singular forms and the third-person plural first (because stems are alike) and the two other plural forms last.

Venir and the *passé récent*

The verb **venir** (*to come*) is irregular.

PRESENT TENSE OF **venir**			
je	**viens**	nous	venons
tu	**viens**	vous	venez
il/elle/on	**vient**	ils/elles	**viennent**

Nous **venons** de Saint-Malo. — *We come from Saint-Malo.*
Viens voir la plage! — *Come see the beach!*

Prononcez bien!

The vowels in *viens* and *viennent*

Note that the vowel in the three singular forms of **venir** (**je viens, tu viens, il vient**) is the same nasal vowel [ɛ̃] as in **bien,** and that the **n** is not pronounced.

[ɛ̃]: **tu deviens, il obtient**

In the third-person plural form (**ils viennent**), however, the presence of **nn** denasalizes the vowel into [ɛ], as in **lait,** and the **nn** is pronounced.

[ɛn]: **ils deviennent, elles obtiennent**

1. **Venir de** + infinitive means *to have just* (*done something*). This is called **le passé récent.**

   Je **viens de nager.** — *I've just been swimming.*
   Mes amis **viennent de téléphoner.** — *My friends have just telephoned.*

2. Verbs conjugated like **venir** include:

   devenir *to become*
   obtenir *to obtain*
   revenir *to come back*

   Ils **reviennent** de vacances. — *They're coming back from vacation.*
   On **devient** expert grâce à l'expérience. — *One becomes an expert with (thanks to) experience.*

Note: Point out that *venir de* is an easy way to indicate a very recent past event.

Suggestion: Point out the two usages of *venir de* (+ infinitive = recent past; + place = origin).

[Allez-y! B-C-D]

Pronunciation practice (1): Have sts. decide whether the following sentences are introduced by *il* or *ils* (i.e., *singulier ou pluriel*): *il vient à la maison, ils obtiennent un rendez-vous chez le dentiste, ils deviennent de bons musiciens, il revient du magasin de sports.*

Pronunciation practice (2): The *Prononcez bien!* section on page 224 of this chapter contains additional activities for practicing these sounds.

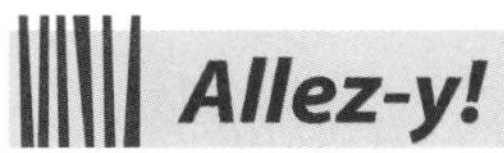

Suggestion: (Preliminary ex.) *Singulier ou pluriel? 1. Ils partent en vacances demain. 2. Elle vient d'obtenir des brochures. 3. Elle sort de l'agence de voyages. 4. Ils reviennent en voiture.*

Additional activity: *Le programme d'une journée de vacances. Faites les substitutions indiquées et les changements nécessaires. 1. Jean-Marie part pour faire du vélo. (les étudiants, nous, tu) 2. Je sors de la caravane à six heures. (vous, Christine et Marie-France, il) 3. Nous sentons les fleurs. (je, on, Jean-Marie et Chantal) 4. Pierre dort jusqu'à midi. (ils, vous, tu)*

A. Que faire? Clara et Philippe, les amis de Romain, désirent sortir ce soir. Romain hésite. Complétez la conversation avec les verbes corrects: **partir, quitter** ou **sortir.**

PHILIPPE: On ______[1] ce soir? Il y a un bon film qui passe au ciné!
ROMAIN: Désolé! Mes cousins sont en vacances chez moi et ils ______[2] demain matin, alors je vais rester avec eux ce soir.
PHILIPPE: Oh allez! Tu les ______[3] pendant deux heures, le temps du film. Ce n'est pas long!
CLARA: Attends. Tes cousins, ils ne ______[4] pas le samedi soir? Ils ont quel âge?
ROMAIN: Si bien sûr, mais quand vous ______[5] la maison à 5 h du matin, est-ce que vous ______[6] tard la veille, vous?
PHILIPPE: Tu ______[7] en vacances demain, toi, Clara?
CLARA: Ben non…
PHILIPPE: Nous ______[8] donc ce soir?
CLARA: Ah oui!
PHILIPPE: O.K., on te raconte le film demain, Romain. Bonne soirée avec tes cousins!

B. Au pays des pharaons. Loïc et Nathalie sont en vacances en Égypte avec le Club Aquarius. Ils envoient (*send*) une carte postale à leur grand-mère. Complétez la carte avec les verbes de la colonne de droite.

Chère mamie,

Nous ______[1] d'arriver en Égypte. Le Club Aquarius, c'est le grand confort. Nous ______[2] dans des chambres immenses et tous les matins on ______[3] le petit déjeuner dans la chambre. Demain nous ______[4] pour le temple de Louxor. Nous ______[5] des experts en égyptologie. Nous ______[6] en France dans quatre jours.

À bientôt et grosses bises.

Loïc et Nathalie

devenir
dormir
partir
revenir
servir
venir

C. La curiosité. Imaginez avec un(e) camarade ce que ces personnes viennent de faire. Donnez trois possibilités pour chaque phrase.

MODÈLE: Albert rentre d'Afrique.→
Il vient de visiter le Sénégal. Il vient de passer une semaine au soleil. Il vient de faire un safari.

1. Jennifer part en vacances.
2. Je sors du magasin de sports.
3. Nous revenons de la montagne.
4. Anthony et Yvon reviennent de la campagne.
5. Aïcha rentre du Canada.

D. Conversation. Engagez avec un(e) camarade une conversation basée sur les questions suivantes. Ensuite, faites un commentaire sur les habitudes (*habits*) ou les attitudes de votre camarade.

1. Tu pars souvent en voyage? Tu vas où? Tu viens d'acheter des vêtements ou d'autres objects nécessaires pour tes vacances? Qu'est-ce que tu viens d'acheter?
2. Tu sors souvent pendant (*during*) le week-end ou tu restes à la maison? Tu sors souvent pendant la semaine? Qu'est-ce que tu portes quand tu sors?
3. Tu aimes la fin des vacances? Tes ami(e)s sentent une différence quand tu rentres chez toi? Tu es plus calme? nerveux/nerveuse? triste? heureux/heureuse?

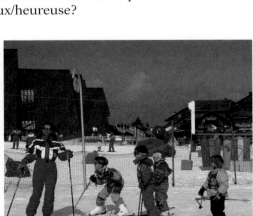

Une école de ski à Méribel en Savoie, en France

Additional activity: *En français, s'il vous plaît. 1. My family is leaving on vacation today. 2. My cousins are leaving New York. 3. My sister is leaving for Brittany tomorrow. 4. My brother has just bought some skis. 5. He's going out with a friend. 6. Why are you leaving? 7. You're going out with my sister now? 8. Let's leave together. 9. I can't go out. I have to work.*

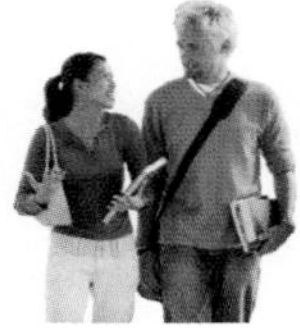

Suggestion: Give sts. a minute to write sentences and then put them on board or check using a digital display.

Suggestion (D): Could be done at end of class hour. Sts. prepare commentary for homework.

Suggestion: Have two sts. read roles of Hector and Juliette. Have sts. talk about how *passé composé* is formed with *être*, from examples of boldfaced verbs.

Le passé composé avec l'auxiliaire *être*

Talking About the Past

De Londres à Cannes

Appel vidéo entre Hector et Juliette.

HECTOR: **Vous êtes arrivées** à Londres?
JULIETTE: En fait, **nous sommes descendues** à Cannes.
HECTOR: À Cannes? Je ne comprends rien. Vous avez changé vos projets? **Vous n'êtes pas parties** en Angleterre?
JULIETTE: **Nous sommes restées** deux jours à Londres. Mais il pleuvait.* Alors, **nous sommes revenues** à Paris et **nous sommes parties** sur la Côte d'Azur.
HECTOR: Vous avez trouvé un petit hôtel?
JULIETTE: Sans problème. C'est facile: **Nous sommes allées** sur TripAdvisor!

*il… *it was raining*

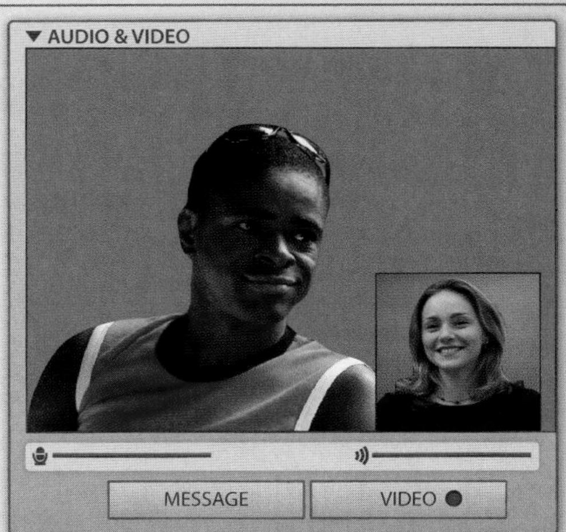

Trouvez la question dans le dialogue.

1. En fait, nous sommes descendues à Cannes.
2. Nous sommes restées deux jours à Londres. Nous sommes revenues à Paris et nous sommes parties sur la Côte d'Azur.
3. Sans problème. Nous sommes allées sur TripAdvisor!

Most French verbs form the **passé composé** with **avoir** as the auxiliary verb. A few, however, require **être** as the auxiliary verb. One of these verbs is **aller.**

Presentation: Model pronunciation of past-tense forms of *aller* using simple sentences. Examples: *Je suis allé(e) en France l'année dernière. Où est-ce que vous êtes allé(e)?* (Question directed to a st. in class, who answers with *je* form). *Ah, il est allé en Californie,* etc.

PASSÉ COMPOSÉ OF **aller**			
je	suis all**é(e)**	nous	sommes all**é(e)s**
tu	es all**é(e)**	vous	êtes all**é(e)(s)**
il/on	est all**é***	ils	sont all**és**
elle	est all**ée**	elles	sont all**ées**

*When **on** clearly represents a plural subject, the past participle agrees with the subject (**on est allés**, **on est allées**). The auxiliary verb will always stay singular.

1. The past participle of verbs conjugated with **être** in the **passé composé** agrees with the subject in gender and number.

Marc est all**é** au Japon.	*Marc went to Japan.*
Agathe est all**ée** en Côte d'Ivoire.	*Agathe went to Ivory Coast.*
Benjamin et Loïc sont all**és** à Chartres.	*Benjamin and Loïc went to Chartres.*
Elles sont all**ées** à Hawaï.	*They went to Hawaii.*

2. The following verbs take **être** in the **passé composé.** Note that most convey motion or a change in state. Irregular past participles are indicated in parentheses.

aller *to go*	**passer** *to pass*
arriver *to arrive*	**rentrer** *to return; to go home*
descendre *to go down; to get off*	**rester** *to stay*
devenir (devenu) *to become*	**retourner** *to return; to go back*
entrer *to enter*	**revenir (revenu)** *to come back*
monter *to go up; to climb*	**sortir** *to go out*
mourir (mort) *to die*	**tomber** *to fall*
naître (né) *to be born*	**venir (venu)** *to come*
partir *to leave*	

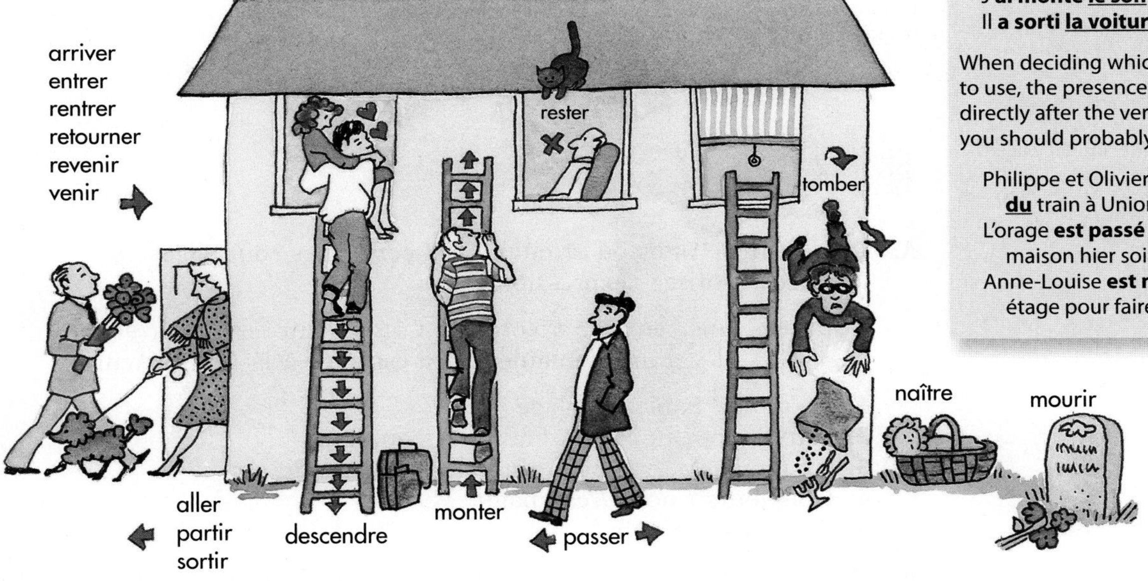

[Allez-y! A-B-C]

Suggestion: Present the acronym DR. and MRS. VANDERTRAMPP (*descendre, rester, monter,* etc.) to help sts. remember these verbs. Note that all verbs except *devenir* are pictured in the drawing.

Suggestion: Emphasize that *rester* means *to stay;* one expresses "to rest" with *se reposer.*

Suggestion: Briefly explain what "direct object" means: It answers the questions *qui? qu'est-ce que?;* there is nothing between the verb and the object.

Vocabulary recycling: Quickly review the presentation of *partir, sortir,* and *quitter* in *Chapitre 8, Leçon 2.* Have sts. go to the board and transform the example sentences in that presentation from present to *passé composé,* making all necessary changes: *Je suis parti(e) lundi,* etc.

Suggestion: Have sts. close books after looking at list of verbs and dictate a half dozen sentences using some of these verbs for immediate written reinforcement.

Mots clés

Avoir ou *être*?

Some of these **"être"** verbs may be followed by a direct object. When this occurs, they take **avoir** in the **passé composé**.

Nous **avons descendu la rivière** en bateau.
Elle **a passé la frontière** (*border*) hier.
J'**ai monté le son** de la radio.
Il **a sorti la voiture** du garage.

When deciding which auxiliary verb to use, the presence of a preposition directly after the verb is one clue that you should probably use **être.**

Philippe et Olivier **sont descendus du** train à Union Station.
L'orage **est passé à côté de** ma maison hier soir.
Anne-Louise **est montée au** 1er étage pour faire ses devoirs.

Grammaire interactive

For more on the **passé composé** with **avoir** and **être**, watch the corresponding Grammar Tutorial and take a brief practice quiz at **Connect French.**

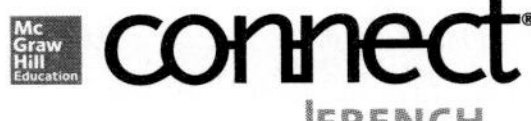

www.mhconnectfrench.com

3. Word order in negative and interrogative sentences in the **passé composé** with **être** is the same as that for the **passé composé** with **avoir.**

Je **ne suis pas** allé au cours.	*I did not go to class.*
Sont-ils arrivés à l'heure?	*Did they arrive on time?*

[Allez-y! D-E]

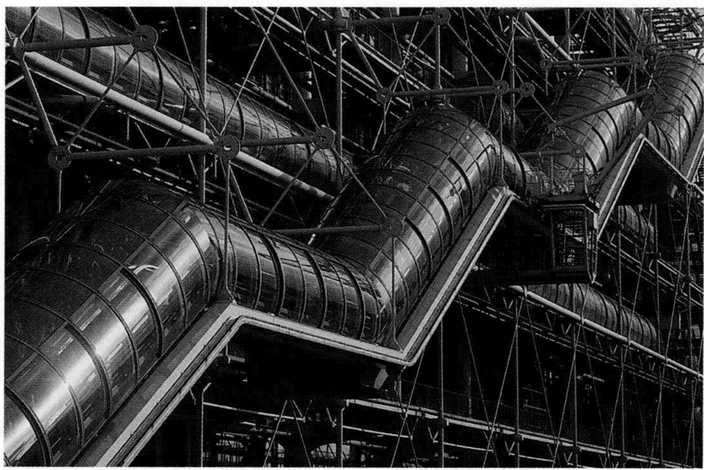

L'année dernière, je suis allée voir le Centre Pompidou à Paris. C'est une usine (*factory*)? une église? un musée?

Mots clés

L'expression *il y a*

The expression **il y a** used with a time period means *ago.* It requires a past tense.

> Ils sont allés au Mexique **il y a** deux ans.
> *They went to Mexico two years ago.*

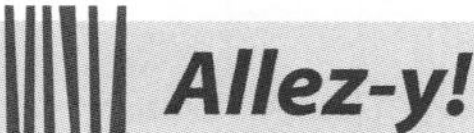

Allez-y!

A. Des sorties. Dites où et quand ces personnes sont allées en vacances. Utilisez l'expression **il y a.**

MODÈLE: une semaine / Nora / la Côte d'Azur →
Il y a une semaine, Nora est allée à la Côte d'Azur.

1. un mois / Fabrice / plage
2. deux jours / tu / forêt / faire du camping
3. six mois / Mme Robert / montagne / faire du ski
4. trois jours / nous / campagne
5. deux ans / je / Nice

Suggestion (B): Give sts. a few minutes to write answers before soliciting oral responses.

Follow-up (B): Ask sts. to invent a similar story, using the following stimuli, which can be dictated or handed out: *Ils vont à la montagne. Ils partent à 6 h du matin. Ils retournent à 6 h 30. Ils entrent dans la maison pour chercher des objets oubliés (leurs skis!). Ils montent dans la voiture. Ils partent de nouveau. Un des skis tombe de la galerie.* Sts. end story as they wish.

B. Départ en vacances. Les Astier, vos voisins, sont partis en vacances ce week-end. Vous racontez maintenant la scène à vos amis. Complétez l'histoire de façon logique et mettez les verbes au passé composé.

Ce matin, mes voisins les Astier ______[1] en vacances. Ils ______[2] à la mer. À 8 h, M. Astier et son fils ______[3] et ______[4] de la maison plusieurs fois avec des sacs et des valises. Mme Astier ______[5] cinq fois dans la maison pour aller chercher des objets oubliés.

Enfin, trois heures plus tard, toute la famille ______[6] dans la voiture et elle ______[7]. Mais pas de chance, une des valises ______[8] de la galerie (*roof rack*). M. Astier ______[9] de la voiture pour la remettre sur la galerie et ils ______[10]. Moi, je ______[11] chez moi.

aller
entrer
partir
retourner
sortir
descendre
monter
partir
repartir
rester
tomber

C. Week-end en Suisse. Valentine et Edgar ont passé le week-end à Genève. Mettez l'histoire au passé composé et faites attention au choix de l'auxiliaire (**avoir** ou **être**).

Edgar vient[1] chercher Valentine pour aller à la gare. Ils montent[2] dans le train. Ils cherchent[3] leur voiture. Le train part[4] quelques minutes plus tard. Il entre[5] en gare de Genève à midi. Edgar et Valentine descendent[6] du train et vont[7] tout de suite à l'hôtel. L'après-midi, ils sortent[8] visiter la ville. Le soir, ils dînent[9] dans un restaurant élégant. Dimanche Valentine va[10] au musée et prend[11] beaucoup de photos de la ville. Edgar reste[12] à l'hôtel. Valentine et Edgar quittent[13] Genève en fin d'après-midi. Ils arrivent[14] à Paris fatigués mais contents de leur week-end.

Qu'est-ce que Valentine a fait qu'Edgar n'a pas fait?

Suggestion: Have sts. write out or give orally the past-tense rendition of this story. Can be done as a short composition, with sts. embellishing story as they wish.

Additional activity: *Alice vous pose des questions sur les activités de vos amis. Répondez à la forme négative. 1. Est-ce que Marianne est déjà montée dans un TGV? 2. Est-ce que son vol est arrivé à l'heure? 3. Sont-ils partis en vacances en train? 4. Êtes-vous allé(e) en France récemment? 5. Sont-ils restés longtemps en Espagne? 6. Es-tu passé(e) par la Suisse? 7. Es-tu rentré(e) en bateau? 8. Sont-elles revenues à San Francisco en septembre?*

D. Les voyageurs. Gaspard, Julien et Arthur ont passé une partie de leurs vacances ensemble (*together*). Ils regardent les photos des vacances et essaient de se souvenir (*try to remember*) des détails. Complétez leur conversation au passé composé.

GASPARD: Tu te souviens quand nous ______[1]? **arriver**
JULIEN: Nous ______[2] dans le train à Metz le 19 avril **monter**
vers 6 h et nous ______[3] à Nice le soir. **partir**
GASPARD: Est-ce que Arthur ______[4] voir sa copine **passer**
de Nice le même (*same*) jour?
JULIEN: Non, il ______[5] chez elle le lendemain **aller**
et ils ______[6] pour l'Italie le 21. **partir**
GASPARD: Arthur et toi, vous ______[7] ensemble **rentrer**
à la fin des vacances, non?
JULIEN: Oui, et toi tu ______[8] à la plage une **rester**
semaine de plus et tu ______[9] en mai. **revenir**
C'est vraiment trop injuste!

E. Souvenirs de vacances. Décrivez les vacances de l'année passée d'un(e) camarade. D'abord, posez les questions suivantes à votre camarade. Si vous voulez, posez encore d'autres questions. Ensuite, présentez à la classe une description de ses vacances.

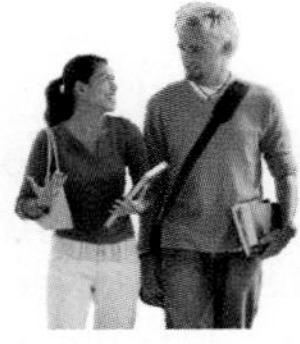

1. Quand es-tu parti(e)? Où es-tu allé(e)? Es-tu resté(e) aux États-Unis ou es-tu allé(e) à l'étranger? As-tu visité un endroit exotique?
2. Es-tu allé(e) voir l'endroit où tes parents sont nés? Où es-tu né(e)?
3. Qu'est-ce que tu as fait pendant les vacances? Est-ce que tu as rencontré des gens (*people*) intéressants?
4. Comment es-tu rentré(e): en avion ou en voiture? Es-tu revenu(e) mort(e) de fatigue?
5. Est-ce que tu prépares déjà tes vacances de l'année prochaine?

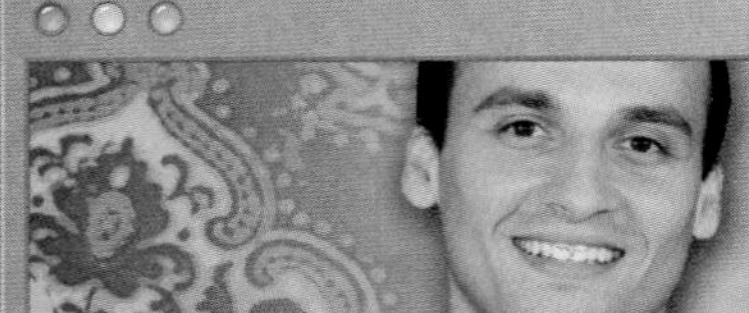

Le blog d'Hassan

Partir!

samedi 13 juin

L'été dernier, j'ai passé des vacances super originales: j'ai fait un échange de logements. Je vous explique: je voulais[1] aller en Louisiane, mais pas comme un simple touriste. Je voulais vivre une expérience authentique. Par Internet, j'ai contacté une famille de La Nouvelle-Orléans qui voulait passer ses vacances à Paris. Et nous avons échangé nos logements: je suis allé chez eux; ils sont venus chez moi.

J'ai découvert La Nouvelle-Orléans, capitale du jazz; j'ai pique-niqué dans le parc Louis Armstrong, j'ai descendu le Mississippi en bateau… Le soir, je rentrais[2] «chez moi» pour cuisiner les spécialités locales. Depuis mon séjour[3] en Louisiane, je suis le champion des haricots rouges avec du riz!

Pendant ce temps, Debby et son mari Scott vivaient[4] dans mon appartement parisien et arrosaient[5] mes plantes!

Maintenant, une amitié est née entre nous.

Et vous? Vous avez déjà pratiqué ce type d'échanges? C'était comment[6]?

Hassan

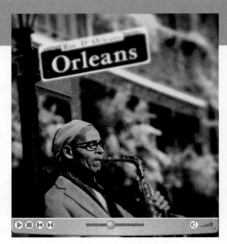

Ça, c'est vraiment La Nouvelle-Orléans!

Suggestion: Model pronunciation and have sts. repeat individually or as a group.

Follow-up: 1. *Expliquez l'expression «pas comme un simple touriste»: que veut dire Hassan?* 2. *Qu'a fait Hassan pendant ses vacances en Louisiane?* 3. *D'après l'expérience d'Hassan, quels sont les avantages d'un échange de logements?* 4. *Quelles sont les objections de Charlotte? Répondez-lui.* 5. *Que propose Poema? Êtes-vous tenté(e)? Expliquez votre réaction.*

Video connection: In the videoblog for this chapter, Hassan and Léa explore various vacation possibilities using an Internet site for house exchanges.

COMMENTAIRES

Alexis

C'était fabuleux: il y a trois ans, j'ai échangé mon appartement de Québec avec un couple de la Réunion. Trésor et moi, nous sommes restés deux semaines chez eux, dans une belle villa avec piscine.[7] On a visité l'île; on a fait de la planche à voile, du ski nautique, de la plongée sous-marine, des randonnées… Eux, ils sont «tombés en amour[8]» pour le Québec!

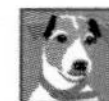

Trésor

Moi, j'ai nagé dans l'océan Indien!

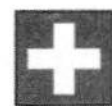

Charlotte

Hassan et Alexis, je pense que vous êtes fous[9]! Des étrangers dorment dans votre lit; ils mangent dans vos assiettes…

Alexis

Et alors? C'est comme à l'hôtel.

Poema

Alexis, est-ce que tu as déjà des projets de vacances pour l'année prochaine? Mes parents ont une jolie villa en Polynésie, à Bora-Bora…

[1]*wanted* [2]*returned* [3]Depuis… *Since my stay* [4]*were living* [5]*were watering* [6]C'était… *How was it?* [7]*pool* [8]tombés… *fell in love (expression used in Quebec)* [9]*crazy*

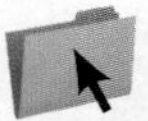

REPORTAGE

France: le pays des grandes vacances

Suggestion: Ask sts. to describe the photo: *Quelles sont les activities des gens sur la plage?*

Chez les Beaufour, on voyage énormément. Mme Beaufour est professeur et a presque[1] quatre mois de congés[2] payés; M. Beaufour, comme tous les salariés, a au minimum cinq semaines de vacances. «À Noël, explique Mme Beaufour, toute la famille part à la neige. Les vacances de février sont généralement consacrées à[3] un petit voyage en Suisse. Pour Pâques, nous passons toujours une semaine chez ma mère qui possède une maison de campagne à Aix-en-Provence. Enfin, pour les vacances d'été, nous aimons le camping.»

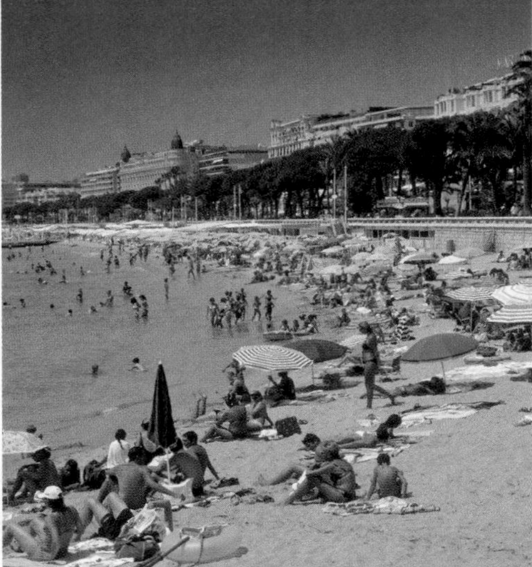

Voilà les vacances! À Cannes, sur la Côte d'Azur, on peut bronzer, nager, faire de la planche à voile ou de la plongée libre et s'amuser.

En France, les vacances sont sacrées et intouchables.

À Noël et en février, les Français privilégient[4] la montagne. À Pâques, on choisit souvent des vacances familiales. En été, on va se faire bronzer sur les plages de la Côte d'Azur ou on pratique le «tourisme vert» à la campagne.

Les jours de départ en vacances sont souvent un vrai cauchemar[5] à cause des embouteillages[6]: pour ne pas perdre une seule minute de leurs précieuses vacances, les Français partent tous le même jour, à la même heure, sur les mêmes autoroutes! Alors voici un bon conseil: en hiver et au printemps, évitez[7] de vous trouver sur les routes du soleil ou de la montagne la veille[8] de Noël ou de Pâques. C'est l'enfer[9]! Et en été, ne partez pas le 1er juillet ou le 1er août: sur l'autoroute du Sud, les vacanciers restent prisonniers de leurs voitures pendant des heures!

[1]*almost* [2]*vacation* [3]consacrées... *devoted to* [4]*favor* [5]*nightmare* [6]à... *because of traffic jams* [7]*avoid* [8]*day before* [9]*hell*

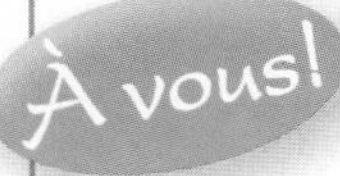

1. Combien de semaines de vacances ont M. et Mme Beaufour? Leur cas est-il unique en France?
2. À quels moments les Français prennent-ils leurs vacances?
3. Comparez les vacances des Français à celles (*those*) des Américains: quelles différences observez-vous? Préférez-vous le système français ou le système américain? Pourquoi?

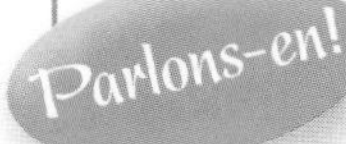

- Dans quelle ville, quelle région, quel pays passez-vous vos vacances?
- Pour combien de temps partez-vous en vacances?
- Quelles sont vos activités pendant les vacances?
- Quels pays rêvez-vous de visiter? Pourquoi?

1. Répondez, par écrit, aux questions ci-dessus (*above*). Écrivez chaque réponse sur une fiche (*index card*) différente.
2. Donnez vos fiches au professeur. Il/Elle va les mélanger (*mix them up*) et les redistribuer.
3. Lisez à voix haute la fiche que vous avez reçue (*received*).
4. Avec l'aide de la classe, devinez qui est l'auteur de la fiche.

CHAPITRE **8**

Leçon 3

STRUCTURES

L'expression impersonnelle *il faut*

Expressing Obligation and Necessity

Des vacances aux Antilles

Poema téléphone à Alexis.

POEMA: Pour aller à la Guadeloupe, est-ce qu'**il faut**[1] un visa?
ALEXIS: Non! La Guadeloupe, c'est la France! **Il faut présenter** une carte d'identité ou un passeport.
POEMA: Je suis toujours anxieuse quand je voyage! J'ai peur d'oublier quelque chose.[2]
ALEXIS: Poema, sois cool! Aux Antilles, **il faut** simplement des lunettes de soleil, une serviette de plage et une crème solaire. C'est tout!
POEMA: Et pour le soir?
ALEXIS: Pour le soir, **il faut avoir** une jolie robe pour aller danser!

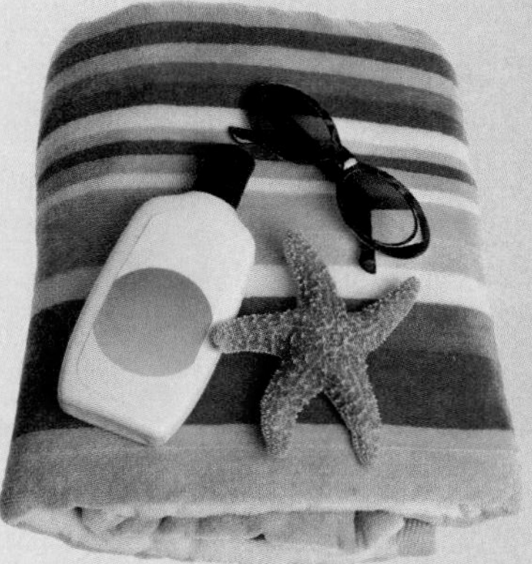
Le bonheur simple à la Guadeloupe

[1]il est nécessaire d'(avoir) [2]d'oublier... *of forgetting something*

Répondez aux questions. Utilisez l'expression **il faut.**

1. Pour aller à la Guadeloupe, quels documents administratifs faut-il?
2. Pour la plage, qu'est-ce qu'il faut?
3. Et pour le soir, qu'est-ce qu'il faut avoir?

Note: *Il faut* is presented again with the subjunctive.

Suggestion: Point out other impersonal forms: *il est tard, il fait, il pleut, il y a*, etc.

1. The expression **il faut** is the impersonal form of the verb **falloir.** Followed by an infinitive, it is used to express general obligation or a necessity.

Il faut étudier pour réussir.	*One has to study to do well.*
Il faut manger pour vivre.	*One has to (It is necessary to) eat to live.*

In the near future (**le futur proche**), **il faut** + infinitive becomes **il va falloir** + infinitive. In the **passé composé,** it becomes **il a fallu.**

Nous avons une réservation pour le train à 8 h: **il va falloir** arriver à l'heure.	*We have a train reservation for 8:00: We will have to be on time.*
Il a fallu réserver très tôt en avance.	*We had to make our reservation very early.*

2. In the negative, the form **il ne faut pas** (*one must not*) expresses a prohibited action.

Il ne faut pas boire d'eau non-potable.	*You must not (should not) drink untreated water.*

3. **Il faut** can also be followed by nouns referring to objects or to qualities to talk about what is needed. The indefinte or partitive article is usually used before the noun in the construction **il faut** + noun.

Pour aller à la Guadeloupe, **il faut** un visa?	*To go to Guadeloupe, do you need a visa?*
Pour faire de la soupe à l'oignon, **il faut** des oignons, du consommé de bœuf, du gruyère et du pain.	*To make onion soup, you need onions, beef broth, Swiss cheese, and bread.*
Il faut du courage pour manger des escargots!	*One needs courage to eat snails!*

Suggestion: You may wish to point out that *il n'est pas nécessaire de/d'...* means "it is not necessary to . . ."

Allez-y!

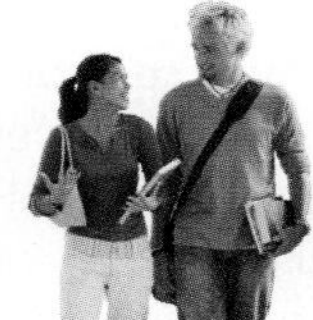

A. **Qu'est-ce qu'il faut?** Répondez aux questions avec un(e) camarade et notez vos conclusions. Répondez avec **il faut** + *infinitif* ou *nom.*

MODÈLE: pour passer une soirée à la française? →
Qu'est-ce qu'il faut pour passer une soirée à la française?
Il faut des amis. (*ou* Il faut aimer la bonne cuisine. / Il faut prendre son temps.)

1. pour passer des vacances parfaites?
2. pour fêter son anniversaire?
3. pour s'amuser (*to have fun*) à une soirée à l'américaine?
4. pour se faire «une bonne bouffe (*a big meal*)»?
5. pour ne pas grossir (*not to gain weight*)?
6. pour être en bonne santé (*health*)?
7. pour bien dormir?

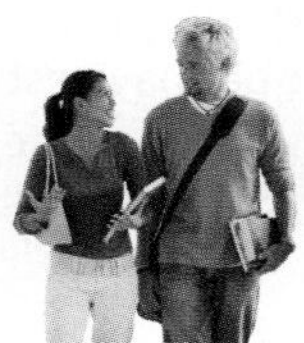

B. **Conversation à trois.** Avec deux autres camarades, vous allez organiser un voyage pour toute la classe. Qu'est-ce que vous voulez faire? Où voulez-vous voyager? Qu'est-ce qu'il faut faire avant de partir? Qu'est-ce qu'il faut acheter? Comment voulez-vous partager le travail? Utilisez les verbes **pouvoir, vouloir** et **devoir** et l'expression **il faut.**

Expressions utiles: devoir acheter, devoir apporter, devoir commander, devoir demander, pouvoir acheter, pouvoir choisir, vouloir bien

Après votre conversation, décrivez le voyage à la classe.

Le parler jeune

avoir la pêche être en forme, de bonne humeur et plein d'énergie
se barrer / se casser partir
s'éclater / se marrer s'amuser
marrant amusant, intéressant
quel pied! exprime le plaisir absolu

Moi, pour **avoir la pêche,** je fais du sport.

La copine de Sébastien n'est pas à la fête, alors il **se casse.**

Les vacances, c'est fait pour **s'éclater.**

C'est **marrant,** la plongée sous-marine, avec tous ces poissons...

Bronzer sur une plage de Tunisie, **quel pied!**

Suggestion (B): Have sts. write out their comments before presenting them orally to the class. One st. can be the note taker.

Vocabulary recycling: Take this opportunity to review intensively the adjectives of nationality from *Chapitre 2, Leçon 1: Un citoyen / Une citoyenne du Japon? C'est un Japonais / une Japonaise,* etc.

Les prépositions devant les noms de lieu

Expressing Location

Soyez extravagants!

Hassan, Abdel et Carole discutent.

Une plage de rêve aux Seychelles

HASSAN: Finalement, vous allez vous marier **à** Paris!

ABDEL: Oui, on va faire un mariage marocain à l'Institut du monde arabe, dans le 5ᵉ arrondissement. Il y a une belle salle au dernier étage, avec une grande terrasse.

CAROLE: Avec ce choix, tout le monde est content: on est à la fois[1] **au** Maroc et **en** France!

ABDEL: Ensuite, on va aller **à** Venise, **en** Italie!

CAROLE: Pour notre voyage de noces[2]!

HASSAN: Venise? Quel conformisme! Pourquoi n'allez-vous pas **à** Tahiti **en** Polynésie française, **à** Zanzibar en Afrique, ou **aux** Seychelles dans l'océan Indien? Soyez extravagants!

CAROLE: Pas question! C'est trop cher! Et puis, j'aime Venise parce que c'est romantique.

ABDEL: … Et moi, j'aime Carole et je veux lui faire plaisir[3]!

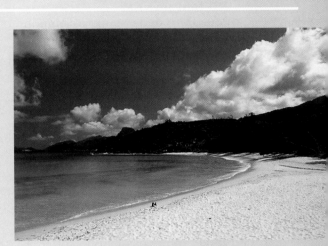

[1]à… *at the same time* [2]voyage… *honeymoon* [3]lui… *make her happy*

Répondez aux questions.

1. Dans quelle ville le mariage va-t-il être organisé?
2. Dans quel pays est l'Institut du monde arabe?
3. Où les futurs mariés vont-ils faire leur voyage de noces?
4. Quels pays et quelles villes Hassan suggère-t-il?

Presentation: Use maps, and ask sts. to give the country name using the article to indicate gender. Later you can use these maps to have sts. say *Je vais en/au/aux… ; Je reviens de/du/des…*

Note: Additional countries not mentioned in this section: *l'Argentine, l'Autriche, la Bolivie, le Brésil, la Bulgarie, le Chili, Cuba, l'Égypte, le Guatemala, l'Indonésie, l'Iran (m.), la Jordanie, le Kenya, le Liban, le Nicaragua, le Nigéria, la Norvège, le Pakistan, le Panama, la Pologne, la République Tchèque, la Roumanie, la Slovaquie, le Soudan, la Thaïlande, la Turquie, le Venezuela.*

Gender of Geographical Nouns

1. In French, most place names that end in **-e** are feminine; most others are masculine. One important exception: **le Mexique.**
2. The names of the continents are feminine: **l'Afrique, l'Amérique du Nord, l'Amérique du Sud, l'Antarctique, l'Asie, l'Europe, l'Océanie** (Australia and the Pacific islands).

3. The names of most states in the United States are masculine regardless of their ending: **le Texas, le Tennessee.** There are nine exceptions:

la Californie	la Louisiane
la Caroline du Nord et du Sud	la Pennsylvanie
la Floride	la Virginie
la Géorgie	la Virginie-Occidentale

Note: Point out that the use of prepositions with the names of states in the U.S. varies. Usually, if the state is feminine, it is preceded by *en* and *de*. Masculine states beginning with a vowel or vowel sound take *en* and *de*. Some islands may also take *en*, e.g., *en Islande* and *en Sicile*. French speakers do not always agree on these points.

Prepositions with Geographical Names

	TO, AT, IN		FROM	
cities islands	**à**	Suzanne habite **à** Lyon. Ils sont allés **à** Cuba.	**de** **(d')**	Elle vient **de** Montréal. Ils arrivent **d'**Hawaï.
continents	**en**	Lidia est née **en** Amérique du Sud.	**de** **(d')**	Je pars **d'**Europe.
feminine countries, states, provinces	**en**	Il y a deux ans, vous avez fait un voyage **en** Suisse. Bâton Rouge est **en** Louisiane. Les explorateurs sont arrivés **en** Nouvelle-Écosse.	**de** **(d')**	Jean arrive **de** Floride. Viviane est **de** Colombie-Britannique.
masculine countries, states, or provinces starting with a vowel		On a voyagé **en** Israël. Il est né **en** Alaska. Elle a travaillé **en** Ontario.		Elle vient **d'**Iran. Ils arrivent **d'**Oregon. Mariane est originaire **d'**Ontario.
masculine countries or provinces starting with a consonant	**au**	**Au** Canada, il y a dix provinces. Je voudrais aller **au** Québec.*	**du**	Ils reviennent **du** Brésil. Il va partir **du** Nouveau-Brunswick.
all plural countries	**aux**	Il y a dix ans, ils sont arrivés **aux** États-Unis.	**des**	Quand sont-ils partis **des** Pays-Bas?
regions masculine states† starting with a consonant	**dans le**	Elle va **dans le** Poitou. J'aime l'automne **dans le** Vermont.	**du** **(de l')**	Nous revenons **du** Sud. Elle vient **du** Colorado.

Suggestion: Review the contractions with *à* and *de*.

Additional activity: *À la chaîne.* St. 1: *En Amérique du Nord* (continent), *il y a les États-Unis* (country). St. 2: *Aux États-Unis, il y a la Californie* (state or province, if possible). St. 3: *En Californie, il y a San Francisco* (city). St. 4: *À San Francisco, il y a le Golden Gate* (object, attraction, etc.).

Pronunciation practice (1): Read the following phrases to sts. and have them decide whether they hear *à* or *au* / *aux: aux États-Unis, à Cleveland, aux Îles Canaries, au Sud, aux Émirats Arabes Unis, à Montréal, au Michigan.*

Pronunciation practice (2): The *Prononcez bien!* section on page 224 of this chapter contains additional activities for practicing these sounds.

*__au Québec__ refers to the province; **à Québec** refers to the city
†Some exceptions: **au / du** Texas
au / du Nouveau-Mexique
dans l'état de / de l'état de New York / Washington (to distinguish the states from the cities)

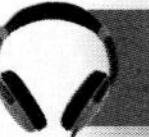

Prononcez bien!

The vowels in *à*, *au*, and *aux*

Make sure you clearly distinguish between [a] and [o] when you pronounce **à** and **au.** Pronounce brief and tense sounds.

Open your mouth wide to say **à.**

[a]: **à Montréal, à La Nouvelle-Orléans**

Close your mouth and round your lips to say **au** and **aux.**

[o]: **au Sénégal, aux Pays-Bas**

Suggestion (A-B): After modeling a few answers, have sts. do activities in pairs for maximum practice. Have sts. come back to whole group periodically to check their answers, or prepare written answer sheets to pass out for correction. If latter idea is used, have 3 sts. in a group, with 1 st. checking answers of others against key. Sts. can take turns using answer key to monitor work of others.

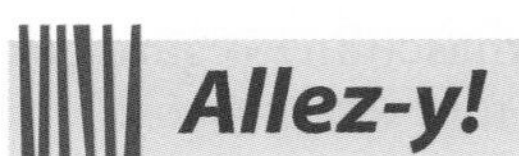

A. Jeu géographique. Voici quelques villes francophones. Dans quels pays se trouvent-elles? (Voir les cartes à la fin du livre.)

MODÈLE: Paris est en France.

1. Rabat	**a.** Haïti
2. Montréal	**b.** la Belgique
3. Kinshasa	**c.** la Tunisie
4. Alger	**d.** la République Démocratique du Congo
5. Dakar	**e.** le Canada
6. Bruxelles	**f.** la Suisse
7. Tunis	**g.** le Maroc
8. Abidjan	**h.** la Côte d'Ivoire
9. Port-au-Prince	**i.** l'Algérie
10. Genève	**j.** le Sénégal

Additional activity: *Pendant son voyage, votre camarade vous envoie des cartes postales. D'où a-t-il/elle envoyé les cartes postales?* MODÈLE: *Afrique / Maroc — Cette carte postale vient-elle d'Afrique? — Oui, il/elle a envoyé cette carte du Maroc.* 1. *Asie / Japon* 2. *Amérique du Nord / Canada* 3. *Asie / Russie* 4. *Afrique / Égypte* 5. *Asie / Inde* 6. *Amérique du Sud / Brésil* 7. *Europe / Suisse*

Continuation (B): *des marrons glacés, des spaghettis, une statue des Pyramides, du whisky, du thé*

B. Retour de vacances. Un groupe de touristes rentre de vacances. D'après ce qu'ils ont dans leurs valises, dites d'où ils arrivent.

MODÈLE: une montre
la Suisse → Ils arrivent de Suisse.

SOUVENIRS	PAYS
1. du parfum	le Cameroun
2. un caméscope (*video camera*)	la Hollande
3. une bouteille de tequila	l'Italie
4. un masque d'initiation	le Mexique
5. des chaussures en cuir (*leather*)	le Japon
	l'Écosse
6. un pull en cachemire	le Maroc
7. des tulipes	la Colombie
8. du café	la Belgique
9. un couscoussier (*couscous maker*)	la France
10. du chocolat	

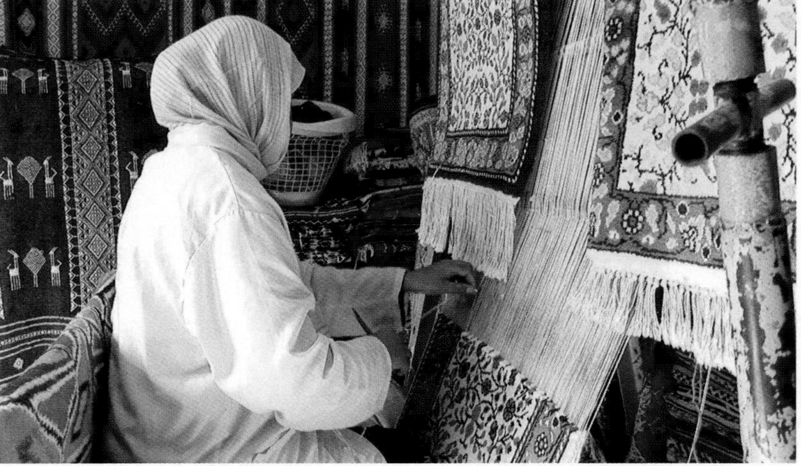

À Tunis, on trouve de beaux tapis.

C. Un(e) jeune globe-trotter. Votre camarade va faire le tour du monde. Vous lui demandez où il/elle va aller.

Continents: l'Afrique, l'Amérique du Nord, l'Amérique du Sud, l'Antarctique, l'Asie, l'Europe, l'Océanie

Pays: l'Algérie, l'Allemagne, l'Australie, le Brésil, le Canada, la Chine, le Danemark, l'Égypte, les États-Unis, la Finlande, la Grèce, l'Inde, l'Italie, le Japon, le Maroc, le Mexique, la Polynésie française, la Norvège, le Vietnam…

MODÈLE: É1: Vas-tu en Asie?
É2: Oui, je vais en Chine (au Japon…).

D. Interview. Posez les questions à un(e) camarade de classe. Ensuite, révélez sa réponse la plus surprenante à la classe.

1. D'où viens-tu? De quelle ville? De quel état? Et tes parents?
2. Où habitent tes parents? Et le reste de ta famille?
3. Dans quels états as-tu voyagé?
4. Est-ce qu'il y a un état que tu préfères? Pourquoi?
5. Dans quel état est-ce qu'il y a de beaux parcs? de beaux lacs? de belles montagnes? de grandes villes? de grands déserts?

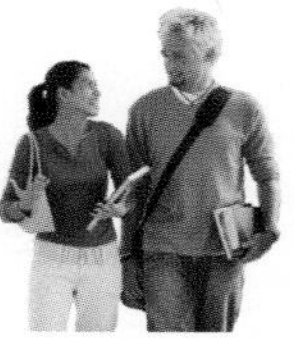

Suggestion (D): Sts. ask questions and take brief notes on classmates' answers in order to report information. Ex. can be done in groups of 3.

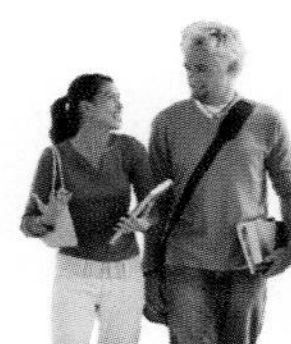

Continuation (D): Sts. can also ask: *Quels pays est-ce que tu as visités? Quelles villes est-ce que tu aimerais* (would you like) *visiter? Pourquoi? Est-ce que tu as déjà visité une île? Laquelle* (Which one)*? Où est-ce que tu aimerais habiter?*

Follow-up (D): Each group reports information about states they come from and states they prefer. Answers are added up to answer final questions of activity.

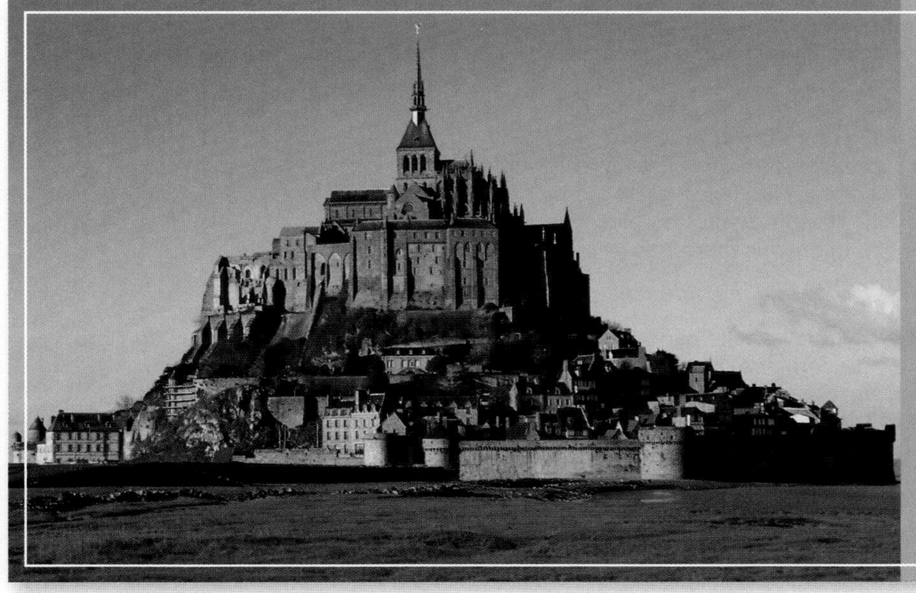

Un peu plus…

Le Mont-Saint-Michel.
C'est un monument avec une histoire riche. Située au large des (*off the*) côtes bretonne et normande, la petite île rocheuse héberge (*shelters*) depuis l'an 966 une abbaye bénédictine dédiée à Saint Michel. Haut lieu de spiritualité, les pèlerinages (*pilgrimages*) au Mont-Saint-Michel ont eu lieu tout au long de son histoire. L'abbaye héberge également des documents précieux qui datent du Moyen Âge. Aujourd'hui, le Mont-Saint-Michel accueille des visiteurs du monde entier. Avez-vous déjà visité un monument avec une histoire riche? Expliquez.

◀ *Le Mont-Saint-Michel, en Normandie*

Prononcez bien!

Script (1A): *1. J'adore pêcher à la ligne. 2. Ma copine Line pêche très bien. 3. C'est la reine de la pêche! 4. Elle règne sur cette activité! 5. Elle finit toujours la journée avec beaucoup de poissons dans son panier. 6. Et le soir, on mange beaucoup de poissons panés!*

Answers (1A): *1. ligne 2. Line 3. reine 4. règne 5. panier 6. panés*

1. The pronunciation of *montagne* (page 202)

A. La pêche. Hugo parle de son activité préférée: la pêche. Choisissez le mot que vous entendez dans chaque phrase.

1.	☐ Line	☐ ligne (*line*)
2.	☐ Line	☐ ligne
3.	☐ reine (*queen*)	☐ règne (*rules* [verb])
4.	☐ reine	☐ règne
5.	☐ panés (*deep-fried*)	☐ panier (*basket*)
6.	☐ panés	☐ panier

B. La pêche (suite). Hugo raconte son meilleur souvenir (*best memory*) de pêche. Avec votre camarade, répétez ses mots. Faites bien attention à la prononciation des mots français en italique.

1. La *dernière* fois (*time*) que j'ai péché à la *ligne*, c'était pendant le voyage que j'ai *gagné* à la loterie.
2. Pour ce voyage, je suis allé à *Cologne*, en *Allemagne*. C'était *magnifique*! Je voudrais bien y retourner (*go back there*)!

Script (2): *1. Il vient samedi prochain. 2. Ils reviennent de vacances à Vienne, en Autriche. 3. Il tient à me présenter sa fiancée. 4. Ils deviennent de plus en plus amoureux. Je suis impatient de rencontrer Lisa!*

Answers (2): *1. Simon 2. Simon et Lisa 3. Simon 4. Simon et Lisa*

2. The vowels in *viens* and *viennent* (page 210)

Un nouveau joueur. Hugo parle de son frère Simon et de la fiancée de Simon. Décidez si Hugo parle uniquement de Simon, ou de Simon et Lisa.

	Simon	**Simon et Lisa**
1. venir samedi prochain	☐	☐
2. revenir de vacances à Vienne, en Autriche	☐	☐
3. tenir à (*to be eager to*) me présenter sa fiancée	☐	☐
4. devenir de plus en plus amoureux (*more and more in love*)	☐	☐

Script (3A): *Je suis allée au Texas, à Hawaï, au Nouveau-Mexique, au Nevada, à New York, à Québec et au Saskatchewan. C'était super!*

Answers (3A): *1. au 2. à 3. au 4. au 5. à 6. à 7. au*

3. The vowels in *à, au,* and *aux* (page 221)

A. Voyage. Isabelle parle des vacances qu'elle a passées en Amérique du Nord l'été dernier. Écoutez et complétez le paragraphe avec ***à*** ou **au.**

Je suis allée _______[1] Texas, _______[2] Hawaï, _______[3] Nouveau-Mexique, _______[4] Nevada, _______[5] New York, _______[6] Québec et _______[7] Saskatchewan. C'était (*It was*) super!

Suggestion: Give sts. the French words for hyphen (*trait d'union*) and exclamation point (*point d'exclamation*) for the spelling of Saint-Louis-du-Ha! Ha!

Culture note: Have students go to the official website of the village of Saint-Louis-du-Ha! Ha! to read about the origins of its unusual name.

B. Voyage. Hugo parle aussi de ses vacances. Il était au Canada. Avec votre camarade, jouez la scène suivante.

HUGO: Moi, j'étais (*I was*) au Canada l'été dernier.
ISABELLE: Ah oui? Où ça?
HUGO: À Saint-Louis-du-Ha! Ha!, au Québec.
ISABELLE: Saint…? Comment est-ce que ça s'écrit? (*How is it spelled?*)
HUGO: S A I N T - L O U I S - D U - H A ! H A ! Ce n'est pas loin du lac Témiscouata dans le sud-est du Québec.
ISABELLE: Ah! Je sais (*know*) comment ça s'écrit! S A I N T - L O U I S - D U - H A ! H A !
HUGO: Exactement!

Leçon 4

Lecture

Avant de lire

Skimming for the gist. Skimming is a useful way to approach any new text, particularly in a foreign language. You will usually find it easier to understand more difficult passages once you have a general idea of the content. At this point, you need not be concerned with understanding everything when reading authentic French texts. Just try to get the gist, then answer the questions that follow the reading to check your overall comprehension.

In the following article, glance at the title and headings. What kind of information do you think the text contains, and how is the information organized? Next, skim the article to get the impression of the major points. Do not attempt to understand every word. Then, read the sections that may have appeared most difficult when you skimmed the article, and guess the meaning based on the rest of the text.

Un peu de pratique. Parcourez rapidement le texte suivant, puis choisissez la ville qui correspond à la description.

1. C'est un centre culturel.
2. C'est le centre politique du Maroc.
3. C'est une ville située près du désert.

Answers: 1. *Fès* 2. *Rabat* 3. *Ouarzazate*

Des vacances au Maroc

À propos de la lecture...
Les auteurs de *Vis-à-vis* ont écrit ce texte.

Prenez votre appareil photo et vos lunettes de soleil. Nous partons pour le Maroc en Afrique du Nord (au Maghreb*). Le Maroc est connu pour son climat exceptionnel et la variété de ses paysages. Villes impériales, oasis sahariennes, marchés extraordinaires: Oui, le Maroc a beaucoup de charme.

À voir

Sur la côte: Casablanca et Rabat, les deux capitales

La ville de Casablanca est la capitale économique du pays. Au bord de l'océan Atlantique, on trouve la mosquée Hassan II, la troisième plus grande mosquée du monde. Quatre-vingt

*Le Maghreb est l'ensemble des pays du nord-ouest de l'Afrique, situés entre la Méditerranée et le Sahara, l'océan Atlantique et le désert de Libye.

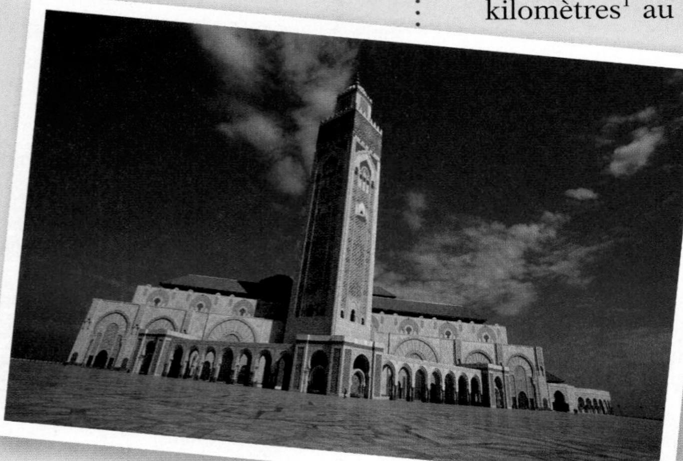

La mosquée Hassan II à Casablanca

kilomètres[1] au nord se trouve la ville de Rabat, une des quatre villes impériales (avec Fès, Marrakech et Meknès) et la capitale administrative et politique du pays. Les anciens quartiers européens aux grandes avenues modernes contrastent avec la médina[2] et ses monuments.

À l'intérieur: Fès, ville d'artisans

Fès est le centre culturel et spirituel du pays. Sa médina est la plus grande au monde avec plus de 9 000 ruelles[3] et de nombreux souks.[4] Les artisans travaillent, les marchands appellent les clients, il y a beaucoup de monde et beaucoup d'ambiance. Fès a une longue tradition de tannage du cuir,[5] d'art du bronze et de poterie bleue.

Au sud: Marrakech et Ouarzazate, les portes du désert

Marrakech, surnommée «la ville rouge», est entourée par une muraille[6] rouge et ocre, et une palmeraie[7] de 100 000 arbres. À l'intérieur des remparts, il y a la médina avec ses charmants ryads.[8] Mais Marrakech est surtout célèbre pour sa Place Jemaa El Fna où on peut voir tous les jours des conteurs,[9] des acrobates, des musiciens et même des charmeurs de serpents.

Située aux portes du Sahara et près des montagnes, Ouarzazate attire de nombreux touristes avec son atmosphère sereine, ses kasbahs[10] et ses paysages extraordinaires. C'est aussi un endroit très populaire avec Hollywood: *La Dernière Tentation du Christ*, *Gladiateur*, *Lawrence d'Arabie*, et *La Momie* ont été tournés[11] dans la région.

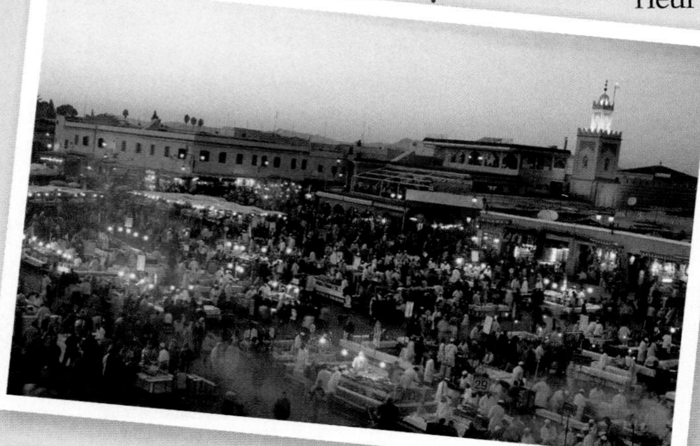

La Place Jemaa El Fna à Marrakech

À faire

Le sport

Au bord de la mer: voile, planche à voile, ski nautique, plongée, pêche, etc.

Dans le désert: planche à sable dans les dunes et excursions à dos de dromadaire.

Les festivals

Les nombreux festivals, en particulier le Festival des Musiques Sacrées du Monde à Fès, le Festival International du Film à Marrakech et la Fête des Roses dans la Vallée du Dadès.

[1]80 km = *about 50 miles* [2]vieille ville arabe [3]*alleys* [4]marchés [5]tannage... *tanning leather* [6]*wall* [7]*palm grove* [8]*villas* [9]*storytellers* [10]quartier fortifié [11]*filmed*

À goûter

Le tajine, c'est le plat national du Maroc. On mange aussi du couscous (le repas traditionnel du vendredi), des pastillas (feuilletés[12] au pigeon) et des pâtisseries à base d'amandes, de noisettes[13] et de dattes. On boit souvent du thé à la menthe. Passez de bonnes vacances!

[12]*flaky pastries* [13]*hazelnuts*

Note: For a description and photo of a *tajine marocain*, see *Reportage* (*Chapitre 7*). Point out to sts. that *tagine* is the name of the dish and the cooking vessel.

Compréhension

La destination de prédilection. Des touristes organisent leur itinéraire. Quel endroit mentionné dans le texte intéresserait (*would interest*) les personnes suivantes?

1. M. Os est passionné par le travail des artisans.
2. Mme Langlois fait une enquête sur le système politique marocain.
3. Mme Léonie aime les paysages désertiques.
4. Les enfants de M. Roman adorent le cirque.
5. Mlle Négoce est une femme d'affaires qui veut créer une entreprise.

Additional activity: *Situez le Maroc en répondant aux questions suivantes. Vocabulaire utile: se trouver; au nord / sud; à l'est / l'ouest.* 1. *Quel pays se trouve au nord, au sud, à l'est du Maroc?* 2. *Quelle est la capitale du pays?* 3. *Où se trouve-t-elle: à l'intérieur du pays ou sur la côte?* 4. *Selon vous, quel est le climat du Maroc (tropical, tempéré, glacial)?* 5. *Quelle est la religion de la majorité de la population?*

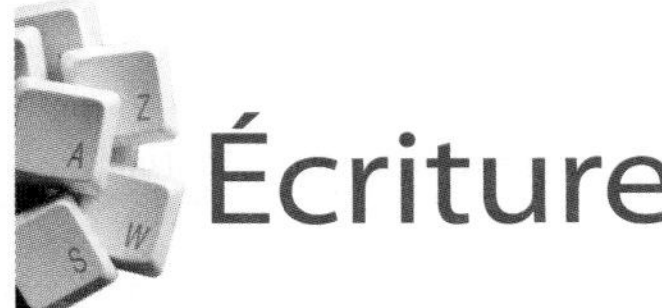

Écriture

The writing activities **Par écrit** and **Journal intime** can be found in the Workbook/Laboratory Manual to accompany *Vis-à-vis*.

Pour s'amuser

Dorothée est en vacances avec sa famille. Sa grand-mère lui téléphone:

—Alors, ces vacances, ça se passe bien?
—Génial!
—Que fais-tu?
—Rien!
—Et ton frère?
—Il m'aide!

La vie en chantant. An activity based on the song "Dans mon île" by Henri Salvador can be found in the Instructor's Manual. The song can be purchased at the iTunes store, or sts. can watch the music video on YouTube.

Le vidéoblog d'Hassan

En bref

Dans cet épisode, Léa et Hassan consultent un site Web qui leur donne des renseignements (*information*) sur des échanges de logement au Québec, au Maroc et à la Martinique. Hassan évoque les activités touristiques à Paris.

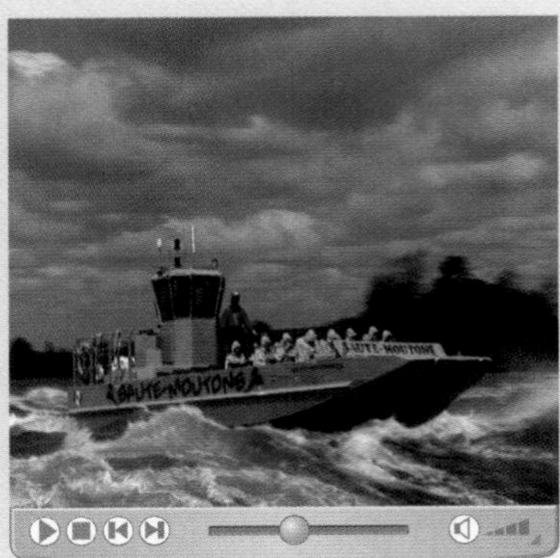

Le Saute-Moutons brave les rapides de Lachine sur le fleuve Saint-Laurent près de Montréal.

Additional vocabulary: Computer terms in this episode include *site Internet, Clique!, page d'accueil, écran.* Other vocabulary you may wish to present before viewing includes *contre, gratuitement, On ne peut pas tout savoir, Tiens, vas-y!*

Vocabulaire en contexte

Où aimez-vous vous loger et qu'est-ce que vous aimez faire quand vous êtes en vacances? Indiquez vos préférences.

Logement
- ☐ une tente et un sac de couchage
- ☐ un appartement en ville
- ☐ une villa **au bord de la mer** (*at the seaside*)
- ☐ un chalet à la montagne
- ☐ un hôtel somptueux dans une capitale **étrangère** (*foreign*)

Activités
- ☐ bronzer à la plage
- ☐ faire des randonnées et du rafting
- ☐ aller dans des musées et des galeries d'art
- ☐ faire de la pêche et de la plongée sous-marine
- ☐ **flâner** (*stroll*); observer la vie **quotidienne** (*everyday*) des gens

Note culturelle

Le Saute-Moutons est une des principales attractions de Montréal. Il consiste à embarquer de 40 à 50 de personnes pour une excursion à travers[1] les rapides de Lachine sur le fleuve Saint-Laurent. Le bateau-jet se lance à toute vitesse[2] dans les eaux agitées du fleuve avec parfois des virages[3] à 360 degrés. Manteau de pluie, bottes et gilet de sauvetage[4] sont indispensables pendant l'expédition.

[1]à… *through* [2]se… *throws itself at top speed* [3]*turns* [4]gilet… *lifejacket*

Visionnez!

Indiquez si les phrases suivantes sont vraies ou fausses.

1. ______ Léa cherche à faire un **échange** de logements.
2. ______ Hassan pense que l'échange de logements est une bonne formule.
3. ______ Le **vacancier** (*vacationer*) à Montréal a apprécié le mélange de sports et de culture.
4. ______ Le vacancier à Marrakech a apprécié les bains de mer.
5. ______ Le vacancier à la Martinique a apprécié la cuisine.

Analysez!

1. Comment l'environnement—paysage (*landscape*) et climat—influence-t-il les activités de vacances proposées dans chaque pays?
2. Quels sont les avantages et les inconvénients de l'échange de logements?

Suggestion: Have sts. post their vacation exchange proposals in the classroom and have other sts. vote on which posting seems the most interesting. They could also make videos for this activity using their phones.

Comparez!

Regardez encore une fois les commentaires des trois vacanciers. Puis, proposez, dans un message éléctronique, un échange de logements à une personne qui habite dans un des trois lieux présentés dans la vidéo. Mentionnez les avantages de votre propre (*own*) domicile et de la ville où vous habitez.

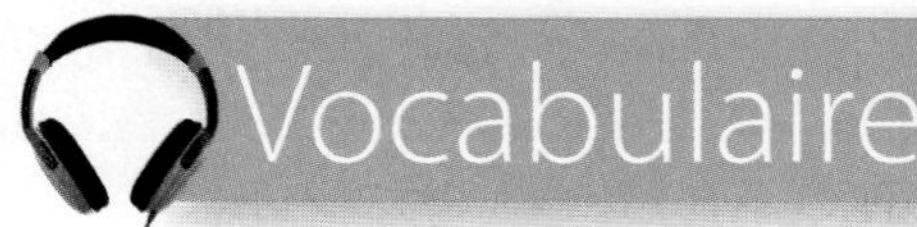

Vocabulaire

Verbes

acheter to buy
aller à la pêche to go fishing
bronzer to get a suntan
devenir to become
dormir to sleep
entrer to enter
faire une randonnée to go hiking
falloir (il faut) to be necessary
monter to go up; to climb
mourir to die
nager to swim
naître to be born
obtenir to obtain, get
oublier to forget
partir (à) (de) to leave (for) (from)
passer (par) to pass (by)
patiner to skate
prendre des vacances to take a vacation
quitter to leave (*someone or someplace*)
rentrer to return; to go home
retourner to return; to go back
revenir to come back to, return (*someplace*)
sentir to feel; to sense; to smell
servir to serve
sortir to leave; to go out
tomber to fall
venir to come
 venir de + *inf.* to have just (*done something*)
voyager to travel

À REVOIR: **descendre, porter, pouvoir, rendre visite à, rester**

Substantifs

l'alpinisme (*m.*) mountaineering
le bateau (à voile) (sail)boat
la campagne country(side)
le camping camping
la carte d'identité ID card
le cheval horse
l'endroit (*m.*) place
l'équitation (*f.*) horseback riding
l'état (*m.*) state
le fleuve (large) river
la forêt forest
le lac lake
la mer sea, ocean
le monde world
la montagne mountain
le parapluie umbrella
le passeport passport
la plage beach
la planche à voile windsurfing
la plongée libre snorkeling
la plongée sous-marine scuba diving
la randonnée hike
la route road
le ski alpin downhill skiing
 ...de fond cross-country skiing
 ...nautique waterskiing
le vélo bicycle
le visa visa

À REVOIR: **la carte postale, le pays, la promenade, les vacances** (*f. pl.*)

Les vêtements et l'équipement sportifs

l'anorak (*m.*) (ski) jacket
le casque helmet
les chaussures (*f.*) **de ski** ski boots
 ...de montagne hiking boots
la crème solaire suntan lotion
l'écran (*m.*) **solaire** sun block
les gants (*m.*) gloves
les lunettes (*f. pl.*) glasses
 lunettes de ski ski goggles
 lunettes de soleil sunglasses
le sac de couchage sleeping bag
la serviette de plage beach towel
le ski ski
la tente tent
la valise suitcase

À REVOIR: **la chaussure, le maillot de bain, la robe**

Expressions temporelles

les années (cinquante) the decade (era) of (the fifties)
il y a ago

Mots et expressions divers

ensemble together
il faut It is necessary to ...; One must ... / One needs ...
Il ne faut pas + *inf.* One must not ...
même same; even
selon according to

Bienvenue...

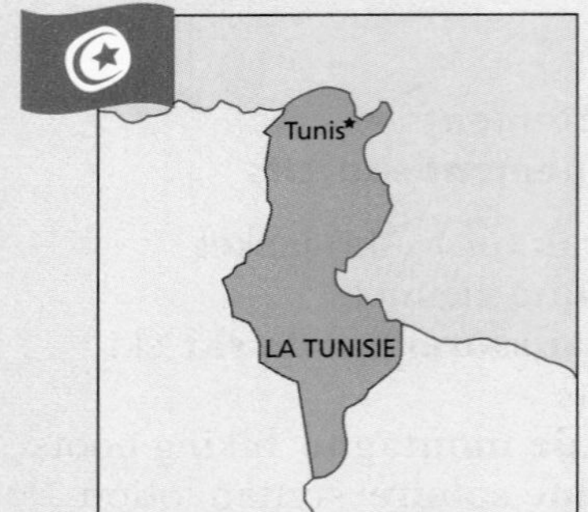

Un coup d'œil sur Tunis, en Tunisie

À quelques heures d'avion de New York, vous pouvez partir à la découverte de la Tunisie en Afrique du Nord. Le désert du Sahara constitue 40 % du territoire, mais il y a aussi 1298 km[1] de côtes qui bordent la Méditerranée. La ville principale est Tunis, la capitale du pays depuis 1159. Il faut absolument voir la médina, avec ses monuments, ses mosquées et ses souks. N'oubliez pas de négocier les prix si vous faites des achats dans ces petites rues remplies[2] de boutiques de tapis, de parfums, d'objets en cuir,[3] de poteries, et cetera. À l'ouest de la ville, visitez le Musée national du Bardo, un musée archéologique particulièrement riche en mosaïques romaines.

Un peu au nord de Tunis: Carthage et Sidi Bou Saïd. Ancienne puissance[4] maritime, commerciale et militaire, Carthage est détruite[5] puis reconstruite[6] par les Romains. Aujourd'hui, on peut admirer les ruines des villas romaines, de l'amphithéâtre et des thermes.[7] Le village de Sidi Bou Saïd est perché sur une falaise[8] dominant Carthage et le golfe de Tunis. Avec ses jolies maisons peintes en bleu et blanc, ses artistes et ses cafés, c'est un endroit pittoresque qui mérite le détour.

[1] 1298 km = *806 miles* [2] *filled* [3] *leather* [4] *power* [5] *destroyed* [6] *rebuilt* [7] *Roman baths* [8] *cliff*

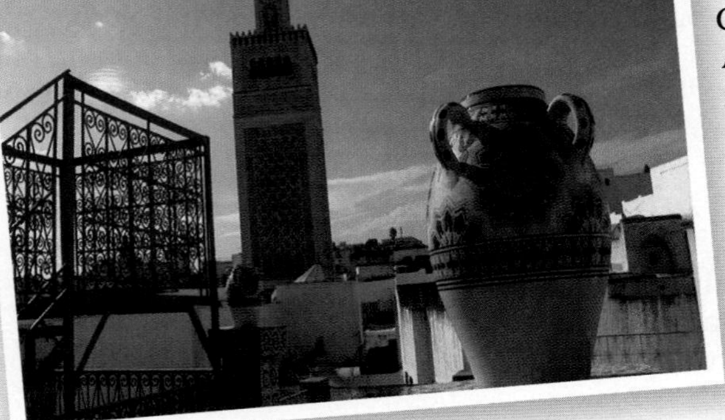

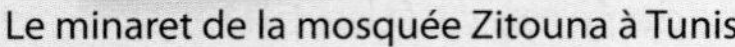
Le minaret de la mosquée Zitouna à Tunis

PORTRAIT Albert Memmi, le droit à la différence

Albert Memmi est né en 1920 à Tunis dans une famille juive de langue arabe. Au début du XX[e1] siècle, la Tunisie est une colonie française majoritairement musulmane. Il existe des tensions entre les Musulmans et les Juifs, alors de nombreux Juifs tunisiens choisissent de s'assimiler à la culture coloniale française. Albert va donc au lycée français de Tunis. Pendant la Deuxième Guerre mondiale, à cause des lois antisémites du gouvernement de Vichy,* on l'envoie dans un camp de travail forcé. Après avoir retrouvé sa liberté, il poursuit des études de philosophie, devient enseignant et épouse une Française. Il s'installe à Paris après l'indépendance de la Tunisie et prend la nationalité française en 1973.

Ces expériences influencent ses œuvres. Ses deux romans les plus célèbres, *La Statue de sel* (1953) et *Agar* (1955), sont autobiographiques et explorent les thèmes de l'aliénation et des mariages mixtes. Memmi écrit aussi plusieurs livres sur le racisme et le colonialisme en Afrique, et des essais où il analyse les effets négatifs de la colonisation. Lauréat de plusieurs prix littéraires prestigieux, Albert Memmi est l'un des plus grands écrivains tunisiens de langue française.

L'écrivain Albert Memmi

[1] vingtième

*The Vichy regime refers to the French government proclaimed by Marshal Philippe Pétain following the military defeat of France. It collaborated with the Germans. Following the liberation of France, General Charles de Gaulle proclaimed a new government recognized by all the allies on October 23, 1944.

en Afrique francophone

Un coup d'œil sur Dakar, au Sénégal

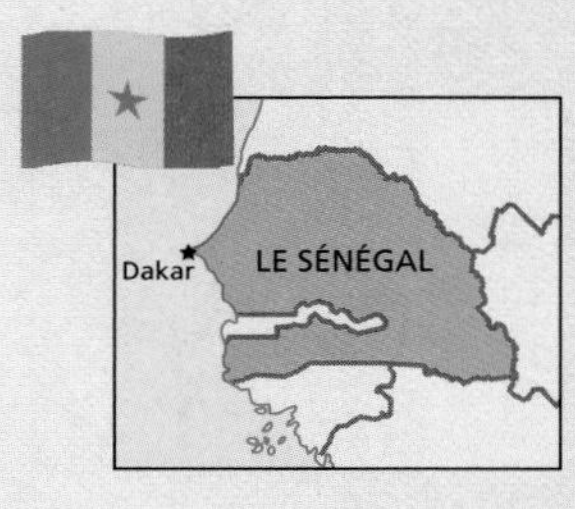

Au Sénégal dont[1] elle est la capitale, Dakar est l'une des pointes[2] les plus avancées de l'Afrique de l'Ouest dans l'océan Atlantique. Les Dakarois vous accueillent toujours avec amitié, «teranga». Visitez avec eux le Marché Sandaga, près de la petite gare, et regardez partir les bateaux qui relient[3] Dakar à la Casamance ou à la Gambie voisines. Dans l'arrondissement du Plateau, vous voyez aussi l'Assemblée nationale et le Palais présidentiel.

Là-bas,[4] on voit dans l'océan l'Île de Gorée, ce joyau[5] de l'architecture coloniale avec ses petites rues et l'ombre[6] fraîche des bougainvillées. Mais, cet endroit tranquille cache[7] un passé terrible: le point de départ de la traite négrière[8] dès le XVI[e9] siècle. La Maison des Esclaves résonne encore de la tragédie de femmes, enfants, hommes, transportés dans des conditions inhumaines vers les Antilles et les Amériques.

[1]*of which* [2]*headlands* [3]*link* [4]*There* [5]*jewel* [6]*shade* [7]*hides* [8]traite... *slave trade* [9]seizième

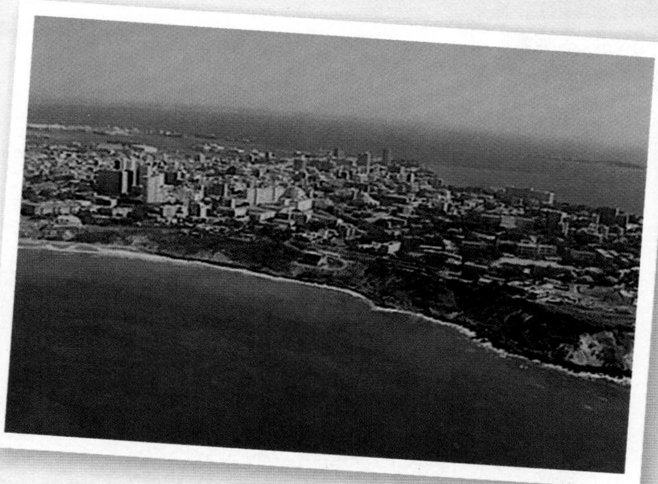

Voici Dakar sur sa péninsule.

PORTRAIT Oumou Sy, la tradition et la modernité

Oumou Sy est née à Podor au nord du Sénégal. Autodidacte, elle ne sait ni lire ni écrire,[1] mais elle ouvre son premier atelier[2] de couture à l'âge de 14 ans. Créatrice de mode, costumière, femme d'affaires, activiste, elle habite aujourd'hui à Dakar. Dans ses collections de haute couture et de prêt-à-porter, elle allie les traditions africaines et la mode européenne. Elle travaille aussi dans le monde du spectacle, où elle crée des costumes pour des chanteurs sénégalais tels que[3] Youssou N'Dour et de grands cinéastes[4] africains comme Ousmane Sembène. En plus, c'est une femme engagée dans le développement de son pays: en 1990, elle ouvre une école chargée d'enseigner les arts traditionnels et modernes du costume et, en 1996, avec son mari, elle ouvre Metissacana, le premier cybercafé de l'Afrique de l'Ouest.

[1]ne... *can neither read nor write* [2]*studio* [3]*such as* [4]*filmmakers*

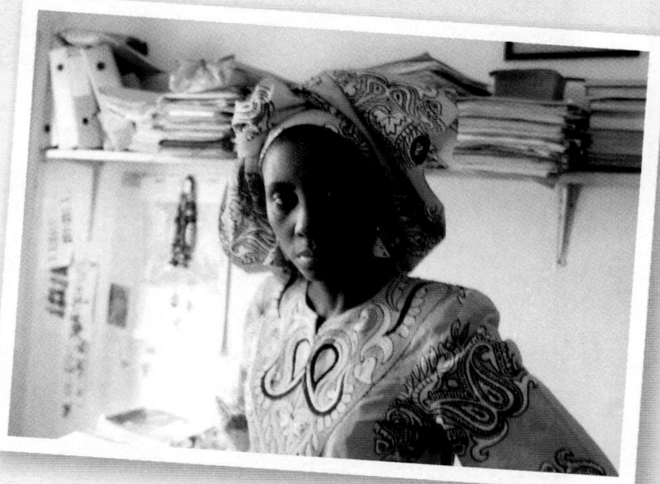

Oumou Sy dans son atelier

YouTube link: You can find footage of Oumou Sy's fashion shows on YouTube.

Note: See the Instructor's Manual for follow-up questions about this *Bienvenue* section.

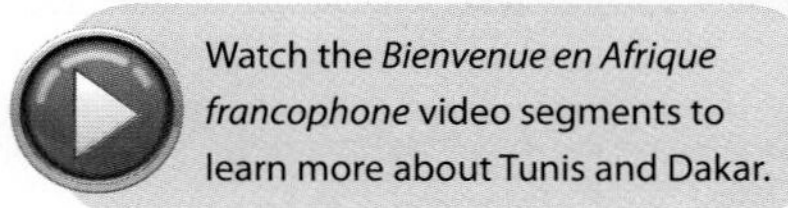

Watch the *Bienvenue en Afrique francophone* video segments to learn more about Tunis and Dakar.

CHAPITRE 9

En route!

Presentation: Ask sts. to imagine what kind of vacation the people in the photo might be taking. Ask questions such as *Où va la voiture? Est-ce que le conducteur est en vacances? Qu'est-ce qu'il va faire pendant ses vacances? Qu'est-ce qu'il a dans la voiture?*

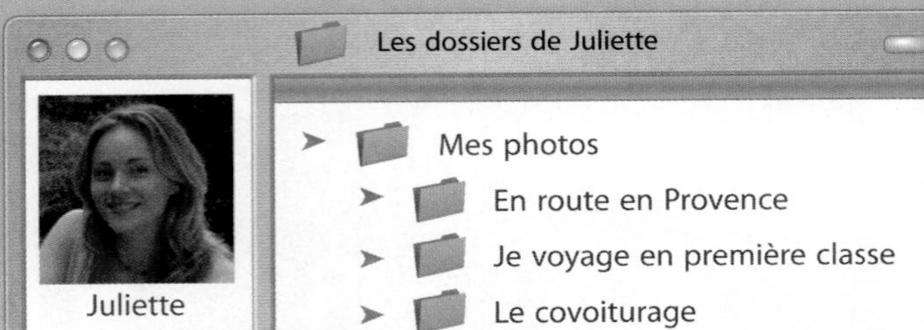

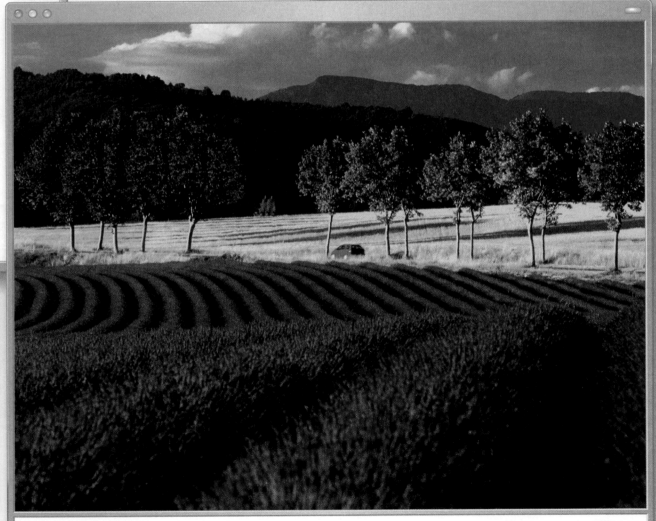

En route parmi les champs de lavande en Provence

Cultural note: *La Provence* in southeastern France is just one of the many regions traversed by the historic *Route Nationale 7*, running from Paris to the French Riviera. This highway, which passes through Lyon, Avignon, Aix-en-Provence, and Nice, is the subject of one of Charles Trenet's most popular songs.

Dans ce chapitre...

OBJECTIFS COMMUNICATIFS

- talking about transportation
- expressing actions
- expressing how long, how long ago, and since when
- talking about the past
- expressing negation
- learning to distinguish between and pronounce selected sounds in French

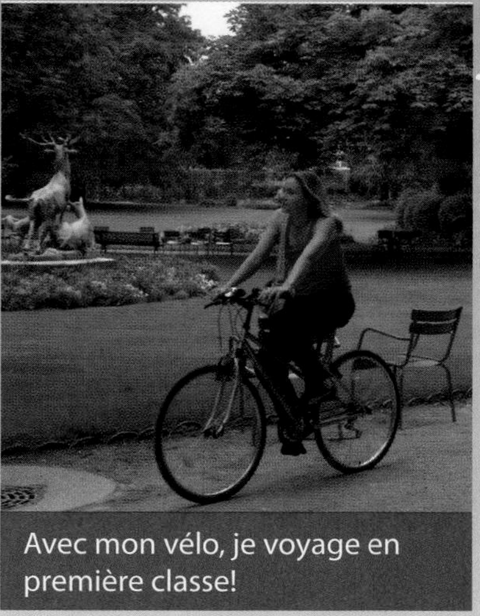

Avec mon vélo, je voyage en première classe!

PAROLES (Leçon 1)

- À l'aéroport
- À la gare
- En route!
- Les points cardinaux

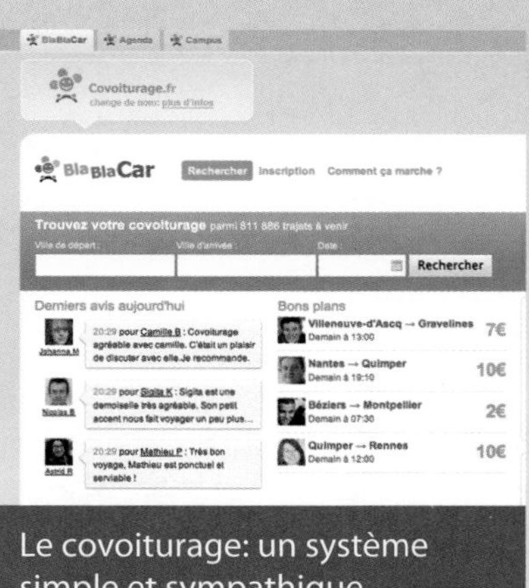

Le covoiturage: un système simple et sympathique

STRUCTURES (Leçons 2 et 3)

- Le verbe **conduire**
- **Depuis** et **pendant**
- Les adverbes affirmatifs et négatifs
- Les pronoms affirmatifs et négatifs

CULTURE

- Le blog de Juliette: *La Rolls du vélo**
- Reportage: *Le covoiturage: quelle bonne idée!*
- Lecture: *Vélib' et Autolib': on innove dans les transports* (Leçon 4)

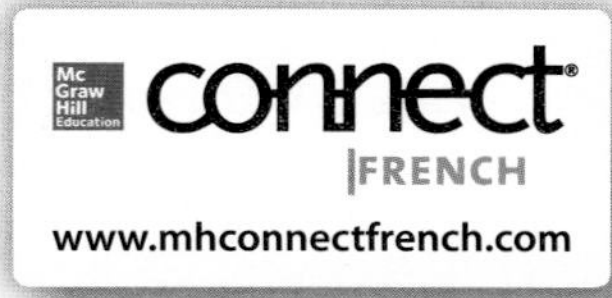

*In **Chapitres 9–12,** Juliette Graf creates a blog and writes about cycling in Paris, the everpresent technologies in Parisian life, the pleasures of living in a city, and her love of art.

Leçon 1

PAROLES

À l'aéroport

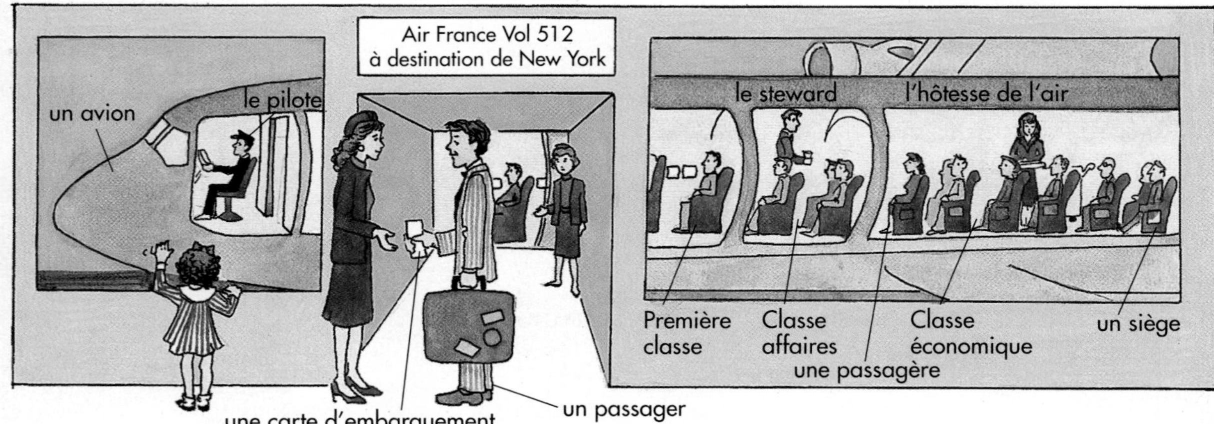

Suggestion: Transform your classroom into an airplane. Give sts. plane tickets. Ask them to find their appropriate place and tell them to find out information about the passenger sitting next to them. Select several sts. and tell them they are in the wrong seat. Encourage them to explain to you that they are actually in the correct seat. You can do this same activity with the train vocabulary on the next page.

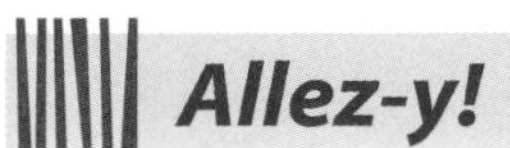

Allez-y!

Suggestion: Point out *monter dans…*, *descendre de…*, *prendre…*

Cultural note: In Quebec, the expression *agent(e) de bord* is used for *steward* and *hôtesse de l'air.*

Additional vocabulary: *à la douane*

Bienvenue à bord! Complétez les phrases d'après le dessin.

1. Le ______ est le conducteur (*driver*) de l'avion.
2. L' ______ apporte les repas.
3. Les gens très riches voyagent en ______.
4. Le ______ sert les boissons.
5. On présente une ______ pour monter dans l'avion.
6. Les hommes et les femmes d'affaires voyagent en ______.
7. Les étudiants voyagent en ______.
8. Le départ du ______ 512 est à 13 h 50.

À la gare

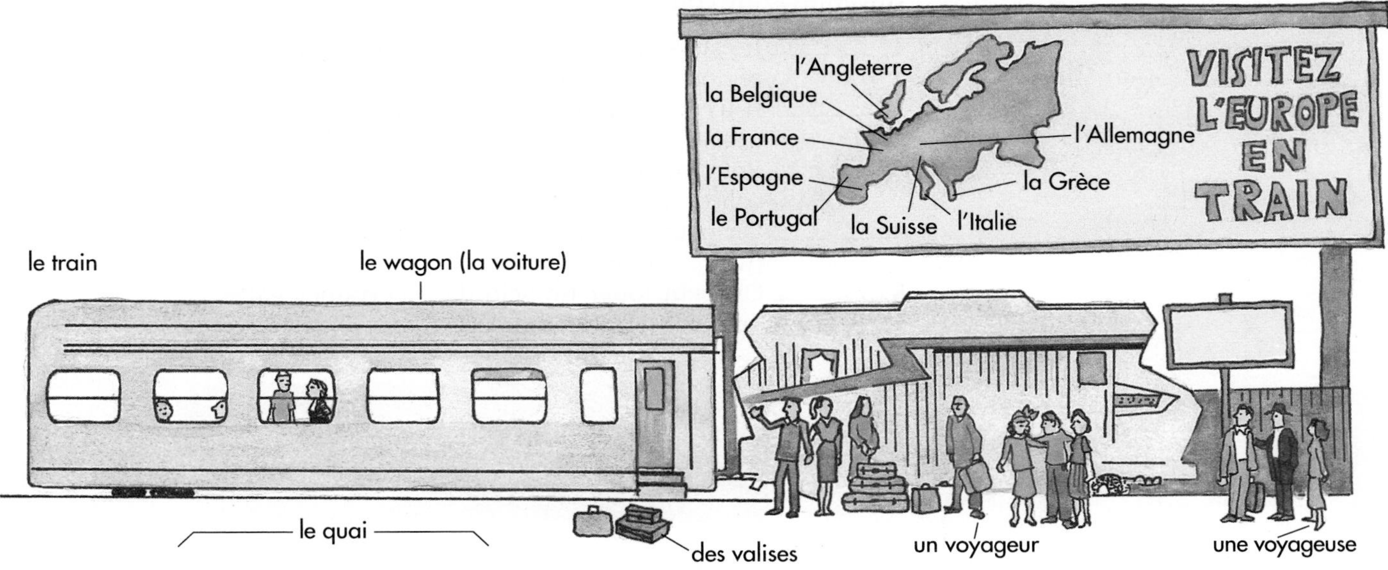

AUTRES MOTS UTILES

un aller-retour	round trip; round-trip ticket
le billet	ticket
le compartiment	compartment
la couchette	berth
le guichet	(ticket) window

Cultural note: Trains are a much more widely used form of transportation in France than in the United States. Since 1938, French railroads have been controlled by the *Société nationale des chemins de fer français* (*SNCF*), a government-regulated monopoly.

Note: The *compartiment* is a space with a door in which six to eight passengers are seated on two facing seats.

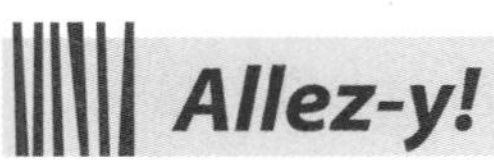

Allez-y!

A. Définitions. Répondez, s'il vous plaît!

1. Quel moyen de transport est-ce qu'on trouve dans une gare?
2. Comment s'appelle chaque voiture d'un train?
3. Comment s'appellent les personnes qui voyagent?
4. Comment s'appelle la partie du wagon où les voyageurs sont assis (*seated*)?
5. Où est-ce que les voyageurs attendent l'arrivée d'un train?
6. Où est-ce qu'on achète les billets?

B. Interview. Demandez à un(e) camarade s'il / si elle a voyagé en train. Est-ce qu'il/elle a mangé dans un wagon-restaurant? Est-ce qu'il/elle a dormi dans un wagon-lit? Quelle ville est-ce qu'il/elle a visitée pendant ce voyage? À qui est-ce qu'il/elle a rendu visite? Ensuite, racontez à la classe le voyage de votre camarade.

Additional vocabulary: *un billet aller-retour, un billet aller simple, un buffet, le couloir, réserver des places, le tableau d'affichage, le TGV, un wagon-bar, un wagon-lit, un wagon-restaurant*

Follow-up: Have sts. create simple definitions of vocab. in drawings. Example: *Ce sont les personnes qui voyagent.* (*passengers*) This can also be done in small groups, with each st. receiving a 3 × 5 card with a word he or she is to define for others who try to identify the word.

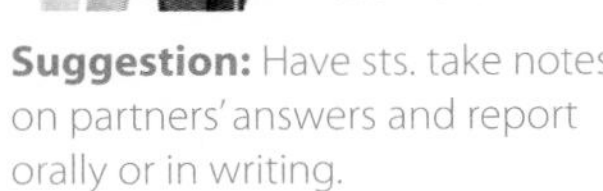

Suggestion: Have sts. take notes on partners' answers and report orally or in writing.

C. **Train + Vélo.** Beaucoup de Français prennent leur vélo avec eux quand ils voyagent en train. Lisez la publicité de la SNCF (Société nationale des chemins de fer français), puis indiquez si les phrases suivantes sont vraies ou fausses.

1. ______ Il est facile de se balader en vélo quand on visite des régions de France.
2. ______ Il n'est pas possible de transporter son vélo dans le train quand on sort du territoire français.
3. ______ Pour voyager en train avec son vélo, il n'y a qu'une seule solution: le prendre avec soi à la gare le jour du départ.
4. ______ On peut laisser son vélo dans certaines gares pendant (*while*) qu'on travaille.
5. ______ On peut louer un vélo dans certaines gares.
6. ______ Toutes les gares de SNCF ont un parc à vélos.

Train + Vélo

Partez avec votre bicyclette à la découverte de nouvelles balades en France comme à l'étranger, grâce à l'espace vélo aménagé par la SNCF à bord de nombreux trains Grandes Lignes (Corail et TGV).
Vous pouvez également vous évader avec votre vélo en profitant d'un transport simple et rapide offert par les trains régionaux (TER et Transilien).

Et si vous désirez voyager plus léger, nous vous proposons notre service Bagages qui expédiera votre vélo là où vous le souhaitez.

Aller à la gare à vélo...
Une bonne façon de partir travailler tout en gardant la forme ! Pour faciliter vos déplacements quotidiens, la SNCF équipe ses gares de parcs à vélos et vous invite également à profiter des services proposés dans certaines gares par les Points Vélos : gardiennage, atelier de réparation, service de location...

À vous de choisir la formule qui vous correspond le mieux pour enfourcher votre bicyclette ! D'autant que cet exercice, bon pour la forme, l'est aussi pour l'environnement.

Source: SNCF, 2010

En route!

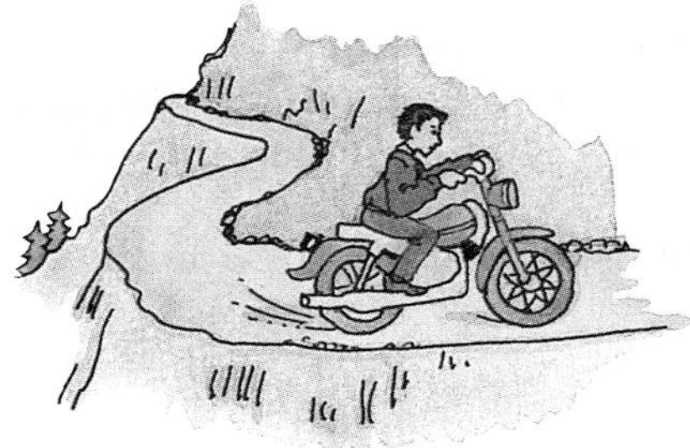

Virgile conduit (*drives*) sa **moto** avec prudence.

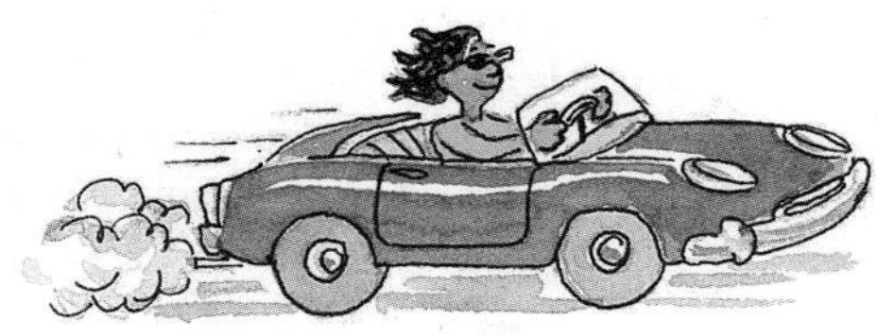

Agathe **roule** toujours très **vite.** Elle préfère **l'autoroute**!

Additional vocabulary: *avoir une crevaison (un pneu crevé), tomber en panne (d'essence).*

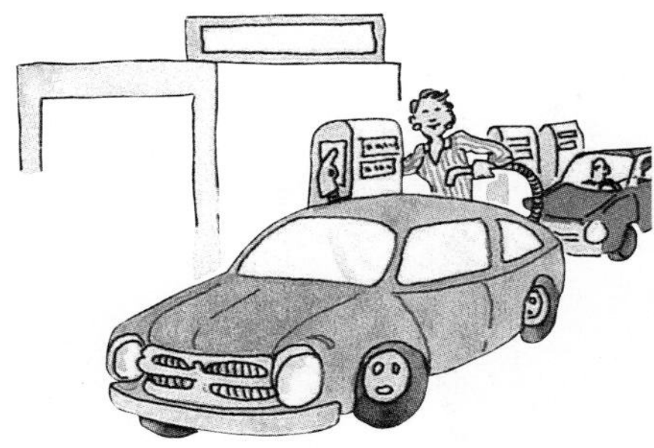

Marianne **fait le plein** d'**essence** (*f.*) à **la station-service.**

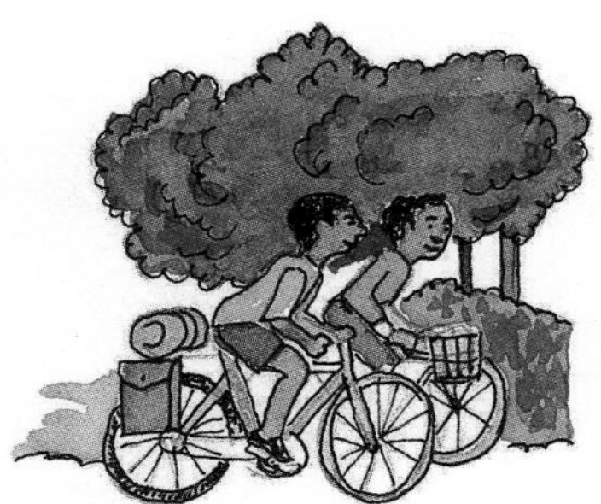

Magali et Anne **traversent** la France **à vélo.**

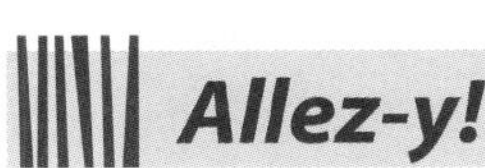

Allez-y!

A. Moyens de transport. Comment vous rendez-vous à (*How do you get to*) votre destination dans les situations suivantes? Utilisez les **Mots clés** et les verbes **aller, voyager,** et cetera.

MODÈLE: Vous voulez aller sur l'autre rive (*shore*) du lac. → Je voyage en bateau.

1. La classe fait une excursion.
2. Il y a des pistes cyclables (*bicycle paths*) dans votre ville.
3. Vous allez en Europe.
4. Vous voulez faire de l'équitation.
5. Vous aimez l'autoroute.
6. Votre famille déménage.
7. Vous voulez vous rendre vite au centre-ville.
8. Vous passez le week-end sur l'île Catalina.

Mots clés

Les prépositions devant les moyens de transport

En is used with means of transportation that you enter.

en autocar, **en** autobus, **en** avion, **en** bateau, **en** camion, **en** métro, **en** train, **en** voiture, et cetera

À is used with means of transportation that you mount or on which you ride. It is also used in the expression **à pied.**

à bicyclette, **à** cheval, **à** moto, **à** vélo, et cetera

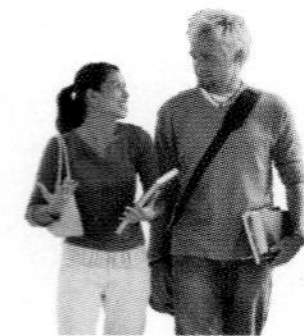

B. Interview. Posez les questions suivantes à un(e) camarade.

1. Comment préfères-tu voyager en vacances? Pourquoi? Est-ce que ça dépend de ta destination?
2. Quels moyens de transport préfères-tu prendre en ville?
3. Nomme des moyens de transport qui correspondent à chacun des adjectifs suivants: **agréable, dangereux, économique, polluant, rapide.**
4. Est-ce qu'il y a des problèmes de transport dans ta ville ou ta région? Si oui, lesquels (*which ones*)?

Les points cardinaux

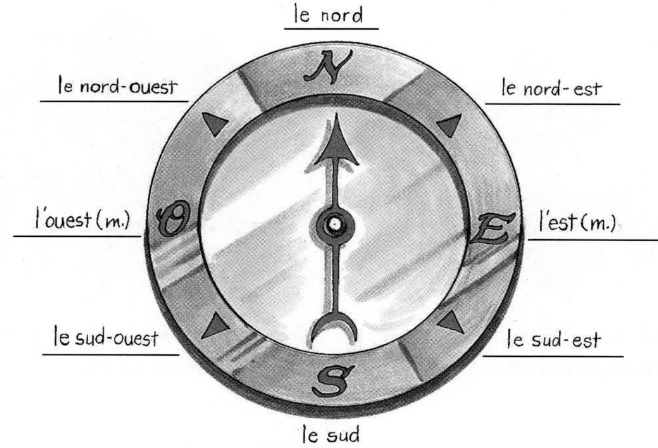

Suggestion: Point out that in the words *sud, est, ouest,* the final consonant is pronounced.

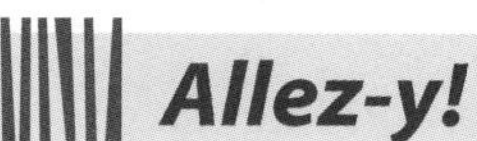

Allez-y!

Suggestions: (1) Can be done as whole-class or small-group activity. (2) It may be useful to have sts. fill in names of countries guessed on a blank map.

Answers: 1. *France: Paris* 2. *Allemagne: Berlin* 3. *Espagne: Madrid* 4. *Portugal: Lisbonne* 5. *Angleterre: Londres* 6. *Italie: Rome* 7. *Suisse: Berne* 8. *Belgique: Bruxelles*

Additional activity: *Maintenant, un(e) camarade décrit la situation géographique d'un pays étranger qu'il/elle a visité ou d'un pays étranger visité par un ami ou un parent. Essayez d'identifier le pays. Puis donnez le nom d'une ville de ce pays. Regardez les cartes à la fin de ce livre.* MODÈLE: *É1: Ma cousine Jessica a visité un pays au nord-ouest de l'Italie. É2: Est-ce que ta cousine a visité la France? É1: Oui. Elle a visité Lille. Voici quelques possibilités: l'Irlande, l'Écosse* (Scotland), *le Danemark, la Suède, l'Autriche* (Austria), *la Grèce, l'Égypte, l'Afrique du Sud, Israël, la Jordanie, l'Arabie Saoudite, l'Iran, l'Australie, l'Argentine, le Venezuela, le Nicaragua.*

Quelques pays européens et leurs capitales. Quel pays est situé dans chacune des régions mentionnées ici? Quelle est sa capitale? (Consultez la carte géographique de l'Europe à la fin de ce livre.)

MODÈLE: au sud-est de l'Italie →
La Grèce est située au sud-est de l'Italie. Capitale: Athènes.

RÉGIONS	CAPITALES
1. au nord-est de l'Espagne	Londres
2. à l'est de la Belgique	Madrid
3. au sud-ouest de la France	Bruxelles
4. à l'ouest de l'Espagne	Berne
5. au nord de la France	Berlin
6. au sud-est de la France	Rome
7. au nord de l'Italie	Lisbonne
8. au nord-est de la France	Paris

Leçon 2

Le verbe *conduire*

Expressing Actions

Comment transporter une table?

Léa et Hector discutent en voiture.

LÉA: **Tu conduis** bien, Hector!
HECTOR: Tu es gentille. Juliette trouve que **je conduis** trop vite…
LÉA: Elle dit* aussi que **je conduis** mal!
HECTOR: En réalité, elle déteste la voiture: elle considère que **ça détruit** l'environnement.
LÉA: Elle a raison, mais les voitures polluantes, c'est bientôt fini: **on produit** maintenant des voitures hybrides. **Elles réduisent** les émissions de CO^2.
HECTOR: Elles sont écologiques!
LÉA: Voiture… métro… bus… train… Moi, je préfère le vélo comme Juliette.
HECTOR: Oui, mais pour transporter une table, ce n'est pas très pratique, n'est-ce pas, Léa!

*says

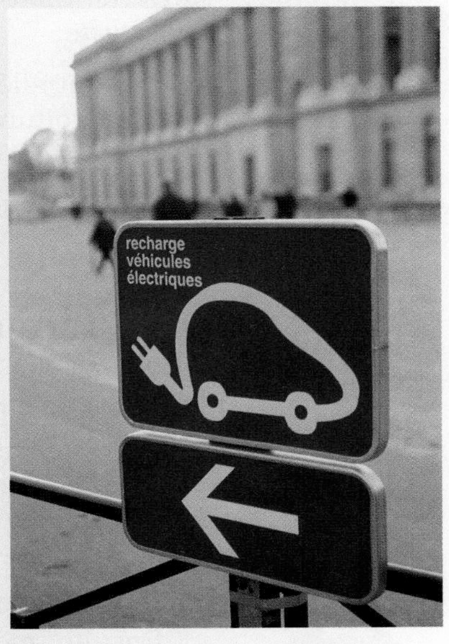

La voiture électrique: une réalité dans Paris

Complétez les phrases en utilisant les verbes du dialogue.

1. Tu ____ bien.
2. Je ____ trop vite.
3. Je ____ mal.
4. Les voitures polluantes, ça ____ l'environnement.
5. On ____ des voitures hybrides.
6. Elles ____ la pollution.

PRESENT TENSE OF **conduire** (*to drive*)			
je	cond**uis**	nous	cond**uisons**
tu	cond**uis**	vous	cond**uisez**
il/elle/on	cond**uit**	ils/elles	cond**uisent**
past participle: **conduit**			

All verbs ending in **-uire** are conjugated like **conduire.**

construire *to construct* — Nous **construisons** une nouvelle ville.

Pronunciation practice: The *Prononcez bien!* section on page 252 of this chapter contains activities for practicing these sounds.

Prononcez bien!

The semivowel in *conduire*

French has three semivowels: [j] as in **travailler,** [w] as in **voiture,** and [ɥ] as in **conduire.** These three sounds are pronounced very rapidly and are linked to the following vowel. To pronounce the sound [ɥ] in **conduire,** start from the [y] in **tu** (with your lips rounded and protruding, and your tongue all the way to the front, pressing against your lower teeth), and immediately pronounce the following vowel.

[ɥ]: **conduire, depuis, duel, suave, buée** (*mist*)

détruire *to destroy*	On **détruit** le vieux pour construire du neuf.
produire *to produce*	Le soleil **produit** de l'énergie.
réduire *to reduce*	**Réduisez** votre vitesse dans les zones scolaires.
traduire *to translate*	**Traduis** cette brochure en espagnol.

Note: *Bien se conduire* (to behave properly), *mal se conduire* (to misbehave)

In French, the verb **conduire** is used to express the physical act of driving. It is used with types of cars, ways of driving, and so on.

Sébastien **conduit** une Peugeot.	*Sébastien drives a Peugeot.*
Les jeunes **conduisent** rapidement.	*Young people drive fast.*

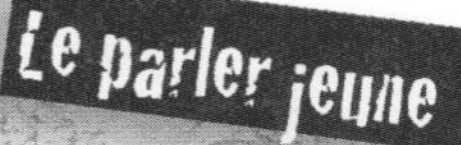

une bagnole	une voiture
une bécane	un vélo, une bicyclette, une moto
une meule	une moto, une mobylette
une valoche	une valise

On peut monter à six dans ma **bagnole.**

Ma **bécane,** c'est une japonaise.

Regarde, elle est belle ma **meule,** hein?

Moi, je voyage léger: une seule **valoche**!

However, the construction **aller en voiture** is used to express *to drive somewhere.*

Ils sont allés en Belgique en voiture.	*They drove to Belgium.*

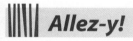

Allez-y!

A. Sur la route. Complétez le texte suivant sur les nouvelles voitures plus écologiques. Utilisez les éléments donnés.

1. ma vieille voiture / produire / trop de pollution
2. les gaz toxiques / détruire / l'environnement
3. nous / conduire / de nouveaux véhicules
4. ils / réduire / le niveau (*level*) de pollution
5. conduire (*impératif, vous*) / avec prudence

Suggestion (B): Have sts. ask questions in pairs and have a few report answers. As a whole-group activity, sts. ask you similar questions.

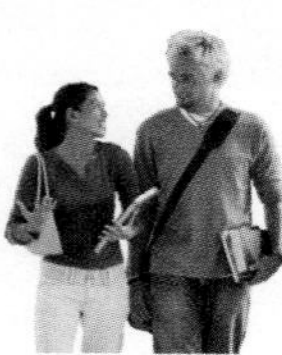

B. Interview. Posez les questions suivantes à un(e) camarade de classe. Ensuite, mentionnez le fait le plus intéressant à la classe.

1. Conduis-tu souvent? Quand tu sors avec des copains, conduisez-vous ou utilisez-vous les transports en commun?
2. Dans ta famille, qui conduit le plus (*the most*) souvent? Qui ne conduit pas?
3. Aimes-tu conduire? Quelle marque de voiture préfères-tu? Pourquoi? Préfères-tu les voitures américaines ou les voitures fabriquées à l'étranger (*abroad*)?
4. Penses-tu que les voitures détruisent la qualité de la vie en ville? Est-ce qu'on construit trop d'autoroutes aux États-Unis?
5. Qu'est-ce que tu penses des motos et des vélos?
6. As-tu déjà traversé les États-Unis en voiture? Si oui, quand et avec qui?

Depuis et *pendant*

Expressing How Long, How Long Ago, and Since When

Pendant les embouteillages

Juliette et Hector discutent en voiture.

JULIETTE: Tu conduis **depuis combien de temps,** Hector?
HECTOR: Je conduis **depuis sept ans**. J'adore les voitures!
JULIETTE: Pas moi… Je n'ai pas mon permis et je n'ai pas de voiture.
HECTOR: C'est pourtant pratique…
JULIETTE: Vraiment? Et qu'est-ce que tu fais **pendant** les embouteillages[1]? Tu danses?
HECTOR: **Pendant** les embouteillages, je chante[2]!
JULIETTE: Moi, je deviens folle.[3]
HECTOR: Fais comme moi. Chante!

[1]*traffic jams* [2]*sing* [3]*crazy*

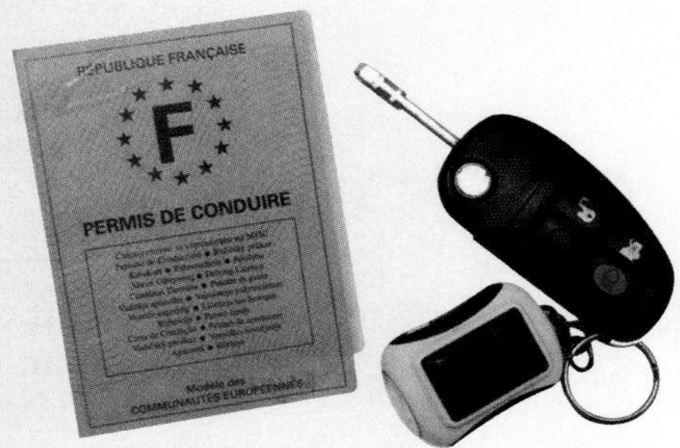

Les objets indispensables du conducteur

Répondez aux questions en utilisant **depuis** et **pendant**.

1. Depuis combien de temps Hector conduit-il?
2. Que fait Hector pendant les embouteillages?
3. Que fait Juliette pendant les embouteillages?

Depuis

Depuis is used with a verb in the present tense to talk about an activity that began in the past and continues in the present time. The most frequent English equivalent is *have been* + -ing.

1. With a starting point that can be a date (day, month, year) or a noun:

Depuis quand… ? + *present tense* = Since when . . . ?
present tense + **depuis** + *starting point in the past* = . . . since . . .

Depuis quand est-ce que tu conduis?	*Since when have you been driving?*
Je conduis **depuis** 2011.	*I have been driving since 2011.*
Je conduis plus lentement **depuis** mon accident.	*I have been driving more slowly since my accident.*

Presentation and Suggestion: Model the pronunciation of the sentences. Give personal examples and ask sts. to give some, too. Example: *J'étudie le français depuis septembre. Je suis à l'université de X depuis trois ans. Nous étudions le français depuis septembre.*

Note: *Depuis que* is followed by a verb clause. The constructions *il y a… que, voilà … que, ça (cela) fait… que* can also be used in this context. However, these expressions are not presented for active use in *Vis-à-vis*.

2. To express a duration:

Depuis combien de temps... ? + *present tense*	= (For) How long . . . ?
present tense + **depuis** + *period of time*	= . . . for (*duration*)

Depuis combien de temps est-ce que vous prenez l'autobus?	*(For) How long have you been taking the bus?*
Je prends l'autobus **depuis** six mois.	*I have been taking the bus for six months.*

[Allez-y! A-B-C]

Pendant

1. Pendant expresses the duration of a habitual or repeated action, situation, or event with a definite beginning and end. It is often used with the **passé composé.**

Suggestion: Point out that *pendant* is often omitted: *Je suis resté à Paris deux semaines.*

Suggestion: (Listening comprehension) Ask sts. to indicate whether the action took place in the past or if it is still going on. 1. *J'étudie le français depuis quatre ans.* 2. *J'ai voyagé en France il y a deux ans.* 3. *J'ai passé un mois en France.* 4. *J'écris* (I write) *des lettres à mes amis français depuis mon retour.* 5. *Ils ont habité à Paris pendant dix ans.* 6. *Depuis le mois de mai ils habitent Lyon.*

Pendant combien de temps... ? + *present or past tense*	= (For) How long . . . ?
present or past tense + **pendant** + *time period*	= . . . for (*duration*)

Pendant combien de temps es-tu resté en Belgique?	*(For) How long did you stay in Belgium?*
Je suis resté en Belgique **pendant** deux semaines.	*I stayed in Belgium for two weeks.*
D'habitude, le matin, j'attends l'autobus **pendant** vingt minutes.	*Usually, in the morning, I wait for the bus for twenty minutes.*

2. Pendant can also mean *during.*

Qu'est-ce que tu as fait **pendant** ce temps?	*What did you do during this time?*

Reminder: **Il y a** + *time period* = ago

J'ai fait mes réservations **il y a** un mois.	*I made my reservations a month ago.*

[Allez-y! B]

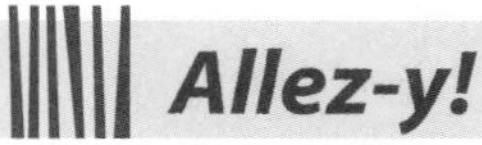

Allez-y!

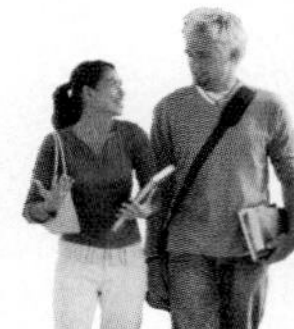

Additional activity: Have sts. ask classmates the following questions. Then decide together who has the most sensible habits. *1. Combien d'heures est-ce que tu dors la nuit? 2. Combien d'heures passes-tu à la bibliothèque le week-end? 3. Pendant combien de temps est-ce que tu étudies le soir, d'habitude? 4. Est-ce que tu fais du sport régulièrement? Pendant combien de temps? Depuis quand?*

A. Le temps passe. Carole (C) et Thomas (T), deux étudiants étrangers à l'université de Lyon, parlent de leur vie en France. Avec un(e) camarade, à tour de rôle, posez les questions et répondez. Utilisez **depuis quand** ou **depuis combien de temps** selon l'indice.

MODÈLE: (C) habiter / Europe (2012) →
CAROLE: Depuis quand est-ce que tu habites en Europe?
THOMAS: J'habite en Europe depuis 2012.

1. (T) travailler / Lyon (deux ans)
2. (C) faire / vélo (mon arrivée en France)
3. (T) étudier / cette université (un an)
4. (C) conduire (2010)
5. (T) être mariée (six mois)
6. (C) étudier l'informatique (l'automne dernier)

B. Expressions de temps. Thomas et Carole continuent leur conversation. Complétez les phrases suivantes en utilisant **depuis, pendant** ou **il y a.**

Thomas a rencontré sa femme Carole ______[1] les vacances. Aujourd'hui, ils sont mariés ______[2] trois ans. Ils aiment partir en voyage ensemble. ______[3] deux mois, Carole a fait un voyage en Tunisie sans Thomas. Elle est restée à Sousse ______[4] trois semaines et Thomas lui a beaucoup manqué. Cet été, ils veulent aller en Belgique ______[5] deux semaines. Et ils veulent partir ensemble! Alors, ______[6] deux jours, ils ont fait leurs réservations sur Internet. Ça n'a pas été facile. Ils ont comparé les prix. Ils ont cherché ______[7] plus de deux heures! Finalement, ils ont trouvé une formule «couple» pas chère. Et c'est fait: ils partent ensemble!

C. Activités. Demandez à vos camarades depuis quand ou depuis combien de temps ils/elles font les activités suivantes.

MODÈLE: être étudiant(e) →
—Depuis combien de temps est-ce que tu es étudiant(e)?
—Je suis étudiant(e) depuis...

1. étudier le français
2. pratiquer son sport préféré
3. être à l'université
4. avoir son ordinateur
5. habiter à ...
6. ?

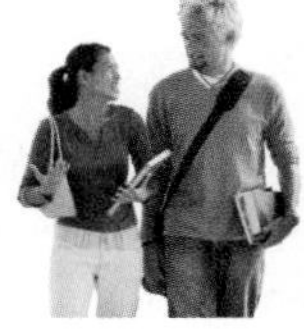

Suggestion (C): After sts. have circulated around the classroom to gather answers to their poll, have each st. present the responses from one of their interviews. Then ask the class to guess the identity of the interviewee.

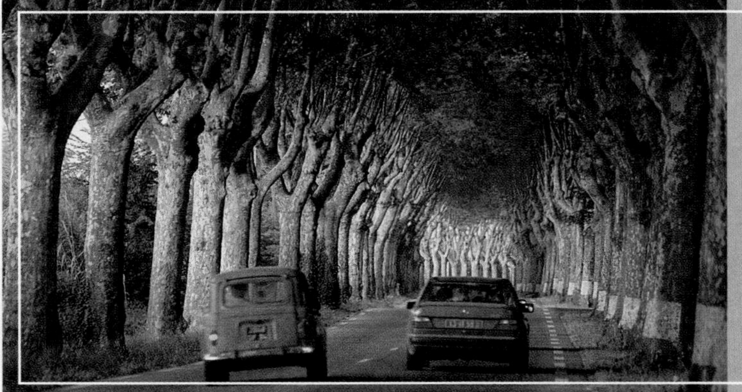

Un peu plus...

En voiture. Voyager en France est facile. Le système ferroviaire (les chemins de fer) et le système routier (les autoroutes) sont très développés. Les voitures en France sont souvent plus petites qu'en Amérique. Ceci facilite la circulation dans les rues étroites des villes médiévales, et la taille modeste des voitures leur permet de consommer moins d'essence, chose indispensable étant donné (*given*) le prix beaucoup plus élevé (*higher*) de l'essence en France. Il y a deux grandes marques de voiture fabriquées en France: PSA Peugeot Citroën et Renault. Quelle marque de voiture préférez-vous?

◄ *Sur la route, dans les environs de Saint-Rémy-de-Provence*

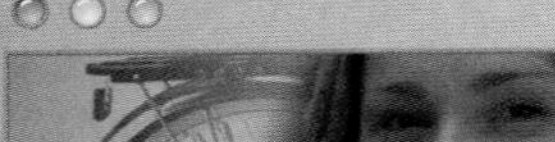
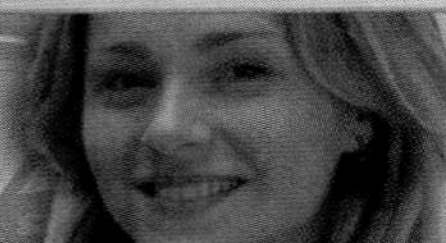

Le blog de Juliette

La Rolls du vélo

vendredi 10 juillet

Salut!

J'espère que vous allez aimer mon blog. Je viens de le créer et j'ai déjà une bonne nouvelle! Depuis longtemps, je rêve d'un vélo! Et voilà! Il est là, mon vélo neuf.[1] C'est un vélo hollandais, la Rolls du vélo: il est solide, élégant, écolo.[2] Regardez la photo!

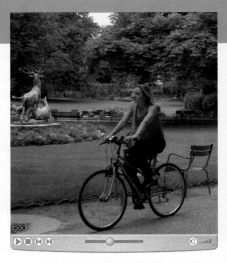

Avec mon vélo, je voyage en première classe!

Moi, j'ai toujours détesté les transports en commun.[3] Mais pendant deux ans—depuis que j'habite Paris—j'ai pris le bus ou le métro. Ces modes de transport ne sont pas très agréables: il y a trop de gens!

Au contraire, Paris à vélo, quel bonheur et quelle liberté! Cet après-midi, j'ai roulé pendant des heures du Quartier latin à La Villette, dans de petites rues, de grandes avenues et sur la piste cyclable du Canal Saint-Martin.

Mais rouler à Paris, c'est vraiment du sport! Ça monte et ça descend constamment! Pour aller à Montmartre, à la Montagne Sainte-Geneviève, à Belleville et Ménilmontant, il faut pédaler dur[4]! Alors, voilà une suggestion: pour faire du vélo à Paris, mangez des vitamines!

Juliette

Follow-up: 1. *Que savez-vous de Juliette? (Regardez sa carte d'identité, page 3.) Qui sont ses amis?* 2. *Quel type de vélo Juliette a-t-elle choisi? Pour vous, l'élégance d'un vélo est-elle importante? Expliquez votre point de vue.* 3. *Pourquoi Juliette est-elle heureuse d'avoir un vélo?* 4. *Est-il facile de rouler à vélo à Paris? Pourquoi?* 5. *Commentez le message de Charlotte. Est-elle pour ou contre le vélo?* 6. *Personnellement, que pensez-vous du vélo dans une grande ville?*

Video connection: In the videoblog for this chapter, Juliette films the arrival of the Tour de France in Paris.

Suggestion: Have sts. use the map on page 292 to trace Juliette's bicycle routes around Paris. The route she describes in her blog is approximately 6 kilometers long.

COMMENTAIRES

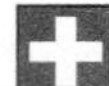

Charlotte

Le vélo, c'est un moyen de transport économique, agréable et excellent pour l'environnement. Mais c'est dangereux, non? Tu roules au milieu des voitures et des gaz toxiques... Tu risques un accident... Il faut porter un casque!

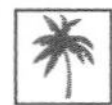

Poema

Moi, je suis une fan du Vélib'[5]! Cést pratique, pas cher et vraiment top.

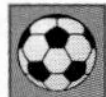

Mamadou

Juliette, tu vas aller sur les Champs-Élysées pour l'arrivée du Tour de France le 23 juillet?

Alexis

Salut, Juliette
Moi aussi, j'ai un vélo. Des balades dans Paname,[6] ça t'intéresse? J'habite à Versailles, mais je peux mettre mon vélo dans le RER.

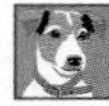

Trésor

Je veux venir!

[1]*new* [2]*ecological (fam.)* [3]transports... *public transportation* [4]*hard* [5]*a public bicycle rental program*
[6]*affectionate name for Paris*

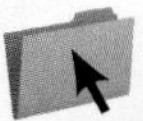

REPORTAGE

Le covoiturage: quelle bonne idée!

Qu'est-ce que le covoiturage? C'est une solution idéale pour réduire la circulation, contrôler la pollution, préserver les ressources naturelles et rencontrer de nouveaux amis. Le principe est simple: vous possédez une voiture. Quand vous faites un voyage, vous proposez d'emmener des gens avec vous en partageant la dépense.[1] Mais ces gens, vous ne les connaissez pas! Alors, comment faire pour leur communiquer votre itinéraire, vos conditions et votre prix?

Encore une fois, Internet nous donne la solution. Il y a, en France, de nombreux sites spécialisés dans le covoiturage. Le propriétaire d'une voiture publie une annonce sur le site et les personnes intéressées le contactent. C'est simple et sympathique.

Le covoiturage: un système simple et sympathique

Voici un exemple d'annonce:

Paris → Lyon

Prix: 25 euros/passager
Départ: jeudi 28 février, à 07 h 00.
Flexibilité horaire: +/− 15 minutes
Durée estimée: 4 h 30
Distance estimée: 480 km
Émissions estimées: 100 kg de CO^2
Cigarette: non

Animaux: non
Bagages: un petit sac
Lieu de rendez-vous: Métro Saint-Paul (75003)
Lieu de dépose:[2] Lyon, gare de la Part-Dieu.
Détours[3]: OK pour détour de 15 minutes si besoin.
Véhicule: Peugeot 507. Couleur: grise.
Confort: Normal

La réputation du conducteur

Après un voyage, le conducteur est évalué par ses passagers: «Conducteur très agréable, prudent et sympathique» (11 févr. 2013); «Bon voyage, bon chauffeur, bonne compagnie» (22 nov. 2013); «Super voyage!!! Merci beaucoup, Brice!» (13 janvier 2014). Ces évaluations aident les futurs passagers à choisir un conducteur prudent, ponctuel et agréable.

Dans toute l'Europe

Inauguré aux USA pendant la Deuxième Guerre[4] mondiale, quand l'essence était très chère, le covoiturage triomphe maintenant en Europe. Avec la crise économique, chaque individu cherche à contrôler ses dépenses. Le covoiturage signifie aussi qu'on limite le nombre des voitures: c'est bon pour l'environnement! Enfin, ce système de transport correspond, chez les Français, à un désir de partager et d'être ensemble.

[1]en... *by sharing expenses* [2]lieu... *drop-off spot* [3]*Side trips* [4]*War*

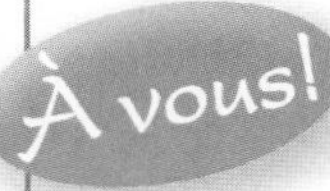

À vous!

1. Quels sont les avantages et les inconvénients du covoiturage?
2. Comment trouve-t-on les passagers?
3. Comment est-ce que les passagers peuvent évaluer les conducteurs?
4. Faites-vous ou aimeriez-vous faire du covoiturage? Expliquez.

Parlons-en!

1. Préparez, avec toute la classe, le texte d'une annonce à publier sur un site Internet de covoiturage.
2. Travaillez à deux. Jouez le rôle du propriétaire (*owner*) de la voiture et d'une personne intéressée par l'annonce. Cette personne pose des questions bizarres et indiscrètes. Par exemple, est-ce vous êtes allergique aux chats? Vous êtes marié(e)? Le dialogue se déroule (*takes place*) au téléphone. Présentez-le devant vos camarades.

Suggestion: To help sts. do step 1 of the activity, you may wish to display ads from French ride sharing sites as additional models. Search "*covoiturage France.*"

Leçon 3

STRUCTURES

Les adverbes affirmatifs et négatifs

Expressing Negation

La pluie sur la tête

Juliette contacte Charlotte, une amie, sur sa page Facebook (Messagerie instantanée).

JULIETTE: Charlotte, le vélo ce n'est pas dangereux. Il faut simplement être prudent.

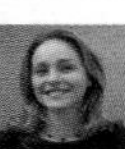
CHARLOTTE: Je **n**'ai **pas encore** adopté cette solution… J'hésite… On est vulnérable à bicyclette. Et je **n'**aime **pas du tout** recevoir la pluie sur la tête!

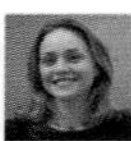
JULIETTE: Il **ne** pleut **pas toujours** à Genève! Quand il fait beau, le vélo c'est le bonheur*! Tu as **déjà** essayé?

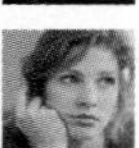
CHARLOTTE: Non, **jamais**… Je prends **souvent** le bus et **parfois** la voiture.

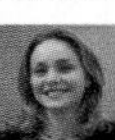
JULIETTE: Et ton mari, comment est-ce qu'il va à son travail?

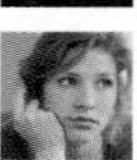
CHARLOTTE: Mon mari: il marche!

*happiness

Trouvez, dans le dialogue, les réponses de Charlotte à ces questions.

1. Est-ce que tu as adopté la solution du vélo?
2. Est-ce que tu aimes recevoir la pluie sur la tête?
3. Est-ce qu'il pleut souvent à Genève?
4. Est-ce que tu as déjà essayé le vélo quand il fait beau?
5. Est-ce que tu prends le bus? la voiture?

The adverbs **toujours, souvent,** and **parfois** (*sometimes*) generally follow the verb in the present tense. The expression **ne (n')... jamais,** constructed like **ne... pas,** is the negative adverb (**l'adverbe de négation**) equivalent to *never* in English.

Henri voyage **toujours** en train.* Marie voyage **souvent** en train.* Hélène voyage **parfois** en train.	Je **ne** voyage **jamais** en train. *I never travel by train.*

Other common adverbs follow this pattern.

AFFIRMATIVE	NEGATIVE
encore *still* Le train est **encore** sur le quai. *The train is still at the platform.*	**ne (n')... plus** *no longer, no more* Le train **n'**est **plus** sur le quai. *The train is no longer at the platform.*
déjà *already* Nos valises sont **déjà** là? *Are our suitcases there already?*	**ne (n')... pas encore** *not yet* Nos valises **ne** sont **pas encore** là. *Our suitcases aren't there yet.*
déjà *ever* Est-ce que tu es **déjà** allé à Lyon? *Have you ever been to Lyon?*	**ne... jamais** *never* Non, je **ne** suis **jamais** allé à Lyon. *No, I have never been to Lyon.*

Suggestion: Point out that *jamais* and *pas encore* can be used without the *ne* as an answer.

Suggestion: Point out that *déjà* meaning "ever" is found only in an interrogative context.

Note: Point out that when a conjugated verb is followed by an infinitive, negative particles surround the conjugated verb, as with *ne... pas: Je ne vais plus acheter de billets.* Also, when the infinitive itself is being negated, the two negative particles precede the infinitive directly: *J'ai l'intention de ne plus voyager dans le Sud.*

1. As with **ne (n')... pas,** the indefinite article and the partitive article become **de (d')** when they follow negative adverbs.

AFFIRMATIVE	NEGATIVE
Je vois **toujours des Américains** dans l'autocar. *I always see Americans on the tour bus.*	Je **ne** vois **jamais de Français** dans l'autocar. *I never see (any) French people on the tour bus.*
Avez-vous **encore des billets** à vendre? *Do you still have (some) tickets to sell?*	Non, je **n'**ai **plus de billets** à vendre. *No, I have no more (I don't have any more) tickets to sell.*
Karen a **déjà des amis** en France. *Karen already has (some) friends in France.*	Vincent **n'**a **pas encore d'amis** aux États-Unis. *Vincent doesn't have any friends in the United States yet.*

2. Definite articles do not change.

   Je ne vois jamais **le** contrôleur (*conductor*) dans ce train.
   Anne ne prend plus **l'**autoroute pour aller à Caen.
   On ne voit pas encore **le** sommet de la montagne.

3. In the **passé composé,** affirmative adverbs are generally placed between the auxiliary and the past participle.

   M. Huet a **toujours** / **souvent** / **parfois** pris l'avion.

Note: The expressions *quelquefois* and *des fois* can be used instead of *parfois.*

*Sentences whose verbs are modified by **toujours** and **souvent** can also be negated by **ne (n')... pas: Henri ne voyage pas toujours en train. Il voyage parfois en avion. Marie ne voyage pas souvent en train. Elle préfère conduire.**

4. **Ne... pas du tout** is used instead of **ne... pas** for emphasis.

Je **n'**aime **pas du tout** les avions!	*I don't like planes at all!*
—As-tu faim? —**Pas du tout!**	*Are you hungry?* *Not at all!*

Additional activity: *Personnalités opposées. Voici le portrait de Monique. Faites le portrait de Joseph en suivant le modèle.*
MODÈLE: Monique a parfois sommeil en cours. → Joseph n'a jamais sommeil en cours.
1. Monique a déjà des problèmes avec ses études. 2. Elle a souvent envie de changer de cours. 3. Elle a parfois peur des professeurs. 4. Elle a déjà besoin de vacances.

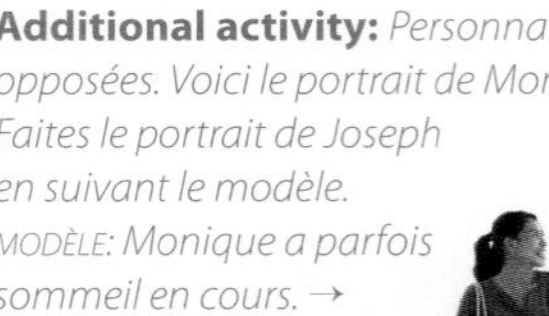

Mots clés

La négation *ne... que*

The expression **ne (n')... que (qu')** is used to indicate a limited quantity of something or a limitation of choices. It has the same meaning as **seulement** (*only*).

Je **n'**ai **qu'**un billet.
J'ai **seulement** un billet.
I have only one ticket.

Hélène **n'**a fait **que** deux réservations.
Hélène a fait **seulement** deux réservations.
Hélène made only two reservations.

Suggestion (C): Model one or two items, and then have sts. do activity in pairs for maximum practice.

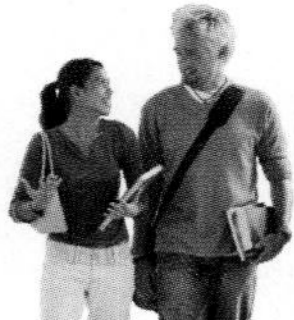

Allez-y!

A. Un voyageur nerveux. Chaque fois qu'il part en vacances, M. Laffont se préoccupe de tout (*worries about everything*). Mme Laffont essaie toujours de le calmer (*calm him down*). Avec un(e) camarade, jouez les rôles de M. et Mme Laffont. Suivez le modèle.

MODÈLE: M. LAFFONT: Tu n'as pas encore trouvé les valises.
MME LAFFONT: Mais si!* J'ai déjà trouvé les valises.

1. Nous ne faisons jamais de voyages agréables.
2. Il n'y a plus de places dans le train.
3. Il n'y a plus de billets en seconde classe.
4. Nous ne sommes pas encore arrivés.
5. Il n'y a jamais de téléphone à la gare.
6. Il n'y a plus de voitures à louer.
7. Tu n'as pas encore trouvé la carte.
8. Nous ne sommes pas encore sur la bonne route (*the right road*).

B. En voyage. Dites ce que font ces personnes quand elles sont en voyage. Remplacez **seulement** par **ne... que.**

MODÈLE: Je prends seulement le train. →
Je ne prends que le train.

1. Martin envoie (*sends*) seulement des cartes postales.
2. Vous achetez seulement des souvenirs drôles.
3. Mes cousins mangent seulement dans les fast-foods.
4. Tu prends seulement une valise.
5. Nous dormons seulement dans des auberges de jeunesse.
6. Sophie regarde seulement les bateaux sur la mer.

C. Préparatifs de voyage. Quand vous partez en voyage, faites-vous les choses suivantes? Utilisez **toujours, souvent, parfois** ou **ne... jamais** dans vos réponses.

MODÈLE: arriver à l'aéroport à la dernière minute →
É1: Est-ce que tu arrives toujours à l'aéroport à la dernière minute?
É2: Moi non, je n'arrive jamais à l'aéroport à la dernière minute! (J'arrive parfois à l'aéroport à la dernière minute.) Et toi?

1. oublier ton passeport (ton billet, ta carte de crédit...)
2. prendre ton appareil photo (un guide, une carte...)
3. acheter de nouveaux vêtements (de nouvelles chaussures, de nouvelles lunettes de soleil...)
4. tracer un itinéraire (à l'avance, au dernier moment...)
5. faire ta valise au dernier moment (la veille [*the day before*], une semaine avant...)

---

*Remember that **si** rather than **oui** is used to contradict a negative question or statement.

D. Voyages exotiques. Interviewez vos camarades.

MODÈLE: camper dans le Sahara

VOUS: N'as-tu jamais fait de camping dans le Sahara?

VOTRE CAMARADE: Non, je n'ai jamais fait de camping dans le Sahara. (*ou* Si, j'ai fait du camping dans le Sahara [l'été passé, il y a deux ans, et cetera].)

1. faire du bateau sur le Nil
2. voir le Sphinx en Égypte
3. faire une expédition en Antarctique
4. passer tes vacances à Tahiti
5. faire de l'alpinisme dans l'Himalaya
6. voir les chutes Victoria (*Victoria Falls*) en Afrique
7. faire un safari-photos au Cameroun
8. ?

Qui dans votre classe a fait le voyage le plus exotique?

Les pronoms affirmatifs et négatifs

Expressing Negation

La grève des transports

Léa et Juliette échangent des textos (SMS).

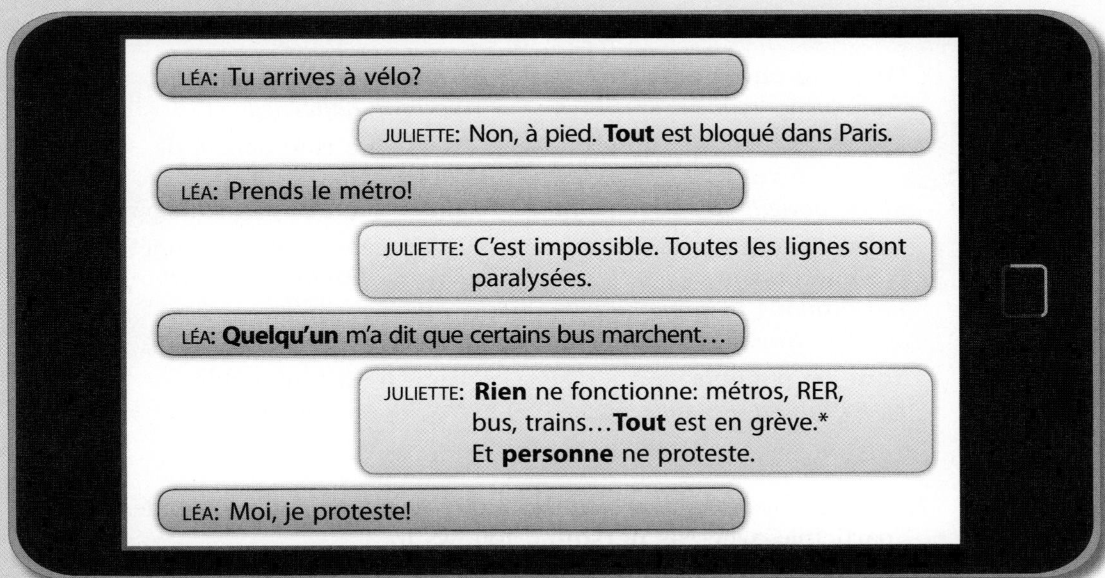
LÉA: Tu arrives à vélo?
JULIETTE: Non, à pied. **Tout** est bloqué dans Paris.
LÉA: Prends le métro!
JULIETTE: C'est impossible. Toutes les lignes sont paralysées.
LÉA: **Quelqu'un** m'a dit que certains bus marchent…
JULIETTE: **Rien** ne fonctionne: métros, RER, bus, trains…**Tout** est en grève.* Et **personne** ne proteste.
LÉA: Moi, je proteste!

*en… *on strike*

Répondez aux questions à l'aide des pronoms indéfinis du dialogue.

1. Qu'est-ce qui est bloqué dans Paris?
2. Qui a dit que certains bus marchent?
3. Qu'est-ce qui fonctionne?
4. Qu'est-ce qui est en grève?
5. Est-ce que les gens protestent?

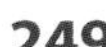

Suggestion: Sts. often confuse the *personne… ne* construction with the noun *une personne.* Point out and compare the examples where the negative pronouns are subjects and objects.

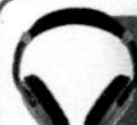

Prononcez bien!

The consonant sounds [p], [t], and [k]

In English, these sounds are aspirated, that is, they are pronounced with a very noticeable puff of air. Hold your hand close to your mouth as you pronounce the English words *pat, tap,* and *cat.* When you pronounce the following French words, the puff of air should be considerably lighter: **pâtes, tape** (*v.* type), **quatre.** Holding your breath to minimize aspiration might help you until you feel more comfortable with these sounds. Notice the spellings of each sound.

[p]: **appeler, personne, porte**

[t]: **attendre, sympathique, tout**

[k]: **classe, d'accord, psychologie, quelqu'un, skier**

Pronunciation presentation: Bring tissues to class and demonstrate the aspiration of English [p], [t], and [k], and lack thereof for their French counterparts, by having sts. hold (1) their hand and (2) a tissue close to their mouth, and pronounce the following English and French words: pat, tap, cat, *pâtes, tape, quatre.*

Pronunciation practice (1): Have sts. hold their hand or a tissue in front of their mouth as they repeat the following words: *peu, taille, paresseux, quarante, quartier, tout le monde, pardon, pays, concert, table, pas, président, tableau, quelque chose, pauvre, père, camarade, cahier, couleur, calme, qu'est-ce que c'est, répétez, d'accord, cinquante.*

Pronunciation practice (2): Have sts. create and pronounce sentences and/or questions using the following elements: 1. *aéroport, passager, présenter, carte d'embarquement* 2. *pilote, conduire, moto, autoroute, rapidement* 3. *parfois, nous, envoyer, cartes postales, quand, nous, être, en vacances* 4. *est-ce que, tu, avoir, tente, pour, faire du camping*

Pronunciation practice (3): The *Prononcez bien!* section on page 252 of this chapter contains additional activities for practicing these sounds.

Just as there are affirmative and negative adverbs (see pages 246–248), there are also affirmative and negative pronouns.

1. **Quelqu'un*** (*Someone*), **quelque chose** (*something*), **tout** (*everything, all*), and **tout le monde** (*everybody*) are indefinite pronouns (**des pronoms indéfinis**). All four can serve as the subject of a sentence, the object of a verb, or the object of a preposition.

   Personne (*No one, nobody, not anybody*) and **rien** (*nothing, not anything*) are negative indefinite pronouns generally used in a construction with **ne** (**n'**). They can be the subject of a sentence, the object of a verb, or the object of a preposition.

AFFIRMATIVE	NEGATIVE
quelqu'un / tout le monde	**personne**
Quelqu'un est monté dans le train. *Someone got on the train.*	**Personne n'**est monté dans le train. *No one got on the train.*
J'ai vu **quelqu'un** sur le quai. *I saw someone on the platform.*	Je **n'**ai vu **personne** sur le quai. *I didn't see anyone on the platform.*
Jacques a parlé avec **quelqu'un.** *Jacques spoke with someone.*	Jacques **n'**a parlé avec **personne.** *Jacques didn't speak with anyone.*
Tout le monde est prêt? *Is everyone ready?*	**Personne n'**est prêt. *No one is ready.*

AFFIRMATIVE	NEGATIVE
quelque chose / tout	**rien**
Quelque chose est arrivé. *Something happened.*	**Rien n'**est arrivé. *Nothing happened.*
Marie a acheté **quelque chose** de bizarre. *Marie bought something strange.*	Marie **n'**a **rien** acheté de bizarre. *Marie didn't buy anything strange.*
Je pense à **quelque chose** d'intéressant. *I'm thinking of something interesting.*	Je **ne** pense à **rien** d'intéressant. *I'm not thinking of anything interesting.*
Tout est possible. *Everything is possible.*	**Rien n'**est impossible. *Nothing is impossible.*

2. As the object of a verb in the **passé composé, rien** precedes the past participle, whereas **personne** follows it.

Marie **n'**a **rien** acheté au buffet de la gare.	*Marie didn't buy anything at the station restaurant.*
Je **n'**ai vu **personne.**	*I didn't see anyone.*

[Allez-y! A-C]

*__Quelqu'un__ is invariable in form: It can refer to both males and females.

3. Like **jamais, rien** and **personne** can be used without **ne** to answer a question.

—Qu'est-ce qu'il y a sur la voie?	*What's on the track?*
—**Rien.**	*Nothing.*
—Qui est au guichet?	*Who's at the ticket counter?*
—**Personne.**	*Nobody.*

4. You may have noticed that when used with adjectives, the expressions **quelque chose, quelqu'un, ne... rien,** and **ne... personne** are followed by **de (d')** plus the masculine singular form of the adjective.

J'ai rencontré **quelqu'un d'intéressant** dans le compartiment d'à côté.	*I met someone interesting in the next compartment.*
Je **n'**ai parlé à **personne d'important.**	*I didn't speak to anyone important.*

[Allez-y! B-C]

Grammaire interactive

For more on negative words, watch the corresponding Grammar Tutorial and take a brief practice quiz at **Connect French.**

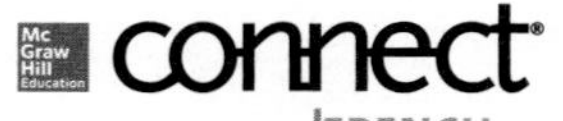

www.mhconnectfrench.com

Allez-y!

A. **À la gare.** Vous avez des ennuis avant de partir en voyage. Transformez les phrases suivantes.

MODÈLE: Tout le monde est prêt! → Personne n'est prêt!

1. Chloé demande l'heure du départ à quelqu'un.
2. Tout est prêt une heure avant le départ.
3. Quelqu'un a pensé à sortir les valises de la voiture sur le parking.
4. Quelqu'un a acheté les billets avant d'arriver sur le quai.
5. Thomas a quelque chose à porter s'il fait froid.
6. Mehdi a tout emporté pour prendre des photos.

Suggestion: Dictate affirmative statements with sts. working at the board or in their seats. Then have them make the sentences negative.

B. **La vie en rose.** Transformez les phrases pessimistes de votre camarade. Suivez le modèle.

MODÈLE: Il n'y a personne à la caisse (*cash register*). →
É1: Il n'y a personne à la caisse.
É2: Mais si! Il y a quelqu'un à la caisse.

1. Il n'y a personne dans ce restaurant. **2.** Il n'y a rien de bon sur le menu. **3.** Il n'y a rien dans ce magasin de sports. **4.** Il n'y a rien de joli ici. **5.** Il n'y a personne dans cette agence de voyages. **6.** Il n'y a rien d'intéressant dans ces brochures. **7.** Il n'y a rien de moderne dans ce quartier. **8.** Il n'y a rien d'intéressant dans les rues.

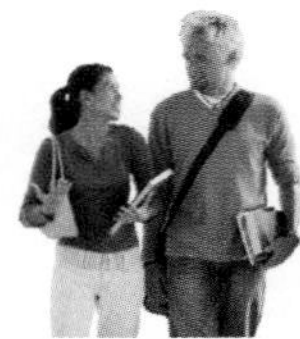

Suggestion: Have sts. play roles of 2 people who don't agree on anything. One person is pessimistic and uses a complaining tone; the other is optimistic and answers with a positive, reassuring tone.

Interaction: Have sts. act out the following situation, using the vocabulary and structures from this chapter.

C. **Trouvez quelqu'un...** Circulez dans la classe et trouvez quelqu'un qui a fait les choses suivantes. Avec un(e) camarade, posez les questions et répondez. (Attention à la question qu'il faut poser!)

1. prendre sa voiture pour aller au marché (hier)
2. avoir quelque chose d'important à faire (la semaine dernière)
3. voir quelqu'un d'intéressant (avant de venir en classe)
4. travailler jusqu'à une heure du matin (hier soir)
5. arriver en classe à 8 heures (ce matin)
6. finir tous les devoirs pour demain (déjà)

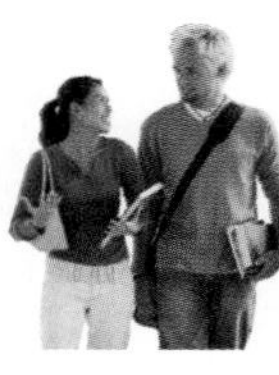

Un mauvais voyage: You are in France. You are so angry with your travel agent that you call him or her to complain. Among other things, mention the following: the plane left late, your hotel room was not reserved (*réservé*), no one is friendly, there is nothing good to eat, there's so much traffic that it's impossible to drive, the phones don't work, etc.

Prononcez bien!

Script (1A): *1. Louis a vingt-trois ans aujourd'hui. 2. C'est un linguiste. 3. Il est idéaliste, et très individualiste aussi. 4. Il est sympa, mais un peu bizarre: il n'aime pas le bruit. 5. En plus, il ne dort pas bien la nuit. 6. Oui, il a des ennuis avec le sommeil.*

Answers (1A): 1. *aujourd'hui* 2. *linguiste* 3. *individualiste* 4. *bruit* 5. *nuit* 6. *ennuis*

Answers (1B): 1. *huit* 2. *cusine* 3. *fruits* 4. *parapluie* 5. *minuit* 6. *cuillère* 7. *huître* 8. *huile*

1. **The semivowel in *conduire*** (page 239)

A. Louis. Louis, le frère de votre colocataire Isabelle, va passer le week-end avec vous. Isabelle parle de lui (*him*). Pour chaque phrase que vous entendez, écrivez le mot qui contient le son [ɥ] comme dans *conduire*.

1. ________ **3.** ________ **5.** ________ **7.** ________
2. ________ **4.** ________ **6.** ________ **8.** ________

B. Révisions. Vous révisez le vocabulaire pour votre prochain examen de français en utilisant les images ci-dessous. Avec votre camarade, identifiez à voix haute les choses représentées.

1. 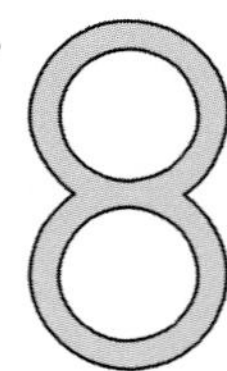

4. 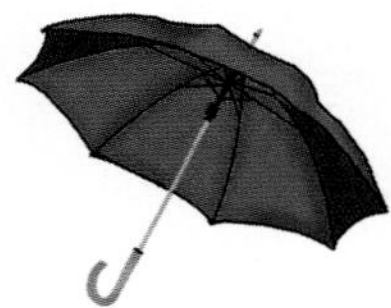

7. 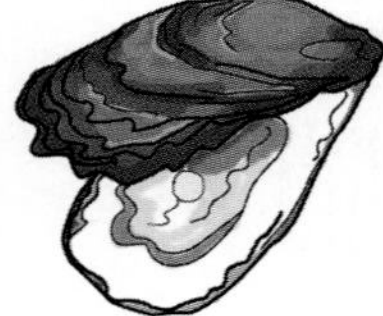

2. 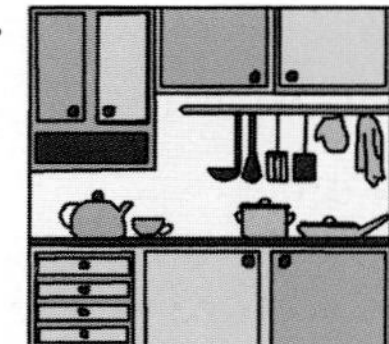

5. 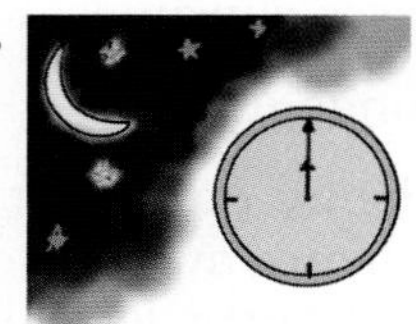

8. 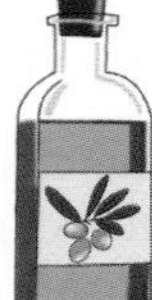

3. 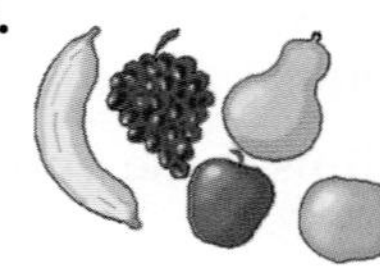

6. 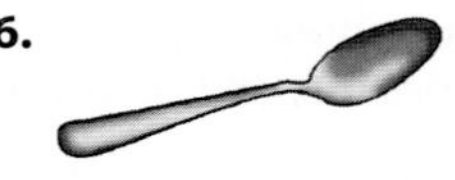

2. **The consonant sounds in [p], [t], and [k]** (page 250)

Dans l'avion. Vous allez passer le week-end en Italie. Pendant le vol, vous entendez discuter les passagers devant vous. Avec votre camarade, jouez la scène. Mettez (*Put*) la main tout près de la bouche (*mouth*) pour faire bien attention à la prononciation des sons [p], [t], et [k].

PASSAGER A: Tu as entendu? Le pilote est une femme. Elle s'appelle Caroline. Je pense qu'elle est québécoise: elle parle avec un accent canadien.
PASSAGER B: Ah oui, je l'ai vue (*I saw her*). Elle est petite avec les cheveux courts sous sa casquette. Elle porte un tailleur kaki.
PASSAGER A: Regarde! Les derniers passagers ont embarqué. On va bientôt partir.
PASSAGER B: Oui. Dans quelques (*a few*) minutes, l'hôtesse de l'air va servir du café aux passagers. Tant mieux (*So much the better*)! Je suis encore un peu fatigué.

Leçon 4

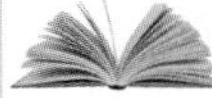

Lecture

Avant de lire

Using background knowledge and knowledge of text type to predict content. Before reading a new text, your general knowledge of the subject matter may help you anticipate important details. Sometimes the type or genre of a text can help you predict its content.

The text you will be reading contains information about two relatively new rideshare programs in France.

Look at the information below from the **Vélib'** website page entitled "**Comment ça marche?**" What can you already predict about the rest of the passage? How might **Autolib'** be different from **Vélib'?** Make a list of two things you will probably learn about each service.

Utiliser Vélib'

Prendre un vélo dans une station, le déposer dans une autre. Vélib' est un système de location en libre-service simple à utiliser, disponible 24 heures sur 24 et 7 jours sur 7.

Retirer un vélo

Pour louer un vélo, identifiez-vous sur la borne, accédez au menu et choisissez un vélo parmi ceux proposés sur l'écran.

GAGNEZ DU TEMPS ET ABONNEZ-VOUS À L'ANNÉE!

Grâce à la carte annuelle Vélib' et au passe NAVIGO©, vous pouvez retirer un vélo directement sur le point d'attache.

Restituer son vélo

Une fois votre trajet terminé, accrochez le vélo sur un point d'attache libre dans n'importe quelle station Vélib'.

Attendez quelques instants, un signal sonore et un voyant lumineux vous confirmeront que le vélo a bien été restitué.

■

Now scan the following reading and look for this information. How accurate were your predictions?

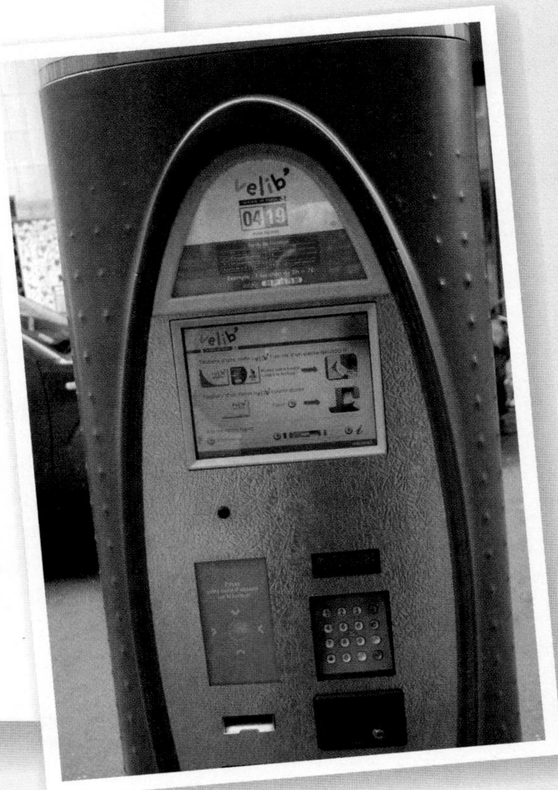

À propos de la lecture...
Les auteurs de *Vis-à-vis* ont écrit ce texte.

Vélib' et Autolib': on innove dans les transports

On les voit partout dans Paris: ce sont les Vélib' et les Autolib', ces bicyclettes et ces mini-voitures que chacun peut utiliser librement selon ses besoins, pour un coût[1] très raisonnable. L'idée, c'est de partager des bicyclettes et des voitures pour lutter[2] contre l'excès de trafic et contre la pollution. En adoptant ces moyens de transport, on fait une bonne action écologique et on économise de l'argent: voilà deux arguments irrésistibles!

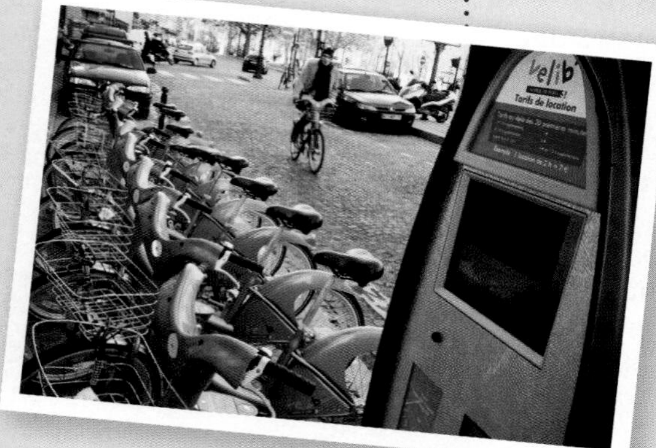

Le vélo pour tous

Vélib': Des vélos pour tout le monde

Vélib' est un système de location[3] de vélos en libre-service,[4] disponible[5] 24 heures sur 24 et 7 jours sur 7. Depuis 2007, plus de 20 000 vélos attendent leurs clients dans 1 500 stations. On les utilise dans la semaine pour aller au travail ou en cours, et le week-end pour se promener dans les rues de la capitale. Le fonctionnement du service est très simple: on prend un vélo dans une station, on va où on veut aller, et on dépose[6] le vélo dans une autre station.

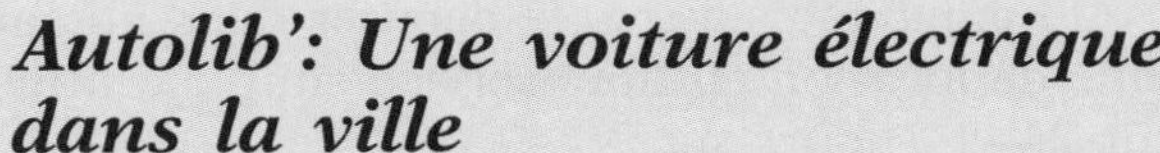

Autolib': Une voiture électrique dans la ville

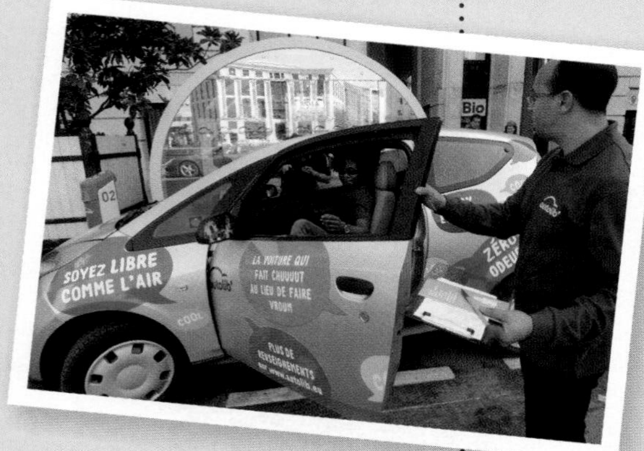

Des petites voitures pour la ville

L'Autolib' obéit au même principe. Depuis 2011, 1 800 mini-voitures électriques disposées dans des centaines[7] de stations proposent une alternative aux Parisiens qui n'aiment pas pédaler. Propre[8] et silencieuse, pratique et facile, l'Autolib' est une voiture sans défaut[9]! La voiture du futur! Elle permet de bouger en ville, d'aller en proche banlieue, de transporter facilement des enfants, des amis... ou des paquets! Et de faire des économies: avec Autolib', pas d'assurance,[10] pas d'entretien,[11] pas de parking!

Comment ça marche?

Pour accéder au service Vélib', on doit acheter un abonnement[12] annuel (29 euros) ou un ticket pour une journée, une semaine ou quelques jours. Dans tous les cas, les 30 premières minutes de chaque trajet[13] sont gratuites.[14] Ensuite, chaque demi-heure coûte à peu près un euro. Toutes les informations sur les prix sont données sur le site Vélib' de la Mairie de Paris. Pour Autolib', plusieurs tarifs et abonnements sont proposés sur leur site.

[1]*cost* [2]*fight* [3]*rental* [4]*en... self-service* [5]*available* [6]*drop off* [7]*hundreds* [8]*Clean* [9]*fault* [10]*insurance* [11]*maintenance* [12]*subscription* [13]*trip* [14]*free*

Quelques critiques

Le Vélib' et L'Autolib' sont aujourd'hui bien installés à Paris. Mais tout n'est pas encore parfait: d'abord, pourquoi ces vélos et ces voitures sont-ils gris? Pourquoi pas jaunes, verts ou bleus? Quel dommage! Les Français tellement attachés à l'esthétique détestent cette absence de couleur: «Ces vélos et ces voitures ressemblent à des tanks de la dernière guerre». Voilà ce qu'on entend! Certains utilisateurs reprochent aussi au Vélib' son poids: 22,5 kilos, c'est très lourd quand vous devez monter à Montmartre ou au parc des Buttes Chaumont! Quant aux[15] mini-voitures, elles sont souvent en panne[16] et les délais de réparation sont trop longs. «Simple défaut de jeunesse» répondent les fans!

[15]Quant... *As for* [16]en... *broken down*

Compréhension

1. Qu'est-ce que le Vélib'? l'Autolib'?
2. Comment est-ce qu'on accède au service Vélib' ou au service Autolib'?
3. Quels sont les avantages du Vélib' et de l'Autolib'?
4. Que disent les critiques? À votre avis, est-ce que leurs objections sont valables? Expliquez.
5. Dans votre ville ou votre pays, est-ce qu'il y a des systèmes de location équivalents? Comparez-le(s) au système Vélib' et Autolib'.

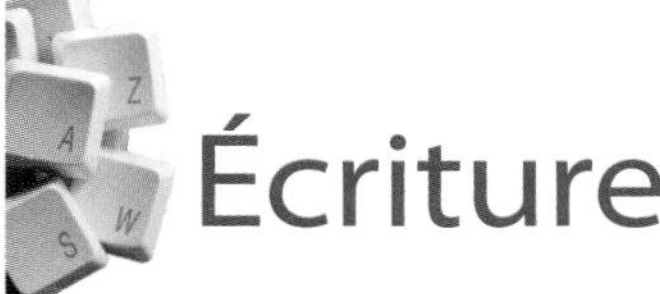

Écriture

The writing activities **Par écrit** and **Journal intime** can be found in the Workbook/Laboratory Manual to accompany *Vis-à-vis*.

La vie en chantant. An activity based on the song "Route nationale 7" by Charles Trenet can be found in the Instructor's Manual. The song can be purchased at the iTunes store, or sts. can watch the music video on YouTube.

Pour s'amuser

Dans le train, le contrôleur parle à une vieille dame:

—Madame, votre billet est pour Bordeaux. Mais ce train va à Nantes!
—Ça c'est ennuyeux, proteste la voyageuse. Moi je vais à Bordeaux!... Et le conducteur* se trompe souvent comme ça?

**driver, engineer*

Le vidéoblog de Juliette

En bref

Dans cet épisode, Juliette a rendez-vous avec Léa au jardin du Luxembourg; elle y arrive sur son nouveau vélo. Les deux amies veulent regarder l'arrivée du Tour de France—la célèbre course cycliste que Juliette décrit dans son vidéoblog.

Vocabulaire en contexte

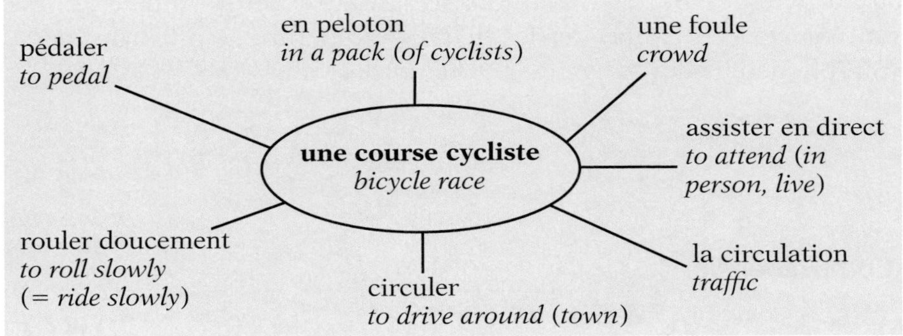

Visionnez!

Indiquez si les phrases sont vraies ou fausses.

1. _______ Juliette va rouler à vélo au lieu d'utiliser (*instead of using*) les transports en commun.
2. _______ Juliette et Léa comptent (*plan on*) regarder l'arrivée du Tour de France ensemble.
3. _______ Juliette préfère regarder l'arrivée du Tour de France à la télé.
4. _______ Le Tour de France passe dans toute la France pendant quatre semaines.
5. _______ Le cycliste victorieux porte un maillot tricolore (bleu, blanc, rouge).

Analysez!

Répondez aux questions suivantes.

1. L'arrivée à Paris du Tour de France est une grande fête populaire. Donnez des exemples.
2. Comment la ville de Paris se prépare-t-elle pour l'arrivée du Tour de France?

Comparez!

Quel est l'événement sportif le plus prestigieux dans votre pays? Où et quand a-t-il lieu? Regardez encore une fois la partie culturelle de la vidéo: en France, le Tour de France est une grande fête populaire. Est-ce que c'est aussi le cas pour le grand événement sportif dans votre pays? Expliquez.

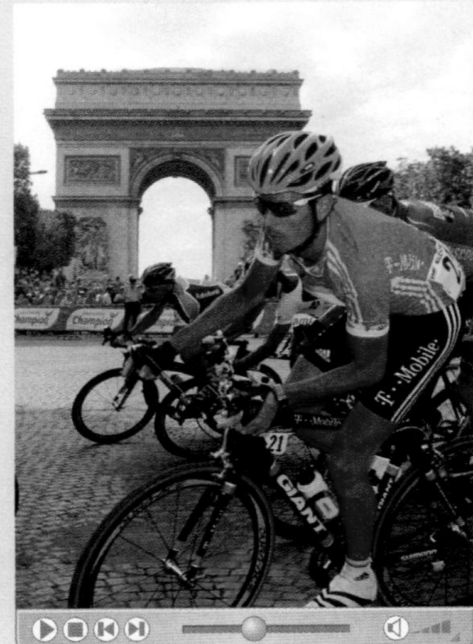

L'arrivée à Paris du Tour de France sur les Champs-Élysées

Suggestion: Ask sts. short-answer questions based on the vocabulary to aid their comprehension of the video episode: *Aimez-vous la vitesse? Roulez-vous vite à vélo? en voiture? Préférez-vous assister à un événement sportif en direct ou le regarder à la télé?* etc.

Additional vocabulary: Other vocabulary you may wish to present before viewing includes *j'en ai marre, tu ne m'as rien dit, j'irai.*

Suggestion: Have sts. correct the false sentences.

Note culturelle

En France, le vélo urbain est un phénomène de société. Moyen de transport écologique, le vélo en libre-service triomphe à Paris avec le Vélib', à Lyon avec le Vélo'v, à Dijon avec le Vélodi, à Bordeaux avec V^3, à Nice avec le Vélobleu. Toutes les villes de France adoptent ce système qui, pour un prix très bas, met à la disposition des habitants des milliers de vélos, 24 heures sur 24, 7 jours sur 7.

Follow-up: Have sts. indicate which sporting event they chose. Is the class in agreement? If not, have sts. defend their choices.

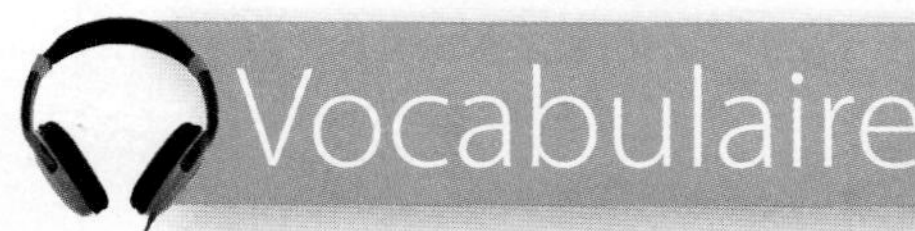

Vocabulaire

Verbes

conduire to drive
construire to construct
détruire to destroy
faire le plein to fill it up (*gas tank*)
produire to produce
réduire to reduce
rouler to roll; to travel (*in a car, on a bike*)
traduire to translate
traverser to cross

À REVOIR: **partir, voyager**

Substantifs

l'aéroport (*m.*) airport
un aller-retour round trip; round-trip ticket
l'arrivée (*f.*) arrival
l'auberge (*f.*) **de jeunesse** youth hostel
l'autocar (*m.*) interurban bus
l'autoroute (*f.*) highway
l'avion (*m.*) airplane
le billet ticket
le camion truck
la carte d'embarquement boarding pass
la classe affaires business class
la classe économique tourist class
le coffre trunk
le compartiment compartment
le conducteur / la conductrice driver
la consigne (automatique) coin locker
la couchette berth
le départ departure
la deuxième classe second class
l'ennui (*m.*) problem, trouble
l'essence (*f.*) gasoline
la gare train station
le guichet (ticket) window
l'hôtesse (*f.*) **de l'air** stewardess
le métro subway
la moto(cyclette) motorcycle
le moyen de transport means of transportation
le passager / la passagère passenger
le pilote pilot
la première classe first class
le quai platform (*at the train station*)
le siège seat
la station-service service station
le steward steward
le train train
le vol flight
le wagon train car

À REVOIR: **l'endroit** (*m.*), **l'état** (*m.*), **la fois, le monde, le pays, la semaine, la valise, la voiture**

Expressions affirmatives et négatives

déjà already; ever
encore still
ne... jamais never
ne... pas du tout not at all
ne... pas encore not yet
ne... personne no one, nobody
ne... plus no longer
ne... que only
ne... rien nothing
parfois sometimes
quelque chose something
quelqu'un someone
seulement only
tout everything
tout le monde everybody, everyone

Les points cardinaux

l'est (*m.*) east
le nord north
le nord-est northeast
le nord-ouest northwest
l'ouest (*m.*) west
le sud south
le sud-est southeast
le sud-ouest southwest

Mots et expressions divers

à by; on (*bicycle, horseback, foot*)
à destination de to, for
à l'est / l'ouest to the east / the west
à l'étranger abroad, in a foreign country
à l'heure on time
à pied on foot
à velo by bike
au nord / sud to the north / south
depuis since, for
  Depuis combien de temps... ? (For) How long . . . ?
  Depuis quand... ? Since when . . . ?
  en in; by (*train, plane, bus*)
  pendant for; during
    Pendant combien de temps... ? (For) How long . . . ?
si yes (*response to a negative question*)
vite quickly

CHAPITRE 10

Comment communiquez-vous?

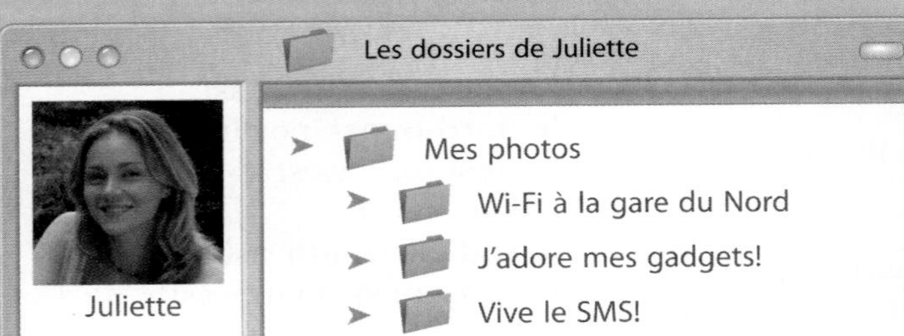

Presentation: *Décrivez la photo. Avez-vous une connexion Wi-Fi sur votre mobile ou sur votre portable? Où y a-t-il des connexions Wi-Fi dans votre ville?*

Les dossiers de Juliette

Juliette

- Mes photos
  - Wi-Fi à la gare du Nord
  - J'adore mes gadgets!
  - Vive le SMS!

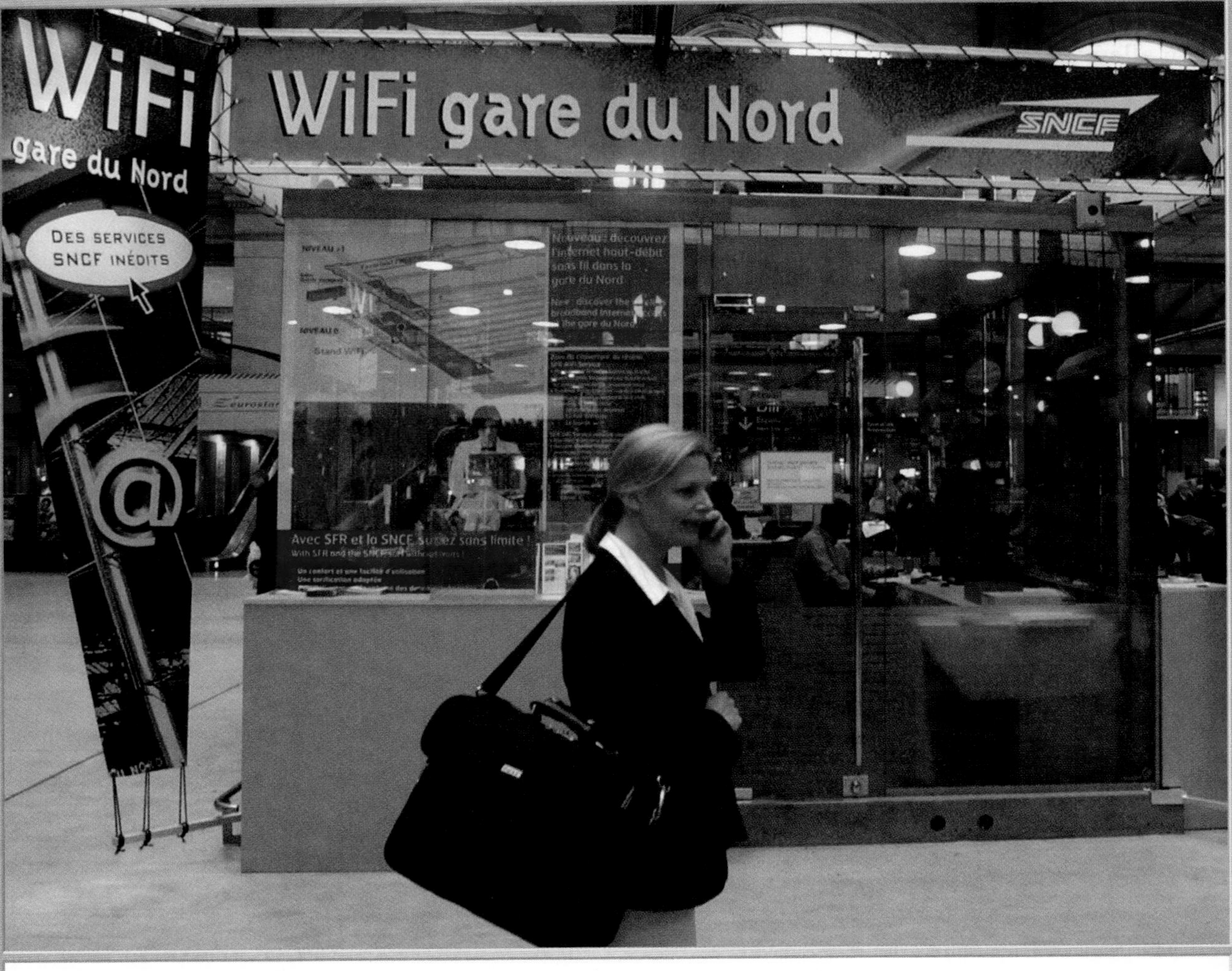

La gare du Nord à Paris: Partout où on va, on est connecté.

Cultural note: The *Gare du Nord* is one of six terminus stations in Paris and the busiest train station in Europe. It serves trains to *la Picardie* and *le Nord-Pas-de-*Calais in northern France as well as those to London, Brussels, and Amsterdam.

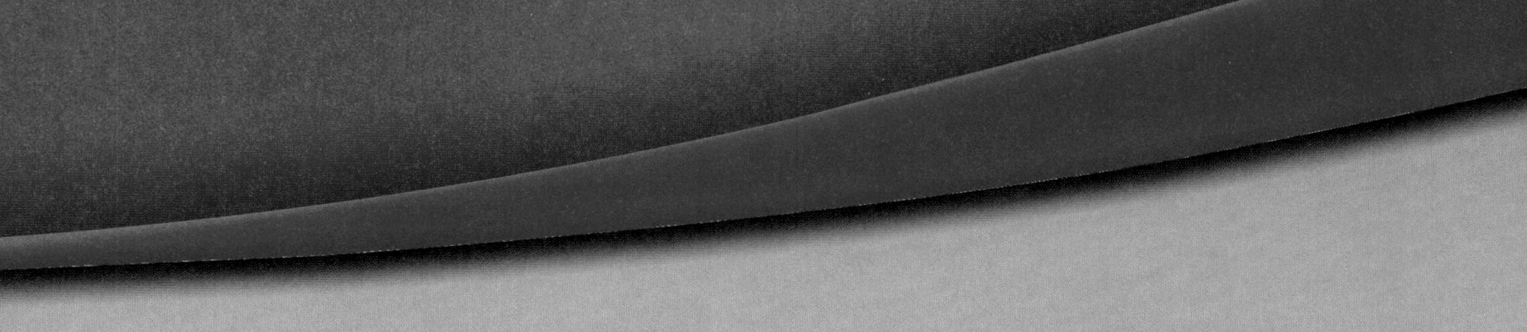

Dans ce chapitre...

OBJECTIFS COMMUNICATIFS

- talking about communication, the media, and modern technology
- describing the past
- speaking succinctly
- expressing observations and beliefs
- learning to distinguish between and pronounce selected sounds in French

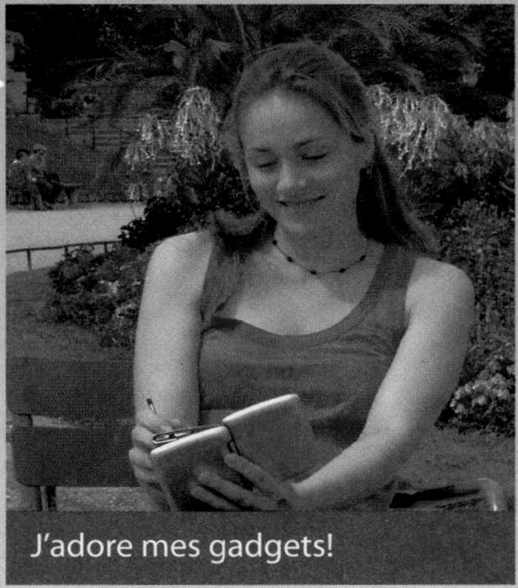

J'adore mes gadgets!

PAROLES (Leçon 1)

- Les nouvelles technologies
- Les médias et la communication
- Quelques verbes de communication

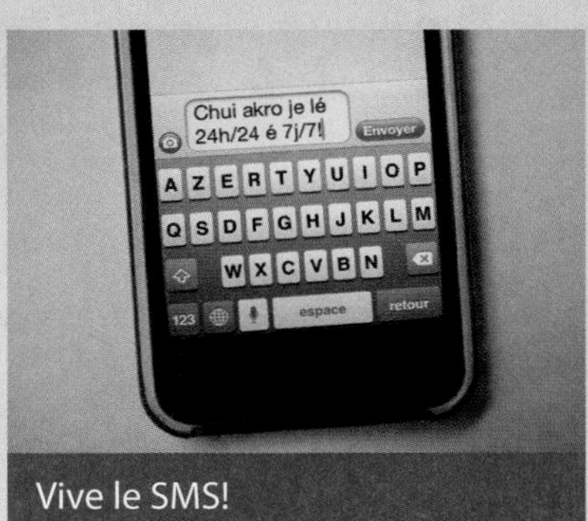

Vive le SMS!

STRUCTURES (Leçons 2 et 3)

- L'imparfait
- Les pronoms d'objet direct
- L'accord du participe passé
- Les verbes **voir, croire** et **recevoir**

CULTURE

- Le blog de Juliette: *Ordinateur, mon amour!*
- Reportage: *Les accros du texto*
- Lecture: *Rencontres en ligne: rendez-vous avec le bonheur* (Leçon 4)

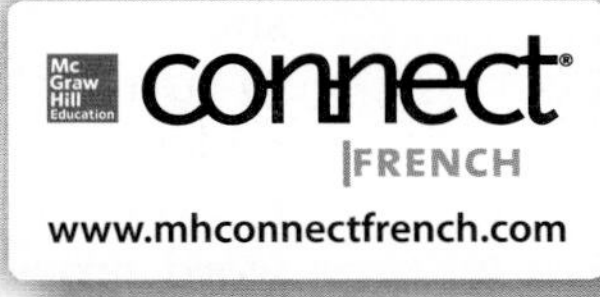

Leçon 1

PAROLES

Les nouvelles technologies

Qu'est-ce que vous voulez comme cadeau (*m.*) (*gift*)?

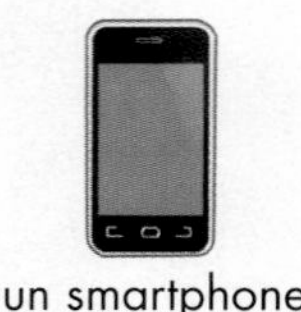
un smartphone

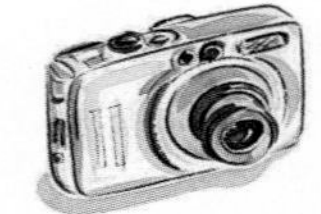
un appareil (photo) numérique

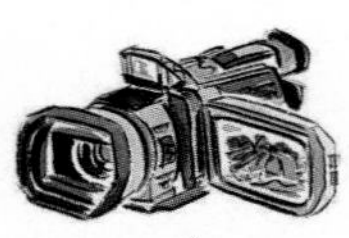
un caméscope

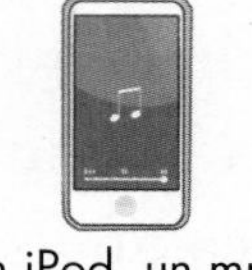
un iPod, un mp3

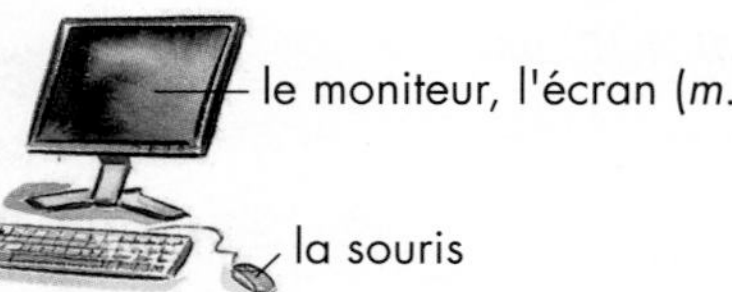
le moniteur, l'écran (*m.*)
le clavier
la souris

un ordinateur de bureau, un micro (micro-ordinateur)

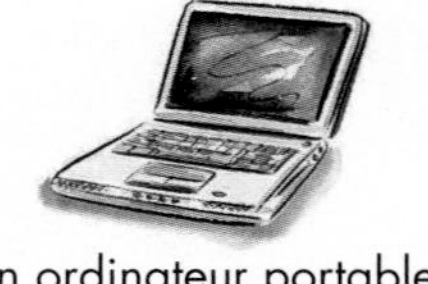
un ordinateur portable (un portable)

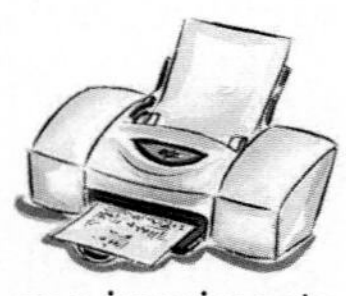
une imprimante

Suggestion: Bring in pages advertising some of these items from a French or Francophone catalogue; use as an authentic reading document. Ask sts. to choose the item they prefer and discuss why they chose it.

Note: Additional technology vocabulary is listed on page 284.

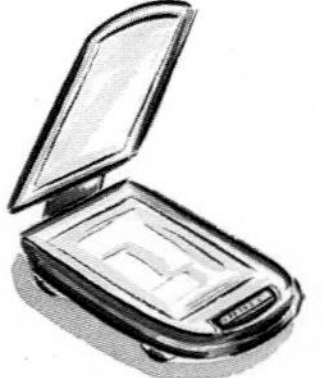
un scanner

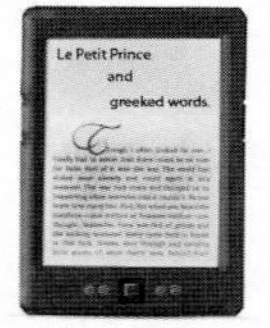

une liseuse
un livre numérique

AUTRES MOTS UTILES

cliquer sur	to click on
une connexion ADSL	DSL connection/line
le courriel, le mél	e-mail message
le fichier	file
Internet (*m.*) **(sur Internet)**	Internet (on the Internet)
le logiciel	software (program)
le navigateur	browser
un photocopieur	photocopy machine
le site	site
surfer sur le Web	to surf the web
une tablette	tablet computer
télécharger	to download
le traitement de texte	word processing
le Web	(World Wide) Web
le Wi-Fi	Wi-Fi, wireless (connection)

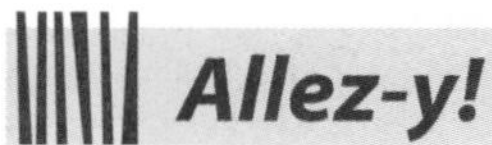

Définitions. Regardez les illustrations et la liste de vocabulaire et trouvez le mot qui correspond à chaque définition. Faites une phrase avec **C'est un(e)...**

1. C'est un appareil qui vous permet d'imprimer vos fichiers.
2. C'est un appareil qu'on utilise pour faire des films.
3. C'est un appareil qui nous permet d'écouter notre musique préférée.
4. Ce sont deux machines qu'on peut utiliser pour copier une image.
5. C'est un message écrit sur l'ordinateur.
6. Avec ces appareils, on prend des photos.
7. Avec ces appareils, on peut regarder des vidéos sur un écran.
8. On fait cette action si on reçoit (*receives*) un fichier avec un mél.
9. Avec ces appareils, on peut lire un livre numérique.
10. Avec ce service, on surfe très vite (*fast*) sur le Web.

Les médias et la communication

1. Nous écrivons (*write*) et nous envoyons*...

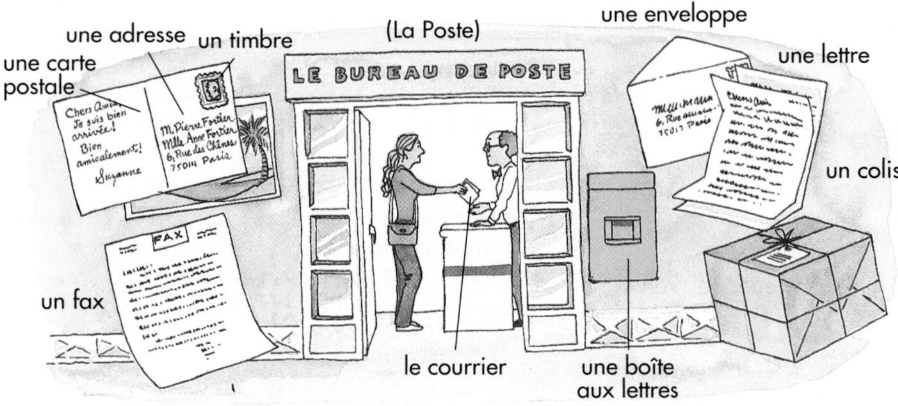

Où est la dame sur l'illustration? Qu'est-ce qu'il y a, en général, sur une enveloppe? Où se trouve la boîte aux lettres? Que fait-on quand on a besoin d'une copie d'un document tout de suite. Qu'est-ce qu'on envoie souvent pendant les vacances? Si vous envoyez un cadeau à quelqu'un, qu'est-ce que vous envoyez?

*The conjugation of **écrire** (*to write*) is presented on page 265. The present-tense conjugation of **envoyer** (*to send*) is **j'envoie, tu envoies, il/elle/on envoie, nous envoyons, vous envoyez, ils/elles envoient.**

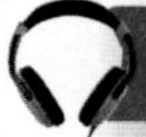

Prononcez bien!

Final consonants and *liaison*

Remember, as a general rule, only final **-c, -r, -f,** and **-l** are pronounced in French.*

lac, ordinateur, bœuf, mél

But

pied, trop, colis, départ, chez

However, when final **-d, -n, -r, -s, -t,** and **-x,** are followed by a word beginning with a vowel or mute **h,** they are pronounced and reattached to that vowel.

-t, -d	→	[t]: **un petit‿appareil numérique, un grand‿écran**
-n	→	[n]: **on‿écrit, un‿annuaire**
-r	→	[R]: **le premier‿homme, le dernier‿étage**
-s, -x	→	[z]: **nous‿avons deux‿ordinateurs**

*For exceptions to this rule, see **Prononcez bien!** on the pronunciation of final consonants, page 69.

Pronunciation presentation (1): Model the pronunciation of sentence 2 in *Allez-y! Définitions* and emphasize the liaison between *c'est* and *un*, between *un* and *appareil* and between *on* and *utilise*.

Pronunciation presentation (2): You may want to teach the expression CaReFuL as a mnemonic device.

Pronunciation practice: The *Prononcez bien!* section on page 281 of this chapter contains activities for practicing these sounds.

Note: Although *fax* and *envoyer par fax* are widely used, *la télécopie* and *envoyer par télécopieur* are the French terms.

Additional vocabulary: *affranchir, poster une lettre, envoyer une lettre aux États-Unis, par avion.*

Note: It would be helpful to show photos from the Internet of post offices (interiors and exteriors), mailboxes, and mail trucks.

Suggestion: Teach sts. the configuration of a typical French phone number, e.g., 01 45 88 69 92. Have sts. pronounce such numbers by expressing the pairs of two digits together.

Additional activity: *Conseils. Vous venez d'arriver en France et vous êtes un peu désorienté(e). Exposez votre problème et donnez des conseils.* MODÈLE: *Je voudrais trouver du travail.* → *Cherche un journal!* 1. *Je voudrais acheter un journal.* 2. *Je voudrais appeler un ami.* 3. *Je voudrais appeler une amie en Afrique.* 4. *Je voudrais acheter un timbre.* 5. *Je voudrais envoyer cette lettre.*

Suggestions: (1) Model pronunciation, with group and individual repetition. (2) *Devinettes.* Indicate objects with definitions or locations, e.g., *Il est sur l'enveloppe* (*le timbre*). *on l'utilise pour chercher un numéro de téléphone* (*l'annuaire électronique*). *Ils sont dans le kiosque* (*les journaux, les magazines,* etc.). *C'est une des chaînes de la télévision française* (*TF1*).

Note: You may wish to bring in several types of French magazines for sts. to compare with North American ones.

Additional vocabulary: *un coup de fil, les Pages blanches* (*bottin des particuliers*), *les Pages jaunes* (*bottin des professionnels*), *le récepteur, décrocher, raccrocher.*

Note: *Faire le numéro* is a common synonym of *composer le numéro.*

Cultural note: In Quebec, *faire un appel à frais renversés ou virés.*

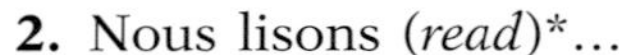

2. Nous lisons (*read*)*...

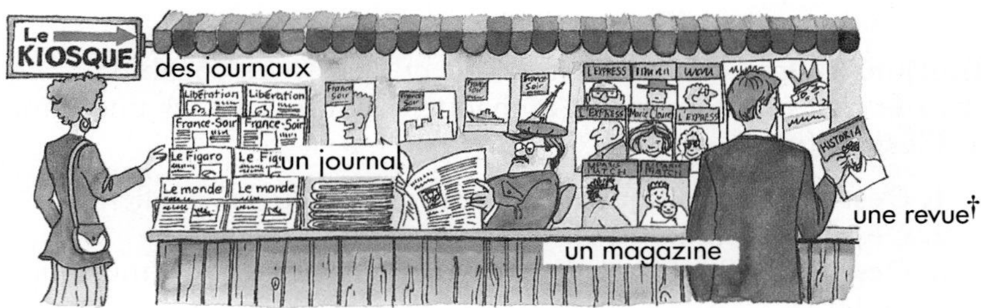

AUTRES MOTS UTILES

les petites annonces (*f.*)	classified ads
un roman	novel

Où est-ce qu'on va pour acheter des journaux? Où se trouvent (*are found*) les petites annonces? Pour quelles raisons est-ce qu'on lit les petites annonces?

3. Nous parlons...

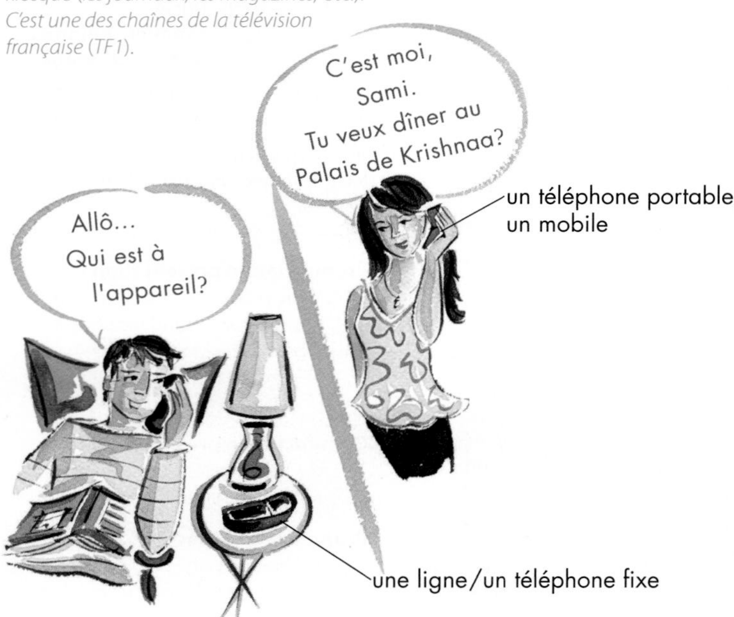

AUTRES MOTS UTILES

l'annuaire (*m.*) **électronique**	online telephone directory
appeler‡	to call
la boîte vocale	voice mail
composer le numéro	to dial the number
consulter l'annuaire électronique	to look up (a phone number) in the online directory
envoyer un SMS, un texto	to send a text message

Comment est-ce qu'on cherche les numéros de téléphone? Qu'est-ce qu'on fait pour appeler un ami? Que dit la personne qui répond? Qu'est-ce qu'on fait si on veut envoyer un message court (*short*)?

---

*The conjugation of **lire** is presented on page 265.

†**Une revue** is generally a monthly publication of a scholarly or informational nature; **un magazine,** on the other hand, contains articles on a wide variety of topics and has many photographs and advertisements.

‡The present-tense conjugation of **appeler** (*to call*) is **j'appelle, tu appelles, il/elle/on appelle, nous appelons, vous appelez, ils/elles appellent. Appeler** takes a direct object: **Il appelle sa petite amie.**

4. Nous écoutons et nous regardons...

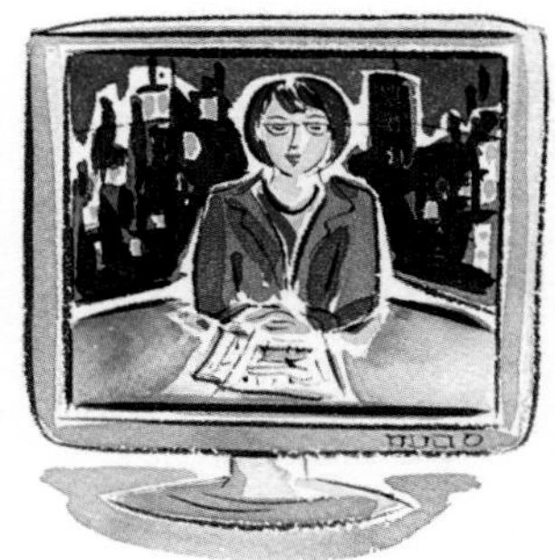

le journal télévisé,
les informations (*f. pl.*)

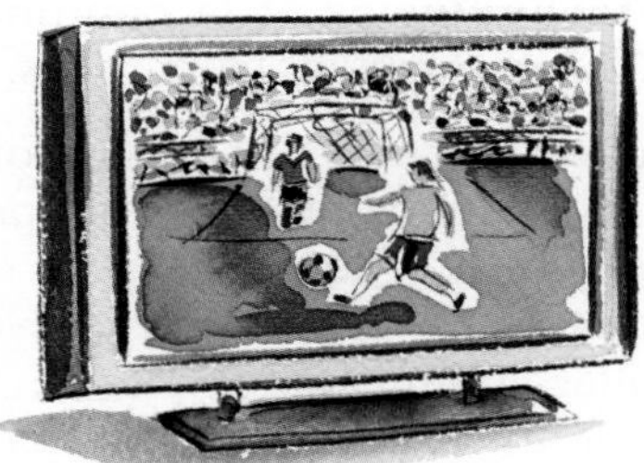

une retransmission sportive

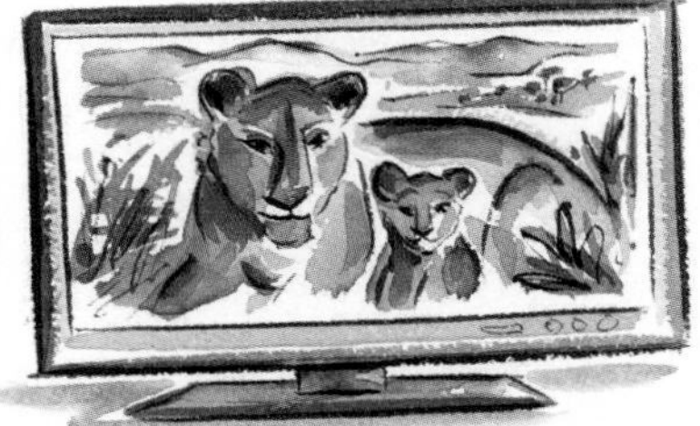

un documentaire

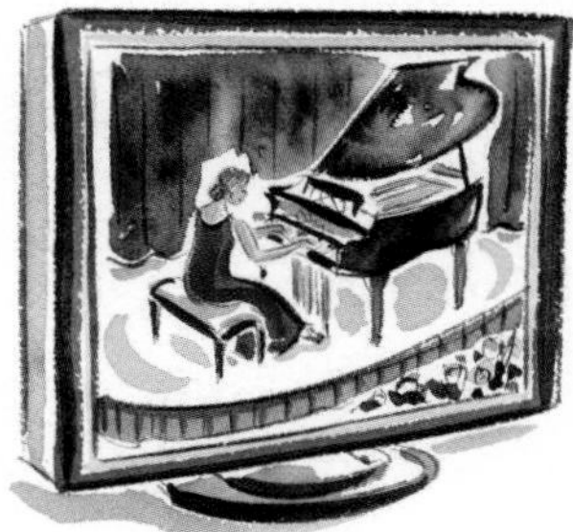

une émission de musique

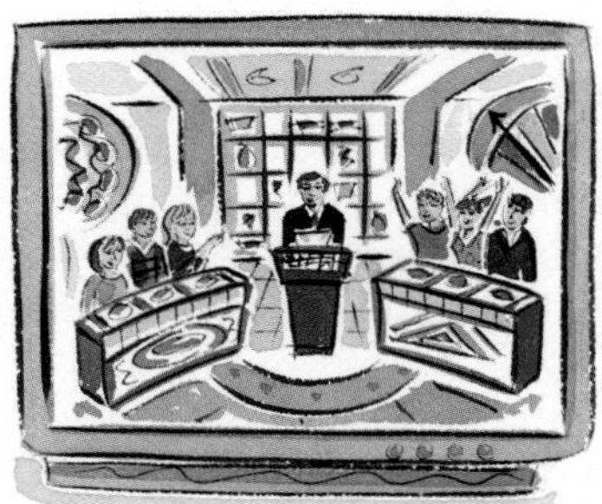

un jeu télévisé

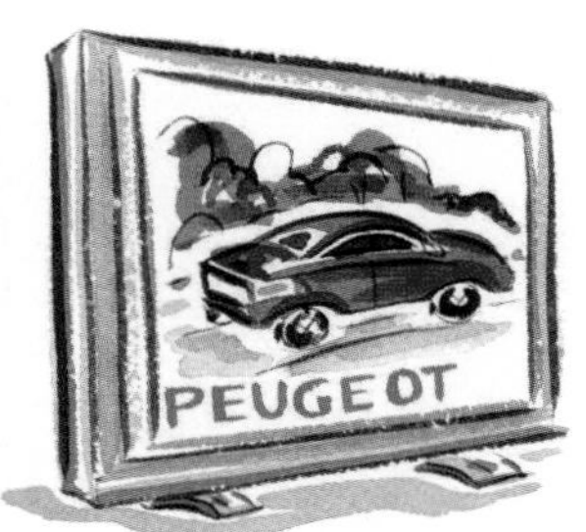

une publicité

AUTRES MOTS UTILES

le câble	cable television
une chaîne	television channel; network
un DVD (des DVD)	DVD
une émission de télé réalité	reality show
un feuilleton	soap opera
un lecteur de DVD	DVD player
une série télévisée	serial drama
une télécommande	remote control
la télévision satellite	satellite television
la TNT (télévision numérique terrestre)	high-definition television

Note: There are many television networks and channels in France. Those that have been in existence for many years include public stations such as *France 2, France 3, la cinq* (*Arte*), and privately owned stations such as *TF1* (*Télévision Française 1*) and *Canal Plus*.

Aimez-vous les émissions de musique classique? les retransmissions sportives? les documentaires? les séries humoristiques? Regardez-vous régulièrement le journal télévisé? Que pensez-vous des publicités? Préférez-vous regarder un film ou une émission télévisée? Pourquoi? Utilisez-vous souvent la télécommande?

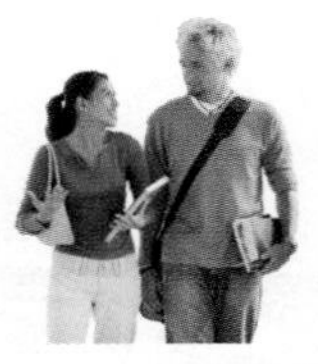

Suggestion: Hand out several copies of a TV schedule showing the program titles and possibly other information. Ask sts. what types of programs different titles might be.

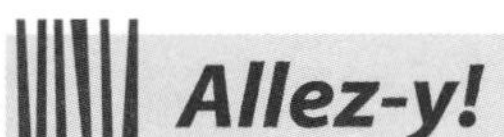

Allez-y!

Les nouvelles technologies et la communication. Posez les questions suivantes à un(e) ou plusieurs camarades.

1. Tu as un ordinateur? Est-ce un portable ou un ordinateur de bureau? Est-ce que tu as ton propre (*own*) site Web? Que fais-tu sur le Web? En général, qu'est-ce que tu fais sur ton ordinateur?
2. Est-ce que tu préfères télécharger des films et les regarder chez toi ou aller au cinéma? Explique.
3. Est-ce que tu as un iPod / un mp3? Décris-le.
4. Tu as un caméscope? Si oui, qu'est-ce que tu aimes filmer?
5. Vas-tu souvent à la poste? Pourquoi (pas)?
6. Quels journaux, magazines ou revues achètes-tu régulièrement?
7. Tu as une ligne fixe et un mobile / un téléphone portable ou un smartphone? Quelles technologies de communication sont indispensables pour toi? Explique.
8. Que fais-tu si tu veux contacter une personne qui n'est pas chez elle (*at home*)? Que fais-tu quand elle est chez elle?
9. Préfères-tu la télé ou Internet? Explique.
10. Quelle est ton émission préférée à la télé? Pourquoi?

Quelques verbes de communication

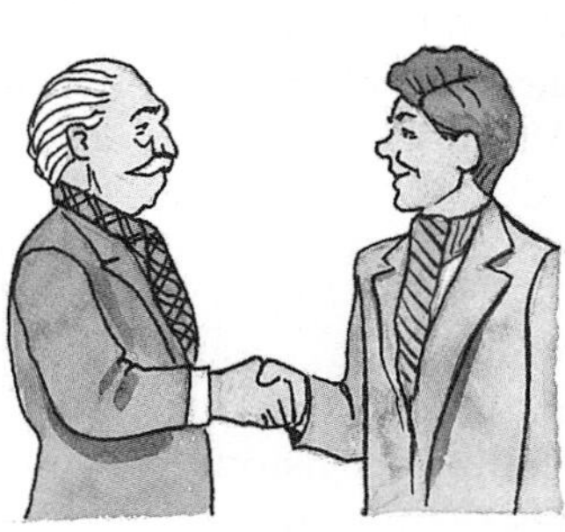

dire bonjour

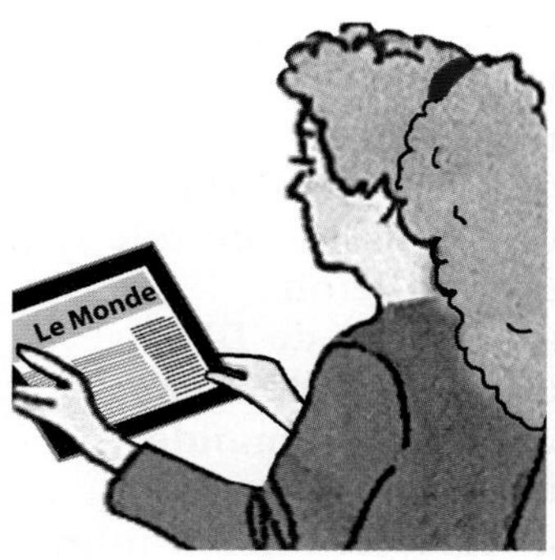

lire le journal

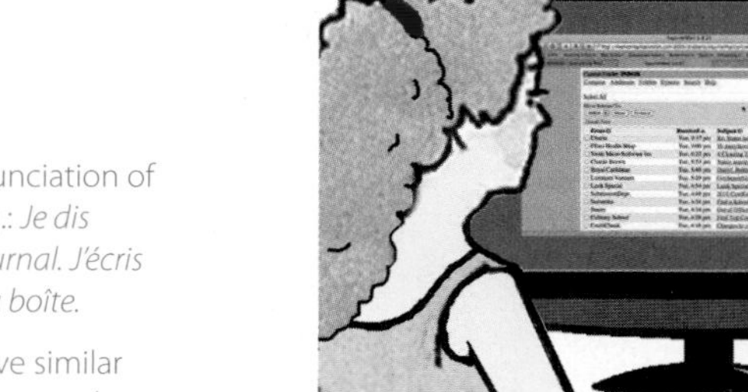

écrire un mél / un courriel

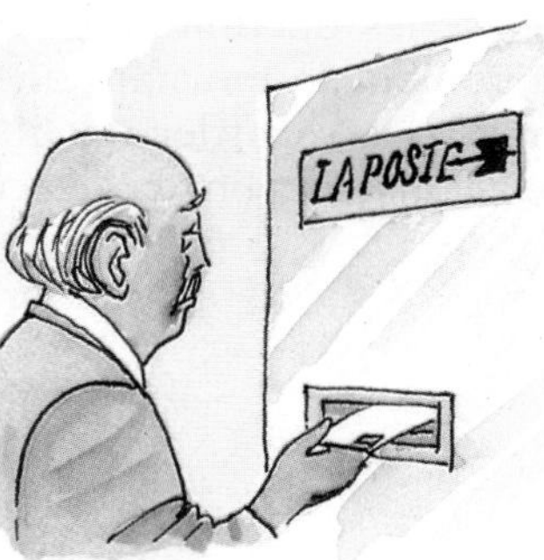

mettre une lettre à la boîte

Presentation: Model pronunciation of verbs in short sentences, e.g.: *Je dis bonjour (tu, il, etc.). Je lis le journal. J'écris une lettre. Je mets la lettre à la boîte.*

Note: *Dire, lire,* and *écrire* have similar conjugations except for the second-person plural (*vous* form) of *dire* and the *v* in the plural stem of *écrire.*

dire (*to say; to tell*)		lire (*to read*)		écrire (*to write*)		mettre (*to place; to put*)	
je	**dis**	je	**lis**	j'	**écris**	je	**mets**
tu	**dis**	tu	**lis**	tu	**écris**	tu	**mets**
il/elle/on	**dit**	il/elle/on	**lit**	il/elle/on	**écrit**	il/elle/on	**met**
nous	**disons**	nous	**lisons**	nous	**écrivons**	nous	**mettons**
vous	**dites**	vous	**lisez**	vous	**écrivez**	vous	**mettez**
ils/elles	**disent**	ils/elles	**lisent**	ils/elles	**écrivent**	ils/elles	**mettent**
Past participle:	**dit**		**lu**		**écrit**		**mis**

Another verb conjugated like **écrire** is **décrire** (*to describe*). **Mettre** can also be used to mean *to put on* (*clothing*). **Mettre le couvert** means *to set the table*. **Mettre une lettre (une carte) à la poste** means *to mail a letter* (*card*).

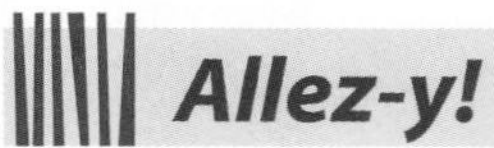

Allez-y!

A. Message aux parents. Vous racontez à un(e) camarade ce que vous mettez dans le mél que vous écrivez à vos parents. Complétez les phrases avec les verbes **décrire, dire, écrire** et **lire,** au présent. Faites tous les changements nécessaires.

Cet après-midi, je/j' ______[1] un long mél à mes parents. Dans mon mél, je ______[2] mes cours et ma vie à l'université. Je donne aussi beaucoup de détails sur mes camarades et mes professeurs parce que mes parents sont très curieux. Ils sont aussi très compréhensifs (*understanding*) et je leur ______[3] toujours la vérité quand j'ai des problèmes. Avant de l'envoyer, je ______[4] mon message une dernière fois (*last time*).

Racontez la même histoire, mais cette fois remplacez **je** par **mon (ma) camarade de chambre,** puis par **Stéphanie et Albane.** Faites tous les changements nécessaires.

B. Interview. Posez les questions suivantes à un(e) camarade, puis inversez les rôles.

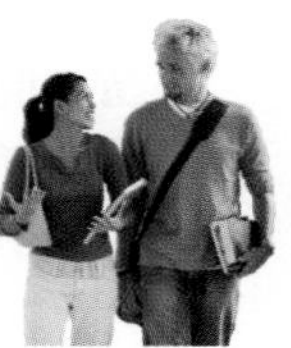

1. Est-ce que tu écris souvent des lettres ou des cartes postales? À qui écris-tu? D'habitude, pour donner de tes nouvelles à tes amis, préfères-tu écrire un texto, un mél ou préfères-tu téléphoner ou contacter les gens sur Facebook?
2. Est-ce que tu aimes lire? Lis-tu le journal tous les jours? Si oui, lequel? As-tu déjà cherché un appartement dans les petites annonces? Quel(s) magazine(s) achètes-tu régulièrement? As-tu lu un bon livre récemment? Quel est le titre de ce livre? Préfères-tu lire des livres papier ou des livres numériques? As-tu une liseuse?
3. Est-ce que tu regardes la télévision tous les soirs? Quelles émissions préfères-tu? Que penses-tu de la télévision américaine? À ton avis, y a-t-il trop de publicité à la télévision?

D'après ses réponses, que pouvez-vous dire de votre camarade et de ses goûts?

Leçon 2

STRUCTURES

L'imparfait

Describing the Past

Une enfant de l'Internet

Appel vidéo entre Charlotte et Juliette.

CHARLOTTE: Tu aimes la technologie?
JULIETTE: Beaucoup! Je prépare un Master[1] multimédia interactif à la Sorbonne.
CHARLOTTE: **Tu avais** un ordinateur quand **tu étais** petite?
JULIETTE: Moi non, mais mon père **possédait** un Mac.
CHARLOTTE: **Tu naviguais** sur le Web?
JULIETTE: Pas exactement! **Je regardais** des films, **je dessinais,**[2] **je faisais** des puzzles, **j'écoutais** des chansons.[3]
CHARLOTTE: **Tu étais** déjà une enfant de l'Internet!

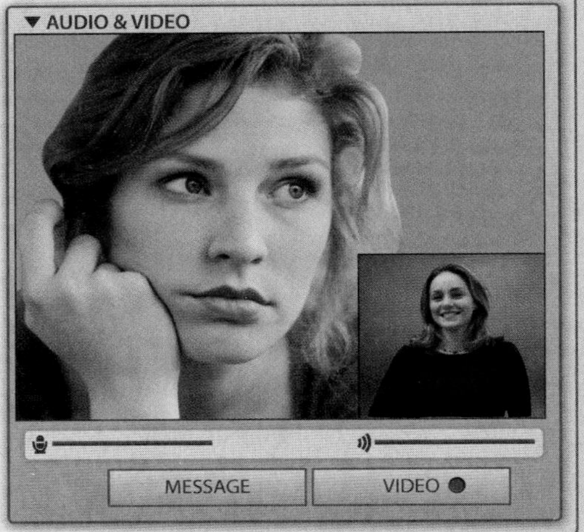

[1]*2-year professional degree* [2]*drew* [3]*songs*

Vrai ou faux? Corrigez les phrases fausses.

Quand Juliette était petite...

1. elle avait un ordinateur.
2. son père possédait un PC.
3. elle naviguait sur le Web.
4. elle ne faisait rien sur Internet.
5. elle était déjà une enfant de l'Internet.

Suggestion: Point out the *imparfait* form of the following impersonal verbs: *il fallait, il neigeait, il pleuvait, il y avait.*

Note: *Si* + *imparfait* is used to express a wish: *Si je pouvais partir!* The use of the *imparfait* in making a hypothesis is explained in *Chapitre 15.*

You are already familiar with one past tense in French: the **passé composé,** used to relate events that began and ended in the past. In contrast, the **imparfait** (*imperfect*) is used to describe continuous, repeated, or habitual past actions or situations.* It is also used in descriptions.

The **imparfait** has several equivalents in English. For example:

Je parlais. { *I talked.* / *I was talking.* / *I used to talk.* / *I would talk.* }

*You will learn more about the differences between the **passé composé** and the **imparfait** in **Chapitre 11, Leçon 2.**

Formation of the *imparfait*

The formation of the **imparfait** is identical for all French verbs except **être.** To find the regular imperfect stem, drop the **-ons** ending from the present-tense **nous** form. Then add the imperfect endings.

nous parl~~ons~~	**parl-**	nous vend~~ons~~	**vend-**
nous finiss~~ons~~	**finiss-**	nous av~~ons~~	**av-**

IMPARFAIT OF **parler**			
je	parl**ais**	nous	parl**ions**
tu	parl**ais**	vous	parl**iez**
il/elle/on	parl**ait**	ils/elles	parl**aient**

J'**allais** au bureau de poste tous les matins. — *I used to go to the post office every morning.*

Mon grand-père **disait** toujours: «L'excès en tout est un défaut.» — *My grandfather always used to say, "Moderation in all things."*

Quand j'**habitais** avec les Huet, je **mettais** souvent la table. — *When I lived with the Huets, I would often set the table.*

1. Verbs with an imperfect stem that ends in **-i** (**étudier: étudi-**) have a double **i** in the first- and second-person plural of the **imparfait: nous étud*ii*ons, vous étud*ii*ez.** The **ii** is pronounced as a lengthened *i* sound, to distinguish the **imparfait** from the present-tense forms **nous étudions** and **vous étudiez.**
2. Verbs with stems ending in **-c** or **-g** have a spelling change when the **imparfait** endings start with **a: je mang*e*ais, nous mangions; elle commen*ç*ait, nous commencions.** In this way, the pronunciation of the stem is preserved.
3. The verb **être** has an irregular stem in the **imparfait: ét-.** The endings, however, are regular.

IMPARFAIT OF **être**			
j'	**étais**	nous	**étions**
tu	**étais**	vous	**étiez**
il/elle/on	**était**	ils/elles	**étaient**

Quand tu **étais** petit, tu aimais bien lire les contes de ma mère l'Oye. — *When you were little, you liked to read Mother Goose stories.*

J'**étais** très heureux quand j'habitais à Paris. — *I was very happy when I lived in Paris.*

Vocabulary recycling: Time for a quick review of present-tense verb forms. Write a series of verbs on the board (*parler, finir, attendre, avoir, aller, faire,* etc.); give sts. a minute or two to write original sentences using those verbs and this chapter's thematic vocabulary: *Je vais au kiosque tous les jours,* etc. Have sts. lead the class in rapid-reponse drills: *Léa? Léa va au kiosque tous les jours,* etc. Emphasize the *nous* forms by wrapping up with an energetic drill: *Faire? Faisons! Vendre? Vendons!* etc.

Suggestion: To practice listening comprehension, ask sts. to indicate whether they hear imperfect or present tense. 1. *Que faites-vous?* 2. *Nous visitons le musée.* 3. *Paul regardait la statue.* 4. *Vous allez à la banque?* 5. *Tu finis ton livre?* 6. *J'allais à la pharmacie.*

Note: Point out that *changer, déranger, juger, nager,* and *voyager* are conjugated like *manger* in the imperfect.

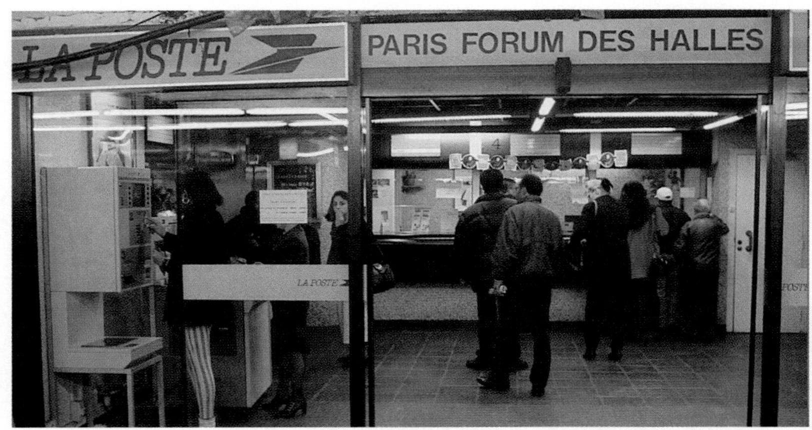

À Paris, j'allais au bureau de poste tous les jours pour envoyer des cartes postales. Est-ce que vous envoyez des cartes postales quand vous voyagez ou est-ce que vous envoyez des photos et des MMS avec votre smartphone?

Uses of the *imparfait*

Suggestion: Model pronunciation of sentences. Point out the pronunciation of *faisait* [fəzɛ].

In general, the **imparfait** is used to describe actions or situations that existed for an indefinite period of time in the past. There is usually no mention of the beginning or end of the event. The **imparfait** is used in the following situations.

1. In descriptions, to set a scene:

C'**était** une nuit tranquille à Paris. Il **pleuvait** et il **faisait** froid. M. Cartier **lisait** le journal. Mme Cartier **regardait** la télévision.	*It was a quiet night in Paris. It was raining and (it was) cold. Mr. Cartier was reading the newspaper. Mrs. Cartier was watching television.*

2. For habitual or repeated actions:

Quand j'étais jeune, j'**allais** chez mes grands-parents tous les dimanches. Nous **faisions** de belles promenades.	*When I was young, I went to my grandparents' home every Sunday. We would take (used to take) lovely walks.*

3. To describe feelings and mental states:

Cécile **était** très heureuse—elle **avait** envie de chanter.	*Cécile was very happy—she felt like singing.*

4. To tell the time of day, the date, and to express age in the past:

C'était un samedi. Il **était** cinq heures et demie du matin.	*It was a Saturday. It was 5:30 A.M.*
C'était son anniversaire; il **avait** 12 ans.	*It was his birthday; he was 12 years old.*

5. To describe appearance and physical traits:

Le suspect **portait** un jean; il **avait** les cheveux blonds et les yeux verts.	*The suspect was wearing jeans; he had blond hair and green eyes.*

6. To describe an action or situation that was happening when another event (usually in the **passé composé**) interrupted it:

Emmanuel **lisait** le journal quand le téléphone a sonné.	*Emmanuel was reading the paper when the phone rang.*

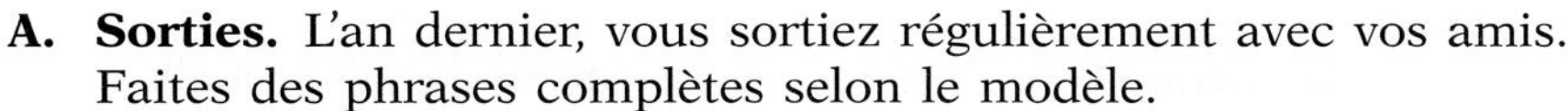

Allez-y!

Suggestion (A): Can be done with books closed.

Suggestion (B): Can be done in small groups or as a writing ex.

A. Sorties. L'an dernier, vous sortiez régulièrement avec vos amis. Faites des phrases complètes selon le modèle.

MODÈLE: dîner ensemble → Nous dînions ensemble.

1. jouer au tennis **2.** prendre un café **3.** faire des promenades l'après-midi **4.** pique-niquer à la campagne **5.** aller en boîte tous les week-ends **6.** partir en vacances ensemble

B. Souvenirs d'enfance. Qui dans votre famille faisait les choses suivantes quand vous étiez petit(e)?
Expressions utiles: mes parents, mon frère / ma sœur, mon meilleur ami / ma meilleure amie et moi

1. Qui lisait le journal tous les matins? **2.** Qui regardait la télévision après le dîner? **3.** Qui aimait écouter la radio le matin? **4.** Qui faisait beaucoup de sport? **5.** Qui étudiait tous les après-midi?

C. Avant la télévision. Marc demande à son arrière-grand-mère (*great grandmother*) Isabelle de parler de sa jeunesse (*youth*). Complétez la conversation avec les verbes appropriés à l'imparfait.

MARC: Est-ce que tu _____[1] la télé tous les soirs quand tu _____[2] jeune?
ISABELLE: Mais non, il n'y _____[3] pas de télévision!
MARC: Et alors, qu'est-ce que vous _____[4] chaque soir?
ISABELLE: D'habitude, nous _____[5] la radio. Mais moi, j' _____[6] lire pendant que (*while*) mon frère _____[7] du piano.
MARC: Dis donc, la vie n' _____[8] pas très intéressante en ce temps-là.
ISABELLE: Ce n'est pas vrai. En général, nous _____[9] très heureux. Toute la famille _____[10] du temps ensemble. Tous les dimanches, nous _____[11] chez mes grands-parents et après le déjeuner nous _____[12] au cinéma ou au parc. Aujourd'hui, il est difficile de trouver du temps pour partager des activités.

aimer
aller
avoir
déjeuner
écouter
être (×3)
faire
jouer
passer
regarder

D. Conversation. Posez les questions suivantes à un(e) camarade. En 2005…

1. Quel âge avais-tu? **2.** Habitais-tu à la campagne, dans une petite ville ou dans une grande ville? Avec qui habitais-tu? **3.** Comment était ta maison ou ton appartement? **4.** Étais-tu bon(ne) élève (*pupil*)? Aimais-tu tes instituteurs (*teachers*)? **5.** Où passais-tu tes vacances? **6.** Faisais-tu du sport?

Maintenant racontez à la classe ce que votre camarade faisait en 2005.

Mots clés

Exprimer une action répétée dans le passé

Use **tous les** (*m.*) or **toutes les** (*f.*) in the following expressions to indicate habitual actions.

tous les jours
every day

tous les après-midi (matins / soirs)
every afternoon (morning / evening)

toutes les semaines
every week

Other adverbs used with the **imparfait** include the following.

d'habitude
as a rule, habitually

en général
generally

souvent
often

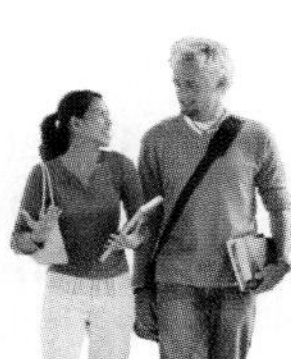

Suggestion: Give sts. other information to find out: *animaux, frères et sœurs, lecture, loisirs.*

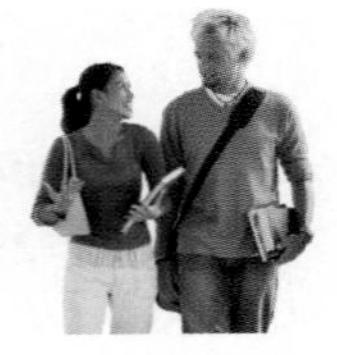

Interaction: Have sts. act out the following situation, using the vocabulary and structures from the chapter. **La soirée:** Call a friend (your partner) to find out why she or he did not come to your party. Tell her or him who was there, what you talked about, and what you did. Describe how the party was. She or he will ask you questions to get a good description.

Presentation: Some sts. have trouble recognizing direct or indirect objects in English. Giving English examples first may be the best preparation for this grammar section. Ask sts. to find direct objects in these sentences: *Robert turns on his phone. He looks for the number in his "Contacts." He calls his friend. He gives him advice. His friend tells him some news. He wrote it in an email, etc.*

E. Mon enfance. D'abord, posez les questions suivantes (et encore d'autres) à un(e) camarade. Ensuite, trouvez quelque chose que vous avez en commun avec ce (cette) camarade et une chose que vous n'avez pas en commun.

1. Quand tu étais petit(e), est-ce que tu voyais beaucoup de films? Quels films est-ce que tu aimais surtout (*especially*)? Avec qui est-ce que tu allais au cinéma?
2. Qu'est-ce que tu regardais à la télé? Quelles étaient tes émissions préférées? Jusqu'à quelle heure est-ce que tu pouvais regarder la télé?
3. Tu lisais beaucoup? Quels livres est-ce que tu aimais? Quelles bandes dessinées (*comic strips*)? Quand est-ce que tu lisais?

Les pronoms d'objet direct

Speaking Succinctly

Nos jouets technologiques

Dans le magasin Apple du Carrousel du Louvre, Juliette et Hector discutent.

HECTOR: Regarde Juliette, le nouvel iPhone! Tu **le** trouves joli?
JULIETTE: Je **le** trouve pas mal. Mais il n'a rien d'exceptionnel. Je préfère le modèle de Samsung.
HECTOR: Pas moi. Quand tu **le** mets dans ta poche,[1] il est trop grand.
JULIETTE: Qu'est-ce que tu penses[2] de cette tablette? Je **la** trouve futuriste.
HECTOR: Elle est belle mais trop chère… Smartphones, tablettes, ordinateurs: tu **les** achètes et ils sont obsolètes trois mois après.
JULIETTE: Et alors?
HECTOR: Et alors, c'est décourageant.[3]

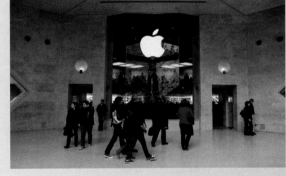

Le magasin Apple du Carrousel du Louvre à Paris

[1]*pocket* [2]*think* [3]*discouraging*

Trouvez dans le dialogue les mots remplacés par le pronom d'objet direct.

1. Hector le trouve joli.
2. Juliette le trouve pas mal.
3. Quand on le met dans sa poche, il est trop grand.
4. Juliette la trouve futuriste.
5. On les achète et ils sont obsolètes trois mois après.

Direct objects are nouns that receive the action of a verb. They usually answer the question *what?* or *whom?* For example, in the sentence *Malik reads the text message.* The noun *text message* is the direct object of the verb *reads.*

Direct object pronouns (**les pronoms complément d'objet direct**) replace direct object nouns: Malik *reads it.*

J'aime bien mon ordinateur. Je **l'**utilise tous les jours.	*I like my computer. I use it every day.*
J'ai écrit ce texto hier: Je **l'**ai envoyé tout de suite.	*I wrote this text yesterday. I sent it right away.*

Suggestion: Provide lots of examples so that sts. get used to hearing sentences with object pronouns. They may find it helpful to have 1–2 simple examples to call to mind as they do later exs. and activities: *Elle veut la pomme. → Elle la veut. / Il veut lire le livre. → Il veut le lire.*

Note: Agreement of past participle is in *Leçon 3* in this chapter.

Forms and Position of Direct Object Pronouns

DIRECT OBJECT PRONOUNS			
me (m')	*me*	**nous**	*us*
te (t')	*you*	**vous**	*you*
le (l')	*him, it*	**les**	*them*
la (l')	*her, it*		

1. Usually, French direct object pronouns immediately precede the verb in the present and the imperfect tenses and the auxiliary verb in the **passé composé.**

   Malik lit **le texto.** → Malik **le** lit.

   Malik lisait **le texto.** → Malik **le** lisait.

   Malik a lu **le texto.** → Malik **l'**a lu.

2. Third-person direct object pronouns agree in gender and in number with the nouns they replace.

—Est-ce que Robin lisait **le journal**?	*Was Robin reading the newspaper?*
—Oui, il **le** lisait.	*Yes, he was reading it.*
—Vois-tu **ma mère?**	*Do you see my mother?*
—Oui, je **la** vois.	*Yes, I see her.*
—Est-ce que vous postez **ces lettres**?	*Are you mailing these letters?*
—Oui, je **les** poste.	*Yes, I'm mailing them.*

3. If the verb following the direct object pronoun begins with a vowel sound, the direct object pronouns **me, te, le,** and **la** become **m', t',** and **l'.**

J'achète la carte postale. Je **l'**achète.	*I'm buying the postcard. I'm buying it.*
Isabelle **t'**admirait. Elle ne **m'**admirait pas.	*Isabelle used to admire you. She didn't admire me.*
Nous avons lu le journal. Nous **l'**avons lu.	*We read the newspaper. We read it.*

Grammaire interactive

For more on direct object pronouns, watch the corresponding Grammar Tutorial and take a brief practice quiz at **Connect French.**

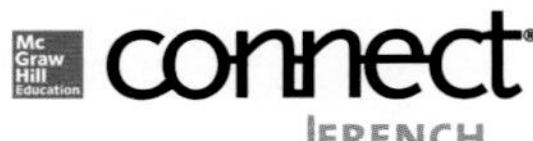

www.mhconnectfrench.com

Suggestion: Have sts. pick out direct object pronouns in the following listening ex. and suggest noun(s) they might be replacing. You might give this as a partial dictation, with sts. writing only the pronoun, along with possible noun(s). 1. *Je ne les cherche pas.* 2. *Est-ce que tu la trouves?* 3. *Ils nous regardent.* 4. *Elle l'admire.* 5. *Nous les admirons aussi.* 6. *Tu vas la regarder?* 7. *Nous allons les acheter.* 8. *Nous ne vous appelons pas.*

4. If the direct object pronoun is the object of an infinitive, it is placed immediately before the infinitive.

Alexandra va **poster la lettre** demain.	*Alexandra is going to mail the letter tomorrow.*
Alexandra va **la poster** demain.	*Alexandra is going to mail it tomorrow.*
Elle allait **la poster.** Elle est allée **la poster.**	*She was going to mail it. She went to mail it.*

5. In a negative sentence, the direct object pronoun always immediately precedes the verb to which it refers.

Nous ne regardons pas **la télévision.** Nous ne **la** regardons pas.	*We don't watch TV. We don't watch it.*
Je ne vais pas acheter **les billets.** Je ne vais pas **les** acheter.	*I'm not going to buy the tickets. I'm not going to buy them.*
Elle n'est pas allée chercher **le journal.** Elle n'est pas allée **le** chercher.	*She did not go to get the newspaper. She did not go to get it.*

6. Direct object pronouns also precede **voici** and **voilà.**

Le voici!	*Here he (it) is!*
Me voilà!	*Here I am!*

Le parler jeune

une bafouille	une lettre
les infos	les informations, les actualités
un ordi	un ordinateur
la pub	la publicité
tchatcher	parler

Je viens de recevoir une petite **bafouille** d'Anna.

Moi, je regarde les **infos** sur TF1.

Mon **ordi** commence à être fatigué.

J'adore la **pub**!

Magali **tchatche** pendant des heures au téléphone.

Allez-y!

A. Eurêka! Suivez le modèle.

MODÈLE: Je cherche le bureau de poste. → Le voilà. (*ou* Le voici.)

1. Où est mon portable?
2. Elle a perdu le numéro de téléphone.
3. Où est le téléphone?
4. Il cherche le kiosque.
5. Il a envie de lire *Le Monde* d'hier.
6. Avez-vous le journal?
7. Où est l'adresse des Thibaudeau?
8. J'ai besoin de la grande enveloppe blanche.
9. Où sont les toilettes?
10. Aïcha et Nathan, où êtes-vous?

B. De quoi parlent-ils? Vous êtes dans un café parisien et vous entendez les phrases suivantes. Trouvez dans la colonne de droite l'information qui correspond à chaque pronom.

1. Je vais les poster cet après-midi.	**a.** l'adresse
2. Elle le consulte.	**b.** les lettres
3. Je l'écris sur l'enveloppe.	**c.** le numéro
4. Nous venons de la lire.	**d.** l'annuaire électronique
5. Je les achète à la poste.	**e.** la revue
6. Je l'ai déjà composé.	**f.** les timbres

Continuation (C): *lire les petites annonces dans le journal; regarder la télévision; acheter la revue* Historia.

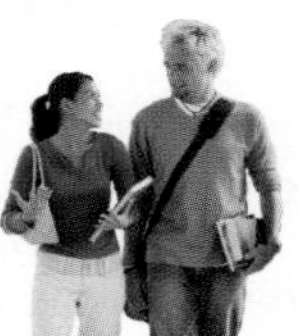

C. Projets de voyage. Luca et Philippe font toujours la même chose. Avec un(e) camarade, parlez de leurs projets selon le modèle.

MODÈLE: étudier le français cette année →
É1: Est-ce que Luca va étudier le français cette année?
É2: Oui, et Philippe va l'étudier aussi.

1. apprendre le français très rapidement
2. prendre l'avion pour Paris en juin
3. lire les journaux le matin
4. admirer la vue du haut de la tour Eiffel
5. prendre ses repas dans de bons restaurants
6. regarder les gens sur les Champs-Élysées
7. essayer de lire les romans de Flaubert

Maintenant imaginez que Luca est l'opposé de Philippe.

MODÈLE: É1: Est-ce que Luca va étudier le français cette année?
É2: Oui, mais Philippe, il ne va pas l'étudier.

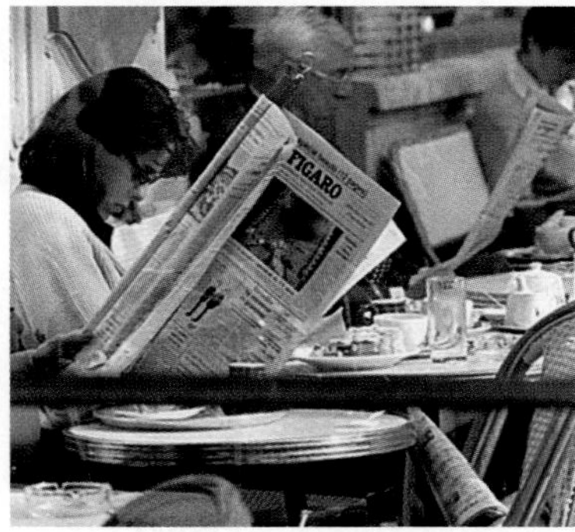

Le Figaro, un petit café crème: un après-midi parisien. Lisez-vous un journal? Quel journal? Quand le lisez-vous?

D. Interview. Interviewez un(e) camarade de classe sur ses préférences. Votre camarade doit utiliser un pronom complément d'objet direct dans sa réponse.

1. Utilises-tu souvent ton portable / ton mobile?
2. Appelles-tu souvent tes camarades de classe? tes professeurs? tes parents?
3. Est-ce que tes parents t'appellent souvent? tes amis?
4. Regardes-tu souvent la télé?
5. Aimes-tu regarder la publicité?
6. Préfères-tu apprendre les nouvelles dans le journal ou à la radio? à la télé ou sur Internet?
7. Lis-tu les bandes dessinées?
8. Tu utilises souvent Internet pour faire des recherches? pour faire des achats?

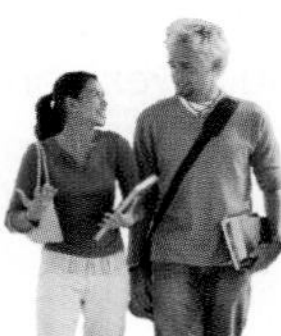

Suggestions (D): (1) Have sts. do interview and report answers as follows: *Doug, est-ce que Suzanne utilise souvent son mobile?* Doug: *Oui, elle l'utilise souvent.* (etc.) (2) Dictate questions at board and have sts. write answers with object pronouns. Then compare individual responses. Example: *Ah, Julia utilise souvent le téléphone, mais Mark ne l'utilise jamais.*

Le blog de Juliette

Ordinateur, mon amour!

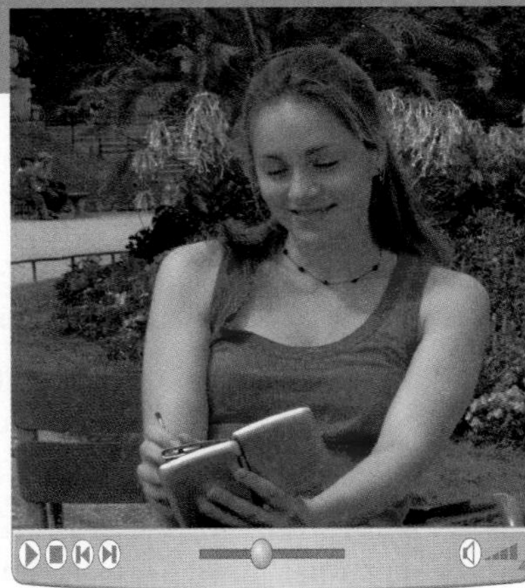
J'adore mes gadgets!

jeudi 18 juin

Salut tout le monde!

Je vous pose une question: «Peut-on vivre aujourd'hui sans ordinateur?»

Ma réponse est NON. Sans mon ordinateur, je suis comme un poisson hors de[1] l'eau. Je meurs[2]!

Avec mon ordinateur, je fais tout: je travaille, j'étudie, je lis, j'écris. Je surfe sur le Web, je lis la presse, je participe à des forums, et, bien sûr, j'écris mon blog! En plus, chaque jour, je reçois[3] et j'envoie des dizaines de courriels, je regarde des films et j'écoute de la musique. Donc, mon ordinateur, c'est mon oxygène.

Pour vous montrer une image exacte de mon univers technologique, je vais vous faire une confession: je vis scotchée[4] à mon smartphone. Je suis la championne des SMS et des textos; j'appelle mes amis cent fois par jour (Léa, 50 fois!).

Chez moi, j'ai une télé, un ordinateur portable avec la Wi-Fi, une imprimante, un appareil photo numérique, un iPod, et, pour Noël, mes parents m'ont offert une tablette! Bon, vous avez compris: je suis une technophile.

Mais j'ai une excuse: la technologie, c'est mon univers! Je prépare un Master multimédia à la Sorbonne.

Juliette

COMMENTAIRES

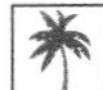
Poema
Est-ce qu'il te reste du temps pour rêver et pour ne rien faire?

Alexis
Tu massacres la langue française avec des textos? Tu me déçois,[5] Juliette…

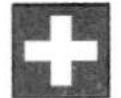
Charlotte
Nos parents, ils n'avaient pas tous ces gadgets technologiques et ils étaient très heureux! Mais j'apprécie ton blog Juliette, et je le lis régulièrement.

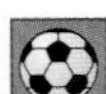
Mamadou
Quand j'étais petit, au Sénégal, on avait rarement la télévision; le téléphone était réservé aux riches; on rêvait de posséder un ordinateur. Aujourd'hui, l'Afrique est entrée dans la société de l'information, comme nous tous.

Follow-up: 1. *Décrivez l'univers technologique de Juliette. Décrivez le vôtre* (yours). 2. *Combien de fois par jour utilisez-vous votre téléphone portable? À qui téléphonez-vous? Qui vous appelle?* 3. *Répondez à la remarque de Poema: êtes-vous d'accord ou non?* 4. *Pourquoi Juliette déçoit-elle Alexis? Qu'en pensez-vous?* 5. *Commentez la remarque de Charlotte.*

Video connection: In the videoblog for this chapter, Juliette and Hector take a «Psycho Quizz» on their technology habits and give an overview of technology use in the Francophone world. Sts. can take the quiz themselves at **Connect French (www.mhconnectfrench.com)**.

[1]hors… *out(side) of* [2]*am dying* [3]*receive* [4]vis… *live glued (slang)* [5]me… *disappoint me*

REPORTAGE

LES ACCROS° DU TEXTO

°*fanatics*

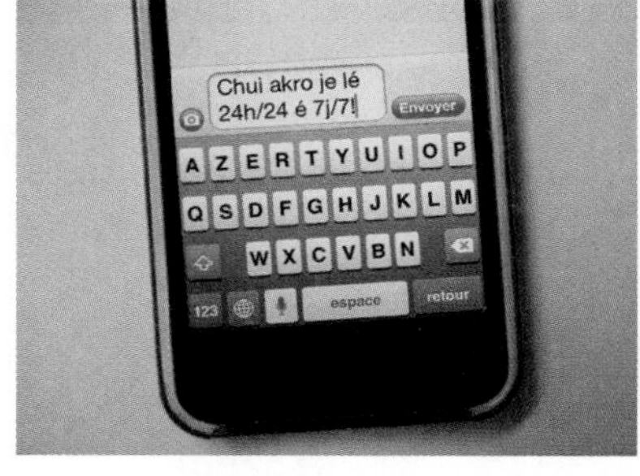

En France, SMS (*Short Message Service*) est très populaire parmi les utilisateurs des portables.

Qu'est-ce qu'un accro du texto? C'est un individu, souvent jeune, qui passe son temps à envoyer des textos (SMS), petits textes de 160 caractères maximum. Seul ou en compagnie, en famille, avec des amis, en classe, au travail, à la maison, dans le métro, dans le bus, l'accro du texto vit en intimité avec son téléphone. Il est encouragé par les offres des opérateurs téléphonie mobile[1] (Free, Orange, SFR et Bouygues) qui proposent des formules «textos illimités». Comment résister dans ces conditions?

Le portable: un inséparable compagnon

Sophie, 17 ans, explique: «J'envoie des messages 24 heures sur 24. Le matin je me lève, j'envoie des messages. Sous la douche, aux WC, pendant que je m'habille, je pianote.[2] Je textote[3] partout, matin, midi, soir, nuit, tout le temps. Oui, je me sens dépendante de mon téléphone, totalement». Sa copine Justine ajoute: «C'est vital pour moi. Dans le bus, dans le train, à la boulangerie, j'échange 12 000 SMS par mois... Non, non, je n'exagère pas; c'est la vérité!»

Caricature? Absolument pas! Car l'accro du texto n'a pas de limites. Il écrit vite et utilise des abréviations. Pour lui, l'orthographe, la ponctuation, la grammaire et les accents ne sont pas importants: «mwa je lach jamè mn port chui akro je lè 24h/24 è 7j/7!!» (Moi, je ne lâche[4] jamais mon portable, je suis accro, je l'ai 24 h sur 24 et 7 jours sur 7); «mon portable c toute ma vie si je lé pa partou ou je vé je meur» (Mon portable, c'est toute ma vie; si je ne l'ai pas partout où je vais, je meurs[5]).

Des mini-messages tellement pratiques!

On doit reconnaître que, dans la vie de tous les jours, les SMS sont très pratiques. Un bref message et tout est dit: on donne un rendez-vous («K penses-tu du resto VIRGILE, vers 20 h? Confirme SVP!»), on avertit[6] qu'on est en retard («trafic +++; j'arrive dans 10 mn»), on donne son avis («C trop top!»), on envoie des félicitations («Congrats pour ton job!»)... Dans les grandes occasions, ils sont indispensables. Pour le Nouvel An, par exemple, les accros ont échangé, cette année, plus de 500 millions de textos! Et détail important, les SMS transmettent aux amoureux des messages enflammés: «Tu é le soleil ki illumine ma vie» (Tu es le soleil qui illumine ma vie); «Je taiiimeee!!!!! » (je t'aime).

[1]opérateurs... *cellphone service providers* [2]*type clumsily* [3]*text (fam.)* [4]*part with* [5]*die* [6]*lets (someone) know*

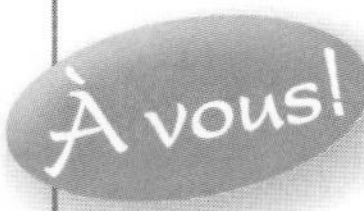

1. Décrivez «un accro du texto» typique, selon l'évocation du *Reportage*. Donnez au moins (*at least*) trois caractéristiques.
2. Dans quels endroits est-ce que les accros aiment échanger leurs messages?
3. Quels sont les caractéristiques du langage des SMS?
4. Quels sont les avantages et les inconvénients des textos?

Parlons-en!

Travaillez en petits groupes et répondez aux questions suivantes.

1. Qui possède un smartphone?
2. Comment communiquez-vous? Par SMS, MMS, Tweet, mél, téléphone? Avec Facebook, BBIM (Blackboard Messagerie instantanée), Skype?
3. Comparez vos habitudes et expliquez vos préférences.

   Qui est l'accro le/la plus fanatique de la classe?

Leçon 3

L'accord du participe passé

Talking About the Past

Facile!

Juliette et Charlotte discutent sur la page Facebook de Juliette.

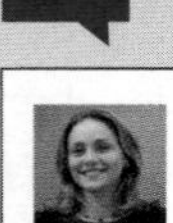
JULIETTE: Alors, Charlotte, ta page Facebook, tu **l'**as **créée**[1]!

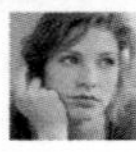
CHARLOTTE: Finalement, oui! J'ai longtemps hésité parce que je n'aime pas beaucoup parler de moi... Mais ça y est,[2] c'est fait! J'ai raconté[3] ma vie, j'ai laissé des messages...

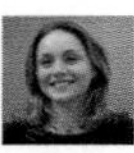
JULIETTE: Et ton profil?

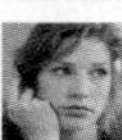
CHARLOTTE: Je **l'**ai **finalisé**! C'est un autoportrait honnête.

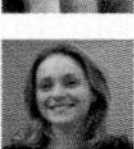
JULIETTE: Tu as retrouvé tes copines du lycée?

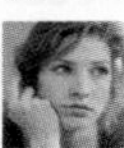
CHARLOTTE: Oui! Je **les** ai **retrouvées** et je **les** ai **contactées**. Nous avons échangé des photos.

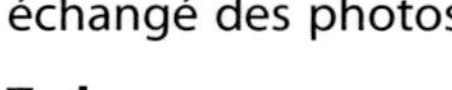

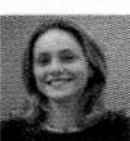
JULIETTE: Tu **les** as **reconnues**[4] sur les photos?

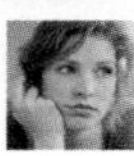
CHARLOTTE: Je **les** ai toutes **identifiées**. Finalement nous n'avons pas tellement[5] changé... Nous sommes toujours[6] jeunes et belles!

[1]*created* [2]*ça... there it is* [3]*told about* [4]*recognized* [5]*so much* [6]*still*

Complétez les réponses aux questions suivantes en utilisant les formes verbales du dialogue.

1. Charlotte a créé sa page Facebook? Oui, ...
2. Elle a finalisé son profil? Oui, ...
3. Elle a retrouvé ses copines du lycée? Oui, ...
4. Elle a contacté ses copines? Oui, ...
5. Elle a reconnu et identifié ses copines sur les photos? Oui, ...

In the **passé composé,** the past participle is generally used in its basic form. However, when a direct object—noun or pronoun—precedes the auxiliary verb **avoir** plus the past participle, the participle agrees with the preceding direct object in gender and number.

Suggestion: Point out that the difference is heard only if the masculine form of the past participle ends with a consonant (*Je l'ai mis—je l'ai mise*). Otherwise, the difference is written only (*Je l'ai appelé—je l'ai appelée*).

J'ai lu le **journal.**	J'ai lu les **journaux.**
Je **l'**ai **lu.**	Je **les** ai **lus.**
J'ai lu **la revue.**	J'ai lu les **revues.**
Je **l'**ai **lue.**	Je **les** ai **lues.**
Quels **amis** avez-vous **appelés?**	Quelles **émissions** avez-vous **regardées?**

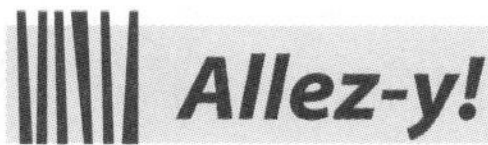

Allez-y!

A. Un nouveau travail. Vous travaillez comme assistant administratif / assistante administrative. Votre patronne (*boss*) vous pose des questions. Répondez à la forme affirmative ou négative.

Suggestion (A): Can be done first with books closed for further practice of object pronouns. As an ex. on agreement of past participle, can be assigned as homework.

MODÈLE: Avez-vous regardé *le calendrier* ce matin? ⟶ Oui, je l'ai regardé. (Non, je ne l'ai pas regardé.)

1. Est-ce que vous avez donné *notre numéro de téléphone* à Mme Milaud?
2. Est-ce que vous avez mis *le nouveau nom de la firme* sur les enveloppes?
3. Avez-vous contacté *la responsable de notre Comité de Direction*?
4. Avez-vous fini *le rapport*?
5. Avez-vous appelé *Georges Dupic et Catherine Duriez*?
6. Avez-vous vu *Anne et Clémentine* ce matin?
7. *M'*avez-vous comprise pendant la réunion (*meeting*) hier?

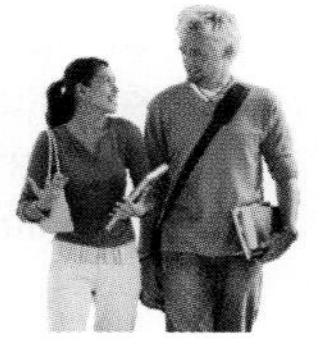

B. Conversation. Posez les questions suivantes à un(e) camarade. Il/elle utilise, quand c'est possible, un pronom complément d'objet direct dans ses réponses.

1. Quand tu étais enfant, aimais-tu l'école? les vacances? les voyages? l'aventure? Quelle sorte d'aventure aimais-tu?
2. L'année dernière, as-tu passé tes vacances à la montagne? à l'étranger? en famille?
3. As-tu déjà essayé le camping? l'alpinisme? le bateau? le ski?
4. As-tu lu le dernier numéro de *Time*? de *People*? de *Sports Illustrated*? de *L'Express*?
5. As-tu lu les romans d'Albert Camus? les livres de Saint-Exupéry?
6. Quand as-tu appelé tes grands-parents? tes parents? ton professeur de francais? Pourquoi?

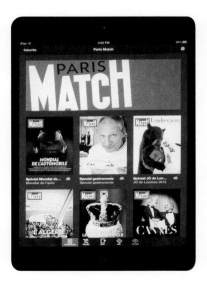

Les verbes *voir, croire* et *recevoir*

Expressing Observations and Beliefs

Être ou ne pas être matérialiste

Hassan téléphone à Juliette.

HASSAN: **Tu crois** qu'Hector* a finalement acheté un iPad?
JULIETTE: Non, **je** ne **crois** pas. Il n'est pas un grand consommateur[1] de technologies.
HASSAN: Pourtant[2] il a un ordinateur. **Il reçoit** et il envoie vingt courriels par jour!
JULIETTE: C'est vrai, mais il est satisfait avec sa vieille machine. **Il** ne **voit** pas l'intérêt de dépenser[3] de l'argent pour une tablette...
HASSAN: Hector est un artiste... Il n'est pas matérialiste...
JULIETTE: **Tu crois** ça? Tu ignores certainement qu'il adore les voitures de luxe!

[1]*consumer* [2]*Nevertheless* [3]*spend*

Un peu bling-bling: la voiture préférée d'Hector!

Trouvez, dans le dialogue, les phrases où...

1. Hassan demande si Hector a acheté un iPad.
2. Juliette suggère qu'Hector n'a pas acheté d'iPad.
3. Hassan explique qu'Hector utilise la messagerie de son ordinateur.
4. Juliette explique qu'Hector n'aime pas dépenser de l'argent pour la technologie.
5. Juliette révèle qu'Hector est matérialiste.

The verbs **voir** (*to see*) and **croire** (*to believe*) are irregular.

voir		croire	
je **vois**	nous **voyons**	je **crois**	nous **croyons**
tu **vois**	vous **voyez**	tu **crois**	vous **croyez**
il/elle/on **voit**	ils/elles **voient**	il/elle/on **croit**	ils/elles **croient**
Past participle: **vu**		*Past participle*: **cru**	

*__Croire__ and **voir** must be followed by **que** (*that*) when they introduce another clause.

J'**ai vu** Michèle à la plage la semaine passée.	*I saw Michèle at the beach last week.*
Est-ce que tu **crois** cette histoire?	*Do you believe this story?*
Je **crois** qu'il va faire beau demain.	*I think the weather is going to be fine tomorrow.*
Tu **crois?**	*You think so? / Are you sure?*

1. **Revoir** (*to see again*) is conjugated like **voir.**

   Je **revois** les Moreau. — *I'm seeing the Moreau family again.*

2. **Croire à** means *to believe in* a concept or an idea.

   Nous **croyons à** la chance. — *We believe in luck.*
   Ils **croient au** Père Noël. — *They believe in Santa Claus.*

3. **Croire en** means *to believe in* a god or to have confidence in someone.

   Vous **croyez en** Dieu? — *Do you believe in God?*

4. **Croire que** means *to think* (*that*), *to believe* (*that*) and is followed by another clause. It is used to express an opinion.

   Je **crois qu'**Internet est la grande invention du XXe siècle. — *I think* (*that*) *the Internet is the great invention of the 20th century.*

Note: The verb **recevoir** (*to receive; to entertain as guests*) is also irregular. The conjugation is similar to the verb **voir** in the singular forms, but differs in the plural forms.

recevoir			
je	**reçois**	nous	**recevons**
tu	**reçois**	vous	**recevez**
il/elle/on	**reçoit**	ils/elles	**reçoivent**
Past participle: **reçu**			

Elle **reçoit** beaucoup de textos tous les jours.

Allez-y!

Suggestion (A): Can be done in groups of 3 as a role-play activity.

Mots clés

Marquer une hésitation ou une pause

Eh bien,...	*Well,...*
Voyons,...	*Let's see,...*
C'est-à-dire que...	*That is / I mean...*
Euh...	*Uhmm...*
Oui, mais...	*Yes, but...*

Suggestion (C): If sts. have not traveled recently, they may have to invent a trip.

Suggestion (B): Ask sts. to prepare a list of their beliefs in order to help conversation flow more smoothly.

Follow-up (B): Ask sts. to volunteer to describe the beliefs of a classmate.

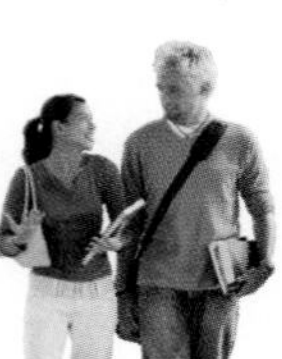

A. Paris dans le brouillard (*fog*). Trois étudiants étrangers sont désorientés. Complétez la conversation avec les verbes **croire** et **voir** au présent, sauf quand le passé composé est indiqué.

JULIE: Tu ______[1] où on est?
KANI: Non, je ne ______[2] pas cette rue sur le plan.
WAN QING: Vous faites confiance à ce vieux plan?
JULIE: Non, nous ______[3] ce que nous a dit Anne, le guide.
KANI: Elle a beaucoup d'expérience et je ______[4] ce qu'elle dit.
WAN QING: Moi, je pense qu'elle ______[5] à la chance!
JULIE: Très drôle... mais dis, Kani, tu ______[6] (*passé composé*) le guide quelque part?
KANI: Oui, j' ______[7] (*passé composé*) Anne, mais il y a environ une heure, au café...
WAN QING: Cette fois, je ______[8] que nous sommes perdus! Heureusement, j'ai mon portable!

B. Interview. Interrogez un(e) camarade sur ses croyances. Est-ce qu'il/elle croit à la chance, à l'amour, au progrès, à une religion, à la perception extra-sensorielle, aux O.V.N.I.* (*UFOs*), à ______? Utilisez les **Mots clés.**

C. Conversation. Avec un(e) camarade, parlez d'une ville qu'il/elle a visitée récemment. Qu'est-ce qu'il/elle a vu? Qui est-ce qu'il/elle a rencontré? Qu'est-ce qu'il/elle veut revoir? Qui veut-il/elle revoir? Ensuite, racontez à la classe l'expérience la plus intéressante (*most interesting*) de votre camarade.

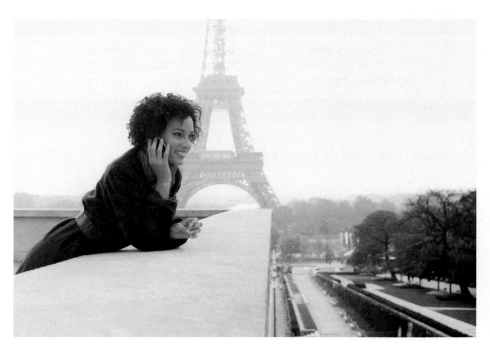

De quoi parle-t-elle?

*Objets volants non identifiés

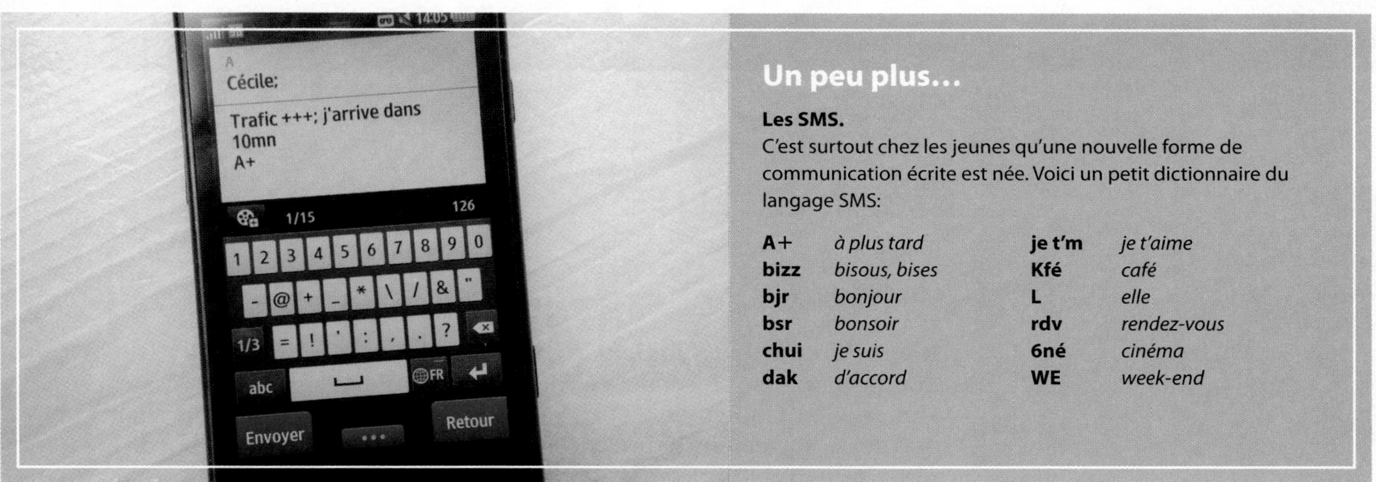

Un peu plus...

Les SMS.
C'est surtout chez les jeunes qu'une nouvelle forme de communication écrite est née. Voici un petit dictionnaire du langage SMS:

A+	*à plus tard*	**je t'm**	*je t'aime*
bizz	*bisous, bises*	**Kfé**	*café*
bjr	*bonjour*	**L**	*elle*
bsr	*bonsoir*	**rdv**	*rendez-vous*
chui	*je suis*	**6né**	*cinéma*
dak	*d'accord*	**WE**	*week-end*

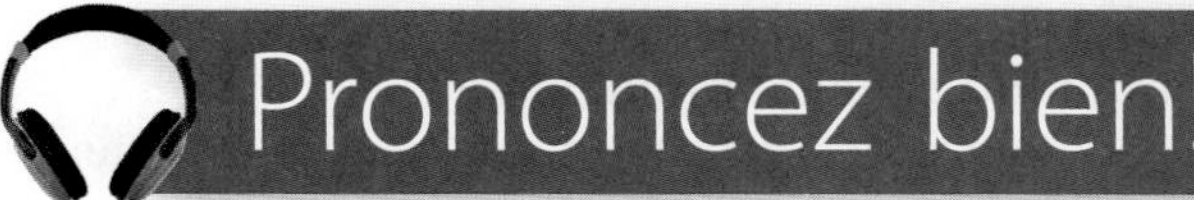

Prononcez bien!

Final consonants and *liaison* (page 261)

L'arrivée de Louis. En rentrant à la maison après les cours, vous trouvez Hugo seul dans le salon. Avec votre camarade de classe, jouez la scène. Faites bien attention aux liaisons.

VOUS: Isabelle n'est pas là?
HUGO: Non, elle est allée chercher Louis, son frère. Elle est née le premier avril et demain c'est son anniversaire. Pour l'occasion, son frère va passer le week-end avec elle et lui faire (*give her*) beaucoup de cadeaux.
VOUS: Il voyage en autobus?
HUGO: Non, en avion.
VOUS: Quand est-ce qu'ils arrivent?
HUGO: Dans deux heures. C'est un grand aéroport et il faut beaucoup de temps pour en (*of it*) sortir!

Leçon 4

PERSPECTIVES

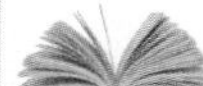

Lecture

Avant de lire

Identifying a text's logical structure. Being able to identify words that authors use to sequence their presentation of ideas, express cause and effect, or qualify an observation will facilitate your comprehension of a text's logical structure. For example, words such as **d'abord, en plus, puis, ensuite, enfin,** and **finalement** may be used to develop an argument or support a point of view. To support the point of view that technology has revolutionized communication, an author might write:

D'abord, Internet facilite la communication.
En plus, on peut communiquer plus rapidement.
Finalement, on peut contacter des gens partout dans le monde.

To affirm a preceding idea, words such as **alors, en effet** (*indeed*), and **effectivement** might be used:

Internet est un outil (*tool*) important dans la vie quotidienne. En effet, il a transformé nos goûts et nos habitudes.

Cependant (*However, Nevertheless*) and **pourtant** (*yet*) qualify a preceding idea or express a reservation:

Cependant, certains pensent qu'Internet a des effets négatifs.

As you read, pay attention to these important words that express logical development and the relationship between ideas.

À propos de la lecture...
Les auteurs de *Vis-à-vis* ont écrit ce texte.

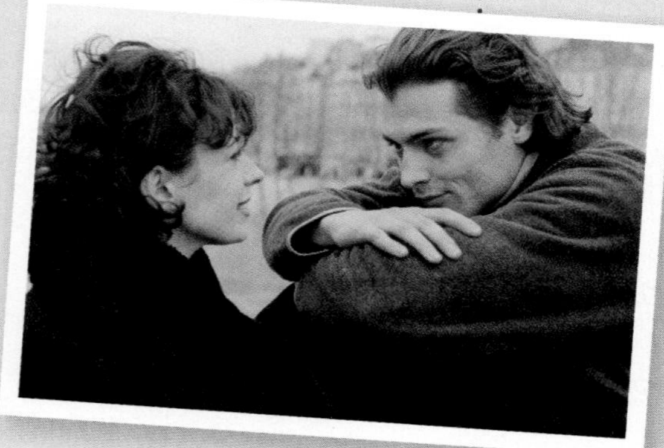

Une histoire d'amour à Paris

Rencontres en ligne°: rendez-vous avec le bonheur

Rencontres... *Online dating*

Vous rêvez de sortir de votre solitude? Vous êtes timide? Vous n'avez tout simplement pas le temps pour la séduction? Internet peut vous aider! Les sites de rencontre vous ouvrent les portes du bonheur. La plupart[1] sont très sérieux et contrôlent la bonne moralité des membres inscrits.[2] Ils attirent[3] un grand nombre de célibataires—jeunes, adultes et même retraités[4]—à la recherche de l'amour. Plusieurs millions de Français fréquentent chaque jour les sites de rencontre sur Internet.

[1]La... *Most* [2]*registered* [3]*attract* [4]*retired people*

Pourquoi ce fabuleux succès?

- D'abord, parce que c'est pratique et facile. Un «clic» et le contact est établi! On choisit un pseudonyme et un mot de passe; on décrit son profil; on définit le partenaire idéal et on peut immédiatement envoyer son premier message. On se présente avec des photos ou une vidéo. C'est déjà une façon[5] de séduire!
- Ensuite, parce que c'est anonyme. Le pseudonyme permet aux candidats de contacter les autres membres en gardant le secret de leur véritable identité.
- En plus, ça favorise le dialogue. Pour séduire, les internautes[6] parlent de leurs sentiments et échangent des idées. Ils écrivent de belles lettres pleines d'humour ou de romantisme.
- Enfin, on augmente ses chances de rencontre. Un seul courrier électronique peut générer plusieurs centaines de réponses, surtout si on décide de mettre une photo avec son profil. C'est vérifié: les candidats qui ont des photos ont beaucoup plus de succès.

Et pourtant, il y a des malchanceux...

Certains n'ont pas de chance sur Internet, comme Marc, un jeune agriculteur[7] de 35 ans. Les jeunes femmes qu'il a rencontrées n'ont pas toléré l'isolement[8] de sa ferme. Elles sont toutes reparties en le laissant seul avec ses vaches[9] et son ordinateur.

Les statistiques confirment ce cas: les rencontres Internet favorisent surtout les citadins.[10] De même, les deux sexes ne sont pas également représentés: sur les sites, on trouve trois hommes pour une femme.

Alors, bonne chance, mesdames!

[5]*way, means* [6]*Internet users* [7]*farmer* [8]*isolation* [9]*cows* [10]*city dwellers*

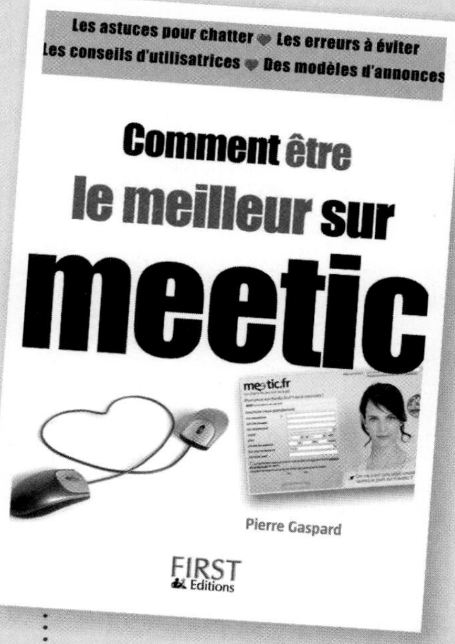

Avez-vous envie de lire ce livre? Pourquoi ou pourquoi pas?

Compréhension

A. Vocabulaire. Pour chaque mot, donnez l'équivalent en anglais.

1. en ligne **2.** un clic **3.** un pseudonyme **4.** un mot de passe **5.** un(e) internaute

B. Vrai ou faux? Si c'est faux, donnez la solution correcte.

1. Il y a peu de sites Web où vous pouvez trouver l'amour en ligne en France.
2. Les sites de rencontre en ligne attirent des gens de tout âge.
3. Le succès des rencontres en ligne est d'abord dû à la facilité de l'usage.
4. D'habitude, les gens qui habitent en ville trouvent plus facilement l'amour sur les sites de rencontre que les gens qui habitent à la campagne.

C. Opinions. Lisez la phrase suivante et donnez votre opinion.

Internet est un outil important dans la vie quotidienne [...], cependant certains pensent qu'il a des effets négatifs.

Internet: un monde vaste!

Voici une liste de quelques autres mots et expressions utiles pour parler des smartphones, des ordinateurs et d'Internet.

appuyer	*press/push a key*
(re)lier	*to link*
un abonnement	*subscription*
une base de données	*database*
une clé USB	*flash drive*
un clic	*click*
un dossier	*document, file*
un fournisseur d'accès	*Internet provider*
un graveur de CD/DVD	*CD/DVD burner*
un identifiant	*username*
un lien	*a link*
le matériel	*hardware*
la mémoire	*memory*
un MMS	*multimedia message*
un mot de passe	*password*
un moteur de recherche	*search engine*
un opérateur	*service provider*
une page d'accueil	*home page*
un port USB	*USB port*
un répertoire	*directory*
un réseau	*network*
le survol	*browsing*

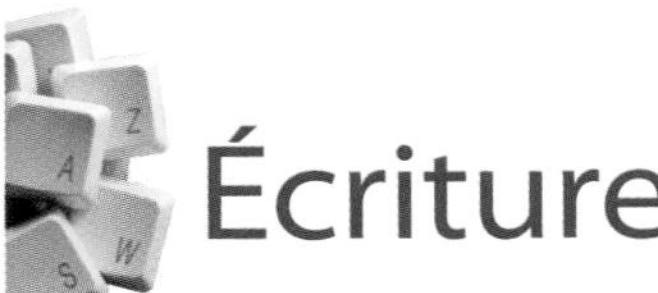

Écriture

The writing activities **Par écrit** and **Journal intime** can be found in the Workbook/Laboratory Manual to accompany *Vis-à-vis*.

La vie en chantant. An activity based on the song "Je ne regrette rien" by Édith Piaf can be found in the Instructor's Manual. The song can be purchased at the iTunes store, or sts. can watch the music video on YouTube.

Pour s'amuser

Y a un copain qui m'a dit:

—Prouve-moi que c'est utile ton Internet.

—Okay, je sais pas quoi faire cet été, je fais une recherche sur le mot «vacances». 7 395 sites à visiter. Ça va m'occuper tout l'été.

—Anne Roumanoff, extrait du sketch *Internet*

 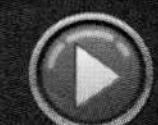

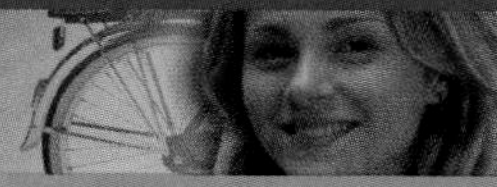

Le vidéoblog de Juliette

En bref

Dans cet épisode, Juliette et Hector répondent aux questions d'un sondage (*survey*) sur l'utilisation des téléphones portables. Dans son vidéoblog, Juliette continue à parler des nouvelles technologies dans le monde francophone.

Vocabulaire en contexte

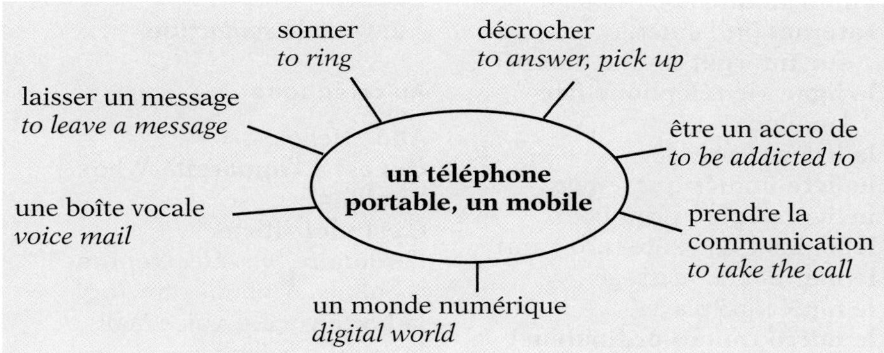

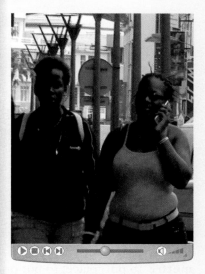

Le mobile: un phénomène universel

Suggestion: Ask sts. short-answer questions based on the vocabulary to aid their comprehension of the video episode: *Avez-vous une boîte vocale? Un(e) ami(e) est en train de vous parler d'un problème très sérieux quand votre téléphone sonne. Que faites-vous?*, etc.

Additional vocabulary: Other vocabulary you may wish to present before viewing includes *un truc, évidemment, c'est fou, dis donc.*

Suggestion: Have sts. respond to questions by supplying the name(s) and conjugating the verbs appropriately.

Visionnez!

Indiquez qui fait les activités suivantes: Juliette, Hector ou les deux.

	Juliette	Hector	les deux
1. téléphoner à quelqu'un avant le petit déjeuner	☐	☐	☐
2. prendre son mobile dans les toilettes	☐	☐	☐
3. décrocher quand le téléphone sonne dans un restaurant	☐	☐	☐
4. annoncer que le mobile symbolise l'amitié	☐	☐	☐
5. avoir son mobile dans son lit la nuit	☐	☐	☐

Analysez!

Répondez aux questions suivantes.

1. Quels éléments, autres que le téléphone portable, font partie de la «culture du multimédia»?
2. Selon la vidéo, nous vivons dans un «monde numérique». Est-ce une bonne chose, selon vous? Pourquoi ou pourquoi pas?

Comparez!

Est-ce que votre propre culture est aussi une culture du multimédia? Expliquez pourquoi (pas). Êtes-vous, comme Juliette et Hector, «accro» du téléphone portable? Regardez encore une fois la partie culturelle de la vidéo: utilisez-vous les nouvelles technologies plus (*more*) ou moins (*less*) souvent qu'une personne typique de votre pays?

Note culturelle

En France, il est interdit[1] de téléphoner dans un hôpital ou dans sa voiture si on n'a pas de kit mains-libres.[2] Dans de nombreux lycées, il est interdit de téléphoner en cours ou dans les couloirs, mais l'utilisation du mobile est permis dans les cours de récréation.[3] En avion, Air France interdit l'utilisation du mobile pendant le vol. Dans le train, il est demandé aux voyageurs d'utiliser leur mobile avec discrétion pour ne pas irriter les autres voyageurs.

[1]*prohibited* [2]kit... *hands-free phone*
[3]cours... *playgrounds*

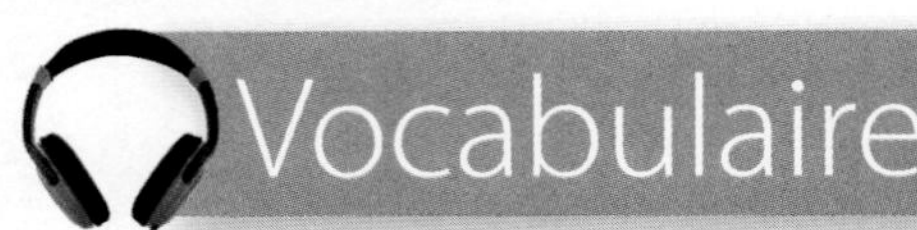

Vocabulaire

Verbes

appeler to call
composer le numéro to dial the number
consulter l'annuaire électronique to look up (a phone number) in the online directory
croire to believe
décrire to describe
dépenser to spend
dessiner to draw
dire to say
écrire (à) to write (to)
envoyer (à) to send (to)
lire to read
mettre to put, place; to put on (clothes)
  mettre le couvert to set the table
mettre une lettre (une carte) à la poste to mail a letter (card)
naviguer to navigate, to browse
penser to think
poster to mail
raconter to tell (a story)
recevoir to receive
revoir to see again
télécharger to download
voir to see

MOTS APPARENTÉS: **cliquer, échanger, payer, posséder, surfer sur le Web**

À REVOIR: **acheter, écouter, entendre, jouer, regarder, rendre**

Substantifs

l'appareil (*m.*) apparatus
le bureau de tabac tobacco store
le cadeau gift
la monnaie coins, change
la poche pocket

Les nouvelles technologies

l'appareil (*m.*) **(photo) numérique** digital camera
le caméscope digital camcorder
le clavier keyboard
la connexion ADSL DSL connection/line
le courriel e-mail message
le fichier file
l'imprimante (*f.*) printer
Internet (*m.*) Internet
  sur Internet on the Internet
la ligne / le téléphone fixe landline
la liseuse e-reader
le livre numérique e-book
le livre papier print book
le logiciel software (program)
le mél e-mail message
le mp3 mp3 player
le micro (micro-ordinateur) desktop computer
le navigateur browser
l'ordinateur (*m.*) **de bureau** desktop computer
  l'ordinateur portable (*fam.* **le portable)** laptop computer
le traitement de texte word processing

MOTS APPARENTÉS: **le moniteur, le photocopieur, le scanner, le site, le Web, le Wi-Fi**

À REVOIR: **l'iPod, l'écran** (*m.*), **l'ordinateur** (*m.*), **la souris, la tablette**

Au bureau de poste

la boîte aux lettres mailbox
le bureau de poste (La Poste) post office
le colis package
le courrier mail
la poste mail
le timbre stamp

MOTS APPARENTÉS: **l'adresse** (*f.*), **la carte postale, l'enveloppe** (*f.*), **le fax, la lettre**

Au kiosque

le journal (les journaux) newspaper; news
le kiosque kiosk; newsstand
les petites annonces (*f.*) classified ads
le roman novel

MOTS APPARENTÉS: **la revue**

À REVOIR: **le magazine**

Au téléphone

Allô. Hello.
Qui est à l'appareil? Who's calling?
C'est moi. It's me.
l'annuaire (*m.*) **électronique** online telephone directory
la boîte vocale voice mail
le mobile cell phone
le numéro (de téléphone) (telephone) number
le téléphone portable cell phone
le texto text message

MOTS APPARENTÉS: **le smartphone**

À REVOIR: **le SMS, le téléphone**

À la télévision

la chaîne televison channel; network
l'émission (*f.*) program; broadcast
  émission de musique music program
  émission de télé réalité reality show
le feuilleton soap opera
les informations (*f. pl.*) news
le jeu télévisé game show
le journal télévisé television news program
la publicité commercial; advertisement; advertising
la retransmission sportive sports broadcast
la série series
  série télévisée serial drama
la télécommande remote control

la TNT (télévision numérique terrestre) high-definition television

MOTS APPARENTÉS: **le câble, le documentaire, la télévision satellite**

À REVOIR: **le DVD (les DVD), le lecteur de DVD, la télé(vision)**

Autres mots et expressions

C'est-à-dire (que)... That is / I mean . . .
Eh bien,... Well, . . .
Euh... Uhmm . . .
là-bas over there
Oui, mais... Yes, but . . .
surtout especially
tous les (jours, après-midi, matins, soirs, et cetera) every (day, afternoon, morning, evening, etc.)
tout, toute, tous, toutes all; every
toutes les semaines every week
Voyons,... Let's see, . . .

À REVOIR: **d'habitude, en général, souvent**

CHAPITRE 11

Vivre en ville

Les dossiers de Juliette

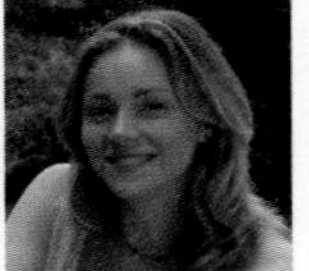
Juliette

- Mes photos
  - La Place du Capitole à Toulouse
  - La campagne à Paris
  - Le village de Riquewihr, en Alsace

Presentation: Use photo to review vocabulary and generate discussion, asking questions such as *Que voyez-vous sur la photo? Croyez-vous que les gens sont des touristes ou des citadins de Toulouse? De quelle année, à votre avis, datent les immeubles? Quel temps fait-il? Préférez-vous habiter en ville, en banlieue ou à la campagne? Pourquoi?*

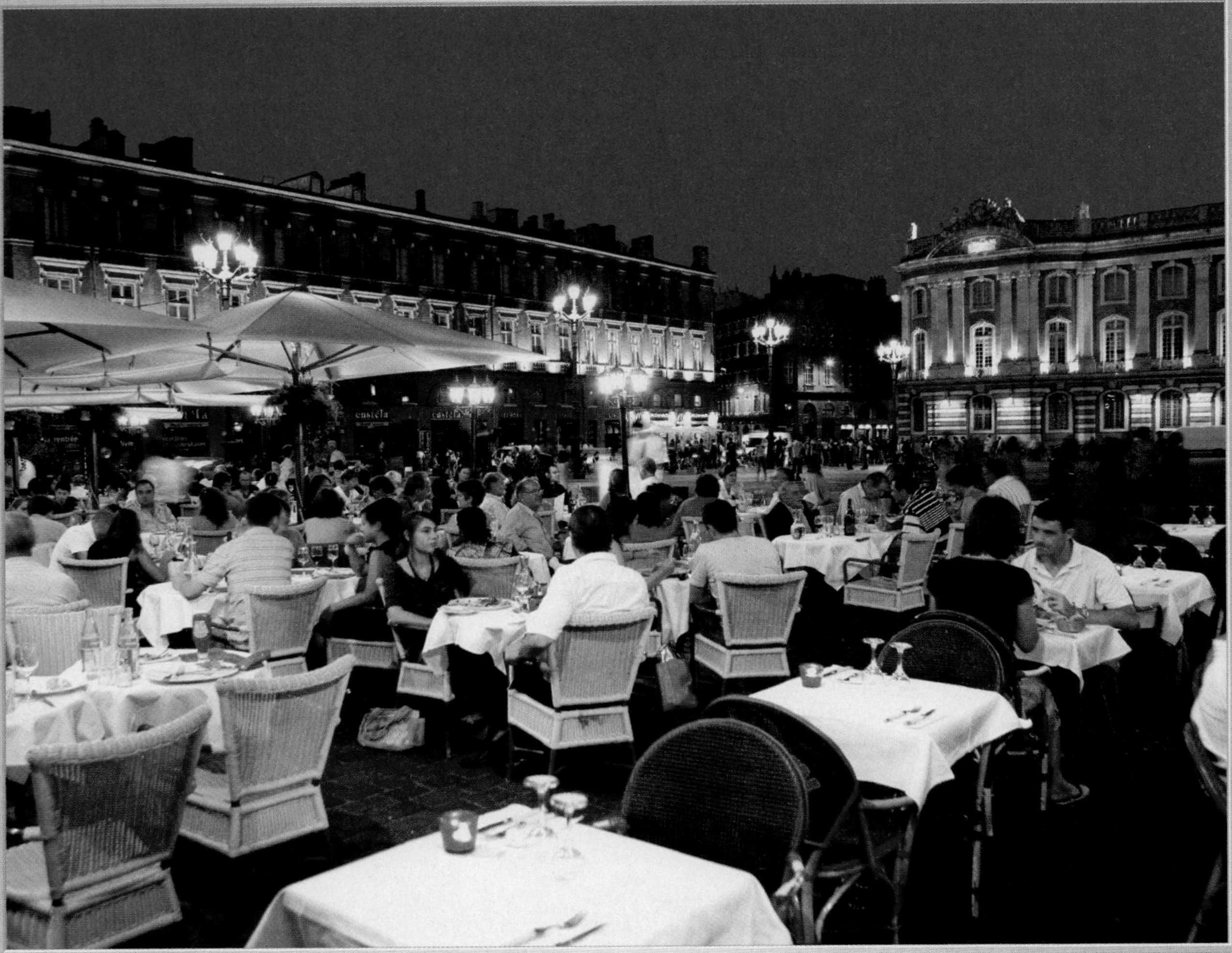

Un restaurant sur la Place du Capitole à Toulouse

Cultural note: Located in southwest France, Toulouse is the *chef-lieu* of the *Haute-Garonne* department in the *Midi-Pyrénées* region. It is the fourth-largest city in France, after Paris, Marseille, and Lyon.

Dans ce chapitre...

OBJECTIFS COMMUNICATIFS

- talking about city life
- describing past events
- speaking succinctly
- expressing what and whom you know
- learning to distinguish between and pronounce selected sounds in French

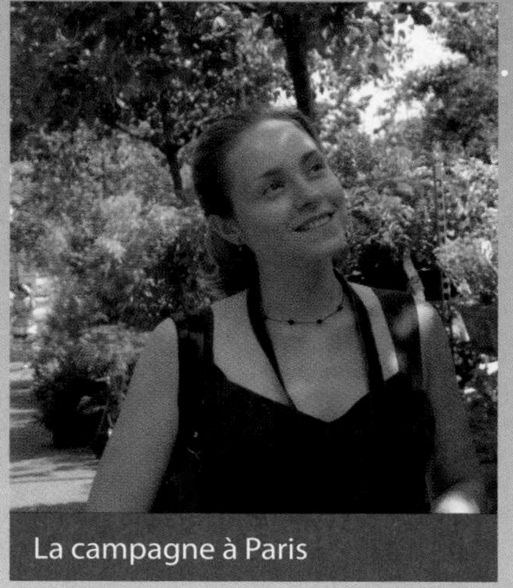

La campagne à Paris

PAROLES (Leçon 1)

- La ville et les directions
- Les arrondissements de Paris et les nombres ordinaux

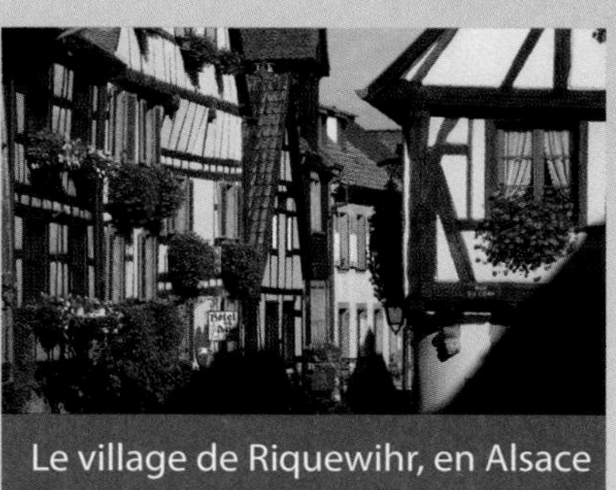

Le village de Riquewihr, en Alsace

STRUCTURES (Leçons 2 et 3)

- Le passé composé et l'imparfait
- Les pronoms d'objet indirect
- Les verbes **savoir** et **connaître**
- Les pronoms **y** et **en**

CULTURE

- Le blog de Juliette: *«Ajoutez deux lettres à Paris: c'est le Paradis.»*
- Reportage: *Jolis villages de France*
- Lecture: «Le chat abandonné» (poème de Paul Degray) (Leçon 4)

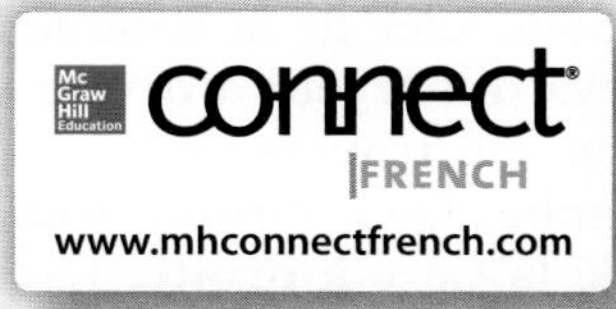

Leçon 1

PAROLES

Une petite ville

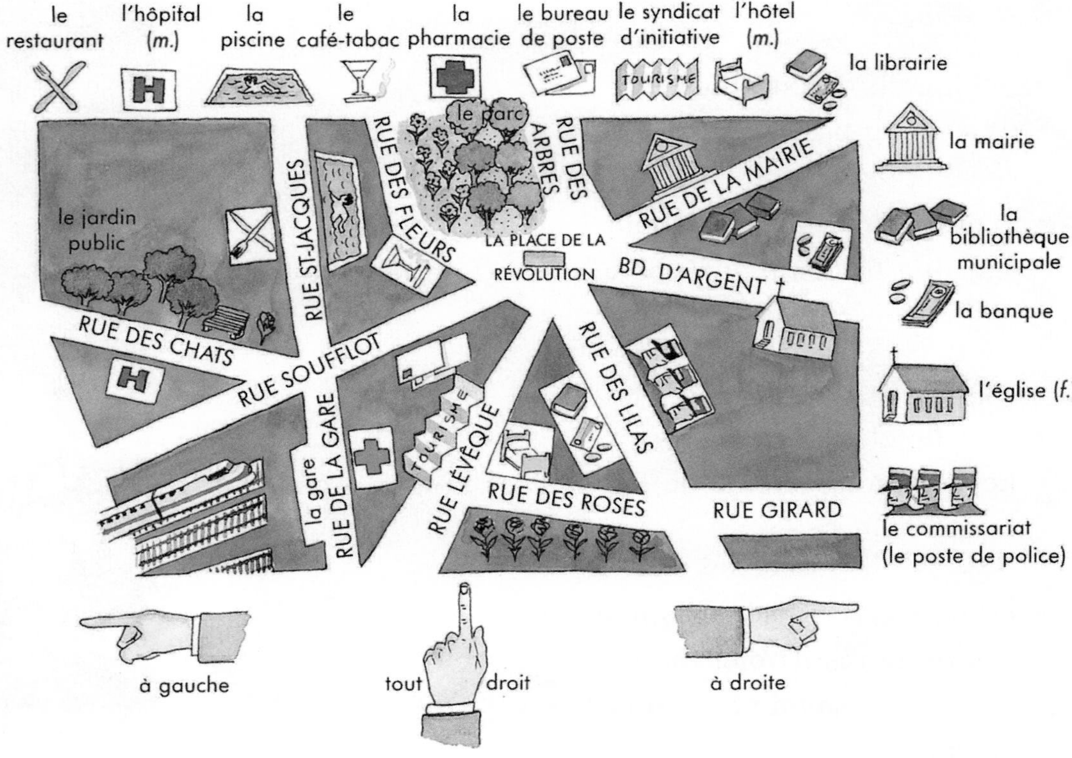

Vocabulary recycling: Emphasize the importance of giving directions. Review expressions such as *à côté de, derrière, devant, en face de, entre, près de, tourner à droite, à gauche.* Teach *Où se trouve… ?* as a fixed expression.

Additional vocabulary: *la biblio, le centre, l'hosto* (slang for *hôpital*), *la mosquée, le synagogue, le temple.*

Suggestion: Emphasize the difference between *à droite* [adʀwat] and *tout droit* [tudʀwa].

Follow-up: Ask sts. to describe a shorter route to the pharmacy from the bank.

AUTRES MOTS UTILES

le bâtiment	building
le carrefour	intersection
le chemin	way; road
le coin	corner
jusqu'à	up to, as far as
le marché en plein air	open-air market
le plan	map (*of a city*)
se trouver	to be located (situated)

—Comment fait-on pour aller de la banque à la pharmacie?
—On **prend** le boulevard d'Argent **à droite** et on va **jusqu'à** la place de la Révolution. On **traverse** la rue des Lilas et on **prend** la rue Lévêque **à gauche.** On **continue tout droit jusqu'au coin** et on **prend** la rue de la Gare **à droite.** La pharmacie est **en face de** la gare.

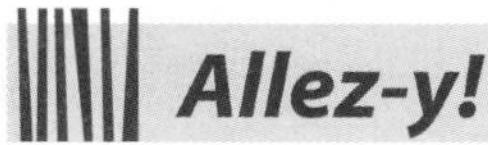

Allez-y!

A. Les endroits importants. Où est-ce qu'on va pour ______?

MODÈLE: acheter des livres →
Pour acheter des livres, on va à la librairie.

1. retirer de l'argent du distributeur automatique (*ATM*) **2.** acheter de l'aspirine **3.** parler avec le maire (*mayor*) de la ville **4.** obtenir des brochures touristiques **5.** nager **6.** admirer des plantes et des fleurs **7.** assister à (*to attend*) des services religieux catholiques **8.** acheter des timbres **9.** prendre une bière

B. Où est-ce? Précisez l'emplacement des endroits suivants selon le plan de la ville à la page précédente.

Suggestion (B): Have sts. describe locations in the same manner using a map of campus or the local town.

MODÈLE: Où est l'hôtel? →
L'hôtel est en face du syndicat d'initiative dans* la rue Lévêque.

1. Où est le jardin public?
2. Où est le commissariat?
3. Où est la bibliothèque?
4. Où est l'église?
5. Où est la librairie?
6. Où est le syndicat d'initiative?

C. Trouvez votre chemin. Regardez le plan de la ville. Imaginez que vous êtes à la gare. Un(e) touriste vous demande où est le bureau de poste; vous lui indiquez le chemin. Jouez les rôles avec un(e) camarade.

MODÈLE: LE/LA TOURISTE: Pardon, madame / monsieur, pourriez-vous me dire où est le bureau de poste?
VOUS: Tournez à gauche. Prenez la rue Soufflot à droite et vous y êtes (*you're there*).
LE/LA TOURISTE: Je tourne à gauche, je prends la rue Soufflot à droite et j'y suis.

1. le café-tabac **2.** le restaurant **3.** l'hôtel **4.** la banque **5.** le poste de police **6.** le parc **7.** la mairie **8.** la pharmacie **9.** le jardin public **10.** la place de la Révolution **11.** la piscine **12.** le syndicat d'initiative

Maintenant, avec un(e) autre camarade de classe, faites une liste de cinq ou six endroits sur votre campus ou dans votre ville. À tour de rôle, indiquez le chemin pour aller à ces endroits. Votre salle de classe est votre point de départ.

Additional activities: (A) Listening comprehension practice. Tell sts. *Vous êtes devant la gare. Vous prenez la rue de la Gare jusqu'à la rue Soufflot, où vous tournez à droite. Continuez jusqu'à la place, et prenez la première rue à gauche. Où êtes-vous?* Continue giving directions to other places on the map. (B) *À pied. Expliquez comment on va de la banque aux endroits suivants. Indiquez le chemin pour aller… 1. à l'hôpital 2. à la piscine 3. à la bibliothèque 4. au syndicat d'initiative*

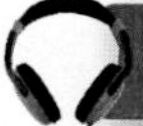

Prononcez bien!

Nasal vowels

Remember to let the air go through both your nose and mouth as you pronounce nasal vowels. Pay attention to the openness of your mouth and the shape of your lips.

For [ɔ̃] as in **bon**, close your mouth and round your lips.

[ɔ̃]: **on, révolution, connexion, feuilleton, voyons**

For [ɛ̃] as in **chemin**, open your mouth and stretch your lips in a smile.

[ɛ̃]: **timbre, jardin, syndicat, Internet, matin**

For [ɑ̃] as in **plan**, open your mouth and relax your lips.

[ɑ̃]: **banque, bâtiment, prend, argent, en**

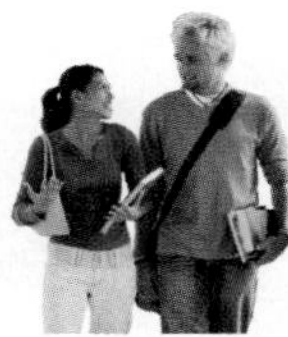

Pronunciation practice (1): Pronounce the following words and have sts. raise their hand when they hear any word that has the same nasal vowel as (1) bon: *sans, main, long, faim, ton, vent*; (2) chemin: *montre, bain, temps, non, blanc, pain*; (3) plan: *plein, champ, oncle, plante, vont, écran.*

Pronunciation practice (2): Write the following words on the board and elicit from sts. pronunciation of words containing the other two nasal vowels. MODÈLE: *fend* → *fin, fond. rein* (*rend, rond*); *long* (*lin, lent*); *saint* (*sans, son*); *pend* (*pain, pont*); *bain* (*banc, bon*); *gond* (*gain, gant*); *ment* (*main, mon*); *teint* (*temps, ton*); *vont* (*vin, vent*).

Pronunciation practice (3): The *Prononcez bien!* section on page 312 of this chapter contains additional activities for practicing these sounds.

Suggestion (C): Teach *Pourriez-vous… ?* (*Could you … ?*) as a fixed expression.

Suggestion (C): Display the map and have sts. in pairs use it to follow the pathway as they describe how to get from place to place.

*One says **dans la rue, sur le boulevard,** and **sur** or **dans l'avenue.**

Les arrondissements° de Paris

districts

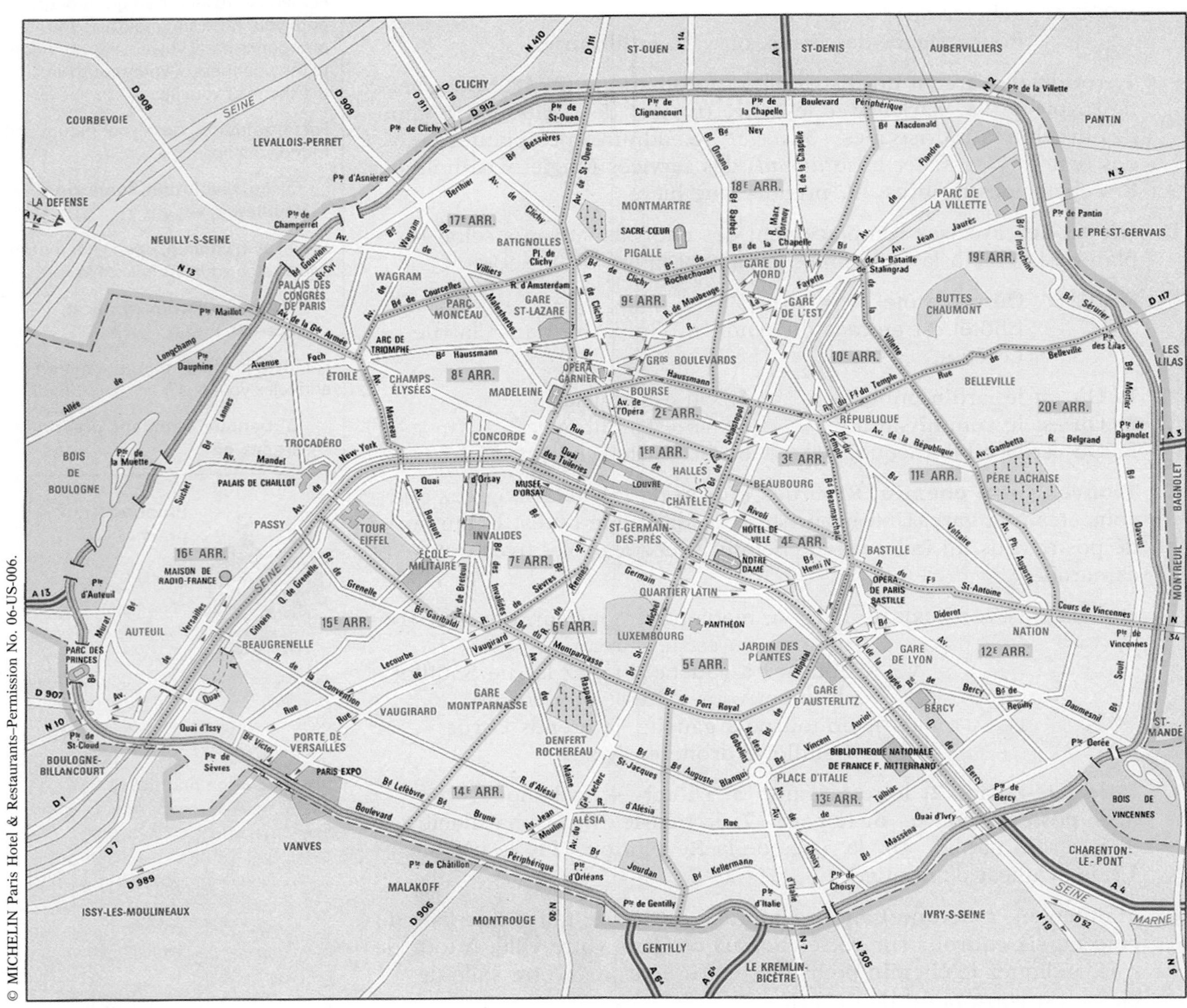

AUTRES MOTS UTILES

la banlieue	suburbs
la carte	map (*of a region, country*)
le centre-ville	downtown
la Rive droite / gauche	Right / Left Bank

Cultural note: Point out that the *arrondissements* are numbered in a spiral pattern, whose center (1er *arr.*) is on the Right Bank and includes *le Louvre*.

Les vingt arrondissements de Paris:

1er le premier	11e le onzième
2e le deuxième	12e le douzième
3e le troisième	13e le treizième
4e le quatrième	14e le quatorzième
5e le cinquième	15e le quinzième
6e le sixième	16e le seizième
7e le septième	17e le dix-septième
8e le huitième	18e le dix-huitième
9e le neuvième	19e le dix-neuvième
10e le dixième	20e le vingtième

Presentation: Model pronunciation. Give other numbers in English and ask sts. to form ordinals: 22nd, 45th, 36th, 57th, 63rd, etc.

Notes: (1) When there are only two elements in a series, the form *second(e)* can be used to replace *deuxième.* (2) The abbreviations for *premier* and *première* are *1er* and *1re*.

Les nombres ordinaux

- Ordinal numbers (*first, second,* and so on) are formed by adding **-ième** to cardinal numbers. Note the irregular form **premier / première,** and the spelling of **cinquième** and **neuvième.**
- **Le** and **la** do not elide before **huitième** and **onzième: le huitième.**
- The superscript abbreviation ^{e} indicates that a number should be read as an ordinal: 7 = **sept;** 7e = **le/la septième.**
- Note the forms **vingt et unième, trente et unième,** and so on.

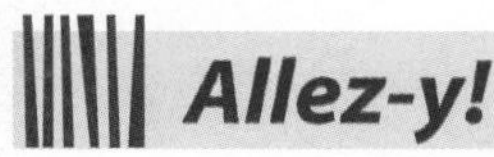

A. Les arrondissements de Paris. Quels arrondissements se trouvent sur la Rive gauche de la Seine? sur la Rive droite? Quel arrondissement est situé au bord du bois de Boulogne? du bois de Vincennes? Où est l'île de la Cité?*

B. Le plan de Paris. Avec un(e) partenaire, situez les endroits suivants.

MODÈLE: É1: la tour Eiffel?
É2: Euh, voyons... La tour Eiffel se trouve dans le septième arrondissement.

1. le Panthéon†
2. Notre-Dame
3. la gare de l'Est
4. le Louvre
5. Montmartre‡
6. Beaubourg§
7. le Sacré-Cœur
8. l'opéra Bastille
9. l'arc de Triomphe

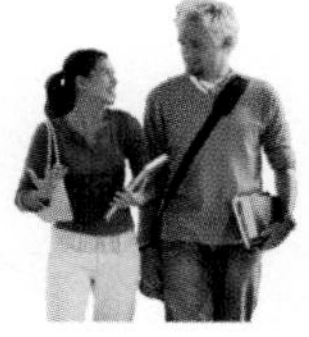

Note: Display photos of Paris to show the chief monuments and parks so that sts. can visualize the places they want to visit. You may also want to use the map of Paris found at the back of the book.

Continuation: *Quels arrondissements constituent le centre-ville? Quels arrondissements constituent les beaux quartiers résidentiels, Paris-Ouest? Quels arrondissements constituent le quartier des affaires sur la Rive droite, dans le centre-ville? Quels arrondissements constituent Paris-Est?*

*The **île de la Cité** is the historical center of Paris; it is one of the two islands on the Seine in Paris. The other is the **île St-Louis.**
†The **Panthéon** is a building in the **5e arrondissement** in Paris where several famous people are buried, including Voltaire, Rousseau, Marie Curie, and Louis Braille.
‡**Montmartre** is a lively area in northern Paris where Sacré-Cœur, a basilica, is located. The name **Montmartre** comes from **Mont des Martyrs** because several church officials were killed there long ago.
§**Beaubourg** is an ultramodern museum in Paris, and is also known as the **Centre Pompidou.** It is often surrounded by street artists and contains a wonderful collection of modern art.

CHAPITRE 11

Leçon 2

STRUCTURES

Presentation: Ask sts. to read roles of minidialogue aloud while others follow in text. After reading, have sts. speculate why verbs in bold are in a given tense. From these ideas, go on to generalize and give explanations.

Le passé composé et l'imparfait

Describing Past Events

Guide touristique à Paris

Alexis téléphone à Poema.

ALEXIS: Finalement **tu es partie** à la Guadeloupe?

POEMA: Mais non! **J'ai** tout **annulé**[1]: au dernier moment, **mes parents** m'**ont annoncé** leur arrivée à Paris. Alors **j'ai joué** les guides touristiques!

ALEXIS: Qu'est-ce que **vous avez fait**?

POEMA: Tous les jours la même chose! Le matin, **nous prenions** le petit déjeuner à la terrasse d'un café; ensuite **nous visitions** la capitale. À pied!

ALEXIS: Et le soir?

POEMA: **J'étais** complètement KO[2]! Maintenant qu'**ils sont partis,** j'ai vraiment besoin de vacances!

[1]*cancelled* [2]*exhausted*

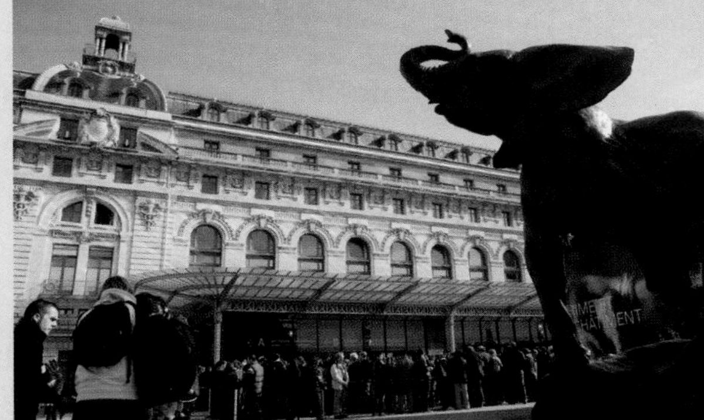

Paris: On fait la queue devant le musée d'Orsay.

Notes: (1) Point out to sts. that, as they learned in Ch 8, Leçon 3, the preposition *à* is used before the name of an island: *à la Guadeloupe / à la Martinique*. However, it is also very common to hear *en Guadeloupe / en Martinique*. (2) Another way to express *jouer les guides touristiques* is *jouer au guide touristique*. These expressions can be used interchangeably.

Répondez aux questions selon le dialogue.

1. Poema est-elle partie à la Guadeloupe?
2. Pourquoi a-t-elle changé ses projets?
3. Quel rôle a-t-elle joué avec ses parents?
4. Qu'est-ce que Poema et ses parents faisaient, tous les jours, à Paris?
5. Le soir, dans quel état était Poema?
6. Où sont ses parents maintenant?

When speaking about the past in English, you choose which past tense forms to use in a given context: *I visited Guadeloupe, I did visit Guadeloupe, I was visiting Guadeloupe, I used to visit Guadeloupe,* and so on. Usually only one of these options will convey exactly the meaning you want to express. Similarly in French, the choice between the **passé composé** and the **imparfait** depends on the kind of past action or condition that is being conveyed, and sometimes on the speaker's point of view with respect to the past event.

As you've learned, the **passé composé** is used to indicate a single completed action, something that began and ended in the past, or a sequence of such actions. The **imparfait,** on the other hand, usually indicates an ongoing or habitual action in the past. It does not emphasize the end of that action.

1. Compare the following sets of examples.

Suggestion: Ask sts. if the examples are an ongoing action, a completed action, or a habitual action.

J'**écrivais** des lettres.	*I was writing letters.*
J'**ai écrit** des lettres.	*I wrote (have written) letters.*
Je **commençais** mon travail.	*I was starting on my assignments.*
J'**ai commencé** mon travail.	*I started (have started) my assignments.*
Elle **allait** au parc le dimanche.*	*She went (used to go) to the park on Sundays.*
Elle **est allée** au parc dimanche.	*She went to the park on Sunday.*

Suggestion: Point out the differences in these examples: the *imparfait* presents scene-setting information, whereas the *passé composé* makes the story progress.

2. The following chart sets out the major differences between these two tenses.

IMPARFAIT	PASSÉ COMPOSÉ
1. *Ongoing action with no emphasis on the completion or end of the action*	*Completed action, or a series of completed events or actions*
J'**allais** en France. Je **visitais** des monuments.	Je **suis allé(e)** en France. J'**ai visité** des monuments.
2. *Habitual or repeated action*	*A single event*
J'**allais** en France tous les ans. Je **visitais** souvent le château de Versailles.	Je **suis allé(e)** en France l'année dernière. J'**ai visité** Versailles un samedi matin.
[Allez-y! A]	
3. *Description or "background" information; how things were or what was happening when . . .*	*. . . an event or events occurred. ("foreground" information)*
Je **visitais** Beaubourg...	...quand on **a annoncé** la projection d'un vieux film de Chaplin.
J'**étais** à Paris...	...quand une lettre **est arrivée.**
[Allez-y! B]	
4. *Physical or mental states of being (general description)*	*Changes in an existing physical or mental state at a precise moment, or for a particular isolated cause*
Ma nièce **avait** peur des chiens.	Ma nièce **a eu** peur quand le chien a aboyé (*barked*).

*Remember the role of the definite article with days of the week: **le dimanche** (*on Sundays*); **dimanche** (*on Sunday*).

Grammaire interactive

For more on the uses of the **imparfait** and the **passé composé,** watch the corresponding Grammar Tutorial and take a brief practice quiz at **Connect French.**

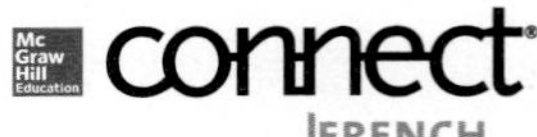

www.mhconnectfrench.com

3. In summary, the **imparfait** is generally used for *descriptions* in the past, and the **passé composé** is generally used for the *narration* of specific events in the past. The **imparfait** also often sets the stage for an event expressed with the **passé composé.** Look over the following passages with these points in mind.

IMPARFAIT	PASSÉ COMPOSÉ
Il **faisait** beau; le ciel (*sky*) **était** clair; les terrasses des cafés **étaient** pleines (*filled*) de gens; c'**était** un beau jour de printemps à Paris.	J'**ai continué** tout droit dans la rue Mouffetard, j'**ai traversé** le boulevard de Port-Royal et j'**ai descendu** l'avenue des Gobelins jusqu'à la place d'Italie.

4. The following indicators of tense can help you determine whether to use the **passé composé** or the **imparfait.**

IMPARFAIT	PASSÉ COMPOSÉ
autrefois (*formerly*) d'habitude de temps en temps le lundi (le mardi…) le week-end pendant que	au moment où lundi (mardi…) plusieurs fois soudain (*suddenly*) tout à coup (*suddenly*) un jour un week-end une fois (*once*), deux fois…
D'habitude, nous **étudiions** à la bibliothèque.	**Un jour,** nous **avons étudié** au café.
Quand j'**étais** jeune, nous **allions** à la plage **le week-end.**	**Un week-end,** nous **sommes allés** à la montagne.

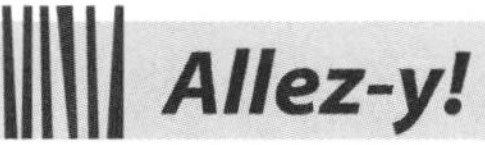

Allez-y!

Suggestion (A): Model a few sentences. Then have sts. do them in pairs for maximum oral practice. After 3–5 minutes, have whole group go over a few examples to make certain everyone has understood.

A. Un dimanche pas comme les autres. Votre voisin Marc Dufour était une personne routinière, mais un dimanche, il a changé ses habitudes. Voici son histoire.

MODÈLE: le dimanche matin / dormir en général jusqu'à huit heures / mais ce dimanche-là / dormir jusqu'à midi →
Le dimanche matin, il dormait en général jusqu'à huit heures, mais ce dimanche-là, il a dormi jusqu'à midi.

1. normalement au petit déjeuner / prendre des céréales et une tasse de café / mais ce matin-là / prendre un petit déjeuner copieux

2. après le petit déjeuner / faire toujours du jogging dans le parc / mais ce jour-là / rester longtemps au téléphone
3. souvent l'après-midi / regarder le match de football à la télé / mais cet après-midi-là / lire des poèmes dans le jardin
4. d'habitude le soir / sortir avec ses copains / mais ce soir-là / sortir avec une jeune fille
5. parfois / aller au cinéma ou / lire un roman / mais ce soir-là / inviter son amie à un restaurant élégant
6. normalement / rentrer chez lui assez tôt / mais ce dimanche-là / danser jusqu'au petit matin (*early morning*)

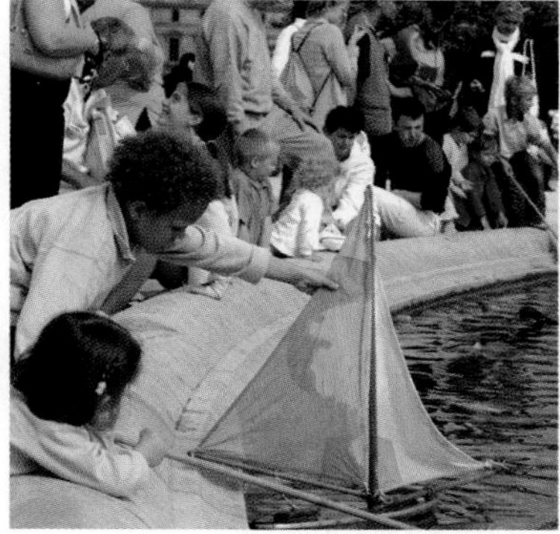

Au jardin du Luxembourg, à Paris. Est-ce que vous aimiez les parcs quand vous étiez petit(e)?

À votre avis, est-ce que Marc est malade (*sick*)? amoureux (*in love*)? déprimé (*depressed*)?... Justifiez votre réponse. Et vous, est-ce qu'il y a des choses que vous faisiez autrefois que vous ne faites plus maintenant? Expliquez.

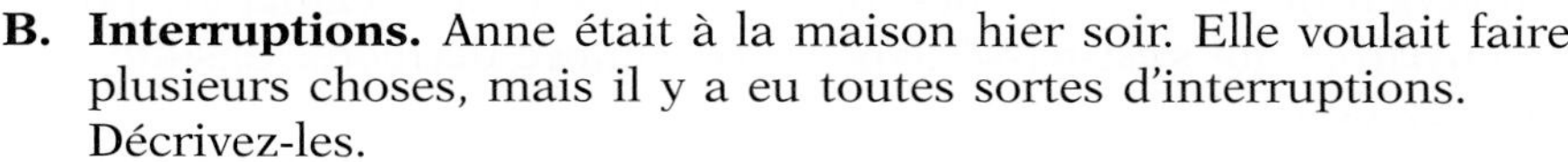

B. Interruptions. Anne était à la maison hier soir. Elle voulait faire plusieurs choses, mais il y a eu toutes sortes d'interruptions. Décrivez-les.

MODÈLE: étudier... téléphone / sonner →
Anne étudiait quand le téléphone a sonné.

Suggestion (B): Have sts. write ex. out on paper while several sts. write sentences on board for verification. Ask sts. why each tense is used in both clauses.

1. parler au téléphone / un ami... l'employé / couper la ligne (*to cut the line*)
2. écouter / iPod... son voisin / commencer à faire / bruit (*m., noise*)
3. lire / journal... le propriétaire / venir demander / argent
4. faire / devoirs... un ami / arriver
5. regarder / informations à la télé... son frère / changer de chaîne
6. dormir... quelqu'un / frapper (*to knock*) à la porte

C. Une année à l'université de Caen. Jérémie a passé un an à Caen, une des grandes villes de Normandie. Il raconte son histoire. Choisissez l'imparfait ou le passé composé pour les verbes suivants.

Suggestions (C): (1) Use as dictation material, with verbs conjugated. Sts. write out story, their books closed, and underline verbs. Then they explain why a given tense was used in each instance. (2) Have sts. write out ex. for homework, with correction next day in class. (3) Have sts. do ex. orally, explaining use of appropriate tense for each item.

Mon année en Normandie a été vraiment super, mais j'ai dû passer beaucoup de temps à étudier. Je (avoir)[1] cours le matin de 8 h à 11 h. L'après-midi, je (étudier)[2] en général à la bibliothèque. Le week-end, avec des amis, nous (faire)[3] du tourisme. Le samedi, nous (rester)[4] en ville et le dimanche, nous (aller)[5] à la campagne. En octobre, nous (faire)[6] une excursion à Rouen. Ce (être)[7] très intéressant. Pour Noël, je (rentrer)[8] chez mes parents. En février, je (faire)[9] du ski dans les Alpes. Nous (avoir)[10] de la chance car (*because*) il (faire)[11] très beau et je (rentrer)[12] bien bronzé (*tanned*). De temps en temps, je (manger)[13] chez les Levergeois, des amis français très sympathiques. Pendant ces dîners entre amis, je (perfectionner)[14] mon français. Finalement, au début du mois de mai, je (devoir)[15] quitter Caen. Je (être)[16] triste de partir.

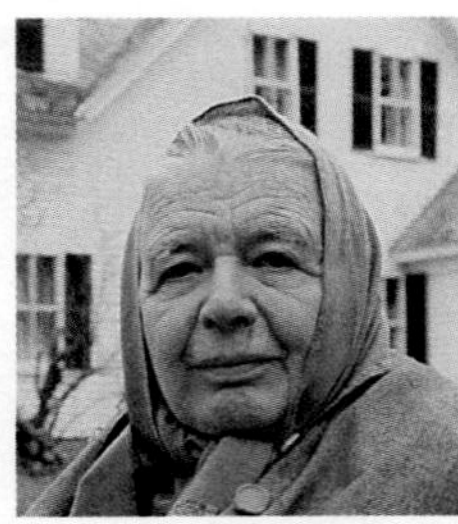

Marguerite Yourcenar

D. Biographie de Marguerite Yourcenar. Voici quelques faits (*facts*) importants de la vie de cette romancière (*novelist*) et historienne de langue française. Mettez-les dans l'ordre chronologique et utilisez les adverbes de temps des **Mots clés.**

1. Elle est allée aux États-Unis en 1958.
2. Elle a écrit son fameux livre *L'Œuvre au noir* en 1968.
3. Elle est née à Bruxelles en 1903.
4. Elle est morte en 1987 à l'âge de 84 ans dans le Maine, aux États-Unis.
5. Elle a été la première femme élue à l'Académie française, en 1980.

Maintenant, faites brièvement (*briefly*) votre autobiographie. Utilisez des adverbes de temps.

Suggestion (D): Have sts. do items silently first. Then solicit completed sentences in correct order.

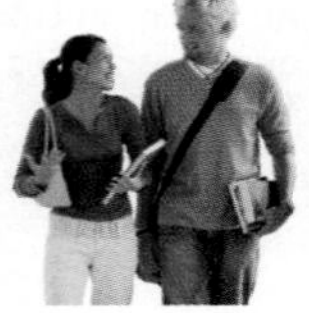

Suggestions (E): (1) Have sts. interview one another and take notes on answers. Ask them to write a *résumé* of responses. Collect for listening comprehension or dictation material. (2) Do as a whole-group activity, eliciting several oral responses for each question.

E. Conversation. Posez les questions suivantes à un(e) camarade pour découvrir ce qui s'est passé dans sa vie l'année dernière. Ensuite, changez de rôle.

1. Où étais-tu? Où as-tu étudié? Qu'est-ce que tu as étudié?
2. Qu'est-ce que tu as fait pendant tes vacances? As-tu fait un voyage? Où es-tu allé(e)? Comment était le voyage?
3. Et tes amis, où étaient-ils l'année dernière? Qu'est-ce qu'ils ont fait pendant les vacances?

F. Il était une fois... (*Once upon a time . . .*) Racontez une histoire que vous avez vécue (*lived*) ou une histoire fantastique (inventez-la!). Utilisez les éléments suggérés pour organiser votre histoire et choisissez le temps convenable (passé composé ou imparfait).

Suggestions: l'heure, le temps, la description de la scène, la description des personnages, la description des sentiments...

Expressions utiles: soudain, tout à coup, d'habitude, en général, puis, ensuite, enfin, alors, autrefois, quand, souvent, parfois, toujours...

Suggestions (F): (1) Ask sts. to write out stories and read them to another group in class or to whole class. (2) Use stories as dictation or listening comprehension material. (3) Make a transparency of a couple of stories, covering the sts.' names, and correct these stories as a group. Ask sts. to explain the corrections they find necessary. Then ask if everyone agrees with them.

Note: Sts. tend to be more engaged when they create stories on their own than when they fill in paragraphs (even though they may make more mistakes). You may want to set up several situations in which sts. creatively use the *passé composé* in conjunction with the *imparfait.*

Mots clés

Mettre les événements par ordre chronologique

d'abord *first of all*
puis *next*
ensuite *and then*
après *after that*
enfin *finally*

Puis and **ensuite** can be used interchangeably.

DÉPANNAGE (*Emergency Repair*)
D'abord, j'ai garé (*parked*) la voiture.
Puis, j'ai téléphoné à un garage dans le quartier.
Ensuite, j'ai tout expliqué au mécanicien.
Après, j'ai attendu dans la voiture.
Enfin, il est arrivé. Maintenant, le carburateur fonctionne à merveille.

Les pronoms d'objet indirect

Speaking Succinctly

Cannes en été

Hector et Hassan discutent au café.

HECTOR: Juliette et Léa **nous** proposent de les rejoindre[1] pour un week-end à Cannes.
HASSAN: Je sais: Elles **m'**ont téléphoné…
HECTOR: Qu'est-ce que tu **leur** as répondu?
HASSAN: Que je devais **te** parler avant de prendre une décision!
HECTOR: Pour moi, c'est «oui»!
HASSAN: Pour moi, c'est «non». Parce que Cannes en été, c'est la foule[2] dans les rues, dans les restaurants, sur la plage. C'est infernal!

[1]*join, accompany* [2]*crowd*

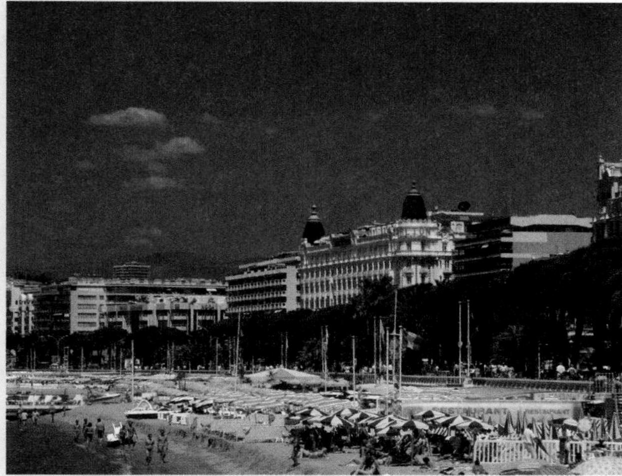

Cannes: un mythe et une délicieuse réalité

Trouvez, dans le dialogue, la phrase équivalente.

1. Hector dit à Hassan qu'ils sont invités pour le week-end à Cannes.
2. Hassan le sait: Juliette et Léa lui ont téléphoné.
3. Hector veut connaître la réponse d'Hassan.
4. Hassan a dit à Juliette et à Léa qu'il voulait consulter Hector.

Indirect Objects

Presentation: Point out that indirect object pronouns refer only to people or animals, never objects. Provide lots of oral examples so that sts. get used to hearing sentences with object pronouns.

1. As you know, direct object nouns and pronouns answer the question *what?* or *whom?* Indirect object nouns and pronouns usually answer the question *to whom?* or *for whom?* In English, the word *to* is frequently omitted: I gave the book *to Paul.* ⟶ I gave *Paul* the book. In French, the preposition **à** is *always* used before an indirect object noun.

J'ai donné des informations **à** Paul.	*I gave information to Paul.*
Elle a écrit une lettre **au** maire.	*She wrote a letter to the mayor.*
Nous montrons l'article **aux** journalistes.	*We show the article to the journalists.*
Elle prête les photos **à** son frère.	*She lends the photos to her brother.*

2. If a sentence has an indirect object, it usually has a direct object as well. Some French verbs, however, take only an indirect object. These include **téléphoner à, parler à,** and **répondre à.**

Je téléphone / parle souvent **à** mes amis.	*I often phone / speak to my friends.*
Elle a répondu **au** professeur.	*She answered the instructor.*

Suggestion: Present the following list of verbs. A. …*quelque chose à quelqu'un:* *acheter, apporter, demander, dire, donner, écrire, emprunter, envoyer, montrer, préparer, prêter, raconter, rendre, vendre;* B. …*à quelqu'un:* *obéir, parler, poser une question, rendre visite, répondre, téléphoner*

Indirect Object Pronouns

1. Indirect object pronouns replace indirect object nouns. They are identical in form to direct object pronouns, except for the third-person forms, **lui** and **leur.**

Note: Point out [ɥ] sound in *lui.*

INDIRECT OBJECT PRONOUNS			
me, m'	*(to/for) me*	nous	*(to/for) us*
te, t'	*(to/for) you*	vous	*(to/for) you*
lui	*(to/for) him, her*	**leur**	*(to/for) them*

Grammaire interactive

For more on indirect obect pronouns, watch the corresponding Grammar Tutorial and take a brief practice quiz at **Connect French.**

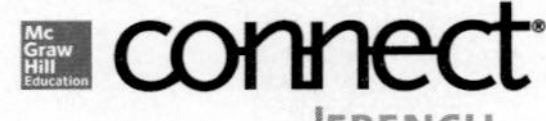

www.mhconnectfrench.com

2. The placement of indirect object pronouns is identical to that of direct object pronouns. However, the past participle does not agree with a preceding indirect object.

Je **lui** ai montré la réception.	*I showed him (her) the (front) desk.*
On **m'**a demandé l'adresse de l'auberge de jeunesse.	*They asked me for the address of the youth hostel.*
Valérie **nous** a envoyé un texto.	*Valérie sent us a text message.*
Nous allons **leur** téléphoner maintenant.	*We're going to telephone them now.*
Je **leur** ai emprunté* la voiture.	*I borrowed the car from them.*
Ils **m'**ont prêté de l'argent.	*They loaned me some money.*

3. In negative sentences, the object pronoun immediately precedes the auxiliary verb in the **passé composé.** If the pronoun is the indirect object of an infinitive, it is placed directly before the infinitive.

Elle **ne lui** a **pas** téléphoné.	*She hasn't telephoned him (her).*
Je **ne** vais **pas leur** écrire.	*I am not going to write to them.*

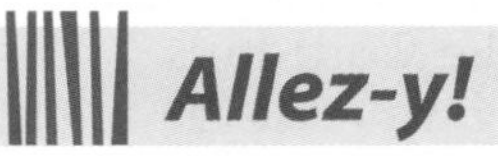

Allez-y!

Suggestion: Give sts. a few minutes to work on this activity individually, before eliciting responses.

A. L'après-midi d'Elsa. Elsa va tous les vendredis après-midi chez sa grand-mère qui habite dans son quartier. Elle nous raconte ce qu'elle a fait vendredi dernier. Complétez son histoire avec les pronoms qui correspondent: **me, te, lui, nous, vous, leur.**

Après les cours, j'ai pris un café avec des amies. Je ______[1] ai montré mon nouvel iPad. Un peu plus tard, j'ai rendu visite à ma grand-mère. Je ______[2] ai apporté ses magazines préférés. Elle était très contente et elle ______[3] a dit: «Je vais ______[4] préparer un bon

*****Emprunter (quelque chose) à (quelqu'un)** means *to borrow (something) from (someone).*

goûter.» En fin d'après-midi, mon frère est arrivé. Il ______[5] a raconté ses aventures avec sa nouvelle moto. Nous avons bien ri. (*We laughed a lot.*)

Au moment de partir, ma grand-mère ______[6] a demandé (à mon frère et à moi): «Je vous revois la semaine prochaine, les enfants?» Nous ______[7] avons répondu, «Bien sûr, à vendredi prochain!»

B. N'oublie pas... Au moment de dire au revoir, la grand-mère d'Elsa se rappelle (*remembers*) plusieurs questions qu'elle voulait lui poser. Jouez le rôle d'Elsa et répondez-lui, en utilisant les pronoms complément d'objet indirect.

1. As-tu téléphoné à ton oncle? **2.** Tu as écrit à ta tante Céline? **3.** Tu as donné le plan de la ville à ton frère pour son voyage? **4.** As-tu répondu à M. et Mme Morin en Espagne? **5.** Est-ce que tu as souhaité (*wished*) «bon anniversaire» à ton petit cousin? **6.** Est-ce que tu as rendu à Nicolas et Virginie le livre qu'ils nous ont prêté?

C. Êtes-vous communicatif / communicative? Posez les questions suivantes à un(e) camarade et créez de nouvelles questions sur le même sujet.

1. À qui as-tu écrit la semaine dernière? Qu'est-ce que tu lui as écrit? Pourquoi? En général, écris-tu souvent?
2. À qui as-tu téléphoné hier soir? Qu'est-ce que tu lui as dit?
3. Tu envoies souvent des textos? À quelle occasion? À qui?

Ensuite, dites à la classe si votre camarade est très ou peu communicatif / communicative. Qui est la personne la plus communicative de la classe?

Continuation (B): *As-tu envoyé la carte postale à ta tante? Est-ce que tu as emprunté la voiture à ta mère? As-tu donné le cadeau au professeur?*

Additional activity: Prepare the following translation activity. *En français, s'il vous plaît. Marc parle de ses vacances à la plage. Il écrit en anglais. Traduisez pour lui.* 1. *My French friends and I are spending our vacation at the beach.* 2. *I showed them the countryside.* 3. *I spoke to them about the region* (région). 4. *I sent photos to my parents with my smartphone.* 5. *I described* (décrire) *the trip to them.* 6. *I telephoned a friend.* 7. *I talked to her about my vacation.* 8. *I sent her a text, too.* 9. *My friends needed money, so I lent them some euros.* 10. *They lent me some clothes.* 11. *I haven't yet had the time to go* (le temps d'aller) *to the beach!*

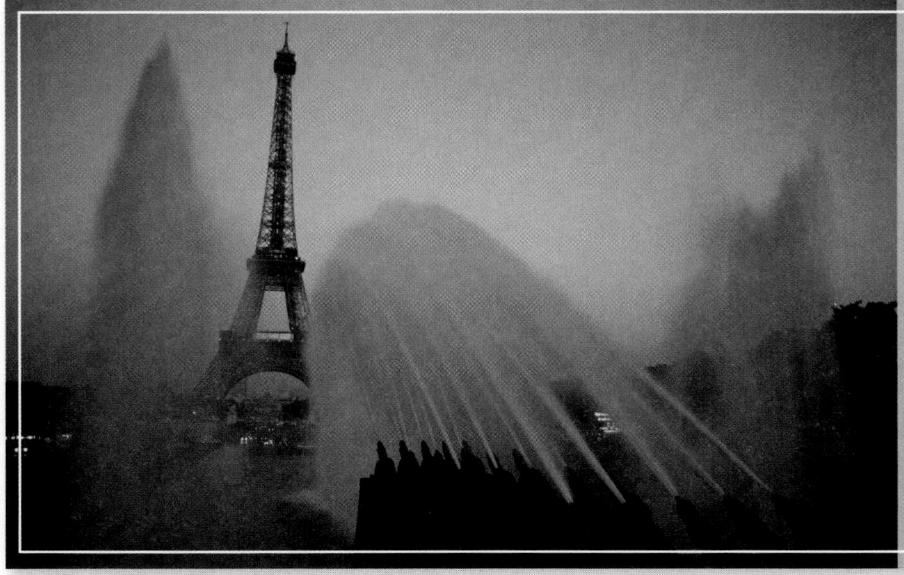

Un peu plus...

Le Trocadéro.
Où trouver, à Paris, un endroit où l'on peut visiter plusieurs grands musées, se rendre dans un théâtre national et profiter d'une vue impressionnante de la tour Eiffel? Place du Trocadéro, bien sûr! Le Trocadéro est une grande place située en face de la tour Eiffel, sur la Rive droite de la Seine. Sur cette place se trouve le Palais de Chaillot qui abrite (*houses*) le musée national de la Marine, le musée de l'Homme et la Cité de l'architecture et du patrimoine. C'est aussi le lieu du Théâtre National de Chaillot.

◄ *Le Trocadéro au crépuscule* (dusk). *Décrivez la scène.*

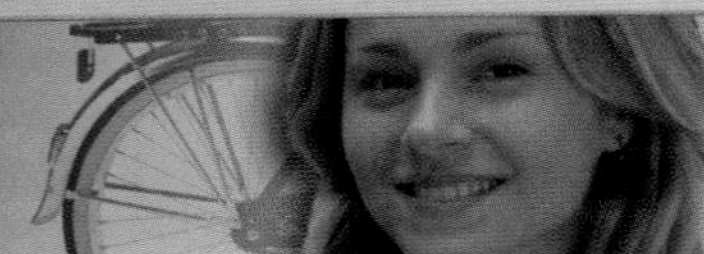

Le blog de Juliette

«Ajoutez deux lettres à Paris: c'est le Paradis.»

—(Jules Renard)

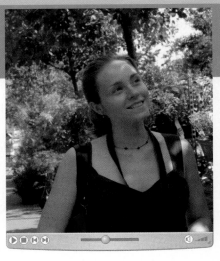

Vous voyez, la campagne à Paris, c'est une réalité!

mardi 21 juillet

Vous rêvez de Paris? Moi, j'y[1] habite depuis trois ans!

Avant, je visitais la capitale comme une touriste: je connaissais[2] tous les monuments, les musées, les promenades, les restaurants.

Maintenant, je sais[3] utiliser les transports en commun et lire un plan; je passe sans problème des cafés de la Rive gauche aux grands magasins de la Rive droite; je fréquente les petits restaurants bobos[4] du 11e. Je connais aussi le vieux Paris, avec ses lieux secrets pleins[5] de charme.

J'ai toujours aimé les grandes villes. Après mon Master, dans un an, je veux aller travailler dans une capitale à l'étranger. Déjà, l'an dernier, j'ai fait un stage[6] de trois mois dans une entreprise à Londres.

Vous avez compris: la banlieue ou les petites villes de province, ce n'est pas ma passion (ou ce n'est pas ma tasse de thé, comme disent les Anglais!).

Bisous quand même[7] à tous les banlieusards[8] et à tous les provinciaux[9]!

Juliette

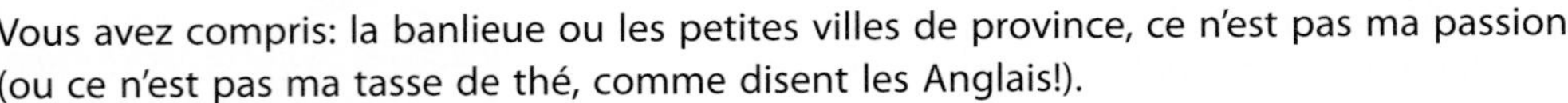

COMMENTAIRES

Alexis

Moi, j'ai passé toute mon enfance à Québec et je connais New York, Chicago, Miami. J'ai aussi visité Rome, Barcelone et Varsovie. Eh bien, je vais te dire: j'aime mieux Versailles! Quand je suis arrivé ici, j'ai compris que je préférais le charme à la grandeur…

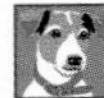

Trésor

Hypocrite! Et le château, c'est du charme ou de la grandeur?

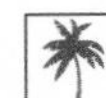

Poema

Personnellement, je suis très attachée à Papeete, la ville de mon enfance. Cette petite capitale de la Polynésie française n'a que 100 000 habitants! Avec ses bateaux à voile blancs, ses palmiers du bord de mer, elle ressemble à une cité balnéaire[10] de la Côte d'Azur.[11]

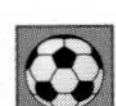

Mamadou

Vous connaissez Dakar, ma ville natale? On y trouve plein de[12] choses à faire.

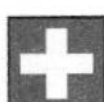

Charlotte

C'est vrai! À Dakar, on trouve des bars, des restaurants, et aussi des musées, une université, des bibliothèques, des galeries d'art, des cinémas! Je le sais, j'y suis allée!

[1]y = *there* [2]*was familiar with* [3]*know how to* [4]*hipster* (*from* **bo**urgeois-**bo**hème) [5]*full* [6]*internship* [7]quand… *nevertheless* [8]*people living in the suburbs* (*pej.*) [9]*city dwellers in other regions of France* (*as opposed to Paris*) (*fam.*) [10]cité.. *summer resort town* [11]Côte… *French Riviera* [12]plein… *plenty of*

Cultural note: Jules Renard was a French writer who lived at the end of the 19th century and died in 1910. He was part of the literary scene in Paris and wrote novels, poems, short stories, and plays. His journal was published in 1925 and is well-known for its introspection and humor.

Video connection: In the videoblog for this chapter, Juliette and Hector discuss the advantages and disadvantages of city life. Juliette posts her video on *Paris caché* and Hector's blog on his hometown, les Anses d'Arlet, in Martinique on her website.

Follow-up: 1. *Quelles nouvelles expériences Juliette a-t-elle faites à Paris?* 2. *Que voulez-vous visiter quand vous allez visiter Paris?* 3. *Quels aspects de leur ville natale Poema et Mamadou aiment-ils particulièrement? Quelle personnalité révèlent-ils à travers leurs commentaires?* 4. *Préférez-vous les grandes villes, les petites villes de province ou la banlieue? Expliquez pourquoi.*

Note: There are photos of Dakar and Papeete in the *Bienvenue* sections after Chapters 8 and 16, respectively.

REPORTAGE

Jolis villages de France

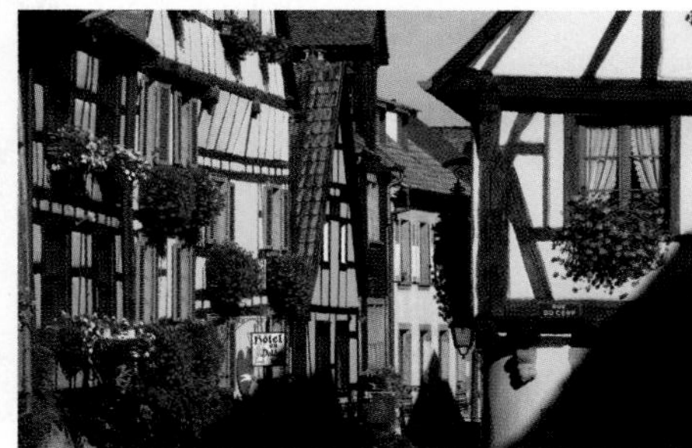

Riquewihr: charme et histoire

Ils sont pittoresques, charmants, perdus dans la nature ou installés au sommet d'une montagne comme une cerise[1] sur un gâteau: Ce sont les 32 000 villages de la campagne française. L'existence y est simple et tranquille. On y vit au milieu des moutons, des vaches et des poules.[2]

Dans un village typique de France, on trouve toujours une église, une mairie, une école, un cimetière, une salle des fêtes. Très anciens, les jolis villages de France ont des visages multiples: villages-forteresses organisés autour d'un château, villages-jardins, villages de pêcheurs,[3] villages-labyrinthes… Chaque village raconte une page de l'histoire de France et définit l'identité d'une région. Par exemple, **Riquewihr**, situé à quelques kilomètres de Colmar dans l'est de la France, est un village médiéval typiquement alsacien. Il est célèbre pour ses maisons aux colombages[4] sculptés, pour ses petites rues tortueuses, pour ses vieux puits[5] et ses fontaines. **Gordes**, avec son château monumental construit au centre du village, est situé au milieu de champs de lavande et des vignes. C'est un centre culturel et artistique qui attire des visiteurs amoureux de la Provence. Dans les Hautes-Alpes, **Saint-Véran** est un adorable village de montagne situé à 2 042 m[6] d'altitude. L'hiver, il se transforme en station de ski; l'été, il propose de merveilleuses randonnées aux amoureux de la nature.

Certains villages construisent leur réputation sur leur production locale: vins, cidres, champagnes, fromages, pâtés, miel,[7] gâteaux, bonbons… Allez à **Pérouges**, près de Lyon: c'est un minuscule village du XIIe siècle, célèbre pour ses galettes[8] au sucre absolument exquises. Arrêtez-vous à **La Roque-Gageac**, ravissant village du Sud-Ouest, construit le long de la Dordogne: On y déguste[9] un foie gras fabuleux fabriqué dans la région. À **Hauvillers**, village du Nord-Est surnommé[10] «La Perle du Champagne», on boit du champagne! Et on visite l'abbaye où repose, pour l'éternité, le fameux moine[11] Dom Pérignon. C'est lui qui a donné son nom à l'un des meilleurs champagnes français: le Dom Pérignon.

Aujourd'hui, les jolis villages vivent essentiellement du tourisme. Avec leurs églises, leurs châteaux, leurs abbayes, leurs fermes et leurs maisons bourgeoises, ils proposent une expérience authentique aux visiteurs. Prendre un petit café au soleil, manger un poulet fermier[12] dans le restaurant local, acheter des œufs frais et des fruits de saison à l'épicerie, se promener dans les rues tranquilles et dire bonjour à tout le monde, voilà les plaisirs uniques qu'on découvre dans les jolis petits villages de France.

[1]*cherry* [2]*chickens* [3]*fishermen* [4]*half-timbers* [5]*wells* [6]*6,636 feet* [7]*honey* [8]*tarts* [9]*tastes* [10]*nicknamed* [11]*monk* [12]*farm-raised*

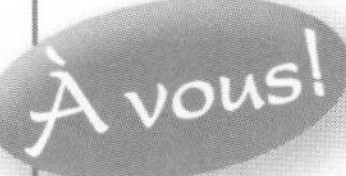

1. Décrivez un petit village typiquement français selon le *Reportage*.
2. Qu'est-ce qu'on trouve dans tous les petits villages typiques de France?
3. Quel village en France est célèbre pour ses galettes? son champagne? son foie gras?
4. Décrivez plusieurs endroits que les touristes aiment visiter dans les petits villages.

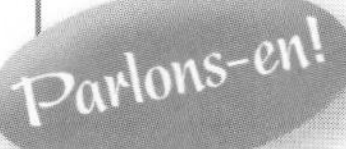

1. Travaillez à deux ou en petits groupes. Allez sur le site Internet de l'association «Les plus beaux villages de France». Parmi les 156 villages remarquables de son répertoire, sélectionnez un village que vous trouvez particulièrement charmant.
2. Situez votre village sur une carte de France. Précisez dans quelle région il se trouve (la Bourgogne, le Centre, la Lorraine…), si c'est un village de campagne, de montagne ou de pêcheurs, s'il propose une activité particulière, etc.
3. Expliquez pourquoi ce village vous intéresse.

Suggestion (Parlons-en!): Alternatively, you may ask sts. to present a beautiful village that they know using the same criteria. In any case, after pairs or groups work together, have them present "their" village to the class.

CHAPITRE **11**

Leçon 3

STRUCTURES

Les verbes *savoir* et *connaître*

Expressing What and Whom You Know

Les mystères du château de Versailles

Alexis téléphone à Poema.

ALEXIS: **Tu connais** le château de Versailles?
POEMA: **Qui ne connaît pas** le château de Versailles? **Nous connaissons** tous le château: c'est un symbole de la France!
ALEXIS: **Tu sais** qu'il reçoit des millions de visiteurs par an?
POEMA: **Je sais**! C'est un monument national. Comme le musée du Louvre ou la tour Eiffel.
ALEXIS: Moi, **je connais** les mystères du château… Si tu veux, je te montre un passage secret entre la chambre du Roi et la chambre de la Reine…
POEMA: Tu crois qu'on va rencontrer le fantôme de Marie-Antoinette?

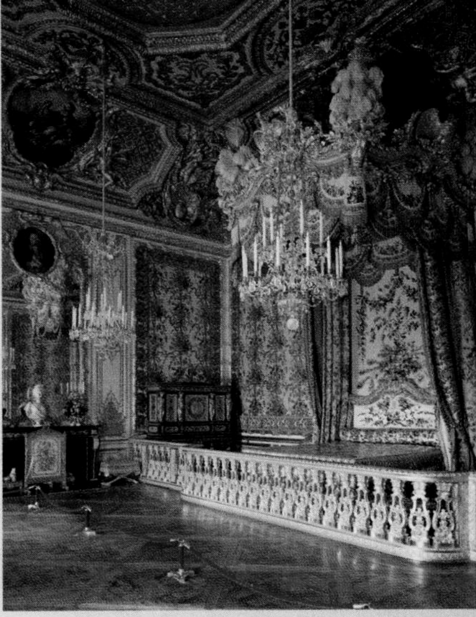

Versailles: la chambre somptueuse de la reine Marie-Antoinette

Suggestion: Point out the difference between *savoir* (intellectual knowledge of a technique) and *pouvoir* (the capacity to act): *Il sait faire du ski—Il ne peut pas faire de ski à cause de son accident.*

Note: You may wish to point out the difference between *Je connais cette chanson—Je la sais par cœur.*

Faites des phrases complètes pour montrer que vous avez compris le dialogue. Choisissez le verbe approprié. **Attention!** il y a parfois plusieurs réponses possibles.

Tout le monde Alexis Poema	{ sait connaît }	le château de Versailles. que c'est un monument national. les mystères du château.

The verbs **savoir** and **connaître** both correspond to the English verb *to know,* but they are used differently.

Forms of *savoir* and *connaître*

PRESENT TENSE OF **savoir**			
je	**sais**	nous	**savons**
tu	**sais**	vous	**savez**
il/elle/on	**sait**	ils/elles	**savent**
Past participle: **su**			

PRESENT TENSE OF **connaître**			
je	**connais**	nous	**connaissons**
tu	**connais**	vous	**connaissez**
il/elle/on	**connaît**	ils/elles	**connaissent**
past participle: **connu**			

Note: You may wish to point out that verbs like *connaître* are spelled with a circumflex on the *i* in each form where *i* precedes *t: elle connaît, il paraît.*

Uses of *savoir* and *connaître*

1. **Savoir** means *to know* or *to have knowledge of* a fact, *to know by heart,* or *to know how to* do something. It is frequently followed by an infinitive or by a subordinate clause introduced by **que, quand, pourquoi,** and so on.

Sais-tu l'heure qu'il est?	*Do you know what time it is?*
Savez-vous où est le bureau de poste le plus proche d'ici?	*Do you know where the closest post office is?*
Je **sais** que le bureau de poste du boulevard Haussmann est fermé.	*I know that the post office on Boulevard Haussmann is closed.*

2. In the **passé composé, savoir** means *learned* or *found out.*

J'**ai su** hier que la mairie allait être démolie.	*I learned yesterday that the city hall is going to be demolished.*

3. **Connaître** means *to know* or *to be familiar* (*acquainted*) *with* someone or something. **Connaître**—never **savoir**—means *to know a person or a place.* **Connaître** is always used with a direct object; it cannot be followed directly by an infinitive or by a subordinate clause.

—**Connais**-tu Lucille?	*Do you know Lucillle?*
—Non, je ne la **connais** pas.	*No, I don't know her.*
Ils **connaissent** très bien Dijon.	*They know Dijon very well.*

4. In the **passé composé, connaître** means *met for the first time.* It is the equivalent of the **passé composé** of **faire la connaissance de.**

J'ai connu Didier à l'université.	*I met Didier at the university.*

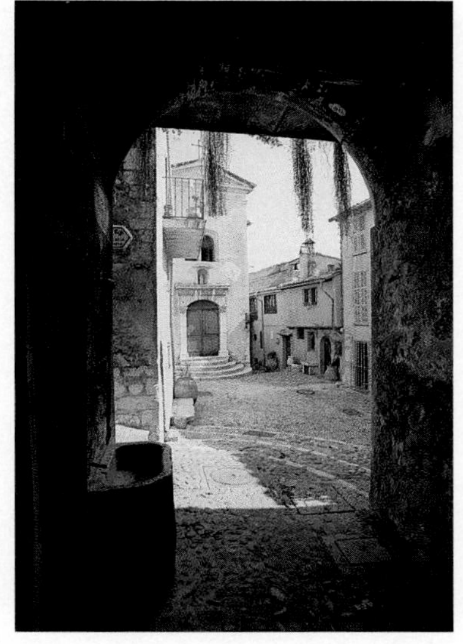

Cagnes-sur-mer, un petit village de la Côte d'Azur. Connaissez-vous la Côte d'Azur? Voulez-vous la visiter? Pourquoi?

Allez-y!

A. Dialogue. Complétez les phrases avec **connaître** ou **savoir.**

MME DUPUY: ______[1]-vous Paris, monsieur?
M. STEIN: Je ______[2] seulement que c'est la capitale de la France.
MME DUPUY: ______[3]-vous quelle est la distance entre Paris et Marseille?
M. STEIN: Non, mais je ______[4] une agence de voyages où on doit le ______[5]. Dans cette agence, ils ______[6] très bien le pays.
MME DUPUY: ______[7]-vous s'il y a d'autres villes intéressantes à visiter?
M. STEIN: Comme je l'ai dit, je ne ______[8] pas bien ce pays, mais hier j'ai fait la connaissance d'un homme qui ______[9] où aller pour passer de bonnes vacances.
MME DUPUY: Je voudrais bien ______[10] cet homme. ______[11]-vous où il travaille?

Suggestion: Give sts. a short time to fill in blanks. Ask for volunteers to read each sentence. Ask another st. why an answer is correct or incorrect.

Suggestion: Slides or pictures of places mentioned would help make this ex. more meaningful to sts.

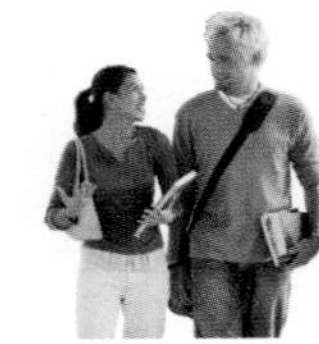

Le parler jeune

une balade	une promenade
se balader	se promener
une manif	une manifestation
quartier bobo	quartier bourgeois-bohème
quartier branché	quartier à la mode

Une **balade** à vélo, ça t'intéresse?

J'aime bien **me balader** sur la croisette (*boardwalk*) à Cannes.

À Paris, les grandes **manifs** populaires passent par République.

Le XIe arrondissement? C'est le **quartier bobo** de Paris.

Le haut Marais, c'est le nouveau **quartier branché** de Paris.

B. Et toi, connais-tu Paris? Avec un(e) camarade, posez des questions et répondez-y.

MODÈLE: l'Opéra-Bastille →

VOUS: Connais-tu l'Opéra-Bastille?

VOTRE CAMARADE: Non, je ne le connais pas, mais je sais qu'on y va pour écouter de la musique.

ENDROITS	DÉFINITIONS
l'Opéra-Bastille	C'est le quartier des étudiants à Paris.
Notre-Dame de Paris	Le président y habite.
le Louvre	On y va pour écouter de la musique.
le Palais de l'Élysée	On y trouve une vaste collection de livres.
la tour Eiffel	C'est une église située dans l'île de la Cité.
la Bibliothèque nationale	C'est la structure en verre (*glass*) devant le Louvre.
le Quartier latin	On y trouve une riche collection d'art.
la Pyramide	Elle a 320 mètres de haut (*tall*) et elle est en fer (*iron*).

Note: The pronoun *y* is presented in the next lesson. Introduce it as a lexical element meaning *there.*

Un peu plus...

L'Opéra-Garnier.
Cet opéra est l'un des édifices les plus somptueux de Paris. L'intérieur est fait de différents marbres et décoré de nombreuses sculptures. La salle de concert est rouge et or. C'est Napoléon III qui a fait construire l'Opéra du palais Garnier. Son décor flamboyant devait représenter le luxe, l'art et le plaisir. De nos jours, on y présente de grands spectacles de danse.

Aimez-vous le luxe? Expliquez.

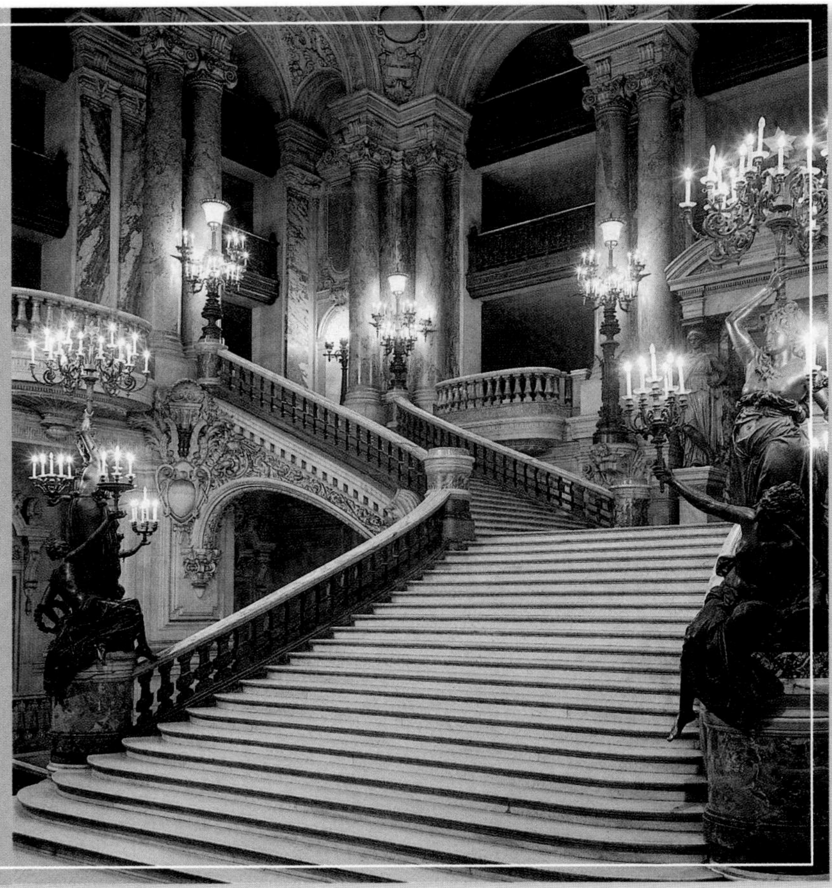

► *Les luxes de la ville: le grand escalier de l'Opéra de Paris.*

C. Vos connaissances. Utilisez ces phrases pour interviewer un(e) camarade. Dans les réponses, utilisez le verbe **savoir** ou **connaître.**

1. Nomme deux choses que tu sais faire.
2. Nomme deux choses que tu veux savoir faire un jour.
3. Nomme deux domaines (*fields*) où tu es plus ou moins compétent(e). (Je connais / ne connais pas bien...)
4. Nomme une personne que tu as connue récemment.
5. Nomme quelqu'un que tu aimerais (*would like*) connaître.

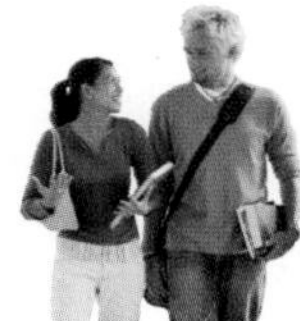

Continuation (C): 6. *Nomme deux villes que tu connais bien.* 7. *Nomme deux villes que tu veux connaître et dis pourquoi.*

D. Une ville. Donnez le nom d'une ville que vous connaissez bien. Ensuite, racontez ce que vous savez sur cette ville.

MODÈLE: Je connais New York. Je sais qu'il y a d'immenses gratte-ciel (*skyscrapers*).

Suggestions (D): (1) Give sts. a moment to reflect. (2) Can be done as a game. St. gives hints: *Je sais qu'il y a d'énormes gratte-ciel dans cette ville. Je sais qu'elle est sur la côte est.* Others guess which city is being described.

Les pronoms *y* et *en*

Speaking Succinctly

Presentation: Model sentences in the grammar sections and have sts. repeat sentences using *y*.

Le musée Picasso

Juliette et Léa discutent au café.

JULIETTE: Tu as un plan d'Antibes sur toi?
LÉA: J'**en** ai un sur mon iPhone. Qu'est-ce que tu cherches?
JULIETTE: Le musée Picasso.
LÉA: C'est au château Grimaldi, dans la vieille ville, face à la mer. J'**y** suis déjà allée.
JULIETTE: J'ai deux billets gratuits.[1] Tu **en** veux un?
LÉA: Si j'**en** veux un? Bien sûr!
JULIETTE: Tu veux **y** retourner?
LÉA: Sans hésitation! C'est tellement[2] beau! On **y** va ensemble!

[1]*free* [2]*so*

Trouvez, dans le dialogue, des phrases équivalentes.

1. J'ai un plan d'Antibes sur mon iPhone.
2. Je suis déjà allée au musée Picasso.
3. Tu veux un billet?
4. Tu veux retourner au musée Picasso?
5. On va ensemble au musée Picasso.

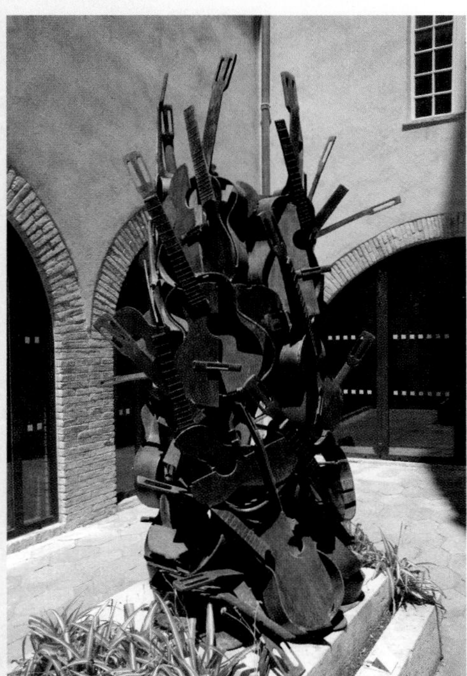

Pour les amateurs d'art

The Pronoun *y*

Note: In informal conversation, *y* is now used frequently to refer to people: *Je pense aux enfants. J'y pense.*

1. The pronoun **y** can refer to a place that has already been mentioned. It replaces a prepositional phrase, and its English equivalent in such cases is *there.*

—Est-ce que Nathalie est déjà allée **au parc Montsouris**?	*Has Nathalie already gone to Montsouris Park?*
—Non, mais elle **y** va samedi.	*No, but she is going there Saturday.*
—Est-ce que Myriam va **au festival** avec elle?	*Is Myriam going to the festival with her?*
—Non, elle n'**y** va pas avec elle.	*No, she isn't going (there) with her.*
—Vont-elles **chez Nathalie** ce week-end?	*Are they going to Nathalie's this weekend?*
—Oui, elles **y** vont ensemble.	*Yes, they're going (there) together.*

Note that *there* is often implied in English, whereas **y** must always be expressed in French.

2. **Y** can replace the combination **à** + *noun* when the noun refers to a place or thing. This substitution most often occurs after certain verbs that are followed by **à: répondre à, réfléchir à, réussir à, penser à** (*to think about someone or something*), **jouer à.** It is not usually applied to the **à** + *noun* combination when the noun refers to a person; in these cases, a stressed or indirect object pronoun is used.

—As-tu répondu **au texto de ta sœur**?	*Did you answer your sister's text message?*
—Oui, j'**y** ai répondu.	*Yes, I answered it.*
—Elle pense déjà **au voyage à Marseille**?	*Is she already thinking about the trip to Marseille?*
—Non, elle n'**y** pense pas encore.	*No, she's not thinking about it yet.*

BUT

—As-tu téléphoné **à ta mère?**	*Did you call your mother?*
—Non, je ne **lui** ai pas téléphoné, mais je pense à **elle.**	*No, I didn't call her, but I'm thinking about her.*

3. The placement of **y** is identical to that of object pronouns: It precedes a conjugated verb, an infinitive, or an auxiliary verb in the **passé composé.**

La ville de Nice? Nous **y** cherchons une maison.	*The city of Nice? We're looking for a house there.*
Mon mari va **y** aller jeudi.	*My husband will go there on Thursday.*
Est-ce qu'il **y** est allé en train ou en avion?	*Did he go there by train or by plane?*

[Allez-y! A]

The Pronoun *en*

1. **En** can replace a combination of a partitive article (**du, de la, de l'**) or indefinite article (**un, une, des**) plus a noun; **en** is then equivalent to English *some* or *any*. Again, whereas these expressions can often be omitted in English, **en** must always be used in French. Like other object pronouns, **en** is placed directly before the verb that refers to it. In the **passé composé,** it is placed directly before the auxiliary verb.

—Est-ce qu'il y a **des musées intéressants** à Avignon?	*Are there interesting museums in Avignon?*
—Oui, il y **en** a.	*Yes, there are (some).*
—Est-ce que vous avez visité **des sites touristiques** à Avignon?	*Did you visit any tourist attractions in Avignon?*
—Oui, nous y **en** avons visité.	*Yes, we visited some (there).*
—Avez-vous acheté **des souvenirs**?	*Did you buy souvenirs?*
—Non, nous n'**en** avons pas acheté.	*No, we didn't buy any.*
—Voici **du vin d'Avignon. En** veux-tu?	*Here's some wine from Avignon. Do you want some?*
—Non merci. Je n'**en** veux pas.	*No, thanks, I don't want any.*

Note: The responses in the first and second examples combine the two pronouns *y* and *en*. The sequence of these two pronouns in *il y en a* in the first example is explained on the next page. The combination of *y* and *en* in the second example is explained in *Chapitre 12, Leçon 2*.

2. **En** can also replace a noun modified by a number or by an expression of quantity such as **beaucoup de, un kilo de, trop de, deux,** and so on. Only **en** (*of it, of them*) and the number or expression of quantity are used in place of the noun.

—Avez-vous **une chambre**?	*Do you have a room?*
—Oui, j'**en** ai **une.***	*Yes, I have one.*
—Vous avez **beaucoup de chambres** disponibles?	*Do you have a lot of rooms available?*
—Oui, j'**en** ai **beaucoup.**	*Yes. I have a lot.*
—**Combien de lits** voudriez-vous?	*How many beds would you like?*
—J'**en** voudrais **deux.**	*I'd like two.*

3. **En** is also used to replace **de** plus a noun and its modifiers (unless the noun refers to people) in sentences with verbs or expressions that use **de: parler de, avoir envie de,** and so on.

—Avez-vous besoin **de ce guide**?	*Do you need this guidebook?*
—Oui, j'**en** ai besoin.	*Yes, I need it.*
—Parliez-vous **des ruines romaines**?	*Were you talking about the Roman ruins?*
—Non, nous n'**en** parlions pas.	*No, we weren't talking about them.*

[Allez-y! B-C]

*In a negative answer to a question containing **un(e)**, the word **un(e)** is not repeated: **Je n'en ai pas.**

Presentation: Model sentences and have sts. repeat sentences with pronoun *en* or *y* and *en* and *y* together where appropriate to reinforce word order.

Y and *en* Together

The combination of **y en** is very common with the expression **il y a.**

—Combien de terrains de camping est-ce qu'il y a?	*How many campgrounds are there?*
—Il **y en** a sept.	*There are seven (of them).*
—Combien de campeurs y avait-il?	*How many campers were there?*
—Il **y en** avait à peu près cent cinquante.	*There were about a hundred fifty (of them).*

[Allez-y! D-E]

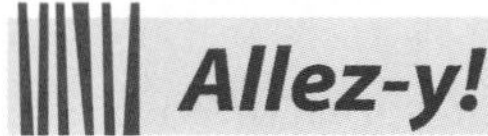

Suggestion (A): Use for oral response, or have a few sts. at board and others at seats write responses for each sentence that you read orally. Assign second part of ex. for homework.

Additional activity (B): *Au café-tabac.* MODÈLE: *revues* (3) → *—Combien de revues voulez-vous?—J'en veux trois.* 1. *cartes postales* (2) 2. *timbres* (6) 3. *films* (2) 4. *tasses de café* (4) 5. *verres de vin* (3) 6. *glaces* (2) 7. *journaux* (1)

Note (B): Make sure sts. are consistent in their answers. *Tu prends un café? Oui, j'en prends un.—Tu prends du café? Oui, j'en prends.*

Suggestion (B): Could be done in groups of 3, with 2 sts. talking and a third taking notes to report back to the class.

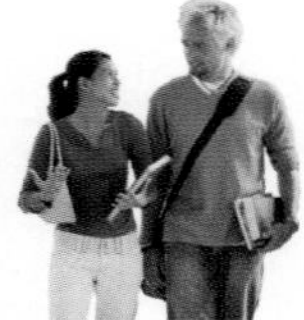

A. Roman policier. Paul Marteau est détective. Il file (*trails*) une suspecte, Pauline Dutour. Doit-il aller partout (*everywhere*) où elle va?

MODÈLE: Pauline Dutour va à Paris. →
Marteau y va aussi. (*ou* Marteau n'y va pas.)

1. La suspecte entre dans un magasin de vêtements.
2. Elle va au cinéma.
3. Elle entre dans une pharmacie.
4. Pauline reste longtemps dans un bistro.
5. La suspecte monte dans un taxi.
6. Elle va chez le coiffeur (*hairdresser*).
7. Elle entre dans un hôtel.
8. La suspecte va au bar de l'hôtel.
9. Finalement, elle va en prison.

Maintenant, racontez les aventures de Marteau au passé composé.

B. Un dîner chez Maxim. Un(e) camarade vous interroge sur votre choix.

MODÈLE: pâté →
É1: Tu as envie de manger du pâté? (Prends-tu du pâté?)
É2: Oui, j'ai envie d'en manger. (Oui, j'en prends.) (*ou* Non, je n'ai pas envie d'en manger. / Non, je n'en prends pas.)

1. hors-d'œuvre	**3.** escargots	**5.** légumes	**7.** dessert
2. soupe	**4.** viande	**6.** vin	**8.** café

C. Mél à ma mère. Lisez le mél et répondez aux questions suivantes. Utilisez le pronom **en** dans vos réponses.

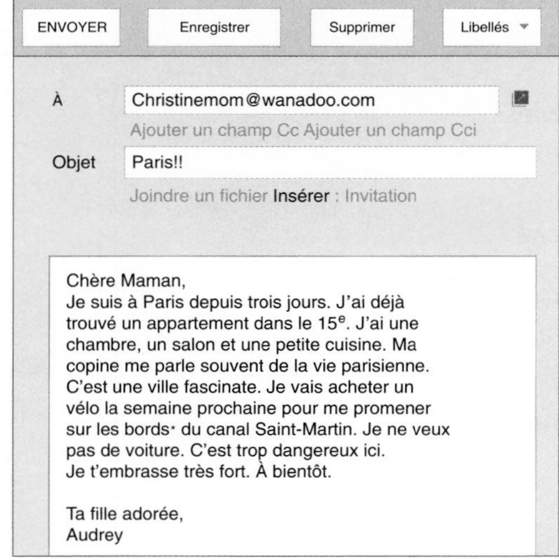
ENVOYER | Enregistrer | Supprimer | Libellés

À: Christinemom@wanadoo.com
Ajouter un champ Cc Ajouter un champ Cci
Objet: Paris!!
Joindre un fichier Insérer : Invitation

Chère Maman,
Je suis à Paris depuis trois jours. J'ai déjà trouvé un appartement dans le 15e. J'ai une chambre, un salon et une petite cuisine. Ma copine me parle souvent de la vie parisienne. C'est une ville fascinate. Je vais acheter un vélo la semaine prochaine pour me promener sur les bords* du canal Saint-Martin. Je ne veux pas de voiture. C'est trop dangereux ici.
Je t'embrasse très fort. À bientôt.

Ta fille adorée,
Audrey

*me... *ride along the banks*

1. Est-ce qu'Audrey a trouvé un appartement?
2. Combien de pièces est-ce qu'il y a?
3. Est-ce qu'Audrey et sa copine parlent souvent de la vie parisienne?
4. Quand va-t-elle acheter un vélo?
5. Pourquoi ne veut-elle pas de voiture?

D. Votre ville. Imaginez qu'un(e) touriste vous pose des questions sur votre ville. Jouez les rôles avec un(e) camarade. Utilisez dans vos réponses le pronom **en** et un nombre ou une expression de quantité. Donnez aussi le plus de détails possible.

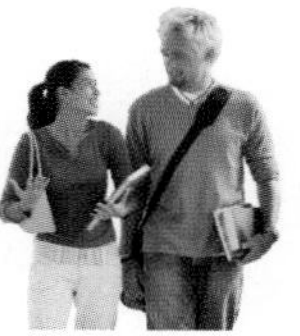

MODÈLE: É1: Il y a des grands magasins dans votre ville?
É2: Oui, il y en a beaucoup—Saks, Macy's, Nordstrom... (Il y en a seulement deux, Macy's et Saks.)

1. Avez-vous une université dans votre ville?
2. Il y a des musées intéressants à visiter?
3. Combien de cinémas et de théâtres avez-vous?
4. Est-ce qu'on peut y faire beaucoup de sport?
5. Combien d'habitants est-ce qu'il y a dans votre ville?
6. On y rencontre beaucoup d'étrangers?

Résumez! Maintenant, votre camarade décrit votre ville à la classe. Il/Elle commence par «Mon/Ma camarade est de ______. Il y a beaucoup de grands magasins à ______... » Est-ce que tout le monde est d'accord avec cette description? Comparez les descriptions d'une même ville. Qui a donné le plus de détails? Qui a été le plus précis / la plus précise?

Mots clés

Demander à quelqu'un son opinion

Que pensez-vous / penses-tu de...*
What do you think of...

Qu'en pensez-vous / penses-tu?
What do you think about that?

À votre/ton avis,...
In your opinion,...

Donnez son opinion

Je pense que...
I think that...

***Penser de** is normally used to ask a person's opinion about something or someone; **penser à** means to think about (to have on one's mind) something or someone.

Suggestion (*Mots clés*): Also teach *Qu'est-ce que vous pensez / tu penses de... ? Qu'est-ce que vous en pensez / tu en penses?*

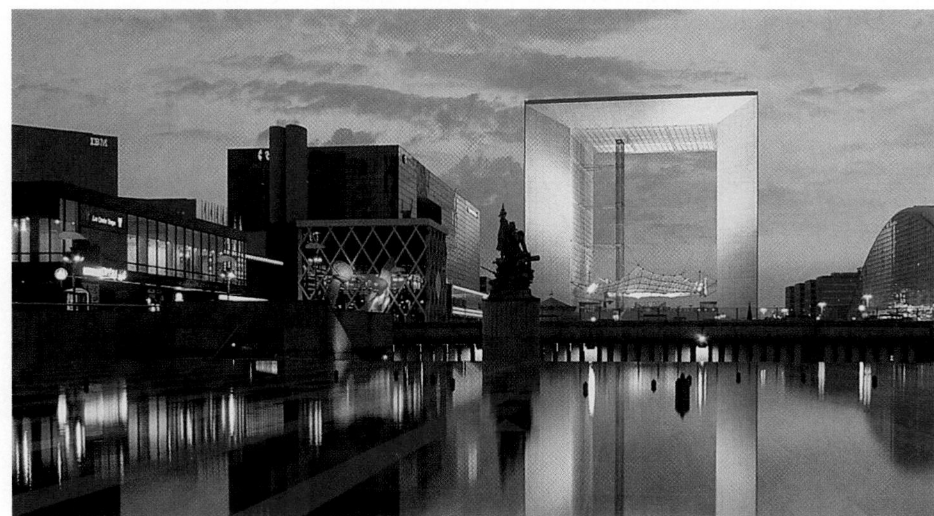

La Grande Arche à la Défense, le centre d'affaires de Paris. Est-ce qu'il y a une arche comme celle-ci (*this one*) dans votre ville?

E. Échange d'opinions. Avec un(e) camarade, donnez des opinions sur des sujets divers. Utilisez les **Mots clés.**

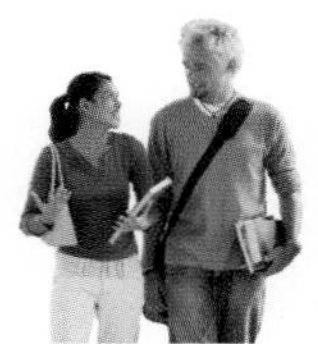

Suggestion (E): Have sts. give an oral *résumé* of some of their partners' opinions.

Continuation (E): *la mode française, les films français, la classe de français,* etc.

Suggestions: les chauffeurs de taxi, les grandes villes américaines, les monuments, les musées, les touristes, les transports en commun...

MODÈLE: É1: Que penses-tu des voitures japonaises?
É2: Elles sont jolies (trop petites, pratiques)... Et toi, qu'en penses-tu?
É1: Je (ne) les aime (pas). Elles (ne) sont (pas)...

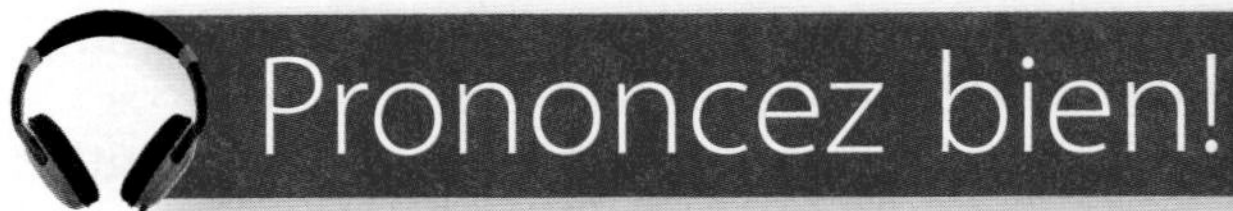

Prononcez bien!

Script (A): 1. Isabelle: *Moi, je vais prendre le saumon au vin blanc, avec un verre de Sancerre. J'adore le poisson!* 2. Louis: *J'ai envie de charcuterie! Pour moi, du saucisson et du pâté de campagne, s'il vous plaît. Et comme boisson, une coupe de champagne!* 3. Hugo: *Et moi, je vais prendre le bœuf bourguignon avec une demi-bouteille de vin rouge et beaucoup de pain pour la sauce!*

Answers (A): 1. a. *saumon* b. *poisson* 2. a. *envie* b. *campagne* c. *champagne* 3. a. *vin* b. *pain*

Nasal vowels (page 291)

A. Un anniversaire au restaurant. Pour fêter l'anniversaire d'Isabelle, vous allez au restaurant avec elle, ses amis et votre camarade de classe. Vous venez de réviser les voyelles nasales en cours de français, alors vous faites attention à leur prononciation pendant que vos amis passent leur commande (*place their order*).

1. Écoutez Isabelle et écrivez les mots contenant la voyelle [ɔ̃] comme dans **bon.**

   a. ________ **b.** ________

2. Écoutez Louis et écrivez les mots contenant la voyelle [ɑ̃] comme dans **plan**.

   a. ________ **b.** ________ **c.** ________

3. Écoutez Hugo et écrivez les mots contenant la voyelle [ɛ̃] comme dans **chemin**.

   a. ________ **b.** ________

B. Un anniversaire au restaurant (suite). Maintenant, votre camarade et vous passez votre commande. Choisissez au moins trois choses sur le menu ci-dessous.

VOUS: Moi, je vais prendre…
VOTRE CAMARADE: Et pour moi…

Aujourd'hui, le chef vous propose…

Entrées

Pâté de campagne • Assiette de jambon • Champignons à la grecque • Saucisson

Plats principaux

Gratin de pommes de terre • Bœuf bourguignon[1] • Saumon au vin blanc • Canard à l'orange

Desserts

Macarons aux amandes • Meringue à la framboise • Far breton[2] • Tarte tatin[3]

Boissons

• Saint-Émilion (vin rouge) • Sancerre (vin blanc) • Champagne
Jus d'orange • Bouteille d'Évian

[1]Bœuf… Beef stew with red wine sauce [2]Far… traditional cake from Brittany
[3]Tarte… Upside down apple tart

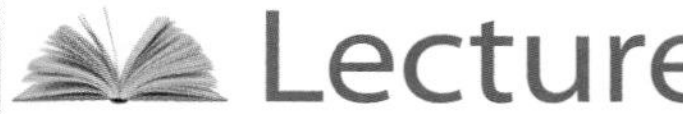

Lecture

Avant de lire

Reading poetry (Part 1). Up until this chapter, you have been reading narrative texts. Depending on the text type, you have used a variety of strategies to facilitate comprehension: anticipating context by the use of titles and visuals, guessing from context, scanning for the gist, and so on.

Reading poetry, on the other hand, requires different skills. To identify these skills, it will be helpful for you to first clarify your expectations in reading poetry. Which of the following statements are true for you?

Poetry ______.

- □ is hard to read and understand
- □ uses abstract and figurative language
- □ must rhyme
- □ is written for the ear as well as for the eye
- □ should be read for the literal meaning
- □ creates a mood
- □ tells a story

Based on your answers, which of the following strategies would be most useful to read poetry effectively and pleasurably?

- □ Poetry should be read aloud.
- □ Be alert to both the literal and figurative meaning of a word.
- □ Skip unimportant details and concentrate on the main idea.
- □ Both the meaning of words and the shape of the text contribute to understanding.
- □ Because poetry is difficult to read, it helps to paraphrase the text.

À propos de la lecture...
«Le chat abandonné» est un poème inédit de Paul Degray, poète et instituteur français contemporain.

«Le chat abandonné»

Je suis le chat de ton quartier
On me dit abandonné.
Ne cherche pas à m'attraper
Car mes griffes sont acérées.[1]

Je me promène sur les toits
Qu'il fasse nuit, qu'il fasse froid.[2]
Je n'ai pas peur de tomber
Car la Lune sait me guider.

Pour manger au restaurant
Je n'ai pas besoin d'argent
Je me sers dans les poubelles[3]
Et ne fais jamais d'vaisselle.

Je suis le chat de ton quartier
On me dit abandonné
Ça ne me fait pas pleurer
Car mon nom est Liberté.

[1]Car... *For my claws are sharp* [2]Qu'il... *Whether it's night, whether it's cold* [3]*garbage cans*

Poème inédit de Paul Degray in Christian Lamblin, *Poésies et Jeux de langage CP/CE1, Éd.* Retz, 2003

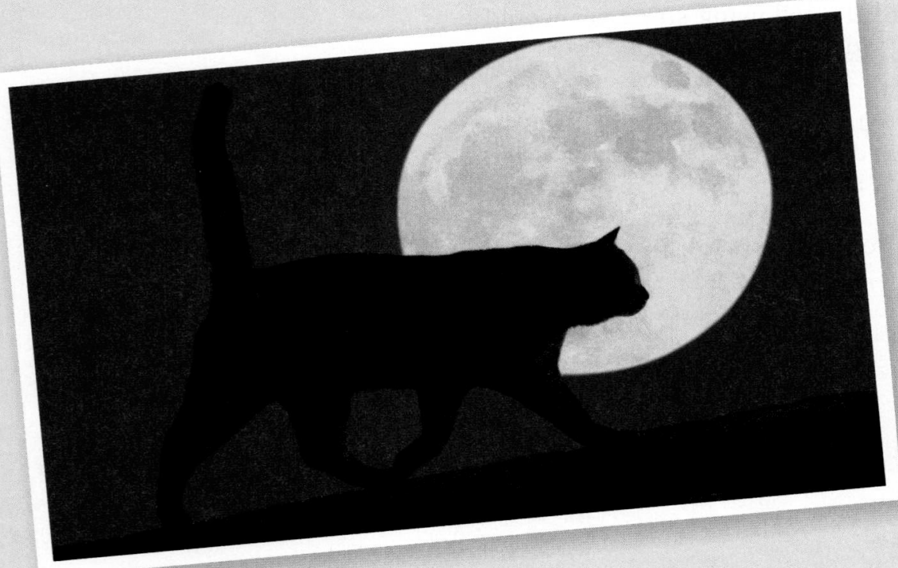

«Mon nom est Liberté»

Compréhension

Complétez les phrases suivantes selon votre compréhension du poème. Justifiez vos réponses.

1. Le chat du quartier est ______.
   a. abandonné
   b. content de sa vie
   c. triste
   d. attrapé
2. La nuit, le chat a ______.
   a. froid
   b. des difficultés à voir les toits
   c. la Lune pour le guider
   d. peur de se promener
3. Pour manger, le chat cherche ______.
   a. un endroit protégé de la pluie
   b. un refuge dans une maison du quartier
   c. un repas dans une poubelle
   d. un restaurant ouvert
4. Le chat du quartier se sent ______.
   a. abandonné
   b. libre
   c. sans amis
   d. énergique

Follow-up: 1. *Quelle est l'image du chat la plus frappante pour vous? Expliquez.* 2. *Que ressentez-vous en lisant le poème?* 3. *Imaginez ce qui est arrivé à ce chat.*

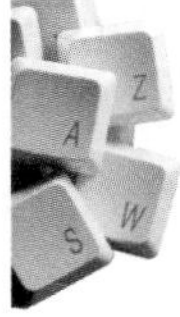

Écriture

The writing activities **Par écrit** and **Journal intime** can be found in the Workbook/Laboratory Manual to accompany *Vis-à-vis*.

Pour s'amuser

Conduire dans Paris c'est une question de vocabulaire.

—Michel Audiard

La vie en chantant. An activity based on the song "Paris" by Camille Dalmais can be found in the *Instructor's Manual.* The song can be purchased at the iTunes store, or sts. can watch the music video on YouTube.

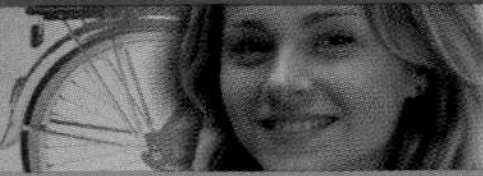

Le vidéoblog de Juliette

En bref

Dans cet épisode, Juliette et Hector font une promenade au jardin du Luxembourg. Les deux amis parlent de leur ville natale et de leur vie actuelle (*present*) à Paris. Dans son vidéoblog, Juliette présente le côté «villageois» de Paris et Hector nous fait visiter son village à la Martinique.

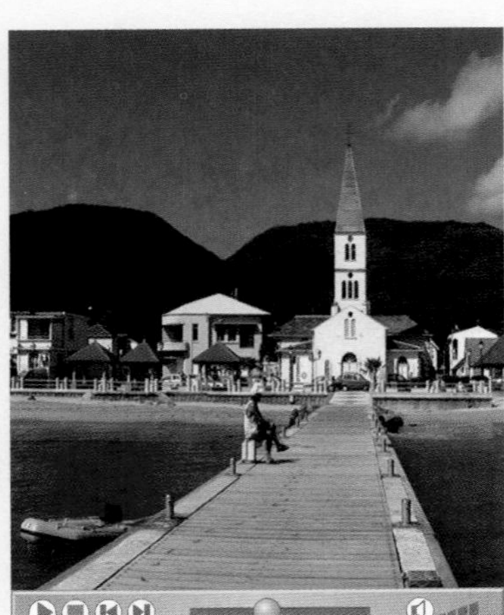

L'église aux Anses d'Arlet, à la Martinique

Additional vocabulary: Other vocabulary you may wish to present before viewing includes *les racines, faire le tour, trésors cachés, les gens sont tellement distants, tout à coup, l'amour fou.*

Vocabulaire en contexte

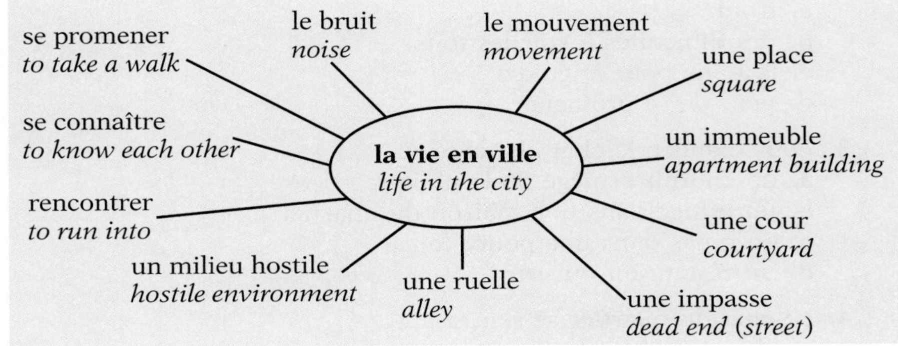

Note culturelle

Le long des côtes de la Martinique, on trouve de nombreux villages de pêcheurs[1] dans de très petites baies appelées «anses». L'Anse Dufour est un village de pêcheurs qui a gardé tout son charme d'origine; les Trois-îlets tiennent[2] leur nom des trois petits îlots rocheux[3] qui émergent au large de[4] la pointe aux Pères; le village des Anses d'Arlet est célèbre pour ses deux plages superbes: la grande Anse et la Petite Anse.

[1]villages… *fishing villages* [2]*take*
[3]îlots… *rocky islands* [4]au… *offshore from*

Visionnez!

Est-ce que les phrases suivantes décrivent Paris ou les Anses d'Arlet à la Martinique?

	Paris	les Anses d'Arlet
1. Il y a toujours du bruit, du mouvement.	☐	☐
2. On rencontre toujours les mêmes gens.	☐	☐
3. On vit (*makes a living*) de la pêche.	☐	☐
4. On est toujours près de la nature.	☐	☐
5. Au cœur (*heart*) de la capitale, il y a de vrai villages.	☐	☐
6. Il y a des villas, des lofts et des ateliers d'artistes.	☐	☐

Analysez!

1. Hector nous dit qu'aux Anses d'Arlet, tout est «à l'échelle (*scale*) humaine». Expliquez pourquoi il a ce sentiment.
2. Quels aspects d'une petite ville trouve-t-on même à Paris?

Comparez!

Décrivez votre ville natale. S'agit-il d'une commune (*town*) rurale ou d'une grande ville? Qu'a-t-elle en commun avec les Anses d'Arlet? Et avec Paris? Regardez encore une fois les parties culturelles de la vidéo: Dans quelle sorte de lieu désirez-vous vivre plus tard (*later*)? Expliquez.

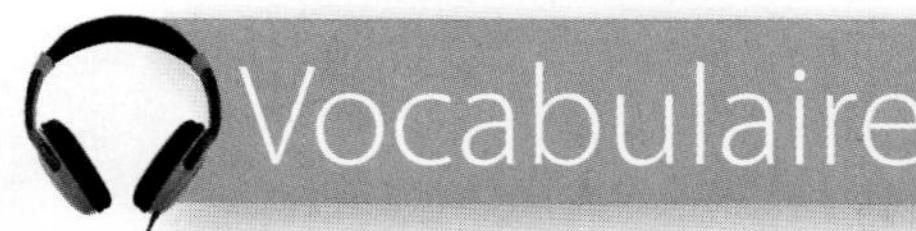

Vocabulaire

Verbes

annuler to cancel
connaître to know, be familiar with
emprunter (à) to borrow (from)
penser à to think of (about)
penser de to think of (about) (to have an opinion about)
poser une question (à) to ask a question
prêter (à) to lend (to)
savoir to know (how, a fact)

À REVOIR: **écrire, envoyer, montrer, prendre, réfléchir (à), rendre visite (à), réussir (à), traverser**

Substantifs

l'arrondissement (*m.*) district, section (*of Paris*)
la banlieue suburbs
le bâtiment building
le bois forest, woods
le boulevard boulevard
le café-tabac bar-tobacconist
le carrefour intersection
la carte map (*of a region, country*)
le centre-ville downtown
le château castle, château
le chemin way (road)
le coin corner
le commissariat police station
l'église (*f.*) church
l'île (*f.*) island
la mairie town hall
le marché en plein air open-air market
la piscine swimming pool
la place square
le plan map (*of a city*)
le poste de police police station
la Rive droite the Right Bank (*in Paris*)
la Rive gauche the Left Bank (*in Paris*)
le syndicat d'initiative tourist information bureau
la tour tower

À REVOIR: **la bibliothèque, le bureau de poste, le jardin, la librairie, la pièce, le quartier, le restaurant, la rue**

Les nombres ordinaux

le premier (la première), le/la deuxième,... , le/la cinquième,... , le/la huitième, le/la neuvième,... , le/la onzième, etc.

Les expressions temporelles

au moment où at the time when
autrefois formerly
d'abord first, first of all, at first
enfin finally
ensuite then, next
pendant que while
puis then, next
soudain suddenly
tout à coup suddenly
une fois once

À REVOIR: **de temps en temps, un week-end**

Mots et expressions divers

À votre (ton) avis,... ? In your opinion, . . . ?
de nouveau (*adv.*) again
en (*pron.*) of them; of it; some; any (*in negatives*)
gratuit (*adj.*) free
jusqu'à up to, as far as
partout (*adv.*) everywhere
plusieurs several
Qu'en penses-tu / pensez-vous? What do you think of that?
Que penses-tu / pensez-vous de... ? What do you think about . . . ?
tellement (*adv.*) so
tout droit (*adv.*) straight ahead
y (*pron.*) there

À REVOIR: **à droite, à gauche**

Mots apparentés

Verbes: **continuer, tourner, traverser**
Substantifs: **la banque, l'hôpital** (*m.*), **l'hôtel** (*m.*), **le monument, le musée, le parc, la pharmacie, la station (de métro)**
Adjectifs: **municipal(e), public / publique**

CHAPITRE 12

La passion pour les arts

Presentation: Ask sts. questions about the photo such as *Connaissez-vous cette sculpture? Où l'avez-vous vue? C'est de quel sculpteur/artiste? Comment s'appelle le bâtiment? Quel personnage célèbre y est enterré?*

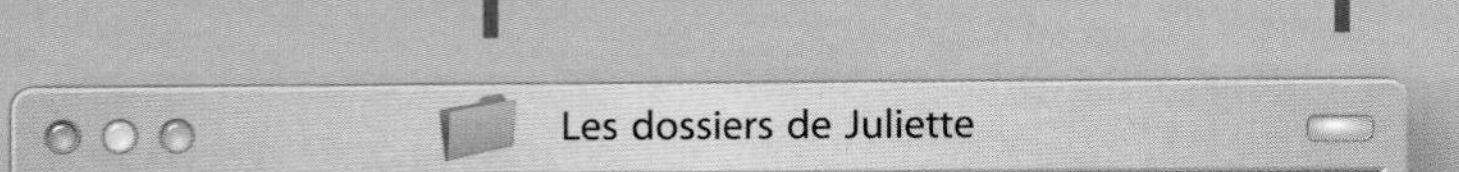

Juliette

- Mes photos
  - *Le Penseur*, de Rodin
  - Grand stabile rouge
  - Au musée d'Orsay

Le Penseur de Rodin, dans le jardin du musée Rodin avec, à l'arrière, le dôme des Invalides

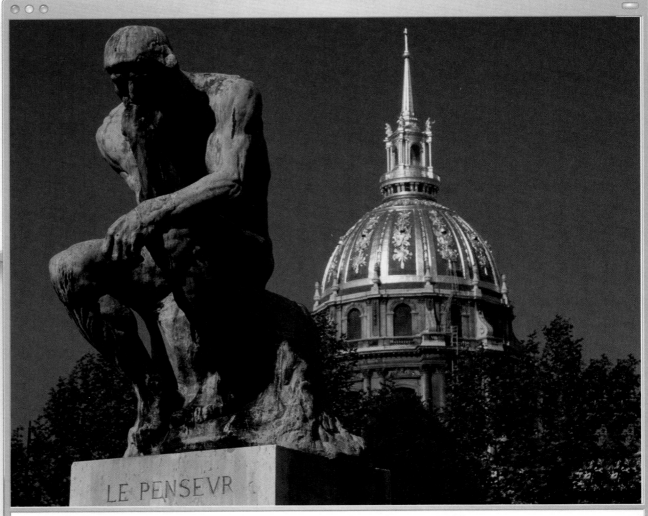

Cultural note: *Les Invalides* and the *musée Rodin* are located in the 7th *arrondissement* of Paris. In addition to housing Napoléon Bonaparte's tomb, the complex also contains a hospital and retirement home for veterans as well as several military museums.

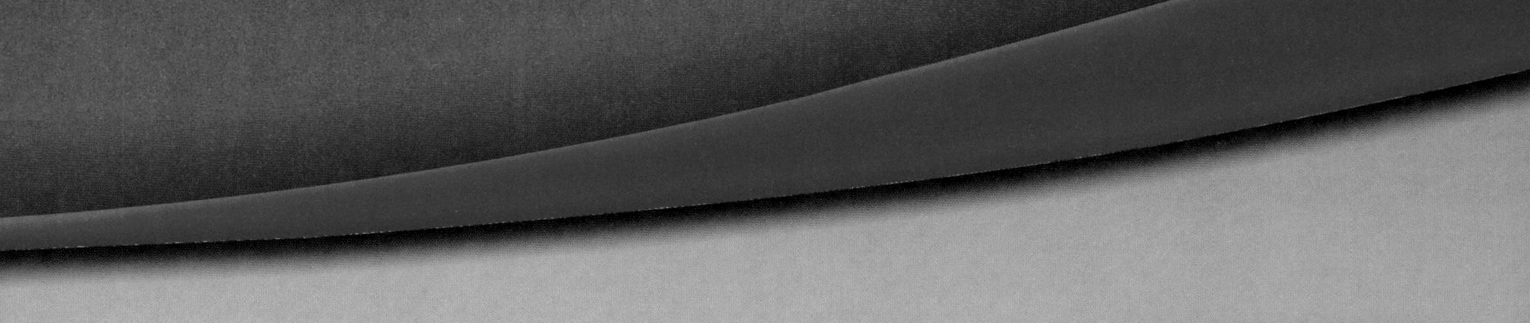

Dans ce chapitre...

OBJECTIFS COMMUNICATIFS

- talking about artistic and historical heritage
- emphasizing and clarifying
- speaking succinctly
- expressing actions
- talking about how things are done
- learning to distinguish between and pronounce selected sounds in French

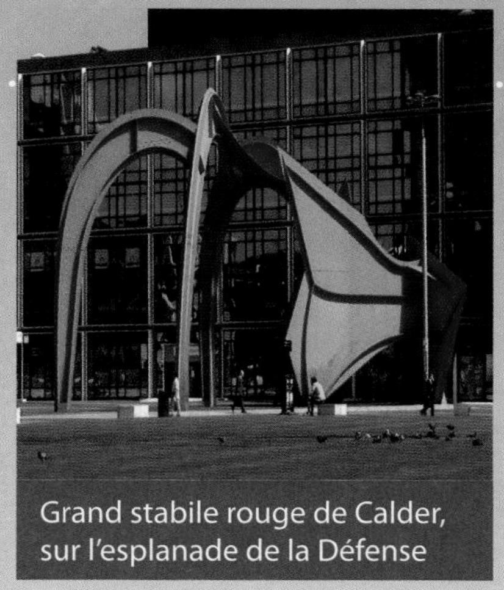

Grand stabile rouge de Calder, sur l'esplanade de la Défense

PAROLES (Leçon 1)

- Le patrimoine historique
- Les œuvres d'art et de littérature
- Les verbes **suivre, vivre** et **habiter**

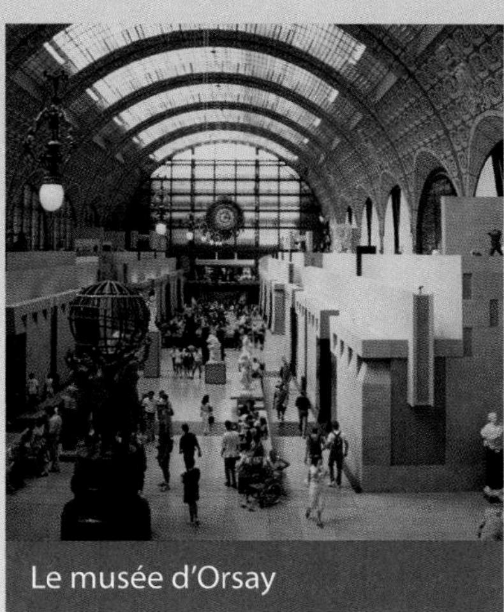

Le musée d'Orsay

STRUCTURES (Leçons 2 et 3)

- Les pronoms accentués
- La place des pronoms personnels
- Les verbes suivis de l'infinitif
- Les adverbes

CULTURE

- Le blog de Juliette: *Pour les amateurs d'art*
- Reportage: *Les musées parisiens*
- Lecture: «Déjeuner du matin» (poème de Jacques Prévert) (Leçon 4)

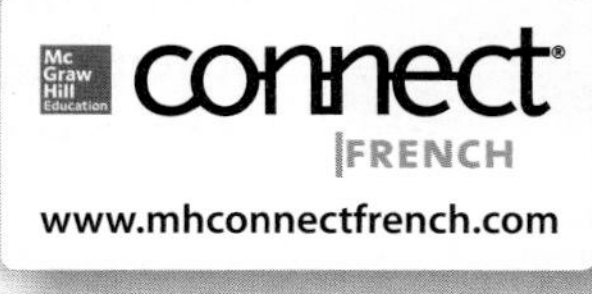

Leçon 1

Suggestion: Throughout the chapter, you will find appropriate occasions to display images from the Internet showing the art and architecture of France.

Le patrimoine historique°

Le... *Historical heritage*

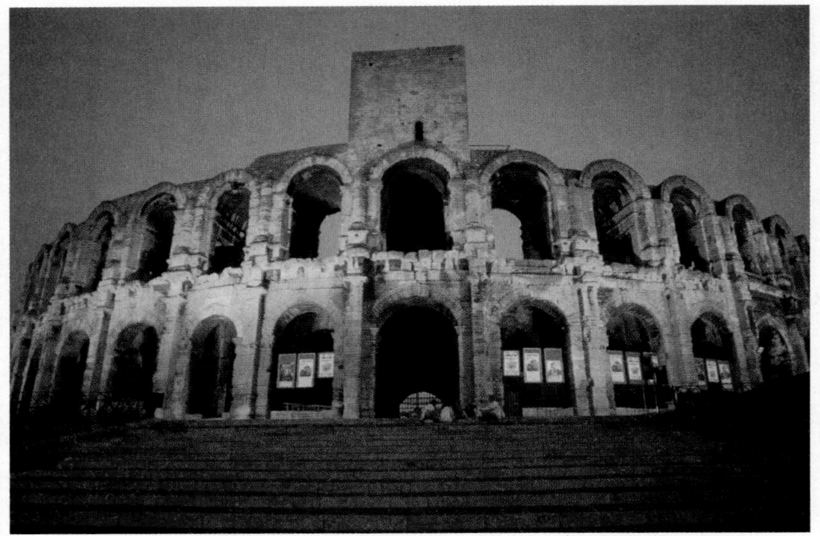
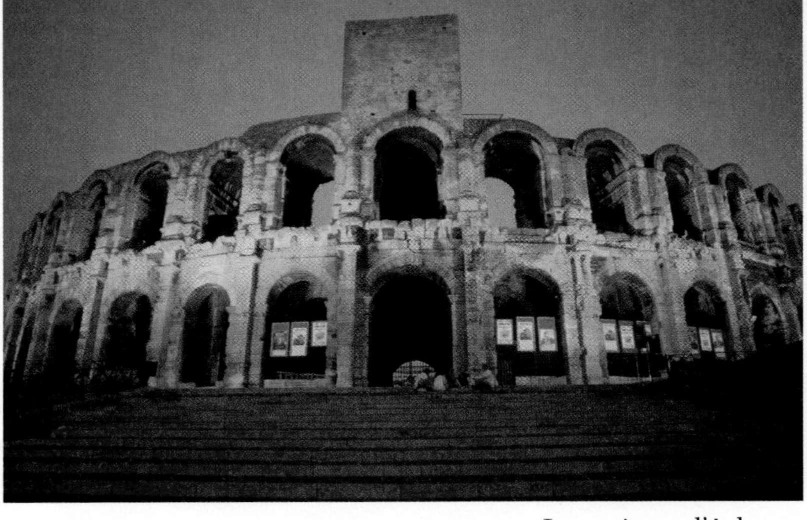

Les arènes d'Arles, monument de l'époque romaine (59 av. J.-C.*–Ve siècle)

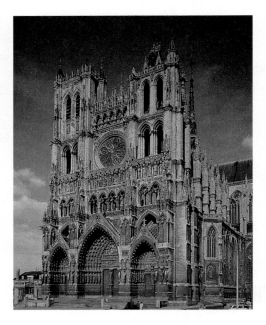

La cathédrale d'Amiens, chef-d'œuvre (*masterpiece*) du Moyen Âge (l'époque médiévale: V^{e}–XVe siècles)

Vocabulary recycling: Review use of ordinal numbers with *siècle*.

Suggestion: On a map, locate Arles, Amiens, Chenonceaux, Versailles.

*avant Jésus-Christ

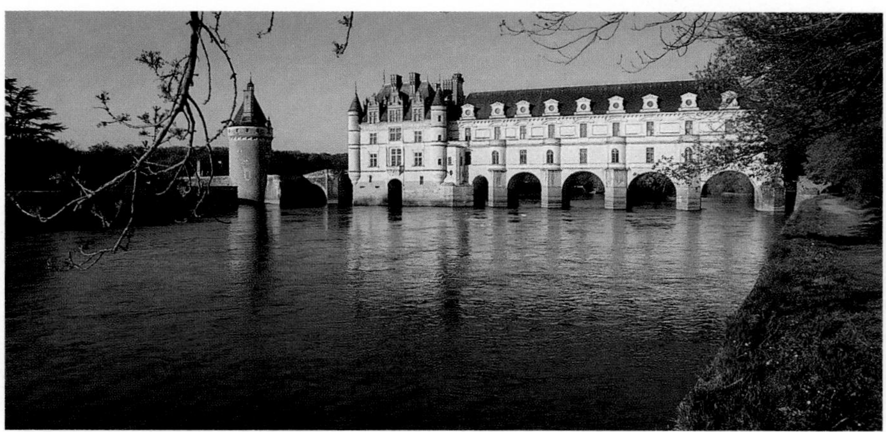

Chenonceaux, château de la Renaissance (XVIe siècle)

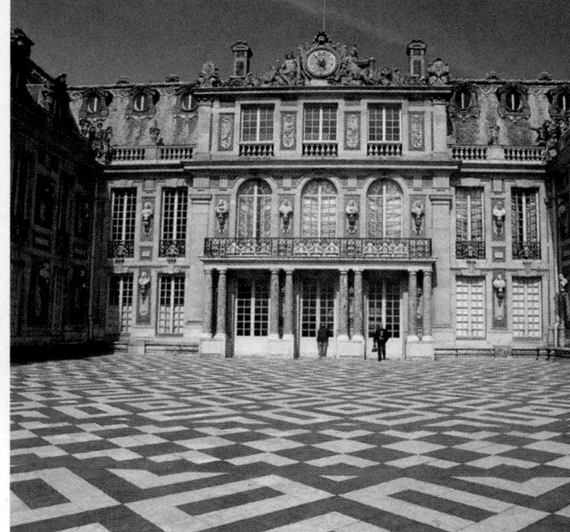

Versailles, château de l'époque classique (XVIIe siècle)

Allez-y!

A. Définitions. Regardez les quatre photos et complétez les phrases.

1. Une période historique, c'est une ______.
2. Une durée de cent ans, c'est un ______.
3. On a bâti (*built*) la cathédrale d'Amiens à l'époque ______.
4. L'époque historique qui se situe entre le Ve et le XVe siècles s'appelle le ______.
5. Le château de Chenonceaux a été bâti au ______.
6. Le château de Versailles date de l'époque ______.
7. Les arènes d'Arles datent de l'époque ______.

B. Leçon d'histoire. Indiquez dans une phrase en quel siècle et à quelle époque chacun des événements suivants s'est passé (*took place*). Remplacez les éléments en italique par des pronoms.

MODÈLE: *Guillaume, duc de Normandie,* a conquis *l'Angleterre* en 1066. → Il l'a conquise au XIe siècle, à l'époque du Moyen Âge.

1. *Blaise Pascal* a inventé *la première machine à calculer* en 1642.
2. On a bâti *les arènes de Nîmes* au premier siècle.
3. *La ville de Paris* s'appelait Lutèce du IIe siècle av. J.-C. jusqu'au IVe siècle après J.-C.
4. *Jacques Cartier* a pris possession *du Canada* au nom de la France en 1534.
5. *Jeanne d'Arc* a essayé de prendre *la ville de Paris* en 1429.
6. *René Descartes* a écrit *sa «Géométrie»* en 1637.
7. *Charlemagne* est devenu roi (*king*) en 768.

Continuation (A): 8. *La Renaissance a commencé au ______ siècle.* 9. *Le ______ a commencé au Ve siècle.* 10. *La cathédrale d'Amiens a été construite au ______.* 11. *La date du début de l'époque romaine, c'est ______.*

Note (A, 5): Mention that this form is the passive voice often used in historical contexts. It can be avoided by using the indefinite pronoun *on* with the *passé composé*. The passive voice is not presented in *Vis-à-vis*.

Suggestion (B): Allow sts. a few minutes to work on answers, either individually or in pairs, before doing the ex. orally.

Additional activity: *L'histoire plus récente. Répondez aux questions suivantes.* MODÈLE: *En quel siècle Thomas Edison a-t-il inventé l'ampoule électrique? → Il l'a inventée au XIXe siècle.* 1. *En quel siècle a-t-on inventé la photographie?* 2. *En quel siècle Neil Armstrong a-t-il marché sur la Lune?* 3. *En quel siècle a-t-on inventé la télévision?* 4. *En quel siècle a-t-on découvert de l'or en Californie?*

Suggestion: Give sts. guidelines for justifying their choice of excursion. Example: *Pour justifier votre choix, dites* (a) *pourquoi vous voulez voir cet endroit;* (b) *ce qui rend cet endroit extraordinaire ou plus intéressant que les deux autres endroits;* (c) *les avantages d'y aller;* (d) *ce que vous espérez apprendre pendant la visite.*

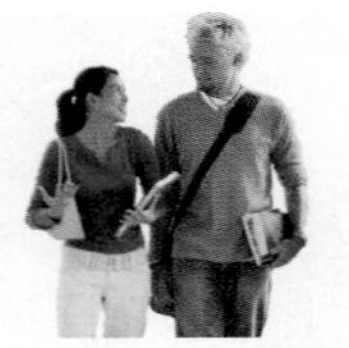

C. À vous! Imaginez que votre classe de français est en visite à Paris. Votre guide vous propose trois sites à visiter. En groupes de trois ou quatre personnes, choisissez un site parmi les suggestions suivantes. Vous devez présenter votre choix à la classe et le justifier. Finalement, on vote pour choisir un seul site pour toute la classe.

Les arènes de Lutèce

Histoire: des arènes romaines de 15 000 places avec une arène séparée pour les combats des gladiateurs

Aujourd'hui: un jardin public très agréable où on peut flâner (*stroll*), pique-niquer ou rêver

À proximité: le Quartier latin

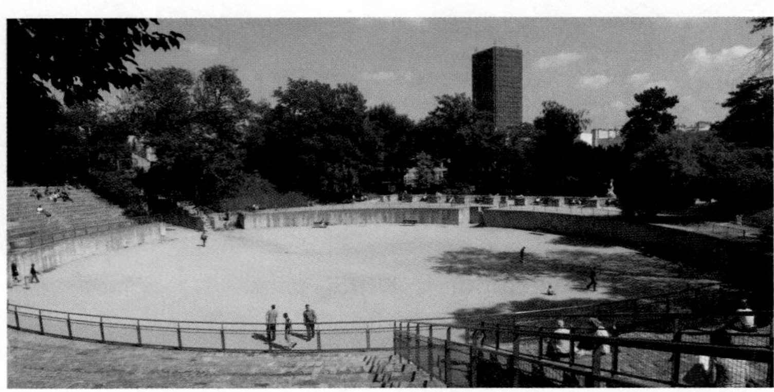

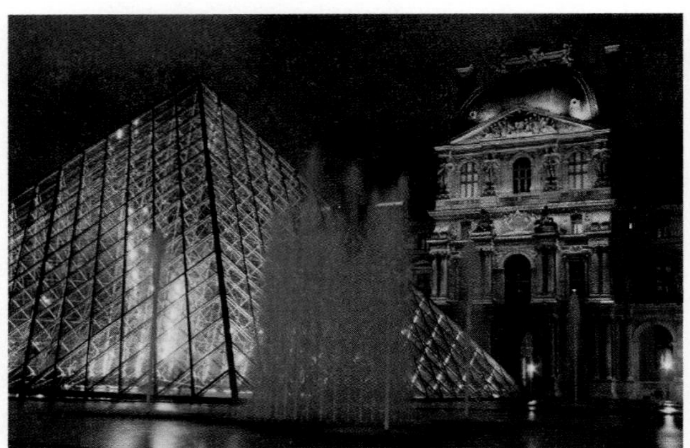

Le palais du Louvre

Histoire: ancienne résidence royale commencée au XIIIe siècle

Aujourd'hui: un magnifique musée d'art

À proximité: le quartier élégant de l'Opéra

Suggestion (C): You may wish to show sts. the *Un coup d'œil sur Paris* video and have them write their own narration for it.

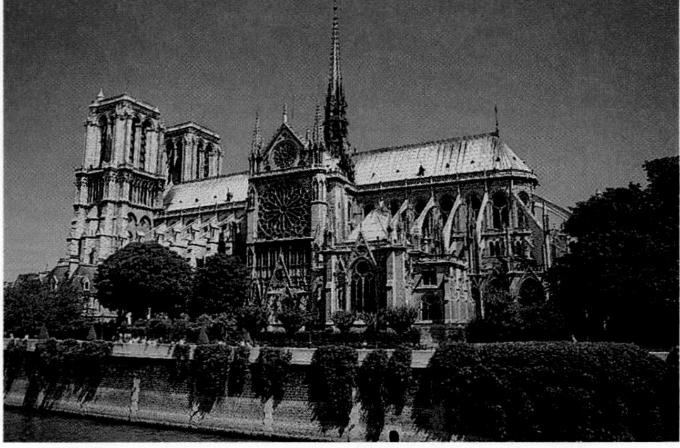

La cathédrale de Notre-Dame

Histoire: Le grand chef-d'œuvre du Moyen Âge. Commencée en 1163 et finie en 1345. Son architecture de style gothique crée une atmosphère de mystère et de beauté.

Aujourd'hui: Toujours une église catholique. On peut monter les 387 marches (*steps*) jusqu'au sommet de sa tour et prendre de splendides photos de Paris.

À proximité: le Quartier latin, l'île Saint-Louis, l'Hôtel de Ville (*City Hall*) de Paris

Les œuvres d'art et de littérature

La littérature

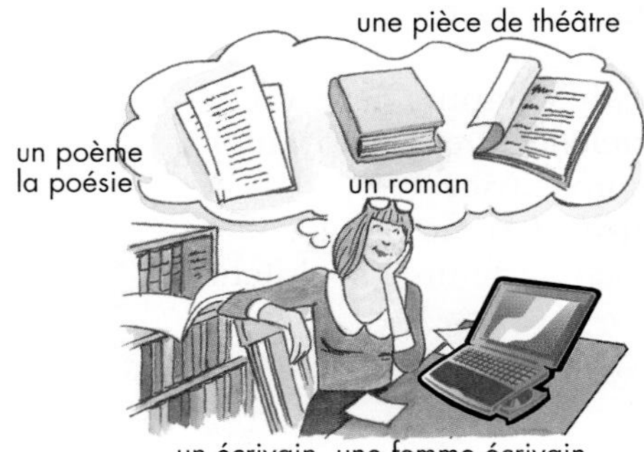

un écrivain, une femme écrivain

La sculpture

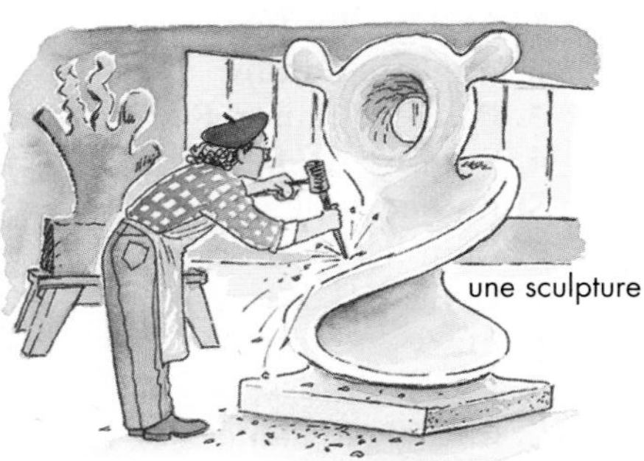

un sculpteur, une femme sculpteur

La peinture

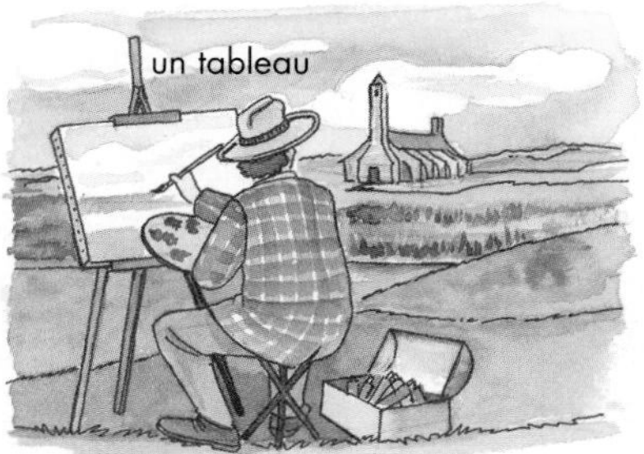

un peintre, une femme peintre

La musique

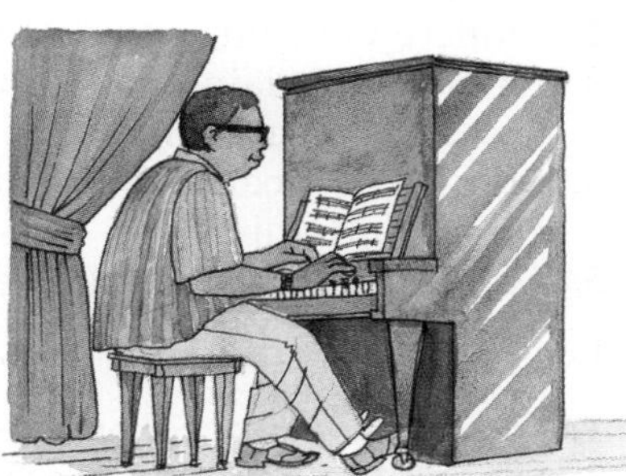

un musicien, une musicienne

Le cinéma

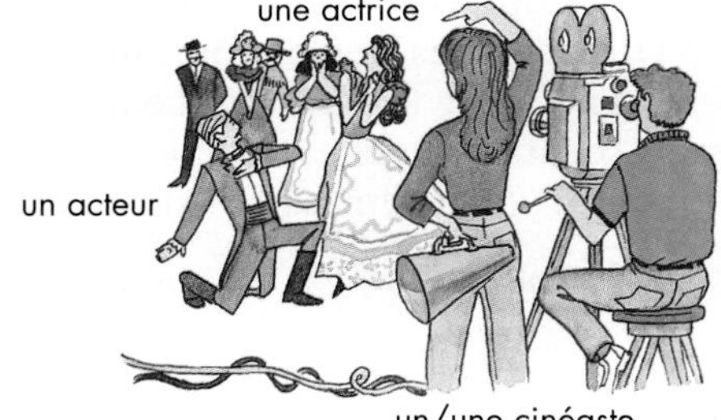

un/une cinéaste

AUTRES MOTS UTILES

un auteur dramatique	playwright
un comédien, une comédienne	stage actor / actress
un compositeur, une compositrice	composer
une œuvre	work, composition
un recueil	collection

Additional vocabulary: *metteur en scène* (director of a stage play), *producteur/productrice* (producer), *réalisateur/réalisatrice* (director of a movie)

Prononcez bien!

The vowel sound in *sculpture*

To pronounce the [y] in **sculpture,** close your mouth and purse your lips. Make sure your tongue is at the front of your mouth, pressed against your lower teeth. If you let it shift to the back of your mouth, you will be pronouncing [u] as in **vous.**

[y]: **sculpture,* littérature, peinture, musique**

*The **p** in **sculpture** is silent. Remember to pronounce the ending as **-ture,** not **-tchure.**

Pronunciation practice (1): Write the words *vous* and *vu* on the board and have sts. decide whether the following words sound like the former or the latter: (1) *bout, bu;* (2) *su, sous;* (3) *lu, loup;* (4) *nous, nu;* (5) *jus, joue.*

Pronunciation practice (2): Have sts. produce the [u] or [y] counterpart of the following words. *MODÈLE: rue → roux. mue* (*mou*); *Q* (*cou*); *fut* (*fou*); *doux* (*du*); *pouls* (*pu*); *nue* (*nous*).

Pronunciation practice (3): The *Prononcez bien!* section on page 344 of this chapter contains additional activities for practicing these sounds.

Additional activity (A): *Trivial Pursuit.* Give names of *expatriés (écrivains ou artistes étrangers qui ont vécu en France)* and ask sts. to name one of their works and country of origin. Examples: Samuel Beckett, Chagall, F. Scott Fitzgerald, Ernest Hemingway, James Joyce, Henry Miller, Picasso, Gertrude Stein, Oscar Wilde. Ask sts. to think of names to stump their classmates.

Follow-up (A): Use as a discussion question: *Pour quelles raisons les artistes vont-ils souvent habiter en France?*

Answer key (A): *Tautou: actrice; Rodin: sculpteur; Renoir: peintre; Beauvoir: femme écrivain; Malle: cinéaste; Claudel: femme sculpteur; Debussy: musicien et compositeur; Cassatt: femme peintre; Matisse: peintre; Deneuve: actrice*

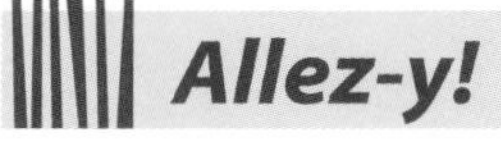

A. Qui sont-ils? Retrouvez la profession de ces artistes. Si vous ne savez pas, devinez ou faites des recherches.

MODÈLE: Jean-Paul Sartre → C'est un écrivain.

1. Audrey Tautou
2. Auguste Rodin
3. Pierre Auguste Renoir
4. Simone de Beauvoir
5. Louis Malle
6. Camille Claudel
7. Claude Debussy
8. Mary Cassatt*
9. Henri Matisse
10. Catherine Deneuve

acteur / actrice
cinéaste
écrivain / femme écrivain
musicien(ne) et compositeur / compositrice
peintre / femme peintre
sculpteur / femme sculpteur

B. Littérature. Complétez les phrases avec la forme correcte des mots suivants: **acteur, écrivain, pièce de théâtre, poème, poésie, roman.**

1. *L'Étranger* est un ______ d'Albert Camus.
2. Molière était un ______ et un ______. Il a écrit des ______.
3. La vie de Verlaine a été turbulente, mais ses ______ font partie des chefs-d'œuvre de la ______ française.
4. Simone de Beauvoir a écrit des ______ et des essais sur la condition féminine.
5. *Les Fleurs du mal* est un recueil de ______ de Charles Baudelaire.

C. Les goûts artistiques. Posez les questions à un(e) camarade.

1. Quel est ton roman préféré? C'est de qui?
2. Qui est ton peintre préféré? Pourquoi?
3. Connais-tu des artistes français? Lesquels (*Which ones*)?
4. Est-ce que tu écoutes de la musique classique? Qui est ton compositeur préféré / ta compositrice préférée?
5. Aimes-tu la poésie? Quels poètes anglais ou américains aimes-tu? Connais-tu un poème par cœur (*by heart*)? Lequel?
6. Vas-tu quelquefois au théâtre? Quelle pièce as-tu vue récemment?
7. Aimes-tu aller au cinéma? Quel film as-tu vu récemment?

Maintenant, décrivez les goûts artistiques de votre camarade à la classe.

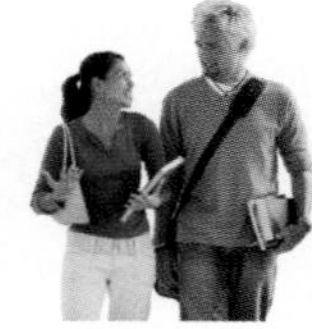

Le parler jeune

un bouquin	un livre
faire un bide	ne pas réussir (pour décrire un spectacle)
faire un carton, cartonner	avoir du succès (pour décrire un spectacle)
un navet	un mauvais film
un tube	une chanson à succès

Lire un **bouquin** sur un écran? Pourquoi pas?

Avec un mauvais scénario, on est sûr de **faire un bide.**

Le prochain film de Tarantino va **cartonner** en Europe.

À ton avis, c'est un bon film ou **un navet**?

Tu l'aimes, le dernier **tube** de Camille?

*Mary Cassatt est née à Pittsburgh, mais elle a vécu (*lived*) à Paris et a participé au mouvement impressionniste.

Les verbes *suivre* et *vivre*

suivre (*to follow*)		vivre (*to live*)	
je **suis**	nous **suivons**	je **vis**	nous **vivons**
tu **suis**	vous **suivez**	tu **vis**	vous **vivez**
il/elle/on **suit**	ils/elles **suivent**	il/elle/on **vit**	ils/elles **vivent**
Past participle: **suivi**		*Past participle:* **vécu**	

Suivre and **vivre** are irregular verbs, and they have similar conjugations in the present tense. **Suivre un cours** means *to take a course.* **Poursuivre** (*to pursue*) is conjugated like **suivre.**

Combien de cours d'art **suis**-tu?	*How many art courses are you taking?*
Suivez mes conseils!	*Follow my advice!*
Monet **a vécu** de nombreuses années à Giverny.	*Monet lived many years in Giverny.*
Est-ce qu'il **a poursuivi** ses études de musique?	*Did he pursue his musical studies?*

Mots clés

Les verbes *vivre* et *habiter*

Use **vivre** to express *to live; to be alive, to exist.* Use it also to express how one lives.

Picasso **a vécu** jusqu'à 92 ans.
Cette artiste ne **vit** pas dans le luxe.
Ils **vivent** toujours dans cette région.

Vivre is also used in certain idiomatic expressions.

Elle est **difficile / facile à vivre.**
She's hard / easy to live with.

Il est parti sans raison apparente, «pour **vivre ma vie**», a-t-il dit.
He left without any apparent reason, to "live my own life," as he put it.

In general, use **habiter** to express *to reside.*

Mary Cassatt **a habité** Paris pendant des années.
Vous **habitez** rue de Rivoli?

Note: Sometimes people say *J'habite à Paris,* using the preposition *à* after *habiter.* It is now more common, however, to exclude the preposition. This also applies to other prepositions with place names.

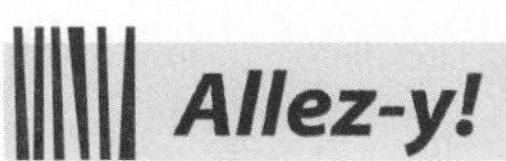

Allez-y!

Suggestion (A): Do as a preliminary activity: *Études ou vacances?* 1. *Qui suit le cours de sociologie? Jean le suit.* (nous, Marie, vous, les Dupont) 2. *Qui ne vit que pour les vacances? Chantal ne vit que pour les vacances.* (je, Marie et François, tu)

A. Van Gogh. Complétez cette biographie en utilisant les verbes suivants: **suivre, poursuivre, vivre, habiter.** Mettez tous les verbes, excepté le numéro 7, au présent.

Vincent Van Gogh est né en 1853 à Groot-Zundert, aux Pays-Bas. En 1877, il ______[1] des cours pour devenir pasteur (*preacher*), mais malheureux, il change d'avis. Il ______[2] des études de dessin anatomique parce qu'il veut devenir artiste. Après des séjours en Belgique et aux Pays-Bas, où il peint *Les Mangeurs de pommes de terre,* il ______[3] à Paris, où il fait la connaissance des peintres impressionnistes comme Monet. C'est Pissarro qui le convainc d'utiliser des couleurs vives (*bright*). À Paris, Van Gogh ne vend aucun* tableau; il ______[4] dans la misère (*poverty*). De 1888 jusqu'à sa mort, Van Gogh ______[5] le sud de la France où il ______[6] sa passion pour la peinture. De plus en plus tourmenté, il se suicide en 1890. Il ______[7] (*passé composé*) seulement jusqu'à l'âge de 37 ans et n'a vendu qu'un seul tableau pendant sa vie.

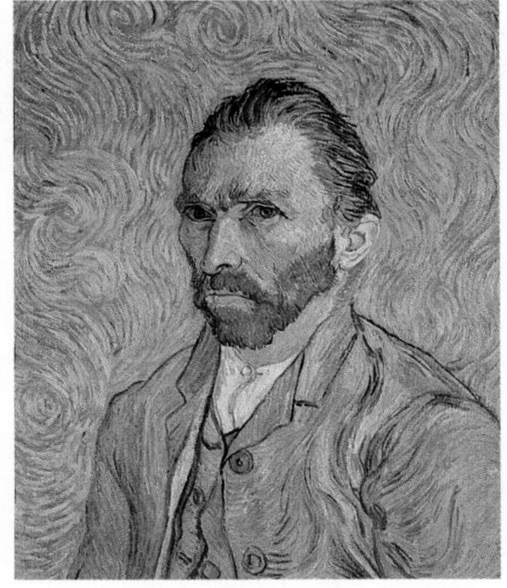

Vincent Van Gogh: *Autoportrait,* 1889–1890 (Musée d'Orsay, Paris)

*__ne... aucun(e)__ is a negative expression meaning *no, not one.*

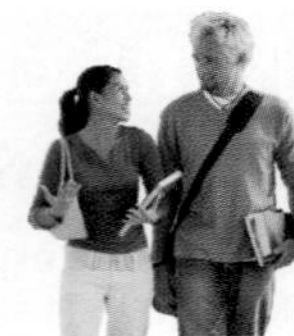

B. Conversation. Avec un(e) camarade, répondez aux questions suivantes.

1. Quelle carrière veux-tu poursuivre? Suis-tu déjà des cours qui mènent à (*lead to*) cette carrière?
2. Est-ce que la plupart (*majority*) des gens basent leur choix de carrière sur ce qui les intéresse? Sinon, comment la choisissent-ils?
3. Comment veux-tu vivre dans dix ans? Dans le luxe en ville, par exemple, ou très simplement à la campagne? Dans quelle sorte de logement veux-tu habiter?
4. À ton avis, est-il plus important de suivre ses passions dans la vie ou de poursuivre la fortune? Pourquoi?

Un peu plus...

Claude Monet. (1840–1926)
Comme ils ne sont pas acceptés dans les galeries traditionnelles, Monet et ses amis peintres décident, en 1874, d'organiser leur propre exposition. La technique de Monet vise (*aims*) à suggérer une expression spontanée de la nature par une application de couleurs vives. C'est la naissance du mouvement impressionniste qui sera (*will be*) reconnu plus tard comme l'un des plus importants mouvements d'art moderne. Vous aimez l'impressionnisme? Expliquez.

► *Claude Monet: Impression, soleil levant, 1873 (Musée Marmottan Monet, Paris)*

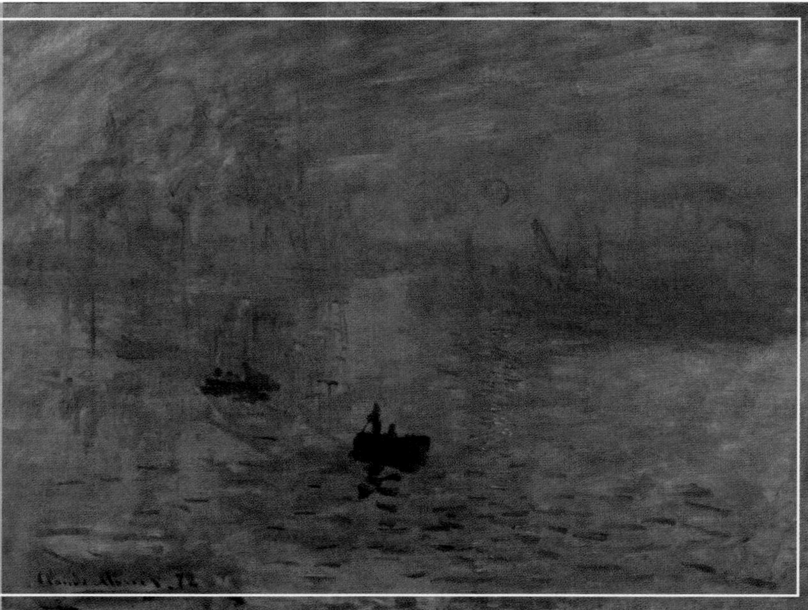

Leçon 2

Presentation: Make sure not to overstress pronouns in minidialogue with your voice. Instead, show how use of form itself creates emphasis in French.

Les pronoms accentués

Emphasizing and Clarifying

Savoir parler d'amour

Hassan, Hector, Juliette et Léa discutent chez Hector.

HASSAN: **Moi**, j'aime la sculpture. Je passe des heures au musée Rodin.
JULIETTE: **Moi**, j'ai une passion pour la peinture, surtout pour Kandinsky. Je le trouve joyeux. Picasso, **lui**, est moins[1] gai.
LÉA: Et **toi**, Hector, qu'est-ce que tu aimes?
HECTOR: **Moi**, j'adore la danse: c'est ma passion, mon métier[2] et ma raison de vivre.[3]
LÉA: **Vous**, vous êtes différents de **moi.** Parce que **moi**, j'aime la poésie et les poètes.
JULIETTE: Pourquoi les poètes?
LÉA: Parce que **eux**, ils savent parler d'amour!

[1]*less* [2]*profession* [3]raison... *reason for living*

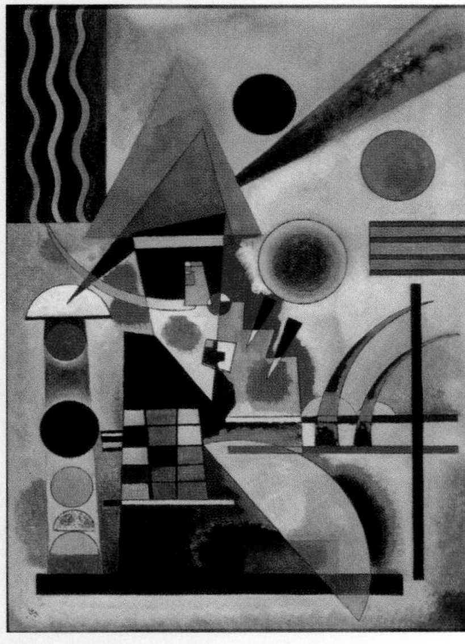

Wassily Kandinsky: *Balançant,* 1925 (Tate Gallery, Londres)

Complétez les phrases suivantes en utilisant **moi, toi, lui, vous** *ou* **eux**.

1. Et ______, vous aimez la sculpture?
2. ______, tu as une passion pour la peinture?
3. Kandinsky est joyeux, Picasso, ______, est moins gai.
4. ______, j'adore la danse.
5. Et ______, tu aimes la poésie et les poètes?
6. Les poètes, ______, ils savent parler d'amour.

Forms of Stressed Pronouns

Stressed pronouns (**les pronoms accentués**) are used as objects of prepositions or for clarity or emphasis. The following chart shows their forms. Note that several are identical in form to subject pronouns.

Suggestion: Point out the forms *moi, toi, lui, soi,* and *eux,* which are different from the subject pronoun forms.

STRESSED PRONOUNS			
moi	*I, me*	**nous**	*we, us*
toi	*you*	**vous**	*you*
lui	*he, him*	**eux**	*they, them* (*m.*)
elle	*she, her*	**elles**	*they, them* (*f.*)
soi*	*oneself*		

***Soi** corresponds to the subjects **on, tout le monde,** and **chacun** (*each one*).

Suggestion: Point out that the stressed pronouns preceded by *c'est à* indicate possession.

Suggestion: Recycle possession: *L'ordinateur? C'est à Luc. C'est à lui. C'est son ordinateur.*

Uses of Stressed Pronouns

Stressed pronouns are used:

1. As objects of prepositions

Nous allons travailler chez **toi** ce soir.	*We're going to work at your house tonight.*
Après **vous**!	*After you!*
Après le concert, tout le monde rentre chez **soi.**	*After the concert, everybody goes back home.*

2. As part of compound subjects

Clara et elle ont lu *À la recherche du temps perdu** en entier.	*She and Clara read the entire* In Search of Lost Time.
Robin et moi avons joué ensemble une sonate de Debussy.	*Robin and I played a Debussy sonata together.*

Note: In many cases, English uses intonation to obtain the same effect of clarity or emphasis.

Presentation: Use pronouns in short sentences to illustrate their use. Have sts. repeat after your model. Examples: *Moi, j'aime le français. Robert, lui, le déteste. Et toi? Que penses-tu du français?* etc.

3. With subject pronouns, to emphasize the subject

Et **lui,** écrit-il un roman?	*What about him? Is he writing a novel?*
Eux, ils ont de la chance.	*As for them, they are lucky.*
Tu es brillant, **toi**!	*You're brilliant!*

When stressed pronouns emphasize the subject, they can be placed at the beginning or the end of the sentence.

[Allez-y! A]

4. After **ce** + **être**

—C'est **vous,** Monsieur Lemaître?	*Is it you, Mr. Lemaître?*
—Oui, c'est **moi.**	*Yes, it's me* (*it is I*).
C'est **lui** qui donnait le cours sur Proust.	*He's the one who was teaching the course on Proust.*

5. In sentences without verbs, such as one-word answers to questions and tag questions

—Qui a visité le musée Delacroix?	*Who has visited the Delacroix Museum?*
—**Toi!**	*You!*
—As-tu pris mon livre d'art?	*Did you take my art book?*
—**Moi?**	*Me?*
Nous allons visionner une vidéo sur la peinture moderne. Et **lui?**	*We're going to see a video on modern painting. What about him?*

*Long novel by Marcel Proust, in seven volumes. The original English translation was titled *Remembrance of Things Past.* A 2003 translation is called *In Search of Lost Time.*

6. In combination with **même(s)** for emphasis

Préparent-ils la vidéo **eux-mêmes**?	*Are they preparing the video themselves?*
Allez-vous choisir les images **vous-même**?	*Are you going to choose the pictures yourself?*

[Allez-y! B-C]

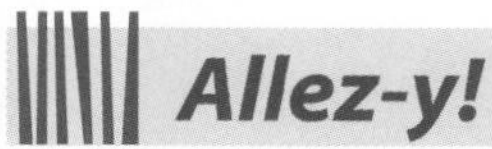

Allez-y!

A. Au théâtre. Vos amis et vous avez présenté une pièce de théâtre devant la classe. Décrivez le comportement des acteurs / actrices avant le commencement de la pièce, à l'aide des pronoms accentués.

MODÈLE: nous / fatigués ⟶ Nous, nous étions fatigués.

1. je / préoccupé(e)
2. Alice / anxieuse
3. Louis / agité
4. Jessica et Anaïs / sérieuses
5. Marc et Angela / calmes
6. nous / heureux

B. Pour monter la pièce. (*To prepare the play.*) D'autres étudiants vous ont aidé(e) à monter la pièce de l'exercice précédent. Dites ce qu'ils ont fait. Remplacez les mots en italique par des pronoms qui correspondent aux mots entre parenthèses. Faites attention à la conjugaison du verbe.

1. Qui a fait les costumes? C'est *moi* qui ai fait les costumes. (Sandrine, Bruno, Pierre et Nassim)
2. Vous avez écrit le scénario vous-mêmes? Oui, *nous* l'avons écrit *nous*-mêmes. (je, une amie et moi, Richard et Florent, les acteurs)

C. Êtes-vous indépendant(e)? Est-ce que vos camarades et vous faites des choses intéressantes, utiles ou inhabituelles? Renseignez-vous sur les activités de quatre camarades. Utilisez les pronoms accentués + **même(s)** et les verbes de la liste suivante.

Verbes utiles: acheter, aller, bâtir* (*to build*), devoir, faire, gagner, jouer, lire, pouvoir, préparer, réparer, travailler, vendre, venir, voir, vouloir

MODÈLES: Moi, je fais toujours le pain moi-même pour les repas à la maison.
J'ai une camarade qui, elle, répare elle-même sa voiture.

Additional activity: *Tempête de neige. Il neigeait hier soir et les étudiants suivants ont dû rester chez eux. Décrivez leurs activités en vous basant sur le modèle.* MODÈLE: *vous → Vous avez fait vos devoirs chez vous. 1. nous 2. je 3. Marie et toi 4. Pierre et Marie 5. tu 6. mon ami Marc 7. les étudiantes en médecine 8. les étudiants de mon cours*

Additional activity: *Quelle aventure! Tout d'un coup il n'y a plus d'électricité à la bibliothèque. On n'y voit plus rien. Chacun essaie de trouver ses camarades dans le noir. En français, s'il vous plaît,* THOMAS: *Nicole, is that you?* N: *Yes, it's me. Where are you?* T: *Me? I'm here, next to Jean-Michel.* VOICE: *I'm not Jean-Michel!* J-M: *I'm near the window. Where's Christophe?* N: *I don't know. Is that him next to the door?* T: *I think that's him. Claude is next to him, isn't he?* J-M: *No, that's not Claude. It's a coatrack (un portemanteau). He was studying with Marlène.* N: *With her? Why is he studying with her?* J-M: *You know why. She always passes the exams.*

*conjugated like **finir**

La place des pronoms personnels

Speaking Succinctly

Pas d'argent entre nous!

Alexis contacte Poema sur sa page Facebook (Messagerie instantanée).

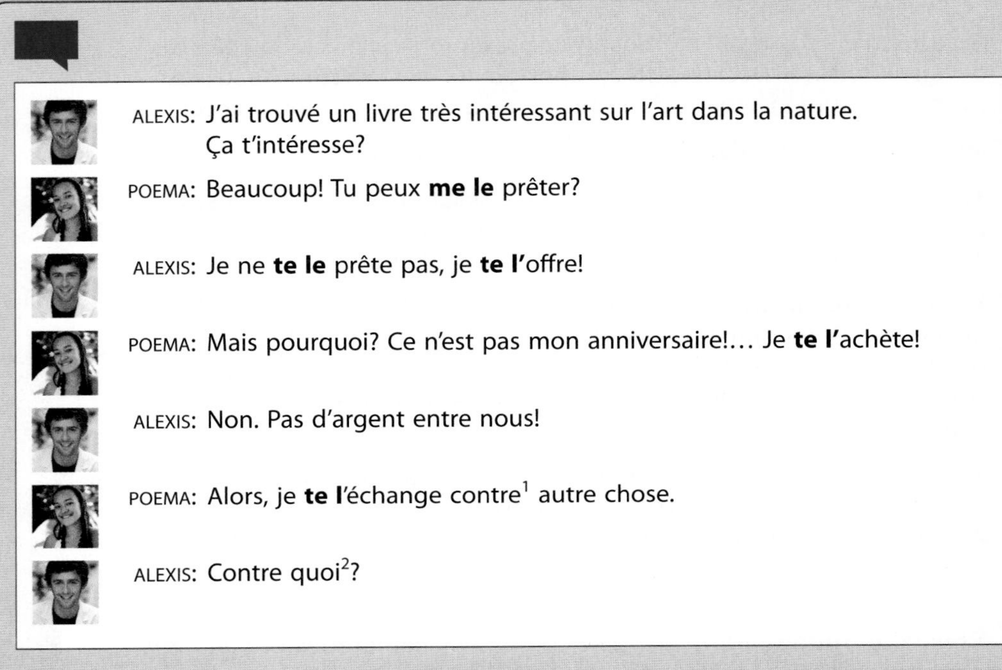

ALEXIS: J'ai trouvé un livre très intéressant sur l'art dans la nature. Ça t'intéresse?
POEMA: Beaucoup! Tu peux **me le** prêter?
ALEXIS: Je ne **te le** prête pas, je **te l'**offre!
POEMA: Mais pourquoi? Ce n'est pas mon anniversaire!... Je **te l'**achète!
ALEXIS: Non. Pas d'argent entre nous!
POEMA: Alors, je **te l'**échange contre[1] autre chose.
ALEXIS: Contre quoi[2]?

[1]échange... *trade for* [2]*what*

Trouvez, dans le dialogue, la phrase équivalente.

1. Tu peux me prêter ton livre?
2. Je ne te prête pas mon livre.
3. Je t'offre mon livre.
4. Je t'achète le livre.
5. Je t'échange le livre.

Order of Object Pronouns in Declarative Statements

When two or more pronouns are used in a declarative sentence, they follow a fixed order. The direct object pronoun is usually **le, la,** or **les. Me, te, nous,** and **vous** precede **le, la,** and **les; lui** and **leur** follow them. The pronouns **y** and **en,** in that order, come last.

DIRECT OR INDIRECT OBJECT	DIRECT OBJECT	INDIRECT OBJECT	**y / en**
me te nous vous	le la les	lui leur	y / en

Note: Orally, when *le, la,* or *les* is combined with *lui* or *leur,* the direct object pronoun might not be heard (*Je vais la lui donner.* → *Je vais lui donner*).

—Le guide vous a expliqué la théorie des peintres impressionnistes?	*Did the guide explain the theory of the Impressionist painters to you?*
—Oui, il **nous l'**a expliquée.	*Yes, he explained it to us.*
—Avez-vous montré le tableau de Manet aux étudiants américains?	*Did you show the Manet painting to the American students?*
—Oui, je **le leur** ai montré.	*Yes, I showed it to them.*
—Est-ce que le guide a donné des livrets sur l'impressionnisme aux autres étudiants?	*Did the guide give booklets on Impressionism to the other students?*
—Oui, il **leur en** a donné.	*Yes, he gave them some.*

It might help you to remember this formula: First and second person before third; direct object before indirect object. Apply the first part if it is relevant, then the second.

1. When the pronouns are objects of an infinitive, they are placed immediately before the infinitive. The same order rules apply.

—Quand est-ce que tu vas donner le cadeau à Line?	*When are you going to give Line the gift?*
—Je vais **le lui** donner à Noël.	*I am going to give it to her at Christmas.*

2. In negative sentences with object pronouns, **ne** precedes the pronouns; when the negative sentence is in the **passé composé, pas** follows the conjugated verb (the auxiliary) and precedes the past participle.

—Ils nous ont envoyé les horaires des autres musées de Paris?	*Did they send us the schedules of the other museums in Paris?*
—Non, ils **ne nous les** ont **pas** envoyés.	*No, they didn't send them to us.*

[Allez-y! A-B]

Commands with One or More Object Pronouns

1. The order of object pronouns in a negative command is the same as the order in declarative sentences: the pronouns precede the verb.

N'**en** parlons pas!	*Let's not talk about it!*
N'**y** pense pas!	*Don't think about it!*
Ne **me** donnez pas le tableau!	*Don't give me the painting!*
Ne **me le** donnez pas!	*Don't give it to me!*
Ne **leur** dites pas que vous êtes venus!	*Don't tell them you came!*
Ne **le leur** dites pas!	*Don't tell them!*

Note: To review the formation of the imperative, see *Chapitre 6, Leçon 3.*

2. In affirmative commands with one object pronoun, the pronoun follows the verb and is attached with a hyphen. When **me** and **te** come at the end of the expression, they become **moi** and **toi.**

La lettre? **Écrivez-la!**	*The letter? Write it!*
Voici du papier. **Prenez-en!**	*Here's some paper. Take some!*
Tes amis? **Donne-leur** des billets!	*Your friends? Give them some tickets!*
Parle-moi des concerts!	*Tell me about the concerts!*

As you know, the final **-s** is dropped from the **tu** form of regular **-er** verbs and of **aller** to form the **tu** imperative: **Parle de tes problèmes! Va à la maison!** However, the **-s** is *not* dropped before **y** or **en** in the affirmative imperative: **Parles-*en*! Vas-*y*!**

3. When there is more than one pronoun in an affirmative command, however, all direct object pronouns precede indirect object pronouns, followed by **y** and **en,** in that order. All pronouns follow the command form of the verb and are attached by hyphens. The forms **moi** and **toi** are used except before **y** and **en,** where **m'** and **t'** are used.

DIRECT OBJECT	INDIRECT OBJECT			**y / en**
le	moi	(m')	nous	
la	toi	(t')	vous	y / en
les	lui		leur	

—Voulez-vous ma carte d'entrée au musée? —Oui, **donnez-la-moi.**	*Do you want my museum entrance card?* *Yes, give it to me.*
—Je t'apporte du papier? —Oui, **apporte-m'en.**	*Shall I bring you some paper?* *Yes, bring me some.*
—Tu veux que je cherche l'horaire du musée? —Oui, **cherche-le-moi.**	*Do you want me to look for the museum schedule?* *Yes, look for it for me.*
—Est-ce que je dis aux autres que l'entrée est gratuite? —Oui, **dites-le-leur.**	*Shall I tell the others that admission is free?* *Yes, tell them that* (lit., *tell it to them*).

[Allez-y! C-D-E]

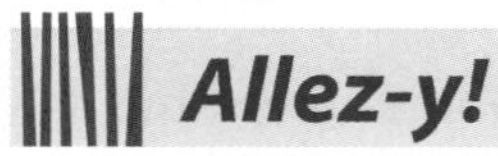

Allez-y!

A. **Travail d'équipe.** Audrey et ses camarades préparent un exposé sur la Fondation Maeght, un musée d'art moderne au sud de la France. Transformez les phrases selon le modèle.

MODÈLE: Audrey donne <u>ses notes</u> <u>à Anaïs.</u> →
Elle les lui donne.

1. Elle prête le livre sur Chagall à Sylvie.
2. Anaïs envoie des photos de la cour Giacometti à Audrey.
3. La prof explique les sculptures de Miró aux trois filles.
4. Sylvie parle à sa prof de l'exposition sur Braque.
5. Audrey et ses camarades présentent leur exposé aux autres étudiants du cours.

B. Détails pratiques. Vous faites une visite artistique de Paris. Répondez par *oui* ou *non* et utilisez des pronoms.

MODÈLE: Achetez-vous vos guides (*guidebooks*) à la librairie?
Oui, je les y achète. (Non, je ne les y achète pas.)

1. Prenez-vous vos repas dans les musées?
2. Achetez-vous vos cartes postales au musée?
3. Emmenez-vous vos amis au musée?
4. Il y a des sculptures au musée du Louvre?
5. Avez-vous rencontré vos amis au ciné-club?
6. Apportez-vous votre appareil photo au musée?
7. Est-ce qu'il y avait beaucoup de visiteurs à l'exposition du Grand-Palais?

C. Pour devenir un écrivain célèbre. Dans les phrases suivantes, remplacez les mots en italique par des pronoms.

MODÈLES: Lisez *beaucoup de romans.* →
Lisez-en beaucoup!

Montrez *vos œuvres à vos amis.* →
Montrez-les-leur!

1. N'oubliez jamais *vos cahiers à la maison.*
2. Prenez *des notes.*
3. Révisez *votre travail.*
4. Envoyez *votre roman à l'éditeur.*
5. Invitez *votre éditeur* à dîner.
6. Après la publication du roman, demandez *à vos amis* d'acheter un exemplaire (*copy*).

D. Situations. Vous entendez des fragments de conversation. Imaginez la situation.

MODÉLE: N'y touche pas! →
La mère de Tristan vient de faire un gâteau, et Tristan essaie d'en manger un morceau.

1. Vas-y! **2.** N'y touche pas! **3.** Ne m'en donne pas! **4.** Ne les regardez pas! **5.** Donne-la-lui! **6.** Ne lui parle pas si fort! **7.** Montre-les-moi! **8.** Ne le lui dis pas!

E. Interview. Interrogez un(e) camarade sur une ville ou une région que vous pensez visiter. Suivez le modèle.
Mots utiles: une cathédrale, le cinéma, un musée, la musique, une pièce de théâtre, la sculpture, les tableaux; des acteurs / actrices célèbres, des compositeurs / compositrices, des cinéastes, des écrivains

MODÈLE: É1: Est-ce qu'il y a une belle cathédrale à Strasbourg?
É2: Oui, il y en a une.

Additional activity (C): Dictate the following sentences as board work, underline the appropriate words, and then have sts. transform the sentences using pronouns. *Pour devenir un étudiant modèle: Dans les phrases suivantes, remplacez les mots soulignés par un pronom.* 1. *Ne parlez pas dans la bibliothèque.* 2. Ne posez pas de questions inutiles. 3. *N'oubliez pas vos notes.* 4. Écrivez *les mots français au tableau.* 5. *À la fin de l'année, invitez votre professeur à dîner.*

Mots clés

Les verbes *apporter* et *emmener*

Apporter (*to bring something*) is used only with objects.

Il apporte ses tableaux à la galerie d'art.

Emmener (*to take someone along; to invite*) is used with people or animals.

Je t'emmène au cinéma?

Note (*Mots clés*): This group of verbs can be very confusing:

1. *apporter* (to bring s.th. with the idea, stated or implied, of where you are coming from): *Le facteur apporte le courrier (du bureau de poste).*
2. *emporter* (to take s.th. with the idea, stated or implied, of where you are going): *Il est parti (pour Paris) et n'a rien emporté.*
3. *amener* (to bring s.o., you leave the person when you arrive at the destination): *Elle amène sa fille à l'école.*
4. *emmener* (to take s.o. or an animal with you, to invite): *J'emporte peu de bagages, mais j'emmène mon chien; Je l'emmène au restaurant.*

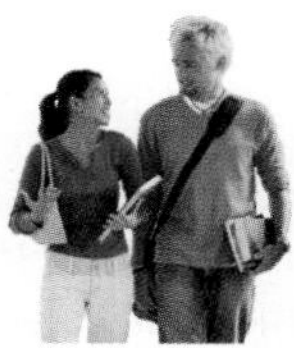

Suggestion (E): Have sts. prepare this activity at home. Assign one French town or city to each st.; sts. look up basic information about famous places to visit or people from that city. In class, sts. can work either in pairs or in groups; each st. is the "expert" on one place, and others ask him/her questions.

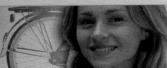

Le blog de Juliette

Pour les amateurs d'art

samedi 2 août

J'aime l'art.

J'ai commencé à aimer la peinture vers[1] l'âge de 12 ans, quand ma mère m'a emmenée voir une exposition du peintre Kandinsky, le peintre des compositions abstraites et des jeux de couleurs.

Ensuite, j'ai appris à peindre. Je rêvais de créer une œuvre, je voulais être le Mozart de la peinture! Mais rapidement, j'ai accepté de reconnaître une vérité absolue: je n'ai aucun talent[2]...

Alors, je me contente[3] d'admirer les œuvres des autres, de voir des expositions et d'explorer des musées. La semaine dernière, par exemple, j'ai visité les musées en plein air[4] de Paris: les œuvres sont exposées dans des lieux publics, sous le vent, la pluie[5] et le soleil! C'est une expérience unique!

Malheureusement, je ne serai jamais[6] une artiste... Je dois l'accepter. Mais j'ai décidé de promouvoir[7] les chefs-d'œuvre des jeunes artistes...

Je vais donc créer une galerie d'art virtuelle sur le net pour encourager les jeunes peintres et sculpteurs à montrer leurs œuvres.

Mes amis du blog sont les premiers informés!

Juliette

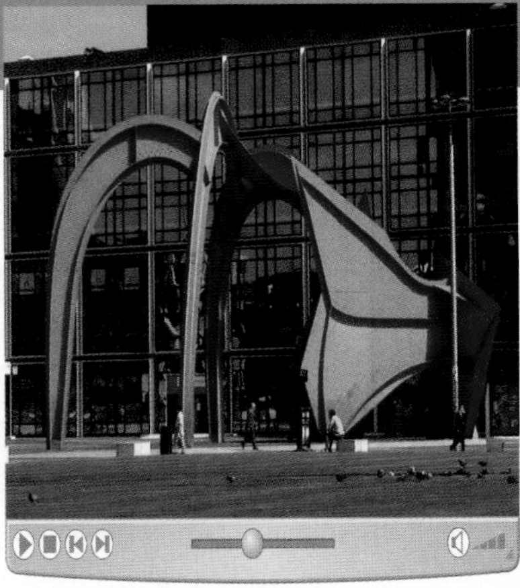

Grand stabile rouge de Calder sur l'esplanade à la Défense

Cultural connection: Alexander Calder (1898–1976) was an American sculptor known for inventing the mobile. He also created stabile sculpture seen in many outdoor venues, in countries around the world.

Follow-up: 1. *À quelle période de sa vie Juliette a-t-elle commencé à aimer la peinture? À quelle occasion?* 2. *Pour quelle raison Juliette a-t-elle renoncé à la peinture? De quelle manière satisfait-elle son amour de l'art?* 3. *Quelle grande nouvelle annonce Juliette dans son blog? Que pensez-vous de son projet?* 4. *Que proposent Alexis, Mamadou et Poema? Que suggère Charlotte? Vous aussi, donnez des conseils à Juliette.* 5. *Quelle forme d'art aimez-vous particulièrement? Qui sont vos artistes préférés? Expliquez pourquoi.*

Video connection: In the videoblog for this chapter, Juliette and Léa take a tour of two outdoor art exhibitions in Paris instead of visiting the musée d'Orsay.

COMMENTAIRES

Alexis

Franchement Juliette, c'est une bonne idée. Mais des galeries virtuelles, il y en a déjà beaucoup sur le Web. Pourtant, si tu veux faire la promotion des jeunes peintres québécois, je peux t'aider...

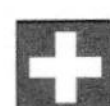

Charlotte

Juliette, je te conseille de poursuivre ton projet. Il faut seulement créer un site différent et original. Toi, tu as une double expertise et tu peux inventer un concept génial: tu connais parfaitement le multimédia et tu connais l'art.

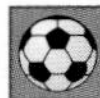

Mamadou

Pourquoi ne pas organiser des expositions d'art africain d'avant-garde? Évidemment, tout le monde connaît les masques, les statuettes et les tissus[8] africains traditionnels, mais en Afrique, il y a aussi des artistes contemporains vraiment exceptionnels. Moi-même, j'en connais et je peux te les présenter.

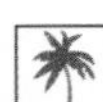

Poema

La plupart des artistes polynésiens ont des difficultés pour exposer leurs tableaux en Europe. Tu peux les aider à réussir sur le marché français!

[1]*around* [2]Je... *I have no talent whatsoever* [3]me... *am satisfied* [4]musées... *open-air museums* [5]*rain* [6]ne... *will never be* [7]*promote* [8]*fabrics*

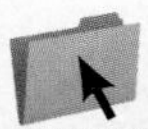

REPORTAGE

Les musées parisiens

Où se trouve *Le Penseur,* la plus fameuse sculpture d'Auguste Rodin? À Paris, au musée Rodin, qui était autrefois l'hôtel Biron où l'artiste a passé beaucoup de temps pendant les dernières années de sa vie. Le jardin qui entoure[1] le musée est une petite merveille. Flânez dans les allées et découvrez les chefs-d'œuvre du grand maître exposés en plein air.

Ensuite, visitez le musée. Imaginez une sorte de petit palais avec des parquets cirés.[2] D'une pièce à l'autre, vous découvrez des sculptures remarquables: *Le Baiser,*[3] *La Main de Dieu*[4]...

Vous sortez de ce musée fasciné par la blancheur du marbre, charmé par ces corps et ces visages[5] sculptés dans la pierre[6] éternelle.

Pour continuer votre visite des musées parisiens, vous devez, bien sûr, aller au Louvre: cette ancienne demeure[7] des rois de France est une pièce majeure du patrimoine français et l'un des plus grands musées d'art du monde. On y trouve notamment la célèbre *Joconde*[8] au sourire mystérieux. Le musée d'Orsay, très riche en tableaux impressionnistes, mérite aussi une visite.

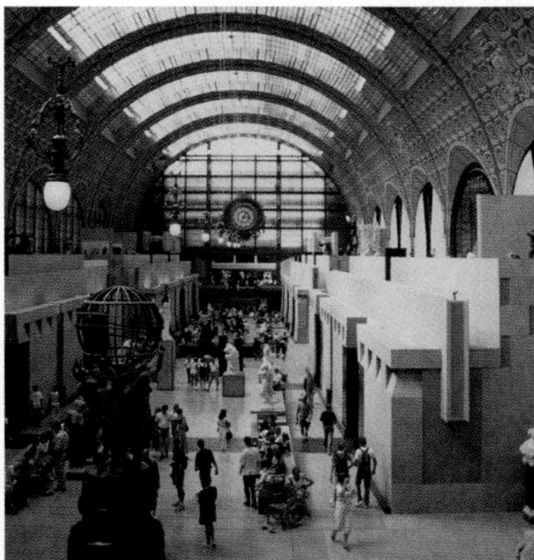

C'est dans l'ancienne gare d'Orsay que le musée d'Orsay s'est installé. Ce bâtiment magnifique, classé monument historique, date de 1900. Construit pour l'Exposition Universelle, il réunit aujourd'hui des chefs-d'œuvre de l'impressionnisme et du post-impressionnisme français, comme *Femme à l'ombrelle* de Monet ou *La Danseuse* de Renoir.

Mais si vous voulez sourire, il faut aller au musée Grévin, qui présente plus de 450 personnages célèbres... en cire,[9] ou au musée de la Poupée,[10] qui va vous rappeler votre enfance. Et si vous aimez la littérature, vous devez absolument visiter la maison de Balzac et la maison de Victor Hugo: dans ces murs, des œuvres immortelles sont nées.

[1]*surrounds* [2]parquets... *waxed wood floors* [3]*Kiss* [4]*Main... Hand of God* [5]*faces* [6]*stone* [7]*residence* [8]*Mona Lisa* [9]en... *in wax* [10]*Doll*

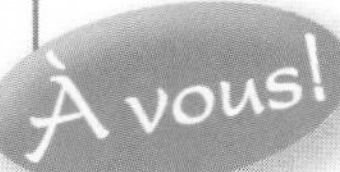

1. Avez-vous envie de visiter le musée Rodin ou un autre musée parisien? Expliquez pourquoi.
2. Est-ce que vous avez visité, aux États-Unis ou dans d'autres pays, des musées originaux et surprenants? Racontez une de ces expériences et expliquez vos réactions.

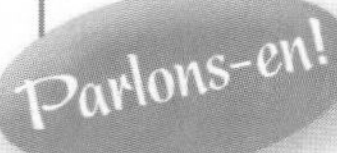

1. Travaillez à deux ou en petits groupes. Préparez un circuit (*tour*) de trois petits musées originaux à Paris. Aidez-vous d'Internet.
2. Pour chaque musée, trouvez deux mots-clés pouvant expliquer votre sélection. Par exemple, pour le musée de la Vie romantique: «ambiance, Chopin».
3. Avec votre camarade ou votre groupe, présentez et expliquez votre circuit de musées à la classe. N'oubliez pas de mentionner les mots clés.

   Quel est le musée le plus intéressant? Votez!

Leçon 3

Les verbes suivis de l'infinitif

Expressing Actions

Provocation?

Mamadou contacte Léa sur sa page Facebook (Messagerie instantanée).

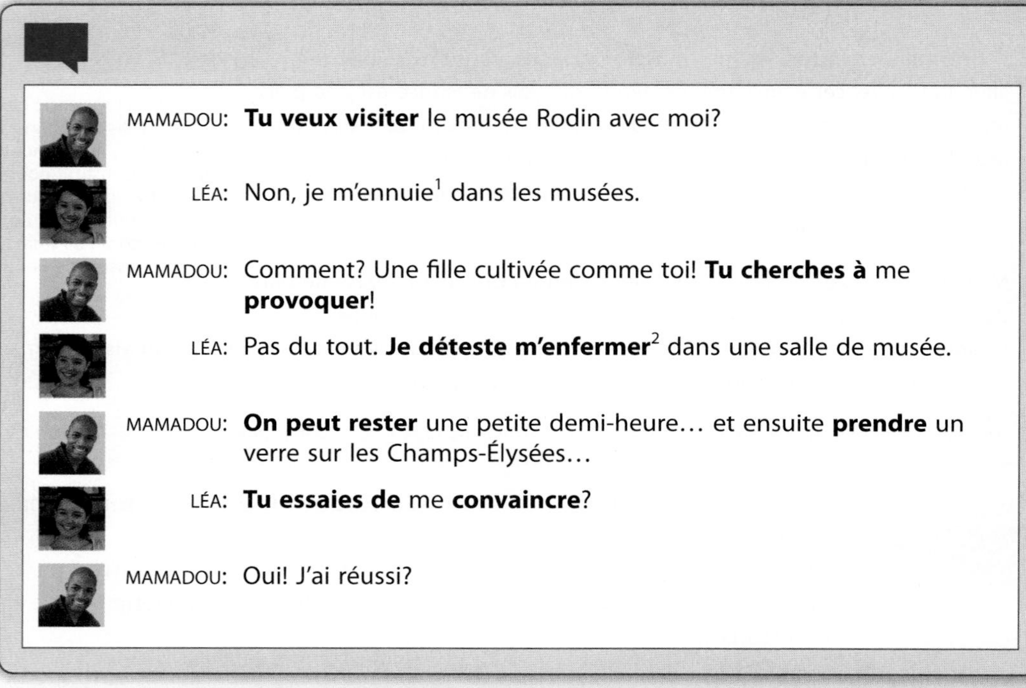

MAMADOU: **Tu veux visiter** le musée Rodin avec moi?

LÉA: Non, je m'ennuie[1] dans les musées.

MAMADOU: Comment? Une fille cultivée comme toi! **Tu cherches à** me **provoquer**!

LÉA: Pas du tout. **Je déteste m'enfermer**[2] dans une salle de musée.

MAMADOU: **On peut rester** une petite demi-heure... et ensuite **prendre** un verre sur les Champs-Élysées...

LÉA: **Tu essaies de** me **convaincre**?

MAMADOU: Oui! J'ai réussi?

[1]*je... I get bored* [2]*shut myself up*

Dans le dialogue, trouvez les verbes à l'infinitif qui suivent les verbes conjugués.

1. Tu veux ______ le musée Rodin avec moi?
2. Tu cherches à me ______?
3. Je déteste ______ dans une salle de musée.
4. On peut ______ une petite demi-heure.
5. Tu essaies de me ______?

1. Some verbs can be followed by an infinitive without an intervening preposition. Among the most common:

aimer	**détester**	**falloir (il faut)**	**savoir**
aller	**devoir**	**pouvoir**	**venir**
désirer	**espérer**	**préférer**	**vouloir**

Je **déteste chanter.** Mais je **sais** très bien **jouer** de la guitare.	*I hate singing, but I know how to play the guitar very well.*
Sophie **ne peut pas aller** au cinéma samedi soir. Elle **doit aller voir** sa grand-mère.	*Sophie cannot go to the movies on Saturday evening. She has to visit her grandmother.*

When **penser** is followed by an infinitive, it means *to count or plan on doing something.*

Je **pense rester** chez moi ce week-end.	*I'm planning on staying home this weekend.*

2. Other verbs require the preposition **à** directly before the infinitive. These include:

aider à	**chercher à**	**continuer à**	**réussir à**
apprendre à	**commencer à**	**enseigner à**	

J'**ai commencé à fumer** quand j'avais 16 ans. Caroline m'**a aidé à arrêter.**	*I started to smoke when I was 16. Caroline helped me quit.*
La semaine prochaine, je vais **apprendre à jouer** au tennis et je **continue à prendre** des cours de yoga deux fois par semaine.	*Next week I will learn how to play tennis, and I will continue to take yoga classes twice a week.*

Note: Encourage sts. to memorize these verbs and prepositions. Warn them, however, of the difficulty of assimilating them immediately without intensive oral, writing, and listening practice.

Suggestion: Make a *Trouvez quelqu'un* ex. using verbs from the lists in this section. Put these verbs and the infinitives that follow in boldface. After sts. complete the activity, ask them why these verbs are in boldface. This can serve as an introduction to this section.

3. Still other verbs require the preposition **de** directly before the infinitive.

accepter de	**décider de**	**finir de**	**rêver de**
arrêter de	**demander de**	**oublier de**	**venir de**
choisir de	**empêcher de**	**permettre de**	
conseiller de	**essayer de**	**refuser de**	

Rachid **a décidé de prendre** des cours d'art dramatique. Il **rêve de devenir** acteur. Il **vient de jouer** un petit rôle dans *Le Cid* à l'université. L'année prochaine, il va **essayer d'entrer** au Conservatoire de Paris.	*Rachid has decided to take drama classes. He dreams of becoming an actor. He just played a small role in* Le Cid *at the university. Next year, he is going to try to get into the Paris Conservatory.*

Suggestion: Have sts. generate clear examples for all the verbs listed in 1–3.

Additional vocabulary: *hésiter à, cesser de, regretter de.*

4. A few verbs change in meaning with different prepositions. **Commencer** regularly takes **à** before an infinitive; **finir** normally takes **de** before an infinitive. However, they can both take **par. Commencer par** is used to talk about what one did first in a series of things; **finir par** means *to end up by doing something.*

   Grégoire **a commencé par** jouer un petit rôle dans une comédie à l'université. Il **a fini par** devenir acteur à Hollywood.

5. Note that the meaning of **venir** changes depending on whether it is followed directly by an infinitive or by **de** plus an infinitive. **Ils viennent dîner** means *They are coming to dinner.* **Ils viennent de dîner** means *They've just had dinner.*

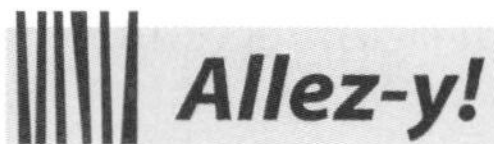

Allez-y!

Suggestion: Give sts. a minute to do the activity alone before eliciting responses.

A. Au cabaret de la Contrescarpe. Deborah, Chuck et Jacques arrivent à la Contrescarpe, dans le quartier Montmartre, à Paris. Classez leurs activités par ordre chronologique de 1 à 8.

_____ Ils décident de commander du champagne.
_____ Ils finissent par s'endormir dans le séjour.
_____ Ils demandent au serveur de leur apporter l'addition.
_____ Ils choisissent de s'asseoir à une table près de la scène.
_____ Ils commencent par regarder la salle.
_____ Ils commencent à chanter en rentrant chez eux.
_____ Ils arrêtent de parler quand le spectacle commence.
_____ Ils n'oublient pas de laisser un pourboire au serveur.

Suggestion: Elicit a variety of answers from several sts., or use in an interview format.

B. Projets et activités. Posez des questions à vos camarades pour vous informer de leurs projets et de leurs activités.

MODÈLE: aller / faire / ce soir →
É1: Qu'est-ce que tu vas faire ce soir?
É2: Je vais sortir avec mes amis.

1. vouloir / faire / ce week-end
2. aller / faire / l'été prochain
3. devoir / faire / demain
4. aimer / faire / après les cours
5. penser / faire / la semaine prochaine
6. détester / faire / le soir
7. espérer / faire / ce soir

Follow-up: *Regardez de nouveau les résolutions que vous avez prises. Lesquelles allez-vous probablement tenir?*

C. Résolutions du Nouvel An. Énumérez quelques-unes de vos résolutions à vos camarades. Complétez les phrases suivantes avec un infinitif.

MODÈLE: Cette année, je vais finir... →
Cette année, je vais finir de lire *La Vie mode d'emploi* de Georges Perec.*

1. Je voudrais apprendre...
2. Je vais commencer...
3. J'ai aussi décidé...
4. En plus, je vais arrêter...
5. Enfin, je rêve...
6. Mais je refuse...

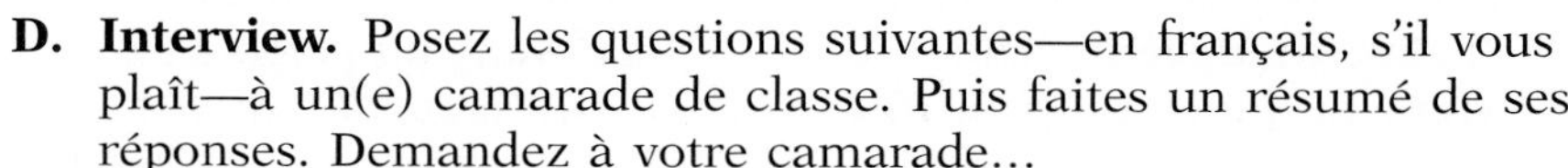

D. Interview. Posez les questions suivantes—en français, s'il vous plaît—à un(e) camarade de classe. Puis faites un résumé de ses réponses. Demandez à votre camarade...

1. what he/she likes to do in the evening
2. what he/she hates to do in the house
3. if he/she is learning to do something interesting, and what it is
4. if he/she has decided to continue to study French
5. what he/she has to do after class
6. if he/she prefers going to a play or to a movie
7. if he/she has just read a good book, and what it was
8. what he/she knows how to do well
9. what he/she tries, but does not always succeed in doing well
10. if he/she forgot to do something this morning, and what it was
11. if he/she has stopped doing something recently, and what it was
12. ?

---

*Perec (1936–1982) était un artiste et écrivain français. *La Vie mode d'emploi,* fruit de neuf années de travail, retrace l'histoire d'un immeuble parisien et de ses habitants.

Les adverbes

Talking About How Things Are Done

L'art et le foot

Léa et Mamadou discutent au café.

LÉA: Une heure au musée, c'est **vraiment** le maximum pour moi!
MAMADOU: Dis la vérité: tu as **beaucoup** aimé les sculptures. Tu étais fascinée!
LÉA: **Franchement,** j'ai apprécié la lumière* naturelle sur les œuvres.
MAMADOU: Tu vois: il faut **toujours** aller au musée avec moi!
LÉA: Et **maintenant,** qu'est-ce qu'on fait?
MAMADOU: On va d'**abord** prendre un verre au Fouquet's.
LÉA: Et **ensuite**?
MAMADOU: **Ensuite,** je t'emmène à un match de foot!

*light

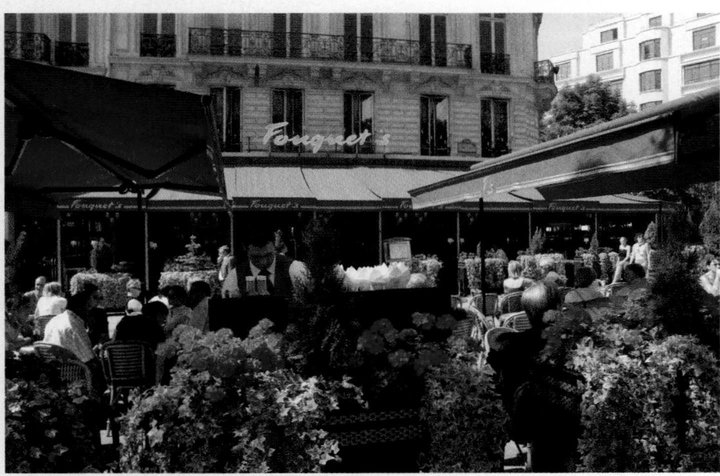

Le célèbre Fouquet's sur les Champs-Élysées

Répondez aux questions en utilisant les adverbes du dialogue.

1. Est-ce que deux heures au musée, c'est le maximum pour Léa?
2. Est-ce que Mamadou pense qu'elle a aimé les sculptures?
3. Qu'est-ce qu'elle a apprécié?
4. Avec qui faut-il aller au musée?
5. Qu'est-ce qu'ils vont faire après leur visite du musée?

Cultural note: Fouquet's, a fashionable brasserie on the Champs-Élysées, opened its doors in 1899. Having a drink or meal there is a chic Parisian tradition.

Forms of Adverbs

Adverbs (**les adverbes,** *m.*) modify a verb, an adjective, or another adverb: She learns *quickly.* He is *extremely* hardworking. They see each other *quite often.* You have already learned a number of adverbs, such as **souvent, parfois, bien, mal, beaucoup, trop, peu, très, vite, d'abord, puis, ensuite, après,** and **enfin.**

Note: Other adverbs sts. have also learned include *toujours, rarement, quelquefois, de temps en temps, déjà, encore, maintenant, aujourd'hui, autrefois, soudain.*

1. Most adverbs are formed by adding **-ment** (often corresponding to *-ly* in English) to the feminine form of an adjective.

FEMININE ADJECTIVE	ADVERB	
franche	**franchement**	*frankly*
active	**activement**	*actively*
(mal)heureuse	**(mal)heureusement**	*(un)fortunately*

Note: Mention irregular adverbs *dur, précisément, profondément, énormément, brièvement,* and *gentiment.*

Suggestion: Point out that these adverbs generally answer the questions *Comment… ? De quelle manière… ?*

2. If the masculine form of the adjective ends in a vowel, **-ment** is usually added directly to it.

MASCULINE ADJECTIVE	ADVERB	
absolu	**absolument**	*absolutely*
poli	**poliment**	*politely*
rapide	**rapidement**	*quickly*
vrai	**vraiment**	*truly, really*

3. If the masculine form of the adjective ends in **-ent** or **-ant,** the corresponding adverbs have the endings **-emment** and **-amment,** respectively. The two endings have the same pronunciation.

Suggestion: Point out the pronunciation of these adverbs [**amã**].

MASCULINE ADJECTIVE	ADVERB	
différent	**différemment**	*differently*
évident	**évidemment**	*evidently, obviously*
constant	**constamment**	*constantly*
courant	**couramment**	*fluently*

One exception to this rule is **lent,** which adds **-ment** to the feminine adjective to form **lentement.**

Note: In English, the adverbial forms of *good* and *bad* are *well* and *badly.* In French, the adverb forms of **bon** and **mauvais** are both irregular.

bon → **bien**	Sonia est une **bonne** actrice; elle joue **bien** son rôle.
mauvais → **mal**	Normand est un **mauvais** cinéaste; il dirige **mal** ses acteurs.

[Allez-y! A-B]

Position of Adverbs

1. When adverbs qualify adjectives or other adverbs, they usually precede them.

Elle est **très** intelligente.	*She is very intelligent.*
Il va au cinéma **assez** souvent.	*He goes to the movies fairly often.*

2. When a verb is in the present or imperfect tense, the qualifying adverb usually follows it. In negative constructions, the adverb comes after **pas.**

Je travaille **lentement.**	*I work slowly.*
Elle voulait **absolument** devenir écrivain.	*She absolutely wanted to become a writer.*
Vous ne l'expliquez pas **bien.**	*You aren't explaining it well.*

3. Short adverbs usually precede the past participle when the verb is in a compound form; they usually follow **pas** in a negative construction.

J'ai **beaucoup** voyagé cette année.	*I've traveled a lot this year.*
Il a **déjà** visité le Louvre.	*He has already visited the Louvre.*
Elle n'est pas **souvent** allée en Bretagne.	*She has not often been to Brittany.*
Je n'ai pas **très** faim.*	*I'm not very hungry.*

4. Adverbs ending in **-ment** follow a verb in the present or imperfect tense, and usually follow the past participle when the verb is in the **passé composé.**

Tu parles **couramment** le français.	*You speak French fluently.*
Il était **vraiment** travailleur.	*He was really hardworking.*
Paul n'a pas répondu **intelligemment.**	*Paul didn't respond intelligently.*

[Allez-y! C-D]

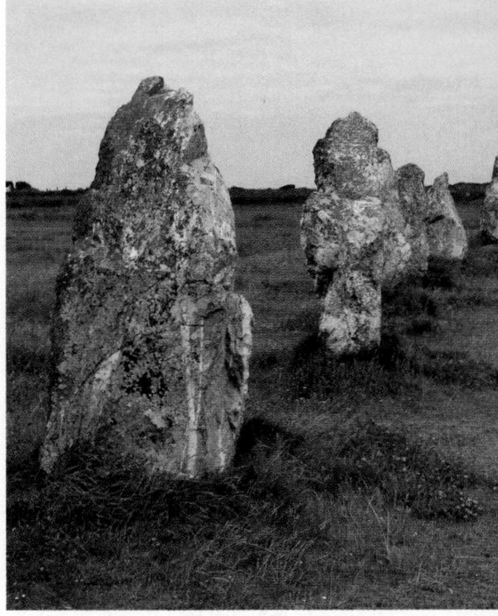

Des menhirs préhistoriques à Carnac, en Bretagne: ces pierres dressées (*standing stones*) sont vraiment mystérieuses!

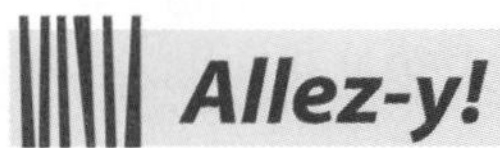

Allez-y!

A. Ressemblances. Donnez l'équivalent adverbial de chacun des adjectifs suivants.

MODÈLE: franc → franchement

1. heureux
2. actif
3. long
4. vrai
5. différent
6. naturel
7. certain
8. constant
9. absolu
10. admirable
11. poli
12. intelligent

Continuation: *lent, évident, seul* (alone), *indépendant*

*In idiomatic expressions with **avoir,** one often uses an adverb: **J'ai très soif; Elle a très chaud,** and so on.

Suggestion: If done in class, give sts. a few minutes to work out answers individually. Then have them complete sentences orally, explaining choices.

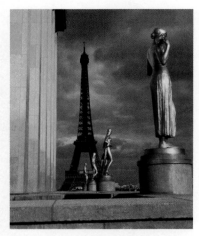

Le Théâtre National de Chaillot se trouve au Palais de Chaillot, à Paris. Décrivez cette photo comme si c'était une œuvre d'art.

B. Carrières. Complétez les paragraphes suivants avec des adverbes logiques.

1. Le linguiste

   Adverbes: bien, bientôt, couramment, ensuite, évidemment, probablement, vite

   Jean-Luc parle ______[1] l'anglais. Il a vécu aux États-Unis. Il est allé au lycée (à l'école secondaire) à New York et il a très ______[2] appris la langue pendant son séjour. ______[3], à l'université il a choisi la section langues étrangères. Il va ______[4] passer sa licence d'anglais. ______[5], il doit ______[6] choisir entre la traduction (*translation*) littéraire et l'enseignement. Ses parents sont professeurs et je pense qu'il va ______[7] choisir de devenir professeur.

2. L'actrice

   Adverbes: absolument, beaucoup, constamment, fréquemment, rarement, seulement, souvent, très

   Marie veut ______[1] devenir une artiste célèbre. Elle travaille ______[2] pour y arriver: le matin, elle arrive ______[3] au Théâtre National de Chaillot après six heures et elle y reste ______[4] jusqu'à neuf heures du soir. Dans la journée, elle travaille ______[5] et prend ______[6] quinze minutes pour déjeuner. ______[7], elle est fatiguée le soir. Mais je pense qu'elle va réussir parce qu'elle est ______[8] travailleuse et ambitieuse.

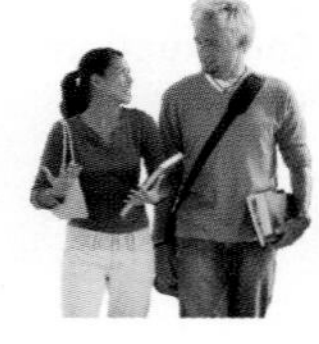

C. Interview. Interviewez un(e) camarade de classe sur ses préférences et ses habitudes. Votre camarade doit utiliser dans sa réponse un adverbe basé sur les mots entre parenthèses. Décidez ensuite quelle sorte de personne il/elle est (calme, énergique, patiente, pratique, travailleuse, et cetera).

MODÈLE: Comment déjeunes-tu d'habitude? (rapide / lent) →
Je déjeune lentement pour me reposer. *ou* Je déjeune rapidement parce que je suis toujours pressé(e).

1. Quand fais-tu la sieste? (fréquent / rare)
2. Comment attends-tu le résultat de ton examen? (patient / impatient)
3. Regardes-tu souvent ta montre? (constant / fréquent / rare / jamais)
4. Comment travailles-tu en général? (bon / mal)
5. Lis-tu souvent les romans policiers? (fréquent / rare / jamais)

Maintenant décrivez le caractère de votre camarade.

Suggestion: Encourage sts. to use several different adverbs.

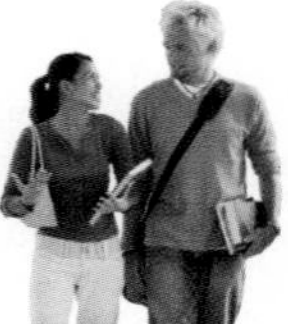

D. Qu'en pensez-vous? Posez les questions suivantes à des camarades. Ils vont répondre en utilisant des adverbes.

Suggestions: absolument, admirablement, constamment, couramment, diligemment, évidemment, franchement, heureusement, intelligemment, lentement, malheureusement, poliment, souvent, tranquillement, vite

MODÉLE: É1: Qu'est-ce qu'on doit faire pour avoir de bonnes notes?
É2: On doit étudier constamment.
É1: On doit travailler intelligemment.

1. Qu'est-ce qu'on doit faire pour être un bon professeur?
2. Qu'est-ce qu'on doit faire pour devenir président(e) des États-Unis?
3. Qu'est-ce qu'on doit faire pour courir dans un marathon?
4. Qu'est-ce qu'on doit faire pour devenir riche?
5. Qu'est-ce qu'on doit faire pour avoir de bons rapports (*a good relationship*) avec une autre personne?

E. Opinions et habitudes. Posez ces questions à un(e) camarade. Dans sa réponse il/elle doit employer des adverbes.

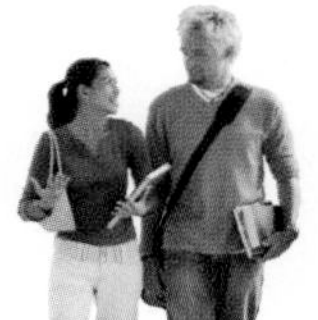

1. À ton avis, est-ce qu'on doit beaucoup travailler pour réussir?
2. Quel est l'aspect le plus important de ta carrière future?
3. Est-ce que l'argent fait le bonheur?
4. Est-ce que l'amitié est plus importante que la réussite?
5. Est-ce que tu rêves de quitter ton pays pour aller vivre sur une île tropicale?

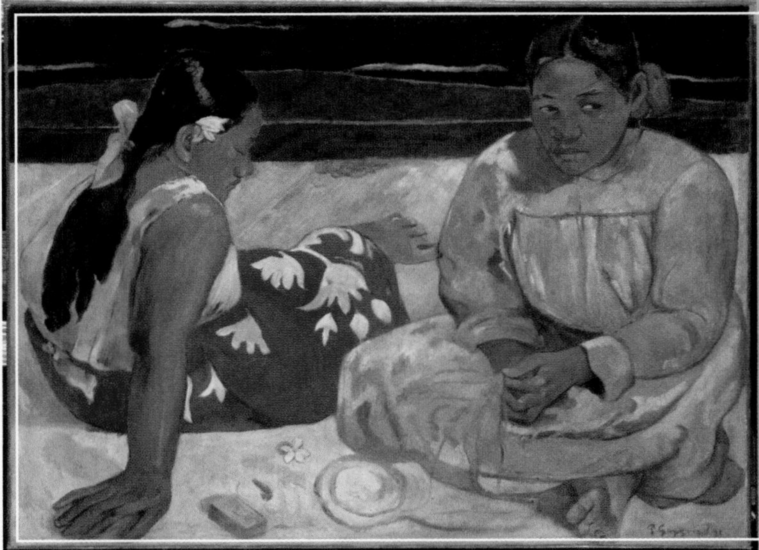

Un peu plus...

Paul Gauguin. (1848–1903)
Après plus de dix ans comme agent de change (*stockbroker*) à Paris, où il fait la connaissance de Camille Pissarro et découvre l'impressionnisme, Gauguin quitte la Bourse (*stock exchange*) pour se consacrer à la peinture. Il privilégie les couleurs vives et les contours clairement démarqués, comme son ami Van Gogh. En 1888, Gauguin et Van Gogh passent neuf semaines ensemble à Arles mais l'amitié tourne mal et se termine avec le drame de l'oreille coupée de Van Gogh. Quelques années plus tard, Gauguin s'installe à Tahiti où il s'inspire de la culture polynésienne et des mythes anciens pour peindre ses plus fameux tableaux. Vous aimez les tableaux de Gauguin? Pourquoi ou pourquoi pas?

◄ *Paul Gauguin: Femmes de Tahiti, 1891 (Musée d'Orsay, Paris)*

Video connection: The video *Bienvenue aux îles francophones,* which follows Chapter 16, has a segment on Tahiti that includes information on Gauguin.

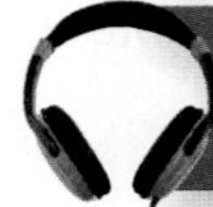

Prononcez bien!

Script (A): 1. *Tout va bien. C'est Pierre, notre voisin. Il a sûrement laissé tomber un objet.* 2. *Il habite au-dessus de chez nous.* 3. *Isabelle et moi, nous l'avons rencontré pendant notre cure l'année dernière.* 4. *C'est quelqu'un qui est très sourd. Alors, ne t'inquiète pas!*

Answers (A): 1. a 2. b 3. b 4. a

The vowel sound in *sculpture* (page 323)

A. Un bruit bizarre... Vous regardez la télévision avec Hugo quand vous entendez un bruit bizarre. Hugo vous rassure. Sélectionnez les phrases qu'il dit.

1. **a.** Tout va bien. C'est Pierre, notre voisin. Il a sûrement laissé tomber un objet. **b.** Tu vas bien. C'est Pierre, notre voisin. Il a sûrement laissé tomber un objet.
2. **a.** Il habite au-dessous de chez nous. **b.** Il habite au-dessus de chez nous.
3. **a.** Isabelle et moi, nous l'avons rencontré pendant notre cours l'année dernière. **b.** Isabelle et moi, nous l'avons rencontré pendant notre cure (*vacation at the hot springs*) l'année dernière.
4. **a.** C'est quelqu'un qui est très sourd (*deaf*). Alors, ne t'inquiète pas! **b.** C'est quelqu'un qui est très sûr (*reliable*). Alors, ne t'inquiète pas!

B. Des photos. Hugo vous montre les photos de ses vacances d'été. Jouez la scène suivante avec votre camarade de classe en faisant attention à la prononciation de [u] comme dans **vous** et de [y] comme dans **sculpture**.

VOUS: C'est qui ça?
HUGO: Ah, c'est Luc, mon cousin.
VOUS: Qu'est-ce qu'il a sur la figure (*face*)?
HUGO: Des gouttes (*drops*) de jus de prune (*plum*). Il faisait très chaud ce jour-là. Une vraie canicule (*heat wave*)! Nous avons beaucoup bu.
VOUS: Et sur cette photo, on dirait qu'il fume.
HUGO: Oui, mais il a arrêté récemment parce qu'il toussait (*was coughing*) beaucoup.
VOUS: Voilà une bonne nouvelle!

Leçon 4

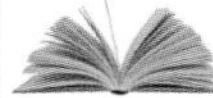

Lecture

Avant de lire

Reading poetry (Part 2). Poetry often remains popular for decades and even centuries. One of the reasons is that it is often based on emotions that are universal over time such as happiness, sadness, love, sorrow, jealousy, fear, and anger. Effective poetry engages the reader emotionally and often articulates one of those inner feelings for him or her. The impact of the poem is often derived from the sounds and the repetition of those sounds along with the rhythm and rhyming used.

In *Déjeuner du matin,* Prévert uses much repetition.

Find...

1. which phrase is repeated at least six times.
2. which phrases contain the word **sans**. Note which ones are repeated more than one time.
3. which verb tense is used repeatedly throughout the poem.

Glance through the text to determine which inner feeling will be engaged. Use the following information to help you guess.

Find out...

1. how many people are involved.
2. where the scene is taking place.
3. what the weather is like.
4. what one character does at the very end.

À propos de la lecture...
La poésie de Jacques Prévert (1900–1977) est accessible à un très large public. Elle traite de justice, de liberté et de bonheur. Ce poème est tiré du recueil *Paroles* (1946).

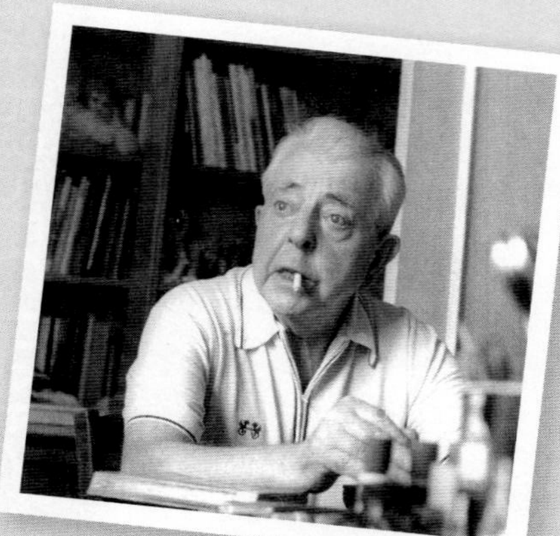

Le poète Jacques Prévert

«Déjeuner du matin»

Il a mis le café
Dans la tasse
Il a mis le lait
Dans la tasse de café
Il a mis le sucre
Dans le café au lait
Avec la petite cuiller
Il a tourné
Il a bu le café au lait
Et il a reposé[1] *la tasse*
Sans me parler
Il a allumé[2]
Une cigarette
Il a fait des ronds
Avec la fumée
Il a mis les cendres
Dans le cendrier
Sans me parler
Sans me regarder
Il s'est levé[3]
Il a mis
Son chapeau sur sa tête
Il a mis
Son manteau de pluie
Parce qu'il pleuvait
Et il est parti
Sous la pluie
Sans une parole
Sans me regarder
Et moi j'ai pris
Ma tête dans ma main
Et j'ai pleuré.[4]

[1]a... *put down again* [2]a... *lit* [3]s'est... *got up* [4]j'ai... *I cried*

Follow-up: (1) Once sts. have read the poem, ask them why they think Prévert repeated certain phrases over and over and to what effect. Ask sts. to come up with some words in French that are evoked by this repetition. Possible answers: *la banalité, la distance émotionnelle, l'ennui, la monotonie, la routine, le silence, la solitude, la tristesse.* (2) Ask sts.: *Quel effet vous a fait ce poème?*

Compréhension

Qu'en pensez-vous? Dites si les phrases suivantes reflètent votre interprétation du poème. Sinon, reformulez-les pour mieux exprimer votre opinion. Justifiez votre point de vue en citant des extraits du poème.

1. Dans ce poème, une mère raconte son petit déjeuner avec son fils.
2. Ces personnes se connaissent (*know each other*) depuis longtemps.
3. On a l'impression que c'est un repas typique entre ces deux personnes.
4. Le narrateur / La narratrice est très satisfait(e) de sa vie.
5. Le poète crée une ambiance de joie.

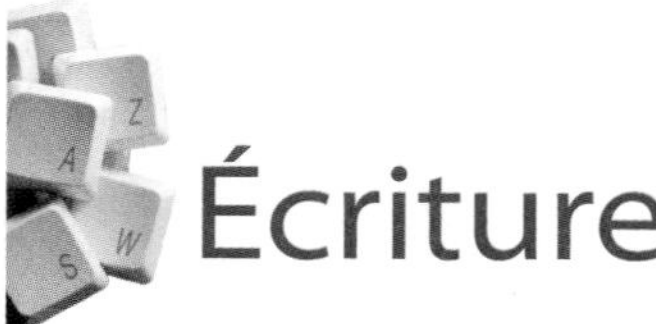

Écriture

The writing activities **Par écrit** and **Journal intime** can be found in the Workbook/Laboratory Manual to accompany *Vis-à-vis*.

La vie en chantant. An activity based on the song "Dans mon rêve" by Zachary Richard can be found in the *Instructor's Manual*. The song can be purchased at the iTunes store, or sts. can watch the music video on YouTube.

Pour s'amuser

Un jeune peintre se passionne pour l'abstraction.

—Ce que les gens préfèrent dans mes tableaux, c'est l'imagination.
—Vraiment?
—Oui. Après avoir regardé mes œuvres, beaucoup me disent: «Si vous appelez ça de l'art, vous avez beaucoup d'imagination!»

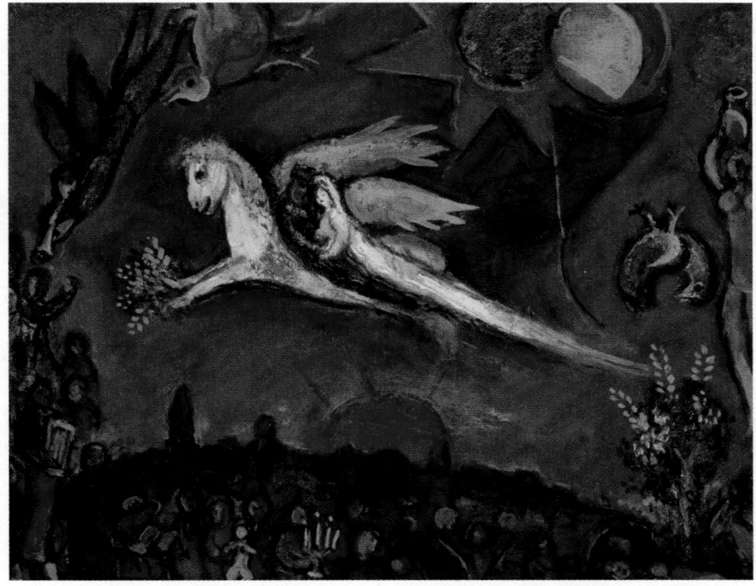

Marc Chagall*: *Le Cantique des cantiques IV*, 1958 (Musée National Message Biblique Marc Chagall, Nice)

*Marc Chagall (1887–1985) est un artiste et peintre né en Bélarussie. Il a vécu principalement en France.

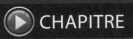

Le vidéoblog de Juliette

En bref

Dans cet épisode, Juliette rencontre Léa sur le pont près du musée d'Orsay. Comme il faut faire la queue pour y entrer, les deux amies décident de passer l'après-midi à découvrir les œuvres des musées «en plein air».

Vocabulaire en contexte

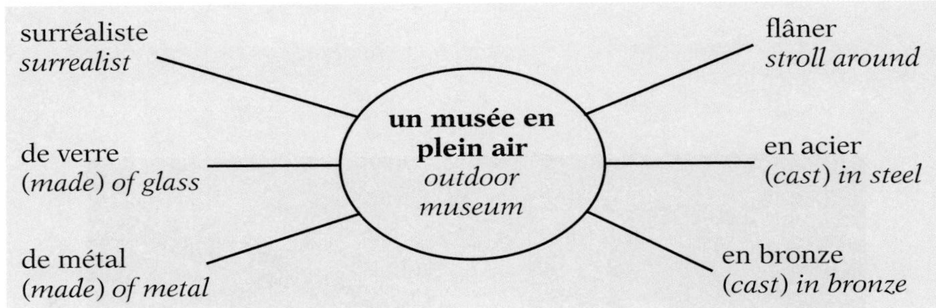

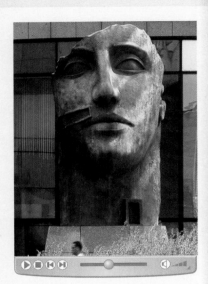

Tête monumentale dans le musée en plein air de la Défense

Additional vocabulary: Other vocabulary you may wish to present before viewing includes *prendre un pot, j'ai changé d'avis, insensible.*

Answers: 1. e, 2. c, 3. a, 4. d, 5. f, 6. b

Follow-up: Sts. can vote in class on which work of art seen in the video they wish to have in their town or on their school campus and explain their choice.

Visionnez!

Trouvez la description qui correspond à chaque œuvre d'art.

ŒUVRES D'ART	DESCRIPTIONS
1. ______ *Le Pouce (The Thumb)*	**a.** un homme qui marche sur une boule de métal
2. ______ *Stabile*	**b.** une œuvre qui célèbre l'amour
3. ______ *Le Somnambule*	**c.** un énorme insecte en acier rouge
4. ______ *Deux personnages fantastiques*	**d.** une composition surréaliste
5. ______ *Tête monumentale*	**e.** une reproduction en bronze par l'artiste César
6. ______ *Le mur des «je t'aime»*	**f.** un visage (*face*) sans émotion par l'artiste Mitoraj

Note culturelle

Le monument «la Défense de Paris», qui commémore les soldats défenseurs de la ville pendant la guerre[1] franco-allemande de 1870, a donné son nom au quartier.

L'œuvre *Tête monumentale* se trouve aujourd'hui sur le parvis[2] de la Défense. Elle est accompagnée d'une soixantaine d'œuvres d'art contemporain, fresques et sculptures monumentales qui forment un musée en plein air.

[1]*war* [2]*square*

Analysez!

1. Comment imaginez-vous un musée parisien typique? Comment est-ce que ces musées en plein air diffèrent de (*differ from*) cette image?
2. Est-ce que les œuvres du musée en plein air à la Défense reflètent bien le quartier dans lequel (*in which*) elles se trouvent? Expliquez pourquoi (pas).

Comparez!

Regardez encore une fois la partie culturelle de la vidéo. Y a-t-il des musées d'art dans votre ville? Trouve-t-on des sculptures à l'extérieur (dans les parcs ou devant les bâtiments, par exemple)? Quelle œuvre présentée dans la vidéo aimeriez-vous (*would you like*) voir dans votre ville? Expliquez.

J'aimerais voir ______ parce que...

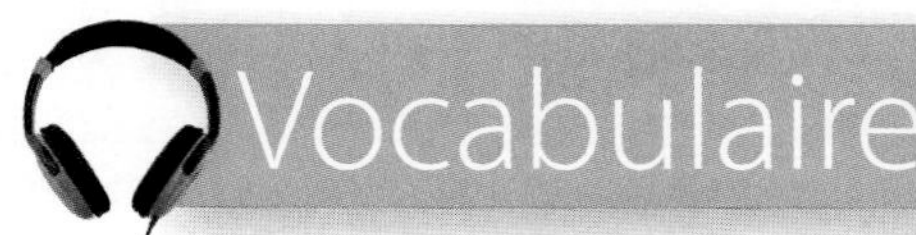

Vocabulaire

Verbes

bâtir to build
dater (de) to date from
deviner to guess
emmener to take someone along; to invite
flâner to stroll
peindre to paint
poursuivre to pursue
suivre to follow; to take (*a course*)
vivre to live

À REVOIR: **apporter, habiter**

Verbes suivis de l'infinitif

accepter (de) to accept (to)
aider (à) to help (to)
arrêter (de) to stop
chercher à to try to
commencer par to begin by (*doing something*)
conseiller (de) to advise (to)
continuer (à) to continue (to)
décider (de) to decide (to)
empêcher (de) to prevent (from)
enseigner (à) to teach (to)
essayer (de) to try (to)
finir par to end up (*doing something*)
permettre (de) to permit, allow (to)
refuser (de) to refuse (to)
réussir (à) to succeed (in)

À REVOIR: **aimer, aller, apprendre à, choisir de, commencer à, demander de, désirer, détester, devoir, espérer, finir de, il faut, oublier de, penser, pouvoir, préférer, rêver de, savoir, venir, venir de, vouloir**

Substantifs

l'acteur / l'actrice actor
les arènes (*f. pl.*) arena
l'artiste (*m., f.*) artist
l'auteur dramatique (*m.*) playwright
la cathédrale cathedral
le chef-d'œuvre (*pl.* **les chefs-d'œuvre**) masterpiece
le/la cinéaste filmmaker
le comédien / la comédienne stage actor
le compositeur / la compositrice composer
la conférence lecture
l'écrivain (*m.*) **/ la femme écrivain** writer
l'époque (*f.*) period (*of history*)
l'événement (*m.*) event
l'exposition (*f.*) exhibit
l'horaire (*m.*) schedule
le Moyen Âge Middle Ages
le/la musicien(ne) musician
l'œuvre (*f.*) **(d'art)** work (of art)
le palais palace
le patrimoine legacy, heritage
le peintre / la femme peintre painter
la peinture painting
la pièce de théâtre play
la place seat
le poème poem
la poésie poetry
le poète / la femme poète poet
le recueil collection
la reine queen
la Renaissance Renaissance
le roi king
le sculpteur / la femme sculpteur sculptor
la sculpture sculpture
le siècle century
le tableau painting
le théâtre theater

À REVOIR: **le cadeau, la carte postale, le château, le cinéma, la littérature, la musique, le roman**

Adjectifs

actif / active active
absolu(e) absolute
classique classical
constant(e) constant
courant(e) common; standard
évident evident, obvious
franc(he) frank
gothique Gothic
historique historical
lent(e) slow
magnifique magnificent
malheureux / malheureuse unhappy; unfortunate
médiéval(e) medieval
poli(e) polite
rapide fast, rapid
romain(e) Roman

À REVOIR: **bon(ne), différent(e), heureux / heureuse, mauvais(e), vrai(e)**

Adverbes

activement actively
absolument absolutely
constamment constantly
couramment fluently
différemment differently
évidemment evidently, obviously
franchement frankly
heureusement fortunately
lentement slowly
malheureusement unfortunately
poliment politely
rapidement rapidly
récemment recently
vraiment really

À REVOIR: **après, beaucoup, bien, d'abord, enfin, ensuite, mal, parfois, peu, puis, souvent, très, trop, vite**

Mots et expressions divers

la plupart de the majority
moi-même myself
toi-même, lui-même...
par cœur by heart

Bienvenue...

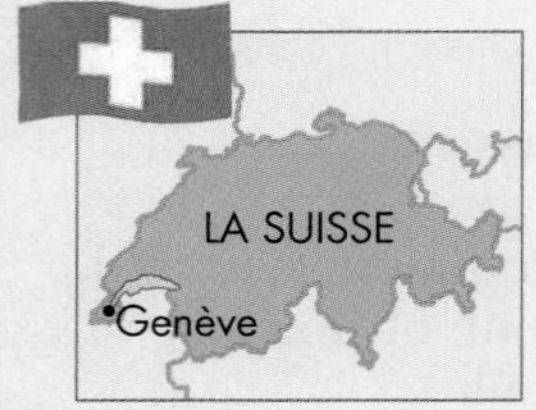

Un coup d'œil sur Genève, en Suisse

Vous avez sans doute déjà entendu parler de Genève, en Suisse, notamment lorsqu'on parle des Conventions de Genève ou du Comité international de la Croix-Rouge.

Genève est une belle ville située dans la partie francophone* de la Suisse, au pied des Alpes.

La Suisse, qui est une des plus anciennes démocraties du monde et un pays politiquement stable et neutre, est donc un lieu privilégié pour de nombreuses organisations internationales. Genève, en particulier, est le siège des Nations Unies en Europe, de l'Assemblée de l'Organisation mondiale de la Santé et du CERN† (Centre européen de recherches nucléaires).

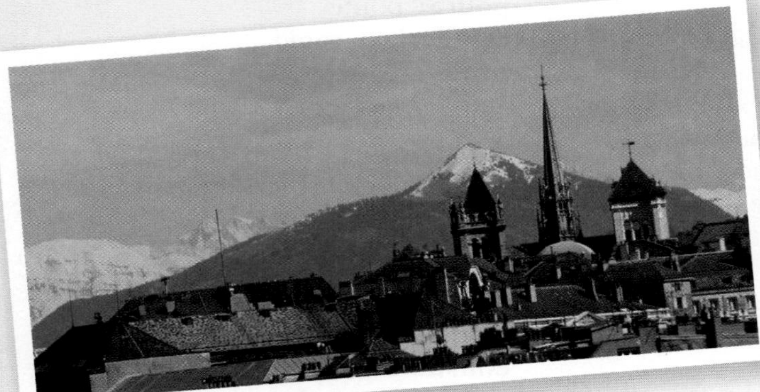

▲ Genève avec, à l'arrière, le mont Blanc, le plus haut sommet des Alpes

PORTRAIT Henri Dunant (1828–1910)

L'une des organisations internationales les plus importantes du monde, le Comité international de la Croix-Rouge, a été fondée à Genève par un Genevois, Henri Dunant.

À l'âge de 18 ans, Henri Dunant allait déjà visiter les pauvres, les malades et les prisonniers. Plus tard, en 1859, alors qu'il se trouvait à Solférino, en Italie du Nord, le lendemain d'une terrible bataille entre 100 000 Français et Italiens d'une part[1] et 100 000 Autrichiens qui occupaient l'Italie‡ d'autre part, Dunant a été horrifié quand il a vu les nombreux hommes blessés, mourants ou morts, abandonnés sur le champ de bataille. Il a immédiatement organisé le secours aux blessés des deux camps avec l'aide des habitants du village.

Il a décrit cette terrible expérience dans son livre, *Un souvenir de Solférino*, et a proposé la création d'une organisation neutre qui apporterait[2] de l'aide à *tous* les soldats blessés, quelle que soit[3] leur nationalité. Une commission a adopté le projet de Dunant et un comité international de secours aux militaires blessés a été créé en 1863. Ce comité est ensuite devenu le Comité international de la Croix-Rouge.

Dunant s'est battu toute sa vie pour ses idées humanitaires. En 1901, il a reçu le premier prix Nobel de la paix pour son rôle dans la fondation du Comité international de la Croix-Rouge et dans la première Convention de Genève, qui, en cas de guerre, protège les militaires blessés ou malades, les ambulances et hôpitaux militaires et le personnel sanitaire. Cette première convention a été le point de départ d'un vaste mouvement humanitaire.

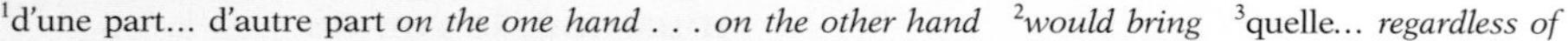

[1]d'une part... d'autre part *on the one hand . . . on the other hand* [2]*would bring* [3]quelle... *regardless of*

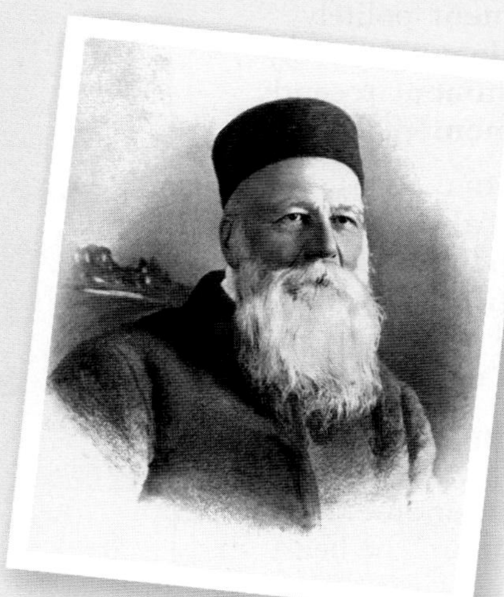

▲ Henri Dunant, foundateur de la Croix-Rouge

*There is no language called "Swiss." Switzerland has four official languages: German (63.7%), French (20.4%), Italian (6.5%), and Romanche (0.5%).

†A scientist at CERN invented the "World-Wide Web" in 1989 to enable the sharing of academic and scientific information. Today, many physicists at CERN research the state of matter at the beginning of the universe, using the largest particle accelerators and detectors in the world.

‡Austria had occupied Italy. The Italians fought back against the Austrian occupation and were aided in the fight by the French.

en Europe francophone

Un coup d'œil sur Bruxelles, en Belgique

Bruxelles
LA BELGIQUE

Capitale du Royaume de Belgique, Bruxelles est aussi l'une des villes-phares[1] de la francophonie depuis le Moyen Âge. On y parle flamand—surtout dans les quartiers historiques du centre—et français. En fait, les Bruxellois se composent de deux groupes linguistiques: les Wallons (ceux[2] qui parlent français) et les Flamands (ceux pour qui le flamand est la langue maternelle). Les Bruxellois sont donc souvent bilingues.

À Bruxelles, le temps est souvent gris, mais on dit que ses habitants ont le soleil dans le cœur. Vous y serez[3] accueilli avec chaleur[4] et bonne humeur. Ses musées, ses églises, ses petites rues commerçantes et ses passages couverts où sont installés confiseries,[5] chocolateries et magasins de dentelles font de Bruxelles une ville de culture et de commerce. Les fêtes se succèdent[6] été comme hiver; à ces occasions, les cortèges,[7] comme celui de Carnaval, convergent vers la Grand-Place, ou *Grote Markt* en flamand. Beaucoup de belles demeures anciennes de la Grand-Place sont maintenant des restaurants où vous pouvez trouver des spécialités culinaires comme les moules-frites ou le célèbre waterzoï.[8] Bruxelles est aussi la capitale politique de l'Union européenne, siège du Parlement européen, ce qui lui donne un caractère cosmopolite.

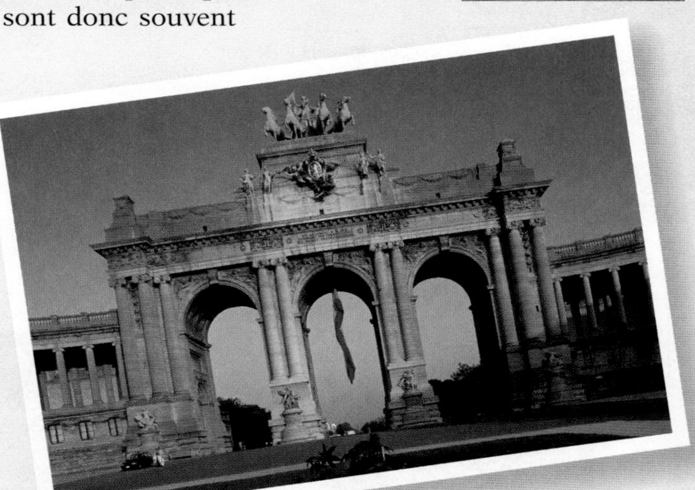

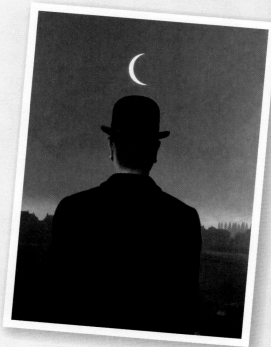

▲ Le triple Arc de Triomphe domine le parc du Cinquantenaire, à Bruxelles.

[1]*beacons* [2]*those* [3]*will be* [4]*warmth* [5]*candy stores* [6]se... *follow each other* [7]*processions* [8]*Belgian speciality made from fish or meat in a cream sauce*

PORTRAIT René Magritte (1898–1967)

René Magritte est le peintre surréaliste par excellence. Ce Belge rivalise dans cet art du XXe siècle avec l'Espagnol Salvador Dali. Ses nombreuses œuvres nous ouvrent un monde inconnu[1] où se mélangent le rêve et une réalité transposée par l'artiste. Il crée des associations étranges et conçoit[2] des personnages extraordinaires et des paysages fabuleux. Son univers est imprévisible,[3] énigmatique, absurde, ironique.

▲ René Magritte: *Le Maître d'école,* 1954 (collection particulière, Genève)

[1]*unknown* [2]*conceives* [3]*unpredictable*

Note: Follow-up questions about this *Bienvenue* section are located in the Instructor's Manual.

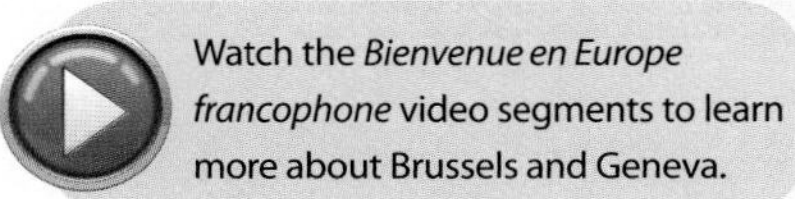

Watch the *Bienvenue en Europe francophone* video segments to learn more about Brussels and Geneva.

CHAPITRE 13

La vie quotidienne

Presentation: Ask sts. to describe what they see in the photo.

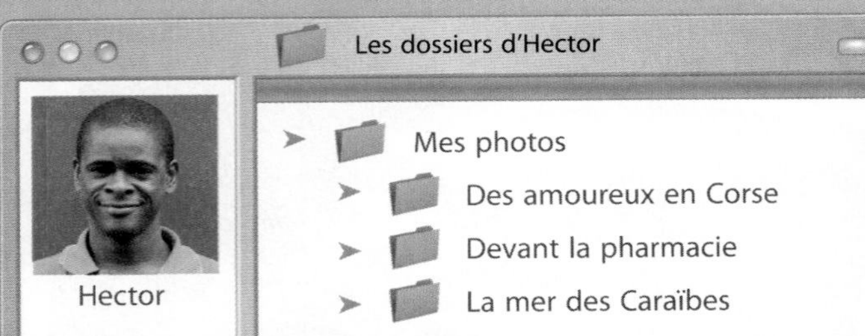

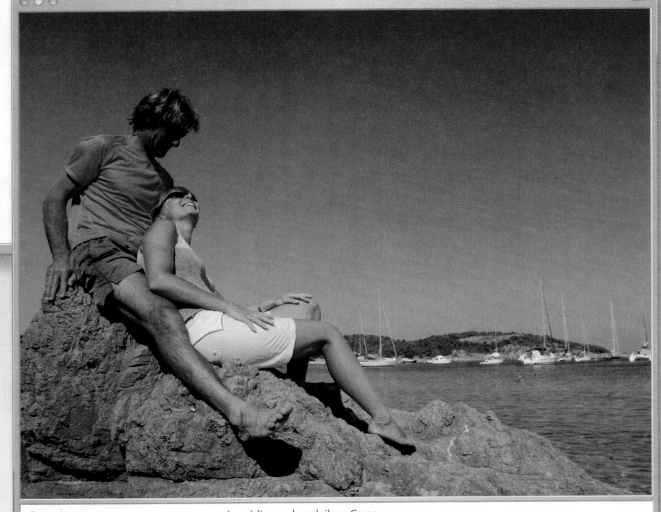

Deux jeunes amoureux passent un après-midi sous le soleil en Corse

Cultural note: The *Baie de Rondinara* is considered to be one of the best beaches in Europe. It is located on the southeastern coast of the island of Corsica, in the *Corse-du-Sud* department.

Dans ce chapitre...

OBJECTIFS COMMUNICATIFS

- talking about love, marriage, the human body, and daily life
- expressing actions
- reporting everyday events
- expressing reciprocal actions
- talking about the past
- giving commands
- learning to distinguish between and pronounce selected sounds in French

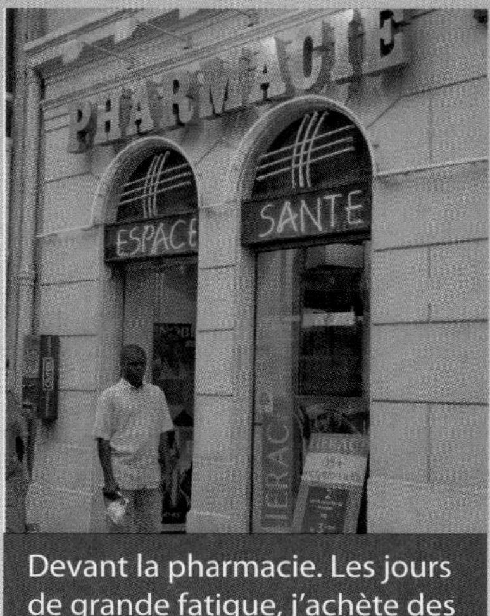

Devant la pharmacie. Les jours de grande fatigue, j'achète des vitamines.

PAROLES (Leçon 1)

- L'amour et le mariage
- Le corps humain
- Les activités de la vie quotidienne

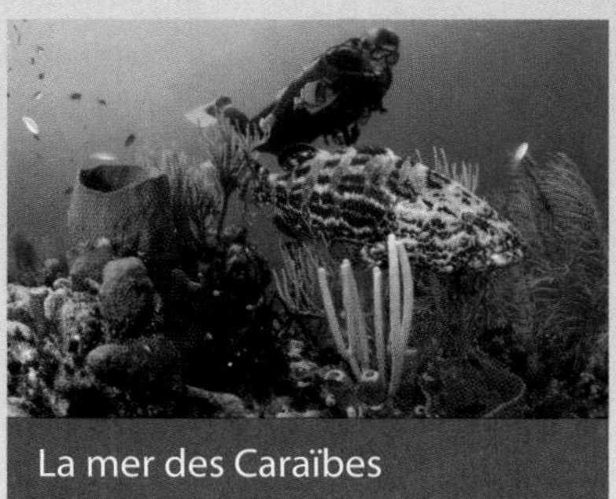
La mer des Caraïbes

STRUCTURES (Leçons 2 et 3)

- Les verbes pronominaux (première partie)
- Les verbes pronominaux (deuxième partie)
- Les verbes pronominaux (troisième partie)
- Les verbes pronominaux (quatrième partie)

CULTURE

- Le blog d'Hector: *Discipline!**
- Reportage: *La Martinique au quotidien*
- Lecture: «Pour toi mon amour» (poème de Jacques Prévert) (Leçon 4)

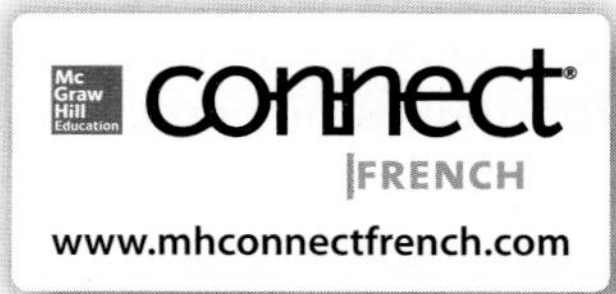

*In **Chapitres 13–16** you will read Hector Clément's blog about his life as a dancer, what he likes to do in his spare time, his efforts to find a new job, and his feelings about the problems of the world.

Leçon 1

PAROLES

L'amour et le mariage

1. Ils se rencontrent. Ils tombent amoureux.

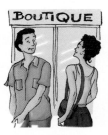

Les amoureux: le coup de foudre*

*****

2. Ils se fiancent.

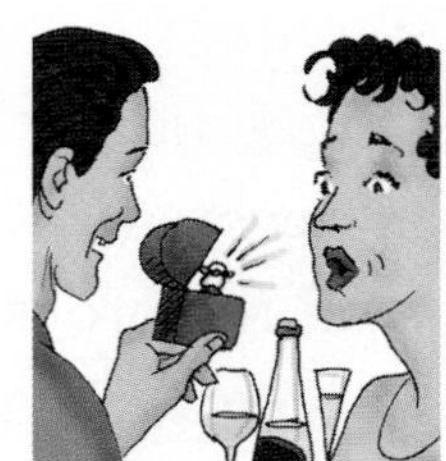

Le couple: les fiançailles (*f. pl.*)

*****

3. Ils se marient.

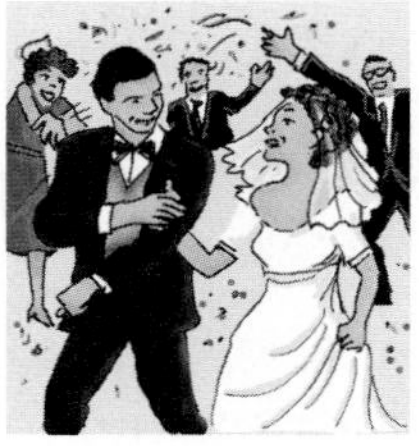

Le couple: la cérémonie

4. Mais ils ne s'entendent pas toujours.

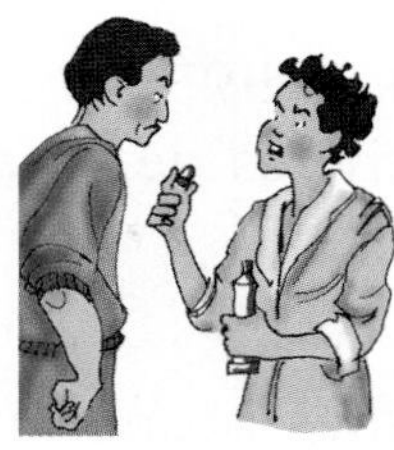

Les nouveaux mariés: parfois, ils se disputent.

Le parler jeune

draguer	essayer de séduire
un dragueur	un séducteur
être accro à	être incapable de vivre sans
être mordu	être amoureux
kiffer	adorer, être fou de
un rencard	rendez-vous

Moi, je ne **drague** pas: je parle d'amour.

Comment décourager un **dragueur**?

Je **suis accro à** Jérôme.

Pour la première fois de ma vie, je suis vraiment **mordu.**

Tu la **kiffes,** Léa?

Ce soir, j'ai un **rencard** avec Juliette.

Cultural note: Nowadays, many couples live together without being married. The following expressions are used to express this state: *cohabiter, être pacsé, vivre en couple, vivre ensemble, vivre en union libre.*

Follow-up: *Couples célèbres. Nommez un couple...* 1. *tragique* 2. *légendaire* 3. *comique* 4. *admirable* 5. *détestable* 6. *idéal* 7. *aventureux*

AUTRES MOTS UTILES

l'amitié (*f.*)	friendship
le/la célibataire	single person
divorcer	to divorce
le voyage de noces	honeymoon

Allez-y!

A. Pour commencer... Quelles phrases de la colonne de droite correspondent aux étapes traditionnelles qui précèdent le mariage?

**love at first sight* (lit., *flash of lightning*)

1. la rencontre
2. le coup de foudre
3. les rendez-vous
4. les fiançailles
5. la cérémonie
6. l'installation (*setting up house*)

a. Ils se marient.
b. Ils sortent ensemble.
c. Ils tombent amoureux.
d. Ils se rencontrent.
e. Ils s'installent.
f. Ils se fiancent.

Note: The verb *se fréquenter* is also used to express *sortir ensemble.*

Follow-up (B): Have sts. pretend they're at *une agence matrimoniale.* Directions: *Vous interviewez un jeune homme ou une jeune fille qui veut se marier. Quelles questions allez-vous lui poser pour pouvoir lui trouver le/la partenaire idéal(e)?* MODÈLE: *Quels sont vos défauts? Quelles sont vos qualités?*

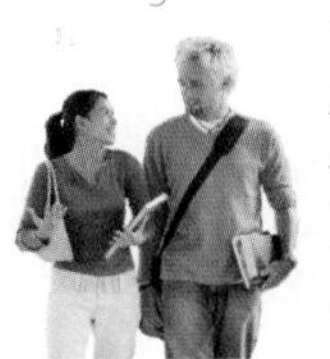

B. Conversation. Posez les questions suivantes à un(e) camarade.

1. Est-ce que tu préfères sortir seul(e), avec un ami / une amie ou avec d'autres couples?
2. Selon toi, est-ce que les jeunes d'aujourd'hui tombent trop vite ou trop souvent amoureux?
3. Est-ce que tu crois au coup de foudre? Pourquoi ou pourquoi pas?
4. Est-ce que tout le monde doit se marier? Pourquoi ou pourquoi pas? Si oui, à quel âge?

Suggestion: Ask sts. to describe their qualities, physical attributes, and likes/dislikes on a card. Collect cards to use as a source of candidates for the *agence matrimoniale* suggested as Follow-up (B).

Prononcez bien!

The vowels in *le* and *la*

Remember to make a clear distinction between [ə] in **le** and [a] in **la.** For **le,** pronounce a brief and tense sound while closing your mouth and rounding your lips. For **la,** open your mouth wide and stretch your lips in a semi-smile.

[ə]: **je, ne, me, de**

[a]: **passif, va, ça, ma**

Le corps humain

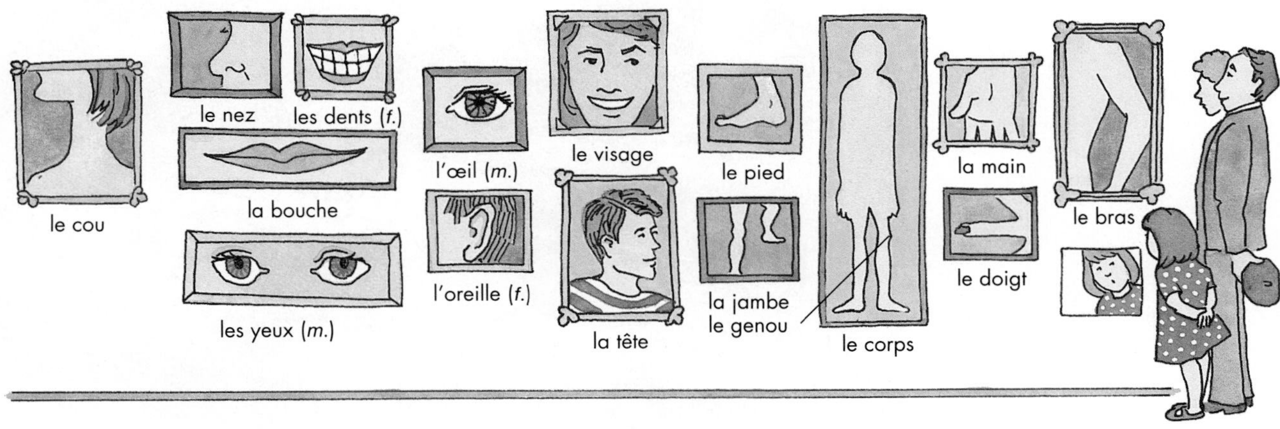

AUTRES MOTS UTILES

avoir mal (à)	to hurt, have a pain (in)
J'ai mal à la tête.	My head hurts. (I have a headache.)
le cœur	heart
le dos	back
la gorge	throat
la santé	health
le ventre	abdomen; stomach
être malade	to be sick

Pronunciation practice (1): Have sts. repeat the following words and precede each with the appropriate article. MODÈLE: *cou → le cou: main, visage, genou, bouche, jambe, nez, dent, pied, tête, corps.*

Pronunciation practice (2): The *Prononcez bien!* section on page 371 of this chapter contains additional activities for practicing these sounds.

Presentation: Model presentation for parts of body. Point to appropriate parts of body or use sketches or pictures from magazines as visual support.

Additional vocabulary: *la cheville, les cils* (*m.*), *la cuisse, l'épaule* (*f.*), les lèvres (*f.*), *le menton, les orteils* (*m.*), *le poignet, la poitrine, les sourcils* (*m.*).

Suggestion: Point out the expressions *avoir mal au ventre* (*to have a stomachache*) and *avoir mal au cœur* (*to feel sick*).

Note (A, 6): *Patrice* is a man's name in French.

Continuation (A): 11. *Martine a lu un livre pendant neuf heures.* 12. *Marc apprenait à faire du ski et il est tombé.* 13. *Vous êtes à un concert de rock et la musique est trop forte.*

Additional activities: (1) *Caractéristiques. Quelle est la caractéristique essentielle des personnages suivants?* MODÈLE: *un géant* → *Il a un très grand corps.* 1. *un vampire* 2. *une girafe* 3. *un cyclope* 4. *un éléphant* 5. *Cléopâtre* 6. *le loup du Petit Chaperon rouge.* (2) *Énigme. Trouvez la partie ou les parties du corps définie(s) par chaque phrase.* 1. *Elle sert à parler.* 2. *Elles servent à écouter.* 3. *Ils servent à faire une promenade.* 4. *Ils servent à regarder.* 5. *Elles servent à toucher.* 6. *Elles servent à manger.* 7. *Il sert à sentir.* 8. *Ils servent à jouer du piano.*

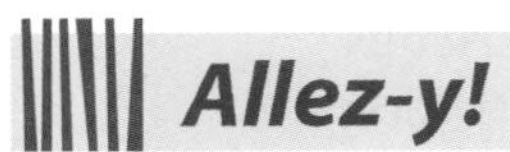

Allez-y!

A. Exercice d'imagination. Où ont-ils mal? Répondez d'après le modèle.

MODÈLE: Il y a beaucoup de bruit chez Judith. →
Elle a mal à la tête / aux oreilles.

1. Vous portez des colis très lourds (*heavy*).
2. Les nouvelles chaussures d'Aurélien sont trop petites.
3. J'ai mangé trop de chocolat.
4. Vous apprenez à jouer de la guitare.
5. Anouk a marché très longtemps.
6. La cravate de Patrice est trop serrée (*tight*).
7. Ils font du ski et il y a beaucoup de soleil.
8. Il fait extrêmement froid et vous n'avez pas de gants (*gloves*).
9. Aïcha va chez le dentiste.
10. Clément chante depuis deux heures.

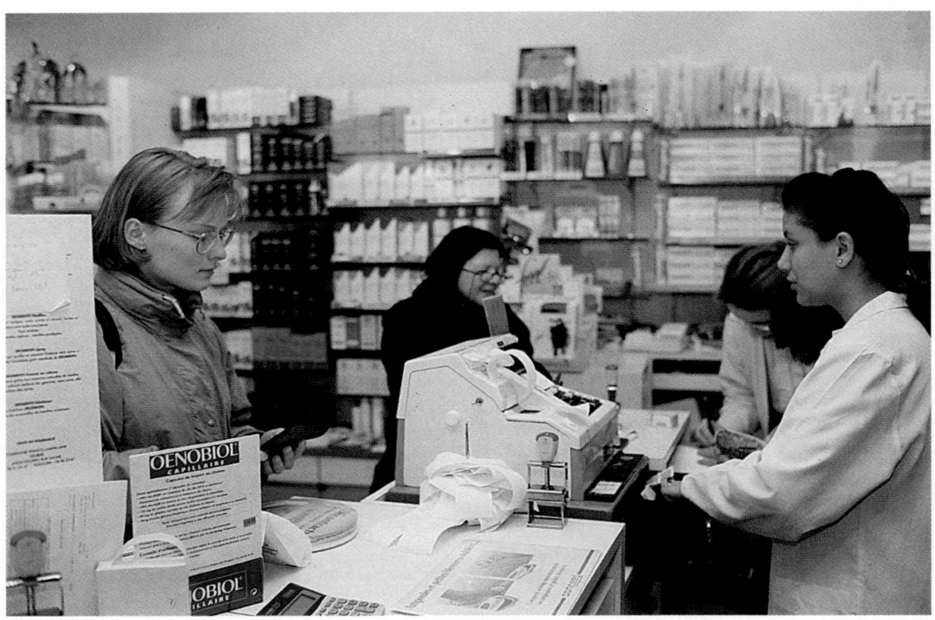

Une pharmacie française. Qu'est-ce que les clientes achètent? Pourquoi? Imaginez.

Suggestion: Play in groups of 4 or 5.

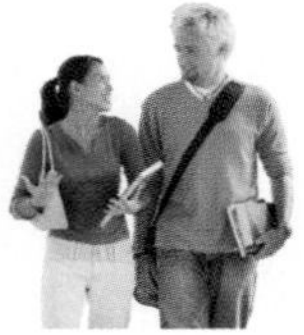

B. Devinettes. Pensez à une partie du corps et donnez-en une définition au reste de la classe. Vos camarades vont deviner de quelle partie il s'agit.

MODÈLE: Vous en avez une. On fait la bise avec cette partie du corps. →
C'est la bouche!

Les activités de la vie quotidienne

Suggestion: Display these illustrations from the e-Book or project similar images from the Internet to preview these verbs. Give the infinitive forms.

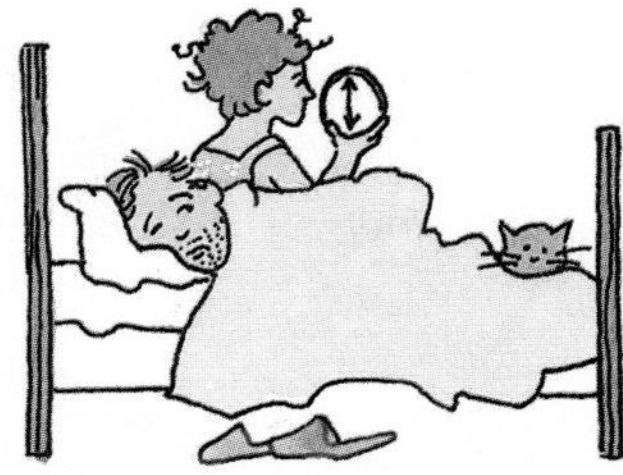

Ils se réveillent et ils se lèvent.

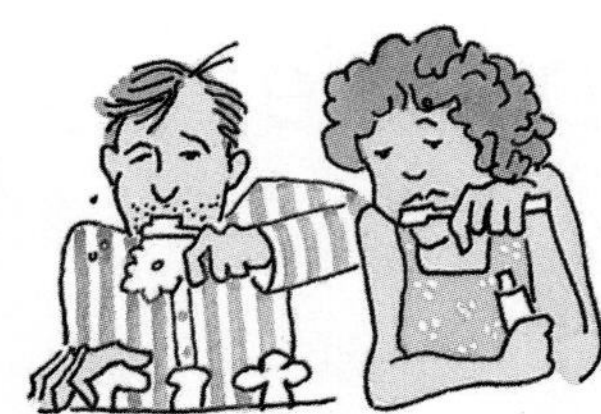

Ils se brossent les dents.

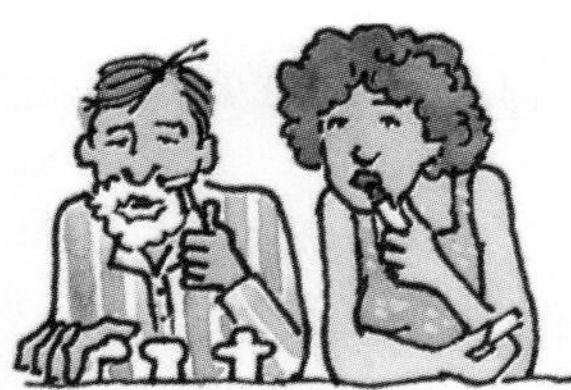

Il se rase et elle se maquille.

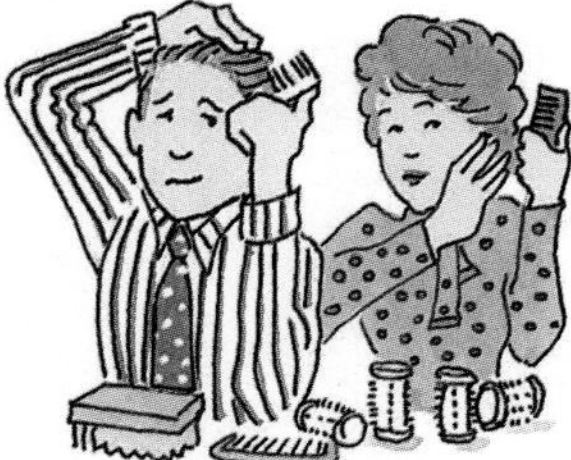

Ils se peignent.

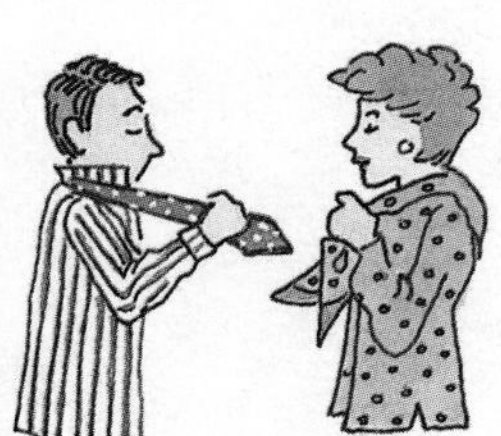

Ils s'habillent.

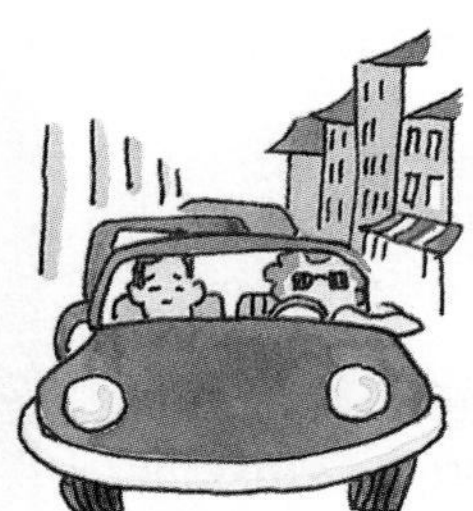

Ils s'en vont.

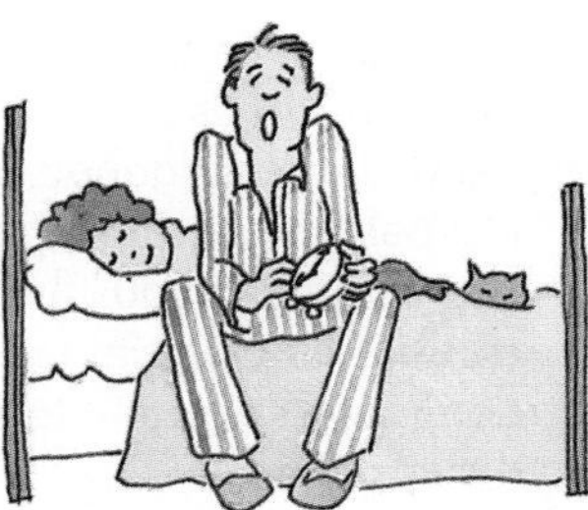

Ils se couchent.

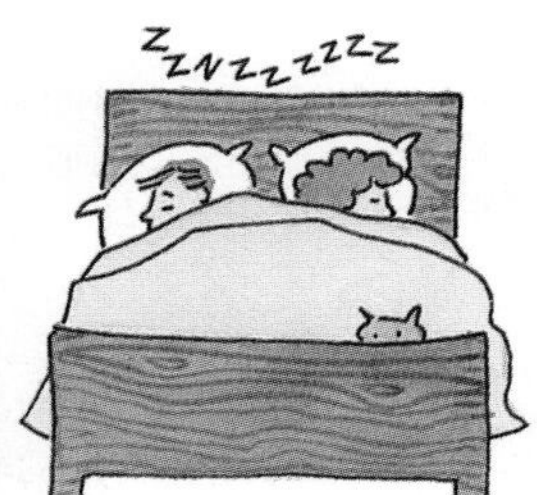

Ils s'endorment.

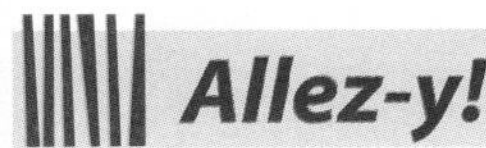

A. Et votre journée? Décrivez votre journée en employant le vocabulaire des illustrations.

Note: Pronominal verbs are explained in *Leçons 2* and *3;* for this ex., present *je me...*

MODÈLE: À ______ heures, je me ______. → À 7 heures, je me réveille.*

B. Habitudes quotidiennes. Dites dans quelles circonstances on utilise les objets suivants.

Mots utiles: se brosser, se coucher, s'en aller, s'endormir, s'habiller, se lever, se maquiller, se peigner, se raser, se réveiller

MODÈLE: une voiture → On utilise une voiture pour s'en aller.

1. un réveil
2. une brosse à dents
3. des vêtements
4. un lit
5. un peigne
6. du rouge à lèvres (*lipstick*)
7. un rasoir (*razor*)
8. un pyjama

*The verbs introduced here are called *pronominal verbs*. To conjugate the **je** form of pronominal verbs, place the pronoun **me** before the first-person conjugation of the verb.

Leçon 2

STRUCTURES

Les verbes pronominaux (*première partie*)

Expressing Actions

Allô, docteur?

Hector téléphone à Hassan.

HECTOR: Hassan, est-ce que tu as un bon médecin?
HASSAN: Excellent. Tu es malade?
HECTOR: J'ai très mal au genou. **Je me demande** si je n'ai pas une tendinite.
HASSAN: Prends rendez-vous! **Le cabinet médical se trouve**[1] au Quartier latin.
HECTOR: Comment **s'appelle le docteur**?
HASSAN: **Il s'appelle** Guy Levi. Il vient juste de **s'installer**.
HECTOR: Je n'ai peut-être pas besoin d'une consultation. Si **je me repose** pendant deux jours…
HASSAN: Quel raisonnement[2] infantile! **Dépêche-toi**[3] de lui téléphoner!
HECTOR: Tu viens avec moi? J'ai peur des piqûres[4]!

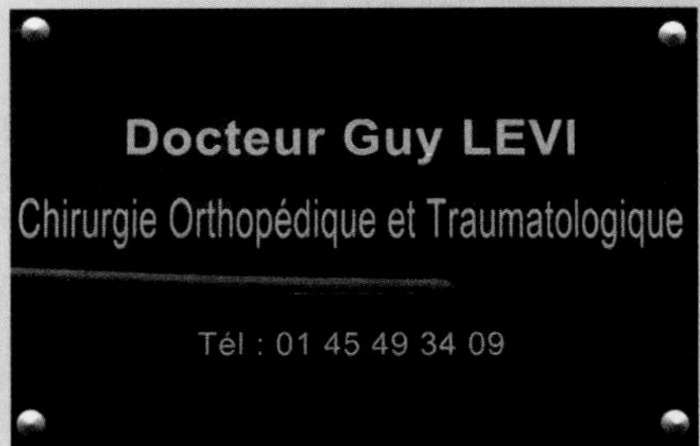

Heureusement, les médecins sont là pour nous soigner!

[1]Le… *the doctor's office is located* [2]*reasoning* [3]*Hurry up* [4]*injections*

Trouvez, dans le dialogue, les phrases qui répondent aux questions suivantes.

1. Quelle question se pose Hector (*does Hector ask himself*)?
2. Où est situé le cabinet médical?
3. Quel est le nom du docteur?
4. Est-ce que le médecin est dans le quartier depuis longtemps?
5. Hector ne veut pas voir le docteur. Quelle est sa solution? Que dit-il?
6. Qu'est-ce qu'Hassan ordonne (*recommend*) à Hector?

Presentation: Use pronominal verbs in list on p. 359 in short, personalized questions, asking several sts. the same question and having sts. remember the responses of classmates. Do a quick transformation ex., having sts. change affirmative verbs to negative or vice versa. *Je me trompe → Je ne me trompe pas*, etc.

Certain French verbs are conjugated with an object pronoun in addition to the subject; consequently, they are called *pronominal verbs* (**les verbes pronominaux**). The object pronoun agrees with the subject of the verb. **Se reposer** (*To rest*) and **s'amuser** (*to have fun*) are two pronominal verbs.

se reposer				s'amuser			
je	**me** repose	nous	**nous** reposons	je	**m'**amuse	nous	**nous** amusons
tu	**te** reposes	vous	**vous** reposez	tu	**t'**amuses	vous	**vous** amusez
il/elle/on	**se** repose	ils/elles	**se** reposent	il/elle/on	**s'**amuse	ils/elles	**s'**amusent

—Est-ce que tu **t'amuses** en général avec tes grands-parents? *Do you usually have fun with your grandparents?*
—Oui, on **s'amuse** bien ensemble. *Yes, we have a good time together.*

1. Note that the object pronouns **me, te,** and **se** become **m', t',** and **s'** before a vowel or a nonaspirate **h.**
2. Common pronominal verbs include:

s'amuser *to have fun*	**s'excuser** *to apologize*
s'appeler *to be named*	**s'installer** *to settle down, settle in*
s'arrêter *to stop*	**se rappeler** *to remember*
se demander *to wonder*	**se reposer** *to rest*
se dépêcher *to hurry*	**se souvenir (de)** *to remember*
se détendre *to relax*	**se tromper** *to make a mistake*
s'entendre (avec) *to get along (with)*	**se trouver** *to be located*

Où **se trouve** l'arrêt d'autobus? *Where is the bus stop?*
L'autobus **s'arrête** devant mon immeuble. *The bus stops in front of my building.*

3. Note that word order in the negative and infinitive forms follows the usual word order for pronouns: the object pronoun precedes the main verb.

Antoine ne **se souvient** pas à quelle heure le musée ouvre. *Antoine doesn't remember what time the museum opens.*
Je vais **me dépêcher** pour arriver à l'heure. *I'm going to hurry to arrive on time.*

Suggestion: Point out that the two pronouns represent the same subject.

Suggestion: Mention that although the infinitive of a pronominal verb is always preceded by *se,* to look up a verb in the dictionary, always look under the first letter of the verb itself.

Suggestion: Refer sts. to the Comprehensive Verb Charts posted at *Connect French* for conjugations of *se rappeler* and *s'appeler.*

Note: *Se souvenir* (conjugated like *venir*) is used with the preposition *de: Je me souviens de votre nom. Se rappeler* is generally used without it: *Je me rappelle son nom.*

Note: *Se tromper de* + noun: *Je me suis trompé de route* means *I took the wrong road.*

Suggestion: Read the following sentences aloud. Have sts. react to them using the negative of one pronominal verb. 1. *Je dis que 37 et 37 font 74.* 2. *Je ne suis pas en retard pour mon cours de français.* 3. *Martine et moi, nous nous disputons tout le temps.* 4. *Tu t'appelles Hervé?* 5. *La tour Eiffel est-elle à Strasbourg?* 6. *J'ai beaucoup de choses à faire ce week-end.*

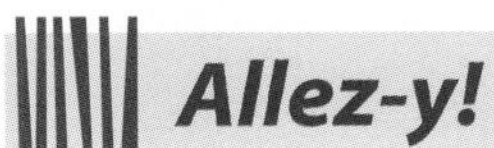

Allez-y!

A. Questions d'amour. Trouvez dans la colonne de droite une réponse logique aux phrases de la colonne de gauche.

1. Je dis que le mariage précède les fiançailles.
2. Demain c'est l'anniversaire de ma femme et je n'ai encore rien acheté.
3. Arthur et moi, nous nous disputons tout le temps. Nous travaillons trop et ne nous amusons jamais.
4. Quelle est la date de l'anniversaire de mariage de vos parents?
5. Toi et moi, nous aimons les mêmes choses! Nous ne nous disputons presque jamais.

a. Désolé(e), mais je ne m'en souviens plus.
b. Tu te trompes!
c. Oui, nous nous entendons bien.
d. Je me demande pourquoi tu n'y as pas pensé!
e. Il faut vous arrêter pour respirer un peu. Prenez le temps de vivre!

Suggestion (B): Ask sts. to work in pairs to complete the activity in writing and then check answers with the whole class.

B. Départ à la hâte. C'est l'heure de partir pour Chartres, mais vous avez un petit problème. Remplacez l'expression en italique par un des verbes pronominaux suivants: **se demander, se dépêcher, se rappeler, se tromper, se trouver.**

Où *est*[1] mon sac à dos? Je ne *me souviens*[2] plus où je l'ai mis. En plus, je dois *faire vite*[3], je suis en retard. Mais je ne peux pas aller à Chartres sans mon appareil photo. Je *veux savoir*[4] si Jean-François l'a mis dans sa valise. Il peut facilement *faire une erreur*[5] quand il est en retard.

Additional activity: *Réflexions sur la personnalité. Complétez les phrases suivantes. Puis comparez vos phrases avec celles de deux camarades de classe. Est-ce que vous vous ressemblez?* 1. *Je me dépêche quand...* 2. *Je ne m'entends pas du tout avec... parce que...* 3. *Quand je pense à mon enfance, je me rappelle surtout...* (nom) 4. *Je me demande souvent si...* 5. *Quand je me trompe, je...* 6. *Pour me détendre, j'aime...* Ask sts. to work in pairs to complete the activity in writing and then check answers with the whole class.

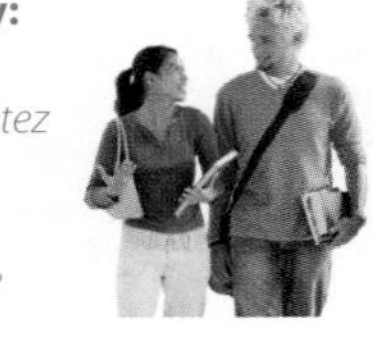

C. Trouvez quelqu'un qui... Circulez dans la classe pour trouver quelqu'un qui fait une des activités suivantes. Ensuite, trouvez quelqu'un qui fait l'activité suivante et ainsi de suite (*so on*).

1. veut s'installer à l'étranger
2. se souvient de son premier jour de classe à l'université
3. se trompe souvent dans ses calculs
4. se détend en regardant (*while watching*) des matchs de foot
5. s'entend bien avec ses frères ou ses sœurs
6. se repose en écoutant (*while listening*) de la musique classique
7. s'arrête tous les jours au café
8. se rappelle son meilleur ami / sa meilleure amie à l'école primaire

Les verbes pronominaux (*deuxième partie*)

Reporting Everyday Events

Tout va bien!

Léa téléphone à Hector.

LÉA: Alors Hector, **tu te sens**[1] mieux?
HECTOR: **Je me sens** très bien; je suis presque guéri[2]!
LÉA: Tu vois: parfois, **on se repose** pendant 24 heures et hop! **La douleur**[3] **s'en va**!
HECTOR: **Tu te trompes. Se détendre** ne suffit pas.[4] J'ai eu une piqûre de cortisone dans le genou... terrible... abominable!
LÉA: Oh! Pauvre Hector! Mais tu peux marcher[5] maintenant?
HECTOR: Je peux marcher, courir[6] et danser!
LÉA: Alors, on va **se promener**[7] ce soir?

Un anti-inflammatoire pour guérir Hector

[1]te... *feel* [2]*cured* [3]*pain* [4]ne... *isn't enough* [5]*walk* [6]*run* [7]se... *to take a walk*

Répondez aux questions selon le dialogue.

1. Hector se sent mieux?
2. Selon Léa, que faut-il faire pendant 24 heures pour aller mieux?
3. Selon Léa, après 24 heures de repos, qu'arrive-t-il?
4. Est-ce qu'Hector pense que Léa a raison ou qu'elle se trompe?
5. Quelle est la théorie d'Hector?
6. Que propose Léa?

Reflexive Pronominal Verbs

1. In reflexive constructions, the action of the verb reflects or refers back to the subject: *The child dressed* ***himself****. Did you hurt* ***yourself****? She talks to* ***herself****.* In these examples, the subject and the object are the same person. In French, common reflexive pronominal verbs include:

se baigner *to bathe; to swim*	**se maquiller** *to put on makeup*
se brosser *to brush*	**se peigner** *to comb one's hair*
se coucher *to go to bed*	**se raser** *to shave*
se doucher *to take a shower*	**se regarder** *to look at oneself*
s'habiller *to get dressed*	**se réveiller** *to wake up*
se laver *to wash oneself*	**se sentir** *to feel*
se lever *to get up*	

Zoé **se réveille** à 6 h. — *Zoé wakes up at 6:00.*
Théo **se douche** et **se rase** pendant que Sarah **se maquille.** — *Théo showers and shaves while Sarah puts on makeup.*

2. Most reflexive pronominal verbs can also be used nonreflexively.

Aujourd'hui, Théo **lave** la voiture. — *Today, Théo is washing his car.*
Le bruit **réveille** tout le monde. — *The noise wakes everyone up.*

3. Some reflexive pronominal verbs can have two objects, one direct and one indirect; this frequently occurs with the verbs **se brosser** and **se laver** plus a part of the body. The definite article—not the possessive adjective, as in English—is used with the part of the body.

Lisa se brosse **les** dents. — *Lisa is brushing her teeth.*
Je me lave **les** mains. — *I'm washing my hands.*

Presentation: Model forms of reflexive pronominal verbs using short sentences. Example: *Je m'habille vite le matin. Tu t'habilles à 7 h,* etc.

Note: See conjugation of *se laver* in Appendix B.

Vocabulary recycling: Take advantage of this opportunity to review various related lexical groups—times of day, sporting goods, clothing, rooms of the house, etc.: *Je me lève à 6 h. Et vous? De quoi a-t-on besoin pour se baigner? pour s'habiller? Je me rase. Où suis-je?,* etc.

Note: *Prendre une douche* is more common than *se doucher;* mention the expression *prendre un bain.*

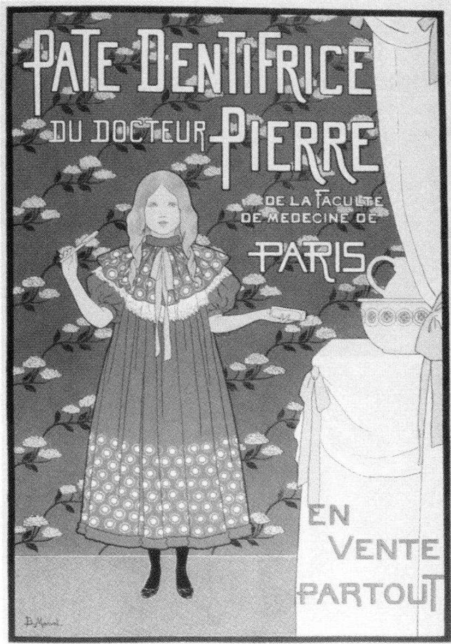

Mon dentifrice, c'est du Docteur Pierre. Et le vôtre?

Suggestion: Ask sts. to produce examples with the verbs listed.

Additional vocabulary: *bien se conduire / mal se conduire* (to behave / to misbehave), *s'habituer à* (to get used to), *se rendre compte (de)* (to realize), *se servir de* (to use).

Idiomatic Pronominal Verbs

When certain verbs are used with reflexive pronouns, their meaning changes.

aller *to go*	→	**s'en aller** *to go away*
appeler *to call*	→	**s'appeler** *to be named*
demander *to ask*	→	**se demander** *to wonder*
endormir *to put to sleep*	→	**s'endormir** *to fall asleep*
ennuyer *to bother*	→	**s'ennuyer** *to be bored*
entendre *to hear*	→	**s'entendre** *to get along*
fâcher *to make angry*	→	**se fâcher** *to get angry*
installer *to install*	→	**s'installer** *to settle in (to a new house)*
mettre *to place, put*	→	**se mettre à** *to begin*
perdre *to lose*	→	**se perdre** *to get lost*
promener *to (take for a) walk*	→	**se promener** *to take a walk*
tromper *to deceive*	→	**se tromper** *to be mistaken*
trouver *to find*	→	**se trouver** *to be located*

Mots clés

Vous parlez français?

You are now at a point where you can answer this question with something else besides **Un peu.** Here are some suggestions:

Je me débrouille. *(I can get by.)*
Oui, couramment.
Bien sûr! Je suis bilingue.

Suggestion: For listening comprehension practice, have sts. indicate whether they hear a pronominal or nonpronominal verb in each of these sentences. Have them write the verb they hear: 1. *Les jeunes mariés s'en vont à la plage.* 2. *Ils la trouvent magnifique.* 3. *Ils s'entendent très bien.* 4. *Martine se met à nager.* 5. *Marc met son maillot de bain.* 6. *Il se demande où est Martine.* 7. *Il entend sa voix.* 8. *Il la voit dans l'eau.* 9. *Il se lève pour aller se baigner avec elle.* This can also be used for a full dictation.

Les jeunes mariés **s'en vont** en voyage de noces.	*The newlyweds are going away on their honeymoon trip.*
Après cela, Véronique va **se mettre à** chercher un appartement.	*Afterward, Véronique is going to start looking for an apartment.*
Tu **te trompes**! Elle en a déjà trouvé un.	*You're wrong! She's already found one.*
Où est-ce qu'il **se trouve**?	*Where is it?*

Suggestion: Can be done as homework and checked during class, at the board, or by displaying the illustrations from the e-Book.

Allez-y!

A. La routine. Que font les membres de la famille Duteil?

Annick

MODÈLE: Annick se lave les mains.

Le matin...

1. Papy

2. 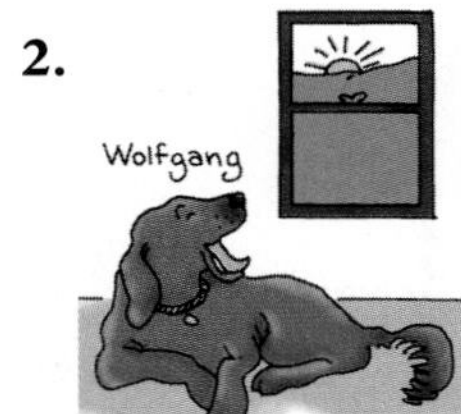

3. 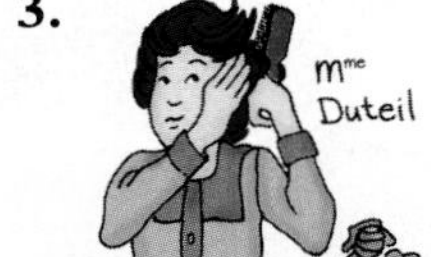
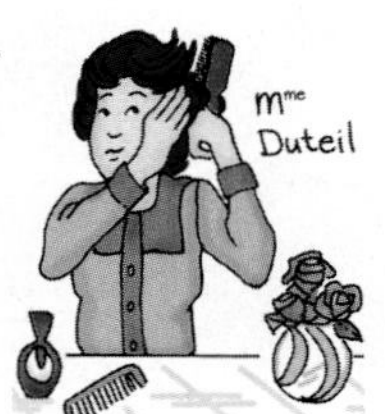

4. 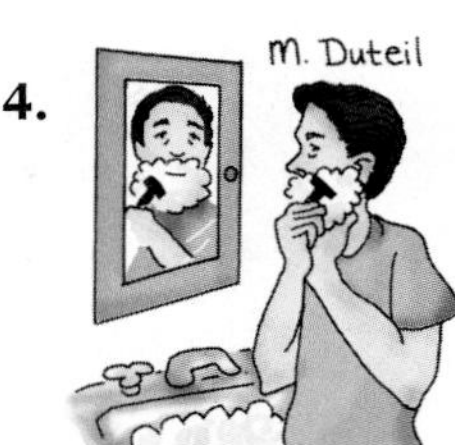

Plus tard...

5. 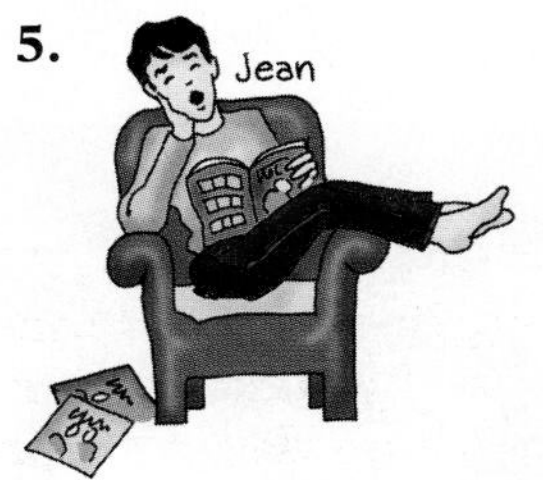

6. 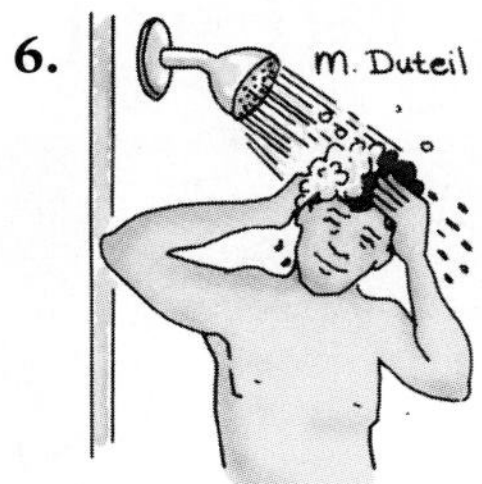

7. 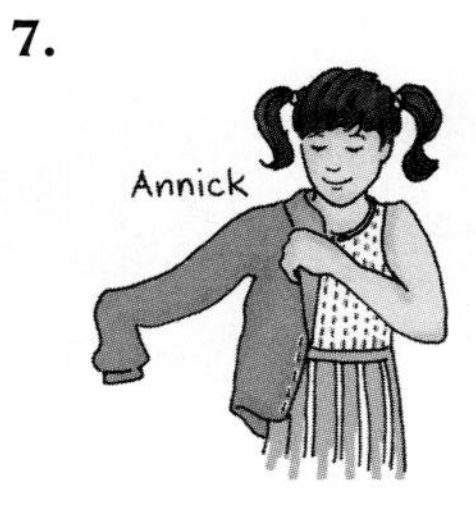

8. 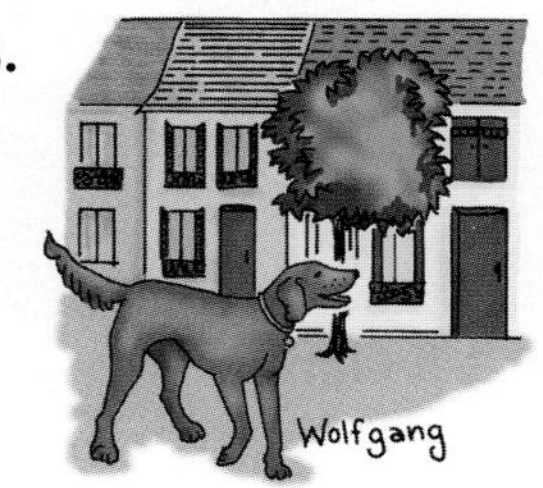

Et vous, parmi ces activités, lesquelles faites-vous régulièrement?

B. Habitudes matinales. Qui dans votre famille a les habitudes suivantes? Faites des phrases complètes. Puis comparez leurs habitudes aux vôtres (*to yours*). Commencez par «Moi aussi, je... » ou «Mais moi, je... ».

mon père	se regarder longtemps dans le miroir
ma mère	se lever souvent du pied gauche*
ma sœur	se réveiller toujours très tôt
mon frère	s'habiller rapidement / lentement
le chien	se maquiller / se raser très vite
le chat	se préparer à la dernière minute
	s'en aller sans prendre de petit déjeuner
	se laver les cheveux tous les jours
	se fâcher quand il n'y a plus de lait
	se tromper de chaussures

Suggestion (B): Can be assigned first as a written activity and then used for discussion.

Additional activities: (1) *La famille Martin. Tous les membres de la famille se couchent à une heure différente. À quelle heure se couchent-ils?* MODÈLE: *Sylvie Martin / 8 h 30 → Sylvie Martin se couche à huit heures et demie.* 1. *les grands-parents / 10 h* 2. *vous / 9 h 30* 3. *tu / 10 h 45* 4. *je / 11 h* 5. *nous / 11 h 15* 6. *M*[me] *Martin / 11 h 30.* 7. *M. Martin / minuit* 8. *Bernard / 1 h du matin*
(2) *Habitudes: Chacun a ses habitudes le matin. Faites des phrases complètes pour les décrire.* 1. *Sylvie / se regarder / longtemps / dans / le miroir* 2. *tu / se brosser / dents / avec / dentifrice (m.)* 3. *nous / se lever / du pied gauche* 4. *je / se réveiller / toujours / très tôt* 5. *Bernard et M. Martin / s'habiller / rapidement* 6. *vous / se préparer / tard / le matin*

C. Synonymes. Racontez l'histoire suivante. Remplacez l'expression en italique par un verbe pronominal.

À sept heures du matin, Sylvie *ouvre les yeux*,[1] elle *sort de son lit*,[2] *fait sa toilette*[3] (*washes up*) et *met ses vêtements*[4]. À huit heures, elle *quitte la maison*.[5] Au travail, elle *commence à*[6] parler au téléphone. Sylvie *finit de*[7] travailler vers 18 h; elle *fait une promenade*[8] et parfois ses amies et elle vont *nager*[9] à la piscine. Le soir, elle *va au lit*[10] et elle *trouve le sommeil*[11] très vite!

D. Interview. Interrogez un(e) camarade sur une de ses journées typiques à l'université. Posez-lui des questions avec les verbes **se réveiller, s'habiller, se dépêcher, s'en aller, s'amuser, s'ennuyer, se reposer, se promener** et **se coucher.** Ensuite, comparez votre journée et celle de votre camarade et présentez les résultats à la classe.

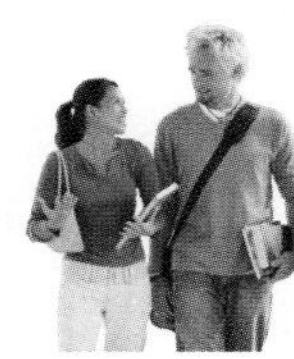

Suggestion (D): Notes taken during interviews can be used in a written composition describing classmate's daily routine, or the activity can be used as stimulus for a composition describing one's daily routine vs. a vacation schedule. If compositions are collected, use them for dictation or listening comprehension material.

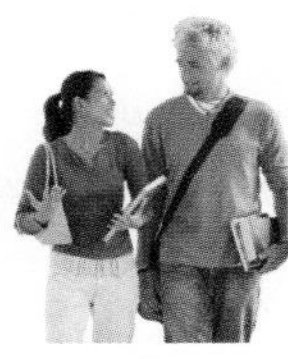

E. Vos habitudes. Comparez vos habitudes avec celles de vos camarades. Trouvez quelqu'un qui...

1. se lève dix minutes avant de partir
2. s'en va sans prendre de petit déjeuner
3. se réveille avant dix heures
4. se lève souvent du pied gauche
5. se promène souvent le soir
6. se douche avant de se coucher
7. se couche souvent après minuit
8. a souvent du mal à† s'endormir

*__Se lever du pied gauche__ is the equivalent of *to get up on the wrong side of the bed.*
†**Avoir du mal à** means *to have difficulty* (*doing something*). It should not be confused with **avoir mal à,** meaning *to have an ache or pain* (*in a part of the body*).

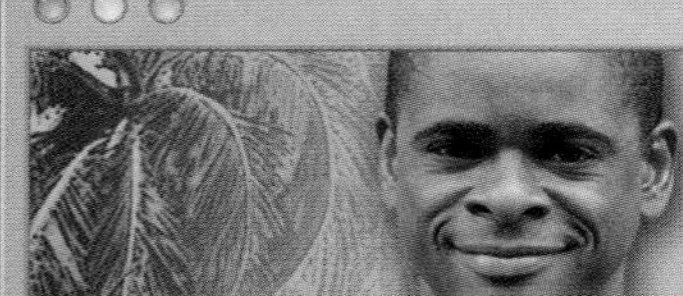

Le blog d'Hector

Discipline!

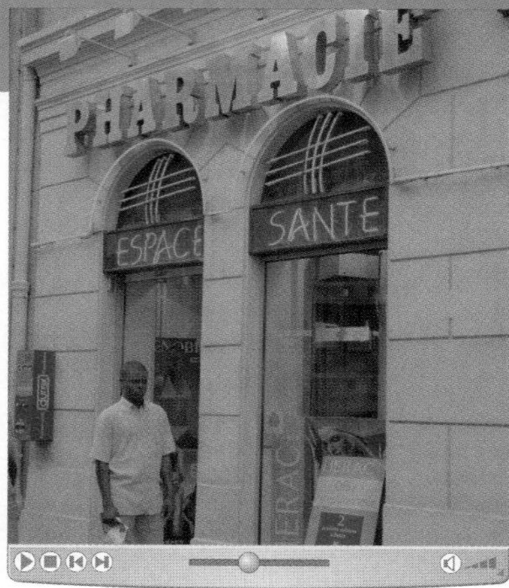

Devant la pharmacie. Les jours de grande fatigue j'achète des vitamines.

vendredi 3 juillet

Salut les amis!

Qui suis-je? Je suis Hector. Je commence mon blog.

Je suis danseur. Danseur, c'est un beau métier, n'est-ce pas? Mais il faut soigner[1] son corps, suivre un régime, avoir de la discipline…

Mes journées sont réglées[2]: je me réveille vers 10 heures. Je me lève, je prends ma douche et je me rase, puis je m'habille. Ensuite, je m'installe devant un petit déjeuner léger avec du thé, des fruits. Si mes colocataires sont là, on s'amuse et on se raconte notre vie! C'est bon pour le moral!

Vers midi, je commence mon entraînement[3] au studio de danse. Quand j'arrive, je mets immédiatement mon tee-shirt et mes collants,[4] puis je m'échauffe[5] seul avant le début du cours de ballet ou la répétition du spectacle.

Je danse jusqu'à 18 heures, mais je m'arrête régulièrement pour manger et pour boire: il faut renouveler[6] les calories et s'hydrater.

Ensuite, je me change et je rentre chez moi. Je me détends avant le spectacle ou je sors avec mes potes. Les jours de grande fatigue, j'achète des vitamines à la pharmacie. Et je retrouve mon énergie.

Elle est belle ma vie d'artiste! C'est vrai. Mais parfois, je désire tout changer et essayer d'autres modes de vie. Mon copain Hassan me parle souvent du Maroc et il me fait rêver…

Hector

Follow-up: 1. *Que savez-vous d'Hector? (Regardez sa carte d'identité, à la page 3.) À quelles occasions avez-vous entendu parler de ce jeune homme?* 2. *Résumez une journée typique d'Hector: quelle place réserve-t-il au travail? aux loisirs et à l'amitié? Présentez une de vos journées ordinaires.* 3. *Comment vivent Alexis, Trésor et Charlotte? Y a-t-il de la place pour la fantaisie et l'improvisation dans leur vie? Justifiez votre réponse.* 4. *Êtes-vous plus attiré(e) par la vie d'Alexis ou de Charlotte? Expliquez vos raisons.*

Video connection: In Hector's videoblog, he posts a segment on daily life in Morocco made by his friend Hassan.

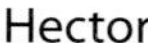

COMMENTAIRES

Alexis

Tout le monde a sa petite routine. Chaque jour, Trésor règle mon train-train.[7] Le matin, il m'appelle: ouah ouah! Impossible de me reposer! Le soir, après mes cours, je me dépêche de rentrer. Il se fâche si j'arrive tard!

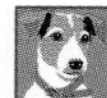

Trésor

Alexis, je m'ennuie tout seul à la maison!

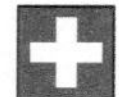

Charlotte

Ma routine est celle[8] d'une mère de famille: je me prépare très tôt le matin; j'accompagne ma fille Gilberte à l'école et je m'en vais au travail. Le soir, mon mari se débrouille[9] pour faire les courses. On se met à table vers 19 h et puis on s'installe devant la télé après avoir couché Gilberte. C'est pas très glamour, tout ça!

[1]*take care of* [2]*well-ordered* [3]*practice* [4]*tights* [5]*warm up* [6]*replenish* [7]*daily routine* [8]*that* [9]se… *manages*

REPORTAGE

La Martinique au quotidien° *daily life*

Vivre dans l'Hexagone[1] ou à la Martinique, est-ce réellement différent? Élisa, qui travaille à Fort-de-France, est catégorique: «Non, car la Martinique est un département d'outre-mer: elle fait partie du territoire français et fonctionne sous la loi[2] française. Ici, nous sommes en France; la vie quotidienne d'un Martiniquais est celle d'un Français du continent: le matin, tout le monde se lève pour aller travailler; les élèves[3] se dépêchent sur le chemin de l'école; les étudiants s'en vont à l'université; les magasins ouvrent[4] leur porte; les ménagères[5] font leurs courses.

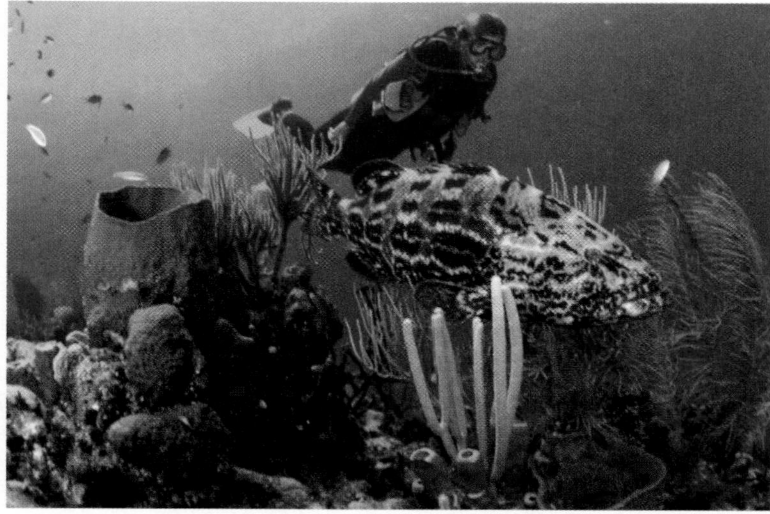

Débutant(e) ou certifié(e) en plongée libre (*snorkeling*) ou avec bouteille (*scuba diving*), vous pouvez découvrir les eaux cristallines et la faune (*animal life*) de la mer des Caraïbes. Vous êtes accueilli(e) par des bancs de poissons multicolores, des barrières de corail (*coral reefs*) intactes et des variétés d'organismes marins uniques.

Mais le week-end, on tire avantage[6] du climat tropical. Comme sur la Côte d'Azur, on reste dehors[7] pour profiter du soleil et de la chaleur.[8] On se promène dans les rues animées de Fort-de-France ou des petits villages cachés[9] dans l'île; on s'installe sur la plage, en famille et avec ses amis; on se repose, on s'amuse, on se baigne, on pique-nique.

Et le soir, on sort, comme à Paris, à Bordeaux ou à Marseille: on va au restaurant goûter quelques plats traditionnels ou manger… un hamburger! Et ensuite, on va au théâtre, au cinéma ou… en boîte. Les Martiniquais adorent la musique: jazz, rock, variétés françaises ou antillaises.

Comme la Guadeloupe, sa voisine,[10] la Martinique réunit[11] tous les ingrédients d'une vie quotidienne tout à fait[12] française sous le soleil des Caraïbes!

[1]*continental France (so called due to its shape)* [2]*law* [3]*pupils* [4]*open* [5]*housewives* [6]tire… *take advantage* [7]*outside* [8]*heat* [9]*hidden* [10]*neighbor* [11]*unites* [12]tout… *completely*

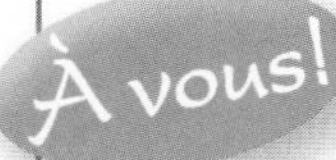

1. Est-ce qu'il y a une différence majeure entre le style de vie d'un Français du continent et d'un Français de la Martinique? Comment vivent-ils leur quotidien?
2. Présentez une journée typique de votre quotidien. Êtes-vous satisfait(e) de votre vie? Que voulez-vous changer?
3. Que faites-vous pour vous détendre? Faites-vous des sports nautiques comme le jeune homme sur la photo? Racontez.

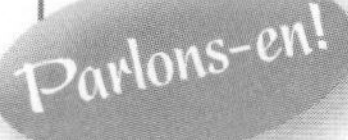

1. Nommez un(e) secrétaire chargé(e) d'écrire au tableau.
2. Quels mots associez-vous au mot «Martinique»? Donnez spontanément vos idées pendant que le/la secrétaire de la classe les enregistre au tableau (ex: «soleil»).
3. Avec tous ces mots, créez, en commun, un petit poème à la gloire de la Martinique.

Leçon 3

Les verbes pronominaux (*troisième partie*)

Expressing Reciprocal Actions

L'amour fou

Poema contacte Alexis sur sa page Facebook (Messagerie instantanée).

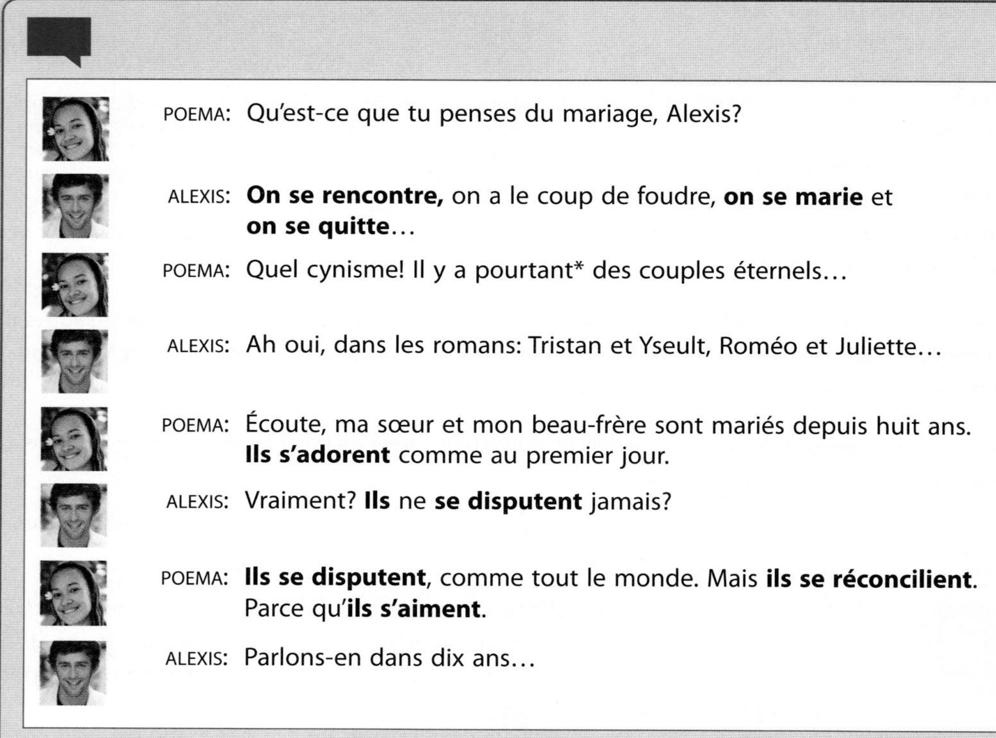

POEMA: Qu'est-ce que tu penses du mariage, Alexis?
ALEXIS: **On se rencontre,** on a le coup de foudre, **on se marie** et **on se quitte**…
POEMA: Quel cynisme! Il y a pourtant* des couples éternels…
ALEXIS: Ah oui, dans les romans: Tristan et Yseult, Roméo et Juliette…
POEMA: Écoute, ma sœur et mon beau-frère sont mariés depuis huit ans. **Ils s'adorent** comme au premier jour.
ALEXIS: Vraiment? **Ils** ne **se disputent** jamais?
POEMA: **Ils se disputent**, comme tout le monde. Mais **ils se réconcilient**. Parce qu'**ils s'aiment**.
ALEXIS: Parlons-en dans dix ans…

**nevertheless*

Répondez aux questions en utilisant les verbes du dialogue.

1. Que pense Alexis du mariage?
2. Que dit Poema sur la relation amoureuse de sa sœur et de son beau-frère?

The plural reflexive pronouns **nous, vous,** and **se** can be used to show that an action is reciprocal or mutual in which two or more subjects interact. Almost any verb that can take a direct or indirect object can be used reciprocally with **nous, vous,** and **se.**

Ils **se** rencontrent par hasard.	*They meet by chance.*
Ils **s'**aiment.	*They love each other.*
Allons-nous **nous** téléphoner demain?	*Are we going to phone each other tomorrow?*
Vous ne **vous** quittez jamais.	*You are inseparable* (*never leave each other*).
Vous **vous** disputez souvent?	*Do you argue often?*

Note: For reciprocal pronominal verbs, the *se* means *each other, one another.*

Suggestion: For listening comprehension practice, ask sts. to indicate whether they hear a pronominal or nonpronominal verb in the following sentences. Ask them to write the verb they hear. 1. *Marie et Marc se parlent pendant les vacances à la mer.* 2. *Marie dit: Dépêche-toi, Marc.* 3. *Marc: Je me brosse les dents.* 4. *Il continue: Tu t'es déjà habillée?* 5. *Marie: Oui, je me prépare vite!* 6. *Marc: Je m'excuse. Je suis en retard.* 7. *Marie: Embrasse-moi.* 8. *Elle continue: Ne nous disputons pas.* 9. *Ils se sourient* (smile). This passage can also be used as a full dictation.

Allez-y!

A. Une amitié sincère. Mme Chabot raconte l'amitié qui unit sa famille à la famille Marnier. Complétez son histoire au présent.

Suggestion (A): Give sts. a few minutes to write out this activity before correcting it with the whole class.

Éva Marnier et moi, nous ______[1] depuis plus de quinze ans. Nous ______[2] tous les jours et nous parlons longtemps. Nous ______[3] souvent en ville. Quand nous partons en voyage, nous ______[4] des cartes postales.

Nos maris ______[5] aussi très bien. Nos enfants ______[6] surtout pendant les vacances quand ils jouent ensemble. Parfois ils ______,[7] mais comme ils ______[8] bien, ils oublient vite leurs différends (*disagreements*).

s'aimer
se connaître
se disputer
s'écrire
s'entendre
se rencontrer
se téléphoner
se voir

B. Une brève rencontre. Racontez au présent l'histoire un peu triste d'un jeune homme et d'une jeune fille qui ne forment pas le couple idéal. Dites quand et où chaque action a lieu.

MODÈLE: se voir → Ils se voient un dimanche matin (au jardin du Luxembourg, à l'Opéra-Garnier, à la gare de Lyon)...

1. se voir
2. se rencontrer
3. se donner rendez-vous
4. se téléphoner
5. s'écrire souvent
6. se revoir
7. se disputer
8. (ne plus) s'entendre
9. se détester
10. se quitter

C. Rapports familiaux. Posez les questions suivantes à un(e) camarade de classe.

1. Avec qui est-ce que tu t'entends bien dans ta famille?
2. Tes parents et toi, quand est-ce que vous vous téléphonez?
3. Tes frères et sœurs et toi, combien de fois par semaine, par mois, par an est-ce que vous vous voyez?
4. Est-ce que tu te disputes souvent avec tes frères et tes sœurs? Quand et pourquoi vous disputez-vous?
5. Tes cousins et toi, est-ce que vous vous connaissez bien? Pourquoi ou pourquoi pas?

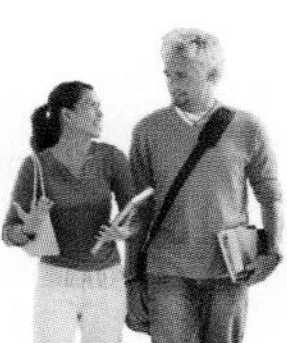

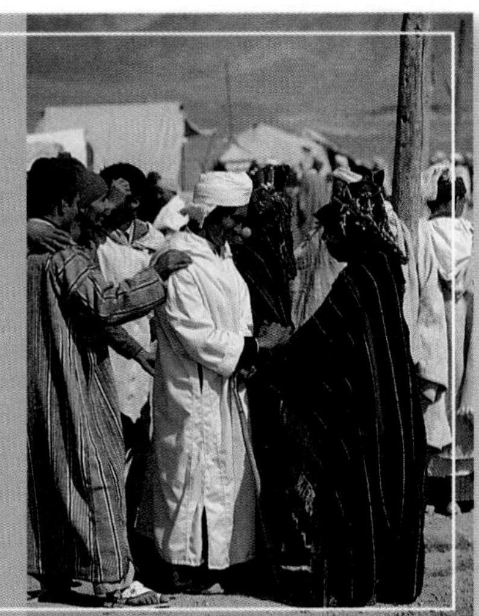

Un peu plus...

Les Berbères.
On retrouve les traces de ce groupe de peuple à diverses époques, de l'Égypte jusqu'à l'Atlantique et du Niger à la Méditerranée. Aussi loin qu'on remonte (*go back*) dans le passé, l'Afrique du Nord est occupée par ce peuple autochtone (*native*). Pasteurs (*Shepherds*), agriculteurs, ils vivaient divisés en tribus; la division reste un fait constant et essentiel de l'histoire berbère.

Des époux (married couple) berbères, au Maghreb. Comparez-les aux époux nord-américains.

Suggestion: Have two sts. read the dialogue aloud. Have others answer comprehension questions, using past-tense forms. For an inductive presentation, have sts. look at examples of past-tense formation and hypothesize about the rules before going over the grammar explanation.

Les verbes pronominaux (*quatrième partie*)

Talking About the Past and Giving Commands

Des petits mots d'amour

Appel vidéo entre Charlotte et Juliette.

CHARLOTTE: Tu es mariée, Juliette?
JULIETTE: Non. Et je ne suis même pas amoureuse!
CHARLOTTE: Moi **je me suis mariée** il y a 10 ans... J'avais 20 ans!
JULIETTE: **Vous vous êtes rencontrés** à la fac?
CHARLOTTE: **On s'est rencontrés** à la bibliothèque.
JULIETTE: **Vous vous êtes aimés** tout de suite?
CHARLOTTE: Pas du tout. **Ne t'imagine pas** que nous avons eu le coup de foudre! Je le trouvais prétentieux et autoritaire!
JULIETTE: Et alors, comment **ça s'est passé?**
CHARLOTTE: C'est inexplicable: **nous nous sommes** tellement **détestés** que nous avons fini par nous aimer!
JULIETTE: Ce sont les paradoxes de l'amour...

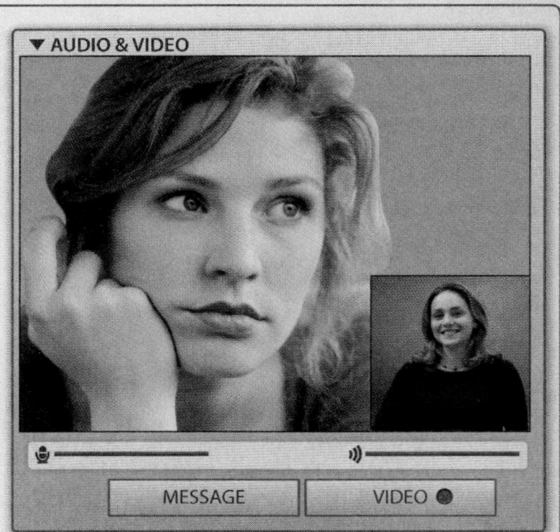

Répondez aux questions suivantes.

1. À quel âge Charlotte s'est-elle mariée?
2. Où Charlotte et son futur mari se sont-ils rencontrés?
3. Est-ce qu'ils se sont aimés tout de suite?

Passé composé of Pronominal Verbs

1. All pronominal verbs are conjugated with **être** in the **passé composé.** The past participle agrees with the reflexive pronoun in number and gender when the pronoun is the *direct* object of the verb.

Note: If you wish, explain structure and rules of agreement for pronominal verbs in *passé composé* where there is both a direct and an indirect object pronoun. Example: *Elle s'est brossé les cheveux. Elle se les est brossés.*

Suggestion: Model verbs in short sentences: *Je me suis baigné(e) dans la mer.*

PASSÉ COMPOSÉ OF **se baigner**			
je	me suis baigné(e)	nous	nous sommes baigné(e)s
tu	t'es baigné(e)	vous	vous êtes baigné(e)(s)
il	s'est baigné	ils	se sont baignés
elle	s'est baignée	elles	se sont baignées
on	s'est baigné(e)(s)		

Nous **nous sommes mariés** en octobre.	*We got married in October.*
Vos parents **se sont fâchés**?	*Did your parents get angry?*
Vous ne **vous êtes** pas **vus** depuis Noël?	*You haven't seen each other since Christmas?*

2. Here are some of the more common pronominal verbs whose past participles do not agree with the pronoun: **se demander, se dire, s'écrire, s'envoyer, se parler, se téléphoner.** The reflexive pronoun of these verbs is *indirect* (**demander à, parler à,** and so on).

Elles se sont **écrit** des textos.	*They wrote text messages to each other.*
Ils se sont **téléphoné** hier soir?	*Did they phone each other last night?*
Vous êtes-vous **dit** bonjour?	*Did you say hello to each other?*

[Allez-y! A-B-D]

Imperative of Pronominal Verbs

Reflexive pronouns follow the rules for the placement of object pronouns. In the affirmative imperative, they follow and are attached to the verb with a hyphen; **toi** is used instead of **te.** In the negative imperative, reflexive pronouns precede the verb.

AFFIRMATIVE		NEGATIVE	
Lève-**toi.**	*Get up.*	Ne **te** lève pas.	*Don't get up.*
Dépêchons-**nous.**	*Let's hurry.*	Ne **nous** dépêchons pas.	*Let's not hurry.*
Habillez-**vous.**	*Get dressed.*	Ne **vous** habillez pas.	*Don't get dressed.*

[Allez-y! C]

Grammaire interactive

For more on pronominal verbs, watch the corresponding Grammar Tutorial and take a brief practice quiz at **Connect French.**

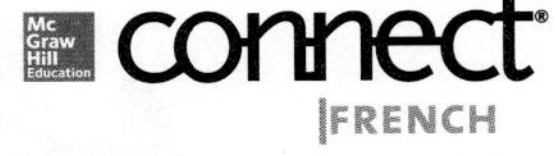

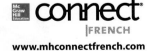

www.mhconnectfrench.com

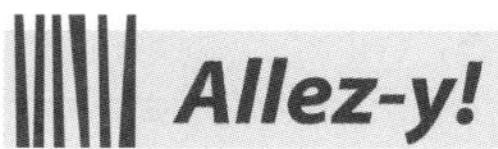

Suggestion: Give sts. a few minutes to write out this activity before correcting it with the whole class.

Additional activity: *Après la soirée. Chacun s'est couché à une heure différente.* MODÈLE: *Sylvie / 11 h → Sylvie s'est couchée à onze heures.* 1. *vous / 11 h 30* 2. *nous / 11 h 45* 3. *tu / 12 h* 4. *Christine / 12 h 35* 5. *je / 1 h 15* 6. *Fabrice et David / 1 h 20*

A. Avant la soirée. Hier, il y avait une fête à la Maison des Jeunes (*youth center*). Décrivez les activités de ces jeunes gens. Faites des phrases complètes au passé composé.

MODÈLE: Fabien / se raser / avant de partir →
Fabien s'est rasé avant de partir.

1. Fabrice / s'habiller / avec soin (*care*)
2. Christine et toi, vous / se reposer
3. Nadia et Thomas / s'amuser / à écouter de la musique
4. Sylvie / s'endormir / sur le canapé
5. David et moi, nous / s'installer / devant la télévision
6. je / se promener / dans le jardin

B. Souvenirs. Rebecca retrouve un vieil album de photos. Lisez son histoire, puis racontez-la au passé composé.

MODÈLE: Rebecca s'interroge sur son passé. →
Rebecca s'est interrogée sur son passé.

1. Elle s'installe pour regarder son album de photos. **2.** Elle s'arrête à la première page. **3.** Elle se souvient de son premier amour. **4.** Elle ne se souvient pas de son nom. **5.** Elle se trompe de personne. **6.** Elle se demande où il est aujourd'hui. **7.** Elle s'endort sur la page ouverte.

Mots clés

Dire à quelqu'un de partir

When you want to tell someone in a firm way that he/she should leave, use the following expression.

Va-t'en! (Allez-vous-en!) *Get going!; Go away!*

C. Un rendez-vous difficile. Bruno a rendez-vous avec quelqu'un qu'il ne connaît pas. Il est très nerveux. Donnez-lui des conseils et utilisez l'impératif.

MODÈLE: Je ne *me suis* pas encore *préparé.* (vite) →
Prépare-toi vite!

1. À quelle heure est-ce que je dois *me réveiller*? (à 5 h)
2. Je n'ai pas envie de *m'habiller.* (tout de suite)
3. Je ne *me souviens* pas de la rue. (rue Mirabeau)
4. J'ai peur de *me tromper.* (ne... pas)
5. Je dois *m'en aller* à 6 h. (maintenant)

Maintenant, utilisez **vous.**

MODÈLE: Je ne *me suis* pas encore *préparé.* (vite) →
Préparez-vous vite!

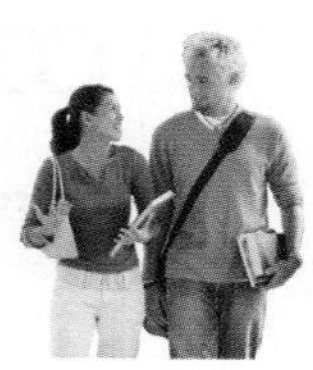

D. Tête-à-tête. Posez les questions suivantes à un(e) camarade. Ensuite, faites une observation intéressante sur votre camarade.

1. Est-ce que tu t'entends bien avec tes amis? avec tes professeurs? avec tes camarades de chambre? (Si votre camarade ne s'entend pas bien avec eux, demandez-lui pourquoi.)
2. Tu as déjà rencontré une personne qui t'a beaucoup impressionné(e)? Comment s'appelle cette personne? De quels traits physiques (yeux, visage, cheveux, taille, et cetera) te souviens-tu?
3. Est-ce que tu te rappelles le moment où tu es tombé(e) amoureux/amoureuse pour la première fois? C'était à quel âge, et avec qui? Ça a été le coup de foudre? C'était l'amour?
4. Tu veux te marier un jour? À quel âge? Où est-ce que tu veux t'installer avec ton mari (ta femme)?

Additional activity: Have sts. recount where, when, and how a couple they know first met.

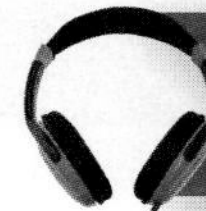

Prononcez bien!

The vowels in *le* and *la* (page 355)

A. Mariage. Hugo est allé à un mariage ce week-end. Il montre les photos à Isabelle. Écoutez ce qu'ils disent et choisissez l'option appropriée.

ISABELLE: Oh! _____[1] a l'air très jeune!
HUGO: Oui, _____[2] aussi: Ils ont tous les deux 22 ans.
ISABELLE: Qui est cette personne?
HUGO: C'est _____[3] de l'ami(e) de mon frère.
ISABELLE: Et où est _____[4]?
HUGO: Là… Ça, c'est une photo de tous les célibataires qui étaient au mariage. _____[5] à gauche des mariés a rencontré _____[6] à leur droite. Ça a été le coup de foudre. Ah! Il y avait beaucoup d'amour dans l'air ce jour-là!

1. a. La mariée **b.** Le marié
2. a. la mariée **b.** le marié
3. a. la fiancée **b.** le fiancé
4. a. la fiancée **b.** le fiancé
5. a. la célibataire **b.** le célibataire
6. a. la célibataire **b.** le célibataire

Script (A): *ISABELLE: Oh! Le marié a l'air très jeune! HUGO: Oui, la mariée aussi : Ils ont tous les deux 22 ans. ISABELLE: Qui est cette personne ? HUGO: C'est la fiancée de l'ami(e) de mon frère. ISABELLE: Et où est le fiancé? HUGO: Là … Ça, c'est une photo de tous les célibataires qui étaient au mariage. Le célibataire à gauche des mariés a rencontré la célibataire à leur droite. Ça a été le coup de foudre. Ah! Il y avait beaucoup d'amour dans l'air ce jour-là!*

Answers (A): 1. b 2. a 3. a 4. b 5. b 6. a

B. Le jeu de la description. Vous êtes chez le médecin avec votre ami(e). Sur les murs, il y a des dessins représentant des personnes avec des traits physiques particuliers. Complétez les phrases suivantes à voix haute en utilisant les articles **le** ou **la** et les parties du corps. Faites bien attention à la forme des adjectifs. Votre camarade va identifier le dessin que vous décrivez.

a.

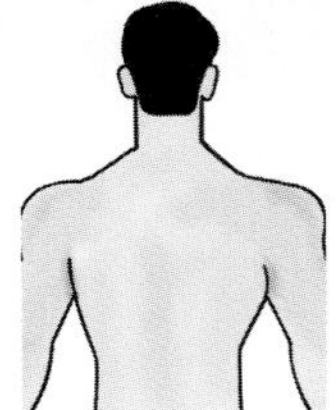

c.

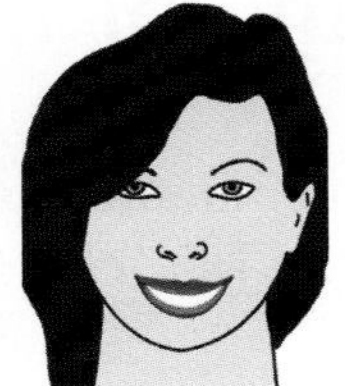

b.

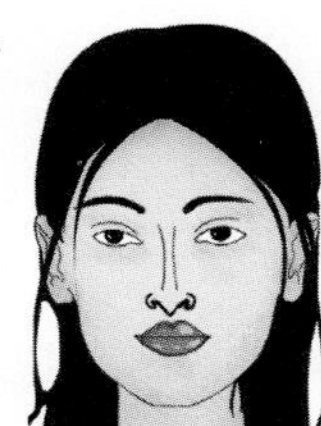

d.

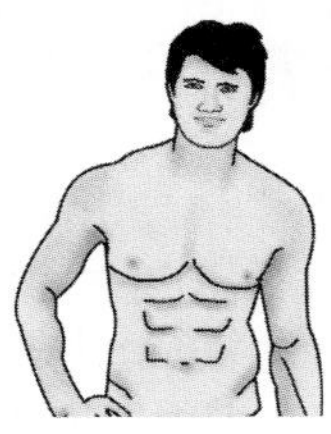

1. La personne dans ce dessin a _____ plat(e) (*flat*) et _____ très rond(e).
2. La personne dans ce dessin a _____ pointu et _____ pulpeux(se) (*fleshy*).
3. La personne dans ce dessin a _____ très long(ue) et _____ très large (*wide*).
4. La personne dans ce dessin a _____ souriant(e) (*smiling*) et _____ large.

Answers (B): 1. d. *le ventre plat, la tête très ronde* 2. b. *le nez pointu, la bouche pulpeuse* 3. a. *le cou très long, le dos très large* 4. c. *le visage souriant, le cou large*

Leçon 4

À propos de la lecture...
Ce poème est tiré du recueil *Paroles* (1946) par Jacques Prévert.

Lecture

Avant de lire

Scanning (Part 2). As noted in **Chapitre 4**, it is helpful to scan a text for specific information before you read it. Scanning is a reading skill that readers use almost every day. The overview you receive from scanning allows you to understand the text better during the first, more thorough reading. Scan the poem to determine the following:

1. *Tense:* Which verb tense is used the most often? What expression is repeated several times?
2. *Structure of the poem:* Which lines are the longest? How do they differ from each other?
3. *Objects:* How many gifts does the author buy for his love? What are those gifts?
4. *Narrative style of the poem:* Is the narrator speaking directly to his love or is he talking about her? How do you know?

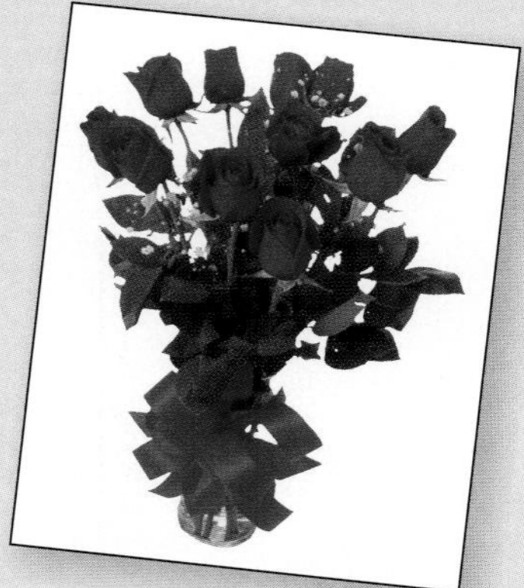

«Pour toi mon amour»

Je suis allé au marché aux oiseaux
Et j'ai acheté des oiseaux
Pour toi
mon amour
Je suis allé au marché aux fleurs
Et j'ai acheté des fleurs
Pour toi
mon amour
Je suis allé au marché à la ferraille[1]
Et j'ai acheté des chaînes
De lourdes chaînes
Pour toi
mon amour
Et puis je suis allé au marché aux esclaves[2]
Et je t'ai cherchée
Mais je ne t'ai pas trouvée
mon amour

[1]*scrap iron, metal* [2]marché... *slave market*

Compréhension

1. Quels cadeaux le poète a-t-il achetés pour son amour?
2. À votre avis, qu'est-ce que chaque cadeau symbolise?
3. Pourquoi est-ce que le poète n'a pas trouvé son amour à la fin du poème?
4. Quel commentaire fait le poète sur les relations entre les hommes et les femmes?

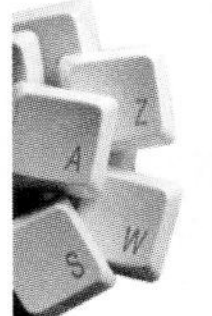

Écriture

The writing activities **Par écrit** and **Journal intime** can be found in the Workbook/Laboratory Manual to accompany *Vis-à-vis*.

La vie en chantant. An activity based on the song "Mon cœur, mon amour" by Anaïs (Croze) can be found in the Instructor's Manual. The song can be purchased at the iTunes store, or sts. can watch the music video on YouTube.

Pour s'amuser

LE MARI: On est mariés depuis cinq ans, et on n'est jamais arrivés à être d'accord sur quelque chose.

LA FEMME: Tu as tort, on est mariés depuis six ans.

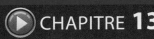

Le vidéoblog d'Hector

En bref

Dans cet épisode, Hassan rencontre Hector devant une pharmacie. Comme Hector ne se sent pas bien, Hassan lui suggère de modifier sa façon de vivre. Il évoque «l'art de vivre» au Maroc.

Vocabulaire en contexte

Qu'est-ce que vous faites pour maintenir (*maintain*) votre santé physique et mentale? Indiquez vos préférences.

- ☐ prendre des **médicaments** (*medications*)
- ☐ ne pas trop **faire la fête** (*to party*)
- ☐ s'arrêter dans un café, un salon de thé
- ☐ boire des jus de fruits
- ☐ se coucher tôt et dormir huit heures
- ☐ prendre des **vitamines**
- ☐ se promener
- ☐ faire du sport, de la gym
- ☐ s'amuser avec des amis
- ☐ **économiser** (*to save, conserve*) son énergie

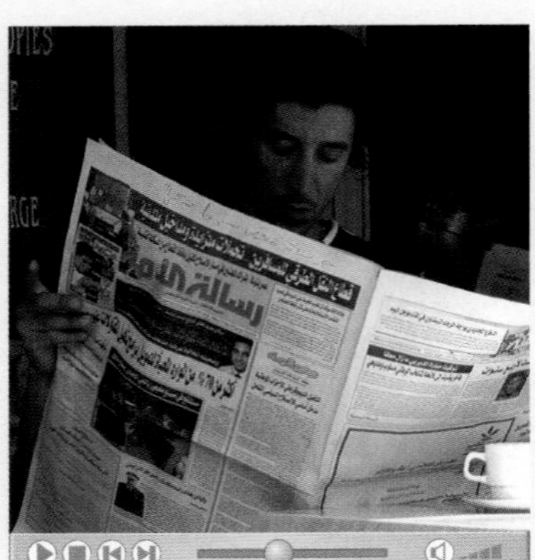

Un Marocain lit le journal le matin au café à Marrakech, au Maroc.

Suggestion: Ask sts. which activities relate more to physical health and which to mental health. Based on the activities they chose, do they tend to think/care more about physical or mental health? To solidify their knowledge of the terms, have sts. create full sentences with *Je* and conjugated verbs.

Additional vocabulary: Other vocabulary you may wish to present before viewing includes *avoir mauvaise mine, avoir du mal à s'endormir, être enrhumé, éternuer, se moucher, être en forme.*

Visionnez!

Choisissez la bonne réponse.

1. Hector se sent fatigué parce qu'il ______.
   a. **s'entraîne** (*practice*) beaucoup **b.** fait trop la fête
2. Hassan lui conseille ______.
   a. de consulter un médecin **b.** d'aller se détendre à la campagne
3. Hassan est content parce qu'il ______ cette semaine.
   a. a du **temps libre** (*free time*) **b.** ferme son restaurant
4. Hassan **trouve que** (*thinks that*) la vie au Maroc est plus (*more*) ______ qu'à Paris.
   a. agréable et **douce** (*gentle*) **b.** ennuyeuse

Analysez!

Répondez aux questions.

1. Quels sont les éléments de «l'art de vivre» au Maroc? Que fait-on, par exemple, pour se détendre le matin, l'après-midi et le soir?
2. À votre avis, est-ce que le climat a une très grande influence sur l'art de vivre au Maroc? Expliquez.

Comparez!

Quels sont les critères de qualité de vie (une vie agréable, douce) dans votre pays? Selon cette définition, avez-vous vous-même une bonne qualité de vie? Regardez encore une fois la partie culturelle de la vidéo: préférez-vous l'art de vivre *à l'américaine* ou *à la marocaine*? Expliquez.

Note culturelle

En France, on distingue les pharmacies des parapharmacies. Les premières sont autorisées à distribuer des médicaments sur présentation d'une ordonnance[1] et à proposer des équivalents génériques. Elles vendent aussi des médicaments accessibles sans ordonnance (ex: l'aspirine) et des produits de santé (ex: un thermomètre). Signalées par une grande croix verte,[2] elles sont, pour certaines, ouvertes[3] la nuit. Les parapharmacies ne peuvent pas vendre de médicaments. Elles distribuent des produits de confort et de beauté (ex: les produits de toilette pour les bébés et pour les femmes). À noter: la publicité pour les médicaments est interdite par la loi.[4]

[1]*prescription* [2]croix... *green cross* [3]*open* [4]interdite... *prohibited by law*

Vocabulaire

Verbes

s'amuser (à) to have fun
s'appeler to be named
s'arrêter to stop
avoir mal (à) to have pain; to hurt
se baigner to bathe; to swim
se brosser (les cheveux, les dents) to brush (one's hair, one's teeth)
courir to run
se coucher to go to bed
se débrouiller to manage
se demander to wonder
se dépêcher to hurry
se détendre to relax
se disputer to argue
divorcer to divorce
se doucher to take a shower
s'embrasser to kiss
s'en aller to go away, go off (*to work*)
s'endormir to fall asleep
s'ennuyer to be bored
s'entendre (avec) to get along (with)
s'excuser to apologize
se fâcher to get angry
se fiancer to get engaged
s'habiller to get dressed
s'installer to settle down, settle in
se laver to wash oneself
se lever to get up
se maquiller to put on makeup
marcher to walk
se marier (avec) to get married (to)
se mettre à (+ *inf.*) to begin to (*do something*)
se peigner to comb one's hair
se perdre to get lost
se préparer to get ready
se promener to take a walk
se rappeler to remember
se raser to shave
se regarder to look at oneself, at each other
se rencontrer to meet
se reposer to rest
se réveiller to awaken, wake up
se souvenir (de) to remember
tomber amoureux / amoureuse (de) to fall in love (with)
se tromper to make a mistake
se trouver to be located

Substantifs

l'amitié (*f.*) friendship
l'amour (*m.*) love
l'amoureux / l'amoureuse lover, sweetheart
la bouche mouth
le bras arm
la brosse brush
  la brosse à cheveux hairbrush
  la brosse à dents toothbrush
le cabinet médical doctor's office
le/la célibataire single person
la cérémonie ceremony
le cœur heart
le corps body
le cou neck
le coup de foudre flash of lightning; love at first sight
le couple (engaged, married) couple
la dent tooth
le doigt finger
le dos back
la douleur pain
les fiançailles (*f. pl.*) engagement
le genou knee
la gorge throat
la jambe leg
la main hand
le mariage marriage
le nez nose
les nouveaux mariés (*m. pl.*) newlyweds
l'œil (*m.*) **(les yeux)** eye(s)
l'oreille (*f.*) ear
les pantoufles (*f.*) slippers
le peigne comb
le pied foot
la piqûre injection, shot
le rasoir razor
la rencontre meeting, encounter
le rendez-vous date
le rouge à lèvres lipstick
la santé health
la tête head
le ventre abdomen; stomach
le visage face
le voyage de noces honeymoon

À REVOIR: **les cheveux** (*m. pl.*), **le réveil**

Adjectifs

amoureux / amoureuse loving, in love
guéri(e) cured, healed
malade sick
quotidien(ne) daily, everyday

Mots et expressions divers

Allez-vous-en! Go away!
Va-t'en! Go away!

CHAPITRE 14

Sur le marché du travail

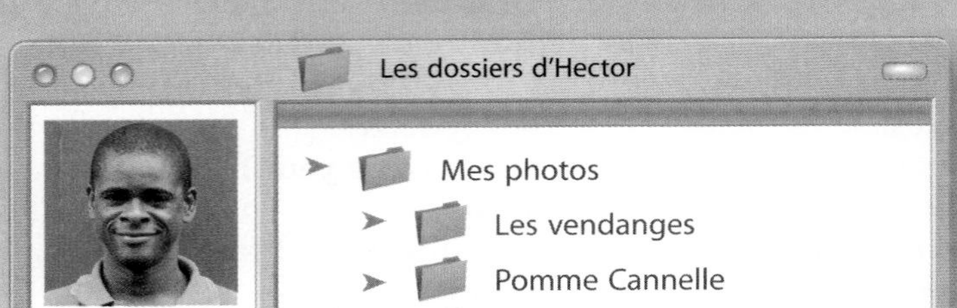

Presentation: *Décrivez les vêtements des deux hommes. Décrivez ce qu'ils ont fait ce matin avant de venir au vignoble. Où est-ce qu'on produit du raisin? Dans quelles régions produit-on du vin en France? Et dans votre pays?*

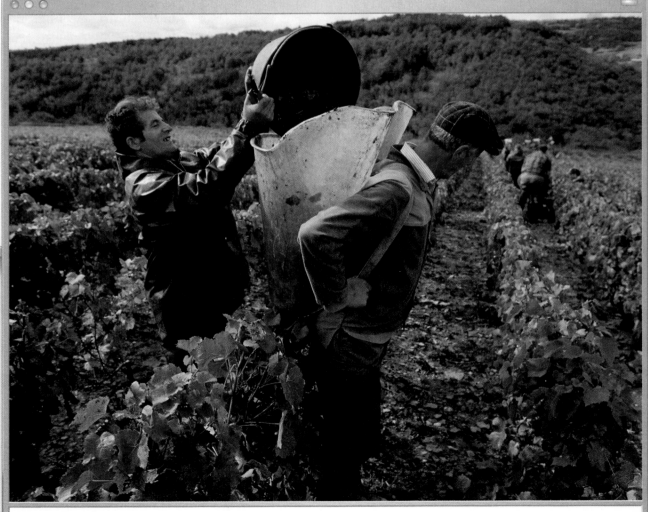

Les vendanges (*Grape harvest*) en Bourgogne

Cultural note: *La Bourgogne*, located in central France, is perhaps best known for its influence on gastronomy. In addition to its famous vineyards, specialities of this region include *escargots, coq au vin*, and, of course, *bœuf bourguignon.*

Dans ce chapitre...

OBJECTIFS COMMUNICATIFS

- talking about jobs and professions
- talking about banking and finances
- talking about the future
- linking ideas
- making comparisons
- learning to distinguish between and pronounce selected sounds in French

PAROLES (Leçon 1)

- Les métiers et professions
- À la banque
- Le budget
- Le verbe **ouvrir**

STRUCTURES (Leçons 2 et 3)

- Le futur simple (première partie)
- Le futur simple (deuxième partie)
- Les pronoms relatifs
- La comparaison de l'adjectif qualificatif

CULTURE

- Le blog d'Hector: *Pas facile, la vie d'artiste!*
- Reportage: *Étudiants: la chasse aux stages et aux petits boulots*
- Lecture: *Des métiers pas ordinaires* (Leçon 4)

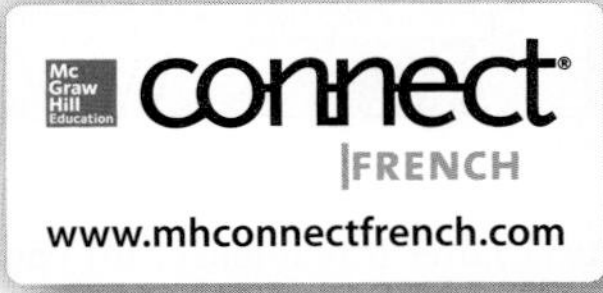

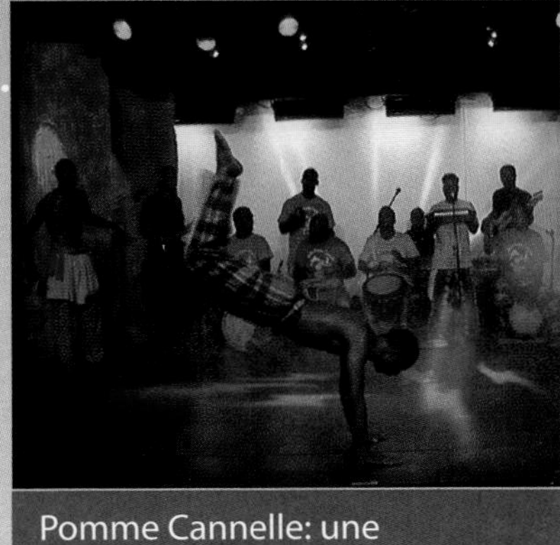
Pomme Cannelle: une troupe de danse antillaise

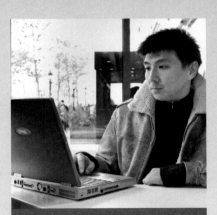
Au CIDJ on propose des milliers (*thousands*) offres d'emploi pour l'été en France

CHAPITRE **14**

Leçon 1

PAROLES

Au travail

Presentation: Model pronunciation of new vocabulary with group repetition. Give names for other professions that sts. are interested in.

1. Les fonctionnaires: ils travaillent pour l'État.

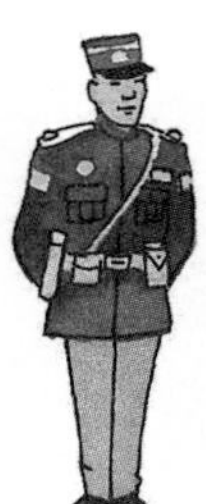
M. Merel, agent de police*

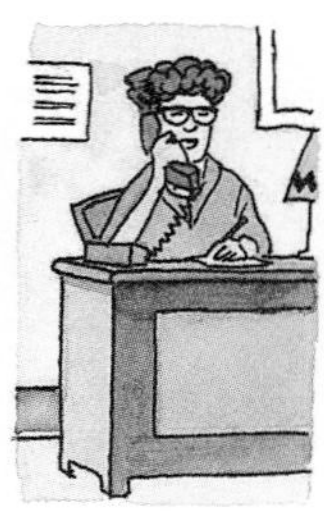
Mlle Drouet, secrétaire‡ de mairie

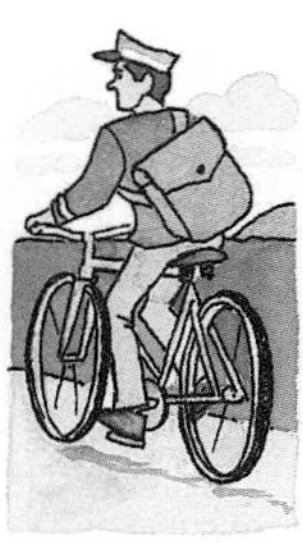
M. Barbier, facteur*

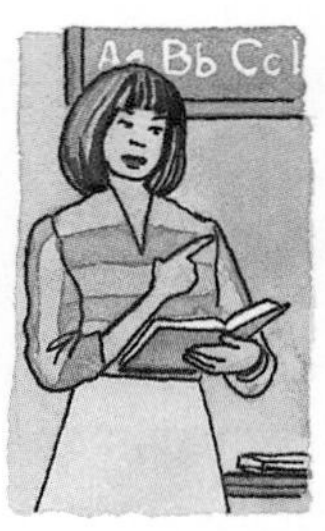

Mme Lambert, professeur des écoles‡

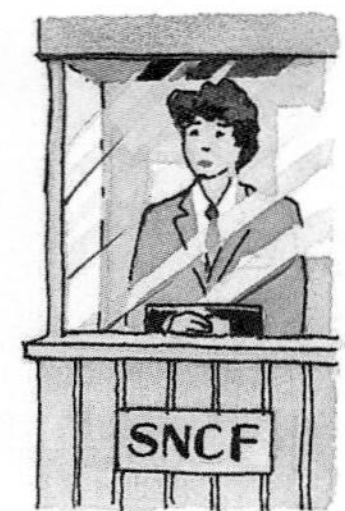

Mme Guilloux, employée† à la SNCF

Suggestion: Emphasize that there is no indefinite article used with professions in the structure noun or subject pronoun + *être* + *profession: Guy est professeur; il est professeur.* However, when the name of the profession is modified, the article is used: *C'est un bon professeur.*

Additional vocabulary: un P.D.G. (président-directeur général).

2. Les travailleurs* salariés: ils travaillent pour une entreprise.

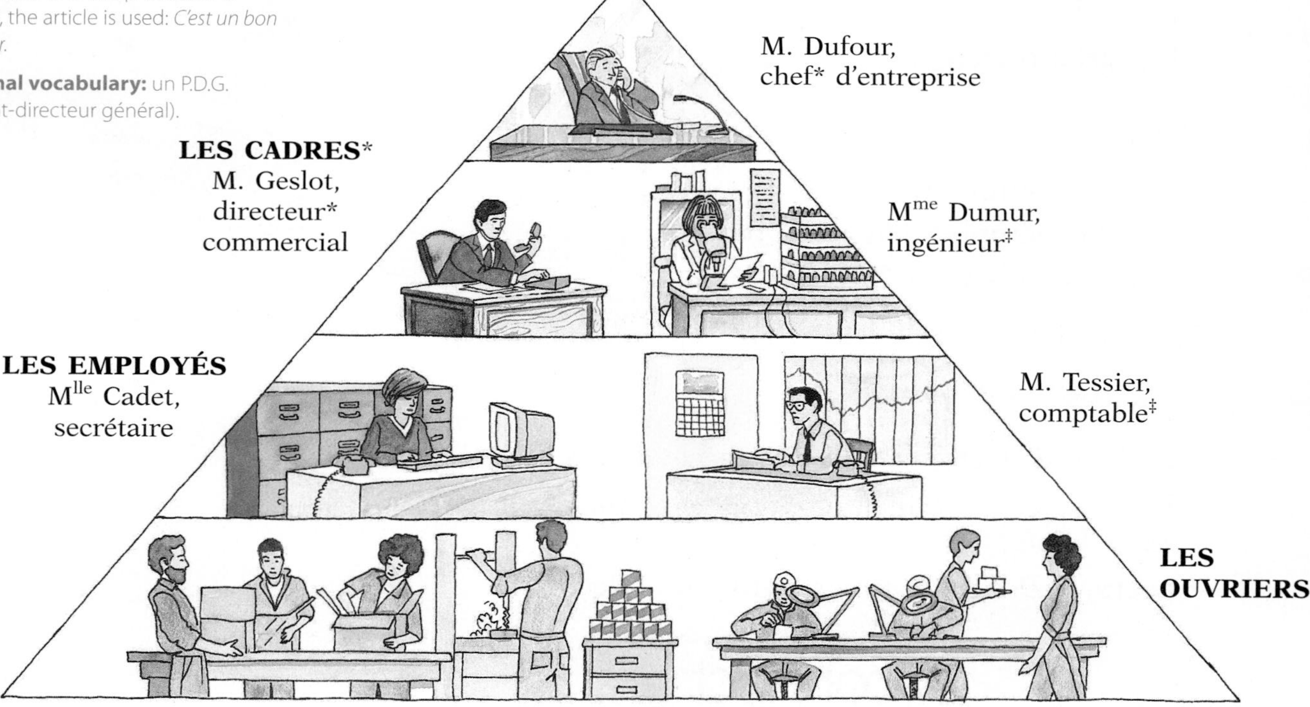
M. Dufour,
chef* d'entreprise
LES CADRES*
M. Geslot,
directeur*
commercial
Mme Dumur,
ingénieur‡
LES EMPLOYÉS
Mlle Cadet,
secrétaire
M. Tessier,
comptable‡
LES OUVRIERS*

**Feminine forms*: un agent, une factrice, une travailleuse, un cadre, un chef, une directrice, une ouvrière

†*Masculine form*: un employé

‡**Secrétaire, professeur,** and **comptable** can be either masculine or feminine. **Ingénieur** is always masculine, even for a woman.

3. **Les travailleurs indépendants:** ils travaillent **à leur compte**.

- **Les artisans**

M. Lepape, plombier*

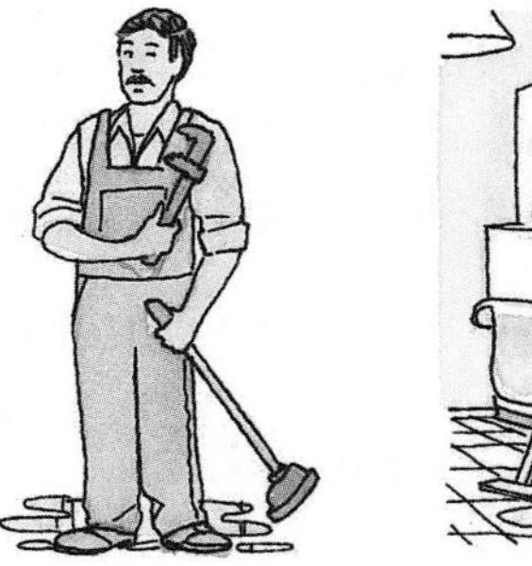

Mme Ngalla, coiffeuse†

AUTRES MOTS UTILES	
un entretien	job interview
un chômeur / une chômeuse	unemployed person
un C.V.	curriculum vitae, résumé
le marché du travail	job market
un stage	internship

- **Les commerçants**

M. Thétiot, boucher‡

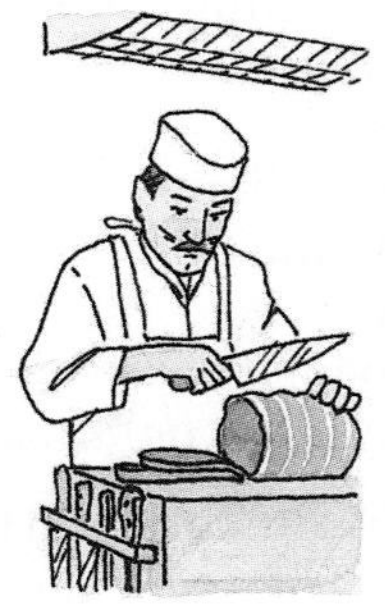

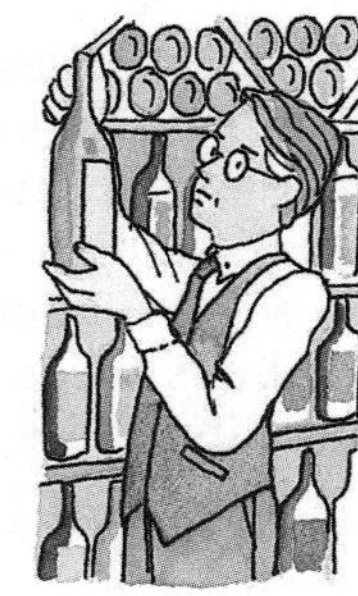

M. Lefranc, marchand‡ de vin

- **Les professions de la santé**

M. Morin, pharmacien‡

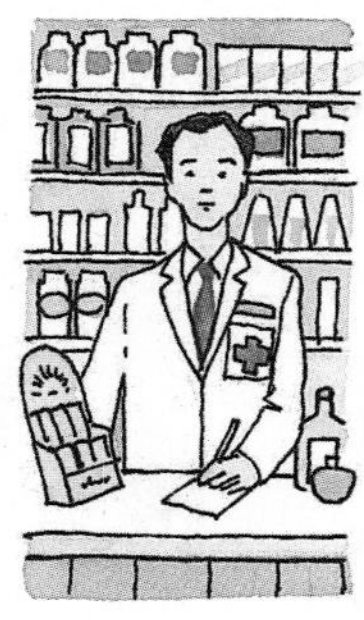

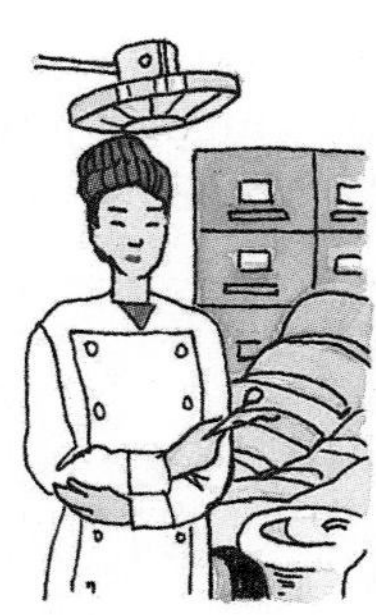

Mlle Wong, dentiste*

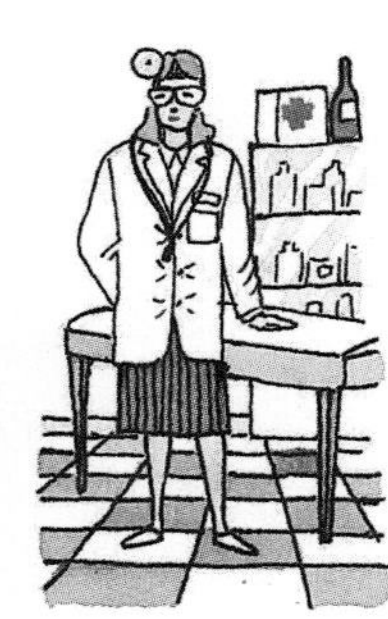

Mme Bouakaz, femme médecin†

- **D'autres professions**

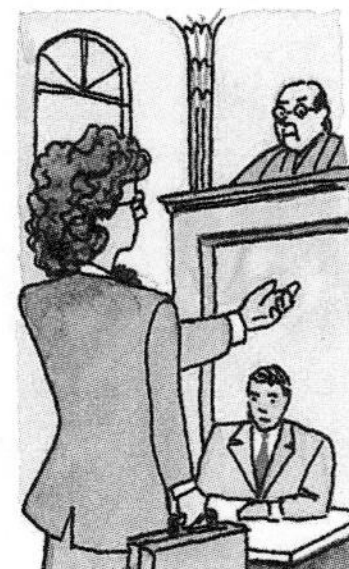

Mme Aubry, avocate†

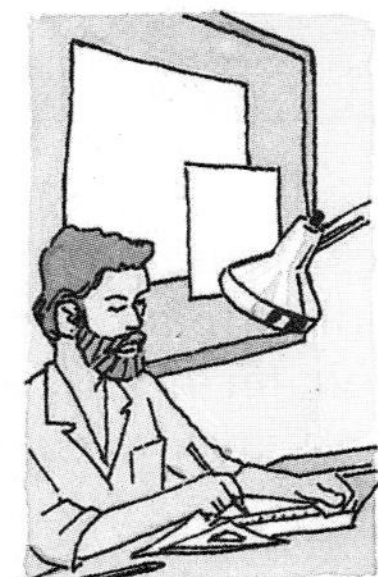

M. Leconte, architecte*

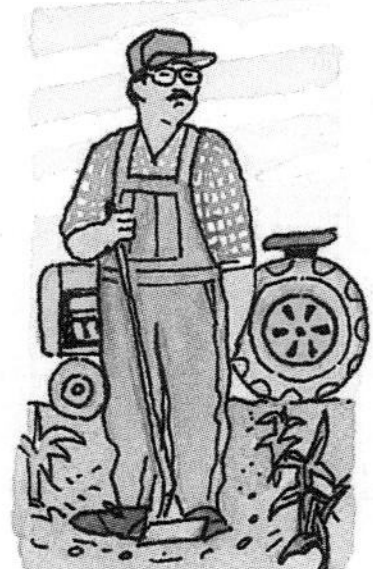

M. Colin, agriculteur‡

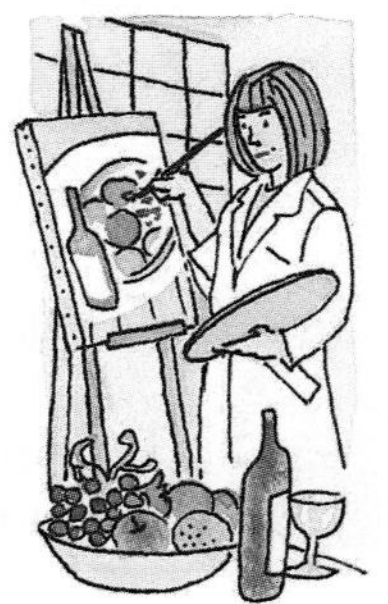

Mlle Cossec, artiste,* peintre*

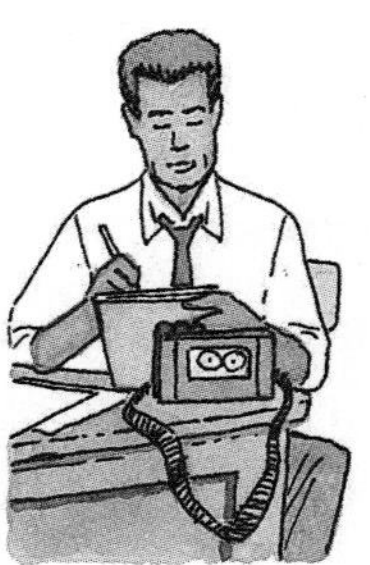

M. Kalubi, journaliste*

***Plombier** is always masculine, even for a woman, but **dentiste, architecte, artiste, peintre,** and **journaliste** can all be either masculine or feminine.

†*Masculine forms*: un coiffeur, un médecin, un avocat

‡*Feminine forms*: une bouchère, une marchande, une pharmacienne, une agricultrice

Suggestions (A): (1) Can be used for listening comprehension. (2) Encourage sts. to give definitions after practicing those in drill. Put names of professions on 3 × 5 cards and have sts. choose cards and then describe profession without naming it while others guess the profession being described.

Vocabulary recycling: An activity to review *les matières: Études. Qu'ont-ils étudié?* MODÈLE: *les avocats* → *Les avocats ont étudié le droit.* 1. *les médecins* 2. *les architectes* 3. *les banquières* 4. *les ingénieurs* 5. *les artistes, peintres* 6. *les interprètes* 7. *les magistrats* 8. *les publicitaires*

Follow-up (A): *Qui sont les collègues des personnes suivantes?* 1. *Jean-Pierre est serveur.* (*Jennifer*) 2. *Julie est cadre.* (*Arthur*) 3. *Denise est comptable.* (*Ahmed*) 4. *Francine est ouvrière agricole.* (Fabien). 5. *Claude est chômeur.* (*Maryse*)

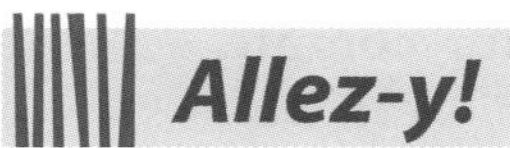

Allez-y!

A. Définitions. Quelle est la profession des personnes suivantes?

MODÈLES: Elle enseigne à l'école primaire. → Elle est professeur des écoles.
Il écrit des articles pour des journaux. → Il est journaliste.

1. Elle soigne les dents de ses patients.
2. Il travaille à la campagne.
3. Il règle la circulation automobile.
4. Elle vend des billets de train.
5. Elle s'occupe de (*takes care of*) la santé de ses patients.
6. Il distribue des lettres et des colis.
7. Il vend de la viande aux clients.
8. Elle coupe (*cuts*) les cheveux des clients.
9. Elle tape des lettres sur un ordinateur.
10. Il vend des vins et des liqueurs.
11. Il prépare et vend des médicaments.
12. Elle fait des portraits et des paysages (*landscapes*).

Suggestion (B): Can be done in small groups.

Follow-up (B): Name other professions and have sts. describe stereotypes (e.g., clothes) of people in those professions.

B. Stéréotypes. Voici quelques dessins du caricaturiste français Jean-Pierre Adelbert. Choisissez la profession qui, selon vous, correspond le mieux à chaque dessin. Expliquez pourquoi.

Professions: architecte, artiste, caricaturiste, chef d'entreprise, chômeur/chômeuse, coiffeur/coiffeuse, comptable, critique de cinéma, critique de cuisine, journaliste de mode, peintre, plombier, vendeur/vendeuse... ?

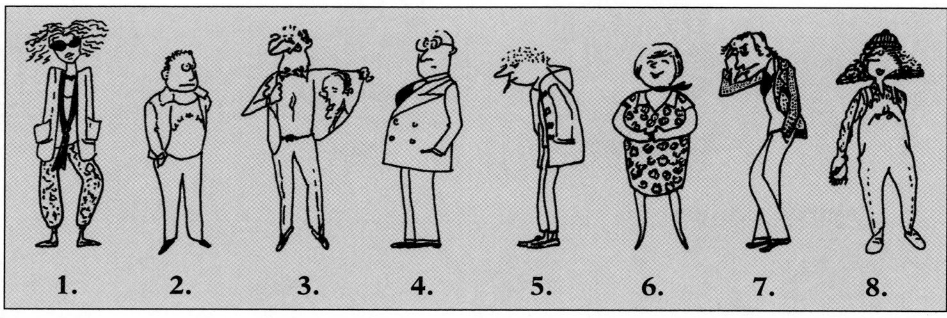

Suggestion (C): Give sts. 5 minutes to interview other sts.

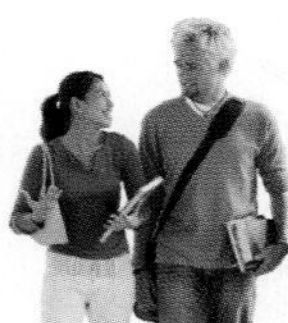

C. Projets d'avenir. Découvrez les futures professions de vos camarades de classe. Interviewez cinq étudiant(e)s pour découvrir quel métier ils/elles désirent faire après avoir terminé leurs études. Ensuite, analysez les résultats. En général, avez-vous des ambitions différentes ou semblables (*similar*)?

MODÈLE: É1: Que veux-tu faire après tes études?
É2: Je veux / Je voudrais devenir avocat(e).
É1: Et pourquoi?...

À la banque

Rebecca Johnson est une architecte américaine.
Elle vient de s'installer en France et va à la banque.

1. Elle ouvre (*opens*) **un compte bancaire** et **un compte d'épargne** pour pouvoir **faire des économies** (*f.*) **(économiser) pour l'avenir** [m.]). Elle a accès à ses comptes sur Internet et peut les gérer (*manage them*) à distance.

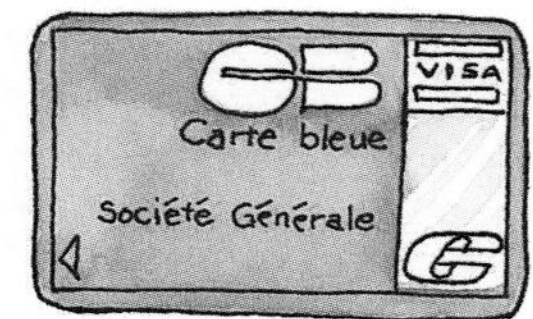

2. Elle prend aussi **une carte bancaire.***
3. Elle regarde **le cours du jour (le taux de change)** et change ses dollars en euros.

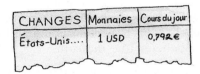

CHANGES	Monnaies	Cours du jour
États-Unis....	1 USD	0,792€

4. Quelques jours plus tard, elle va au **guichet automatique.** Avec sa carte bancaire, elle **retire** du **liquide** et **dépose** un chèque.

AUTRES MOTS UTILES

un bureau de change exchange office
compter to count
contrôler ses relevés (*m.*) check one's bank statements
une dépense expenditure
un emprunt loan
des frais (*m. pl.*) expenses, costs
la monnaie change; currency
un montant sum
payer par prélèvement automatique to make automatic payments
réaliser un virement to transfer money
un reçu receipt
toucher to cash (a check)

Allez-y!

A. Les services bancaires. Assane, un étudiant sénégalais, vient d'obtenir un permis de travail (*work permit*) en France. Complétez les phrases suivantes en utilisant le vocabulaire que vous venez d'apprendre.

1. Pour changer ses francs sénégalais en euros, il consulte ______.
2. Il va à la banque pour ouvrir un ______ et un ______ afin de (*in order to*) pouvoir faire des économies.
3. Quand il veut retirer du ______ ou ______ un chèque sur son compte, il peut aller au ______ et utiliser sa ______.

*__Carte bancaire__ is a general term that refers to both **cartes de crédit** and **cartes de débit.**

Suggestion: Display the illustrations from the e-Book or use images from the Internet to preview the vocab. as you model pronunciation.

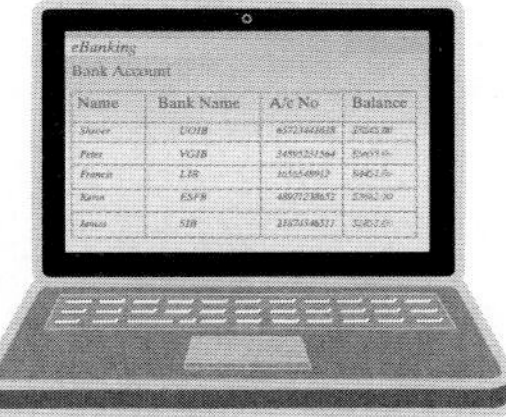

Suggestion: Point out the expression *faire un chèque* (not *écrire*).

Additional activity: Provide the current *taux de change* and have sts. convert $US to euros.

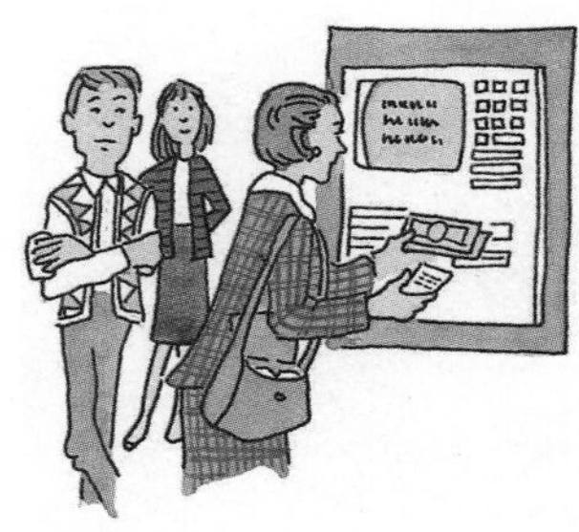

Additional activities: (1) *À la banque. Définitions. Complétez les phrases suivantes. 1. Quand on a accès à ses comptes sur Internet, on peut les ______ à distance. 2. On paie beaucoup de choses (son électricité, son loyer) par ______ automatique. 3. Chaque mois, on reçoit de sa banque un relevé de compte qui indique les sommes d'argent qu'on a ______ sur un compte et les sommes qu'on a ______ 4. L'argent déposé sur un compte d'______ augmente automatiquement parce que la banque paie des intérêts.* (2) Ask personalized questions using the vocab. *Quelles sortes de comptes avez-vous? Touchez-vous souvent des chèques? À quelles occasions? Quelles cartes de crédit avez-vous? Quels en sont les avantages et les inconvénients? Combien de cartes bancaires avez-vous? Quels sont les avantages et les inconvénients des guichets automatiques?*

Follow-up: Ask some sts. to play the roles in the *bureau de change.*

B. Une globe-trotter. Audrey vient d'arriver à Paris. Elle est à l'aéroport Charles-de-Gaulle et veut changer de l'argent. Indiquez dans quel ordre elle doit faire les choses suivantes.

_____ prendre sa carte bancaire et du liquide avec elle
_____ prendre le reçu
_____ compter l'argent
_____ se présenter à un bureau de change avec son passeport
_____ vérifier le montant sur le reçu
_____ dire combien d'argent elle veut changer

Suggestion: Point out that *gagner* means both *to win* and *to earn.*

Le budget de Marc Convert

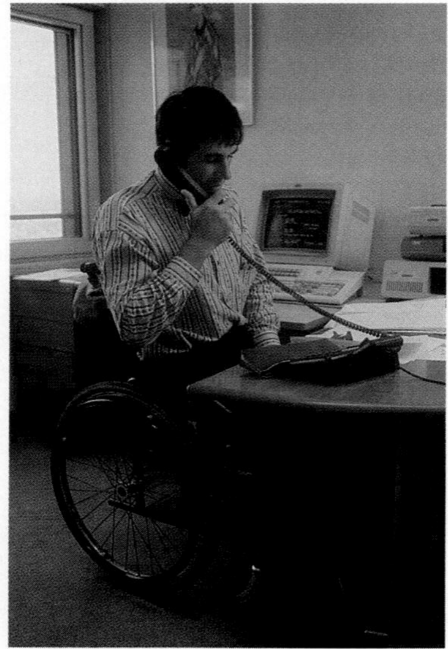

Voulez-vous travailler dans une petite société ou une grande entreprise?

Marc travaille dans une petite **société** (*company*) près de Marseille où il est responsable (*director*) commercial.

Il **gagne** 1 800 euros par mois.

Il **dépense** presque tout ce qu'il gagne pour vivre; le **coût de la vie** est très **élevé** dans les villes françaises. Mais il espère avoir une **augmentation de salaire** dans six mois. En ce moment, il lui est difficile de **faire des économies** pour acheter une maison.

Marc est content de son travail. Il sait qu'il a de la chance **car le taux de chômage** est très élevé en France: 10,4% en juillet 2013.

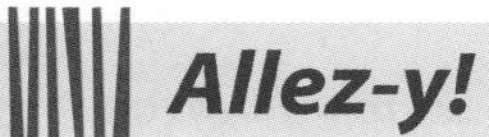

A. Frais et revenus. Complétez les phrases en utilisant le vocabulaire que vous venez d'apprendre.

1. Manon _____ pour acheter une voiture.
2. Les employés demandent souvent des _____.
3. Le _____ est moins élevé dans les petites villes.
4. Dayan est très économe: il _____ très peu.
5. Mme Reich? Elle travaille dans une _____ d'assurance (*insurance*).
6. Irène a un emploi sympa; elle est contente même si elle _____ relativement peu.

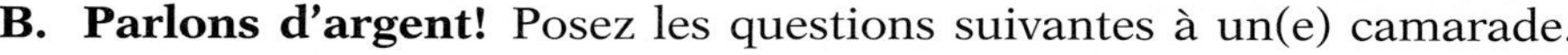

B. Parlons d'argent! Posez les questions suivantes à un(e) camarade.

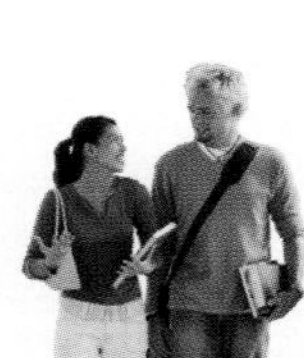

1. Est-ce que tu travailles en ce moment? Si oui, qu'est-ce que tu fais comme travail?
2. Est-ce que tu as un compte bancaire, un compte d'épargne, une carte de crédit?
3. Est-ce que tu gères tes comptes à distance?
4. Comment est-ce que tu paies ton électricité et ton loyer? par prélèvement automatique? par chèque?
5. Qu'est-ce que tu fais pour économiser de l'argent?
6. Est-ce que tu as un budget ou est-ce que tu vis au jour le jour (*from day to day*)? Pourquoi?

Le verbe *ouvrir*

Suggestion: Model the verb in short sentences: *J'ouvre un compte d'épargne*, etc.

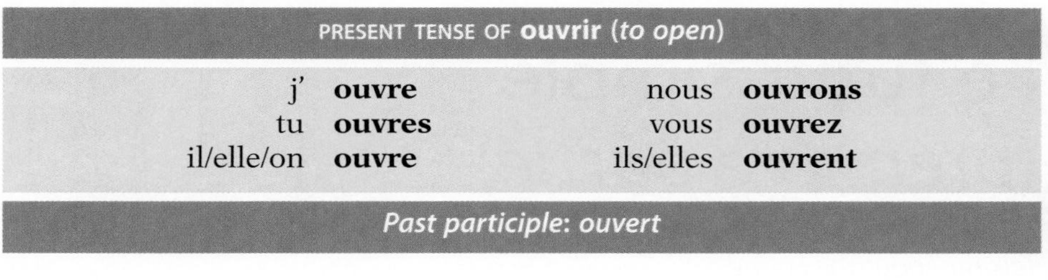

PRESENT TENSE OF **ouvrir** (*to open*)			
j'	**ouvre**	nous	**ouvrons**
tu	**ouvres**	vous	**ouvrez**
il/elle/on	**ouvre**	ils/elles	**ouvrent**
Past participle: *ouvert*			

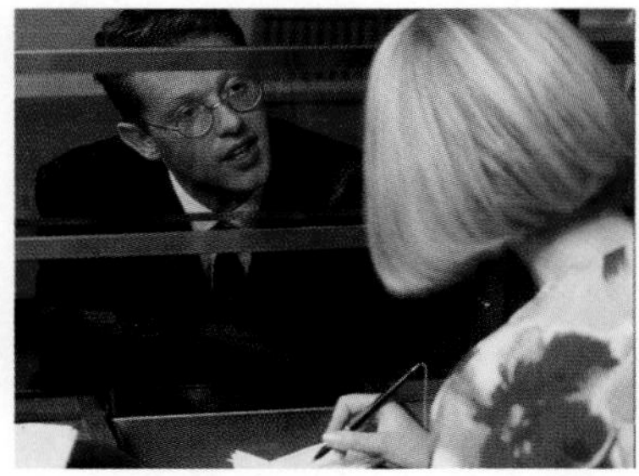

«J'aimerais ouvrir un compte, s'il vous plaît.» Avez-vous un compte bancaire?

The verb **ouvrir** is irregular. Verbs conjugated like **ouvrir** include **couvrir** (*to cover*), **découvrir** (*to discover*), **offrir** (*to offer*), and **souffrir** (*to suffer*). Note that these verbs are conjugated in the present tense like **-er** verbs.

The opposite of **ouvrir** is **fermer** (*to close*).

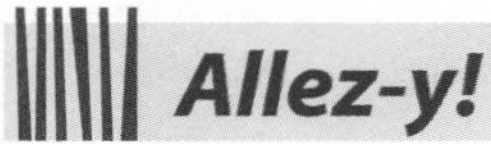

Allez-y!

A. Finances. Ce mois-ci, Jason a des problèmes d'argent. Racontez cette histoire en utilisant les verbes suivants: **ouvrir, couvrir, découvrir, offrir, souffrir.** Utilisez le passé composé (*p.c.*) où c'est indiqué.

Le mois dernier, Jason ______[1] (*p.c.*) un compte bancaire et un compte d'épargne. Sa grand-mère lui ______[2] toujours de l'argent pour son anniversaire, mais il l'utilise pour ses frais scolaires. Jason est très économe. Il ______[3] toujours ses dépenses. Mais ce mois-ci, il a acheté une nouvelle moto et il ______[4] parce qu'il ne peut pas sortir aussi souvent. Alors, il ______[5] les plaisirs de la lecture!

Suggestion: Use the following as a preliminary activity. *De l'argent.* 1. *Jason ouvre un compte d'épargne.* (*nous, je, tu*) 2. *Hier, Sylvie a ouvert un compte bancaire.* (*Paul et Henri, vous, je*) 3. *Comment couvres-tu ces dépenses?* (*elles, on, vous*) 4. *Je vous offre cent euros.* (*nous, il, elles*) 5. *Il m'a offert de l'argent!* (*vous, Claudine et Marie*) 6. *Il souffre d'être trop riche.* (*je, ils, tu*) 7. *A-t-on beaucoup souffert après la crise mondiale économique de 2008?* (*nos parents, vous, les Grecs*)

B. Profil psychologique. Demandez à un(e) camarade ______.

1. s'il / si elle a un compte bancaire
2. s'il / si elle couvre toujours ses dépenses
3. s'il / si elle fait des économies et pourquoi
4. s'il / si elle souffre quand il/elle est obligé(e) de faire des économies
5. combien de fois par semaine, ou par mois, il/elle doit retirer de l'argent de son compte et combien de fois il/elle doit déposer de l'argent
6. si quelqu'un lui a récemment offert de l'argent et ce qu'il/elle en a fait

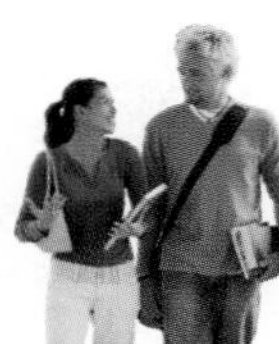

Suggestion: Point out *si + il(s) = s'il(s)*, but there is no elision with *elle(s)*.

Maintenant, dites ce que vous avez découvert et faites un petit portrait psychologique de votre camarade. Ou si vous préférez, lisez l'histoire de Jason dans l'exercice précédent et faites un portrait psychologique de Jason.

Mots utiles: économe, impulsif/impulsive, généreux/généreuse, (im)prudent(e), un magnat des affaires (*tycoon*)

CHAPITRE 14

Leçon 2

STRUCTURES

Suggestion: Ask sts. to comment on the tenses of verbs in bold. Ask them to infer how the future is formed, using these examples.

Le futur simple (*première partie*)

Talking About the Future

La vie d'artiste

Appel vidéo entre Juliette et Hector,

JULIETTE: Tu as signé un nouveau contrat?
HECTOR: Non. Avec la crise,[1] les artistes ont la vie dure[2]! Si ça continue, **je changerai** de métier!
JULIETTE: Tu as des idées?
HECTOR: Oui! **J'enseignerai.** Avec mes potes,[3] **on proposera** des cours de hip-hop pour les enfants. Les gosses[4] adorent ça!
JULIETTE: Alors **tu travailleras** à ton compte?
HECTOR: Exactement. Et **je serai** enfin indépendant.

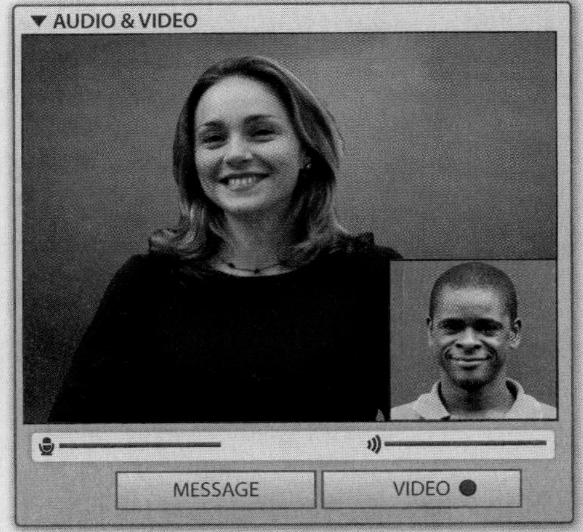

[1]*crisis* [2]la… *a hard life* [3]*buddies, pals* [4]*kids*

Dans les phrases suivantes, identifiez les verbes au futur proche. Puis remplacez-les par les verbes au futur utilisés dans le dialogue.

1. Je vais changer de métier.
2. Je vais enseigner.
3. On va proposer des cours de hip-hop.
4. Tu vas travailler à ton compte?
5. Je vais être indépendant.

Presentation: Model pronunciation of verb forms, using short sentences.

Note: Verbs like *préférer* do not have a spelling change in the *futur simple;* verbs like *acheter, appeler, payer* keep their spelling change in the *futur simple.* This topic is treated in the next grammar point.

Expressing the Future in French

In French, there are three ways of expressing future actions or events:

PRESENT	**J'arrive** à 2 h.	*I arrive at 2:00.*
NEAR FUTURE	Je **vais arriver** demain.	*I'm going to arrive tomorrow.*
FUTURE TENSE	**J'arriverai** en janvier.	*I will arrive in January.*

Verbs with Regular Future Stems

Suggestion: Point out that (1) the future stem always ends with *-r;* (2) the future endings are the same as the *avoir* endings in the present tense.

The future is a simple tense, formed with the infinitive plus the endings **-ai, -as, -a, -ons, -ez, -ont.** The final **-e** of the infinitive of **-re** verbs is dropped.

parler		finir		vendre	
je	parler**ai**	je	finir**ai**	je	vendr**ai**
tu	parler**as**	tu	finir**as**	tu	vendr**as**
il/elle/on	parler**a**	il/elle/on	finir**a**	il/elle/on	vendr**a**
nous	parler**ons**	nous	finir**ons**	nous	vendr**ons**
vous	parler**ez**	vous	finir**ez**	vous	vendr**ez**
ils/elles	parler**ont**	ils/elles	finir**ont**	ils/elles	vendr**ont**

Demain nous **parlerons** avec le conseiller d'orientation. — *Tomorrow we will talk with the job counselor.*
Il te **donnera** des conseils. — *He will give you some advice.*
Ces conseils t'**aideront** peut-être à trouver du travail. — *Maybe this advice will help you find a job.*
La réunion **finira** vers cinq heures. — *The meeting will end around five o'clock.*

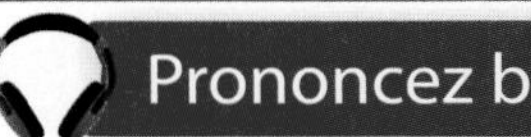

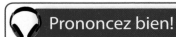

Prononcez bien!

The consonant *r*

Pronounce [ʀ] as you would an *h* in English, but raise the back of your tongue so that the distance between it and the back of your palate is much narrower than for *h*. When in between two vowels, **r** is pronounced more softly than when it occurs next to a consonant sound, especially [p], [t], and [k].

aiderons, arriver, étudiera, Paris

BUT

herbe, Marseille, près, secret, sucre, travail

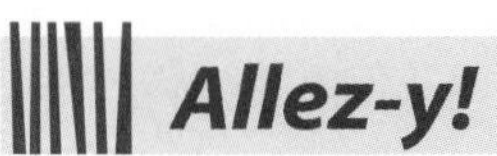

Allez-y!

A. Stratégies. Marie cherche du travail pour cet été. Elle doit se présenter demain à un entretien. Dites ce qu'elle fera.

MODÈLE: se lever très tôt → Elle se lèvera très tôt.

1. se coucher tôt ce soir
2. s'habiller avec soin
3. prendre un petit déjeuner léger
4. mettre son curriculum vitæ dans sa serviette (*briefcase*)
5. prendre le métro pour éviter les embouteillages (*traffic jams*)
6. y arriver un peu en avance
7. se présenter brièvement
8. parler calmement
9. répondre avec précision aux questions de l'employeur
10. remercier l'employeur avant de partir

Maintenant répétez l'exercice en utilisant le sujet **Marie et Loïc.**

MODÈLE: se lever très tôt → Ils se lèveront très tôt.

Additional activity: *Stratégies: Mettez les verbes au futur. 1. Je cherche du travail. 2. Mon frère m'aide à chercher. 3. Il en parle à son directeur. 4. Mes parents m'offrent leur aide. 5. Nous mettons une petite annonce. 6. Tu m'aides à préparer un entretien. 7. L'entretien se passe bien. 8. Je trouve un poste. 9. Nous fêtons ce succès ensemble.*

Suggestion (A): For oral or written practice. Can be done as a rapid-response ex., or sts. can write a short paragraph in future tense using sentences given.

Pronunciation presentation: To review the [ʀ] sound, see *Prononcez bien!*, p. 401, or *Leçon 4* in *Chapitre 7* of the Workbook/Laboratory Manual.

Pronunciation practice (1): Using visuals from *Au travail* in *Leçon 1* and other illustrations, elicit the pronunciation of (1) soft [ʀ]: *amoureux, marié, oreille, salarié, directeur;* (2) stronger [ʀ]: *ouvriers, marchand, pharmacien, architecte, agriculteur, artiste, journaliste*; and (3) strongest [ʀ]: *secrétaire, entreprise, peintre.*

Pronunciation practice (2): The *Prononcez bien!* section on page 401 of this chapter contains additional activities for practicing these sounds.

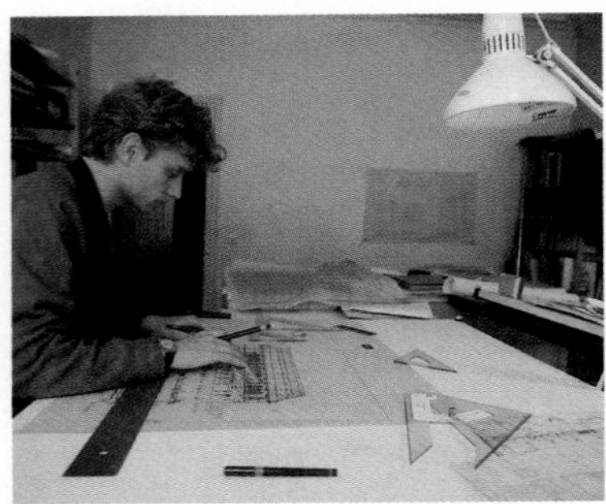

L'architecture: un travail de précision. Est-ce que vous travaillerez comme architecte? comme professeur? comme cadre?

B. Jeu de société. À une soirée, vous jouez à la voyante (*fortune-teller*) et prédisez la carrière de chacun(e) de vos ami(e)s. Choisissez le verbe convenable pour présenter vos prévisions.

Verbes: écrire, enseigner, jouer, s'occuper, participer, travailler, vendre, voyager

1. Vous ______ des bijoux à Alger.
2. Vous ______ le rôle de Hamlet à Londres.
3. Vous ______ à la construction d'un stade à Mexico.
4. Vous ______ des articles pour le *New York Times*.
5. Vous ______ souvent à l'étranger.
6. Vous ______ des malades à Dakar.
7. Vous ______ dans une école primaire à Seattle.
8. Vous ______ comme cosmonaute.

Le futur simple (*deuxième partie*)

Talking About the Future

La grande aventure

Léa téléphone à Juliette.

LÉA: Quand est-ce que **tu feras** ton stage de fin d'études?
JULIETTE: En janvier prochain.
LÉA: **Tu seras** en stage combien de temps?
JULIETTE: Six mois. Ensuite, **je devrai** trouver un emploi. Je veux être chef de projet multimédia.
LÉA: **Tu obtiendras** peut-être un poste dans l'entreprise où **tu feras** ton stage… C'est fréquent, tu sais!
JULIETTE: C'est possible, mais je veux travailler à l'étranger. **J'enverrai** des C.V. dès[1] février.
LÉA: Au Canada, il y a plein d'opportunités[2]! Et on parle français!
JULIETTE: Oui, mais je rêve d'une grande aventure: **j'irai** en Australie! **Tu viendras** me voir?

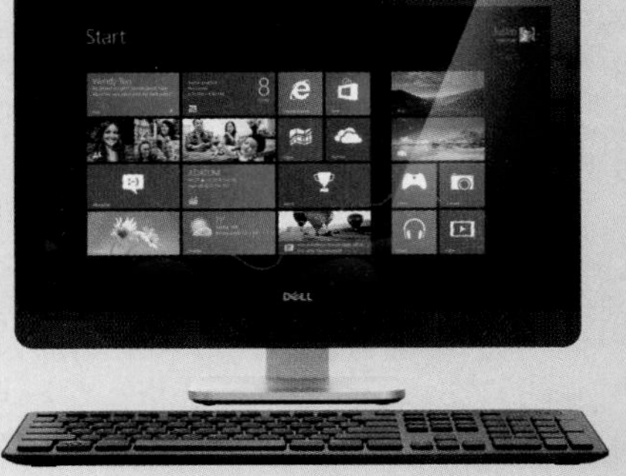

L'avenir appartient aux champions du Web

[1]*beginning in* [2]plein… *lots of opportunities*

Dans les phrases suivantes, identifiez les verbes au futur proche. Puis remplacez-les par les verbes au futur utilisés dans le dialogue.

1. Tu vas faire ton stage?
2. Tu vas être en stage combien de temps?
3. Ensuite, je vais devoir trouver un emploi.
4. Tu vas peut-être obtenir un poste dans l'entreprise où tu vas faire ton stage.
5. Je vais envoyer des C.V. dès février.
6. Je vais aller en Australie. Tu vas venir me voir?

Verbs with Irregular Future Stems

Some verbs have irregular future stems.

aller: **ir-**	faire: **fer-**	recevoir: **recevr-**
avoir: **aur-**	falloir: **faudr-**	savoir: **saur-**
devoir: **devr-**	mourir: **mourr-**	venir: **viendr-**
envoyer: **enverr-**	pleuvoir: **pleuvr-**	voir: **verr-**
être: **ser-**	pouvoir: **pourr-**	vouloir: **voudr-**

J'**irai** au travail la semaine prochaine. — *I'll go to work next week.*

Et toi, quand **enverras**-tu ta demande d'emploi? — *And you? When will you send in your job application?*

Pas de problème! **J'aurai** bientôt un poste. — *No problem! I will have a position soon.*

Alors, vous **devrez** tous les deux vous lever très tôt le matin. — *So both of you will have to get up very early in the morning.*

C'est vrai. Mais demain on **devra** célébrer cela! — *It's true. But tomorrow we should celebrate!*

Verbs with spelling irregularities in the present tense also have irregularities in the future tense. These include verbs such as **acheter, appeler,** and **payer.** See Appendix B: **-er** Verbs with Spelling Changes, at the end of the book.

Note: Remind sts. that verbs like *venir* (*obtenir,* etc.) have the same type of future stem as *venir.*

Suggestion: Model future-tense stems by giving sts. short sentences to repeat in which the verbs listed are used: *Nous irons en France l'année prochaine. Il fera si beau là-bas. Il ne pleuvra pas,* etc.

Suggestion: As a review activity (the following day, perhaps), bring in flash cards with verbs in the infinitive. Line the class up in two teams. Show the first st. in each line an infinitive and a subject pronoun. The first one to conjugate the verb correctly orally in the future tense moves on to play against the next st. Play for 5–7 minutes, or until all sts. have had a turn.

Follow-up: Give additional practice with substitutions: *Les étudiants parlent de leur avenir.* 1. *J'aurai une profession intéressante.* (*nous, tu, Thierry*); 2. *Juliette sera avocate.* (*vous, Jean-Pierre et Francis, je*); 3. *Tu iras travailler en France.* (*mes amies, Claudine, nous*); 4. *Nous devrons beaucoup travailler.* (*vous, Sylvain, je, elles*)

Uses of the Future Tense

1. As you can see from the preceding examples, the use of the future tense parallels that of English. This is also true of the tense of verbs after an *if*-clause in the present tense.

   Si je pose ma candidature pour ce poste, j'**aurai** peut-être des chances de l'obtenir. — *If I apply for this position, I may (will maybe) have some chance of getting it.*

   Mais si tu ne te présentes pas, tu ne l'**auras** sûrement pas! — *But if you don't apply in person, you surely will not get it!*

2. However, in dependent clauses following words such as **quand, lorsque** (*when*), **dès que** (*as soon as*), or **aussitôt que** (*as soon as*), the future tense is used in French if the action is expected to occur at a future time. English uses the present tense in this case.

   Je te **téléphonerai** *dès que* j'**arriverai.** — *I'll phone you as soon as I arrive.*

   Nous **pourrons** en discuter *lorsque* l'avocat **sera** là. — *We'll be able to discuss it when the lawyer arrives.*

   La discussion **commencera** *dès que* tout le monde **sera** prêt. — *The discussion will begin as soon as everyone is ready.*

Note: Although the expression *Les si mangent les r* (after *si,* never use the future or the conditional) is generally true, when *si* is translated by "whether," the *futur simple* (or the conditional) is used after *si: Je me demande si elle viendra.*

Mots clés

Exprimer le futur

All the expressions mentioned in the **Mots clés** of **Chapitre 5, Leçon 2** are also applicable to the **futur simple.** The following expressions are mostly used with the **futur simple:**

à l'avenir *from now on; in the future*
un jour *some day*
à partir de maintenant *from now on*

À l'avenir, nous ferons des économies.
Un jour, nous n'aurons plus de dettes.
À partir de maintenant, je te montrerai toutes mes dépenses.

Note: Explain that the *futur proche* cannot be used interchangeably in time clauses with the simple future.

Note: *si* clause + *imparfait* is covered in *Chapitre 15.*

3. The **futur simple** can also be used to politely express a command, a request, or a piece of advice.

Tu me **donneras** ton adresse avant de partir.	*Give me your address before you leave.*
Vous **finirez** de taper ces documents pour demain.	*Finish typing these documents for tomorrow.*

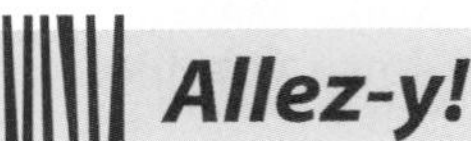

Allez-y!

A. Les exigences du milieu de travail. Transformez les phrases en utilisant le futur simple.

MODÈLE: Téléphone à ton collègue! → Tu téléphoneras à ton collègue!

1. Va poster ce colis!
2. Venez nous voir pendant les vacances!
3. Sois patient(e) avec tes collègues!
4. Envoyez des références!
5. Fais ton possible!

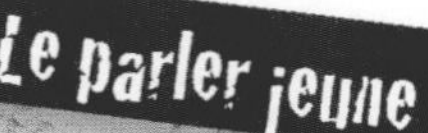

Le parler jeune

le blé, le fric	l'argent
bosser	travailler
un boulot	un travail
claquer	dépenser
être fauché	ne plus avoir d'argent

Pour gagner du **blé,** il faut éviter les métiers intellectuels.

Je préfère **bosser** la nuit.

Moi, j'aime mon **boulot.**

Je viens de **claquer** 100 euros en DVD!

Depuis les vacances, Delphine **est** complètement **fauchée.**

B. Problème urgent. Les membres d'une équipe au travail organisent une réunion pour essayer de trouver une solution à un problème. Utilisez le futur.

MODÈLE: (vous) expliquer le problème / quand / tout le monde / être là → Vous expliquerez le problème quand tout le monde sera là.

1. (tu) commencer la réunion / dès que / la patronne / arriver
2. (Nils) montrer les photos / aussitôt que / il / les recevoir
3. (nous) discuter nos options / quand / le problème / être clair pour tous
4. (je) téléphoner au client / quand / nous / pouvoir répondre à ses questions
5. (Nathalie et Octave) écrire une lettre au client / dès que / nous / être tous d'accord

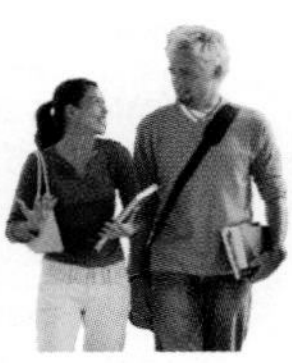

C. Interview. Vous voulez savoir ce que votre camarade pense de l'avenir, et vous lui posez les questions suivantes. Mais malheureusement, il/elle ne vous prend pas au sérieux! L'interviewé(e) utilise toute son imagination et tout son humour pour répondre. À la fin, inversez les rôles.

MODÈLE: dès que tu auras ton diplôme →
É1: Qu'est-ce que tu feras dès que tu auras ton diplôme?
É2: Moi, plus tard, je vendrai des légumes biologiques (*organic*) à Athènes.

1. quand tu seras vieux/vieille
2. si un jour tu es acteur/actrice
3. dans dix ans
4. lorsque tu te marieras
5. dès que tu pourras réaliser un de tes rêves
6. si tu n'obtiens pas tout ce que tu veux
7. lorsque tu auras des enfants

À votre avis, parmi toutes les réponses, laquelle (*which one*) est la plus originale, la plus amusante et la plus bizarre?

Suggestion: Ask sts. to work in groups of 3: Two will discuss, and the third will listen to determine which answers are the most original, funny, and bizarre. This person will report back to the class.

D. Conversation. Posez les questions suivantes à un(e) camarade, qui vous les posera à son tour.

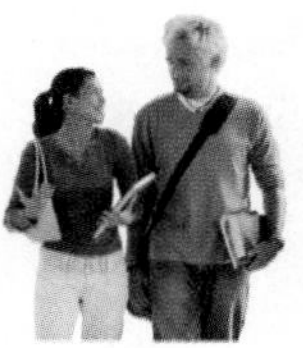

L'été prochain, ______?

1. qu'est-ce que tu écriras?
2. qu'est-ce que tu liras?
3. qu'est-ce que tu achèteras?
4. qui verras-tu?
5. où iras-tu?
6. que feras-tu? Auras-tu un job?

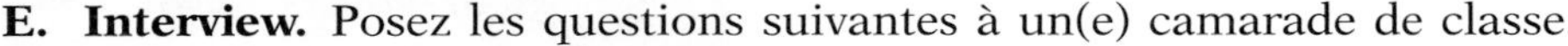

E. Interview. Posez les questions suivantes à un(e) camarade de classe.

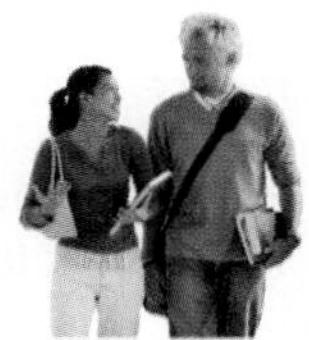

1. Qu'est-ce que tu feras quand l'année scolaire sera terminée? Continueras-tu tes études, iras-tu en vacances ou travailleras-tu?
2. Qu'est-ce que tu feras après tes études? Tu choisiras une profession indépendante? salariée? Seras-tu fonctionnaire? commerçant(e)? artisan(e)?
3. Tu voyageras souvent? Si oui, dans quels pays? Pour quelles raisons?
4. Tu gagneras beaucoup d'argent? Est-ce que cela sera important pour toi?
5. Où est-ce que tu vivras si tu en as le choix? Pourquoi?

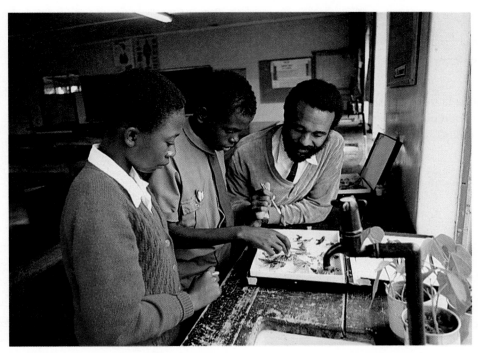

Être professeur: une profession prestigieuse et satisfaisante. Avez-vous un professeur que vous aimez beaucoup? Expliquez.

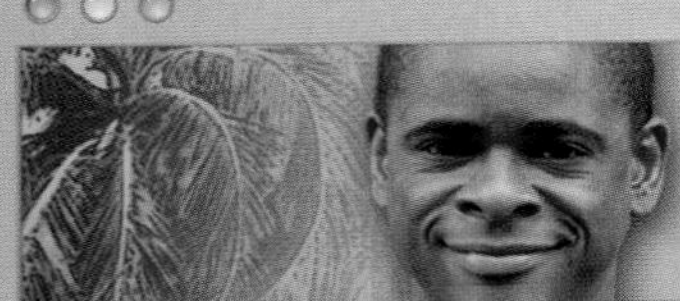

Le blog d'Hector

Pas facile, la vie d'artiste!

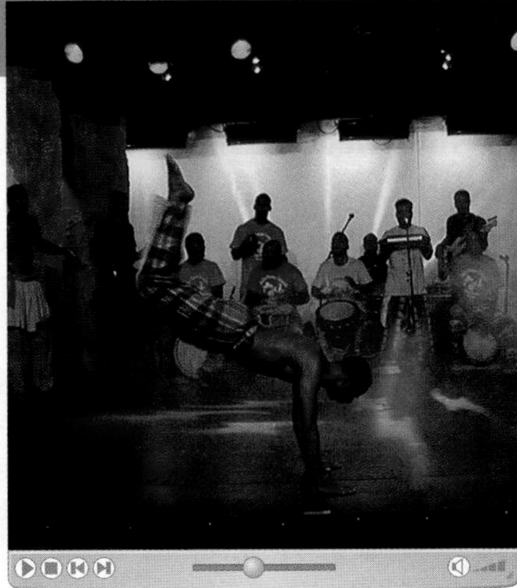

Pomme Cannelle: une troupe de danse antillaise

lundi 6 juillet

La semaine commence mal... Je suis angoissé[1]!

Quelquefois, je regrette de ne pas être plombier, dentiste, ou comptable! Ces professions sont moins fatigantes et plus rassurantes que le métier de danseur. Parce que, vous savez, c'est beau, la vie d'artiste, mais c'est avant tout des concessions, des efforts, des sacrifices, beaucoup de discipline et de courage.

Je ne suis pas un travailleur salarié. Je suis un danseur moderne indépendant. Alors, j'ai toujours des incertitudes[2] sur mon avenir; je me pose mille questions: «Est-ce que j'aurai un contrat cet été? Qu'est-ce que je ferai si je n'ai pas de contrat? Comment est-ce que je paierai mes frais? Serai-je obligé d'emprunter de l'argent à ma banque?»

Dans ma profession, le taux de chômage est élevé et il faut savoir faire des économies pour les mauvais jours. Il faut aussi avoir une bonne relation avec son banquier en cas de problème!

Je vais envoyer une candidature à la troupe antillaise Pomme Cannelle pour un poste de Directeur de spectacles. Je rêve d'un emploi stable et j'aimerais bien partir travailler au soleil: ça me changerait les idées[3]!

Hector

COMMENTAIRES

Alexis

Salut, Hector!
Dans ta prochaine vie, tu seras fonctionnaire! Tu seras moins angoissé!

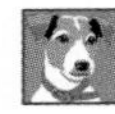

Trésor

Mon métier, c'est d'être le chien d'Alexis. Ce n'est pas toujours facile non plus...

Poema

Les problèmes dont tu parles ne sont pas spécifiques aux artistes. Les travailleurs indépendants n'ont aucune sécurité d'emploi! Je le sais parce que mon père est dentiste.

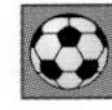

Mamadou

Poema, les gens auront toujours mal aux dents, et ils auront toujours besoin d'un dentiste!

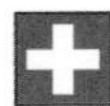

Charlotte

Hector, si tu obtiens ton poste de Directeur de spectacles, tu pourras retourner aux Antilles. Et tu seras un artiste salarié: c'est l'idéal, non?

[1]*anxious* [2]*uncertainties* [3]*ça... that would give me a change of pace*

Follow-up: 1. *Pourquoi Hector est-il angoissé?* 2. *Quelles sont les difficultés du métier d'artiste? Et vous, quel métier comptez-vous exercer plus tard? Quels sont les avantages et les inconvénients de ce métier?* 3. *Comment gérer son argent quand on n'a pas de salaire régulier comme Hector?* 4. *Parmi les commentateurs du blog, qui est le plus encourageant?* 5. *Hector aime-t-il son travail? Et vous, préférez-vous étudier ou travailler? Racontez vos premières expériences professionnelles* (*stages* [internships], *petits boulots*, etc.).

Video connection: In the videoblog for this chapter, Hector shows Léa a film of a performance by the Pomme Cannelle ballet troupe from Martinique, with which he is applying for a job.

Note: See the *Note culturelle* on the videoblog page in this chapter for more information on music and dance in the islands.

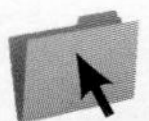

REPORTAGE

Étudiants: la chasse aux stages et aux petits boulots

En France, l'accès à l'université est gratuit.[1] Mais ensuite, comment couvrir vos dépenses et gagner l'argent du loyer, de la nourriture, des livres, des sorties et des vacances? Il n'y a qu'une solution: trouver un petit boulot.

Vous voulez un travail intéressant, pas trop fatigant et, en plus, bien payé? Première règle: si vous désirez travailler en été, commencez vos recherches dès le mois de janvier. Deuxième règle: faites l'inventaire des entreprises qui embauchent[2] des étudiants; parlez de vos projets à votre boucher, à votre dentiste, à votre facteur, à votre pharmacien, aux membres de votre famille, à tout le monde. Troisième règle: envoyez des lettres de motivation personnalisées et des C.V. attractifs qui mettent en valeur[3] vos points forts.

Attention, il ne faut pas confondre petit boulot et stage en entreprise. Aurélie, qui vient de terminer un stage de relations publiques chez Air France, explique: «Un stage en entreprise vous donne une compétence professionnelle. Souvent obligatoire, il complète votre formation universitaire dans le domaine de vos études. Et s'il dure plus de huit semaines, il donne droit à une indemnité.[4] C'est le meilleur argument sur un C.V. au moment de la recherche d'un emploi.» Comment a-t-elle trouvé son stage? «J'ai consulté les petites annonces du CIDJ (Centre d'information et de documentation de la jeunesse) sur Internet et j'ai posé ma candidature sur des sites spécialisés comme Apec.fr et Letudiant.fr. À la fin, j'ai eu plusieurs propositions!»

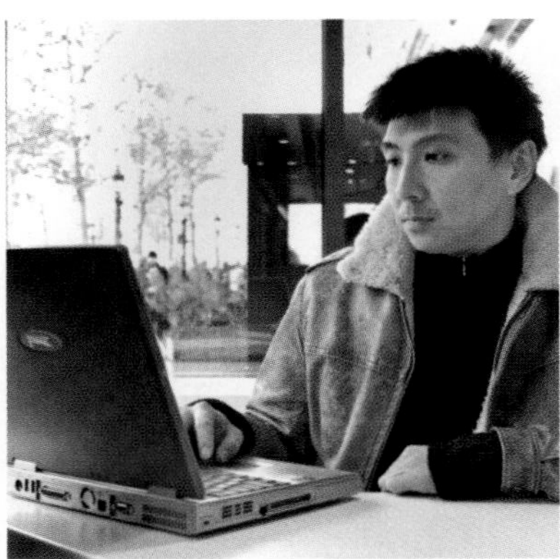

Le CIDJ propose aux étudiants plus de des milliers offres d'emplois pour l'été en France et dans les autres pays d'Europe. Tous les secteurs sont représentés: la vente, l'hôtellerie, le sport, les nouvelles technologies… N'hésitez pas à consulter son site Internet. Comme ce jeune homme, vous y trouverez sûrement le stage ou le petit boulot de vos rêves!

[1]*free* [2]*hire* [3]mettent… *emphasize* [4]*compensation*

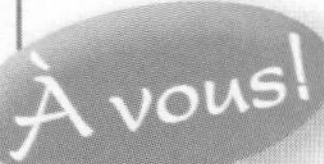

1. En France, quel est le meilleur moyen de trouver un petit boulot pour l'été? En Amérique, comment procédez-vous?
2. Expliquez la différence entre un petit boulot et un stage en entreprise.
3. Avez-vous l'expérience de petits boulots? Avez-vous déjà fait un stage en entreprise? Décrivez votre expérience. Sinon, décrivez l'expérience d'un ami / d'une amie.
4. Quel emploi cherche le jeune homme sur la photo? Imaginez.

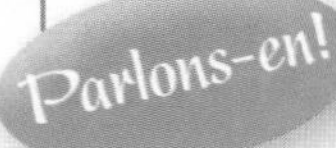

1. Travaillez en groupes de quatre et rédigez (*write up*) une proposition de stage destinée à un étudiant qui vient de terminer ses études. (Vous pouvez vous inspirer des petites annonces publiées sur le site du CIDJ.)
2. Dans votre petite annonce, présentez l'entreprise, précisez la durée du stage et la rémunération. Énumérez, au futur, les tâches à accomplir.
3. Lisez votre offre devant la classe. Vos camarades discuteront les détails de l'offre.
4. Demandez qui, parmi vos camarades, est intéressé par votre stage et pourquoi.
5. Les camarades qui ne sont pas intéressés expliqueront leur point de vue.

Qui propose le stage le plus intéressant? Votez!

CHAPITRE 14

Leçon 3

STRUCTURES

Suggestion: Ask sts. to read the minidialogue and make hypotheses about the referent and meaning of the relative pronouns.

Les pronoms relatifs

Linking Ideas

Ça m'intéresse!

Appel vidéo entre Mamadou et Léa.

MAMADOU: Léa, tu veux toujours écrire des articles pour la presse?
LÉA: Bien sûr! Tu connais un journal **qui** cherche des journalistes en free-lance?
MAMADOU: Oui…
LÉA: Les C.V. **que** j'ai envoyés n'ont pas eu de succès… Si tu as une piste,[1] ça m'intéresse!
MAMADOU: Le journal **dont** je te parle veut une rédactrice[2] **qui** maîtrise parfaitement[3] la langue française: C'est toi!
LÉA: Tu es bien indulgent… Mais donne-moi des précisions: les articles **qu'**il faudra écrire concernent la littérature? la mode[4]? l'actualité[5]?
MAMADOU: Non. Le football.
LÉA: Tu te moques de[6] moi?

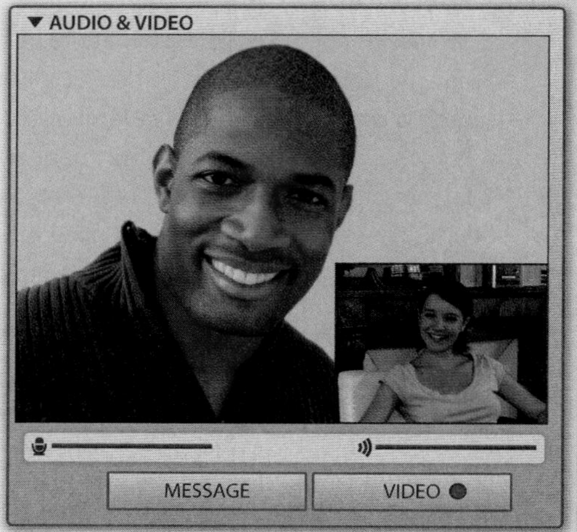

[1]*lead* [2]*editor* [3]maîtrise… *has a command of* [4]*fashion* [5]*current events* [6]Tu… *You're making fun of*

Trouvez, dans le dialogue, les phrases équivalentes.

1. Tu connais un journal cherchant (*looking for*) des journalistes?
2. Mes C.V. envoyés n'ont pas eu de succès.
3. Le journal en question veut une rédactrice.
4. Le journal veut une rédactrice maîtrisant (*with a command of*) la langue française.
5. Les articles à écrire concernent la littérature?

Presentation: Model sentences in each grammar section and have sts. repeat the transformations.

Note: Stress that relative pronouns are never omitted in French as they often are in English.

A relative pronoun (*who, that, which, whom, whose*) links a dependent (relative) clause to a main clause. A dependent clause is one that cannot stand by itself—for example, the italicized parts of the following sentences: The suitcase *that he is carrying* is mine; There is the store *in which we met.*

	PERSON	THING
subject	qui	qui
object	que	que
with preposition	qui	lequel*
with **de**	dont	dont

Qui

1. The relative pronoun used as a subject of a dependent clause is **qui** (*who, that, which*). It can refer to both people and things.

    J'ai un emploi. **Il** me plaît.

    J'ai un emploi **qui** me plaît.

    Je vois la femme. **Elle** vous a parlé.

    Je vois la femme **qui** vous a parlé.

    In the first example, **qui** replaces the subject **il** in the dependent clause. Because it is the subject of the clause, **qui** will always be followed by a conjugated verb (**qui... plaît**). Note that in the second example, **vous** is not a subject but an object pronoun; **elle** is the subject of **a parlé.**

2. **Qui** does not elide when followed by a vowel sound.

    L'architecte **qui** est arrivé ce matin vient du Japon.

3. **Qui** can also be used as the object of a preposition to refer to people.

    Le comptable **avec qui** je travaille est agréable. *The accountant with whom I work is pleasant.*
    L'ouvrier **à qui** j'ai donné du travail est très spécialisé. *The worker to whom I gave some work is highly specialized.*

[Allez-y! A]

Que

1. The relative pronoun used as a direct object of a dependent clause is **que** (*whom, that, which*). It also can refer to both people and things.

    C'est une entreprise. Je connais bien **cette entreprise.**

    C'est une entreprise **que** je connais bien.

    Voici une amie. J'ai rencontré **cette amie** au travail.

    Voici une amie **que** j'ai rencontrée au travail.

    In the second example, **que** replaces the direct object **cette amie. Que** is always followed by a subject and a conjugated verb (**que j'ai rencontrée**). Note that the past participle agrees with the preceding feminine direct object **que** (**une amie**). You may want to review the section on the agreement of past participles in **Chapitre 10, Leçon 3.**

Note: This direct object is called *l'antécédent.*

Suggestion: Use the following as a grammatical sensitivity ex. Have sts. number from 1 to 7; they write *S* for *sujet* when they hear relative pronoun *qui*, and *O* for *objet* when they hear relative pronoun *que* in the following sentences. 1. *Voici les voyageurs qui arrivent.* 2. *Les valises qu'ils portent sont lourdes.* 3. *Le train qui les a amenés ici est déjà parti.* 4. *Le voyageur qui a cette valise verte est mon oncle.* 5. *C'est la valise que je lui ai donnée.* 6. *La femme qui l'accompagne est gentille.* 7. *C'est le premier voyage qu'ils font ensemble.* As follow-up activity, put sentences on board or project them using a digital display, then underline and explain the function of the relative pronouns.

*__Lequel__ is not discussed in this chapter. Refer to **Chapitre 15, Leçon 2** and Appendix E.

2. **Que** elides with a following vowel sound.

L'architecte **qu'**elle a rencontré vient du Japon.

Dont

1. The pronoun **dont** is used to replace the preposition **de (du, de la, de l', des)** plus its object. If the verb of the dependent clause requires the preposition **de** (as in **parler de, avoir besoin de,** etc.) before an object, use **dont.**

Où est le reçu? J'ai besoin **du reçu.**	*Where is the receipt? I need the receipt.*
Où est le reçu **dont** j'ai besoin?	*Where is the receipt that I need?*

2. **Dont** is also used to express possession.

C'est la passagère. Ses valises sont à la douane.	*That's the passenger. Her suitcases are at the customs office.*
C'est la passagère **dont** les valises sont à la douane.	*That's the passenger whose suitcases are at the customs office.*
Aziz est écrivain. On peut acheter ses livres à la librairie.	*Aziz is a writer. You can buy his books at the bookstore.*
Aziz est l'écrivain **dont** on peut acheter les livres à la librairie.	*Aziz is the writer whose books you can buy at the bookstore.*

When **dont** is used, there is no need for a possessive adjective. Note the use of the definite article (**les**).

Où

Où is the relative pronoun of time and place. It can mean *where, when,* or *which.*

Le guichet **où** vous changez votre argent est là-bas.	*The window where you change your money is over there.*
Le 1er janvier, c'est le jour **où** je commence mon nouveau travail.	*The first of January, that's the day (when) I begin my new job.*
L'aéroport d'**où** vous êtes partis est maintenant fermé.	*The airport from which you departed is closed now.*

[Allez-y! B-C-D-E]

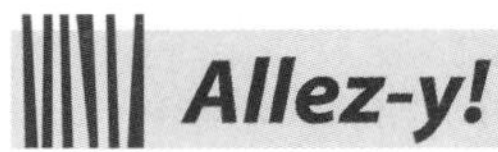

A. À la recherche d'un emploi. Max raconte comment il a passé sa semaine à chercher du travail. Reliez les phrases suivantes avec **qui.**

MODÈLE: Dimanche, j'ai téléphoné à une amie. Elle est directrice d'un journal. →
Dimanche, j'ai téléphoné à une amie qui est directrice d'un journal.

1. Lundi, j'ai déjeuné avec un ami. Il connaît beaucoup de comptables.
2. Mardi, j'ai eu un entretien à la BNP (Banque Nationale de Paris) Paribas. Elle est près de la place de la Concorde.
3. Mercredi, j'ai parlé à un employé du Crédit Agricole. Il m'a beaucoup encouragé.
4. Jeudi, j'ai pris rendez-vous avec un membre de la Chambre de commerce. Il est expert-comptable.
5. Enfin samedi, j'ai reçu une lettre d'une société belge. Elle m'offre un poste de comptable à Bruxelles.
6. Et aujourd'hui, je prends l'avion. Il me conduit vers ma nouvelle vie.

B. **Promenade sur la Seine.** Cet été, Clarisse travaille comme guide sur un bateau-mouche* à Paris. Complétez ses explications avec les pronoms relatifs **qui, que** et **où.**

Ce bâtiment _____[1] vous voyez à présent dans l'île de la Cité, c'est la Conciergerie. Autrefois une prison, c'est l'endroit _____[2] Marie-Antoinette a passé ses derniers jours. Et cette église _____[3] se trouve en face de nous, c'est Notre-Dame. Voici le musée d'Orsay _____[4] vous pourrez admirer les peintres impressionnistes et _____[5] je vous recommande de visiter. Et un peu plus loin, le musée du Louvre _____[6] vous trouverez *la Joconde* et *la Vénus de Milo.* Et enfin, voici la tour Eiffel _____[7] est le symbole de notre ville. Est-ce que vous voyez cette statue _____[8] ressemble à la Liberté éclairant (*lighting*) le monde? Eh bien, c'est l'original de la statue _____[9] la France a donnée aux Américains.

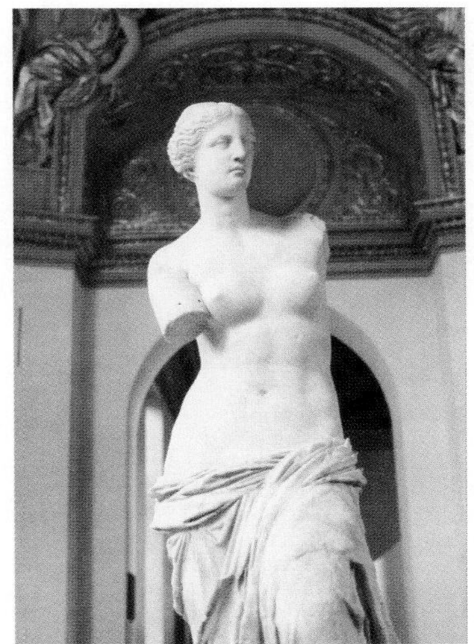

La Vénus de Milo au Louvre

Suggestion: (1) Have sts. write out new sentences first and then give orally.
(2) Ask sts. to write 2 sentences at board and then link them, as in model.

C. **Photos de vacances.** Jade a passé un mois dans un village d'artistes dans le Midi. Elle y a rencontré beaucoup de gens intéressants. Elle montre maintenant ses photos de vacances à ses amis.

MODÈLE: Voici un artisan. Ses poteries sont très chères. →
Voici un artisan **dont les** poteries sont très chères.

1. Charlie est un jeune artiste. On peut admirer ses tableaux au musée de Marseille.
2. Voici Yann. Ses sculptures sont déjà célèbres dans le milieu artistique.
3. Et voilà Clara. On vend ses bijoux à Saint-Tropez.
4. Octave est un jeune écrivain. Son premier roman vient d'être publié.

*The **bateaux-mouches** are cruise boats that take tourists along the Seine in Paris, offering historical commentaries on the various monuments that can be seen during the trip. They serve about five million passengers per year.

D. Travail et vacances. Racontez les projets de Sabine en reliant les deux phrases avec un pronom relatif. Le symbole ▲ indique le début (*beginning*) d'une proposition relative.

MODÈLE: Je travaille au tribunal (*court*). ▲ Je suis avocate au tribunal. →
Je travaille au tribunal où je suis avocate.

1. Je prendrai bientôt des vacances. ▲ J'ai vraiment besoin de ces vacances.
2. Ma camarade de chambre ▲ viendra avec moi. Elle s'appelle Élise.
3. Elle travaille avec des comptables. ▲ Ces comptables sont très exigeants (*demanding*).
4. Nous irons à Genève. ▲ Les parents d'Elise ont une maison à Genève.
5. Hier Élise a téléphoné à son père. ▲ Le père d'Élise nous a invitées.
6. Élise a envie de voir sa mère. ▲ Elle pense souvent à sa mére.
7. J'ai acheté une nouvelle valise. ▲ Je mettrai tous mes vêtements de ski dans cette valise.
8. Nous resterons deux jours à Strasbourg. ▲ Nous visiterons le Palais de l'Europe à Strasbourg.
9. Nous rentrerons trois semaines plus tard, prêtes à reprendre le travail. ▲ Ce travail se sera accumulé (*piled up*).

Maintenant, cherchez l'information demandée dans le récit de Sabine.

1. saison
2. durée des vacances
3. nationalité probable d'Élise
4. état d'esprit (*mental state*) de Sabine

Suggestion: Give sts. a few minutes to create an *énigme* before soliciting individual responses. Or have sts. create one or two *énigmes* as homework to be presented orally during next class. Can be done in groups of five sts.

E. Énigme. Décrivez un objet, une personne ou un endroit à vos camarades. Utilisez des pronoms relatifs. Vos camarades vont essayer d'identifier la chose dont vous parlez.

Catégories suggérées: une classe, un gâteau, un pays, une personne, un plat, une profession, une ville…

MODÈLE: É1: Je pense à un gâteau qui est français et dont le nom commence par un *é*.
É2: Est-ce que c'est un éclair?

Maintenant, continuez ce jeu avec une différence. Cette fois, vous ne donnez que la catégorie d'un objet ou d'une personne. Vos camarades vous demandent des précisions. Répondez-leur par *oui* ou *non*.

Autres catégories suggérées: un acteur / une actrice, un chanteur / une chanteuse, une émission de télévision, un film, une pièce de théâtre…

MODÈLE: É1: Je pense à un film.
É2: C'est un film que tu as vu il y a longtemps?
C'est un film dont l'action se passe à New York?
C'est un film où un animal a joué le rôle principal?
C'est un film dont l'action se déroule (*takes place*) en 1933?
C'est *King Kong*.

La comparaison de l'adjectif qualificatif

Making Comparisons

Vie professionnelle ou développement personnel?

Poema et Alexis discutent au café.

POEMA: Tu travailleras en France ou au Québec après ton diplôme?

ALEXIS: Au Québec. Le marché de l'emploi y est **meilleur**[1] qu'en France et les salaires y sont **plus élevés**.[2]

POEMA: Oui, mais les conditions de travail y sont **moins bonnes**: en France, tu travailles 35 heures par semaine et tu as cinq semaines de vacances payées!

ALEXIS: Je sais. Mais moi, je trouve que **le plus important**, c'est d'aimer son travail. Je ne compterai pas mes heures de présence si j'occupe un poste intéressant.

POEMA: Tu es **plus idéaliste** que moi! Je considère que la vie professionnelle est **moins essentielle** que le développement personnel.

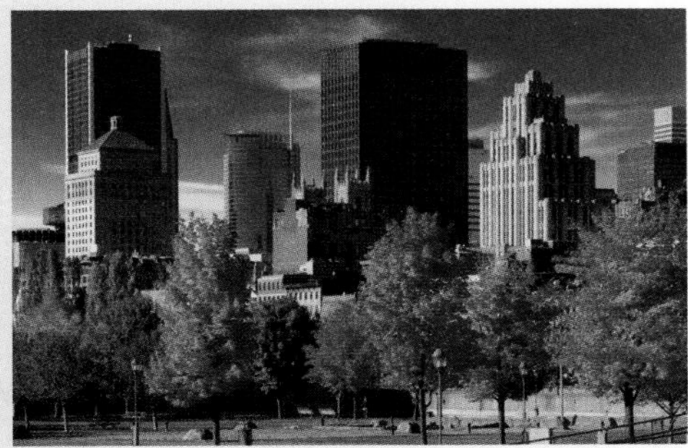

Montréal, au Québec: un marché de l'emploi très dynamique

[1]*better* [2]plus... *higher*

Choisissez la bonne réponse selon le dialogue.

1. Au Québec, le marché de l'emploi est meilleur / moins bon qu'en France.
2. Les salaires y sont plus bas / plus élevés.
3. Les conditions de travail sont meilleures / moins bonnes.
4. Alexis considère que le plus important / le moins important, c'est d'aimer son travail.
5. Poema trouve Alexis plus / moins idéaliste qu'elle.
6. Elle pense que la vie professionnelle est plus / moins essentielle que le développement personnel.

Comparison of Adjectives

Presentation: (1) Magazine pictures or drawings that can be easily compared are useful in presenting these concepts. (2) Use names of famous people to further engage sts.' interest: *Bill Gates est plus riche que moi. Jennifer Lopez a les cheveux plus longs que moi…* etc.

1. In French, the following constructions can be used with adjectives to express a comparison. It is not always necessary to state the second term of the comparison.

plus... que (*more . . . than*)

Chez l'épicier, les produits sont **plus** chers (**qu'**à Carrefour*).	*The products at the grocer's are more expensive (than at Carrefour).*

*supermarché très populaire

moins... que (*less . . . than*)	
Franck pense que Carrefour est **moins** cher (**que** Trouvetout).	*Franck thinks Carrefour is less expensive (than Trouvetout).*

aussi... que (*as . . . as*)	
Pour Laure, l'accueil est **aussi** important **que** la qualité des produits.	*For Laure, the friendly service is as important as the quality of the products.*

2. Stressed pronouns (**Chapitre 12, Leçon 2**) are used after **que** when a pronoun is required.

Elle est plus intelligente que **lui.** — *She is more intelligent than he is.*

[Allez-y! A]

Superlative Form of Adjectives

1. To form the superlative of an adjective, use the appropriate definite article with the comparative form of the adjective.

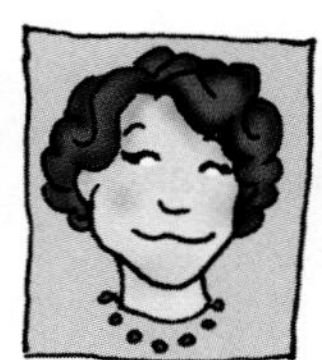
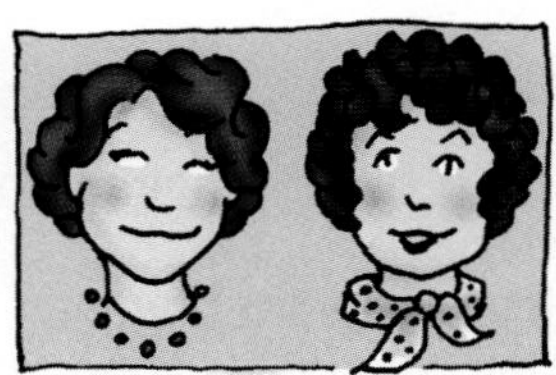
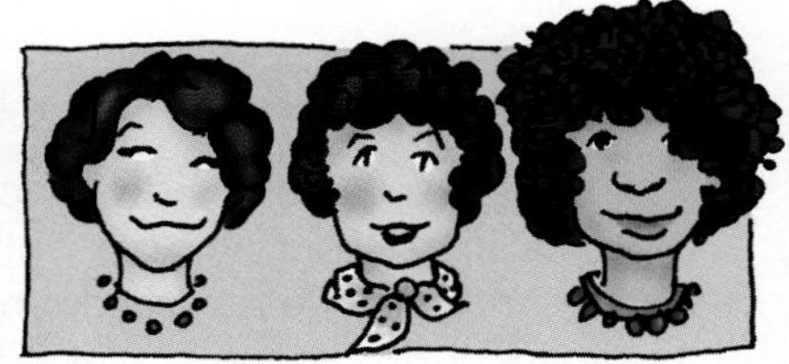

Deborah est frisée. → Juliette est plus frisée que Deborah. → Alice est **la** plus frisée des trois.

OU

Alice est frisée. → Juliette est moins frisée qu'Alice. → Deborah est **la** moins frisée des trois.

2. Superlative adjectives normally follow the nouns they modify, and the definite article is repeated.

Alice est **la** femme **la plus frisée** des trois. — *Alice is the woman with the curliest hair of the three.*

3. Adjectives that usually precede the nouns they modify can either precede or follow the noun in the superlative construction. If the adjective follows the noun, the definite article must be repeated.

la plus petite maison

OU

la maison **la** plus petite

4. The preposition **de** expresses *in* or *of* in a superlative construction.

Note: Stress the use of *de* in the superlative construction; sts. tend to use *dans*.

Alice et Grégoire habitent la plus belle maison **du** quartier.	*Alice and Grégoire live in the most beautiful house in the neighborhood.*
C'est le quartier le plus cher **de** la ville.	*It's the most expensive neighborhood in town.*

Irregular Comparative and Superlative Forms

The adjective **bon(ne)** has irregular comparative and superlative forms. **Mauvais(e)** has both regular and irregular forms.

Note: Model pronunciation of *meilleur.*

	COMPARATIVE	SUPERLATIVE
bon(ne)	meilleur(e)	le meilleur / la meilleure
mauvais(e)	plus mauvais(e)	le plus mauvais / la plus mauvaise
	pire	le/la pire

Les légumes à Carrefour sont bons, mais les légumes à Trouvetout sont **meilleurs.**	*The vegetables at Carrefour are good, but the vegetables at Trouvetout are better.*
Ce grand magasin est **le meilleur** de la ville.	*This department store is the best (one) in town.*
Ce détergent-ci est **plus mauvais (pire)** que ce détergent-là.	*This detergent is worse than that detergent.*
C'est **le plus mauvais (le pire)** des produits.	*It's the worst of products.*

[Allez-y! B-C-D]

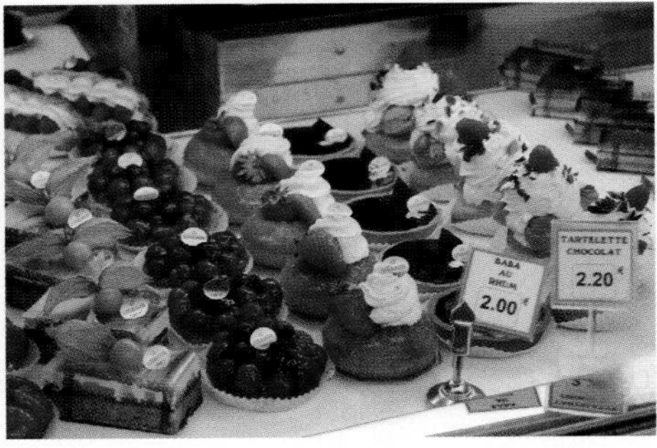

Ces pâtisseries sont les meilleures du quartier!

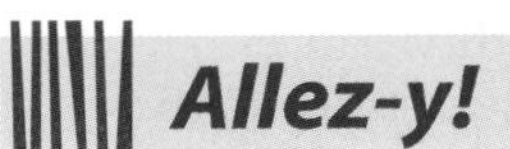

Allez-y!

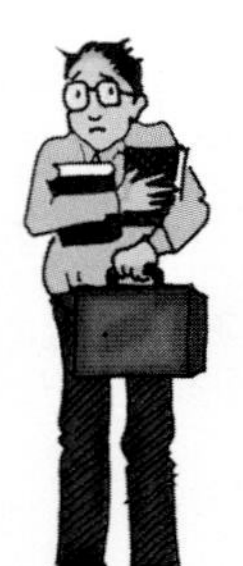

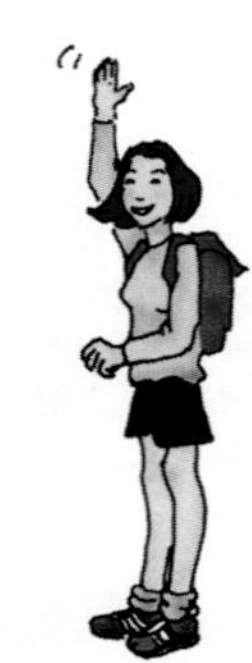

A. Comparaisons. Regardez les deux dessins et répondez aux questions suivantes.

MODÈLE: Qui est moins nerveux, le jeune homme ou la jeune fille?
La jeune fille est moins nerveuse (que le jeune homme).

1. Qui est plus grand, le jeune homme ou la jeune fille? Qui est plus mince?
2. Est-ce que la jeune fille a l'air aussi dynamique et sympathique que le jeune homme?
3. Qui est plus timide? plus bavard (*talkative*)?
4. Est-ce que le jeune homme est aussi studieux que la jeune fille?
5. Est-ce que le jeune homme est plus ou moins travailleur que la jeune fille?
6. Qui est le plus ambitieux des deux? Qui est le plus sportif des deux?

B. Un couple de francophiles. M. et Mme Cohen adorent tout ce qui est français, et ils ont tendance à exagérer. Donnez leur opinion en transformant les phrases selon le modèle.

MODÈLE: Le français est une très belle langue. →
Le français est la plus belle langue du monde.

1. La cuisine française est bonne.
2. Les vins de Bourgogne sont sophistiqués.
3. La civilisation française est très avancée.
4. Paris est une ville intéressante.
5. Les Français sont un peuple cultivé.
6. La France est un beau pays.

C. Opinions. Changez les phrases suivantes, si nécessaire, pour indiquer votre opinion personnelle: **plus / moins / aussi... que; meilleur(e) / plus mauvais(e) que.** Regardez d'abord les expressions de **Mots clés.** Utilisez ces mots et justifiez vos opinions.

1. Le sport est aussi important que les études.
2. Les rapports humains sont aussi importants que les bonnes notes.
3. Grâce à la technologie, la vie des étudiants est meilleure qu'il y a vingt ans.
4. Les cours universitaires sont plus intéressants que les cours à l'école secondaire.
5. Comme étudiant(e), je suis plus sérieux/sérieuse que la plupart de mes ami(e)s.

D. Mais ce n'est pas possible! Vous aimez exagérer. Donnez votre opinion sur les sujets suivants. Pour chaque catégorie, proposez aussi d'autres exemples si possible.

1. Le président ______ / bon ou mauvais / président / le XXe ou XXIe siècle
2. Les Américains / les gens / généreux / le monde
3. Le manque (*lack*) d'éducation / le problème / sérieux / le monde actuel
4. ______ / le problème / grand / ma vie
5. ______ / la nouvelle / intéressant / l'année
6. ______ / l'athlète / bon / l'année

Mots clés

Pour insister

Like **très,** the adverbs **bien** (*much*) and **fort** (*very, mostly*) are used to emphasize a point.

Faire des économies est **bien** plus important qu'on le pense.

Cette employée a une personnalité **fort** agréable.

Suggestion: Ask sts. to work in pairs to compare their answers.

Follow-up: Elicit responses from many sts. Ask them to react to each other's comments.

Continuation: 6. *Les études sont moins importantes que les amis.* 7. *Je suis moins heureux/heureuse que mes parents.* 8. *L'expérience est plus importante que les études.*

Suggestion: Ask sts. to work in pairs to compare their answers.

Follow-up: Elicit responses from many sts. Ask them to react to each other's comments.

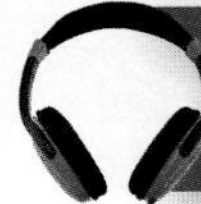

Prononcez bien!

The consonant *r* (page 385)

A. La famille d'Hugo (1). Hugo vous parle de sa famille. Complétez chaque phrase avec le mot qui manque et décidez si le premier *r* dans ce mot est un *r* doux ou un *r* fort.

	***r* doux**	***r* fort**
1. Mon père travaille dans un ______.	☐	☐
2. Ma mère aussi: elle y est ______.	☐	☐
3. C'est une petite ______.	☐	☐
4. Il n'y a que dix ______.	☐	☐
5. Le ______ est un homme honnête et juste.	☐	☐
6. Mais il est un peu ______.	☐	☐
7. Mais dans l'ensemble, mes ______ sont satisfaits de leur métier.	☐	☐

B. La famille d'Hugo (2). Hugo vous parle encore de sa famille. Avec votre camarade, répétez ce qu'il dit. Faites bien attention à la prononciation des *r* dans les mots **en caractères gras**. Dans les phrases 1 et 2, ils sont forts; dans les phrases 3 et 4, ils sont doux.

1. Je suis le plus jeune de la famille! **Patrick,** mon **frère**, a **trente-quatre** ans. Il est **peintre**.
2. Et **Christelle**, ma sœur, a **trente-trois** ans. Elle **travaille** dans le monde de la **traduction**: elle est **interprète**.
3. Mes **parents** sont **mariés** depuis **quarante** ans! Ils vont fêter **leur** long **mariage** à **Paris** dans deux semaines.
4. Il y **aura** beaucoup de gens (*people*) à cette fête. Nous allons bien manger. Et nous **boirons** beaucoup aussi! Je pense que ça **plaira** à mes **parents** de passer la **soirée** avec tout ce monde!

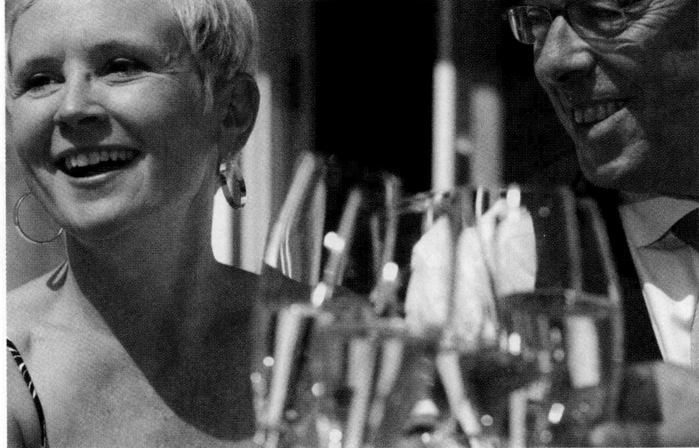

On fête le long mariage des parents d'Hugo. Félicitations!

Script (A): 1. *Mon père travaille dans un garage.* 2. *Ma mère aussi: elle y est secrétaire.* 3. *C'est une petite entreprise.* 4. *Il n'y a que dix salariés.* 5. *Le directeur est un homme honnête et juste.* 6. *Mais il est un peu stricte.* 7. *Mais dans l'ensemble, mes parents sont satisfaits de leur métier.*

Answers (A): *r* doux: 1. *garage* 4. *salariés* 5. *directeur* 7. *parents*; *r* fort: 2. *secrétaire* 3. *entreprise* 6. *stricte*

Leçon 4

 Lecture

Avant de lire

Using the dictionary. As you know, you can figure out from context the meaning of many unfamiliar words that you encounter in readings. Sometimes, however, you will need to consult a dictionary. When you do, keep in mind the following guidelines.

1. If possible, use a good hardback French–English dictionary; paperback dictionaries often do not provide all the common equivalents for a word, nor do they offer examples of usage.
2. Read through *all* the meanings and examples. Make sure the meaning you choose corresponds to the part of speech (noun, verb, etc.) of the French word you are looking for and, of course, that it makes sense in context.
3. Later on, try consulting a monolingual dictionary: one in which French words are defined in French. This may present a bit of a challenge at first, but you will find it of great benefit in terms of vocabulary enrichment and increased range of expression.

The following sentence appears in the middle of the third paragraph of the reading selection: "Au XVIIe siècle, à l'abbaye d'Hautvillers, le moine bénédictin Dom Pérignon perfectionne la création d'un vin qui mousse,… " Look for the meaning of **mousser** in the following excerpt from the *Larousse French Dictionary* (bilingual dictionary):

> **mousser** [muse] *vi* [écumer-champagne, cidre] to bubble, to sparkle; [bière] to froth; [savon, crème à raser] to lather; [détergent, shampooing] to foam, to lather

Which meaning is closest to the use of **mousser** in the sentence quoted from the article? Now, take a look at the definition of **mousser** from the *Nouveau Petit Robert* (monolingual dictionary):

> **1♦** Produire de la mousse. *Boisson qui mousse. Shampooing qui mousse beaucoup.*
> **2♦** Fig. et Fam. *Faire mousser:* vanter, mettre exagérément en valeur (une personne, une chose) ⟶ **valoir.** *Se faire mousser*.

What extra information did you get from the monolingual dictionary?

Des métiers pas ordinaires

À propos de la lecture...
Les auteurs de *Vis-à-vis* ont écrit ce texte.

Les métiers originaux, il y en a plus que vous ne pensez! En voilà quelques exemples.

Si le vin vous intéresse...

Un œnologue est un spécialiste des vins. Il les goûte, les évalue et les classe. Il partage[1] son temps entre le vignoble,[2] la cave[3] et le laboratoire. Conseiller des producteurs, des marchands et des restaurateurs, c'est un expert formé à l'université: quatre ans d'études après le bac sont nécessaires pour obtenir le Diplôme National d'Œnologie.

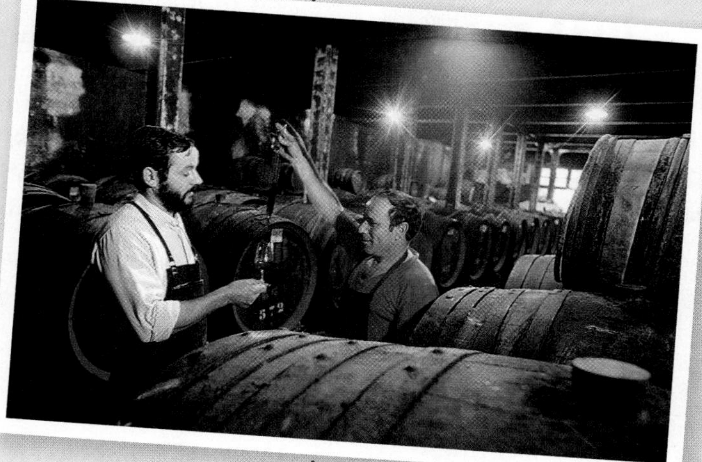

Les œnologues dans leur cave, à Bourgogne, en France. Que feront ces hommes après leur travail?

Le père du champagne

Au XVIIe siècle, à l'abbaye d'Hautvillers, le moine[4] bénédictin Dom Pérignon perfectionne la création d'un vin qui mousse, le prestigieux champagne. L'abbaye doit sa prospérité à cet œnologue subtil et au «seul vin qui rend les femmes plus belles après qu'elles l'aient bu», selon la Marquise de Pompadour.[5]

Si vous préférez les parfums, devenez aromaticien!

Comme l'œnologue, l'aromaticien doit faire confiance à son nez. D'ailleurs, on l'appelle aussi un «Nez». C'est lui qui invente des parfums. Le «Nez» a fait des études de chimie, mais il a surtout une mémoire des odeurs et un instinct de création extrêmement rares. C'est pourquoi il n'y a que 250 «Nez» dans le monde.

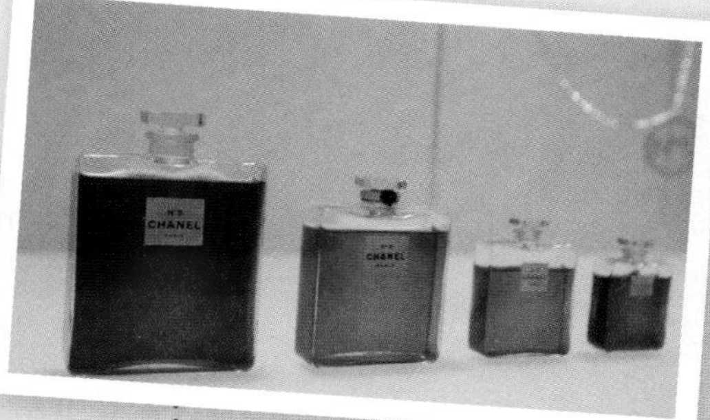

Le parfum le plus célèbre du monde. Aimez-vous les parfums?

Un «Nez» et un parfum célèbres

Le «Nez» en question s'appelle Ernest Beaux. En 1920, il propose à sa patronne, Coco Chanel, différentes créations qu'il a numérotées. Le numéro 5 plaît à Mademoiselle. Elle décide de ne pas changer son nom. Le parfum le plus célèbre du monde, Chanel N°5, vient de naître!

[1]*divides* [2]*vineyard* [3]*cellar* [4]*monk* [5]Marquise... la confidente du roi Louis XV, connue pour sa beauté et son esprit au XVIIIe siècle

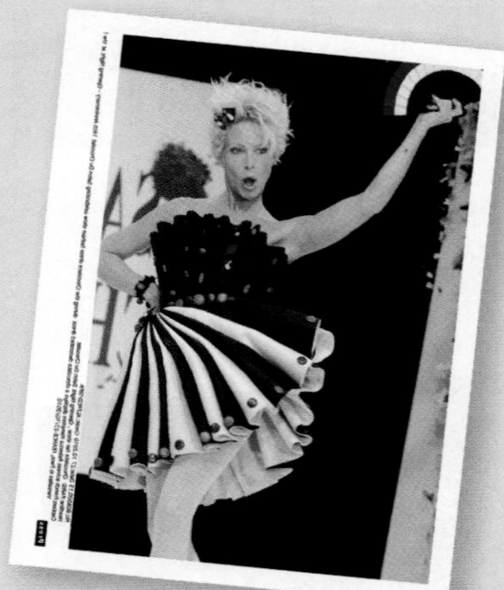

Comment trouvez-vous cette robe en chocolat du Salon du Chocolat 2013?

Un autre parfum: le chocolat

Qui dit chocolat dit chocolatier. Un chocolatier est un spécialiste diplômé d'un lycée professionnel. Il peut devenir célèbre s'il gagne le concours[6] annuel du Meilleur Ouvrier de France. Pour réussir, l'artisan chocolatier doit être aussi doué[7] et travailleur qu'imaginatif.

La mode au chocolat

Le chocolat a toujours inspiré les passions. Sous Louis XIV, on disait «La Reine a deux passions, le Roi et... le chocolat!» La passion du chocolat a aujourd'hui son propre Salon. Une fois par an, au Salon du Chocolat de Paris, des chocolatiers s'associent avec de grands couturiers pour créer une mode absolument délicieuse. Le défilé des robes en chocolat fait fondre[8] les spectateurs de plaisir!

[6]*competition* [7]*gifted* [8]*fait... melts*

Compréhension

Follow-up: 1. Quelle profession préférez-vous: œnologue, aromaticien ou chocolatier? Expliquez. 2. Avez-vous un vin préféré, un parfum préféré ou un chocolat préféré? Lequel?

Un métier pour vous? Répondez aux questions suivantes.

1. Combien d'années d'études sont nécessaires pour devenir œnologue?
2. Qui est Dom Pérignon? Qu'est-ce qu'il a fait?
3. Qu'est-ce que l'aromaticien étudie à l'université?
4. Pourquoi est-ce que le chocolat est aussi populaire en France?

La vie en chantant. An activity based on the song "Chômage" by Zebda can be found in the Instructor's Manual. The song can be purchased at the iTunes store, or sts. can watch the music video on YouTube.

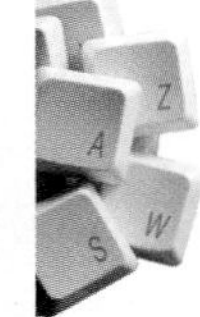

Écriture

The writing activities **Par écrit** and **Journal intime** can be found in the Workbook/Laboratory Manual to accompany *Vis-à-vis*.

Pour s'amuser

Un jeune diplômé se présente pour un poste de cadre dans une entreprise. Le directeur des Ressources humaines insiste:

—Pour ce poste, nous avons besoin d'une personne très responsable.
—C'est parfait! Dans mon poste précédent, chaque fois qu'il se passait quelque chose, on disait que c'était moi!

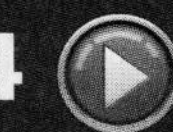

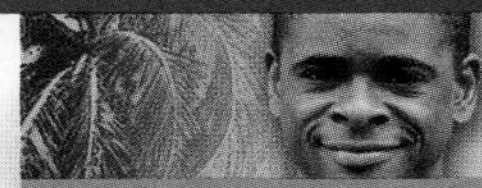

Le vidéoblog d'Hector

En bref

Dans cet épisode, Hector parle au téléphone à Léa d'un emploi qu'il veut obtenir chez Pomme Cannelle. Son entretien s'est bien passé et il attend maintenant un coup de fil du directeur. Pendant leur conversation, Léa et Hector regardent un extrait du spectacle de Pomme Cannelle sur leur site Web.

Vocabulaire en contexte

Mettez les étapes de la recherche d'un emploi en ordre chronologique en les numérotant de 1 à 7.

Étapes de la recherche d'un emploi

______ poser sa candidature
______ négocier son salaire
______ accepter le rendez-vous de l'employeur
______ rédiger (*to write*) un bon C.V.
______ faire bonne impression sur le patron (*boss*)
______ envoyer une lettre de remerciement
______ recevoir une proposition d'embauche (*job offer*)

Visionnez!

Choisissez le mot ou l'expression qui complète le mieux chaque phrase.

1. Hector est optimiste / pessimiste en ce qui concerne (*about*) cet emploi.
2. Pomme Cannelle présente son spectacle en France / dans le monde entier.
3. Pomme Cannelle a un style traditionnel / particulier.
4. Hector gagnerait (*would earn*) au minimum 1 200 / 1 800 euros par mois.
5. Si Hector n'obtient pas ce poste, il restera à Paris / repartira pour la Martinique.

Analysez!

1. Décrivez les étapes qu'Hector a suivies pour obtenir son poste chez Pomme Cannelle.
2. Quel numéro de Pomme Cannelle vous plaît (*do you like*) le plus ou le moins? Expliquez.

Comparez!

Regardez encore une fois la partie culturelle de la vidéo. Y a-t-il des troupes de danse traditionnelle ou des groupes de musique traditionnelle comme Pomme Cannelle dans votre pays ou dans votre culture? Décrivez-les. Où montent-ils leurs spectacles? Qui va les voir? Est-ce que vous aimez ces spectacles? Expliquez.

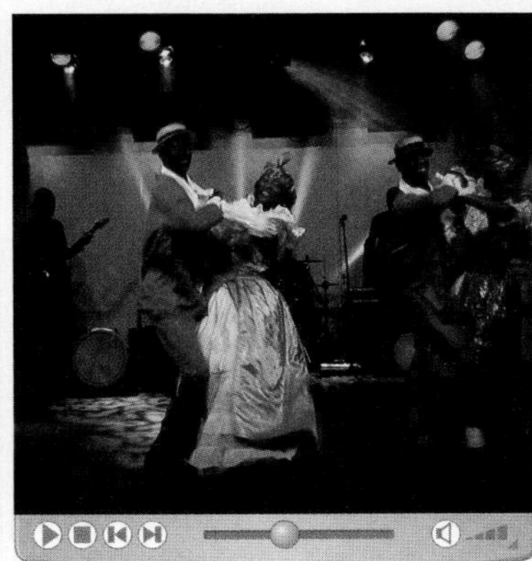

La musique et la danse sont essentielles à la vie antillaise.

Suggestion: Ask sts. short-answer questions based on the vocabulary to aid their comprehension of the video episode: *Avez-vous déjà posé votre candidature en personne pour un emploi? Qu'est-ce qui est difficile quand on rédige un C.V.? Comment est-ce que vous allez gagner votre vie?*, etc.

Additional vocabulary: Other vocabulary you may wish to present before viewing includes *se passer, un cocotier, un succès fou, un talent fou, vous n'aurez aucune dépense, virer un salaire directement sur un compte bancaire, faire partie de la troupe.*

Note culturelle

La musique et la danse sont essentielles à la culture des îles. Elles traduisent des influences européennes, africaines et américaines. Inspirée du rythme des orchestres de jazz de La Nouvelle Orléans, la biguine[1] symbolise aujourd'hui les sons et les rythmes des Antilles françaises. Mais depuis 1980, le zouk a pris la première place dans le folklore euro-antillais. Très rythmé, très sensuel, il existe aussi en version douce[2] et lente: on l'appelle le «zouk-love»!

[1]une danse [2]*soft, gentle*

CHAPITRE 14

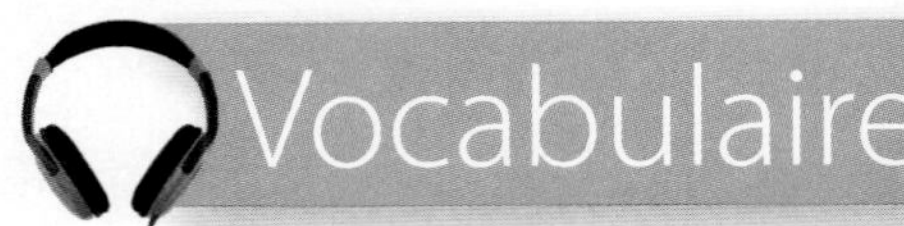

Vocabulaire

Verbes

changer to change
compter to count
contrôler to check, monitor
couvrir to cover
découvrir to discover
dépenser to spend (*money*)
déposer to deposit
diriger to direct
économiser to save money
faire des économies (*f. pl.*) to save (up) money
faire un chèque to write a check
fermer to close
gagner to earn; to win
gérer to manage
intéresser to interest
maîtriser to master, have a command
se moquer de to make fun of
offrir to offer
ouvrir to open
poser sa candidature to apply
proposer to propose
réaliser to make (happen), carry out
recruter to recruit
retirer to withdraw
soigner to treat
souffrir to suffer
toucher to touch; to cash (*a check*)
travailler à son compte to be self-employed

Substantifs

l'actualité (*f.*) current events
l'argent (*m.*) **liquide** cash
l'augmentation (*f.*) increase
  l'augmentation de salaire raise
l'avenir (*m.*) future
le bijou jewel
le budget budget
le bureau de change money exchange (office)
la carte bancaire bank (ATM/credit) card
la carte de crédit credit card
la carte de débit debit card
le chèque check
le chômage unemployment
le chômeur / la chômeuse unemployed person
le compte bancaire bank
le compte d'épargne savings account
le cours exchange rate
le coût de la vie cost of living
le curriculum vitæ (C.V.) résumé
la demande d'emploi job application
la dépense expense
l'emploi (*m.*) job
l'emprunt (*m.*) loan
l'entreprise (*f.*) company
l'entretien (*m.*) job interview
le guichet automatique automatic teller machine (ATM)
les frais (*m. pl.*) expenses, costs
le marché de l'emploi job market
le métier trade, profession
la monnaie change; currency
le montant sum, amount
la piste lead
le prélèvement automatique automatic payment/withdrawal
le reçu receipt
le relevé bank statment
le salaire salary
la societé company
le stage internship
le taux de change exchange rate
le taux de chômage unemployment rate
le virement transfer (money)

À REVOIR: **l'horaire** (*m.*), **la santé**

Les professions

l'agent (*m.*) **de police** police officer
l'agriculteur / l'agricultrice farmer
l'architecte (*m., f.*) architect
l'artisan(e) artisan, craftsperson
l'artiste (*m., f.*) artist
l'avocat(e) lawyer
le boucher / la bouchère butcher
le cadre middle or upper manager
le chef d'entreprise company head, top manager, boss
le coiffeur / la coiffeuse hairdresser
le/la commerçant(e) shopkeeper
le/la comptable accountant
le/la dentiste dentist
le directeur / la directrice manager, head
le directeur / la directrice commercial(e) business manager
l'employé(e) employee
le facteur / la factrice letter carrier
le/la fonctionnaire civil servant
l'ingénieur (*m.*) engineer
le/la journaliste reporter
le marchand / la marchande (de vin) (wine) merchant
le médecin / la femme médecin doctor
l'ouvrier / l'ouvrière (manual) worker, laborer
le/la peintre painter
le/la pharmacien(ne) pharmacist
le plombier plumber
le/la professeur des écoles primary school teacher

le rédacteur / la rédactrice editor
le/la secrétaire secretary
le travailleur / la travailleuse worker
  le travailleur indépendant self-employed worker
  le travailleur salarié salaried worker

À REVOIR: **l'acteur / l'actrice; l'écrivain / la femme écrivain; le serveur / la serveuse**

Mots et expressions divers

à l'avenir from now on, in the future
à partir de maintenant from now on
à son compte for oneself
aussi... que as . . . as
aussitôt que as soon as
car because
dès que as soon as
dont whose, of whom, of which
élevé(e) high
fort (*adv.*) very
un jour someday
lorsque when
meilleur(e) better
moins... que less . . . than
où where; when
parfaitement perfectly
pire worse
plus... que more . . . than
que whom, that, which
qui who, that, which

À REVOIR: **quand**

CHAPITRE 15

Les loisirs

Presentation: *Décrivez la scène. Où sont les acteurs? Devant quel bâtiment? Y a-t-il beaucoup de spectateurs? À votre avis, de quelle époque date la pièce?*

Les dossiers d'Hector

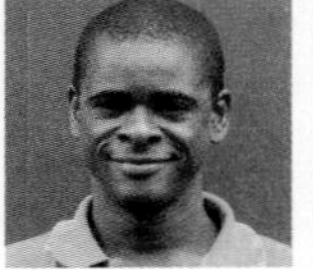

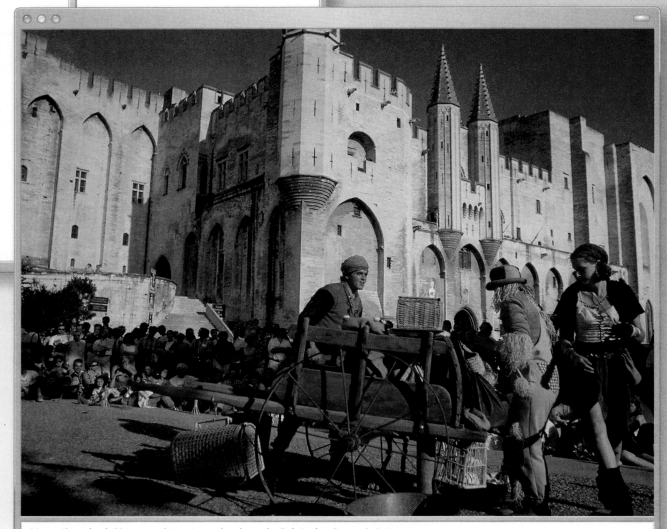

Hector

➤ Mes photos

➤ 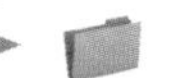 Du théâtre à Avignon

➤ 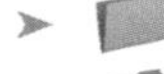 Paris-Plages en été

➤ Deux amies s'amusent au café

Une pièce de théâtre en plein air sur la place du Palais des Papes à Avignon

 **Cultural note:** Located on the *Rhône* river in southeastern France, Avignon is the *chef-lieu* of the *Vaucluse* department in the region of *Provence-Alpes-Côtes d'Azur.*

Dans ce chapitre...

OBJECTIFS COMMUNICATIFS

- talking about leisure-time activities
- getting information
- being polite
- speculating
- making comparisons
- talking about quantity
- learning to distinguish between and pronounce selected sounds in French

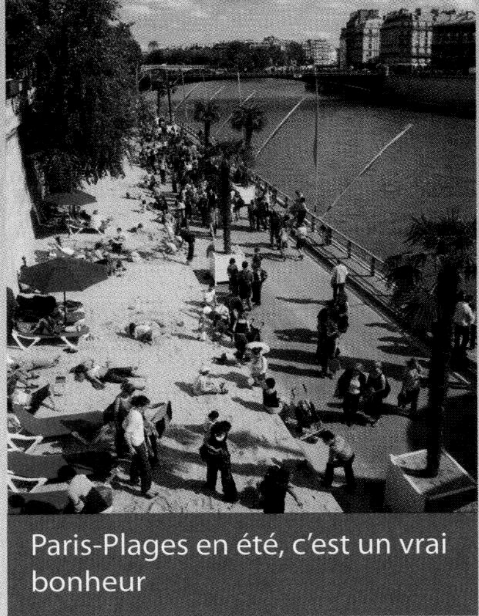
Paris-Plages en été, c'est un vrai bonheur

PAROLES (Leçon 1)

- Les loisirs
- Les verbes **courir** et **rire**

STRUCTURES (Leçons 2 et 3)

- Les pronoms interrogatifs
- Le présent du conditionnel
- La comparaison de l'adverbe et du nom
- Les adjectifs et les pronoms indéfinis

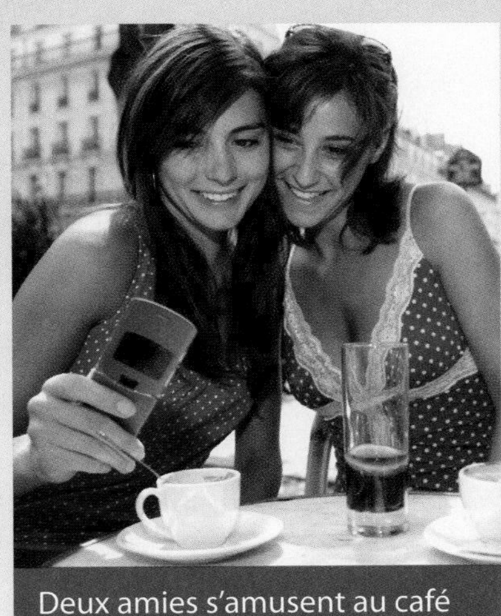
Deux amies s'amusent au café

CULTURE

- Le blog d'Hector: *Le temps de vivre*
- Reportage: *Étudier ou s'amuser?*
- Lecture: *Traversée de l'Atlantique en solitaire* (Leçon 4)

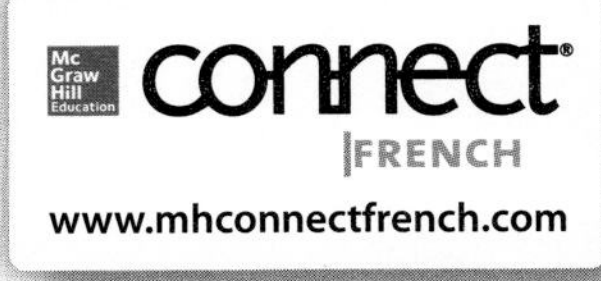

CHAPITRE 15

Leçon 1

Suggestion: Model pronunciation of new vocab. Then ask sts. to describe in as much detail as possible the actions depicted in the drawings. Ask questions to expand on ideas presented. Examples: *Quelles chansons aimez-vous le mieux? Quel film avez-vous vu récemment? Quels sports aimez-vous jouer en plein air? Quels jeux de société préférez-vous?*, etc.

PAROLES

Quelques loisirs°

°(*m.*) *leisure activities*

Cultural note: You may wish to bring in magazines on sports and leisure: *Auto-Moto, Bateaux, France-Football, Mondial, La Voix des Sports, Tennis de France*, etc., and ask sts. to look them over.

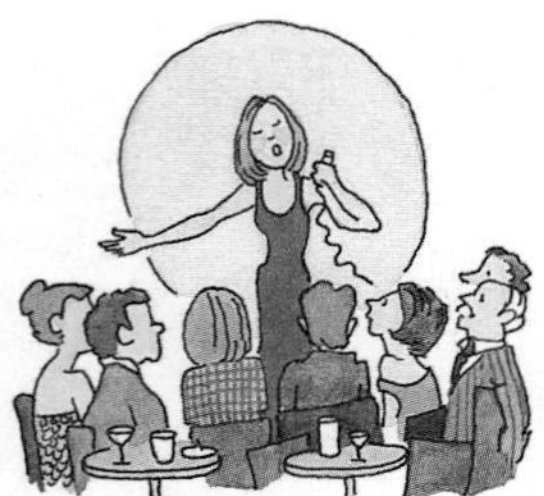

Les spectacles (*m.*)
le spectacle de variétés
le cinéma
l'opéra (*m.*)
le théâtre

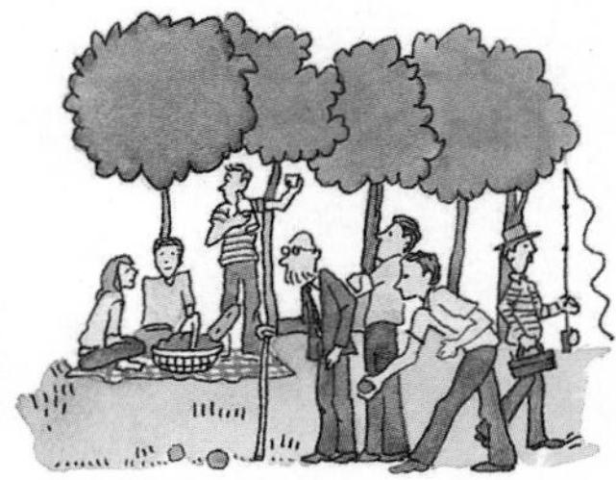

Les activités (*f.*) **de plein air**
le pique-nique
la pétanque*
la pêche
la marche
le ski

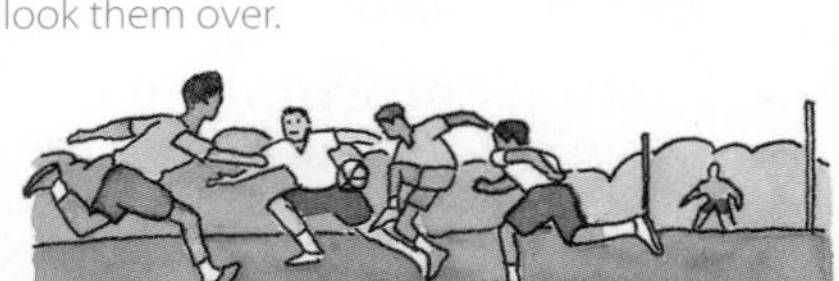

Les sports (*m.*)
le football
le cyclisme
les matchs (*m.*) (de football)

Additional vocabulary: *aller en boîte, l'aérobic, le jogging, la planche à roulettes, la planche à voile, les sorties*

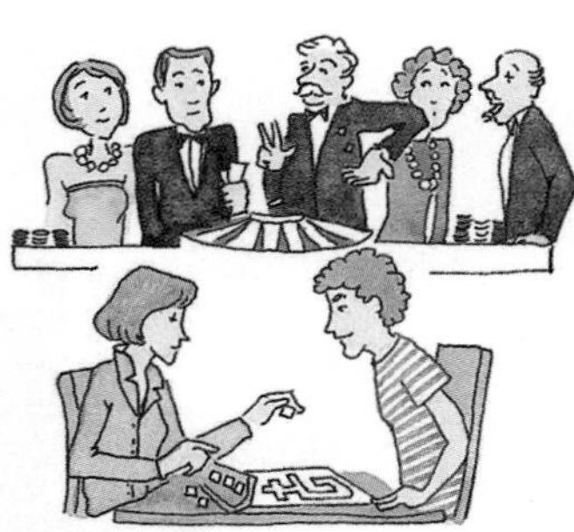

Les jeux (*m.*)
les jeux de hasard
les jeux de société

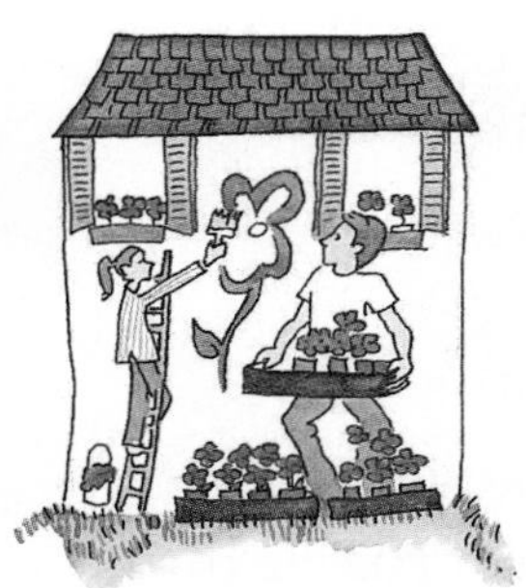

Le bricolage
le jardinage

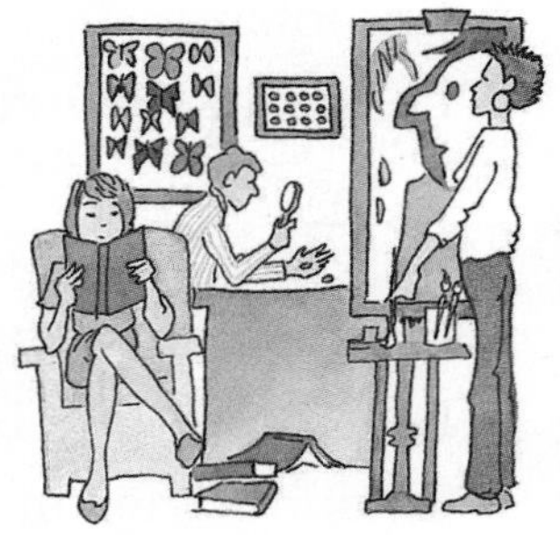

Les passe-temps (*m.*)
la lecture
les collections (*f.*)
la peinture

Vocabulary recycling: *pratiquer un sport, faire de, jouer à, la pièce de théâtre*

Qu'est-ce qu'on est en train de faire? Est-ce qu'on fait un pique-nique? Est-ce qu'on joue au football? Est-ce qu'on assiste à† un concert?

AUTRES MOTS UTILES

bricoler	to putter around, do odd jobs
une chanson‡	song
une équipe	team

*__La pétanque__ is a Provençal game similar to Italian bocce ball.
†**Assister à** means *to attend;* **aider** means *to assist, help.*
‡**Une chanson de variété** is a popular song, frequently associated with a particular singer and sung in a music hall or a small nightclub.

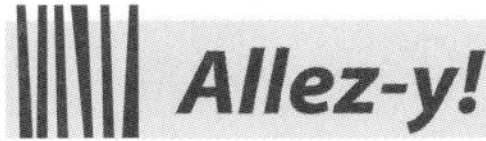

Allez-y!

A. Catégories. Le ballet et l'opéra sont des spectacles. Dans quelle(s) catégorie(s) de distractions classez-vous ______?

MODÈLE: la marche ⟶ La marche, c'est une activité de plein air.

1. un match de football
2. une collection de timbres
3. le jardinage
4. la pêche
5. la roulette
6. la lecture
7. un pique-nique
8. le poker
9. le cinéma
10. la pétanque
11. le cyclisme
12. un concert de jazz

B. Interview. Posez les questions suivantes à un(e) camarade. Demandez-lui ______.

1. quelles sortes de chansons il/elle aime (les chansons d'amour, les chansons folkloriques, le rap, le hip hop?)
2. s'il / si elle a déjà joué à la pétanque
3. à quelles sortes de spectacles il/elle assiste souvent et à quel spectacle il/elle a assisté récemment
4. s'il / si elle préfère faire du sport ou assister à des manifestations sportives; à quel événement sportif il/elle a assisté récemment
5. quel jeu de société il/elle préfère (le bridge, le Scrabble, le Monopoly?)
6. à quels jeux de hasard il/elle a joué, où il/elle y a joué et combien il/elle a gagné ou perdu
7. s'il / si elle aime bricoler et quels objets il/elle a réparés ou fabriqués
8. s'il / si elle collectionne quelque chose

Résumez! D'après ses réponses, parlez brièvement du caractère ou de la personnalité de votre camarade.

Expressions utiles: actif/active, adroit/adroite, audacieux/audacieuse, créateur/créatrice, énergique, être un homme (une femme) à tout faire (*handy*), (im)prudent(e), (n')avoir (pas) le goût du risque, paresseux/paresseuse, (peu) doué(e) (*gifted*) pour les sports, sentimental(e), sportif/sportive, terre à terre (= prosaïque, ordinaire), et cetera

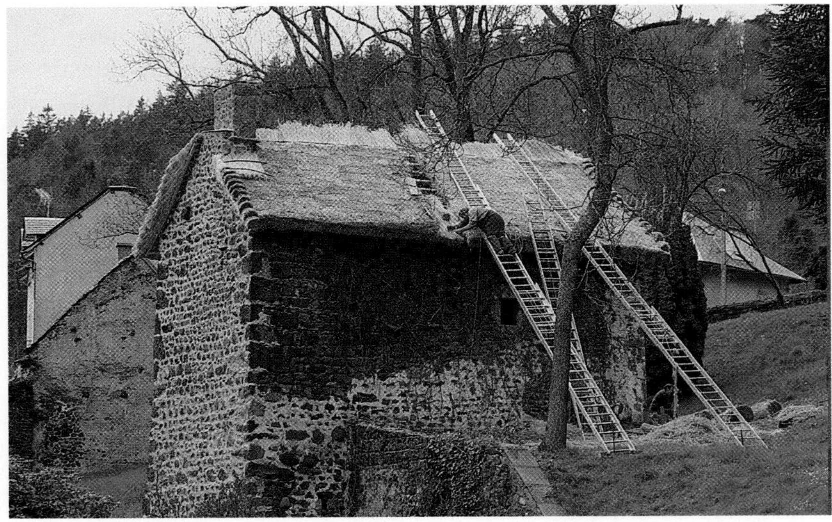

Du travail ou du bricolage? À vous de décider! Expliquez votre réponse.

Suggestion (A): Can be done as a free-association activity or game, where sts. name the first thing they think of. Word-association chains can be made from new words. Example: (1) *le base-ball; les hot-dogs, le stade, les Yankees,* etc.

Continuation (A): *le base-ball, l'opéra, la réparation d'une porte, la sculpture, une collection de tableaux.*

Follow-up (A): *Les loisirs. Le jardinage et la construction d'un barbecue sont deux formes de bricolage. Nommez deux formes de loisirs pour chaque catégorie.* 1. *les manifestations sportives* 2. *les jeux de société* 3. *les spectacles* 4. *les activités de plein air* 5. *les passe-temps*

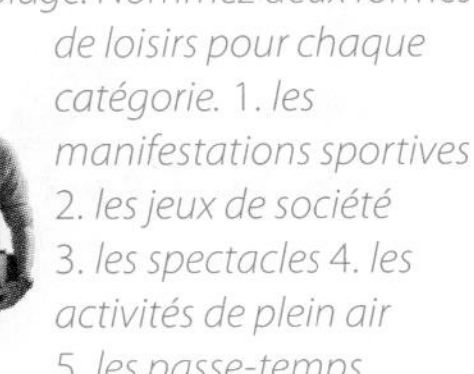

Suggestion (B): Have sts. write a *résumé* of some of the answers of classmates and report to class, or hand *résumé* in as a written assignment.

Suggestion (B): Ask sts. to work in small groups and report back to the class after doing the activity.

Additional activity: Make several sets of flash cards with a variety of vocabulary. Working in pairs, one st. describes the leisure activity on the flash card and the other guesses it. (This game is very similar to the TV game show *$100,000 Pyramid.*) After pairs have gone through their set of flash cards, you may want to have a bonus round between the two best groups.

Les verbes *courir* et *rire*

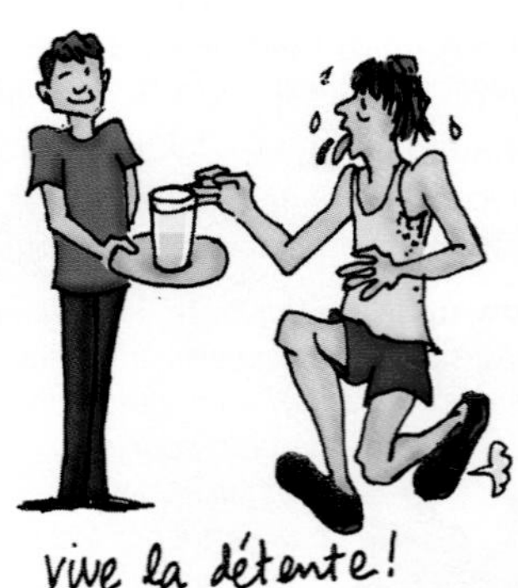

PRESENT TENSE OF **courir** (*to run*)		**rire** (*to laugh*)	
je	cour**s**	je	ri**s**
tu	cour**s**	tu	ri**s**
il/elle/on	cour**t**	il/elle/on	ri**t**
nous	cour**ons**	nous	ri**ons**
vous	cour**ez**	vous	ri**ez**
ils/elles	cour**ent**	ils/elles	ri**ent**
Past participle:	**couru**		**ri**
Future stem:	**courr-**		**rir-**

Suggestion: Model pronunciation of verb forms in short sentences: *Je cours vite. Tu ris pendant le film.*

A verb conjugated like **rire** is **sourire** (*to smile*).

Allez-y!

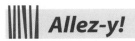

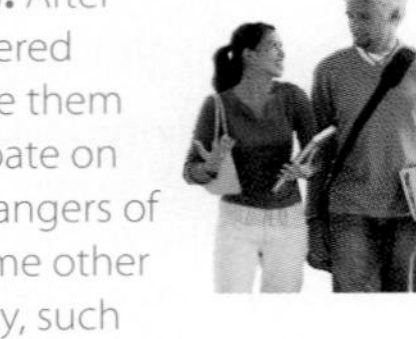

Follow-up (A): After sts. have answered questions, have them organize a debate on the joys and dangers of jogging, or some other exercise activity, such as aerobics (*l'aérobic*) or bicycling. Give them help in forming arguments, either on board or on a handout: *POUR: bon pour la santé, un excellent exercice cardiovasculaire, bon pour la santé mentale, bon pour la circulation du sang, un bon moyen de perdre des kilos, un sport très bon marché; CONTRE: dangereux pour la santé, une vraie obsession, jugé dangereux pour les gens âgés, peut provoquer des accidents cardiaques, peut faire mal aux jambes et aux pieds.*

A. Sondage sur le jogging. De plus en plus de gens sont des adeptes du jogging.

1. Demandez à un(e) camarade s'il / si elle fait du jogging.

Si oui, demandez-lui ______.

2. combien de fois par semaine il/elle court
3. pendant combien de temps il/elle court ou combien de kilomètres il/elle fait (1 mile = 1,6 kilomètres)
4. depuis quand il/elle fait du jogging

Sinon, demandez-lui ______.

5. pourquoi il/elle ne court pas
6. s'il / si elle pratique un autre sport
7. ce qu'il/elle pense des gens qui font du jogging régulièrement

Suggestion (B): (1) Have sts. do in small groups or in pairs. (2) Ask each st. to write down a short joke or riddle in French. It may be easiest if sts. have a model. Example: *Pourquoi l'éléphant s'est-il assis sur la table?* (*Parce que la chaise était trop petite.*) Collect the jokes and read a few at random.

Follow-up: To increase sts.' awareness of cultural aspects of humor, bring in several cartoons from French magazines and have sts. examine them and explain the humor.

B. Le rire. Le rire est le passe-temps préféré de beaucoup de gens. Et vous? Aimez-vous rire? Avec un(e) camarade, répondez aux questions suivantes. Chaque fois que vous répondez que oui, donnez un exemple.

1. Racontez-vous des blagues (*jokes*)? **2.** Faites-vous souvent des jeux de mots (*puns*)? **3.** Avez-vous un comique préféré / une comique préférée? **4.** Est-ce qu'il y a un film ou une pièce de théâtre que vous trouvez particulièrement intéressant(e)? **5.** Est-ce que vous riez quelquefois en cours de français? Quand et pourquoi?

Leçon 2

Les pronoms interrogatifs

Getting Information

C'est quoi, le temps libre?

Juliette téléphone à Charlotte.

JULIETTE: **Que** fais-tu pendant ton temps libre[1]?
CHARLOTTE: C'est **quoi** le temps libre? Je n'ai pas une minute à moi!
JULIETTE: **Qu'est-ce que** tu racontes[2]? **Qu'est-ce qui** t'empêche de prendre quelques heures par semaine pour toi? Il faut être un peu égoïste[3] dans la vie!
CHARLOTTE: Mais **qui** va s'occuper de[4] la maison?
JULIETTE: Charlotte, c'est une blague! J'ai l'impression d'entendre mon arrière-grand-mère! Réserve un après-midi pour toi.
CHARLOTTE: **Lequel**[5]? Je suis super occupée.
JULIETTE: Le samedi après-midi, par exemple: tu pourras faire du sport, du shopping, prendre un café avec une copine…
CHARLOTTE: Tu as raison! Je dois penser à moi.

[1]*free* [2]Qu'est-ce que… *What are you talking about?* [3]*selfish* [4]s'occuper… *take care of* [5]*Which one*

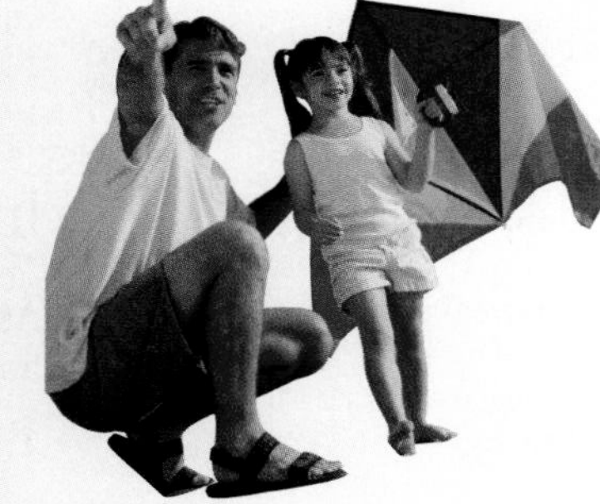

Père et fille sur la plage

Trouvez, dans le dialogue, les questions qui correspondent aux situations suivantes.

1. Juliette interroge Charlotte sur ses loisirs.
2. Charlotte ne comprend pas l'expression «temps libre».
3. Juliette demande des précisions à Charlotte.
4. Charlotte demande comment la maison va fonctionner sans elle.
5. Charlotte demande quel après-midi elle pourrait libérer.

Forms of Interrogative Pronouns

Interrogative pronouns—in English, *who? whom? which? what?*—are used to ask questions. They can play several roles in questions, serving as subjects, as objects of verbs, or as objects of prepositions. You are already familiar with the French interrogative pronouns **qui** and **qu'est-ce que.** Following is a more detailed list of French interrogative pronouns. Note that different pronouns are used for people and for things, and that several pronouns have a short and a long form.

Suggestion: Ask sts. to compare these to the relative pronouns so they do not become confused.

Note: The long and short forms are presented. Sts. at this level should be encouraged to use the form they are most comfortable with, as long as they can recognize both.

USE	PEOPLE	THINGS
Subject of a question	qui qui est-ce qui	—— qu'est-ce qui
Object of a question	qui qui est-ce que	que qu'est-ce que
Object of a preposition	à qui	à quoi

Interrogative Pronouns as the Subject of a Question

As the *subject* of a question, the interrogative pronoun that refers to people has both a short and a long form. The pronoun that refers to things has only one form. Note that **qui** is always followed by a singular verb.

PEOPLE	THINGS
Qui fait du jogging ce matin? **Qui est-ce qui** fait du jogging ce matin?	**Qu'est-ce qui** se passe? (*What's happening?*)

Suggestion: When sts. have reviewed forms and uses of interrogative pronouns, have them go back and analyze use of each pronoun in minidialogue (i.e., why a particular form is used in each case).

Interrogative Pronouns as the Object of a Question

As the *object* of a question, the interrogative pronouns referring to people, as well as those referring to things, have both a long and a short form.

1. Long forms

   PEOPLE: **Qui est-ce que**
   THINGS: **Qu'est-ce que** + *subject* + *verb* + (*other elements*)?

   Qui est-ce que tu as vu sur le court de tennis ce matin? — *Whom did you see on the tennis court this morning?*
   Qu'est-ce que Marie veut faire ce soir? — *What does Marie want to do this evening?*

   Remember that **qu'est-ce que (qu'est-ce que c'est que)** is a set phrase used to ask for a definition: *What is* ______?

   Qu'est-ce que la pétanque? — *What is pétanque?*

2. The short form **qui** can follow the subject and verb in questions using an intonation change.

   Tu cherches **qui?** — *You're looking for whom?*
   Aurélien a vu **qui** au théâtre? — *Whom did Aurélien see at the theater?*

   The short form **qui** can also be followed by an inverted subject and verb.

   Qui (+ *noun subject*) + *verb-pronoun* + (*other elements*)?

   Qui as-tu vu au club de gym? — *Whom did you see at the gym?*
   Qui Marie a-t-elle vu sur le court de tennis? — *Whom did Marie see on the tennis court?*

3. The short form **que** is followed by an inverted subject and verb. This is true for both noun and pronoun subjects.

que + *verb* + *subject* (*noun or pronoun*) + (*other elements*)?

Que cherches-tu?	*What are you looking for?*
Que cherche Justine?	*What is Justine looking for?*

[Allez-y! A]

Note: As with *qui*, the short form *quoi* is often used following the subject and verb in conversational French: *Tu dis quoi?*

Suggestion: Point out that *quoi* can be used by itself as an exclamation or an interrogation: *Quoi! Il a déjà fini?—Quoi? Qu'est-ce que tu dis?* Also mention the expression *Quoi de neuf?* (*What's new?*).

Suggestion: As a listening comprehension activity, ask sts. to indicate whether the following questions are about people or things. It may help to have them imagine they are hearing only one side of a telephone conversation. 1. *Qui est arrivé?* 2. *De quoi avez-vous parlé?* 3. *Qu'est-ce qu'elle a dit?* 4. *Qu'est-ce qui s'est passé ce week-end?* 5. *Qui as-tu vu au match?* 6. *À qui as-tu parlé?* 7. *Que vas-tu faire ce soir?* 8. *Qui est-ce que tu as invité?* 9. *Qui est-ce qui va venir?* If this set of questions is used as dictation, ask sts. to act out conversation, giving answers to each question after they ask it.

Use of *qui* and *quoi* after Prepositions

After a preposition or as a one-word question, **qui** is used to refer to people, and **quoi** is used to refer to things.

À qui est-ce que Djamel parle?	*Whom is Djamel speaking to?*
De qui est-ce que tu parles?	*Whom are you talking about?*
À quoi est-ce que Raphaëlle réfléchit?	*What is Raphaëlle thinking about?*
De quoi est-ce que vous parlez?	*What are you talking about?*

[Allez-y! B-C-D]

Note: You may wish to introduce the forms of *lequel* for recognition only.

Lequel

Lequel, laquelle, lesquels, and **lesquelles** (*which one*[*s*]?) are used to ask about a person or thing that has already been mentioned. These pronouns agree in gender and number with the nouns to which they refer.

—Avez-vous vu cet opéra?	*Have you seen this* (*that*) *opera?*
—**Lequel?**	*Which one?*
—Vous rappelez-vous cette pièce de théâtre?	*Do you remember this* (*that*) *play?*
—**Laquelle?**	*Which one?*
—**Lequel** des chanteurs américains préférez-vous?	*Which American singer do you prefer?*

[Allez-y! E]

Pronunciation presentation: To review *l*, see *Leçon 4* in *Chapitre 7* of the Workbook/Laboratory Manual.

Pronunciation practice (1): Bring in illustrations of the following words and have sts. name them, reminding them of the shape and position of their tongue: *cheval, lac, vélo, lunettes, valise, courriel, téléphone, colis, enveloppe, journal, île, librairie, hôtel, cathédrale, palais.*

Prononcez bien!

The consonant *l*

To pronounce a French **l** [l], remember to keep the body of your tongue flat and shifted to the front of your mouth, with the tip pressing against your upper front teeth. Refrain from (1) lowering the back of your tongue, (2) letting it shift to the back of your mouth, and (3) curling up the tip of your tongue, especially when you pronounce a final **-l.**

[l]: **il, lequel, pâle, Jules, sol**

Pronunciation practice (2): The *Prononcez bien!* section on page 431 of this chapter contains additional activities for practicing these sounds.

Allez-y!

A. À la Maison des jeunes et de la culture.* Posez des questions sur les activités des jeunes à la MJC. Utilisez **qui** ou **qui est-ce qui,** en remplaçant les mots en italique.

MODÈLE: *Pierrot* apprend à jouer du piano. → Qui (Qui est-ce qui) apprend à jouer du piano?

1. *Astrid* est en train de lire (*is reading*) un roman.
2. *Hakim* apprend à faire un portrait dans le cours de peinture.
3. *Alexandre* écoute un concert de musique vietnamienne.
4. *Le professeur* choisit les meilleures œuvres à exposer.

Additional activity: *Posons des questions. Remplacez le(s) mot(s) souligné(s) par un pronom interrogatif.* MODÈLE: *Claire invite le professeur.* → *Qui Claire invite-t-elle? (Qui est-ce que Claire invite?)* 1. *Marie court après le bus.* 2. *Jean court après Marie.* 3. *Marie court après sa sœur.* 4. *Mme Dulac fabrique des étagères.* 5. *M. Dulac fabrique une table.* 6. *M. Leroux a ouvert la bouteille.* 7. *Jean a ouvert la porte.* 8. *Gautier rit avec Jean.* 9. *Paulette a appris à faire de la poterie.* 10. *Jean-Paul a étudié la peinture.*

*The **Maison des jeunes et de la culture (MJC)** is a recreational center supported by the French government. **MJC**s offer courses in many hobbies and sports and sponsor cultural events.

Maintenant, posez des questions avec **que** ou **qu'est-ce que.**

MODÈLE: Colombe regarde *un film de François Truffaut* au ciné-club. →
Que regarde Colombe au ciné-club? (Qu'est-ce que Colombe regarde au ciné-club?)

5. Les jeunes font *des vases* dans le cours de poterie.
6. On joue *un air de Jacques Brel* dans le cours de guitare.
7. Grégory a fabriqué *des étagères* dans l'atelier de bricolage.
8. Marie a travaillé *son service* pendant son cours de tennis.

B. Exposition à la MJC. Vous êtes chargé(e) d'organiser une exposition à votre MJC, et vous donnez des instructions à un groupe de volontaires. Quelles questions vous posent-ils? Choisissez l'interrogatif correct.

MODÈLE: (qui / qu'est-ce que) William nous prêtera une... →
Qu'est-ce que William nous prêtera?

1. (qui / qu'est-ce qui) le directeur a invité...
2. (qui / qu'est-ce que) Joséphine va nous apporter une...
3. (qui / qui est-ce qui) nous devons téléphoner à...
4. (à quoi / de quoi) vous voulez nous parler...
5. (qui est-ce qui / qui) Aurore viendra avec son...
6. (quoi / que) vous pensez beaucoup à la...

Suggestion: Put correct answers on board or overhead as sts. give them.

C. Une matinée de bricolage. Ce matin, il y a eu beaucoup d'animation chez les Fontanet. À son retour de la maternelle (*kindergarten*), la petite Émilie veut tout savoir. À l'aide des mots en italique, formulez les questions.

MODÈLE: Papa a invité *un ami.* →
Qui est-ce que papa a invité?

1. *Maman* fabriquait une petite table.
2. Florent faisait *de la poterie.*
3. Papa parlait avec *son ami.*
4. *Florent* a ouvert la porte.
5. Le chien a vu *le facteur.*
6. Maman a crié après *le chien.*
7. Le chien a couru après *le facteur.*
8. *La poterie* est tombée par terre.
9. *Papa* a rattrapé (*caught*) le chien.
10. Le chien a cassé (*broke*) *la petite table de maman.*

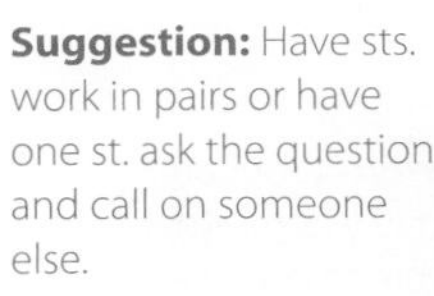
Suggestion: Have sts. work in pairs or have one st. ask the question and call on someone else.

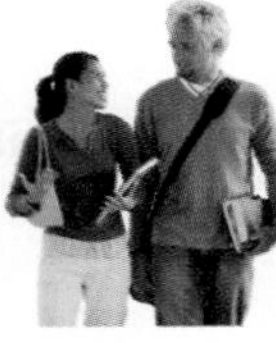

D. Interview. Avec un(e) camarade de classe, posez des questions et répondez-y à tour de rôle.

MODÈLE: acteurs comiques: Will Ferrell, Steve Carell →
É1: Lequel de ces acteurs comiques préfères-tu, Will Ferrell ou Steve Carell?
É2: Je préfère Steve Carell. Et toi, lequel préfères-tu?
É1: Je préfère...

1. actrices: Angelina Jolie, Jennifer Lawrence
2. peintres: le Français Gauguin, l'Espagnol Picasso
3. chanteuses: Taylor Swift, Alicia Keys
4. loisirs: le bricolage, le jardinage
5. spectacles: les manifestations sportives, les spectacles de variétés
6. chansons: les chansons de Green Day, de Coldplay

Que pouvez-vous dire des goûts de votre camarade?

Le présent du conditionnel

Being Polite, Speculating

Note: *Le conditionnel* is a *mode* (mood) and not a tense. Because *le conditionnel passé* is not covered in *Vis-à-vis*, the term *conditionnel* refers to the *conditionnel présent*. An explanation of the formation of the past conditional can be found in Appendix C.

Qu'est-ce qu'on pourrait faire?

Alexis contacte Poema sur sa page Facebook (Messagerie instantanée).

ALEXIS: Poema, qu'est-ce qu'**on pourrait** faire ce week-end?

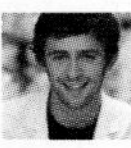
POEMA: Si j'avais le choix,[1] **j'aimerais** bien aller à la pêche.

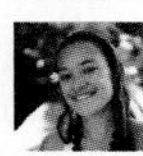
ALEXIS: Ah non! Attendre le poisson toute la journée: **Je m'ennuierais** à mourir! Tu as d'autres idées?

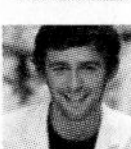
POEMA: **J'adorerais** aller pique-niquer au bord de la Seine. **Nous mangerions** plein de bonnes choses. Après, si tu voulais, **nous irions** nous promener dans la nature. **Trésor viendrait** avec nous…

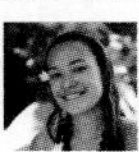
ALEXIS: Bof… Manger sur l'herbe,[2] c'est assez inconfortable… Si on allait plutôt[3] à la piscine? **On nagerait** et **on bronzerait.**

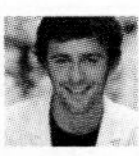
POEMA: Non: Je n'aime pas bronzer: c'est mauvais pour la peau.[4]

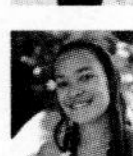
ALEXIS: Finalement, **je préférerais** faire quelque chose de culturel: un musée, un film, une exposition…

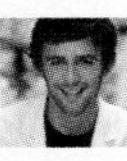
POEMA: Je ne suis pas d'accord: la culture, c'est pour les jours de pluie[5]! Et ce week-end, il va faire beau!

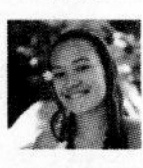
ALEXIS: Alors, qu'est-ce qu'on fait?

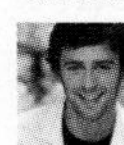

[1]*choice* [2]sur… *on the grass* [3]*instead* [4]*skin* [5]*rain*

Répondez aux questions en utilisant des phrases du dialogue.

1. Que demande Alexis?
2. Quelles sont les suggestions de Poema?
3. Quelles activités préfère Alexis?

Note: Point out the difference in pronunciation between the future ending (*-ai*) [e] and conditional endings (*-ais*) [ɛ].

Presentation: Model pronunciation in short sentences. Examples: *Je parlerais français. Nous finirions la leçon. Ils vendraient le livre.*

Forms of the Conditional

1. In English, the conditional is a compound verb form consisting of *would* plus the infinitive: *He would travel, we would go.* In French, the **conditionnel** is a simple verb form. The imperfect-tense endings **-ais, -ais, -ait, -ions, -iez, -aient** are added to the infinitive. The final **-e** of **-re** verbs is dropped before the endings are added.

parler		finir		vendre	
je	parler**ais**	je	finir**ais**	je	vendr**ais**
tu	parler**ais**	tu	finir**ais**	tu	vendr**ais**
il/elle/on	parler**ait**	il/elle/on	finir**ait**	il/elle/on	vendr**ait**
nous	parler**ions**	nous	finir**ions**	nous	vendr**ions**
vous	parler**iez**	vous	finir**iez**	vous	vendr**iez**
ils/elles	parler**aient**	ils/elles	finir**aient**	ils/elles	vendr**aient**

Elle **passerait** son temps à faire de la peinture. — *She'd spend her time painting.*
Elle **habiterait** dans une grande maison à la campagne. — *She'd live in a big house in the country.*

Suggestion: Point out that the *imparfait* and not the *conditionnel* is used in the context of a past habit: *Quand j'habitais en banlieue, je prenais le train tous les jours.* (*When I lived in the suburbs, I would take the train every day.*)

Suggestion: Review the irregular verb forms.

Note: *Pouvoir* (*could*) and *devoir* (*should*) have special meanings in the conditional.

2. Verbs with irregular stems in the future tense (**Chapitre 14, Leçon 2**) have the same irregular stems in the conditional.

S'il ne pleuvait pas, nous **irions** tous à la pêche. — *If it weren't raining, we would all go fishing.*
Elle **voudrait** venir avec nous. — *She would like to come with us.*
Est-ce que tu **aurais** le temps de m'aider à tout préparer? — *Would you have time to help me prepare everything?*

Suggestion: For listening comprehension practice, ask sts. to indicate whether they hear the verb in the conditional or the future. Ask them to imagine that the conversation is with a travel agent. 1. *Pourriez-vous m'aider?* 2. *Nous serons à Québec au mois de juillet.* 3. *Mon ami Marc voudrait l'adresse d'une école de langues.* 4. *Noémie préférerait visiter les musées.* 5. *Nous aurons tous envie de visiter la campagne.* 6. *Noémie et Marc reviendront après un mois.* 7. *Mais moi, j'y passerai une semaine de plus si j'ai le temps.* Note: Passage can be used for a partial or full dictation.

Uses of the Conditional

1. In both English and French, the conditional is used to make polite requests or inquiries. It gives a softer, more deferential tone to statements that might otherwise seem abrupt (see **Mots clés** of **Chapitre 6, Leçon 2** and **Chapitre 7, Leçon 3**).

Auriez-vous la gentillesse de m'aider? — *Would you be so kind as to help me?*
Je **pourrais** poser une question? — *Could I ask a question?*
Jean **voudrait** venir avec moi. — *Jean would like to come with me.*
Tu **devrais** faire plus de sport. — *You should be more active.*
Nous **aimerions** commander. — *We would like to order.*

[Allez-y! A-B]

2. The conditional is used in the main clause of sentences containing **si** (*if*) clauses to express what *would* happen if the hypothesis of the *if*-clause were true. The imperfect is used in the *if*-clause.

Si j'**avais** le temps, je **jouerais** au tennis.	*If I had time, I would play tennis.*
Si nous **pouvions** pique-niquer tous les jours, nous **serions** contents.	*If we could go on a picnic every day, we would be happy.*
Elle **irait** avec vous au bord de la mer si elle **savait** nager.	*She would go to the seashore with you if she knew how to swim.*

The **si** clause containing the condition is sometimes understood and not directly expressed.

Je **viendrais** avec grand plaisir… (si tu m'invitais, si j'avais le temps, et cetera).	*I would like to come . . . (if you invited me, if I had the time, etc.).*

3. Remember that an *if*-clause in the present expresses a condition that, if fulfilled, will result in a certain action (stated in the future).

Si j'**ai** le temps, je **jouerai** au tennis cet après-midi.	*If I have the time, I'll play tennis this afternoon.*

Note that the future and the conditional are *never* used in the dependent clause (after **si**) of an *if*-clause sentence.

4. The present conditional of the verb **devoir** is used to give advice and corresponds to the English *should.*

—J'aime bien les jeux de hasard.	*I like games of chance.*
—Vous **devriez** aller à Monte-Carlo.	*You should go to Monte-Carlo.*
—Elle a besoin d'exercice.	*She needs some exercise.*
—Elle **devrait** faire du jogging.	*She should go jogging.*

[Allez-y! C-D-E-F]

Suggestion: Point out the similarity between the French and English structures: *J'irais si j'avais le temps.* (*I would go if I had the time.*)

Mots clés

Exprimer un désir et suggérer

The construction **si** + **imparfait** (without the conditional) is used to express a wish or to make a suggestion.

Si seulement **j'étais** riche!
If only I were rich!

Si on dansait?
Shall we dance?

Allez-y!

A. S'il vous plaît. Michael passe ses vacances en France. Il a rencontré une jeune Française et veut l'inviter à sortir avec lui. Il veut faire bonne impression au téléphone. Aidez-le en mettant ses phrases au conditionnel et en ajoutant **s'il vous plaît / s'il te plaît** quand c'est possible.

MODÈLE: Bonjour, madame. Puis-je parler à Manon? → Bonjour, madame. Pourrais-je parler à Manon, s'il vous plaît?

1. Je veux inviter votre fille à venir avec moi au cinéma.
2. Pouvez-vous lui dire que je suis au téléphone?…
3. Salut Manon. Est-ce que tu veux aller voir un film ce soir?
4. Est-ce que nous pouvons partir vers 18 h?
5. Tes parents préfèrent peut-être faire ma connaissance…
6. Tu peux me donner ton adresse?

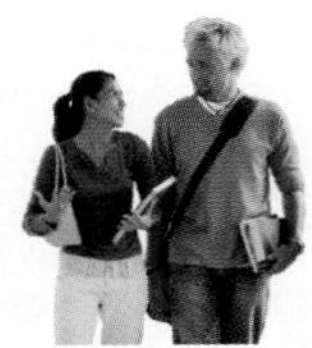

B. Soyons diplomates. Vous avez un ami / une amie qui donne toujours des ordres. Indiquez-lui deux façons de demander la même chose, mais poliment.

MODÈLE: L'AMI(E): Dites-moi à quelle heure le film commence!
VOUS: Non! Pourriez-vous me dire à quelle heure le film commence? (Je voudrais savoir à quelle heure le film commence.)

1. Donnez-moi un billet!
2. Expliquez-moi pourquoi les billets sont si chers.
3. Faites-moi de la monnaie de cinquante euros.
4. Dites-moi dans quelle salle on passe ce film.
5. Dites-moi si je dois réserver des places pour le film.

C. Un après-midi de loisir. Si vous pouviez choisir, laquelle de ces activités feriez-vous cet après-midi? Posez les questions à un(e) camarade.

MODÈLE: faire une promenade en ville ou à la campagne →
É1: Est-ce que tu ferais une promenade en ville ou à la campagne?
É2: Je ferais une promenade à la campagne.

1. jouer au tennis ou au football
2. aller au cinéma ou au café
3. passer une heure au musée ou au parc
4. manger une pizza ou un sandwich
5. boire un café ou un coca-cola
6. faire des courses ou la sieste
7. écouter de la musique classique ou du rock
8. acheter des vêtements ou des livres
9. lire des bandes dessinées ou un roman
10. se reposer ou faire du sport

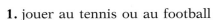

Le parler jeune

une boîte	une discothèque
ça baigne	tout va bien
délirer	s'amuser
faire la bombe	faire la fête
trop/top délire	génial, formidable

On va en **boîte,** samedi soir?

Allô? Oui, il fait très beau! **Ça baigne**!

Avec Léo, on **a** bien **déliré** l'été dernier sur la côte!

Pour ton anniversaire, c'est décidé, on **fait la bombe.**

Regardez cette vidéo, c'est **trop délire**!

D. À l'office du tourisme. Vous êtes de passage dans une ville que vous ne connaissez pas, et vous demandez à l'employé(e) de l'office de tourisme de vous donner des idées de choses à faire. Complétez ses phrases de façon logique.

MODÈLE: VOUS: J'aime profiter de la nature tôt le matin.
L'EMPLOYÉ(E): À votre place, j'irais à la pêche. Il y a un beau lac pas très loin.

1. VOUS: En milieu de matinée, j'aime faire des courses.
L'EMPLOYÉ(E): Si j'étais vous, __________.
2. VOUS: À midi, j'aime manger dehors quand il fait beau.
L'EMPLOYÉ(E): À votre place, __________.
3. VOUS: Quand j'ai fini de manger, j'aime faire un peu de sport.
L'EMPLOYÉ(E): À mon avis, __________.
4. VOUS: L'après-midi, j'aime bien faire quelque chose de culturel.
L'EMPLOYÉ(E): Selon notre guide, __________.
5. VOUS: Et pour entendre de la bonne musique, que me suggérez-vous?
L'EMPLOYÉ(E): À mon avis, __________.
6. VOUS: J'ai besoin de rencontrer des gens le soir, sinon je me sens seul(e).
L'EMPLOYÉ(E): À votre place, __________.

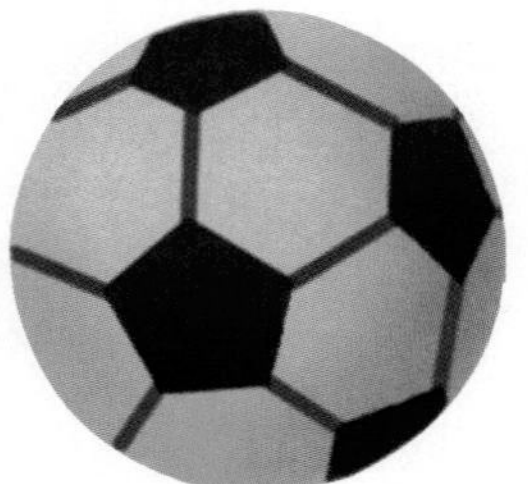

E. Nommez trois choses... Donnez par écrit votre réaction spontanée aux questions suivantes. Écrivez des phrases complètes. Puis, comparez vos réponses avec celles d'un(e) camarade de classe. Lesquelles sont identiques?

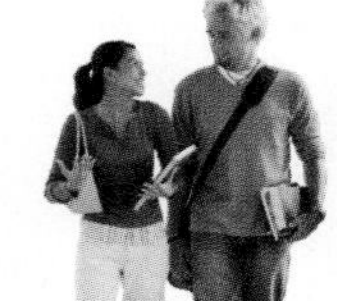

1. Nommez trois choses que vous feriez si vous étiez riche.
2. Donnez trois raisons pour lesquelles vous vous battriez (*you would fight*) si c'était nécessaire.
3. Nommez trois instruments de musique dont vous aimeriez jouer.
4. Nommez trois sports que vous aimeriez bien pratiquer.
5. Nommez trois personnes qui vous font souvent rire.
6. Nommez trois chanteurs (ou chanteuses) que vous admirez.
7. Nommez trois choses que vous feriez ce week-end si vous aviez le temps.

F. De beaux rêves. Imaginez ce que vous feriez dans les situations suivantes. Justifiez vos choix.

MODÈLE: si vous gagniez un voyage →
Si je gagnais un voyage, j'irais à Tahiti.

1. si vous receviez un chèque de 100 000 dollars **2.** si vous deviez vivre dans une autre ville **3.** si vous pouviez avoir la maison de vos rêves **4.** si vous preniez de longues vacances **5.** si vous veniez de finir vos études

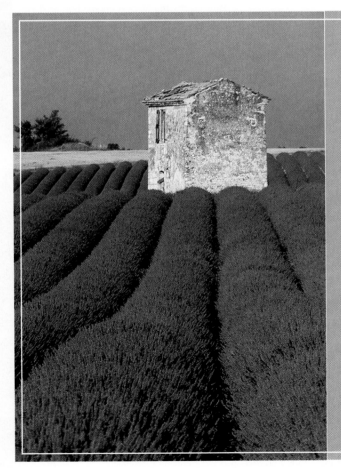

Un peu plus...

En Provence.
La lavande est une plante indigène de la région des Alpes, et différentes variétés poussent (*grow*) partout en Provence. Les fleurs de lavande s'épanouissent (*bloom*) de juin à octobre et colorent de violet les champs (*fields*). Ces fleurs peuvent être séchées (*dried*) et utilisées en cuisine ou pour parfumer le linge (*laundry*). On utilise l'essence de lavande dans les parfums et les savons.

Nommez une plante indigène de votre région.

◄ *Et si on allait en Provence? Que ferait-on?*

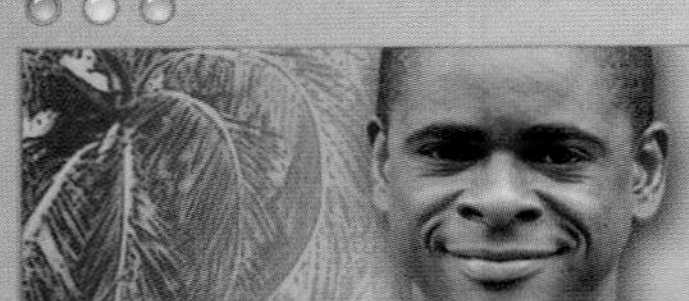

Le blog d'Hector

Le temps de vivre

jeudi 9 juillet

Si j'avais du temps à moi, qu'est-ce que je ferais?

Il y a un Hector paresseux qui dit: «Je resterais des journées entières devant la télé; je surferais toute la nuit sur Internet; je bavarderais pendant des heures au téléphone.»

Il y a un Hector aventurier qui rêve: «Je jouerais au poker, je ferais le commerce des diamants.»

Il y a un Hector intellectuel qui jure[1]: «J'irais au cinéma, au théâtre, à l'opéra; je lirais deux livres par semaine; j'écouterais plus de musique classique que de musique techno; je jouerais du saxophone et j'écrirais des poèmes!»

Il y a un Hector raisonnable qui pense: «Je ferais du bricolage dans l'appartement; je téléphonerais plus souvent à mes parents; je dépenserais moins d'argent… »

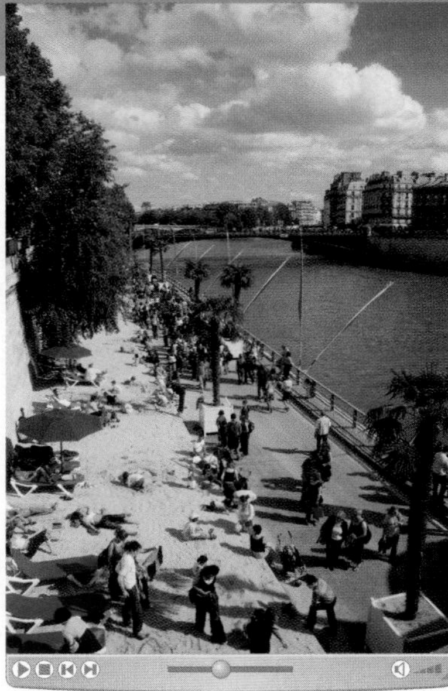

Paris-Plages en été, c'est un vrai bonheur!

Il y a un Hector généreux qui promet: «Je ferais du bénévolat[2] aussi souvent que possible et je donnerais mon temps à des associations de défense de l'environnement.»

Et pour dire la vérité, il y avait, ce week-end, un Hector particulièrement glandeur[3] qui est allé se détendre à Paris-Plages avec Léa. Ce soir, le même Hector assistera au concert en plein air du chanteur Corneille: «Tant mieux[4] pour Hector!»

Hector

Follow-up: 1. *De tous les «Hector» mentionnés dans le blog, lequel vous est le plus sympathique? Pourquoi? À quel Hector vous identifiez-vous le plus facilement?* 2. *Finalement, qui est le véritable Hector? Faites son portrait à partir des éléments donnés dans son blog du 9 juillet.*

Cultural notes: Cornelius (aka Corneille) Nyungura, a Hutu singer now a Canadian citizen, resides in Quebec. His first album, *Parce qu'on vient de loin*, brought him fame. His talent and velvety voice, as well as the story of his escape from the war in Rwanda (where his entire family was killed), appeal to his fans. Isabelle Boulay is a native of Quebec. Born in 1972, she is a star in her own country as well as in France. She sings the standards with modesty and talent. The Olympia music hall is the oldest music hall in Paris, established in 1888 by Joseph Oller, also the founder of the Moulin Rouge. Located at 28, boulevard des Capucines in the 9th *arrondissement* (Métro: Opéra-Madeleine), it is a venue for musicians from all over the world.

COMMENTAIRES

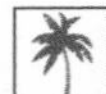

Poema

Corneille, c'est le plus beau, le plus généreux, le moins prétentieux des chanteurs francophones. Si je pouvais, je l'écouterais 24 heures sur 24.

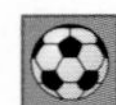

Mamadou

Poema, j'ai deux billets pour le concert de Corneille: ça te dirait de venir avec moi?

Alexis

Qui est-ce qui apprécie Isabelle Boulay? C'est la plus sublime des chanteuses québécoises! Elle va passer à l'Olympia cet automne. Je pourrais avoir des billets…

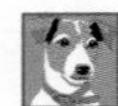

Trésor

Houuuu! Alexis est amoureux de la belle Isabelle!

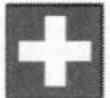

Charlotte

Si j'habitais Paris, j'aimerais bien aller au concert de Corneille ou à Paris-Plages.

Suggestion: Have sts. use the structure of the blog as a model to describe different aspects of their own personalities using the conditional.

Video connection: In the Videoblog for this chapter, Léa and Hector decide to visit *Paris-Plages*.

[1]*swears* [2]*volunteer work* [3]*idle* (fam.) [4]Tant… *So much the better*

REPORTAGE

Étudier ou s'amuser?

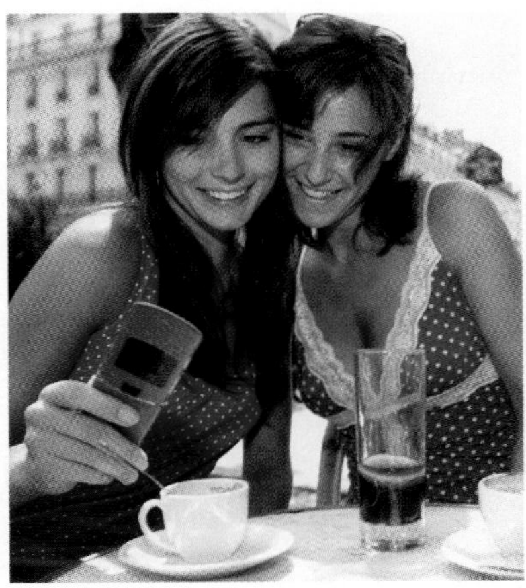

Deux amies s'amusent au café

Est-ce qu'on a le temps de se détendre quand on est étudiant? Entre les cours, les révisions et les examens, peut-on se permettre des loisirs?

«Il n'y a pas que les études dans la vie», répond Élisabeth avec conviction. Cette étudiante brillante concilie[1] sans problème études et loisirs: «Je travaille un maximum pendant la semaine. Mais le week-end, je m'éclate[2]! Il faut savoir faire la fête, non?» À la question «Quelles sont vos activités de loisirs?», elle répond: «Je fais les boutiques avec mes copines, je pratique le judo, j'écoute de la musique rap, je vais en boîte et j'écris des poèmes!»

«Évidemment, je pourrais ne pas lever la tête de mes livres et rester scotché devant mon ordinateur, mais ça ne serait pas efficace,[3] ajoute Saïd, étudiant en médecine. En fait, chacun s'organise en fonction de sa personnalité. Certains travaillent sept jours sur sept et attendent les vacances pour se détendre. D'autres, pour être plus performants, ont besoin de se détendre pendant une heure ou deux chaque jour. C'est mon cas. Alors un jour je vais au ciné, un autre jour je me réserve une soirée avec mes potes. Quand c'est possible, je vais à un concert. Et toutes les semaines, j'ai mon entraînement au foot… Je dois dire aussi que je suis accro[4] aux jeux vidéo… »

Une vie d'étudiant à cent à l'heure[5] n'empêche pas[6] la détente et les loisirs. Quels loisirs? Les jeunes passent leur temps libre avec leurs amis. Ils font du sport, ils écoutent de la musique et ils font la fête. Mais surtout, ils passent des heures sur Internet!

[1]*reconciles* [2]*have fun* (*lit. blow up*) [3]*effective, efficient* [4]*hooked, addicted* [5]à cent… *at 100 miles per hour* [6]n'empêche… *doesn't preclude*

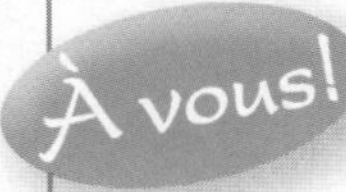

1. Comment Élisabeth organise-t-elle son temps? Quels sont ses loisirs?
2. Comment Saïd se détend-il?
3. Parmi les loisirs préférés des jeunes Français, lequel préférez-vous? Pourquoi?
4. Pour se détendre, que font les deux étudiantes représentées sur la photo?

Parlons-en!

1. Dites quelles activités vous pratiquez pendant votre temps libre. Un(e) étudiant(e) va les inscrire au tableau.
2. Quelle est l'activité la plus populaire auprès des étudiants de la classe? Quelle est la moins pratiquée? La plus originale?
3. Imaginez que vous avez 40 ans. Quels seront alors vos loisirs préférés? Un(e) étudiant(e) va les inscrire au tableau.
4. Discutez: quel changement majeur observez-vous?

CHAPITRE **15**

Leçon 3

STRUCTURES

La comparaison de l'adverbe et du nom

Making Comparisons

Et si on essayait?

Hector, Hassan, Juliette et Léa discutent au restaurant.

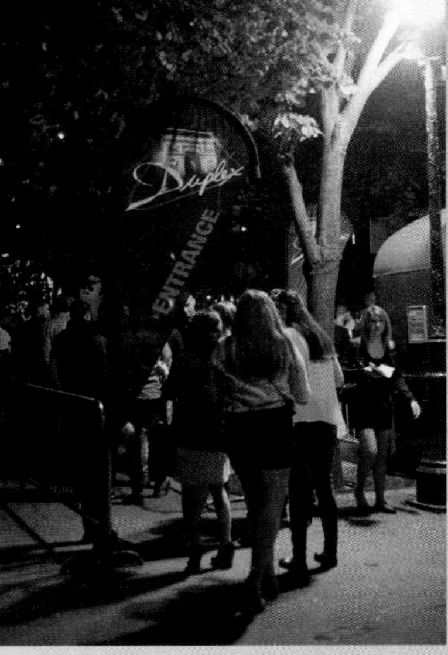

Le Duplex: une boîte de nuit pour les jeunes

LÉA: On va en boîte[1] samedi?

HECTOR: J'aime **mieux** une fête à la maison **qu**'une sortie en boîte: Déjà, ça coûte moins cher.

LÉA: Oui, mais en boîte, on rencontre **plus de gens que** dans une fête privée.

HASSAN: C'est vrai mais, **le plus souvent,** les gens qu'on rencontre en boîte n'ont aucun intérêt[2]…

JULIETTE: Hassan, tu as **plus de préjugés que** d'expérience: Il y a **autant de**[3] **gens** bien dans une boîte **qu**'ailleurs.[4] Moi, j'ai rencontré des gens supers en boîte. Des gens comme nous…

HASSAN: Des gens beaux, intelligents et drôles comme nous? C'est impossible! (*Il rit.*)

HECTOR: Moi, j'avoue[5] que j'irais **plus facilement** dans un bar sympa pour boire un coup entre potes…

JULIETTE: **Le mieux**, c'est d'essayer! On va au Duplex!

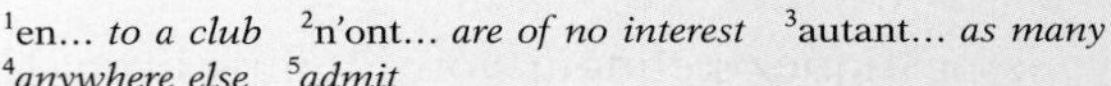

[1]en… *to a club* [2]n'ont… *are of no interest* [3]autant… *as many* [4]*anywhere else* [5]*admit*

Vrai ou faux? Découvrez les phrases fausses et remplacez-les par les phrases du dialogue.

1. Hector préfère une sortie en boîte à une fête à la maison.
2. Hector pense qu'une fête à la maison coûte plus cher.
3. Hassan trouve que, la plupart du temps, les gens qui vont en boîte ne sont pas intéressants.
4. Hassan a moins d'expérience que de préjugés.
5. Selon Juliette, il y a des gens bien partout.
6. Hector irait plus facilement dans un bar.
7. Juliette propose d'essayer une sortie en boîte.

Comparative and Superlative Forms of Adverbs

Vocabulary review: Review formation of comparative and superlative of adjectives (*Chapitre 14, Leçon 3*).

1. The same constructions you learned in **Chapitre 14, Leçon 3** for the comparative forms of adjectives are used for the comparative forms of adverbs.

Jeanne écoute du jazz **plus** souvent (**que** moi).	*Jeanne listens to jazz music more often (than I).*
On écoute la musique **moins** attentivement dans les boîtes de nuit **que** dans les bars de jazz.	*People listen to the music less attentively at discos than at jazz bars.*
Nous allons danser **aussi** souvent **que** possible.	*We go dancing as often as possible.*

plus... que (*more . . . than*)

moins... que (*less . . . than*)

aussi... que (*as . . . as*)

[Allez-y! C]

2. To form the superlative of an adverb, place **le** in front of the comparative form (**le plus...** or **le moins...**). Because adverbs are invariable, the definite article will always be **le.**

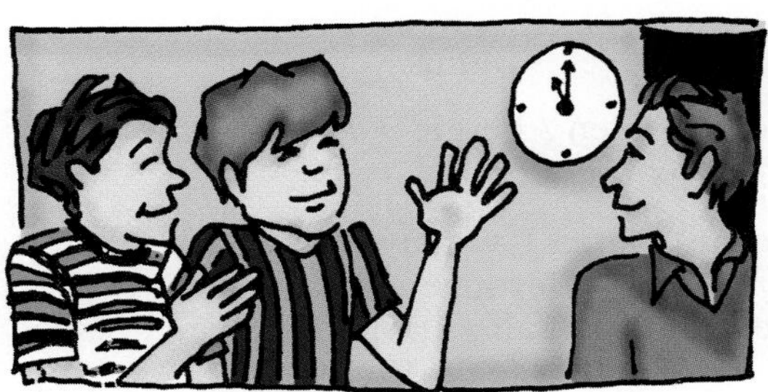
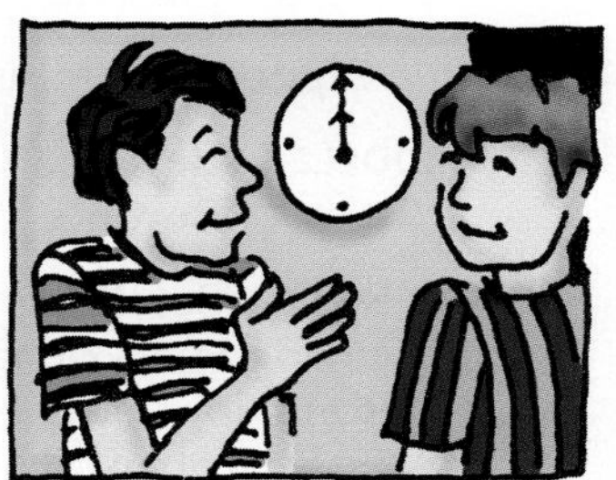
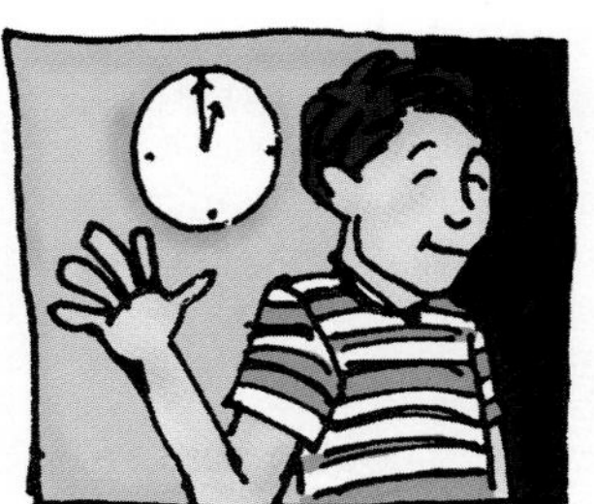

Romain s'en va tard. Louis s'en va plus tard. Sacha s'en va **le plus tard.**

Bien and *mal*

The comparative and superlative forms of **bien** are irregular. The comparative and superlative forms of **mal** are regular.*

	COMPARATIVE	SUPERLATIVE
bien	mieux	le mieux
mal	plus mal	le plus mal

Tu parles français **mieux** que moi.	*You speak French better than I.*
Mais c'est Mehdi qui le parle **le mieux.**	*But Mehdi speaks it best.*
Augustin joue **plus mal** au tennis que moi.	*Augustin plays tennis worse than I.*
Mais c'est Marc qui y joue **le plus mal.**	*But Marc plays the worst.*

[Allez-y! A]

Note: Review irregular forms for comparative and superlative of *bon* and *mauvais*, presented in *Chapitre 14, Leçon 3*.

Note: The structure (*le*) *moins bien* is often preferred over (*le*) *plus mal*.

Mots clés

Tant mieux, tant pis

The expressions **tant mieux** (*so much the better*) and **tant pis** (*that's too bad*) are commonly used in everyday conversation.

Si tu viens, **tant mieux;** si tu ne viens pas, **tant pis.**

Il ne veut pas nous accompagner? **Tant pis** pour lui!

*Irregular comparative and superlative forms of **mal (pis, le pis)** exist, but the regular forms are much more commonly used.

Presentation: Magazine pictures or drawings that can be easily compared are useful in presenting these notions. Use names of famous people to further engage sts.' interest. Examples: *Bill Gates a plus d'argent que nous. J'ai moins de problèmes que le président des États-Unis.*

Comparisons with Nouns

Plus de... (que), moins de... (que), and **autant de... (que)** express quantitative comparisons with nouns.

Ils ont **plus d'**argent (**que** nous), mais nous avons **moins de** problèmes (**qu'**eux).	*They have more money (than we do), but we have fewer problems (than they do).*
Je suis **autant de** cours **que** toi ce semestre.	*I'm taking as many courses as you this semester.*

[Allez-y! B-C]

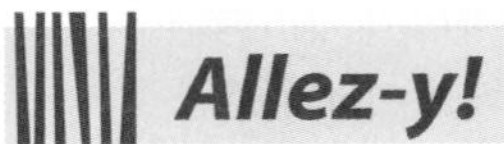

Suggestion (A): Ask sts. to write out responses in class. Have several sts. put sentences on board for correction.

Suggestion (B): Ask sts. to write out 3 or more comparisons first before you elicit oral responses.

Suggestion (C): Type up the 7 questions on 2 halves of a sheet, 3–4 questions on each half. Assign one st. in a group of 3 to ask the first set of questions, one to ask the second set, and the third to act as group monitor, checking the forms of questions asked by the 2 classmates. When a st. asks a question, the other should answer, as in an interview. The monitor can take notes on answers, if desired.

A. Les comparaisons. Formez des phrases pour comparer ces personnes célèbres en vous aidant des signes donnés. Mettez les verbes au présent.

Signes: + plus = aussi − moins

MODÈLE: Beyoncé / danser / + bien / Fergie ⟶ Beyoncé danse mieux que Fergie.

1. Steven Spielberg / aller au cinéma / = souvent / Woody Allen
2. Taylor Swift / chanter / − bien / Beyoncé
3. Ronaldo / jouer / + bien / au football / David Beckham
4. Josh Groban / chanter / = bien / Plácido Domingo
5. Tout le monde / jouer / − bien / au basket-ball / LeBron James

B. Les Français et les loisirs. Regardez le tableau et faites au moins trois comparaisons entre les hommes et les femmes en ce qui concerne les loisirs.

Des millions d'artistes

Pratiques artistiques amateurs au cours des douze derniers mois par sexe et âge (en % de la population de 15 ans et plus):

	Hommes	Femmes
Jouer d'un instrument musical	15	11
Faire de la musique en groupe	11	9
Tenir un journal	6	11
Écrire des poèmes, nouvelles, romans	5	7
Faire de la peinture, sculpture, gravure	9	11
Faire de la poterie, céramique, reliure, artisanat d'art	3	5
Faire du théâtre	2	2
Faire du dessin	16	16
Faire de la danse	5	10

MODÈLE: Les hommes font moins de danse que les femmes, mais ils font plus de musique en groupe que les femmes.

C. Interview. Posez les questions suivantes en français à un(e) camarade. Ensuite, résumez ses réponses.

1. Who in class has more leisure time than you? Why?
2. What sport would you like to be able to play better?
3. Which American plays tennis best?
4. Which athlete (**athlète,** *m., f.*) would you like to speak to the most?
5. Who in the class runs faster than you? How do you know?
6. Who in the class goes to the library as often as you?
7. Who in the class needs to study the least in order to (**pour**) have good grades (**notes,** *f.*)?

D. Les habitudes. Demandez à un(e) camarade combien de fois par semaine, par jour, par mois ou par an il/elle fait quelque chose, puis comparez sa réponse avec vos propres habitudes.

Possibilités: faire du sport, lire le journal, partir en voyage, regarder la télévision…

MODÈLE: É1: Combien de fois par semaine vas-tu au cinéma?
É2: Une ou deux fois par semaine.
É1: J'y vais plus (moins, aussi) souvent que toi.

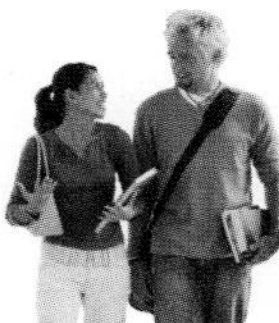

Suggestions (D): *prendre le bus / par semaine; faire du jogging / par semaine; aller à la bibliothèque / par semaine; téléphoner à ses parents / par mois; sortir avec des amis / par semaine; regarder la télévision / par semaine; écrire à ses parents / par mois; se regarder dans un miroir / par jour; se brosser les dents / par jour; se laver les cheveux / par semaine*

Les adjectifs et les pronoms indéfinis

Talking About Quantity

L'influence du soleil

Mamadou téléphone à Léa.

MAMADOU: Alors, ces vacances avec Juliette?
LÉA: **Tout** s'est très bien passé. Après **quelques** heures à Londres, nous sommes allées chercher le beau temps sur la Côte d'Azur.
MAMADOU: Vous vous êtes bien amusées?
LÉA: On a fait **chaque** jour **quelque chose** de différent: un jour la plage, **un autre** les musées, et **plusieurs** fois des randonnées.
MAMADOU: **Tout** est super dans le Midi[1]! Les gens sont tellement cools!
LÉA: Ça, c'est un cliché! Il y a des gens désagréables même sous le soleil de la Côte d'Azur et surtout en été: **certains** sont exaspérés par les touristes, **d'autres** sont furieux à cause des embouteillages.[2] **Les uns** protestent parce qu'il faut faire la queue dans les supermarchés, **les autres** détestent la foule[3] sur la plage…
MAMADOU: Je suis sûr que ce sont des Parisiens!

[1]*South (of France)* [2]*à… because of the traffic jams* [3]*crowds*

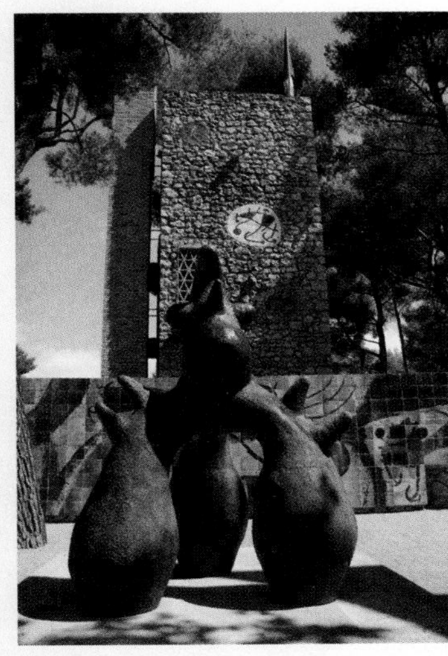

Sculpture sous le soleil de la Côte d'Azur (Fondation Maeght, Saint-Paul-de-Vence)

Répondez aux questions en utilisant les expressions du dialogue.

1. Qu'est-ce qui s'est bien passé?
2. Combien de temps Juliette et Léa sont-elles restées à Londres?
3. Qu'est-ce qu'elles ont fait sur la Côte d'Azur?
4. Pour Mamadou, qu'est-ce qui est super dans le Midi?
5. Que font les gens désagréables sur la Côte d'Azur?

Forms and Uses of *tout*

1. The adjective **tout (toute, tous, toutes)**

   As an adjective, **tout** can be followed by an article, a possessive adjective, or a demonstrative adjective.

Nous avons marché **toute la journée** pour arriver au sommet du volcan.	*We hiked all day to reach the summit of the volcano.*
Nous étions là-haut avec **tous nos amis.**	*We were up there with all our friends.*
Tu as apporté **toutes ces provisions**?	*Did you bring all those supplies?*

[Allez-y! A]

2. The pronoun **tout**

As a pronoun (masculine singular), **tout** means *all, everything.*

Tout va bien!	*Everything is fine!*
Tout est possible dans ce pays.	*Everything is possible in this country.*

3. Tous and **toutes** mean *everyone, every one (of them), all of them.* When **tous** is used as a pronoun, the final **-s** is pronounced: **tous** [tus].

Tu vois ces jeunes gens? Ils veulent **tous** faire une danse traditionnelle.	*Do you see those young people? They all want to do a traditional dance.*
Ces photos sont magnifiques! Sur **toutes,** on voit des costumes traditionnaux.	*These photos are gorgeous! In all of them, you see traditional costumes.*

Presentation: After the charts have been studied and discussed, have sts. go back to the minidialogue to classify the indefinite adjectives and pronouns according to type.

Other Indefinite Adjectives and Pronouns

Indefinite adjectives and pronouns refer to unspecified things, people, or qualities. They are also used to express sameness (the same one) and difference (another). Here is a list of the most frequently used indefinite adjectives and pronouns in French.

ADJECTIVES	PRONOUNS	
quelques* (+ *noun*) *some, a few*	**quelqu'un** (*invariable*)	*someone, anyone*
	quelqu'un de (+ *masc. adj.*)	*someone, anyone* (+ *adj.*)
	quelque chose	*something, anything*
	quelque chose de (+ *masc. adj.*)	*something, anything* (+ *adj.*)
	quelques-uns / quelques-unes (*pl.*)	*some, a few*
chaque (+ *noun*) *each, every*	**chacun(e)**	*each (one)*

Follow-up: For a synthesis of this section, use the following as a full or partial dictation, with only underlined words left out. *Je connais plusieurs personnes qui ont la même passion que moi pour la nature. Quelques-uns préfèrent la plage; d'autres passent leur temps libre à faire du camping à la montagne. Certains de mes amis aiment faire quelque chose de différent chaque week-end. Moi, j'aime faire du camping. J'ai tout l'équipement nécessaire pour tous les temps: la pluie, les tempêtes, la neige, la chaleur! J'ai quelques amis qui ont le même enthousiasme que moi pour la vie en plein air, mais ils ont d'autres idées sur le confort: chaque fois qu'ils font une randonnée, ils la font en voiture! À chacun ses goûts!*

EXPRESSIONS USED AS ADJECTIVES AND PRONOUNS	
un(e) autre *another*	**certain(e)s*** *certain, some*
d'autres[†] *other(s)*	**le/la même; les mêmes** *the same*
l'autre / les autres *the other(s)*	**plusieurs (de)** *several (of)*

***Quelques** and **certain(e)s** can both mean *some* but are used in different ways. **Quelques** is used to indicate a small, non-specific number. **Certain(e)s** is more often used to indicate some as opposed to others. Compare these two examples:

Je lis généralement **quelques** poèmes (*some / a few poems*) avant de m'endormir.

Il y a **certains** poèmes (*some specific poems*) que je lis tous les soirs avant de m'endormir.

[†]Note that **de** is used without an article before **autres** whether **autres** modifies a noun or stands alone as a pronoun.

ADJECTIVES		PRONOUNS
J'ai **quelques** amis à Tahiti.	}	**Quelques-uns** sont agriculteurs. **Quelqu'un** m'a envoyé un livre sur Tahiti.
Nous avons **plusieurs** choix.	→	**Plusieurs** de ces choix sont extrêmement difficiles.
Chaque voyageur voudrait un circuit différent.	→	**Chacun** des voyageurs visitera une île différente.
Tu veux **une autre** tasse de thé?	→	Non, si j'en prenais **une autre,** je ne pourrais pas dormir.
Où est **l'autre** autocar?	→	**L'autre** est parti.
Les autres passagers sont partis.	→	**Les autres** sont partis.
J'ai **d'autres** problèmes.	→	J'en ai **d'autres**.
Ce sont **les mêmes** voyageurs.	→	**Les mêmes** sont en retard.

The indefinite pronouns **quelqu'un** and **quelque chose** are singular and masculine. Remember that adjectives that modify these pronouns follow them and are introduced by **de.**

Je connais **quelqu'un d'intéressant** dans la capitale.	*I know someone interesting in the capital.*
Il a toujours **quelque chose de drôle** à dire.	*He always has something amusing to say.*

[Allez-y! B-C-D]

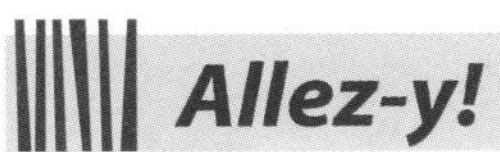

Allez-y!

A. À Dakar. Jeanne-Marie a passé quelque temps à Dakar, capitale du Sénégal. Jouez le rôle de Jeanne-Marie et répondez aux questions avec **tout, toute, tous** ou **toutes.**

MODÈLE: Tu as visité les marchés? → Oui, j'ai visité tous les marchés.

1. Tu as vu le musée anthropologique?
2. Tu as photographié les églises de la ville?
3. Est-ce que tu as visité les bâtiments de l'université?
4. Tu as vu la vieille ville?
5. Tu as lu l'histoire du Sénégal?
6. Est-ce que tu as fait le tour des plantations?

Additional activity: *Excursion. Faites les substitutions indiquées et tous les changements nécessaires. 1. Jean-Paul a vu tout le paysage. (fermes, champs, arbres) 2. Tous mes camarades ont pris des photos. (amis, professeurs, amies) 3. Nous avons apporté tous les appareils photo. (provisions, tentes, vêtements)*

Suggestion: Remind sts. to look for clues other than meaning, such as gender and number of pronouns.

B. L'île de la Martinique. Estelle a passé de nombreuses années à la Martinique. Elle y pense toujours avec nostalgie. Complétez les phrases.

J'aime la Martinique. On y trouve encore (quelques / d'autres)[1] belles maisons coloniales. (Chacun / Certains)[2] jours, à Fort-de-France, je me promenais dans les marchés en plein air, près du port. (Certaines / D'autres)[3] fois, je restais sur la place de la Savane pendant de longues heures. Il y a, tout près de la place, (quelques / quelques-unes)[4] maisons décorées avec du fer forgé (*wrought iron*) qui me rappellent La Nouvelle-Orléans.

(Certaines / Quelques)[5] choses ont changé, il est vrai, mais on trouve encore les (plusieurs / mêmes)[6] gommiers (*gum trees*) et ces bateaux pittoresques aux couleurs vives, que Gauguin* aimait tant.

C. Projets de vacances. Complétez le dialogue suivant avec un des adjectifs ou des pronoms indéfinis à droite.

JULIEN: ______[1] les ans, c'est la ______[2] chose. ______[3] fois que je propose un voyage au Sénégal, tu as d' ______[4] suggestions.

BÉNÉDICTE: Mais j'ai rencontré ______[5] qui m'a dit que ______[6] touristes ont eu des problèmes de santé au Sénégal. D'ailleurs, cette année je voudrais faire ______[7] de différent. J'aimerais faire de l'alpinisme en Suisse.

JULIEN: De l'alpinisme! Mais c'est très dangereux! Bon, eh bien, cette année ______[8] fera ce qu'il voudra. Moi, je pars au Sénégal.

autres
chaque
même
tous
chacun
plusieurs
quelque chose
quelqu'un

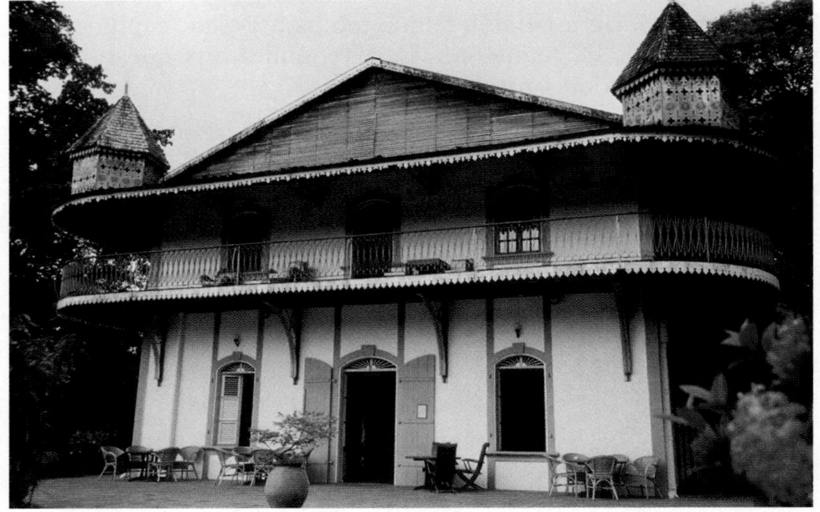

Une maison coloniale à la Martinique. Décrivez-la.

*Le peintre français Paul Gauguin a vécu brièvement à la Martinique et plus tard à Tahiti.

D. La première chose qui vient à l'esprit (*mind*). Avec un(e) camarade de classe, posez des questions—en français, s'il vous plaît—à partir des indications suivantes. Votre camarade doit donner la première réponse qui lui vient à l'esprit.

MODÈLE: *someone important* →
É1: Est-ce que tu as déjà rencontré quelqu'un d'important?
É2: Non, mais une fois mon frère a rencontré le Président.

1. *something important*
2. *something stupid*
3. *something funny*
4. *someone funny*
5. *all the large cities in Quebec*
6. *a few of the Francophone countries in Africa*
7. *several French cities*
8. *other French cities*
9. *another Canadian city*

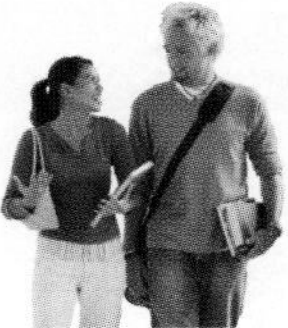

Suggestion: Give sts. a few minutes to prepare questions. Have sts. circulate, asking their questions to 5 or 6 people. Afterward, have them report their findings, using the following expressions: *Certains étudiants disent… Quelqu'un pense… La même personne ajoute… Les autres trouvent que…*

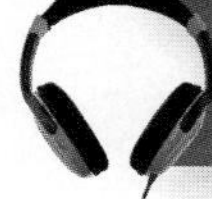

Prononcez bien!

The consonant *l* (page 415)

A. Isabelle. Vous parlez d'Isabelle avec un autre étudiant étranger. Avec votre camarade, lisez la description d'Isabelle en faisant bien attention à la prononciation du **l**.

1. Ma meilleure amie ici s'appelle Isabelle. C'est l'amie idéale! Elle vient de Montréal.
2. Elle parle le français, l'anglais, et l'espagnol.
3. C'est elle qui est venue me chercher à l'hôtel et qui m'a montré la ville quand je suis arrivé(e) ici.
4. En avril, nous allons partir en Italie pour un week-end. J'ai hâte!

B. Virelangue. (*Tongue twister.*) Isabelle vous apprend le virelangue suivant. Écoutez Isabelle et puis, avec votre camarade, entraînez-vous à le prononcer.

«Lulu a lu la lettre à Lyon et Lola a lu le livre à Lille où Lala liait[1] le lilas.[2]»

[1]*was binding* [2]*lilac*

Suggestion: Before beginning the activities with sts., go over the explanation in the *Prononcez bien!* box on page 415.

Leçon 4

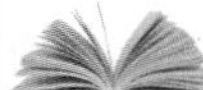 Lecture

Avant de lire

Reading journalistic texts. News reporting, as found in the daily paper and news sites on the Internet, represents a special kind of text. Because of their focus on detail, these texts require intensive reading skills in order to respond to the so-called five questions: *Who* is newsworthy? *What* is the event itself? *Where* and *when* did the event occur? and *Why* did it occur?

The first paragraph of this reading answers four of the five questions. Read through this paragraph and supply these details:

- Who is the person creating the news event?
- What is the news event?
- Where did it take place?
- When did the event occur?

As you read the text, locate other details that deepen your understanding of the event—in particular, the answer to the question *why?*

À propos de la lecture...
Cet article est tiré et adapté d'un article sur le site Web d'**An Tour Tan,** le serveur de la diaspora bretonne.

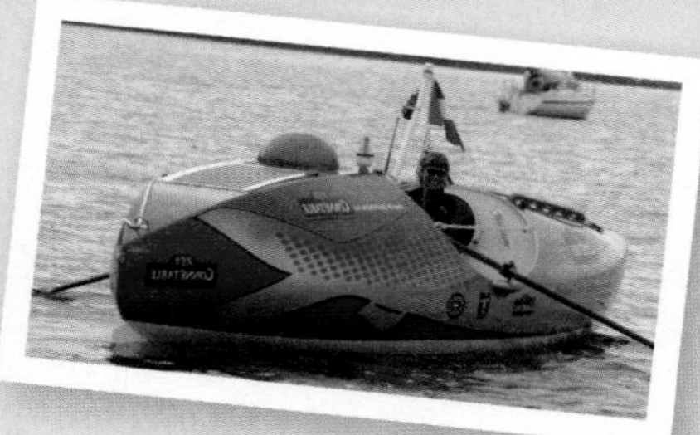
Anne Quéméré dans son bateau «Connétable»

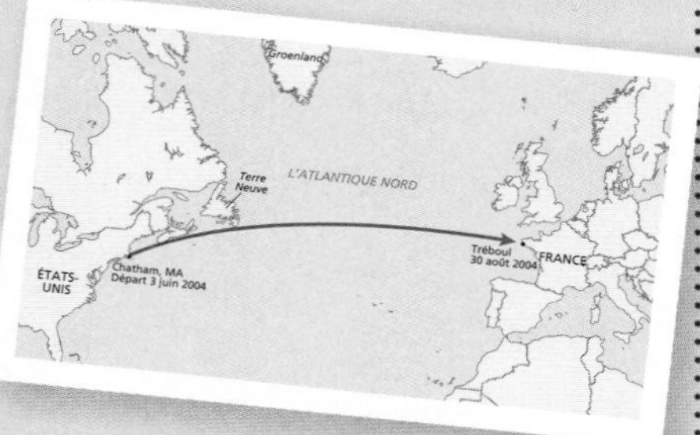

Le voyage d'Anne Quéméré dans un bateau à rame, 2004

Traversée de l'Atlantique en solitaire

Anne Quéméré: une championne

Le lundi 30 août 2004 à 5 h 15 (heure locale), Anne Quéméré a franchi[1] la ligne d'arrivée, près de Rochefort, après avoir traversé l'Atlantique nord à la rame[2] en solitaire et sans assistance en 87 jours, 12 heures et 15 minutes. Elle avait déjà le record féminin de traversée de l'Atlantique sud depuis 2003; elle a maintenant le record féminin de la traversée de l'Atlantique nord.

La traversée

Partie de Chatham (Cape Cod, USA) le 3 juin à 15 h GMT, elle a parcouru environ 5 052 kilomètres (3,139 miles) dans des conditions météo difficiles. Pour mettre toutes les chances de son côté, Anne Quéméré avait préparé[3] avec précision une route idéale. Avec des vents d'ouest dominants et un Gulf Stream qui devait l'aider à progresser, cette route avait plusieurs avantages, mais aussi de nombreux inconvénients: une eau extrêmement froide près de Terre-Neuve, des tempêtes violentes et fréquentes et des vents contraires

[1]a... *crossed* [2]à... *rowing in a rowboat* [3]avait... *had prepared*

susceptibles de faire reculer[4] ou chavirer[5] le bateau. Les conditions météorologiques l'ont d'ailleurs forcée à modifier ses plans. Elle a eu des moments difficiles, particulièrement pendant l'ouragan Alex. «J'ai vu défiler ma vie»,[6] dit-elle avec encore beaucoup d'émotion.

L'arrivée

«J'ai ramé comme une cinglée[7] les derniers 67 km,[8] heureusement aidée par un bon vent de nord-ouest qui m'a permis d'atteindre la ligne d'arrivée. Mon bonheur immédiat a tout effacé,[9] jusqu'au souvenir des heures difficiles.» Accueillie[10] dans le port de Tréboul comme une reine, incapable de se tenir debout seule, Anne Quéméré, très émue, a retrouvé sa petite fille, qui est restée juste à côté de sa maman toute l'après-midi.

Anne Quéméré recherchait la confrontation avec des réalités fondamentales et authentiques: la mer, les vents, le risque de chavirer... Ce dialogue difficile avec la nature lui a permis d'apprendre de nouvelles leçons et de porter un regard différent sur l'existence. Tout est possible: Anne l'a fait et le refera encore, parole de Bretonne!

[4]*move backward* [5]*capsize* [6]J'ai... *I saw my life pass in front of me* [7]*fool, crazy person* [8]*approx. 41 miles* [9]tout... *wiped it all away* [10]*Welcomed*

Note: Anne Quéméré made another crossing, in a boat powered only by a kite that she controlled, in the summer of 2006. She has continued with more adventures, including in 2011, when she sailed in her kite boat from Peru to French Polynesia in 78 days. In 2013 she began an attempt to traverse the Northwest Passage. Her website talks about the effects of global warming on the passage. But she interrupted this project in order to help search for three missing French sailors who had put out a distress signal near the Azores.

Compréhension

Les cinq questions. Testez votre compréhension du texte en utilisant les cinq questions comme points de départ.

1. Qui a établi la route du Connétable? Qui en particulier a accueilli Anne à son retour?
2. Qu'est-ce qu'Anne a trouvé comme obstacles pendant son voyage? Qu'est-ce qui a aidé Anne à arriver à sa ligne d'arrivée?
3. D'où est-elle partie? Où se trouvait la ligne d'arrivée?
4. Quand (À quels moments) Anne s'est-elle sentie désespérée?
5. Selon le texte, pourquoi Anne a-t-elle entrepris un tel voyage? À votre avis, est-ce qu'il s'agit d'un acte purement égoïste?

Suggestion: Review the five questions from *Avant de lire* before doing the comprehension questions: *Qui, Qu'est-ce que, Où, Quand, Pourquoi.*

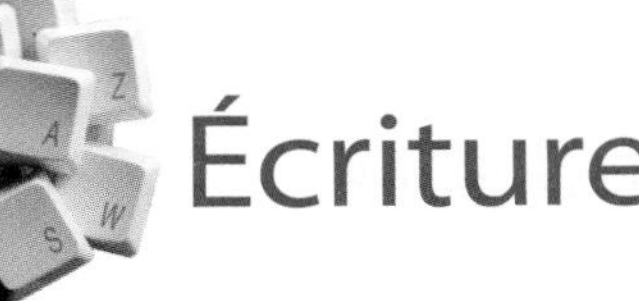

Écriture

The writing activities **Par écrit** and **Journal intime** can be found in the Workbook/Laboratory Manual to accompany *Vis-à-vis*.

La vie en chantant. An activity based on the song "Tes vacances avec moi" by Sonia Dersion can be found in the Instructor's Manual. The song can be purchased at the iTunes store, or sts. can watch the music video on YouTube.

Pour s'amuser

Le travail, c'est la santé; ne rien faire c'est la conserver. —Henri Salvador

Note: Henri Salvador, a singer born in French Guyana, is the subject of the *La vie en chantant* feature in the Instructor's Manual.

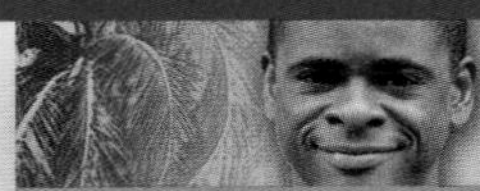

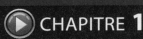

Le vidéoblog d'Hector

En bref

Dans cet épisode, Hector et Léa voudraient passer l'après-midi ensemble, mais ils ont du mal à choisir une activité. Ils finissent par décider d'aller à Paris-Plages, un grand événement de l'été à Paris.

Vocabulaire en contexte

Imaginez qu'un ami / une amie vous propose les activités suivantes. Indiquez les activités que vous feriez volontiers (avec plaisir) et expliquez pourquoi les autres ne vous tentent pas.

Activités

- ☐ aller sur une belle plage de **sable** (*sand*) blanc
- ☐ aller au ciné l'après-midi
- ☐ aller **prendre un verre**
- ☐ **se baigner** à la piscine
- ☐ **se balader** (*stroll*) à vélo
- ☐ se faire **bronzer** (*to tan*)
- ☐ faire de **l'escalade** (*rock/wall climbing*)
- ☐ faire un jogging au parc
- ☐ pique-niquer
- ☐ **se promener** au bord de l'eau

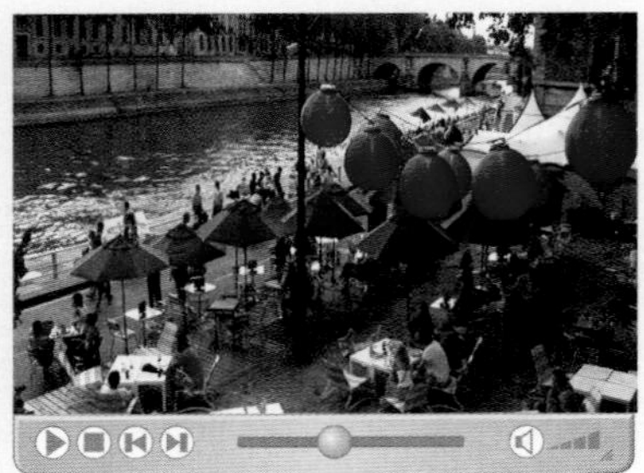

Un café à Paris-Plages, au bord de la Seine

Suggestion: After sts. have made their selections, put them in groups to compare responses. Who in each group is most compatible? Who is most different? Which activities did everyone in the group choose? What did no one choose?

Additional vocabulary: Other vocabulary you may wish to present before viewing includes *tu n'es pas convaincu, insupportable, plein d'enfants, de mauvaise humeur, des palmiers, une foule, les paresseux, l'accrobranche, le trempoling, se refraîchir, gratuit.*

Visionnez!

Pourquoi Hector ne veut-il pas faire les activités suivantes? Choisissez la bonne réponse.

1. Il ne veut pas aller au ciné parce qu'il ______.
   a. n'a plus d'argent **b.** préfère être dehors l'après-midi
2. Il ne veut pas faire un jogging parce qu'il ______.
   a. ne veut pas courir après un repas **b.** ne trouve pas ses tennis
3. Il ne veut pas faire du vélo et aller prendre un verre parce qu'il ______.
   a. n'aime pas le vin **b.** fait trop chaud
4. Il ne veut pas aller à la piscine parce qu'il ______.
   a. y aura trop d'enfants **b.** ne sait pas nager

Analysez!

Répondez aux questions.

1. Quelles activités font de Paris-Plages une vraie plage?
2. À quoi bon (*What good is it*) avoir une plage en centre-ville? Pourquoi, à votre avis, la Mairie de Paris organise-t-elle ce grand événement de l'été?

Comparez!

Y a-t-il beaucoup d'endroits dans votre ville ou votre région où vous pouvez vous amuser? Est-il plus facile de passer son temps libre à l'intérieur (dans un cinéma ou un musée) ou à l'extérieur? Regardez encore une fois la partie culturelle de la vidéo: est-ce que votre ville ou votre région a besoin d'organiser quelque chose comme Paris-Plages?

Note culturelle

Depuis 2001, la Ville de Paris organise avec succès «Paris-Plages» le long de la Seine. Cette opération municipale, qui coûte plus de 1,5 millions d'euros, est financée par la Ville et par des sponsors privés. En 2012, «Paris-Plages» a attiré[1] presque 5 millions de visiteurs, dont 50 % parisiens. L'opération a nécessité 2 plages de 800 mètres; 5 000 tonnes de sable; 900 pièces de mobilier (matelas,[2] transats,[3] parasols, tables, chaises, etc.); 44 palmiers et 74 oriflammes[4]; 60 secouristes[5] et 55 plagistes.[6]

[1]*attracted* [2]*(air) mattresses* [3]*beach chairs* [4]*banners* [5]*first aid workers* [6]*beach attendants*

Vocabulaire

Verbes

assister à to attend
bricoler to putter, do odd jobs
courir to run
désirer to desire, want
indiquer to show, point out
se passer to happen, take place
rire to laugh
sourire to smile

À REVOIR: **aider, emmener, faire du sport, gagner, jouer à, jouer de, perdre**

Substantifs

les activités (*f.*) **de plein air** outdoor activities
la bande dessinée cartoon
la blague joke
le bricolage do-it-yourself work, puttering around
la chanson song
la chanson de variété popular song
la collection collection
le cyclisme cycling
l'équipe (*f.*) team
la foule crowd
le jardinage gardening
le jeu (les jeux) game
le jeu de mot pun
le jeu de hasard game of chance
le jeu de société board game
la lecture reading
les loisirs (*m.*) leisure activities
la manifestation sportive sporting event
la marche walking
le match game
l'opéra (*m.*) opera
le passe-temps hobby
la pêche fishing
la pétanque bocce ball, lawn bowling
le pique-nique picnic
le spectacle show, performance
le spectacle de variétés variety show; floor show (in a restaurant)
le temps libre free time

À REVOIR: **le théâtre**

Expressions interrogatives

lequel, laquelle, lesquels, lesquelles, qu'est-ce qui, qui est-ce que, qui est-ce qui, qui, quoi

Adjectifs et pronoms indéfinis

un(e) autre another
d'autres other(s)
l'autre / les autres the other(s)
certain(e)(s) certain, some
chacun(e)(s) each (one)
chaque each
le/la même (les mêmes) the same one(s)
plusieurs (de) several
quelque chose (de) something
quelques (*adj.*) some, a few
quelqu'un someone, anyone
quelques-uns / quelques-unes (*pron.*) some, a few
tout(e) all, everything
tous / toutes everyone, every one (of them), all of them

Mots et expressions divers

à ta place... if I were you . . .
aller en boîte to go clubbing
autant (de)... que as much (many) . . . as
bien, mieux, le mieux well, better, best
en train de in the process of; in the middle of
je devrais I should
Qu'est-ce que tu racontes / vous racontez? What are you talking about?
Qu'est-ce qui se passe? What's happening? What's going on?
tant mieux so much the better
tant pis that's too bad

À REVOIR: **je pourrais**

CHAPITRE 16

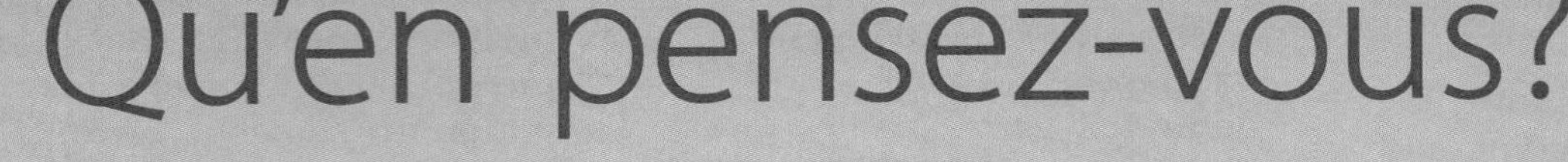

Qu'en pensez-vous?

Presentation: *Décrivez la photo. Feriez-vous de la planche à voile si près d'une centrale nucléaire? Expliquez.*

Les dossiers d'Hector

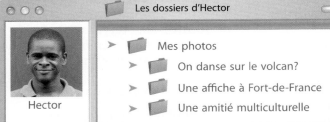

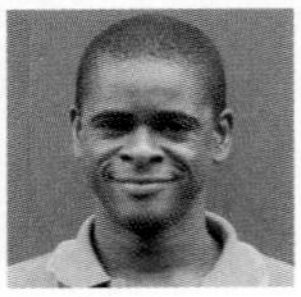

Hector

- Mes photos
  - On danse sur le volcan?
  - Une affiche à Fort-de-France
  - Une amitié multiculturelle

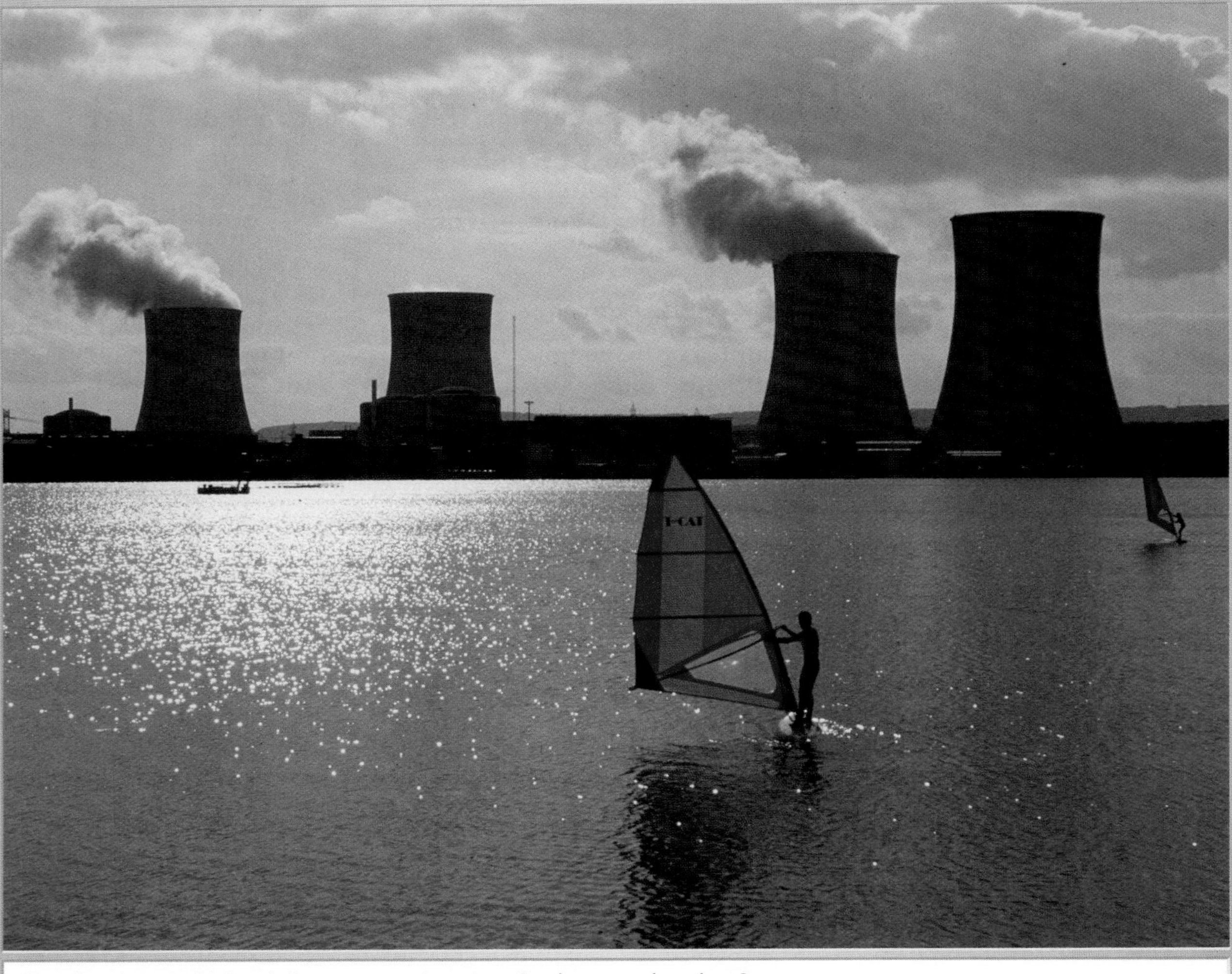

Des réacteurs nucléaires à Cattenom, en Lorraine: On danse sur le volcan?

Cultural note: Cattenom is located in the *Moselle* department in *Lorraine* in northeastern France.

Dans ce chapitre…

OBJECTIFS COMMUNICATIFS

- talking about environmental and social problems
- expressing attitudes, wishes, necessity, possibility, emotions, doubt, and uncertainty
- learning to distinguish between and pronounce selected sounds in French

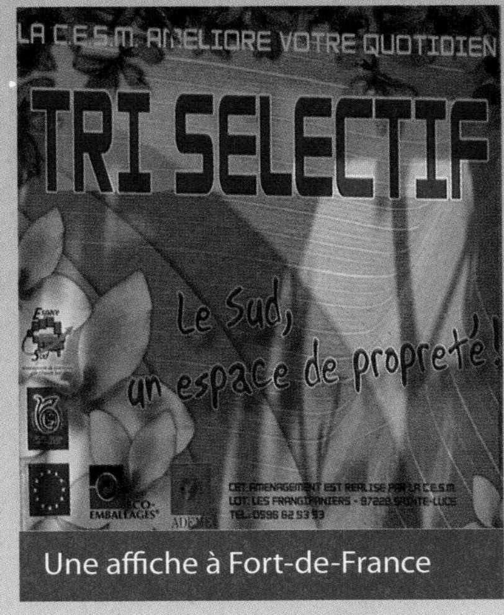

Une affiche à Fort-de-France

PAROLES (Leçon 1)

- L'environnement
- Les problèmes de la société moderne

STRUCTURES (Leçons 2 et 3)

- Le subjonctif (première partie)
- Le subjonctif (deuxième partie)
- Le subjonctif (troisième partie)
- Le subjonctif (quatrième partie)

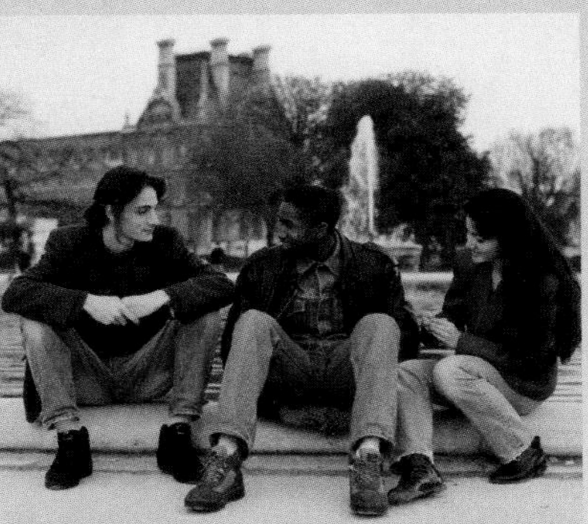
Une amitié multiculturelle

CULTURE

- Le blog d'Hector: *Moi d'abord?*
- Reportage: *La France multiculturelle*
- Lecture: *La Réclusion solitaire* (extrait) de Tahar Ben Jelloun (Leçon 4)

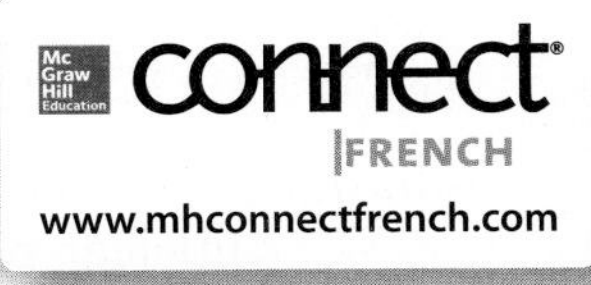

Leçon 1

Presentation: (1) Have sts. repeat the phrases and sentences. Ask them to find cognates and words of the same family. (2) Ask sts. to describe/comment on the illustrations on this page using the vocab. given. Encourage use of complete sentences. Have sts. write their descriptions first, then have a few of them presented to class.

Additional vocabulary: *une catastrophe nucléaire, les combustibles fossiles, la disparition des espèces, les émissions de carbone, une explosion, une fuite de gaz, la marée noire, menacer la santé, un nuage de gaz toxique, protéger les forêts, des rayons ultra-violets.*

L'environnement

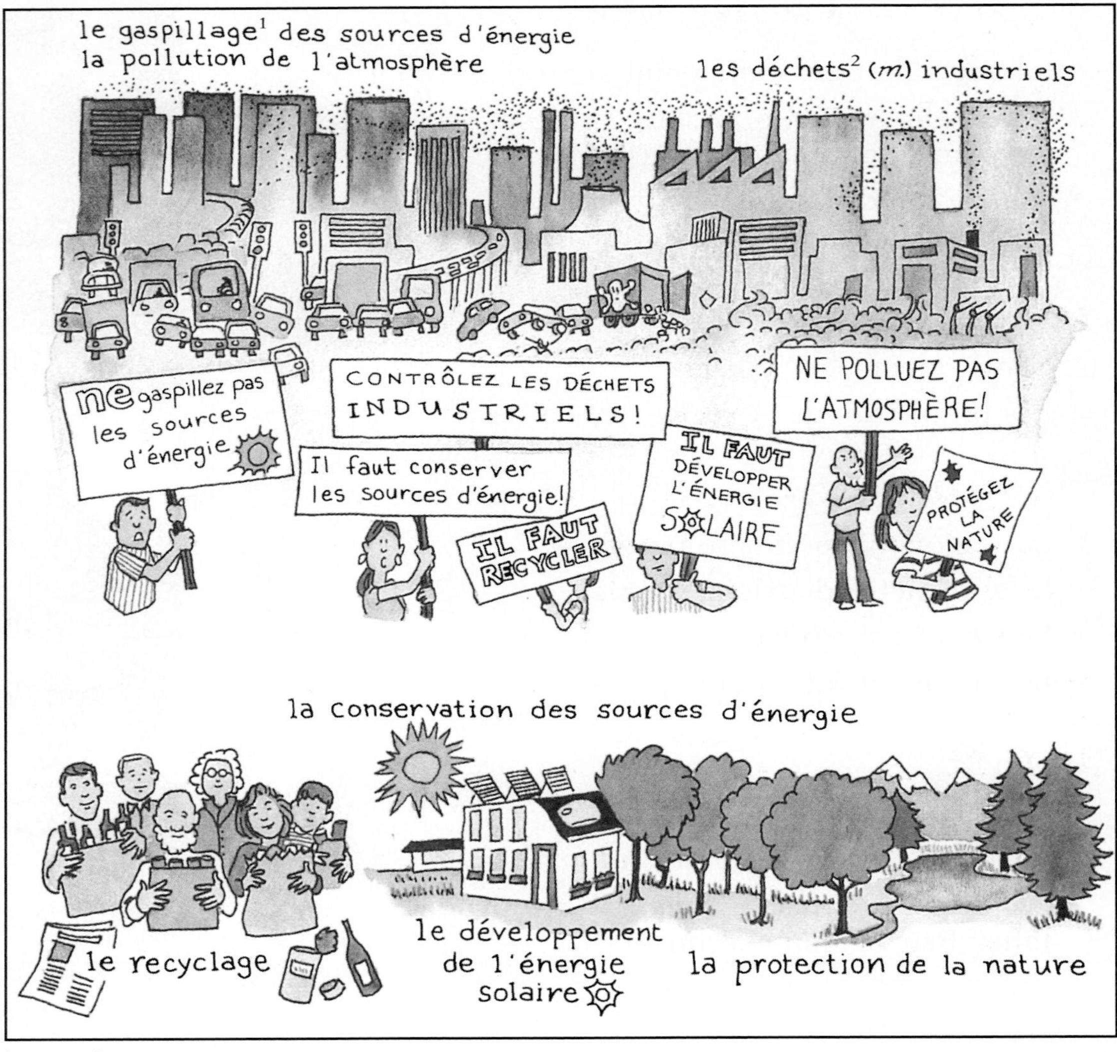
le gaspillage[1] des sources d'énergie
la pollution de l'atmosphère
les déchets[2] (*m.*) industriels
ne gaspillez pas les sources d'énergie
CONTRÔLEZ LES DÉCHETS INDUSTRIELS!
Il faut conserver les sources d'énergie!
IL FAUT RECYCLER
IL FAUT DÉVELOPPER L'ÉNERGIE SOLAIRE
NE POLLUEZ PAS L'ATMOSPHÈRE!
PROTÉGEZ LA NATURE
la conservation des sources d'énergie
le recyclage
le développement de l'énergie solaire
la protection de la nature

[1]*wasting* [2]*waste, refuse*

AUTRES MOTS UTILES

une centrale nucléaire	nuclear power plant
consommer	to consume
le covoiturage	carpooling
épuiser	to use up, exhaust
le réchauffement de la planète	global warming
sauver	to save
la surpopulation	overpopulation
une voiture hybride	hybrid car

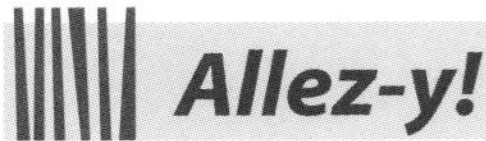

Allez-y!

A. Association de mots. Quels problèmes écologiques associez-vous avec les verbes suivants?

MODÈLE: gaspiller → le gaspillage des sources d'énergie

1. conserver **2.** protéger **3.** polluer **4.** recycler **5.** développer

B. Remèdes. Expliquez quelles sont les actions nécessaires pour sauver notre planète. Utilisez **Il faut** ou **Il ne faut pas** suivi d'un infinitif.

MODÈLES: le contrôle des déchets industriels →
Il faut contrôler les déchets industriels.
le gaspillage de l'énergie →
Il ne faut pas gaspiller l'énergie.

1. la pollution de l'environnement
2. la protection de la nature
3. le développement de l'énergie solaire
4. la conservation des sources d'énergie
5. le gaspillage des ressources naturelles
6. le développement des transports en commun

C. Rendez-vous des Verts. Vous êtes pour une ville plus verte où il y a moins de voitures et plus de gens qui circulent à pied ou à vélo. En résumant le plaidoyer (*defense*) dans le *Manuel du cycliste urbain,* faites une petite présentation pour comparer les voitures aux vélos. Parlez des avantages du vélo, mais n'oubliez pas ses inconvénients.

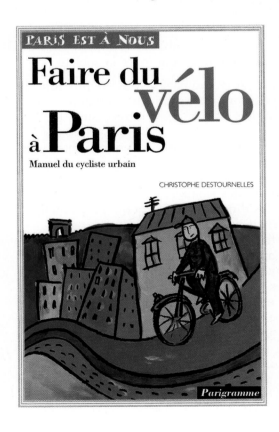

Petit plaidoyer pour le vélo à Paris

Il ne pollue pas
Il est silencieux
Il est très maniable[1]
Il occupe un espace restreint
Il ne demande pas beaucoup d'infrastructures
Il est économique (il revient en moyenne à 100 euros par an, quand une voiture réclame 800 euros par mois, et une Carte orange 125 euros chaque année)
Il se gare[2] *relativement facilement (adieu les soucis de stationnement gênant, les PV,*[3] *les parkings et les horodateurs*[4]*...)*
Il est très bien adapté aux petits parcours en ville[5]
Il est bon pour la santé
Il est bon pour le moral
Il n'est pas aussi dangereux qu'on veut bien le dire
Il expose moins à la pollution que l'habitacle[6] *d'une voiture*
Il permet de découvrir Paris...

[1]*easy to steer* [2]se... *is parked* [3]*tickets* [4]*parking ticket machines* [5]parcours... *trips around town* [6]*interior*

Note: The information in the chart is taken from a 2013 article in *Le Monde*.

Les problèmes de la société moderne

Suggestion: Ask sts. what they perceive to be our society's most serious problems. Do not limit them to the list given. This can be done as a brainstorming activity in pairs or small groups. You can also ask them to suggest solutions to these problems or to compare the problems listed here to those they perceive today, using comparative and superlative constructions (*plus important que, moins important que, le plus grave, le moins pressant,* etc.)

Voici les résultats d'une enquête réalisée pour le journal *Le Monde*.

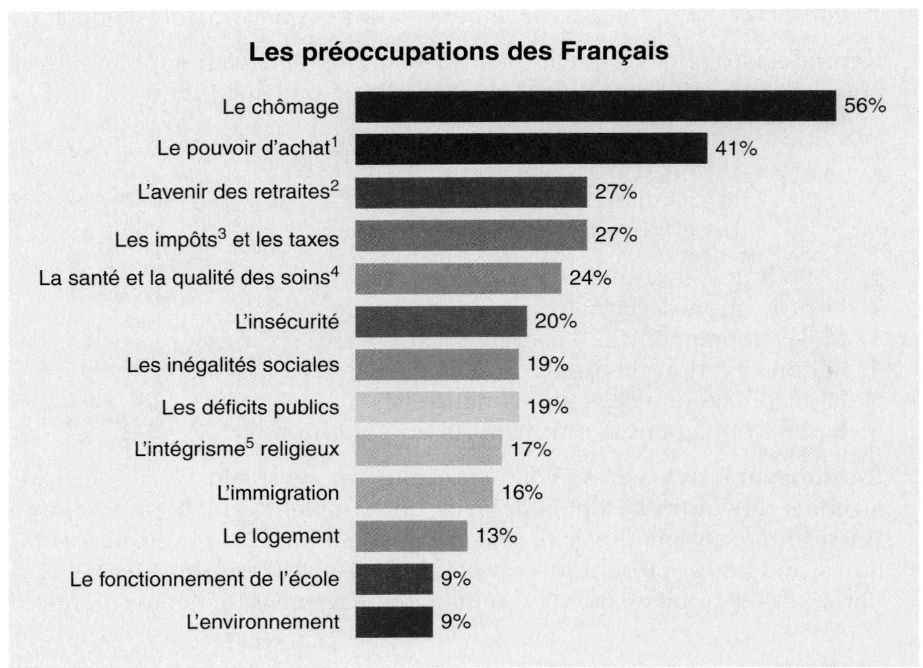

Source: Adapté d'une enquête IPSOS / CGI Business Consulting pour *Le Monde,* Fondation Jean Jaurès et le Cevipof. Janvier 2013.

Les Français sont préoccupés. Le futur leur semble incertain; la crise économique crée un climat d'instabilité qui affecte toute la société.

- Le gros problème de la France, c'est le chômage. «Mes enfants font de longues études: est-ce qu'ils trouveront du travail?» se demandent avec angoisse[6] les parents. Rien de moins sûr car, avec la récession, les entreprises n'embauchent pas.[7]
- Le pouvoir d'achat et les retraites inquiètent. Tout le monde s'interroge: «Comment maintenir mon niveau de vie[8]?» En réalité, les Français sont obligés de réduire leur consommation parce que les impôts augmentent massivement, mais pas les salaires. Et les seniors savent que le montant[9] de leurs retraites diminuera. Pourquoi? Parce qu'il faut, en priorité, réduire un déficit public colossal.
- On a peur aussi de devoir sacrifier le meilleur système social du monde notamment l'accès gratuit à la santé et à l'école, et les aides au logement.[10]
- Dans une société en pleine mutation, les Français perdent leurs repères[11]: les inégalités sociales s'amplifient, l'insécurité et l'intégrisme religieux créent une névrose[12] collective; l'immigration pose le problème de l'identité française.
- Enfin l'environnement devient une question sensible: on sait qu'il faut modifier les comportements et encourager le développement durable[13] pour préserver les ressources naturelles.

---

[1]pouvoir... *purchasing power* [2]*penisons* [3]*taxes* [4]*care* [5]*fundamentalism* [6]avec... *anxiously* [7]n'embauchent... *aren't hiring* [8]niveau... *standard of living* [9]*amount* [10]aides... *housing subsidies* [11]perdent... *are losing their points of reference* [12]*neuroses* [13]développement... *sustainable development*

AUTRES MOTS UTILES

le citoyen / la citoyenne citizen
les droits (*m.*) **civils** civil rights
l'écologiste (*m., f.*) environmentalist
l'électeur / l'électrice voter
l'élection (*f.*) election
la guerre war
l'homme / la femme politique politician
les idées extrémistes extremist ideas
les impôts (*m.*) taxes
le parti political party
la politique politics; policy
la réussite success
le/la sans-abri homeless person
le terrorisme terrorism
augmenter to raise, increase
diminuer to lower, reduce
élire to elect
s'engager (dans) to get involved (in) (*a public issue, cause*)
exiger to require; to demand
exprimer une opinion to express an opinion
faire grève to strike
manifester (pour/contre) to demonstrate (for/against)
poser sa candidature to run for elected office; to apply (for a job)
soutenir to support

Suggestion: Ask questions such as *Et dans votre pays, est-ce que les citoyens sont las? Est-ce qu'ils ont peur? Expliquez.*

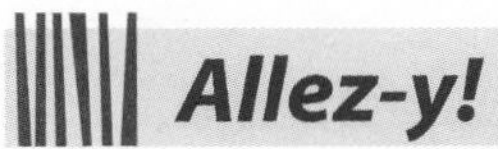

Allez-y!

A. Autrement dit. Choisissez la bonne définition.

_____ **1.** exiger	**a.** prendre publiquement position
_____ **2.** la grève	**b.** encourager
_____ **3.** soutenir	**c.** participer à une manifestation
_____ **4.** élire	**d.** demander, réclamer
_____ **5.** s'engager	**e.** la cessation collective du travail
_____ **6.** manifester	**f.** une personne sans domicile
_____ **7.** la guerre	**g.** choisir
_____ **8.** le/la sans-abri	**h.** le contraire de la paix

B. L'actualité. Lisez à la page précédente les résultats de l'enquête faite pour *Le Monde*. Puis répondez aux questions.

Suggestion (B-C): Assign for homework so sts. have time to prepare their thoughts.

1. Quelles sont les préoccupations des citoyens de votre pays?
2. Parmi ces préoccupations, laquelle considérez-vous comme la plus importante ou la moins importante?
3. Sélectionnez trois problèmes qui, selon vous, affectent gravement la société dans laquelle vous vivez. Proposez des solutions pour les résoudre.
4. Quels autres problèmes pourrait-on ajouter au sondage français?

C. À mon avis. Choisissez une des expressions des **Mots clés** pour exprimer votre point de vue.

MODÈLE: possible / contrôler le problème des déchets nucléaires → Personnellement, je crois qu'il est (qu'il n'est pas) possible de contrôler le problème des déchets nucléaires, parce que…

1. essentiel / développer de nouvelles sources d'énergie
2. impossible / empêcher les accidents nucléaires
3. important / respecter l'image de la femme dans les publicités
4. indispensable / faire attention aux problèmes de la jeunesse
5. inutile / limiter l'immigration
6. essentiel / augmenter les impôts
7. utile / aider les chômeurs (les gens qui sont au chômage)
8. essentiel / protéger et maintenir (*maintain*) les droits civils

Mots clés

Exprimer son opinion

To express a personal point of view, use the following expressions:

Moi, / **Pour ma part,** / **Personnellement,** { **je crois que…** / **je pense que…** / **j'estime que…** / **je trouve que…**

À mon avis…
Selon moi…

Your point will be more convincing if you give examples or refer to other people's opinions. Use the following expressions:

Par exemple…
On dit que…
J'ai entendu dire que…

Leçon 2

Le subjonctif (*première partie*)

Expressing Attitudes

Je rêve, n'est-ce pas?

Juliette téléphone à Charlotte.

JULIETTE: Pourquoi as-tu choisi de travailler pour l'OMS[1] plutôt que pour une administration suisse?

CHARLOTTE: Par idéalisme, je crois. **Je veux que** tous les pays **coordonnent** leurs efforts pour le bien commun;[2] **je désire que** la santé **soit** une priorité universelle. Je rêve, n'est-ce pas?

JULIETTE: Mais non, tu ne rêves pas! La santé est un droit fondamental. Moi aussi, **j'aimerais que** nous **soyons** tous égaux[3] devant la maladie!

CHARLOTTE: À l'OMS, **nous souhaitons**[4] **que** chaque enfant **arrive** à l'âge adulte en bonne santé. **Nous insistons pour que** tous les pays du tiers-monde[5] **établissent** une excellente politique de santé publique.

JULIETTE: C'est un des grands défis[6] du XXIe siècle. Mais moi je parle, je fais des commentaires… alors que toi, tu agis! Cela me fait réfléchir…

CHARLOTTE: J'ai toujours été engagée dans des causes humanitaires. À mon petit niveau,[7] **je veux que** mon travail **puisse** aider les plus vulnérables. C'est juste, non?

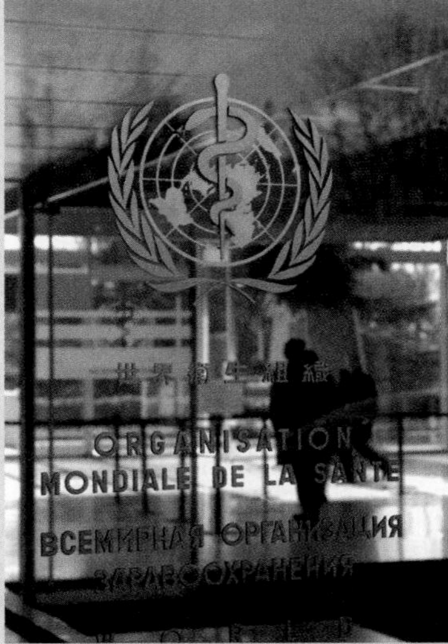

L'OMS: la santé pour tous

[1]Organisation Mondiale de la Santé *WHO* (*World Health Organization*) [2]le… *the common good* [3]*equal* [4]*hope* [5]*third world* [6]*challenges* [7]À… *In my small way*

Trouvez, dans le dialogue, la phrase équivalente.

1. Les pays doivent coordonner leurs efforts pour le bien commun.
2. La santé doit être une priorité universelle.
3. Nous devons tous être égaux face à la maladie.
4. Tous les enfants doivent arriver à l'âge adulte avec un bon capital santé.
5. Les pays du tiers-monde doivent établir une très bonne politique de santé publique.
6. Mon travail doit aider les gens défavorisés.

The Subjunctive Mood

The verb tenses you have learned so far have been in the *indicative* mood (**présent, passé composé, imparfait, futur**), in the *imperative* mood (used for direct commands or requests), or in the *conditional* mood (used to express hypothetical situations). In this chapter, you will learn about the *subjunctive* mood.

The subjunctive is used to present actions or states as subjective or doubtful, instead of as facts. It appears most frequently in dependent clauses, and is used infrequently in English. Compare the following examples.

INDICATIVE	SUBJUNCTIVE
He *goes* to Paris.	I insist that he *go* to Paris for the meeting.
We *are* on time.	They ask that we *be* on time.
She *is* the president.	She wishes that she *were* the president of the group.

In French, the subjunctive is used more frequently than it is in English. It almost always appears in a dependent clause introduced by **que.** In such cases, the main clause contains a verb expressing desire, emotion, uncertainty, or some other subjective view of the action in the dependent clause. For now, you will focus on the use of the subjunctive in dependent clauses introduced by **que** after verbs of volition (wanting), including **aimer bien, désirer, insister (pour), préférer, souhaiter** (*to want, to wish*), and **vouloir.**

Suggestion: Point out that although all subjunctives are preceded by *que*, *que* is not always followed by a subjunctive.

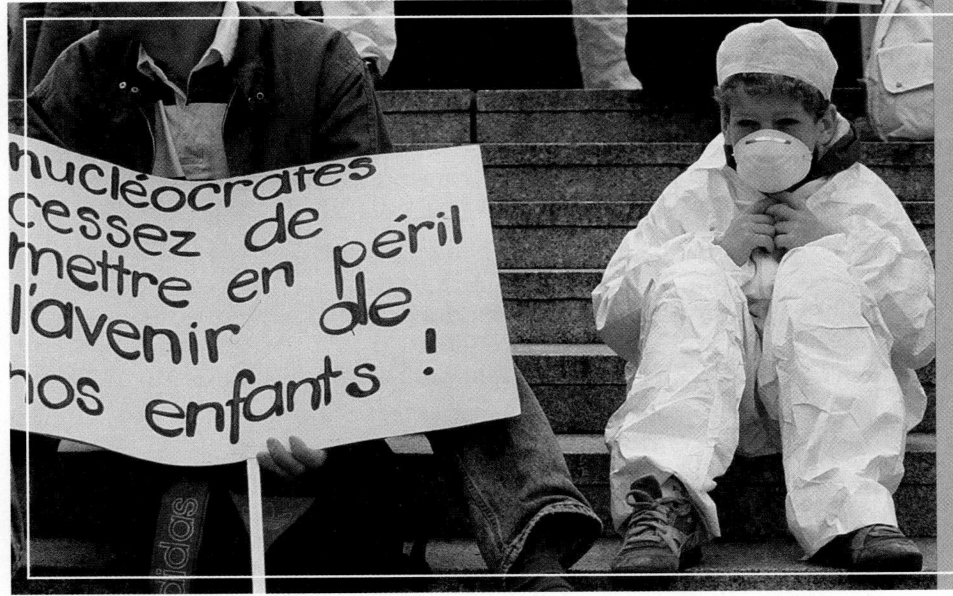
nucléocrates
cessez de
mettre en péril
l'avenir de
nos enfants !

Un peu plus...

Les manifestations.
En France, 75 % de l'énergie nécessaire aux entreprises et aux particuliers (*individuals*) est produite par des centrales nucléaires. Bien que les Français soient généralement en faveur de la production d'énergie nucléaire, le problème des déchets nucléaires les inquiète. Dans les années 80, de violentes émeutes (*riots*) ont éclaté (*broke out*) dans les régions rurales où l'on voulait enfouir (*to bury*) ces déchets. Aujourd'hui, le gouvernement cherche une solution.

◄ *Pour ou contre l'énergie nucléaire? Et vous?*

Usually, the subjects of the main and dependent clauses are different.

MAIN CLAUSE *Indicative*	DEPENDENT CLAUSE *Subjunctive*
Je veux	**que** vous **partiez.**

Note that French constructions with the subjunctive have many possible English equivalents.

que je parle → *that I speak, that I'm speaking, that I do speak, that I may speak, that I will speak, me to speak*

De quoi veux-tu **que je parle**? — *What do you want me to talk about?*

Il préfère **que je parle** des déchets nucléaires. — *He prefers that I speak about nuclear waste.*

L'agent ne croit pas **que le suspect parle**. — *The police officer doesn't believe that the suspect will speak.*

Presentation: Model the pronunciation of the verbs in short sentences: *Il veut que je parle français, que je finisse la leçon,* etc.

Suggestion: Point out that all regular *-er, -ir,* and *-re* verbs have only one stem for the subjunctive, taken from the third-person plural.

Forms of the Present Subjunctive

For most verbs, including many irregular verbs (e.g., **conduire, connaître, écrire, lire, ouvrir, mettre, suivre**) the stem for the forms of the subjunctive is found by dropping the **-ent** of the third-person plural (**ils/elles**) form of the present indicative and by adding the subjunctive endings: **-e, -es, -e, -ions, -iez,** and **-ent.**

	parler	finir	vendre	sortir
	(ils) **parl**/ent	(ils) **finiss**/ent	(ils) **vend**/ent	(ils) **sort**/ent
...que je	parl**e**	finiss**e**	vend**e**	sort**e**
...que tu	parl**es**	finiss**es**	vend**es**	sort**es**
...qu'il/elle/on	parl**e**	finiss**e**	vend**e**	sort**e**
...que nous	parl**ions**	finiss**ions**	vend**ions**	sort**ions**
...que vous	parl**iez**	finiss**iez**	vend**iez**	sort**iez**
...qu'ils/elles	parl**ent**	finiss**ent**	vend**ent**	sort**ent**

Verbs with Two Stems in the Subjunctive

Some verbs that have two stems in the present indicative also have two stems in the subjunctive: One stem is taken from the **ils** form of the present (for **je, tu, il/elle/on,** and **ils/elles**), and the other, from the **nous** form (for **nous** and **vous**). Some verbs of this type are **acheter, apprendre, boire, préférer, prendre,** and **venir.**

boire			
ils boivent nous buvons			
...que je	**boiv**e	...que nous	**buv**ions
...que tu	**boiv**es	...que vous	**buv**iez
...qu'il/elle/on	**boiv**e	...qu'ils/elles	**boiv**ent

[Allez-y! A-B]

Presentation: Model pronunciation in short phrases. Example: *Le chef veut qu'elle soit à l'heure… que nous sachions la vérité.*

Suggestion: Compare the imperative forms of *être* and *avoir* with the subjunctive.

Irregular Subjunctive Verbs

Some verbs have irregular subjunctive stems. The endings themselves are all regular, except for some endings of **avoir** and **être.**

	aller *aill-/all-*	faire *fass-*	pouvoir *puiss-*	savoir *sach-*	vouloir *veuill-/voul-*	avoir *ai-/ay-*	être *soi-/soy-*
...que je/j'	aille	fasse	puisse	sache	veuille	aie	soi**s**
...que tu	ailles	fasses	puisses	saches	veuilles	aies	soi**s**
...qu'il/elle/on	aille	fasse	puisse	sache	veuille	ai**t**	soi**t**
...que nous	allions	fassions	puissions	sachions	voulions	a**yons**	so**yons**
...que vous	alliez	fassiez	puissiez	sachiez	vouliez	a**yez**	so**yez**
...qu'ils/elles	aillent	fassent	puissent	sachent	veuillent	aient	soient

Le professeur veut que nous **allions** au débat. — *The professor wants us to go to the debate.*

Son parti veut que le gouvernement **fasse** des réformes. — *His (Her) party wants the government to make reforms.*

Le président préfère que les sénateurs **soient** présents. — *The president prefers the senators to be there.*

[Allez-y! C-D-E]

Pronunciation practice (1): Draw a table on the board, with *aller* in the left column and *avoir* in the right column. Pronounce the following subjunctive forms and have students decide under which column each falls: *tu aies, ils aient, j'aille, il ait, nous allions, vous ayez.*

Pronunciation practice (2): Have students fill in the blanks with the appropriate subjunctive forms of *aller* and *avoir*: (1) *Il faut que Marc* ________ *au supermarché pour faire les courses;* (2) *Je veux que vous* ________ *de bonnes notes à l'examen;* (3) *Ma mère insiste pour que j'* ________ *un travail cet été;* (4) *Les gens exigent que le gouvernement* ________ *une meilleure politique de contrôle des déchets industriels.*

Pronunciation practice (3): The *Prononcez bien!* section on page 460 of this chapter contains additional activities for practicing these sounds.

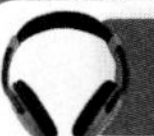

Prononcez bien!

The subjunctive of *aller* and *avoir*

When using the subjunctive, be sure to distinguish between the pronunciation of **aller** and **avoir.** For the **je, tu, il,** and **ils** forms of **aller,** pronounce [aj], somewhat like the English pronoun *I*.

[aj]: ...que j'**aille,** tu **ailles,** il **aille**

For the corresponding persons for **avoir,** pronounce a single sound [ɛ], as in **est.**

[ɛ]: ...que j'**aie,** tu **aies,** elle **ait**

Remember that the **nous** and **vous** forms start with the sound [a] for **aller** and [ɛ] for **avoir.**

[aljɔ̃]: ...que nous **allions**
[alje]: ...que vous **alliez**
[ɛjɔ̃]: ...que nous **ayons**
[ɛje]: ...que vous **ayez**

Additional activity: For listening comprehension practice, ask sts. to listen for indicative or subjunctive in the following sentences. They are to imagine that they are at a political rally where part of the candidates' speeches are made inaudible by cheers of the crowd. 1. *. . .que nous votons socialistes.* 2. *. . .que nous nous rappelions les problèmes des pauvres.* 3. *. . .que vous choisissiez les meilleurs candidats.* 4. *. . .que je suive vos conseils.* 5. *. . .que nous prenions le pouvoir.* 6. *. . .que vous parlez avec les candidats.*

Suggestion: For listening comprehension practice, ask sts. to listen for subjunctive or indicative form of irregular verbs. They are to imagine that they are talking on their cell phones and that the reception is poor. 1. *. . .que j'aille à la réunion.* 2. *. . .que Marc a le temps de faire cela.* 3. *. . .que tu sois présente.* 4. *. . . que nous pouvons poser des questions.* 5. *. . .que vous sachiez la vérité.* 6. *. . .que la candidate fasse le nécessaire.*

Suggestion (B): Do as a rapid-response ex.

Additional activities: (1) *Stratégie. Un groupe d'étudiants prépare la campagne pour élire son candidat au Conseil de l'université. Que dit leur chef, Jean-Michel?* 1. *Jean-Michel veut que vous choisissiez un candidat. (les étudiants, nous, le secrétaire)* 2. *Il préfère que nous agissions tout de suite. (tu, vous, je)* 3. *Il voudrait que Michel finisse les affiches. (Martine et Paulette, tu, vous)* 4. *Il souhaite que tu réfléchisses à notre budget. (la trésorière, je, elles)* 5. *Il désire qu'elles réussissent à obtenir des votes. (tu, nous, vous)* (2) *Dictature. M. Lamoureux dirige son entreprise en véritable dictateur. Voici les ordres qu'il a donnés ce matin. Exprimez-les avec je veux que. . .* MODÈLE: *Vous devez écouter votre chef de service.* → Je veux que vous *écoutiez votre chef de service.* 1. *Vous devez mieux travailler.* 2. *Elle doit arriver à l'heure.* 3. *Ils doivent trouver une solution.* 4. *Nous devons envoyer ce mél.* 5. *Tu dois m'expliquer tes problèmes.* 6. *Il doit s'excuser de son erreur.* 7. *Nous devons convoquer les employés.* 8. *Ils doivent taper plus vite.* 9. *Vous devez appeler un inspecteur.* 10. *Tu dois te rappeler le nouvel horaire.*

Suggestion (C): Do as written transformation at the board or using a digital display.

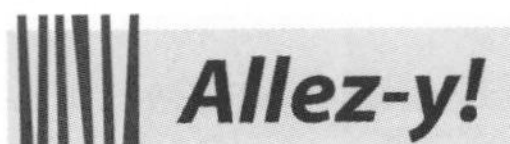

A. Stratégie électorale. Laure accepte de poser sa candidature au Conseil universitaire. Avec un groupe d'étudiants, elle prépare sa campagne. Que veut Laure?

MODÈLE: Elle veut que les étudiants / choisir / des délégués responsables →
Elle veut que les étudiants choisissent des délégués responsables.

1. Elle veut que tout le monde / réfléchir / aux problèmes de l'université
2. Elle aimerait que nous / préparer / tout de suite / une stratégie électorale
3. Elle préfère que vous / finir / les affiches aujourd'hui
4. Elle veut que Luc et Simon / organiser / un débat
5. Elle souhaite que la trésorière / établir / un budget
6. Elle insiste pour que je / convoquer (*to ask to attend*) / tous les bénévoles (*volunteers*) ce soir

B. Discours politique. Ce soir, Laure fait son premier discours de la campagne électorale. Voici ce qu'elle dit aux étudiants.

MODÈLE: Je voudrais que nous / trouver / tous ensemble des solutions à nos problèmes →
Je voudrais que nous trouvions tous ensemble des solutions à nos problèmes.

1. Je veux que le Conseil universitaire / agir / en faveur des étudiants
2. Je souhaite que vous / participer / aux décisions du Conseil
3. Je préfère que nous / discuter / librement des mesures à prendre
4. Je désire que l'université / prendre / nos inquiétudes / en considération
5. Je voudrais que les professeurs / comprendre / nos positions
6. Je souhaite enfin que tous les candidats / se réunir / bientôt pour mieux exposer leurs idées

C. Revendications. (*Demands.*) Les délégués du Conseil universitaire donnent leurs directives aux étudiants. Remplacez les sujets en italique par **vous,** puis par **les étudiants** et faites tous les changements nécessaires.

Nous ne voulons pas que *tu* ailles[1] en cours aujourd'hui. Nous préférons que *tu* sois[2] présent(e) à la manifestation et que *tu* fasses[3] grève. Nous désirons que *tu* aies[4] une affiche lisible (*legible*). Naturellement, nous voudrions que *tu* puisses[5] exprimer tes opinions librement.

D. Engagement politique. Les Legrand ont des opinions libérales. Quels conseils donnent-ils à leurs enfants? Suivez les modèles.

MODÈLES: Arnaud / être réactionnaire →
Nous ne voulons pas que tu sois réactionnaire.
Arnaud et Fabrice / être courageux →
Nous voulons que vous soyez courageux.

1. Jacob / être actif en politique
2. Albane et Jacob / avoir le courage de leurs opinions
3. vous / avoir des amis intolérants
4. Arnaud / être bien informé
5. Joachim / être violent
6. vous / être tolérant
7. Fabrice / avoir de l'ambition politique
8. Arnaud et Joachim / avoir des idéaux pacifistes

E. Exprimez-vous! Composez votre propre slogan. Complétez les phrases suivantes et donnez votre opinion. Commencez avec **Je voudrais que.**

1. notre gouvernement ______
2. les écologistes ______
3. les hommes et les femmes politiques ______
4. nous ______
5. les pays industrialisés ______
6. ?

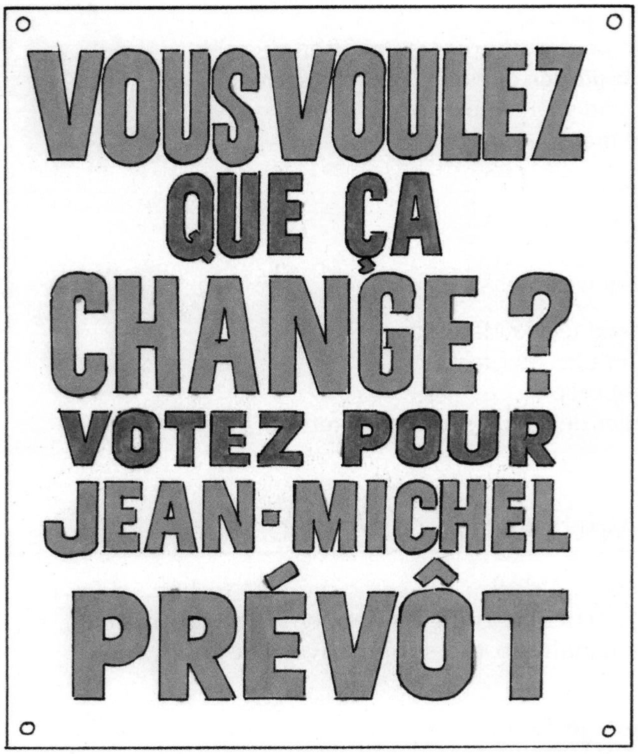

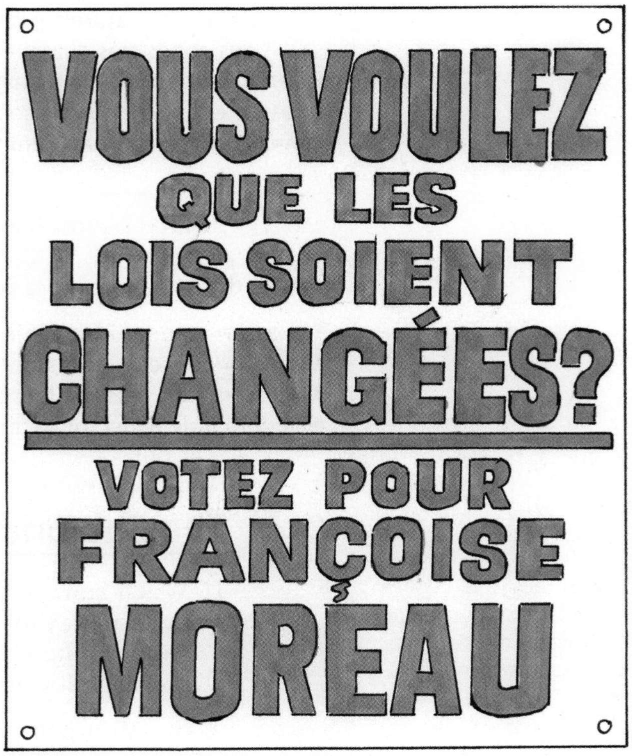

Suggestion (E): Give sts. a moment to write their slogans. Ask some sts. to read theirs and have the class choose the most interesting ones.

VOUS VOULEZ
QUE ÇA
CHANGE ?
VOTEZ POUR
JEAN-MICHEL
PRÉVÔT

VOUS VOULEZ
QUE LES
LOIS SOIENT
CHANGÉES?
VOTEZ POUR
FRANÇOISE
MOREAU

Le subjonctif (*deuxième partie*)

Expressing Wishes, Necessity, and Possibility

Un petit coin de paradis

Appel vidéo entre Hassan et Hector.

HASSAN: **Il est possible que** je **vienne** fin août à la Martinique! Je vais fermer mon restaurant une semaine et j'ai envie d'aller dans les Caraïbes.[1]

HECTOR: Ça serait génial[2]! Mais une semaine, c'est trop court! **Je préfère que** tu **restes** plus longtemps! Il y a tellement de choses à voir et à faire sur cette île sublime!

HASSAN: Oh, tu sais... **Il est** surtout **essentiel que** je **me repose**... Je veux vivre quelques jours loin de la civilisation et de la pollution: pas d'ordinateur, pas de téléphone... l'air pur... le silence...

HECTOR: La plage... la mer transparente... À la Martinique, il y a 22 000 hectares[3] d'espaces naturels protégés! On trouve des zones très solitaires où on peut vivre comme Robinson Crusoé!

HASSAN: **Il faut** absolument **que** tu m'**indiques** quelques endroits secrets.

HECTOR: Je connais un petit coin de paradis...Tu veux savoir où c'est?

HASSAN: Qui dirait non au Paradis? Pas moi!

[1]*Caribbean* [2]*great* [3]*hectare (One hectare is slightly less than 2.5 acres.)*

Trouvez, dans le dialogue, la phrase équivalente.

1. Hassan va peut-être venir une semaine à la Martinique.
2. Hector conseille à Hassan de rester plus longtemps.
3. Hassan veut essentiellement se reposer.
4. Il demande à Hector de lui indiquer de beaux endroits secrets.

The Subjunctive with Verbs of Volition

Note: Conjunctions followed by the subjunctive are not covered in *Vis-à-vis.* Here are the most common: *à moins que, bien que, avant que, jusqu'à ce que, pour que.*

1. When someone expresses a desire for someone else to behave in a certain way, or for a particular thing to happen, the verb in the subordinate clause is usually in the subjunctive. The following construction is used.

Mon père **veut que je fasse** les études aux USA.	*My father wants me to study in the USA.*
Ma mère **préfère que j'étudie** en France.	*My mother prefers that I study in France.*

Note that an infinitive construction is sometimes used in English to express such a desire.

2. Verbs of volition are followed by an infinitive in French when there is no change in subject, as in the first example.

Je veux finir mes études.	*I want to finish my studies.*
Et **ma mère veut** aussi **que** je les **finisse.**	*And my mother wants me to finish them too.*

3. Verbs expressing desires include **aimer bien, désirer, exiger, insister (pour), préférer, souhaiter, vouloir,** and **vouloir bien.** These verbs take the subjunctive. The verb **espérer,** however, takes the indicative.

Suggestion: Point out that most of these verbs are often used in the conditional.

Je souhaite que tu **aies** de bonnes vacances.	*I hope you have a good vacation.*
J'espère que tu **as** mon numéro de téléphone.	*I hope you have my telephone number.*

[Allez-y! A]

The Subjunctive with Impersonal Expressions

1. An impersonal expression is one in which the subject does not refer to any particular person or thing. In English, the subject of an impersonal expression is usually *it: It is important that I go to class.* In French, many impersonal expressions—especially those that express will, necessity, judgment, possibility, or doubt—are followed by the subjunctive in the dependent clause.

Presentation: Go over expressions in the chart, using short sentences to model each one. Have sts. repeat after your model.

Suggestion: Have sts. make up short completions for selected expressions from the chart.

IMPERSONAL EXPRESSIONS USED WITH THE SUBJUNCTIVE	
WILL OR NECESSITY	POSSIBILITY, JUDGMENT, OR DOUBT
il est essentiel que	il est normal que
il est important que	il est peu probable que†
il est indispensable que	il est possible / impossible que
il est nécessaire que	il se peut que (*it's possible that*)
il est préférable que	il semble que (*it seems that*)
il faut que*	
il vaut mieux que* (*it's better that*)	

Il est important que le racisme **disparaisse.**	*It's important that racism disappear.*
Il faut que vous **soyez** au courant de la politique.	*You must (It's necessary that you) keep up with politics.*
Il est peu probable que le sexisme **soit** tout à fait éliminé.	*It's not likely that sexism will be (is) totally eliminated.*
Il se peut que d'autres pays **possèdent** des armes nucléaires.	*It's possible that other countries possess nuclear weapons.*

Grammaire interactive

For more on the subjunctive with **il faut,** watch the corresponding Grammar Tutorial and take a brief practice quiz at **Connect French.**

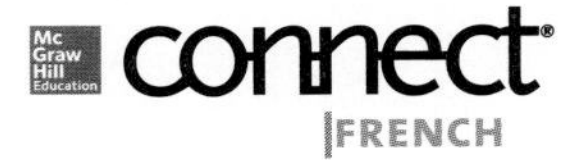

www.mhconnectfrench.com

*The infinitive of the verb conjugated in the expression **il faut que** is **falloir** (*to be necessary*). The infinitive of the verb in **il vaut mieux que** is **valoir** (*to be worth*).
†Although **il est peu probable que** takes the subjunctive because it conveys a lack of certainty, the expression **il est probable que** takes the indicative because it conveys probability or more certainty. For more information on this difference, see page 458.

Except for **il faut que, il vaut mieux que,** and **il semble que,** these impersonal expressions are usually limited to writing and formal discourse.

2. When no specific person or thing is mentioned, impersonal expressions are followed by the infinitive instead of the subjunctive. Compare the following sentences.

Il vaut mieux **attendre.**	*It's better to wait.*
Il vaut mieux **que nous attendions.**	*It's better for us to wait.*
Il est important **de voter.**	*It's important to vote.*
Il est important **que vous votiez.**	*It's important for you to vote.*

Note that the preposition **de** is used before the infinitive after impersonal expressions that contain **être.**

[Allez-y! B-C-D-E]

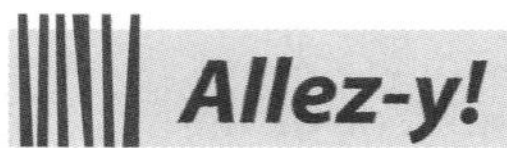

A. À la table de négociations. Faites des phrases pour exprimer des souhaits et des exigences.

MODÈLE: les écologistes / vouloir / le gouvernement / contrôler les déchets industriels →
Les écologistes veulent que le gouvernement contrôle les déchets industriels.

1. les hommes politiques / vouloir (*cond.*) / nous / payer plus d'impôts
2. les Verts / exiger / on / consommer moins d'essence
3. je / aimer (*cond.*) / tout le monde / faire du recyclage
4. vous / vouloir bien (*cond.*) / il y avoir moins de pollution atmosphérique
5. nous / vouloir / les richesses mondiales / être partagées

Continuation: Have sts. think of a few more *conseils.*

Follow-up: Have sts. give advice for the following statements: *Je veux vivre longtemps. Je veux perfectionner mon français. Je veux être riche. Je veux m'amuser ce week-end.*

B. Comment gagner? Donnez des conseils à Jeanne Laviolette, candidate à la mairie de Dijon, en suivant le modèle.

MODÈLE: Il est important de savoir écouter les gens. →
Il est important que vous sachiez écouter les gens.

1. Pour être maire, il faut être dynamique et responsable.
2. Il est essentiel de ne pas avoir peur d'agir.
3. Il est nécessaire de rester calme en toutes circonstances.
4. Il est préférable de parler souvent aux électeurs.
5. Il faut faire attention aux problèmes des jeunes.
6. Il est indispensable de gagner la confiance des commerçants.

C. La routine de tous les jours. Posez des questions à un(e) camarade de classe. Suivez le modèle.

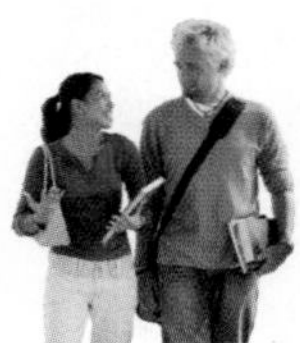

MODÈLE: nécessaire / faire la cuisine chaque soir
É1: Est-il nécessaire que tu fasses la cuisine chaque soir?
É2: Oui, il est nécessaire que je fasse la cuisine chaque soir. (Non, il n'est pas nécessaire que je fasse la cuisine chaque soir; mes copains m'aident souvent.)

1. vaut mieux / aller au cours de français tous les jours
2. préférable / faire ton lit chaque matin
3. faut / nettoyer ta chambre tous les jours
4. normal / pouvoir dormir tard le matin
5. indispensable / étudier chaque soir
6. important / lire le journal chaque jour

Suggestion (D): With whole class, elicit several individual reactions to statements. For second part, where sts. propose solutions to problems, have sts. brainstorm in pairs or in small groups. Compare group contributions.

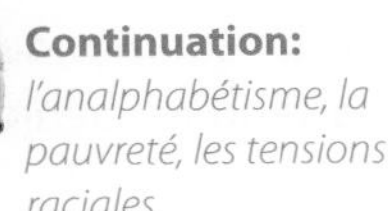

Continuation: *l'analphabétisme, la pauvreté, les tensions raciales.*

D. Problèmes contemporains. Discutez des problèmes suivants avec un(e) camarade. Suggérez des solutions en utilisant les expressions suivantes: **il est important que, il faut que, il est nécessaire que, il est indispensable que, il est essentiel que, il est préférable que.**

1. l'immigration clandestine dans votre pays
2. l'abus de la drogue chez les jeunes
3. la pollution
4. le chômage
5. le gaspillage des sources d'énergie
6. la violence dans votre pays
7. le terrorisme
8. l'intégrisme

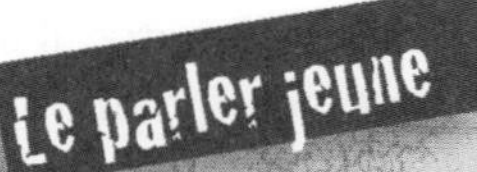

furax	furieux
le hic	le problème
kif-kif	équivalent
ne pas mâcher ses mots	dire ce que l'on pense
râler	protester

Le sondage révèle que les électeurs sont **furax** contre le gouvernement.

Le hic, c'est que les voitures électriques sont trop chères.

En réalité, la «droite» et la «gauche», c'est **kif-kif.**

Tu as entendu son discours sur les droits de l'homme? Il **n'a pas mâché ses mots!**

Arrête de **râler** tout le temps!

E. Nécessités et probabilités. Quelle sera votre vie? Répondez aux questions suivantes. Dans chaque réponse, utilisez une de ces expressions: **il se peut que, il est peu probable que, il est impossible que, il est possible que, il est essentiel que, il faut que, il est nécessaire que.**

MODÈLE: Ferez-vous une découverte (*discovery*) importante? → Il est peu probable que je fasse une découverte importante.

1. Vous marierez-vous?
2. Apprendrez-vous une langue étrangère?
3. Voyagerez-vous beaucoup?
4. Deviendrez-vous célèbre?
5. Serez-vous riche?
6. Saurez-vous jouer du piano?
7. Écrirez-vous un roman?
8. Ferez-vous la connaissance d'un homme / d'une femme d'état?
9. Irez-vous en Chine?
10. Vivrez-vous jusqu'à l'âge de cent ans?

Suggestion (E): Give sts. a minute to reflect before writing the sentences. Ask several sts. to write their sentences at the board.

Maintenant, utilisez ces questions pour interviewer un(e) camarade de classe.

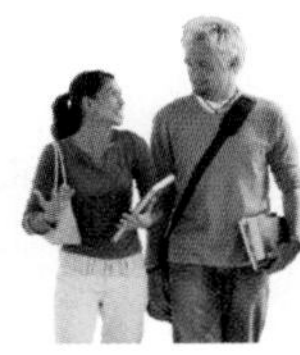

MODÈLE: É1: Feras-tu une découverte importante?
É2: Oui, il est possible que je fasse une découverte importante. (Non, il est peu probable que je fasse une découverte importante.)

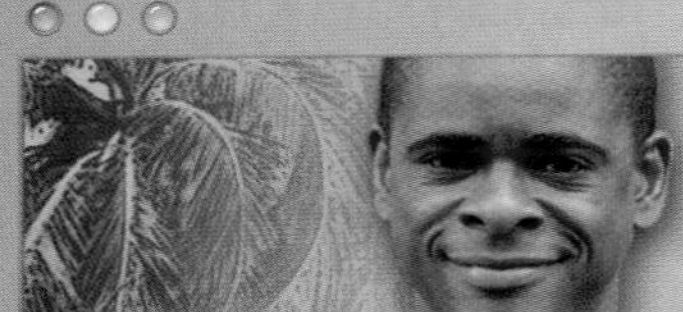

Le blog d'Hector

Moi d'abord?

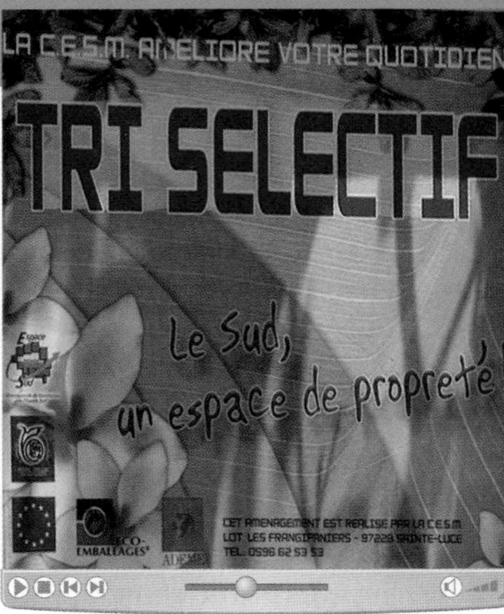
LA C.E.S.M. AMELIORE VOTRE QUOTIDIEN
TRI SELECTIF
Le Sud, un espace de propreté!

Le tri sélectif[3]: une façon d'être un bon citoyen!

lundi 13 juillet

Salut les amis!

Est-ce que nous sommes tous fous, vous, moi et nos hommes politiques?

J'ai 25 ans, et j'appartiens à la génération «Moi d'abord!»: Ce qui compte avant tout, c'est mon plaisir et comme tous les Français, je veux «profiter de la vie» surtout maintenant que je suis à la Martinique! Mais l'autre jour, j'ai vu une émission à la télé qui m'a fait froid dans le dos. C'était sur l'état du monde dans 50 ans. J'aurai 75 ans. Eh bien, savez-vous ce qui attend le «Senior» Hector?

Il est certain que la terre aura épuisé la majeure partie de ses ressources naturelles en pétrole et en gaz. Il est probable que nos réserves d'eau seront très insuffisantes. Il est sûr que le réchauffement de la planète aura changé nos climats et notre géographie: les glaciers auront fondu,[1] Venise sera sous les eaux, il fera aussi chaud à Paris qu'au Sahara. Dans le monde, le choc des cultures et des religions aura provoqué des conflits apocalyptiques.

Alors, qu'est-ce qu'on fait? On réagit ou on danse sur le volcan? Dites-moi ce que vous pensez de tout ça: votre opinion m'intéresse!

Hector

COMMENTAIRES

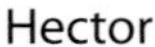

Alexis

Il se peut que ces prévisions[2] soient complètement fausses! Dansons!

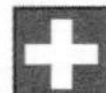

Charlotte

Il faut qu'on réagisse: je propose que chacun fasse attention à sa consommation d'eau et d'électricité. Il faut qu'on arrête de gaspiller l'essence et qu'on prenne les transports en commun. C'est ça être un bon citoyen.

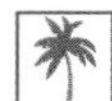

Poema

Tu as raison, Charlotte! Exprimer publiquement son opinion, manifester, faire la grève pour soutenir les grandes causes internationales, c'est inutile. Il semble que nos hommes politiques soient incapables de prendre des décisions radicales. Nous devons nous engager individuellement pour sauver notre belle planète!

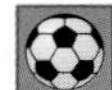

Mamadou

En France, nous avons plus de 1 000 associations engagées dans des actions en faveur de l'écologie du développement durable.

Follow-up: 1. *Définissez la génération «Moi d'abord». Appartenez-vous à cette génération? Comment réagissez-vous aux problèmes de la société et du monde?* 2. *Comment Hector envisage-t-il l'avenir? Quels sont, d'après vous, les problèmes majeurs que le monde devra résoudre dans les 20 prochaines années?* 3. *Expliquez l'expression «danser sur le volcan».* 4. *Expliquez le point de vue d'Alexis, de Charlotte, de Poema et de Mamadou. De qui vous sentez-vous le plus proche?* 5. *Que faites-vous personnellement en faveur de la protection de la nature?*

Video connection: In the videoblog for this chapter, Hassan, Juliette, and Léa discuss their personal efforts to protect the planet. They also look at Hector's blog about Martinique.

[1]*melted* [2]*predictions* [3]tri... *sorting of household trash (for recycling)*

REPORTAGE

La France multiculturelle

Corneille est une star de la chanson française. Il est né au Rwanda. Grâce au chanteur algérien Cheb Khaled, le raï, musique populaire algérienne, a donné au public français le goût des sons et des rythmes orientaux. Dans des salles de spectacles archi-comble,[1] des humoristes de talent comme Gad El Maleh, Smaïn ou Jamel Debbouze font la satire de la société française. Au stade de France, Mapou Yangambiva, né en République centrafrique, ou Steve Mandanda, qui vient de la République démocratique du Congo, font la fierté[2] de l'équipe de France de football.

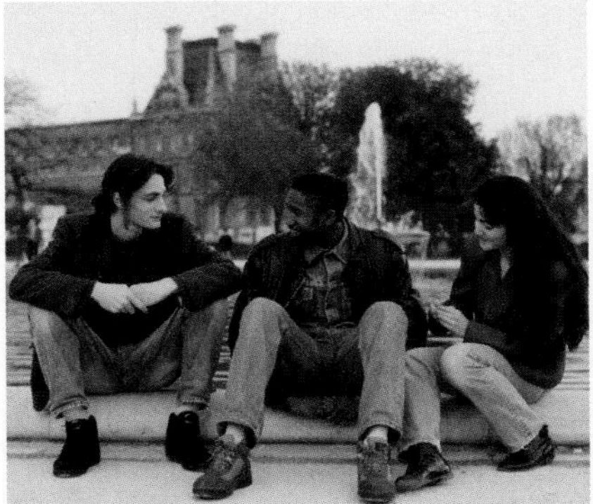

Une amitié multiculturelle. Oui, la France multiculturelle est une réalité!

En littérature, Shan Sa, auteur de *La joueuse de go,* et Dai Sijie, qui a écrit *Balzac et la petite tailleuse chinoise*, sont devenus des écrivains célèbres. Nés en Chine, ils apportent à la littérature française une inspiration asiatique. Avant eux, le Russe Andreï Makine a donné à la littérature de l'Hexagone des œuvres de première qualité comme *Le Testament français* (1995).

En hommage à la France, ces écrivains ont écrit leurs œuvres… en français. Mixité,[3] mélange, altérité,[4] diversité: tous ces termes nobles traduisent la réalité de la société française. Regardez les rues de Paris, de Lyon, de Marseille: on y rencontre toutes les nationalités, on y entend tous les accents. La rue française est algérienne, tunisienne, marocaine, turque, sénégalaise, ivoirienne, chinoise, vietnamienne, polonaise… La France multiculturelle existe: elle associe à ses traditions, des manières de penser, d'agir et de créer complètement nouvelles.

Mais elle veut, avant tout, que les immigrés qui ont choisi de vivre sur son territoire s'assimilent à la société française, seule garantie pour que les différentes communautés vivent en paix les unes avec les autres. Car il n'est pas toujours facile de vivre ensemble. Et il arrive que la diversité ethnique crée en France des tensions difficiles à gérer. Mais au pays des Droits de l'homme, il est important que le désir de s'unir pour un enrichissement mutuel soit plus fort que la tentation de l'exclusion. Et face aux problèmes du monde contemporain, n'est-il pas évident que l'on est plus forts si l'on est unis? C'est ce que pensent les sages…

[1]*full of people* [2]*pride* [3]*Mix of populations* [4]*otherness*

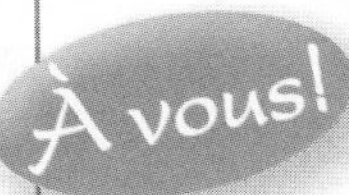

1. Qu'est-ce que «la France multiculturelle»? Donnez une image globale de la société française à partir du **Reportage.**
2. Comment la France accueille-t-elle (*welcome*) les immigrés? Que demande-t-elle aux immigrés qui ont choisi de vivre en France?
3. Comment vivent les immigrés en Amérique du Nord? Gardent-ils les coutumes de leur pays d'origine? Citez quelques exemples.

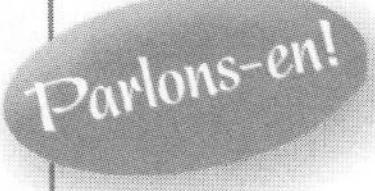

1. Travaillez en petits groupes. Chacun à votre tour, citez, au choix, un personnage représentatif de la France ou de l'Amérique multiculturelle—un artiste, un chanteur, un musicien, un acteur, un sportif, un écrivain, un homme ou une femme politique. Précisez son domaine d'excellence.
2. D'après (*Based on*) cette liste, comment le multiculturalisme transforme-t-il une société? Discutez!

Leçon 3

Suggestion: Ask sts. to comment on the highlighted expressions and say why they might require the subjunctive.

Le subjonctif (*troisième partie*)

Expressing Emotion

Le job de mes rêves

Hassan, Hector, Juliette et Léa discutent au restaurant.

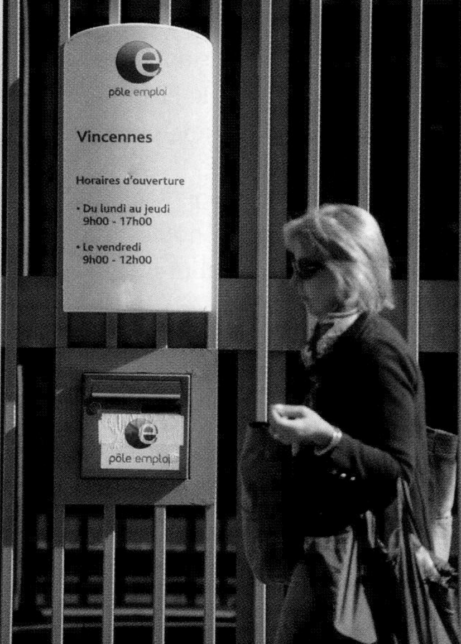
pôle emploi
Vincennes
Horaires d'ouverture
• Du lundi au jeudi
9h00 - 17h00
• Le vendredi
9h00 - 12h00
pôle emploi

Le Pôle Emploi: un établissement public chargé de mettre en relation demandeurs et offreurs d'emplois

HASSAN: Le chômage, c'est quand même[1] le problème essentiel de la société française. **Il est injuste que** nous **fassions** des études et **que** nous ne **trouvions** pas d'emploi!

HECTOR: Toi Hassan, tu as trouvé la solution: tu es ton propre patron.

HASSAN: Oui, et **je regrette que** la plupart des jeunes diplômés **veuillent** devenir fonctionnaires!

JULIETTE: L'époque est difficile! Moi, **je** ne **suis** pas **étonnée que** les jeunes **cherchent** un emploi stable et un salaire garanti.

HASSAN: Personnellement, j'ai l'âme[2] d'un entrepreneur! **Je suis heureux que** mon avenir ne **soit** pas dessiné à l'avance.

HECTOR: Tu es indépendant, travailleur, audacieux: c'est exactement le profil d'un créateur d'entreprise!

HASSAN: **Je suis content que** tu **penses** ça! **Et je regrette que** si peu de jeunes Français **prennent** des risques.

JULIETTE: Mais les jeunes ne refusent pas l'aventure! **Il est bizarre que** tu ne le **saches** pas! Par exemple, beaucoup partent à l'étranger. Moi-même, j'ai l'intention d'aller travailler en Australie!

LÉA: **Nous sommes tristes que** tu **partes,** Juliette… Dans les nouvelles technologies, tu pourrais aussi bien trouver un emploi en France…

JULIETTE: C'est sans[3] doute vrai, mais **il est bon que** les jeunes diplômés **jouent** la carte de l'international. Après tout, on est dans la mondialisation, non?

[1]quand… *even so, anyway* [2]*soul* [3]*without*

Complétez les phrases selon le dialogue.

1. Pour Hassan, il est injuste que les jeunes ____ des études et qu'ils ne ____ pas d'emploi.
2. Hassan regrette que la plupart des jeunes diplômés ____ devenir fonctionnaires.
3. Juliette n'est pas étonnée que les jeunes ____ un emploi dans la fonction publique.
4. Hassan est heureux que son avenir ne ____ pas dessiné à l'avance.
5. Il est content qu'Hector ____ qu'il a le profil d'un créateur d'entreprise. Et il regrette que peu de Français ____ des risques.
6. Juliette s'étonne qu'Hassan ne ____ pas que beaucoup de jeunes acceptent l'aventure.
7. Léa et ses amis sont tristes que Juliette ____.
8. Mais selon Juliette, il est bon qu'on ____ la carte de l'international.

1. The subjunctive is frequently used after expressions of emotion.

EXPRESSIONS OF EMOTION	
happiness:	**être content(e), être heureux / heureuse**
regret:	**être désolé(e), être triste, regretter** (*to be sorry*)
surprise:	**être surpris(e), être étonné(e)**
fear:	**avoir peur**
relief:	**être soulagé(e)**
anger:	**être furieux / furieuse**

Le président **est content** que les électeurs **aient** confiance en lui.	*The president is pleased that the voters have confidence in him.*
Les électeurs **ont peur** que l'inflation **soit** un problème insoluble.	*The voters are afraid that inflation is an insurmountable problem.*
Les écologistes **sont furieux** que les lois contre la pollution des forêts et des rivières **soient** tellement faibles.	*The environmentalists are angry that the laws against polluting the forests and rivers are so weak.*

2. As with verbs of volition, there must be different subjects in the main and dependent clauses. Otherwise, an infinitive is used.

Le président est content de rencontrer le Premier ministre du Canada.	*The president is happy to meet the prime minister of Canada.*

3. The subjunctive is also used following impersonal expressions of emotion.

IMPERSONAL EXPRESSIONS OF EMOTION	
il est bizarre que	il est juste / injuste que
il est bon que*	il est stupide que*
il est dommage que (*it's too bad that*)	il est utile / inutile que

Il est dommage que la guerre y **continue.**	*It's too bad that war is continuing there.*
Est-il bon que les enfants aussi **expriment** leurs opinions?	*Is it good that children also express their opinions?*
Il est stupide que tant de citoyens ne **votent** pas.	*It is stupid that so many citizens do not vote.*

*In everyday conversation, the French often say **c'est stupide que, c'est bon que,** and so on.

Additional activity (A): *Problèmes sociaux. Donnez votre réaction aux idées suivantes. Utilisez des expressions que vous avez apprises dans ce chapitre.* (Suggestion: After a st. reads a sentence, ask *Êtes-vous d'accord?* and have sts. change sentence to conform with their beliefs.) *MODÈLE: La technologie change la vie. → À mon avis, il est évident que la technologie change la vie.* 1. *On gaspille très peu d'énergie aujourd'hui.* 2. *L'atmosphère est moins polluée maintenant qu'il y a dix ans.* 3. *Le gouvernement est en train de développer l'énergie solaire.* 4. *Il n'est pas nécessaire de conserver l'énergie.* 5. *Les déchets industriels ne posent plus de problèmes.* 6. *On n'a plus besoin d'économiser l'essence.* 7. *Les femmes sont toujours respectées dans les publicités.* 8. *Les médias ont trop de liberté.* 9. *La guerre existera toujours.* 10. *La faim n'existe plus dans le monde.*

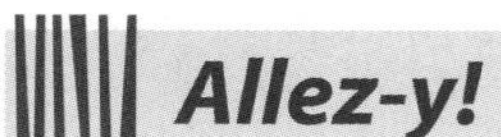

Allez-y!

A. Opinions. Complétez chaque phrase de façon logique en mettant une des expressions en italique au subjonctif.

MODÈLE: Nous sommes furieux / *les leaders politiques se sentent responsables face aux électeurs / la télévision n'analyse pas les problèmes actuels.* →
Nous sommes furieux que la télévision n'analyse pas les problèmes actuels.

1. Je suis vraiment désolé(e) / *les grandes puissances mondiales ne sont pas d'accord sur la protection de l'environnement / le gouvernement prend des mesures pour encourager le développement de l'énergie solaire.*
2. Les gens ont peur / *les hommes politiques font de mauvais choix / les hommes politiques prennent de bonnes décisions.*
3. Je regrette / *il y a encore des dictateurs dans certains pays / on donne tant d'importance à la liberté dans ce pays.*
4. Mon amie Gaëlle est soulagée / *les Européens sont de plus en plus sensibles* (more and more sensitive) *aux questions liées à la protection de l'environnement / le taux de chômage en Europe est élevé cette année.*
5. Les sénateurs sont étonnés / *le public ne veut pas payer plus d'impôts / le public veut payer plus d'impôts.*

Suggestion (B): Give sts. a few minutes to prepare.

B. Le journal. Voici des titres (*headlines*) adaptés de divers journaux français. Donnez votre réaction à chaque situation en utilisant les expressions suivantes: **être content(e), heureux / heureuse, désolé(e), triste, surpris(e), étonné(e), soulagé(e), fâché(e), furieux / furieuse, regretter, avoir peur, il est stupide (bizarre, bon, dommage, juste, injuste, utile, inutile) que.**

MODÈLE: **Les femmes et les chômeurs fument davantage** (*more*) →
Il est dommage que les femmes et les chômeurs fument davantage.

1. **Le Club Méditerranée ouvre son premier village en Chine**
2. **L'Europe aime la France** (La majorité des Européens choisiraient la France comme terre d'accueil [*country where they would settle*].)
3. **Le froid tue** (*kills*) **5 sans-abri** (Des centres d'hébergement [*shelters*] exceptionnels ont ouvert leurs portes aux victimes du froid.)
4. **Les Français disent «non» à la drogue** (68 % des Français sont favorables au maintien de l'interdiction totale des ventes et de la consommation de drogues, selon un sondage.)
5. **L'industrie textile va supprimer** (*to eliminate*) **un emploi sur sept** (L'industrie textile a annoncé qu'elle comptait supprimer 750 emplois.)

Suggestion: To prepare ex., ask sts. to make a list of 5 current events to bring to class.

C. Émotions. Donnez votre opinion personnelle sur les problèmes de la société américaine.

MODÈLE: Je suis heureux / heureuse que… →
Je suis heureux / heureuse que les États-Unis aident plusieurs pays en voie de développement (*developing*).

1. Je suis heureux / heureuse que...
2. Je regrette que...
3. Il est injuste que...
4. Il est bon que...
5. Il est bizarre que...
6. Il est stupide que...

D. Encore des émotions. Reprenez les *trois premières* phrases de l'exercice C. Maintenant demandez à cinq camarades comment ils/elles ont complété ces phrases. Pouvez-vous trouver quelqu'un qui a les mêmes opinions que vous?

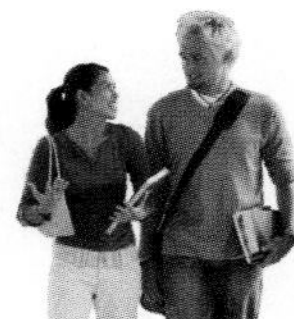

Suggestion (D): Have several sts. read their answers.

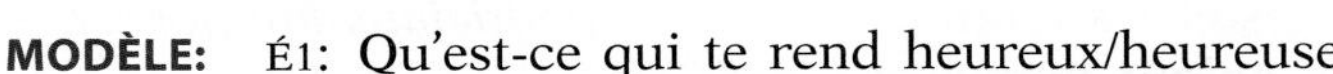

MODÈLE: É1: Qu'est-ce qui te rend heureux/heureuse?
É2: Je suis heureux/heureuse que le maire fasse quelque chose pour aider les sans-abri.

Le subjonctif (*quatrième partie*)

Expressing Doubt and Uncertainty

Parlons de la Francophonie

Mamadou contacte Léa sur sa page Facebook (Messagerie instantanée).

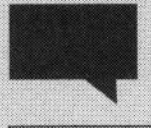

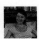

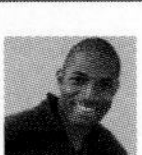

MAMADOU: **Crois-tu que** la Francophonie **ait** un bel avenir?

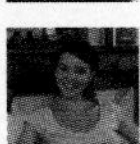

LÉA: J'en suis sûre; elle est si belle la langue française!

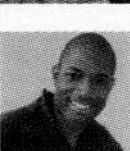

MAMADOU: Je ne suis pas aussi optimiste que toi. Avec la mondialisation, on uniformise tout: on parle anglais partout!

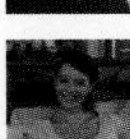

LÉA: **Je ne pense pas que** tout le monde **veuille** ressembler à tout le monde... La Francophonie, c'est un refus d'uniformiser la planète.

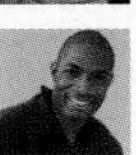

MAMADOU: **Je ne suis pas certain que** les 220 millions de Francophones **tiennent à**[1] être différents du reste du monde. Ils parlent français sans se poser des questions, tout simplement parce que c'est la langue de leur pays.

LÉA: Tu as tort! La Francophonie, c'est bien plus qu'un idiome[2] commun: c'est une culture, c'est un idéal, c'est une passion!

[1]tiennent... *are keen about* [2]*langue*

Trouvez, dans le dialogue, les phrases équivalentes.

1. Mamadou demande si la Francophonie a un bel avenir.
2. Léa pense que les gens veulent être différents les uns des autres.
3. Selon Mamadou, les Francophones ne sont pas attachés à leur singularité.

1. The subjunctive is used—with a change of subject—after expressions of doubt and uncertainty, such as **je doute, je ne suis pas sûr(e),** and **je ne suis pas certain(e).**

Beaucoup de femmes **ne sont pas sûres** que leur statut **soit** égal au statut des hommes.	*Many women aren't sure that their status is equal to the status of men.*
Les jeunes **doutent** souvent que les hommes et les femmes politiques **soient** honnêtes.	*Young people often doubt that politicians are honest.*

2. In the affirmative, verbs such as **penser** and **croire** are followed by the indicative. In the negative and interrogative, they express a degree of doubt and uncertainty and can then be followed by the subjunctive. In spoken French, however, the indicative is more commonly used.

Je **pense** que la presse **est** libre.	*I think the press is free.*
Pensez-vous que la presse **soit** libre? **Pensez**-vous que la presse **est** libre?	*Do you think the press is free?*
Je **ne crois pas** que la démocratie **soit** en danger. Je **ne crois pas** que la démocratie **est** en danger.	*I don't think that democracy is in danger.*

3. The following impersonal expressions are followed by the *indicative* because they imply certainty or probability.*

IMPERSONAL EXPRESSIONS USED WITH THE INDICATIVE	
il est certain que	il est probable que
il est clair que	il est sûr que
il est évident que	il est vrai que

Il est probable que l'Europe et les États-Unis **feront** plus d'échanges culturels et commerciaux.	*It's probable that Europe and the U.S. will engage in more cultural and commercial exchanges.*
Il est vrai que les Québécois **veulent** préserver leur propre identité.	*It's true that the Quebecois want to preserve their own identity.*

*In everyday conversation, you will often hear **c'est,** rather than **il est,** with these expressions.

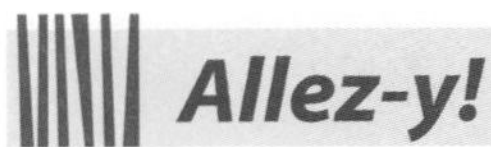

Allez-y!

A. Réflexions sur l'Afrique francophone. Complétez les phrases avec le subjonctif ou l'indicatif des verbes, selon le cas.

1. Il est sûr que le Burkina Faso _____ (être) un pays très, très pauvre.
2. Pensez-vous que le Mali _____ (être) un pays où l'intervention militaire est justifiée?
3. Les observateurs diplomatiques ne croient pas que l'assistance étrangère _____ (pouvoir) améliorer la crise économique et sociale de l'Afrique centrale.
4. On ne doute pas que les Sénégalais _____ (vouloir) multiplier les échanges commerciaux avec les pays voisins.
5. Il est évident que la République de Guinée _____ (avoir) des ressources minières importantes.
6. Je ne crois pas que les autres nations _____ (devoir) intervenir dans les affaires africaines.

B. Discussion. Avec un(e) camarade, discutez des idées suivantes. Choisissez une phrase et posez une question. Votre camarade répond selon sa conviction.

MODÈLE: L'homme politique est honnête. →
É1: Crois-tu que l'homme politique soit honnête?
É2: Oui, je crois qu'il est honnête. (Non, je ne crois pas qu'il soit honnête.)

Idées à discuter:

1. Nous avons besoin d'une armée plus moderne.
2. Les citoyens de ce pays savent voter intelligemment.
3. Le gouverneur de votre état/province a de bonnes idées.
4. On doit limiter l'immigration dans ce pays.
5. L'enseignement bilingue est une bonne idée.

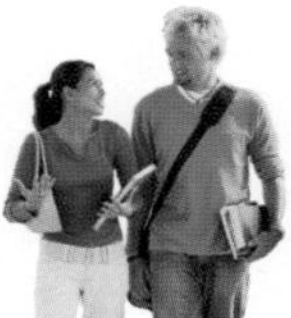

Suggestion (B): Can be done as a whole-class discussion: one st. makes up a sentence and several others react.

Follow-up (B): Ask sts. working in pairs to make a brief statement about their political ideas, using sentences as guides. They may also wish to add political slogans.

C. Opinions et croyances. Complétez les phrases de façon logique. Exprimez une opinion personnelle.

Vocabulaire utile: le covoiturage, les droits civils, la guerre, les impôts, le recyclage, les sans-abris

MODÈLE: Je ne pense pas que… →
Je ne pense pas que les jeunes soient informés sur la contraception.

1. C'est vrai que… **2.** Personne ne croit que… **3.** Je ne suis pas sûr(e) que… **4.** Il est probable que… **5.** Beaucoup d'étudiants trouvent que…

Mots clés

Éviter l'emploi du subjonctif

Espérer, followed by the indicative, can be used instead of **souhaiter** and other constructions that require the subjunctive.

J'**espère** qu'il gagnera les élections.

Devoir + infinitive can sometimes be used instead of **il faut que** and **il est nécessaire que.**

Tu **dois** afficher les prospectus.

In general statements, the infinitive can replace the subjunctive.

Il faut que nous contrôlions les déchets industriels.

Il faut **contrôler** les déchets industriels.

Prononcez bien!

The subjunctive of *aller* and *avoir* (page 445)

Script (A): 1. HUGO: *Cet après-midi, il faut que j'aille à la bibliothèque pour faire des recherches pour mon cours de philosophie.* 2. ISABELLE: *Ah oui! Il faut que tu aies une très bonne note pour réussir à ce cours, non?* 3. HUGO: *Oui, c'est ma dernière chance! Et toi, est-ce qu'il faut que tu y ailles aussi?* 4. ISABELLE: *Non. Ma mère aimerait que mon frère et moi allions voir notre grand-mère cet après-midi.* 5. ISABELLE: *Elle est vieille et ma mère dit toujours: « Je ne voudrais pas que vous ayez des regrets quand votre grand-mère ne sera plus là!» Elle a raison: nous devons en profiter maintenant!*

Answers (A): 1. a 2. b 3. a 4. a 5. b

Answers (B): 1. alliez 2. aient 3. ayez 4. allions

A. Cet après-midi. Hugo et Isabelle discutent de leurs projets pour l'après-midi. Écoutez leur conversation et indiquez si les verbes au subjonctif sont une forme du verbe **aller** ou du verbe **avoir**.

1.	**a.** ☐ aille	**b.** ☐ aie
2.	**a.** ☐ ailles	**b.** ☐ aies
3.	**a.** ☐ ailles	**b.** ☐ aies
4.	**a.** ☐ allions	**b.** ☐ ayons
5.	**a.** ☐ alliez	**b.** ☐ ayez

B. Ce soir. Hugo veut aussi faire des projets pour la soirée. D'abord, complétez les phrases avec la forme appropriée des verbes **aller** et **avoir** au subjonctif. Ensuite, avec votre camarade, lisez la conversation à voix haute, en faisant bien attention à la prononciation de ces verbes.

HUGO: Est-ce que ton frère et toi, vous allez dîner ici ce soir?
ISABELLE: Oui, si tu veux bien.
HUGO: Bien sûr! Mais j'aimerais que vous ________[1] au supermarché pour acheter de la salade. Nous n'en avons plus.
ISABELLE: Pas de problème! Ce serait bien qu'ils ________[2] de la romaine. C'est ma salade préférée.
HUGO: D'accord. Je préfère que vous ________[3] ce que vous aimez!
ISABELLE: Hmmm, finalement, je pense que ce serait mieux que nous ________[4] à l'épicerie: elle est sur notre chemin.
HUGO: Comme vous voulez. À tout à l'heure!

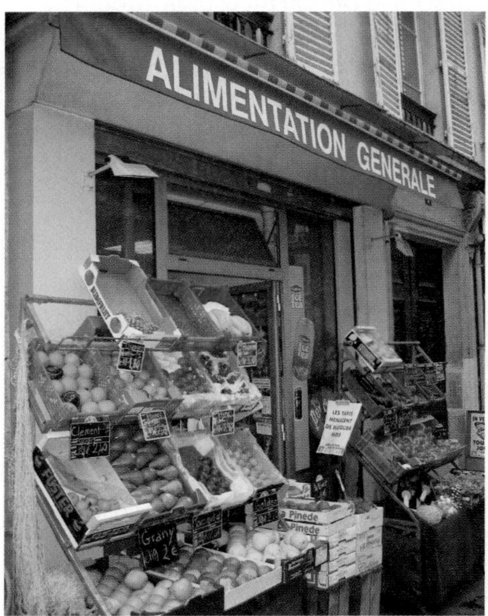

Leçon 4

Lecture

Avant de lire

Inferring an author's point of view. Approximately 8% of the French population is composed of immigrants, chiefly from former French colonies in North and West Africa, as well as Spain, Portugal, and Eastern European countries. These immigrants came to France to seek greater economic opportunities and social freedoms. However, immigrants have not been universally welcomed. Some of the French have associated immigration with increased violence and crime and with a disruption of the French way of life.

You will be reading an excerpt from the novel *La Réclusion solitaire,* written in 1976 by the Moroccan novelist and poet Tahar Ben Jelloun (1944–). In this work, Ben Jelloun draws on his personal experience to describe the sometimes difficult conditions Arabs experience in French society. The narrator, a North African worker, lives in a room with three others. In this excerpt, he describes some of the arbitrary and discriminatory rules imposed upon the residents.

Examine carefully the wording of these rules, as illustrated in the following examples. Which words and structures are repeated?

> Il est interdit de faire son manger dans la chambre...
> Il est interdit de recevoir des femmes; [...]

The repetition of the impersonal expression **Il est interdit de** followed by the infinitive is an example of parallelism.

Now compare the following two rules. You will note that although they are parallel in structure, they do not express parallel ideas. (In what ways are the ideas dissimilar?)

> Il est interdit d'écouter la radio à partir de neuf heures.
> Il est interdit de vous peindre en bleu, en vert ou en mauve.

In the first case, the restriction is of a realistic nature, a rule one might find in places such as workers' housing. In the second, the rule is absurd, a behavior that would never occur and consequently expresses a useless regulation.

As you read the text, pay particular attention to the nature of the behavior forbidden by the repeated formula **Il est interdit de.** Which rules are plausible? Which seem ridiculous? Which criticize the behaviors of immigrants? Which express hostility toward the presence of immigrants in French society?

À propos de la lecture...
Cet extrait est tiré du roman *La Réclusion solitaire* de Tahar Ben Jelloun.

La Réclusion solitaire (extrait) de Tahar Ben Jelloun

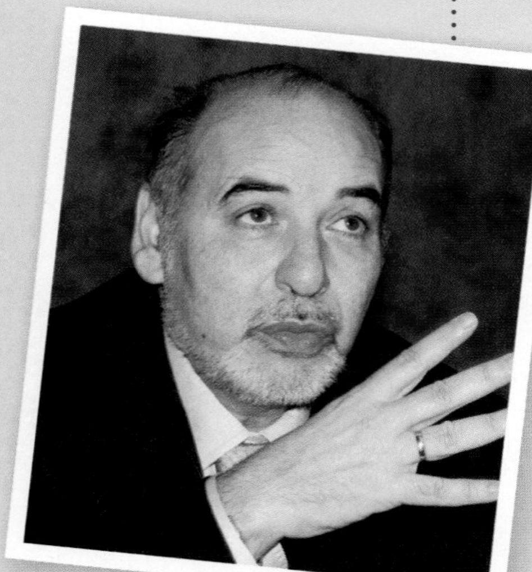

Tahar Ben Jelloun

À l'entrée du bâtiment, on nous a donné le règlement:
—Il est interdit de faire son manger dans la chambre (il y a une cuisine au fond du couloir);
—Il est interdit de recevoir des femmes;...
—Il est interdit d'écouter la radio à partir de neuf heures;
—Il est interdit de chanter le soir, surtout en arabe ou en kabyle;[1]
—Il est interdit d'égorger[2] un mouton dans le bâtiment;...
—Il est interdit de faire du yoga dans les couloirs;
—Il est interdit de repeindre les murs, de toucher aux meubles, de casser les vitres,[3] de changer d'ampoule,[4] de tomber malade, d'avoir la diarrhée, de faire de la politique, d'oublier d'aller au travail, de penser à faire venir sa famille,... de sortir en pyjama dans la rue, de vous plaindre[5] des conditions objectives et subjectives de vie,... de lire ou d'écrire des injures[6] sur les murs, de vous disputer, de vous battre,[7] de manier[8] le couteau, de vous venger.
—Il est interdit de mourir dans cette chambre, dans l'enceinte de[9] ce bâtiment (allez mourir ailleurs: chez vous, par exemple, c'est plus commode);
—Il est interdit de vous suicider (même si on vous enferme à Fleury-Mérogis[10]): votre religion vous l'interdit, nous aussi;
—Il est interdit de monter dans les arbres;
—Il est interdit de vous peindre en bleu, en vert ou en mauve;
—Il est interdit de circuler en bicyclette dans la chambre, de jouer aux cartes, de boire du vin (pas de champagne);
—Il est aussi interdit de... prendre un autre chemin pour rentrer du boulot. Vous êtes avertis. Nous vous conseillons de suivre le règlement, sinon,... ce sera le séjour dans un camp d'internement en attendant votre rapatriement.

[1] *language spoken in Kabylia, a rugged mountain region in northeastern Algeria* [2] *slit the throat of* [3] *windows* [4] *lightbulb* [5] vous... *complain* [6] *insults* [7] vous... *fight* [8] *wield* [9] dans... *within the boundary of* [10] prison près de Paris

Compréhension

Classez. Choisissez sept des règles énumérées dans le texte. Ensuite, classez-les en utilisant les catégories suivantes.

C'est une règle...

- qui convient à la situation.
- qui exprime le racisme.
- qui semble critiquer des pratiques musulmanes.
- ridicule.
- qui exprime de l'hostilité envers la présence maghrébine.
- qui suggère que les Maghrébins sont impliqués dans la criminalité.

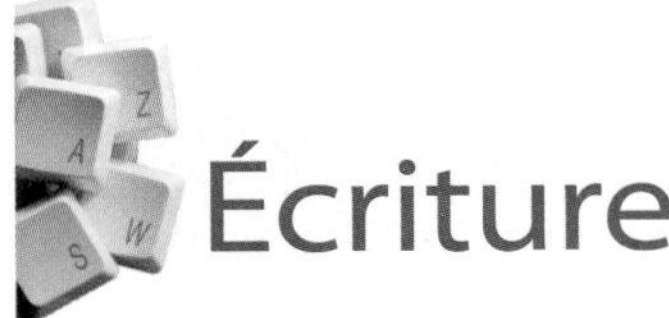

Écriture

The writing activities **Par écrit** and **Journal intime** can be found in the Workbook/Laboratory Manual to accompany *Vis-à-vis*.

Pour s'amuser

Quelques mots sur les hommes politiques:

> «Le mois de l'année où le politicien dit le moins de conneries (*stupid things, tr. fam.*), c'est le mois de février, parce qu'il n'y a que vingt-huit jours.»
>
> —Coluche

> «En politique, on succède à des imbéciles et on est remplacé par des incapables.»
>
> —Georges Clémenceau

La vie en chantant. An activity based on the song "Le pays va mal" by Tiken Jah Fakoly can be found in the Instructor's Manual. The song can be purchased at the iTunes store, or sts. can watch the music video on YouTube.

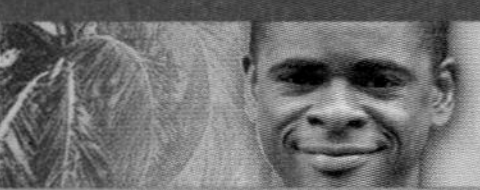

Le vidéoblog d'Hector

En bref

Dans cet épisode, Léa, Juliette, et Hassan discutent de la protection de l'environnement. À la fin de leur conversation, ils regardent le blog d'Hector sur la Martinique.

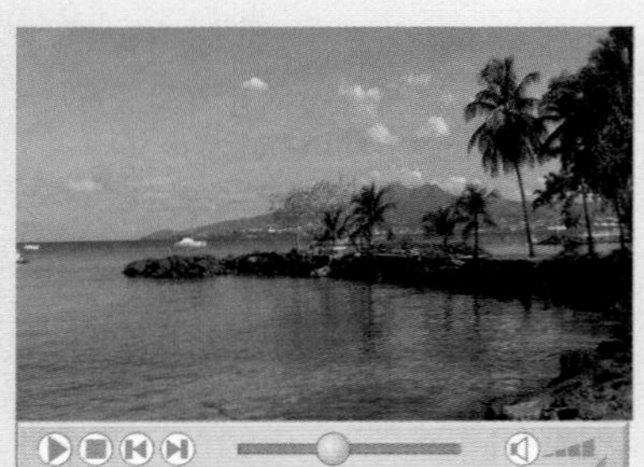

Une belle plage martiniquaise

Suggestion: After sts. have made their selections, put them in groups to compare responses, determining who does the most. Have them provide explanations for why they *don't* undertake certain activities. Afterward, make note of the fact that the activities in the lefthand column are social activist activities, whereas those in the right-hand column are more personal activities. Determine which activity type is the most prevalent among sts. and discuss why.

Additional vocabulary: You may wish to present the verb *agir* before viewing the video.

Vocabulaire en contexte

Indiquez ce que vous faites ou ce que vous avez fait pour protéger l'environnement.

Comment protéger l'environnement

- ☐ **créer** un groupe ou organiser une journée «environnement»
- ☐ écrire aux sénateurs/députés de votre état pour **lutter** (*fight*) contre **la pollution**
- ☐ faire du bénévolat (*volunteer*) pendant une journée «Plages **propres** (*clean*)»
- ☐ participer à une manifestation contre la pollution
- ☐ participer à la **Journée mondiale de la biodiversité**
- ☐ imprimer vos dissertations des deux côtés d'une feuille de papier
- ☐ prendre des douches rapides pour économiser l'eau
- ☐ recycler vos bouteilles, vos boîtes, le papier, le plastique, et cetera
- ☐ réduire vos déchets
- ☐ rouler à vélo ou aller à pied pour économiser l'essence

Visionnez!

Quel personnage dans la vidéo dirait les phrases suivantes?

	Léa	Hassan	Juliette	Hector
1. «Il est préférable de rouler à vélo.»	☐	☐	☐	☐
2. «Il est essentiel de prendre des douches très rapides.»	☐	☐	☐	☐
3. «Il vaut mieux recycler le verre et le papier.»	☐	☐	☐	☐
4. «Il est important de nettoyer (*clean*) nos plages.»	☐	☐	☐	☐
5. «Il faut lutter contre la pollution de l'eau.»	☐	☐	☐	☐

Analysez!

1. Des quatre camarades, quelle est la personne la plus «verte»? Expliquez.
2. Hector est très engagé dans la protection de la nature. Qu'est-ce qu'il fait personnellement? Imaginez pourquoi.

Comparez!

Qu'est-ce qu'on fait dans votre pays pour protéger l'environnement? Y a-t-il des endroits qui ont particulièrement besoin d'être protégés? Quelles actions ont été organisées? Est-ce que vous êtes plus (ou moins) «vert(e)» que les quatre blogueurs? Expliquez.

Note culturelle

En 1971, la France a créé[1] un Ministère de l'environnement. Il est devenu le Ministère de l'Écologie, du Développement durable et de l'Énergie. Ses principaux objectifs sont les suivants: la lutte contre le changement climatique; la préservation de la biodiversité, de l'environnement et des ressources; la cohésion sociale et la solidarité entre territoires et entre générations; les modes de production et de consommation[2] responsables. Initiée par Jacques Chirac, la «Charte de l'environnement» est, en France, un texte à valeur constitutionnelle stipulant le droit[3] de chacun à vivre dans un environnement favorable.

[1]*created* [2]*consumption* [3]*right*

Suggestion: Have sts. return to the phrases in the vocabulary section and create sentences based on their choices using an expression of will/necessity, as modeled in the *Visionnez!* activity.

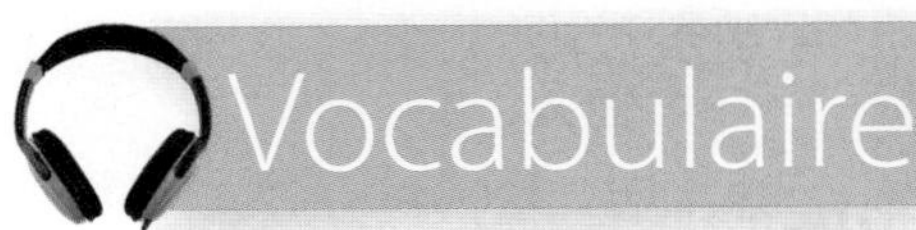

Vocabulaire

Verbes

abolir to abolish
augmenter to raise, increase
conserver to conserve
consommer to consume
contrôler to inspect, monitor
développer to develop
diminuer to lower, reduce, diminish
douter to doubt
élire to elect
embaucher to hire
s'engager (dans) to get involved (in) (*a public issue, cause*)
épuiser to use up, exhaust
estimer to consider; to believe; to estimate
établir to establish
exiger to require; to demand; to necessitate
exprimer une opinion to express an opinion
faire grève to strike
gaspiller to waste
manifester (pour/contre) to demonstrate (for/against)
paraître to appear
polluer to pollute
poser sa candidature to run for elected office; to apply (*for a job*)
protéger to protect
reconnaître to recognize
recycler to recycle
regretter to regret, be sorry
sauver to save, rescue
souhaiter to wish, desire
soutenir to support
tenir à to be keen about
valoir to be worth

Substantifs

le bien commun the common good
la centrale nucléaire nuclear power plant
le citoyen / la citoyenne citizen
le covoiturage carpooling
les déchets (*m. pl.*) waste (*material*)
le défi challenge
les droits (*m.*) **civils** civil rights
l'écologiste (*m., f.*) environmentalist
l'électeur / l'électrice voter
le gaspillage wasting
la grève strike
la guerre war
l'homme / la femme politique politician
les idées (*f.*) **extrémistes** extremist ideas
les impôts (*m. pl.*) taxes
l'intégrisme fundamentalism
la mondialisation globalization
le niveau de vie standard of living
le parti political party
la politique politics; policy
le pouvoir d'achat purchasing power
le réchauffement de la planète global warming
le recyclage recycling
la retraite pension
la réussite success
le/la sans-abri homeless person
le sondage survey
la surpopulation overpopulation
une voiture hybride hybrid car

À REVOIR: **la banlieue, l'essence**

Substantifs apparentés

l'accident (*m.*), **l'atmosphère** (*f.*), **le budget (militaire), le développement, l'élection** (*f.*), **l'énergie** (*f.*) **nucléaire / solaire, l'environnement** (*m.*), **le gouvernement, l'inflation** (*f.*), **la légalisation, la liberté d'expression, les médias** (*m.*), **la nature, l'opinion** (*f.*) **publique, la pollution, le problème, le progrès, la prolifération, la protection, la réduction, la réforme, les ressources naturelles, le rythme, la sécurité, le sexisme, la solitude, la source, le terrorisme**

Adjectifs

désolé(e) sorry
égal(e) equal
étonné(e) surprised
fâché(e) angry
furieux / furieuse furious
grave serious
industriel(le) industrial
préoccupé(e) preoccupied
soulagé(e) relieved
sûr(e) sure, certain
surpris(e) surprised

Expressions impersonnelles

il est... it is . . .
il est vrai que... it's true that . . .
dommage too bad
étrange strange
fâcheux unfortunate
(in)utile useless / useful
il se peut que... it is possible that . . .
il semble que... it seems that . . .
il vaut mieux (que)... it is better (that) . . .

Expressions impersonnelles apparentées

il est... certain, clair, essentiel, évident, important, (im)possible, indispensable, (in)juste, nécessaire, normal, peu probable, préférable, probable, stupide, sûr, urgent

Mots et expressions divers

j'ai entendu dire que... I heard that . . .
par exemple for example
personnellement personally
pour ma part in my opinion, as for me
quand même even so, anyway
sans doute without a doubt

Bienvenue...

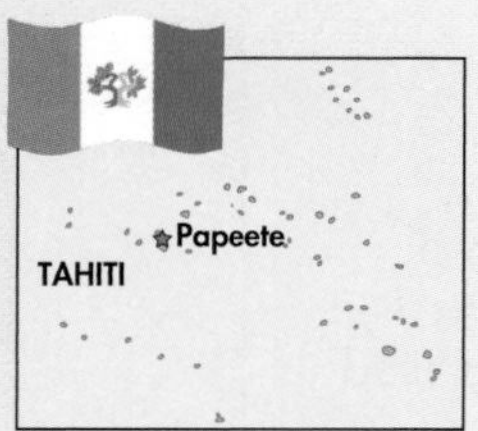

Un coup d'œil sur Papeete, en Polynésie française

La Polynésie, composée de 118 îles et atolls au cœur de l'océan Pacifique, devient une colonie de la France en 1880 et un «Territoire d'Outre-mer» en 1946, ce qui lui donne plus d'indépendance. En 2004, elle devient encore plus autonome. Elle est maintenant un «Pays d'Outre-mer au sein de[1] la République» et se gouverne librement et démocratiquement.

Papeete est la capitale de Tahiti, la plus grande île de la Polynésie. C'est aussi le centre économique de l'île. Malgré d'importants problèmes de pollution, Papeete est une ville agréable à vivre. Le marché de Papeete est un endroit animé et authentique: on peut y trouver de la nourriture, des fleurs, de l'artisanat,[2] des tissus,[3] et même des tatoueurs[4] qui exercent leur art dans des petits studios. Les grandes festivités du *Heiva i Tahiti* (Jeux de Tahiti) ont lieu en juillet. Les compétitions sportives, les chants, les danses polynésiennes et la foire[5] artisanale attirent[6] un grand nombre d'habitants des différentes îles de la Polynésie française. Un événement annuel à ne pas manquer!

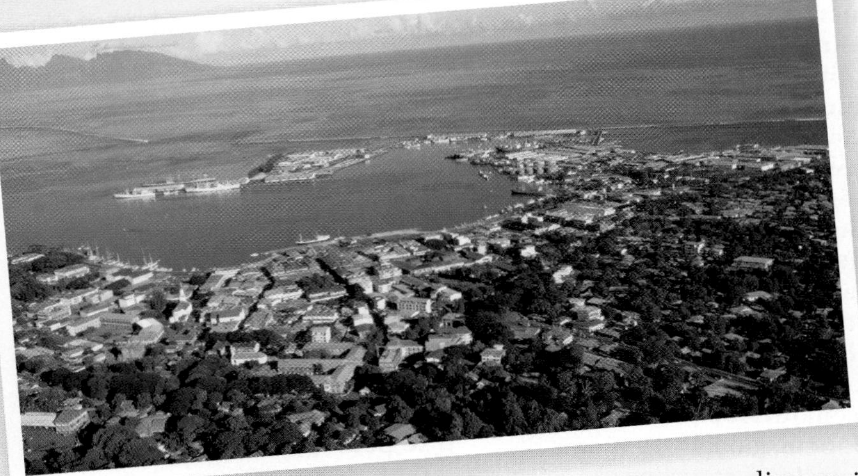

La ville de Papeete

[1]au... *within* [2]*crafts* [3]*fabrics* [4]*tattooers* [5]*fair* [6]*attract*

PORTRAIT Pouvanaa a Oopa (1895–1977)

Né en 1895 en Polynésie, Pouvanaa a Oopa participe à la Première Guerre mondiale aux côtés de la France et joue un rôle important dans le ralliement[1] de la Polynésie à la France libre en 1940. Mais il accuse vite l'Administration française de ne pas respecter les droits des Polynésiens. Il consacre alors le reste de sa vie à lutter en faveur de l'autonomie du territoire polynésien.

Élu député en 1949, il encourage le «Non» lors du[2] référendum de 1958 sur l'attachement de la Polynésie à la France, mais la population vote «Oui». Peu après, il est accusé d'avoir ordonné un incendie[3] à Papeete. Rien n'est prouvé, mais il est condamné à l'exil jusqu'en 1968. Il devient sénateur en 1971 et continue à proclamer son innocence pour les faits de 1958. Pouvanaa meurt avant que la France n'accorde[4] le statut d'autonomie de gestion[5] à la Polynésie française le 12 juillet 1977. Considéré comme le «Metua», ou «Père» des Polynésiens, il reste aujourd'hui encore un symbole du nationalisme polynésien.

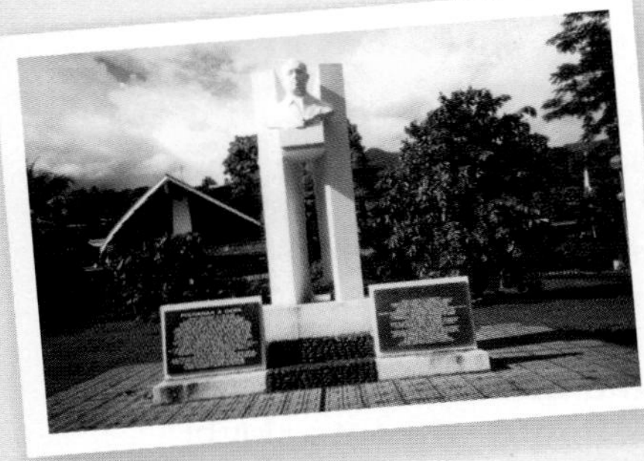

Une statue de Pouvanaa a Oopa à Papeete

[1]*uniting* [2]lors... *at the time of the* [3]*fire* [4]avant... *before France granted* [5]autonomie... *self-government*

dans les îles francophones

Un coup d'œil sur Fort-de-France, à la Martinique

LA MARTINIQUE
Fort-de-France

Tournée vers[1] la mer des Caraïbes, Fort-de-France est la capitale de «l'île aux Fleurs» découverte par Christophe Colomb en 1502. C'est un port où font escale[2] les bateaux de croisière[3] venus d'Amérique et d'Europe. La Martinique est un département français depuis 1946. Le souffle bienfaisant[4] des vents alizés[5] vous accueille pour une visite du centre-ville, avec le marché aux poissons près du canal Levassor, la bibliothèque Schœlcher (du nom de l'abolitionniste du XIXe siècle) dans la rue de la Liberté et la Cathédrale Saint-Louis dans la rue Schœlcher. Ces deux bâtiments sont construits en fer et en acier,[6] comme la tour Eiffel à Paris!

Ici le créole est la langue maternelle et tout le monde apprend le français à l'école, même les Békés. Les Békés, qui sont les descendants blancs des premiers colons français, contrôlent à peu près toute l'économie de l'île. Ils possèdent plus de 50 % des richesses de l'île et sont les propriétaires des plantations de canne à sucre, qu'on appelle des «habitations». Mais la vraie richesse de la Martinique vient de sa culture ainsi que[7] de ses femmes et de ses hommes qui forment une société solidaire.

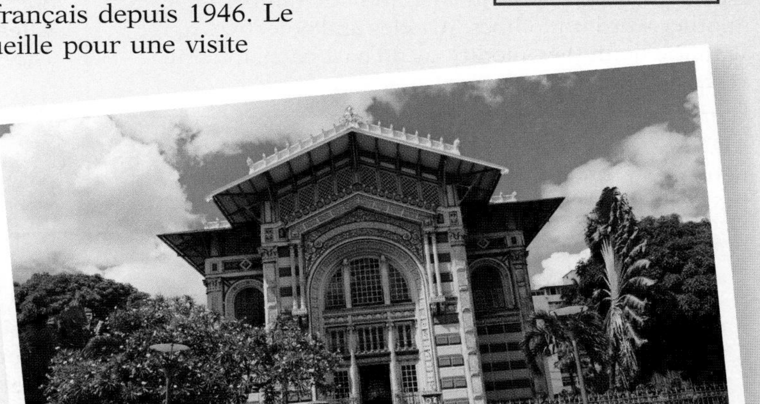

La bibliothèque Schœlcher à Fort-de-France

[1]Tournée… *Facing* [2]font… *stop over* [3]bateaux… *cruise ships* [4]souffle… *refreshing breath* [5]vents… *trade winds* [6]*steel* [7]ainsi… *as well as*

PORTRAIT Aimé Césaire (1913–2008)

Poète et homme politique (Maire de Fort-de-France pendant cinquante ans), il personnifie la théorie de la «négritude».* La littérature mondiale lui doit des œuvres majeures comme *Cahier d'un retour au pays natal,* écrit après sa rencontre avec Léopold Sédar Senghor,† et *La Tragédie du roi Christophe,* sur les difficultés de la libération psychologique des anciens esclaves devenus maîtres[1] d'Haïti.

[1]*masters*

Note: See the Instructor's Manual for follow-up questions about this *Bienvenue* section.

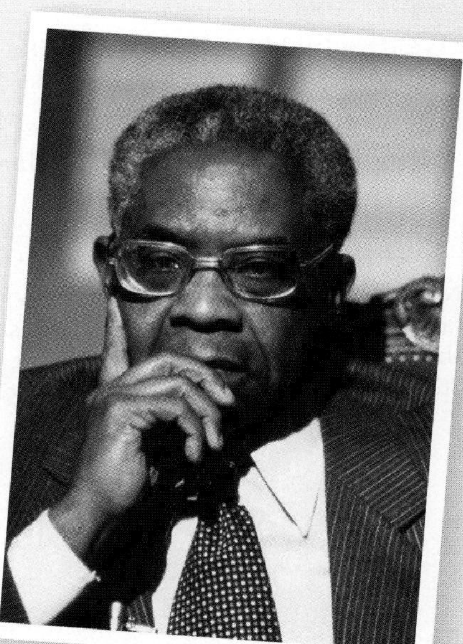

Aimé Césaire

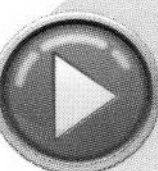

Watch the *Bienvenue dans les îles francophones* video segments to learn more about Fort-de-France and Papeete.

*_Négritude_ was the movement to restore the cultural identity of Africans around the world by rejecting European values and affirming the history and personality of African peoples.

†Léopold Senghor (1906–2001): poet and founding president of Senegal who was an early leader of the Black consciousness movement and who coined the term *négritude.*

Appendix A

Glossary of Grammatical Terms

ACCORD (*m.*) (*AGREEMENT*) There is agreement when a word takes the gender and the number of another word it modifies. Articles and adjectives agree with the noun they modify, as do past participles of verbs conjugated with **être**.	C'est **une femme indépendante.** *She is an independent woman.* **Elles sont arrivées** à temps. *They arrived in time.*
ADJECTIF (*m.*) (*ADJECTIVE*) A word that describes a noun or a pronoun. It agrees in number and gender with the word it modifies.	
Adjectif démonstratif (*Demonstrative adjective*) An adjective that points out a particular noun.	**ce** garçon, **ces** livres ***this*** boy, ***these*** books
Adjectif interrogatif (*Interrogative adjective*) An adjective used to form questions.	**Quelles** affiches cherchez-vous? ***What*** *posters are you looking for?* **Quel** livre? ***Which*** *book?*
Adjectif possessif (*Possessive adjective*) An adjective that indicates possession or a special relationship.	**leur** voiture, **ma** sœur ***their*** *car,* ***my*** *sister*
Adjectif qualificatif (*Descriptive adjective*) An adjective that specifies size, color, or other qualities.	Elles sont **intelligentes**. *They are* ***smart***. C'est une **grande** maison. *It's a* ***big*** *house.*
ADVERBE (*m.*) (*ADVERB*) A word that describes an adjective, a verb, or another adverb.	Il écrit **très bien**. Elle est **plus** efficace. *He writes* ***very well***. *She is* ***more*** *efficient.*
Adverbe interrogatif (*Interrogative adverb*) An adverb that introduces a question about time, place, manner, or quantity (amount).	**Combien** ça coûte? ***How much*** *is it?* **Quand** est-ce que vous partez? ***When*** *are you leaving?*
ANTÉCÉDENT (*m.*) A word, usually a noun, that is replaced by a pronoun in the same or a subsequent sentence. In the example, **Manon** is the antecedent of **elle,** and **un gant** is the antecedent of **le**.	**Manon** a perdu **un gant** et **elle** ne **le** retrouve plus. *Manon lost a glove, and she can't find it anymore.*

ARTICLE (*m.*) A determiner that sets off a noun.	
Article défini (*Definite article*) An article that indicates a specific noun.	**le** pays, **la** chaise, **les** femmes ***the*** *country,* ***the*** *chair,* ***the*** *women*
Article indéfini (*Indefinite article*) An article that indicates an unspecified noun.	**un** garçon, **une** ville, **des** carottes ***a*** *boy,* ***a*** *city,* ***some*** *carrots*
Article partitif (*Partitive article*) In French, an article that denotes part of a whole. *Some* is not always expressed in English, but the partitive is almost always expressed in French.	**du** chocolat, **de la** tarte, **de l'**eau (***some***) *chocolat,* (***some***) *pie,* (***some***) *water*
COMPARATIF (*m.*) (*COMPARATIVE*) The form of adjectives and adverbs used to compare two nouns or actions.	Léa est **moins** bavarde **que** Julien. *Léa is* ***less*** *talkative* ***than*** *Julien.* Elle court **plus** vite **que** lui. *She runs* ***faster than*** *he does.*
CONDITIONNEL (*m.*) (*CONDITIONAL*)	*See* **Mode**.
CONJUGAISON (*f.*) (*CONJUGATION*) The different forms of a verb for a particular tense or mood. A present indicative conjugation:	je parle — *I speak* tu parles — *you speak* il/elle/on parle — *he/she/it/one speaks* nous parlons — *we speak* vous parlez — *you speak* ils/elles parlent — *they speak*
CONJONCTION (*f.*) (*CONJUNCTION*) An expression that connects words, phrases, or clauses.	Christophe **et** Diane *Christophe* ***and*** *Diane* Il fait froid, **mais** il fait beau. *It's cold,* ***but*** *nice.*
CONTRACTION (*f.*) (*CONTRACTION*) Two words combine to form one. In French, this phenomenon happens with **à** and **de** combined with the definite articles **le** or **les**.	Ils parlent **aux** étudiants. *He's talking to the students.* C'est le livre **du** professeur. *It's the teacher's book.*
ÉLISION (*f.*) (*ELISION*) The replacement of the final vowel of a word by an apostrophe before the initial vowel or vowel sound of the following word.	Il arrive à **l'**université à 8 h. *He arrives at the university at 8:00.* J'ai compris **qu'**il reviendrait. *I understood that he would come back.*
GENRE (*m.*) (*GENDER*) A grammatical category of words. In French, there are two genders: feminine and masculine. Gender applies to nouns, articles, adjectives, and pronouns.	(masc. / fem.) articles and nouns — **le** film / **la** vidéo adjectives — **lent, beau** / **lente, belle** pronouns — **il, celui** / **elle, celle**

IMPARFAIT (*m.*) (*IMPERFECT*) In French, a verb tense that expresses a past action with no specific beginning or end.	Nous **nagions** souvent. *We* ***used to swim*** *often.*
IMPÉRATIF (*m.*) (*IMPERATIVE*)	*See* **Mode**.
INDICATIF (*m.*) (*INDICATIVE*)	*See* **Mode**.
INFINITIF (*m.*) (*INFINITIVE*)	*See* **Mode**.
LIAISON (*f.*) (*LIAISON*) A speech-sound redistribution in which an otherwise silent final consonant is articulated with the initial vowel or vowel sound of the following word.	C'est‿un‿animal. [sɛtœ̃nanimal] aux‿États‿Unis [ozetazyni]
MODE (*m.*) (*MOOD*) A set of categories for verbs indicating the attitude of the speaker toward what he or she is saying.	
Mode conditionnel (*Conditional mood*) A verb form conveying possibility.	J'**irais** si j'avais le temps. *I* ***would go*** *if I had time.*
Mode impératif (*Imperative mood*) A verb form expressing a command.	**Allez**-y! ***Go*** *ahead!*
Mode indicatif (*Indicative mood*) A verb form denoting actions or states considered facts.	Je **vais** à la bibliothèque. *I* ***am going*** *to the library.*
Mode infinitif (*Infinitive mood*) A verb form introduced in English by *to*. In French dictionaries, this form appears as the main entry.	**jouer, vendre, venir** ***to play, to sell, to come***
Mode subjonctif (*Subjunctive mood*) A verb form, uncommon in English, used primarily in subordinate clauses after expressions of desire, doubt, or emotion. French constructions with the subjunctive have many possible English equivalents.	Je veux que vous y **alliez**. *I want you to go there.* J'ai peur qu'elle **dise** non. *I'm afraid she will say no.*
MOT APPARENTÉ (*m.*) (*COGNATE*) In two languages, words spelled similarly with similar meaning.	**état, ordre, sérieux** ***state, order, serious***
NOM (*m.*) (*NOUN*) A word that denotes a person, place, thing, or idea. Proper nouns are capitalized names.	**avocat, journal, ville, Louise** ***lawyer, newspaper, city, Louise***
NOMBRE (*m.*) (*NUMBER*) A grammatical category of words. It indicates whether a noun, article, adjective, or pronoun is singular (**singulier**) or plural (**pluriel**).	singular: Le fromage est bon. plural: Les fromages sont bons.
Nombre cardinal (*Cardinal number*) A number that expresses an amount.	**deux** bureaux, **quatre** ans ***two*** *desks,* ***four*** *years*
Nombre ordinal (*Ordinal number*) A number that indicates position in a series.	le **deuxième** bureau, la **quatrième** année *the* ***second*** *desk, the* ***fourth*** *year*

<table>
<tr><td>PARTICIPE PASSÉ (m.) (PAST PARTICIPLE) The form of a verb used in a compound tense (such as the passé composé) with forms of to have in English, and with avoir and être in French.</td><td>mangé, fini, perdu
eaten, finished, lost</td></tr>
<tr><td>PASSÉ COMPOSÉ (m.) In French, a verb tense that expresses a past action with a definite ending. It consists of the present indicative of the auxiliary verb (avoir or être) and the past participle of the conjugated verb. There are several equivalent forms in English.</td><td>J'ai mangé
I ate, I did eat, I have eaten
Elle est tombée
She fell, she did fall, she has fallen</td></tr>
<tr><td>PERSONNE (f.) (PERSON) The form of a pronoun or a verb that indicates the person involved in an action.</td><td><table><tr><td></td><td>singular</td><td>plural</td></tr><tr><td>1st pers.</td><td>je / I</td><td>nous / we</td></tr><tr><td>2nd pers.</td><td>tu / you</td><td>vous / you</td></tr><tr><td>3rd pers.</td><td>il, elle, on / he, she, one, it</td><td>ils, elles / they</td></tr></table></td></tr>
<tr><td>PRÉPOSITION (f.) (PREPOSITION) A word or phrase that specifies the relationship of a word (usually a noun or a pronoun) to another. The relationship is usually spatial or temporal.</td><td>près de l'aéroport, avec lui, avant 11 h
near the airport, with him, before 11:00</td></tr>
<tr><td>PRONOM (m.) (PRONOUN) A word used in place of one or more nouns.</td><td></td></tr>
<tr><td>Pronom accentué ou disjoint (Stressed or disjunctive pronoun) In French, a pronoun used for emphasis or as the object of a preposition.</td><td>Toi, tu es incroyable!
You are unbelievable!
Je travaille avec lui.
I work with him.</td></tr>
<tr><td>Pronom complément (d'objet) (Object pronoun) A pronoun that replaces a direct object noun or an indirect object noun.</td><td>direct: Je vois Alain. Je le vois.
I see Alain. I see him.
indirect: Je donne le livre à Daniel. Je lui donne le livre.
I give the book to Daniel. I give him the book.</td></tr>
<tr><td>Pronom démonstratif (Demonstrative pronoun) A pronoun that singles out a particular person or thing.</td><td>Voici deux livres: celui-ci est intéressant, mais celui-là est ennuyeux.
Here are two books: this one is interesting, but that one is boring.</td></tr>
<tr><td>Pronom interrogatif (Interrogative pronoun) A pronoun used to ask a question.</td><td>Qui parle? Qu'est-ce que vous voulez?
Who is speaking? What do you want?</td></tr>
<tr><td>Pronom réfléchi (Reflexive pronoun) A pronoun that represents the same person as the subject of the verb.</td><td>Je me regarde dans le miroir.
I am looking at myself in the mirror.</td></tr>
<tr><td>Pronom relatif (Relative pronoun) A pronoun that introduces an independent clause and denotes a noun already mentioned.</td><td>On parle à la femme qui habite ici.
We're talking to the woman who lives here.
C'est le stylo que vous cherchez?
Is it the pen (that) you're looking for?</td></tr>
<tr><td>Pronom sujet (Subject pronoun) A pronoun representing the person or thing performing the action of the verb.</td><td>Ils travaillent bien ensemble.
They work well together.</td></tr>
</table>

PROPOSITION (*f.*) (*CLAUSE*) A construction that contains a subject and a verb.	
Proposition principale (*Main clause*) A clause that stands on its own and expresses a complete idea.	**Je cherche la femme** qui joue au tennis. ***I'm looking for the woman*** *who plays tennis.*
Proposition subordonnée (*Subordinate clause*) A clause that cannot stand on its own because it does not express a complete idea.	Je cherche la femme **qui joue au tennis**. *I'm looking for the woman* ***who plays tennis***.
SUJET (*m.*) (*SUBJECT*) The word(s) denoting the person, place, or thing performing an action or existing in a state.	**Mon ordinateur** est là-bas. ***My computer*** *is over there.* **Marc** arrive demain. ***Marc*** *arrives tomorrow.*
SUBJONCTIF (*m.*) (*SUBJUNCTIVE*)	*See* **Mode**.
SUPERLATIF (*m.*) (*SUPERLATIVE*) The form of adjectives or adverbs used to compare three or more nouns or actions. In English, the superlative is expressed by using *most* or *-est*.	Elle a choisi la robe **la plus** chère. *She chose* ***the most*** *expensive dress.* Béatrice court **le plus** vite. *Béatrice runs the fast****est***.
TEMPS (*m.*) (*TENSE*) The form of a verb indicating time: present, past, or future.	
VERBE (*m.*) (*VERB*) A word that reports an action or state.	Elle **est arrivée** hier. *She* ***arrived*** *yesterday.* Elle **était** fatiguée. *She* ***was*** *tired.*
Verbe auxiliaire (*Auxiliary verb*) A verb used in conjunction with an infinitive or a participle to convey distinctions of tense and mood. In French, the main auxiliaries are **avoir** and **être**.	J'**ai** fait mes devoirs. *I did my homework.* Nous **sommes** allés au cinéma. *We went to the movies.*
Verbe impersonnel (*Impersonal verb*) Always accompanied by the impersonal pronoun **il,** impersonal verbs are divided into two categories: verbs reporting natural phenomena and verbs with special meaning.	**Il fait** beau aujourd'hui. ***It is*** *nice today.* **Il faut** travailler fort. ***One has*** *to work hard.*
Verbe pronominal (*Pronominal verb*) In French, a verb with a reflexive pronoun as well as a subject pronoun in its conjugated form. Its infinitive is preceded by **se**.	**se souvenir, je me souviens** *to remember, I remember* **Il se coupe** quand **il se rase**. *He* ***cuts himself*** *when he shaves* (***himself***).

Verb Charts

More complete verb charts that include the conjugations of the pluperfect and the past conditional are available at **Connect French (www.mhconnectfrench.com).** The formation of these tenses and other perfect tenses are explained in **Appendix C.**

Verbes réguliers

INFINITIF ET PARTICIPE PRÉSENT	PRÉSENT	PASSÉ COMPOSÉ	IMPARFAIT	FUTUR	CONDITIONNEL	SUBJONCTIF	IMPÉRATIF
1. **chercher**	je cherche	j'ai cherché	je cherchais	je chercherai	je chercherais	que je cherche	cherche
cherchant	tu cherches	tu as cherché	tu cherchais	tu chercheras	tu chercherais	que tu cherches	cherchons
	il/elle/on cherche	il/elle/on a cherché	il/elle/on cherchait	il/elle/on cherchera	il/elle/on chercherait	qu'il/elle/on cherche	cherchez
	nous cherchons	nous avons cherché	nous cherchions	nous chercherons	nous chercherions	que nous cherchions	
	vous cherchez	vous avez cherché	vous cherchiez	vous chercherez	vous chercheriez	que vous cherchiez	
	ils/elles cherchent	ils/elles ont cherché	ils/elles cherchaient	ils/elles chercheront	ils/elles chercheraient	qu'ils/elles cherchent	
2. **répondre**	je réponds	j'ai répondu	je répondais	je répondrai	je répondrais	que je réponde	réponds
répondant	tu réponds	tu as répondu	tu répondais	tu répondras	tu répondrais	que tu répondes	répondons
	il/elle/on répond	il/elle/on a répondu	il/elle/on répondait	il/elle/on répondra	il/elle/on répondrait	qu'il/elle/on réponde	répondez
	nous répondons	nous avons répondu	nous répondions	nous répondrons	nous répondrions	que nous répondions	
	vous répondez	vous avez répondu	vous répondiez	vous répondrez	vous répondriez	que vous répondiez	
	ils/elles répondent	ils/elles ont répondu	ils/elles répondaient	ils/elles répondront	ils/elles répondraient	qu'ils/elles répondent	
3. **finir**	je finis	j'ai fini	je finissais	je finirai	je finirais	que je finisse	finis
finissant	tu finis	tu as fini	tu finissais	tu finiras	tu finirais	que tu finisses	finissons
	il/elle/on finit	il/elle/on a fini	il/elle/on finissait	il/elle/on finira	il/elle/on finirait	qu'il/elle/on finisse	finissez
	nous finissons	nous avons fini	nous finissions	nous finirons	nous finirions	que nous finissions	
	vous finissez	vous avez fini	vous finissiez	vous finirez	vous finiriez	que vous finissiez	
	ils/elles finissent	ils/elles ont fini	ils/elles finissaient	ils/elles finiront	ils/elles finiraient	qu'ils/elles finissent	
4. **dormir***	je dors	j'ai dormi	je dormais	je dormirai	je dormirais	que je dorme	dors
dormant	tu dors	tu as dormi	tu dormais	tu dormiras	tu dormirais	que tu dormes	dormons
	il/elle/on dort	il/elle/on a dormi	il/elle/on dormait	il/elle/on dormira	il/elle/on dormirait	qu'il/elle/on dorme	dormez
	nous dormons	nous avons dormi	nous dormions	nous dormirons	nous dormirions	que nous dormions	
	vous dormez	vous avez dormi	vous dormiez	vous dormirez	vous dormiriez	que vous dormiez	
	ils/elles dorment	ils/elles ont dormi	ils/elles dormaient	ils/elles dormiront	ils/elles dormiraient	qu'ils/elles dorment	
5. **se laver**†	je me lave	je me suis lavé(e)	je me lavais	je me laverai	je me laverais	que je me lave	lave-toi
(se) lavant	tu te laves	tu t'es lavé(e)	tu te lavais	tu te laveras	tu te laverais	que tu te laves	lavons-nous
	il/elle/on se lave	il/elle/on s'est lavé(e)	il/elle/on se lavait	il/elle/on se lavera	il/elle/on se laverait	qu' il/elle/on se lave	lavez-vous
	nous nous lavons	nous nous sommes lavé(e)s	nous nous lavions	nous nous laverons	nous nous laverions	que nous nous lavions	
	vous vous lavez	vous vous êtes lavé(e)(s)	vous vous laviez	vous vous laverez	vous vous laveriez	que vous vous laviez	
	ils/elles se lavent	ils/elles se sont lavé(e)s	ils/elles se lavaient	ils/elles se laveront	ils/elles se laveraient	qu' ils/elles se lavent	

*Traditionally, only verbs ending in **-ir** like **finir** are considered one of the three regular verb groups. However, verbs like **dormir** also end in **-ir** and are conjugated following their own "regular" pattern, though they are many fewer in number than **-ir** verbs like **finir.** Verbs from this group include: **s'endormir, mentir, partir, sentir,** and **sortir.** Note that **s'endormir, partir,** and **sortir** are conjugated with **être** in the compound tenses.

†All pronominal verbs are conjugated with **être** in the compound tenses.

Verbes réguliers avec changements orthographiques

INFINITIF ET PARTICIPE PRÉSENT	PRÉSENT	PASSÉ COMPOSÉ	IMPARFAIT	FUTUR	CONDITIONNEL	SUBJONCTIF	IMPÉRATIF	AUTRES VERBES
1. **commencer** commençant	je commence tu commences il/elle/on commence nous commençons vous commencez ils/elles commencent	j'ai commencé	je commençais nous commencions	je commencerai	je commencerais	que je commence que nous commencions	commence commençons commencez	divorcer, lancer, remplacer
2. **manger** mangeant	je mange tu manges il/elle/on mange nous mangeons vous mangez ils/elles mangent	j'ai mangé	je mangeais nous mangions	je mangerai	je mangerais	que je mange que nous mangions	mange mangeons mangez	changer, encourager, engager, exiger, mélanger, nager, partager, voyager
3. **préférer** préférant	je préfère tu préfères il/elle/on préfère nous préférons vous préférez ils/elles préfèrent	j'ai préféré	je préférais	je préférerai	je préférerais	que je préfère que nous préférions	préfère préférons préférez	espérer, répéter, s'inquiéter, sécher
4. **payer** payant	je paie tu paies il/elle/on paie nous payons vous payez ils/elles paient	j'ai payé	je payais	je paierai	je paierais	que je paie que nous payions	paie payons payez	employer, envoyer, essayer
5. **appeler** appelant	j' appelle tu appelles il/elle/on appelle nous appelons vous appelez ils/elles appellent	j'ai appelé	j'appelais	j'appellerai	j'appellerais	que j'appelle que nous appelions	appelle appelons appelez	s'appeler, se rappeler
6. **acheter** achetant	j' achète tu achètes il/elle/on achète nous achetons vous achetez ils/elles achètent	j'ai acheté	j'achetais	j'achèterai	j'achèterais	que j'achète que nous achetions	achète achetons achetez	se lever, se promener

Verbes irréguliers

INFINITIF ET PARTICIPE PRÉSENT	PRÉSENT	PASSÉ COMPOSÉ	IMPARFAIT	FUTUR	CONDITIONNEL	SUBJONCTIF	IMPÉRATIF	AUTRES VERBES
1. **aller*** allant	je vais tu vas il/elle/on va nous allons vous allez ils/elles vont	je suis allé(e)	j'allais	j'irai	j'irais	que j'aille que nous allions	va allons allez	
2. **avoir** ayant	j' ai tu as il/elle/on a nous avons vous avez ils/elles ont	j'ai eu	j'avais	j'aurai	j'aurais	que j'aie que nous ayons	aie ayons ayez	
3. **boire** buvant	je bois tu bois il/elle/on boit nous buvons vous buvez ils/elles boivent	j'ai bu	je buvais	je boirai	je boirais	que je boive que nous buvions	bois buvons buvez	
4. **conduire** conduisant	je conduis tu conduis il/elle/on conduit nous conduisons vous conduisez ils/elles conduisent	j'ai conduit	je conduisais	je conduirai	je conduirais	que je conduise que nous conduisions	conduis conduisons conduisez	construire, détruire, produire, réduire, traduire
5. **connaître** connaissant	je connais tu connais il/elle/on connaît nous connaissons vous connaissez ils/elles connaissent	j'ai connu	je connaissais	je connaîtrai	je connaîtrais	que je connaisse que nous connaissions	connais connaissons connaissez	apparaître, disparaître, paraître, reconnaître

*Verbs followed by an asterisk * are conjugated with **être** in the compound tenses.

Verbes irréguliers

INFINITIF ET PARTICIPE PRÉSENT	PRÉSENT		PASSÉ COMPOSÉ	IMPARFAIT	FUTUR	CONDITIONNEL	SUBJONCTIF	IMPÉRATIF	AUTRES VERBES
6. **croire** croyant	je crois tu crois il/elle/on croit	nous croyons vous croyez ils/elles croient	j'ai cru	je croyais	je croirai	je croirais	que je croie que nous croyions	crois croyons croyez	
7. **devoir** devant	je dois tu dois il/elle/on doit	nous devons vous devez ils/elles doivent	j'ai dû	je devais	je devrai	je devrais	que je doive que nous devions	dois devons devez	
8. **dire** disant	je dis tu dis il/elle/on dit	nous disons vous dites ils/elles disent	j'ai dit	je disais	je dirai	je dirais	que je dise que nous disions	dis disons dites	
9. **écrire** écrivant	j' écris tu écris il/elle/on écrit	nous écrivons vous écrivez ils/elles écrivent	j'ai écrit	j'écrivais	j'écrirai	j'écrirais	que j'écrive que nous écrivions	écris écrivons écrivez	décrire
10. **être** étant	je suis tu es il/elle/on est	nous sommes vous êtes ils/elles sont	j'ai été	j'étais	je serai	je serais	que je sois que nous soyons	sois soyons soyez	
11. **faire** faisant	je fais tu fais il/elle/on fait	nous faisons vous faites ils/elles font	j'ai fait	je faisais	je ferai	je ferais	que je fasse que nous fassions	fais faisons faites	
12. **falloir**	il faut		il a fallu	il fallait	il faudra	il faudrait	qu'il faille	—	
13. **lire** lisant	je lis tu lis il/elle/on lit	nous lisons vous lisez ils/elles lisent	j'ai lu	je lisais	je lirai	je lirais	que je lise que nous lisions	lis lisons lisez	
14. **mettre** mettant	je mets tu mets il/elle/on met	nous mettons vous mettez ils/elles mettent	j'ai mis	je mettais	je mettrai	je mettrais	que je mette que nous mettions	mets mettons mettez	permettre, promettre
15. **mourir*** mourant	je meurs tu meurs il/elle/on meurt	nous mourons vous mourez ils/elles meurent	je suis mort(e)	je mourais	je mourrai	je mourrais	que je meure que nous mourions	meurs mourons mourez	

*Verbs followed by an asterisk * are conjugated with **être** in the compound tenses.

Verbes irréguliers (*suite*)

INFINITIF ET PARTICIPE PRÉSENT	PRÉSENT		PASSÉ COMPOSÉ	IMPARFAIT	FUTUR	CONDITIONNEL	SUBJONCTIF	IMPÉRATIF	AUTRES VERBES
16. **naître*** naissant	je nais tu nais il/elle/on naît	nous naissons vous naissez ils/elles naissent	je suis né(e)	je naissais	je naîtrai	je naîtrais	que je naisse que nous naissions	nais naissons naissez	
17. **ouvrir** ouvrant	j' ouvre tu ouvres il/elle/on ouvre	nous ouvrons vous ouvrez ils/elles ouvrent	j'ai ouvert	j'ouvrais	j'ouvrirai	j'ouvrirais	que j'ouvre que nous ouvrions	ouvre ouvrons ouvrez	couvrir, découvrir, offrir, souffrir
18. **plaire** plaisant	je plais tu plais il/elle/on plaît	nous plaisons vous plaisez ils/elle plaisent	j'ai plu	je plaisais	je plairai	je plairais	que je plaise que nous plaisions	plais plaisons plaisez	
19. **pleuvoir** pleuvant	il pleut		il a plu	il pleuvait	il pleuvra	il pleuvrait	qu'il pleuve	—	
20. **pouvoir** pouvant	je peux[†] tu peux il/elle/on peut	nous pouvons vous pouvez ils/elles peuvent	j'ai pu	je pouvais	je pourrai	je pourrais	que je puisse que nous puissions	—	
21. **prendre** prenant	je prends tu prends il/elle/on prend	nous prenons vous prenez ils/elles prennent	j'ai pris	je prenais	je prendrai	je prendrais	que je prenne que nous prenions	prends prenons prenez	apprendre, comprendre
22. **recevoir** recevant	je reçois tu reçois il/elle/on reçoit	nous recevons vous recevez ils/elles reçoivent	j'ai reçu	je recevais	je recevrai	je recevrais	que je reçoive que nous recevions	reçois recevons recevez	
23. **savoir** sachant	je sais tu sais il/elle/on sait	nous savons vous savez ils/elles savent	j'ai su	je savais	je saurai	je saurais	que je sache que nous sachions	sache sachons sachez	
24. **suivre** suivant	je suis tu suis il/elle/on suit	nous suivons vous suivez ils/elles suivent	j'ai suivi	je suivais	je suivrai	je suivrais	que je suive que nous suivions	suis suivons suivez	poursuivre
25. **venir*** venant	je viens tu viens il/elle/on vient	nous venons vous venez ils/elles viennent	je suis venu(e)	je venais	je viendrai	je viendrais	que je vienne que nous venions	viens venons venez	appartenir, contenir, devenir,* obtenir, revenir,* tenir
26. **vivre** vivant	je vis tu vis il/elle/on vit	nous vivons vous vivez ils/elles vivent	j'ai vécu	je vivais	je vivrai	je vivrais	que je vive que nous vivions	vis vivons vivez	survivre
27. **voir** voyant	je vois tu vois il/elle/on voit	nous voyons vous voyez ils/elles voient	j'ai vu	je voyais	je verrai	je verrais	que je voie que nous voyions	vois voyons voyez	revoir
28. **vouloir** voulant	je veux tu veux il/elle/on veut	nous voulons vous voulez ils/elles veulent	j'ai voulu	je voulais	je voudrai	je voudrais	que je veuille que nous voulions	veuille veuillons veuillez	

*Verbs followed by an asterisk * are conjugated with **être** in the compound tenses.
[†]If **je peux** is inverted to form a question, it becomes **puis-je... ?**

Appendix C

Perfect Tenses

In addition to the **passé composé,** French has several other perfect verb tenses (conjugated forms of **avoir** or **être** + the past participle of a verb). Following are the most common perfect tenses.

Le plus-que-parfait (*The Pluperfect*)
The pluperfect tense (also called the past perfect) is formed with the imperfect of the auxiliary verb (**avoir** or **être**) + the past participle of the main verb.

parler		sortir		se réveiller	
j'	avais parlé	j'	étais sorti(e)	je	m'étais réveillé(e)
tu	avais parlé	tu	étais sorti(e)	tu	t'étais réveillé(e)
il/elle/on	avait parlé	il/elle/on	était sorti(e)	il/elle/on	s'était réveillé(e)
nous	avions parlé	nous	étions sorti(e)s	nous	nous étions réveillé(e)s
vous	aviez parlé	vous	étiez sorti(e)(s)	vous	vous étiez réveillé(e)(s)
ils/elles	avaient parlé	ils/elles	étaient sorti(e)s	ils/elles	s'étaient réveillé(e)s

The pluperfect is used to indicate an action or event that occurred before another past action or event, either stated or implied: *I had already left for the country* (*when my friends arrived in Paris*).

Quand j'ai téléphoné aux Dupont, ils **avaient** déjà **décidé** d'acheter la ferme.	*When I phoned the Duponts, they had already decided to buy the farm.*
Marie **s'était réveillée** avant moi. Elle **était** déjà **sortie** à sept heures.	*Marie had awakened before me. She had already left by seven o'clock.*

Le futur antérieur (*The Future Perfect*)
The future perfect is formed with the future of the auxiliary verb (**avoir** or **être**) + the past participle of the main verb.

parler		sortir		se réveiller	
j'	aurai parlé	je	serai sorti(e)	je	me serai réveillé(e)
tu	auras parlé	tu	seras sorti(e)	tu	te seras réveillé(e)
il/elle/on	aura parlé	il/elle/on	sera sorti(e)	il/elle/on	se sera réveillé(e)
nous	aurons parlé	nous	serons sorti(e)s	nous	nous serons réveillé(e)s
vous	aurez parlé	vous	serez sorti(e)(s)	vous	vous serez réveillé(e)(s)
ils/elles	auront parlé	ils/elles	seront sorti(e)s	ils/elles	se seront réveillé(e)s

The future perfect is used to express a future action that will already have taken place when another future action occurs. The subsequent action is always expressed by the simple future.

Je publierai mes résultats quand j'**aurai terminé** cette expérience.	*I'll publish the results when I finish this experiment.*
Aussitôt que mes collègues **seront revenus,** ils liront mon rapport.	*As soon as my colleagues return, they'll read my report.*

Le conditionnel passé (*The Past Conditional*)

A. Formation of the Past Conditional

The past conditional (or conditional perfect) is formed with the conditional of the auxiliary verb (**avoir** or **être**) + the past participle of the main verb.

	parler		**sortir**		**se réveiller**
j'	aurais parlé	je	serais sorti(e)	je	me serais réveillé(e)
tu	aurais parlé	tu	serais sorti(e)	tu	te serais réveillé(e)
il/elle/on	aurait parlé	il/elle/on	serait sorti(e)	il/elle/on	se serait réveillé(e)
nous	aurions parlé	nous	serions sorti(e)s	nous	nous serions réveillé(e)s
vous	auriez parlé	vous	seriez sorti(e)(s)	vous	vous seriez réveillé(e)(s)
ils/elles	auraient parlé	ils/elles	seraient sorti(e)s	ils/elles	se seraient réveillé(e)s

The past conditional is used to express an action or event that would have occurred if some set of conditions (stated or implied) had been present: *We would have worried* (*if we had known*).

B. Uses of the Past Conditional

The past conditional is used in the main clause of an *if*-clause sentence when the verb of the *if*-clause is in the pluperfect.

Si j'**avais eu** le temps, j'**aurais visité** Nîmes.	*If I had had the time, I would have visited Nîmes.*
Si les Normands n'**avaient** pas **conquis** l'Angleterre en 1066, l'anglais **aurait été** une langue très différente.	*If the Normans had not conquered England in 1066, English would have been a very different language.*

The underlying set of conditions (the *if*-clause) is sometimes not stated.

À ta place, j'**aurais parlé** au guide.	*If I were you, I would have spoken to the guide.*
Nous **serions allés** au lac.	*We would have gone to the lake.*

C. The Past Conditional of *devoir*

The past conditional of **devoir** means *should have* or *ought to have.* It expresses regret about something that did not take place in the past.

J'**aurais dû prendre** l'autre chemin.	*I should have taken the other road.*
Nous **aurions dû acheter** un plan.	*We should have bought a map.*

Le subjonctif passé (*The Past Subjunctive*)

The past subjunctive is formed with the present subjunctive of the auxiliary verb (**avoir** or **être**) + the past participle of the main verb.

PAST SUBJUNCTIVE OF **parler**		PAST SUBJUNCTIVE OF **venir**	
que j'	aie parlé	que je	sois venu(e)
que tu	aies parlé	que tu	sois venu(e)
qu'il/elle/on	ait parlé	qu'il/elle/on	soit venu(e)
que nous	ayons parlé	que nous	soyons venu(e)s
que vous	ayez parlé	que vous	soyez venu(e)(s)
qu'ils/elles	aient parlé	qu'ils/elles	soient venu(e)s

Je suis content que tu **aies parlé avec Léa**.	*I'm glad you spoke with Léa.*
Il est dommage qu'elle ne **soit** pas encore **venue**.	*It's too bad that she hasn't come yet.*

The past subjunctive is used following the same expressions as the present subjunctive except that it indicates that the action or situation described in the dependent clause occurred *before* the action or situation described in the main clause. Compare these sentences:

Je suis content que tu **viennes**.	*I'm happy that you are coming.*
Je suis content que tu **sois venu(e)**.	*I'm happy that you came.*
Je doute qu'ils le **comprennent**.	*I doubt that they understand it.*
Je doute qu'ils l'**aient compris**.	*I doubt that they have understood it.*

Appendix D

Le passé simple

1. The **passé simple** is a past tense often used in literary texts; it is not a conversational tense. Verbs that would be used in the **passé composé** in informal speech or writing are in the **passé simple** in formal writing. You may want to learn to recognize the forms of the **passé simple** for reading purposes. The **passé simple** of regular **-er** verbs is formed by adding the endings **-ai, -as, -a, -âmes, -âtes, -èrent** to the verb stem. The endings for **-ir** and **-re** verbs are: **-is, -is, -it, -îmes, -îtes, -irent**. The endings for **-oir** verbs are: **-us, -us, -ut, -ûmes, -ûtes, -urent**.

parler		**finir**		**perdre**		**vouloir**	
je	parlai	je	finis	je	perdis	je	voulus
tu	parlas	tu	finis	tu	perdis	tu	voulus
il/elle/on	parla	il/elle/on	finit	il/elle/on	perdit	il/elle/on	voulut
nous	parlâmes	nous	finîmes	nous	perdîmes	nous	voulûmes
vous	parlâtes	vous	finîtes	vous	perdîtes	vous	voulûtes
ils/elles	parlèrent	ils/elles	finirent	ils/elles	perdirent	ils/elles	voulurent

2. Here are the third-person forms (**il, elle, on; ils, elles**) of some verbs that are irregular in the **passé simple.**

INFINITIVE	PASSÉ SIMPLE
avoir	il eut, ils eurent
dire	il dit, ils dirent
être	il fut, ils furent
faire	il fit, ils firent

Appendix E

Les pronoms

Les pronoms démonstratifs (*Demonstrative Pronouns*)
Demonstrative pronouns such as *this one* and *that one* refer to a person, thing, or idea that has been mentioned previously. In French, they agree in gender and number with the nouns they replace.

	SINGULAR		PLURAL	
Masculine	**celui**	*this one, that one, the one*	**ceux**	*these, those, the ones*
Feminine	**celle**	*this one, that one, the one*	**celles**	*these, those, the ones*

French demonstrative pronouns cannot stand alone. They must be:

1. used with the suffix **-ci** (to indicate someone or something located close to the speaker) or **-là** (for someone or something more distant from the speaker)

    Voici deux affiches. Préférez-vous **celle-ci** ou **celle-là**? — *Here are two posters. Do you prefer this one or that one?*

2. followed by a prepositional phrase (often a construction with **de**)

    Quelle époque t'intéresse, **celle** du Moyen Âge ou **celle** de la Renaissance? — *Which period interests you, that of the Middle Ages or that of the Renaissance?*

3. followed by a dependent clause introduced by a relative pronoun

    On trouve des villages anciens dans plusieurs parcs: **ceux** qui sont dans le Parc de la Brière sont en ruine; **ceux** qui sont dans les parcs de la Lorraine et du Morvan ont été restaurés. — *One finds very old villages in several parks: Those that are in Brière Park are in ruins; those that are in the Lorraine and Morvan parks have been restored.*

Indefinite Demonstrative Pronouns

Ceci (*this*), **cela** (*that*), and **ça** (*that,* informal) are indefinite demonstrative pronouns; they refer to an idea or thing with no definite antecedent. They do not show gender or number.

Cela (Ça) n'est pas important.	*That's not important.*
Regarde **ceci** de près.	*Look at this closely.*
Qu'est-ce que c'est que **ça**?	*What's that?*

Les pronoms relatifs (*Relative Pronouns*)

A. *Ce qui* and *ce que*

Ce qui and **ce que** are indefinite relative pronouns similar in meaning to **la chose qui (que)** or **les choses qui (que);** the first serves as the subject of a dependent clause, and the second as the object. They refer to an idea or a subject that is unspecified and has neither gender nor number, often expressed as *what.*

—Dites-moi **ce qui** est arrivé au touriste américain.	*Tell me what happened to the American tourist.*
—Je ne sais pas **ce qui** lui est arrivé.	*I don't know what happened to him.*
—Dites-moi **ce que** vous avez fait à Reims.	*Tell me what you did in Reims.*
—Je n'ai pas le temps de vous dire tout **ce qu'**on a fait.	*I don't have time to tell you everything we did.*

B. *Lequel*

Lequel (laquelle, lesquels, lesquelles) is the relative pronoun used as an object of a preposition to refer to things and people. **Lequel** and its forms contract with **à** and **de**.

Où est l'agence de voyages **devant laquelle** il attend?	*Where is the travel agency in front of which he's waiting?*
L'hôtel **auquel** j'écris est à la Guadeloupe.	*The hotel to which I am writing is in Guadeloupe.*
Je connais bien l'homme **près duquel** elle est assise.	*I know well the man next to whom she is sitting.*

Les pronoms possessifs (*Possessive Pronouns*)
Possessive pronouns replace nouns that are modified by a possessive adjective or other possessive construction. In English, the possessive pronouns are *mine, yours, his, hers, its, ours,* and *theirs.* In French, the appropriate definite article is always used with the possessive pronoun.

	SINGULAR		PLURAL	
	MASCULINE	FEMININE	MASCULINE	FEMININE
mine	le mien	la mienne	les miens	les miennes
yours	le tien	la tienne	les tiens	les tiennes
his/hers/its	le sien	la sienne	les siens	les siennes
ours	le nôtre	la nôtre	les nôtres	
yours	le vôtre	la vôtre	les vôtres	
theirs	le leur	la leur	les leurs	

POSSESSIVE CONSTRUCTION + NOUN		POSSESSIVE PRONOUN
Où sont **leurs bagages**?	→	**Les leurs** sont ici.
C'est **mon frère** là-bas.	→	Ah oui? C'est **le mien** à côté de lui.
La **voiture de Frédérique** est plus rapide que **ma voiture**.	→	Ah oui? **La sienne** est aussi plus rapide que **la mienne**.

Lexiques

Lexique français-anglais

This end vocabulary provides contextual meanings of French words used in this text. It does not include proper nouns (unless presented as active vocabulary or unless the French equivalent is quite different in spelling from English), most abbreviations, exact cognates, most near cognates, past participles used as adjectives if the infinitive is listed, or regular adverbs formed from adjectives listed. Adjectives are listed in the masculine singular form; feminine endings or forms are included when irregular. An asterisk (*) indicates words beginning with an aspirate *h*. Active vocabulary is indicated by the number of the chapter in which it is activated.

ABBREVIATIONS

A.	archaic	*indic.*	indicative (mood)	*p.p.*	past participle
ab.	abbreviation	*inf.*	infinitive	*prep.*	preposition
adj.	adjective	*interj.*	interjection	*pron.*	pronoun
adv.	adverb	*interr.*	interrogative	*Q.*	Quebec usage
art.	article	*inv.*	invariable	*s.*	singular
colloq.	colloquial	*irreg.*	irregular	*s.o.*	someone
conj.	conjunction	*m.*	masculine noun	*s.th.*	something
fam.	familiar or colloquial	*n.*	noun	*subj.*	subjunctive
f.	feminine noun	*neu.*	neuter	*tr. fam.*	very colloquial, slang
Gram.	grammatical term	*pl.*	plural	*v.*	verb

à *prep.* to; at; in (2); by, on (*bicycle, horseback, foot*) (9); **à bientôt** see you soon (1); **à côté de** beside (4); **à destination de** to, for (9); **à droite (de)** on the right (of) (4); **à gauche (de)** on the left (of) (4); **à l'est/l'ouest** to the east/west (9); **à l'étranger** abroad, in a foreign country (9); **à l'heure** on time (9); **à pied** on foot (9); **à son compte** for oneself (14); **au nord/sud** to the north/south (9); **au printemps** in spring (5); **au revoir** good-bye (1); **à vélo** by bike (9)

abandonné *adj.* abandoned

abats *m. pl.* giblets, offal

abbaye *f.* abbey

abîme *m.* abyss

abolir to abolish (16)

abominable *adj.* appalling

abondance *f.* abundance

abonnement *m.* subscription

abonner to subscribe

abord: d'abord *adv.* first, first of all, at first (11)

abordable *adj.* approachable; reasonable

aboutissement *m.* end, outcome

aboyer (il aboie) to bark (*dog*)

abréger (j'abrège, nous abrégeons) to cut short, shorten

abréviation *f.* abbreviation

abri *m.* shelter; **sans-abri** *m., f.* homeless person (16)

abriter to house

absolu *adj.* absolute

abstrait *adj.* abstract

abus *m.* abuse, misuse

académicien(ne) *m., f. member of the* **Académie française**

Académie française *f.* French Academy (*official body that rules on language questions*)

accéder (j'accède) to access

accent *m.* accent; **accent aigu (grave, circonflexe)** acute (grave, circumflex) accent

accentué: pronom accentué *Gram.* stressed or disjunctive pronoun

accepter (de) to accept (to) (12); to agree to

accès *m.* access; **fournisseur** (*m.*) **d'accès** (*Internet*) service provider (ISP)

accessoire *m.* accessory

acclamé *adj.* cheered

accompagner to accompany, go along (with)

accomplir to perform, accomplish, carry out

accord *m.* agreement; **d'accord** all right, O.K., agreed (2); **être d'accord** to agree, be in agreement

accorder to grant, bestow, confer

accourir to run, rush up

accro à *inv., fam.* addicted to **être un accro de** to be addicted to

accrocher to hang

accroître (*p.p.* **accru**) *irreg.* to increase, add to

accueil *m.* greeting, welcome; **page** (*f.*) **d'accueil** homepage; **terre** (*f.*) **(pays** [*m.*]**) d'accueil** country of settlement (*immigration*)

accueillir (*p.p.* **accueilli**) *irreg.* to greet, welcome

acculer to drive (*s.o.*) back

s'accumuler to accumulate

acéré *adj.* sharp

achat *m.* purchase; **pouvoir** (*m.*) **d'achat** purchasing power (16)

acheter (j'achète) to buy (8)

acheteur/euse *m., f.* buyer, purchaser

s'achever (il s'achève) to end; to come to an end

acier *m.* steel

acquérir (*like* **conquérir**) *irreg.* to acquire

acteur/trice *m., f.* actor, actress (12)

actif/ive *adj.* active; working

action *f.* action; gesture

activé *adj.* activated

activité *f.* activity; **activités de plein air** outdoor activities (15)

actualisé *adj.* updated

actualité *f.* piece of news; present-day event; current events (14)

actuel(le) *adj.* present, current

actuellement *adv.* currently, at the present time

adapter to adapt; **s'adapter à** to adapt oneself to

addition *f.* bill, check (*in a restaurant*) (7)

adepte *m., f.* enthusiast, follower

adieu *interj.* good-bye

adjectif *m., Gram.* adjective

admettre (*like* **mettre**) *irreg.* to admit, accept

administratif/ive *adj.* administrative; **assistant(e)** (*m., f.*) **administratif/ive** administrative assistant

administration *f.* administration; Civil Service

admirer to admire

adolescent(e) *m., f., adj.* adolescent, teenager

adopter to adopt
adorer to love, adore (2)
adresse *f.* address (10)
s'adresser (à) to be intended (for), aimed (at)
ADSL DSL
adulte *m., f., adj.* adult; **âge** (*m.*) **adulte** adulthood
adverbe *m., Gram.* adverb
adverse *adj.* opposing; opposite
aérobic *f.* aerobics; **faire de l'aérobic** to do aerobics (5)
aéroport *m.* airport (9)
affaire *f.* affair; business matter; *pl.* belongings; business; **chiffre** (*m.*) **d'affaires** turnover (*in business*); **classe** (*f.*) **affaires** business class (9); **homme (femme) d'affaires** *m., f.* businessman (-woman)
affectueux/euse *adj.* affectionate; fond
affiche *f.* poster; billboard (4)
afficher to post, put up; to display, show; **s'afficher** to be displayed
affirmatif/ive *adj.* affirmative
affirmation *f.* declaration
affirmer to affirm, state
affreux/euse *adj.* awful
afin de *prep.* to, in order to
africain *adj.* African; **Africain(e)** *m., f.* African (*person*)
Afrique *f.* Africa; **Afrique de l'ouest (Afrique occidentale)** West Africa; **Afrique du Nord** North Africa
âge *m.* age; epoch; **Moyen Âge** *m. s.* Middle Ages (12); **quel âge avez-vous?** how old are you?
agence *f.* agency; **agence de voyages** travel agency
agenda *m.* engagement book, pocket calendar
agitation *f.* bustle
agent *m.* agent; **agent de police** police officer (14)
agir to act (4); **il s'agit de** it's about, it's a question of
agité *adj.* agitated, restless; rough, choppy (*sea*)
agneau: côte (*f.*) **d'agneau** lamb chop
agrandir to make bigger
agréable *adj.* agreeable, pleasant, nice (3)
agricole *adj.* agricultural
agriculteur/trice *m., f.* farmer (14)
ah bon? *interj.* oh, really?
aide *f.* help, assistance; **à l'aide de** with the help of
aider to help (12)
aigreur *f.* sourness; bitterness
aigu: accent (*m.*) **aigu** acute accent **(é)**
aiguille *f.* needle
ail *m.* garlic (7)
ailleurs elsewhere; **d'ailleurs** besides, moreover
aimable *adj.* likable, friendly
aimer to like; to love (2); **aimer bien** to like; **aimer mieux** to prefer (2); **j'aimerais** + *inf.* I would like (*to do s.th.*); **je n'aime... pas du tout** I don't like . . . at all
ainsi *conj.* thus, so; **ainsi que** as well as; **et ainsi de suite** and so on
air *m.* air; look; tune; **activités** (*f. pl.*) **de plein air** outdoor activities (15); **avoir l'air (de)** to seem, look (like) (3); **de plein air** outdoor; **en plein air** outdoors, in the open air; **hôtesse** (*f.*) **de l'air** flight attendant (9)
aise: à l'aise at ease
ajouter to add
album *m.* (photo) album; picture book
alcool *m.* alcohol
alcoolisé *adj.* alcoholic
Alger Algiers
Algérie *f.* Algeria (2, 8)
algérien *adj.* Algerian; **Algérien(ne)** *m., f.* Algerian (*person*) (2)
aligné: faire du patin à roues alignées to do in-line skating
aliment(s) *m.* food, nourishment (6)
alimentaire *adj.* alimentary, pertaining to food
alimentation *f.* food, feeding, nourishment; **magasin** (*m.*) **d'alimentation** food store
alizé: vent (*m.*) **alizé** trade wind
allée *f.* path, walk
allégé *adj.* light, low-fat (*foods*)
Allemagne *f.* Germany (2, 8)
allemand *adj.* German; *m.* German (*language*) (2); **Allemand(e)** *m., f.* German (*person*) (2)
aller *irreg.* to go (5); **aller** + *inf.* to be going (*to do s.th.*) (5); **aller à la pêche** to go fishing (8); **aller en boîte** to go clubbing (15); **aller mal** to feel bad (ill) (4); **allez-vous-en!** go away! (13); **allez-y!** go ahead!; **billet** (*m.*) **aller-retour** round-trip ticket; **ça peut aller** all right, pretty well (1); **ça va?** how's it going? (1); **ça va** fine (things are going well) (1); **ça va bien (mal)** fine (bad[ly]) (things are going well [badly]) (1); **comment allez-vous? (comment vas-tu?)** how are you? (1); **s'en aller** to go away, go off (*to work*) (13); **va-t'en!** go away! (13)
allergique *adj.* allergic
allier to combine
allô *interj.* hello (*phone greeting*) (10)
allumer to light
alors *adv.* so; then, in that case (4)
alouette *f.* lark
alpin *adj.* Alpine; **ski** (*m.*) **alpin** downhill skiing (8)
alpinisme *m.* mountaineering, mountain climbing; **faire de l'alpinisme** to go mountain climbing (8)
alsacien(ne) *adj.* Alsatian
altérité *f.* otherness
amande *f.* almond
amants *m. pl.* lovers
amateur (*m.*) **de** lover of
ambiance *f.* atmosphere, surroundings
ambitieux/euse *adj.* ambitious
âme *f.* soul; spirit
amélioration *f.* improvement
améliorer to improve, better
amener (j'amène) to bring (along)
américain *adj.* American; **à l'américaine** American-style; **Américain(e)** *m., f.* American (*person*) (2)
Amérique *f.* America
ameublement *m. s.* furnishings
ami(e) *m., f.* friend (2); **petit(e) ami(e)** *m., f.* boyfriend, girlfriend
amical *adj.* (*m. pl.* **amicaux**) friendly
amitié *f.* friendship (13)
amour *m.* love (13); love affair
amoureux/euse *adj.* loving, in love (13); *m., f.* lover, sweetheart, person in love (13); **tomber amoureux/euse (de)** to fall in love (with) (13); **vie** (*f.*) **amoureuse** love life
amphithéâtre (*fam.* **amphi**) *m.* lecture hall, amphitheater (2)
ampoule *f.* light bulb
amusant *adj.* amusing, fun (3)
s'amuser (à) to have fun, have a good time (13)
an *m.* year; **avoir (vingt) ans** to be (twenty) years old (3); **l'an dernier (passé)** last year; **par an** per year, each year
analyser to analyze
ananas *m.* pineapple
ancêtre *m., f.* ancestor
ancien(ne) *adj.* old, antique; former (4); ancient; **anciens** *n. m. pl.* elders
ange *m.* angel; **je suis aux anges** I'm in seventh heaven
anglais *adj.* English; *m.* English (*language*) (2); **Anglais(e)** *m., f.* Englishman (-woman) (2)
Angleterre *f.* England (2, 8)
angoissé *adj.* anxious, anxiety-prone
animal *m.* animal; **animal domestique** pet
animateur/trice *m., f.* host, hostess (*radio, TV*); motivator (*in marketing*)
animé *adj.* animated
année *f.* year; **l'année prochaine (dernière [passée])** next (last) year; **les années (cinquante)** the decade (era) of the (fifties) (8)
anniversaire *m.* anniversary; birthday; **bon anniversaire** *interj.* happy birthday; **carte** (*f.*) **d'anniversaire** birthday card
annonce *f.* announcement, ad; **petites annonces** (classified) ads (10)
annoncer (nous annonçons) to announce, declare; **s'annoncer** to look; to promise to be
annuaire *m.* telephone directory (10); **annuaire électronique** online (telephone) directory (10); **consulter l'annuaire** to look up a phone number (10)
annuel(le) *adj.* annual
annuler to cancel (11)
anonyme *adj.* anonymous
anorak *m.* (ski) jacket, wind-breaker (8)
anticiper (sur) to anticipate
anticonformiste *m., f.* nonconformist
antillais *adj.* West Indian; **Antillais(e)** *m., f.* West Indian (*person*)
Antilles *f. pl.* West Indies
antipathique *adj.* disagreeable, unpleasant (3)
anxieux/euse *adj.* anxious
août August (1)
apaiser to appease; to soothe
aperçu *adj.* noticed
apéritif (*fam.* **apéro**) *m.* cocktail
apparaître (*like* **connaître**) *irreg.* to appear
appareil *m.* apparatus (10); device; appliance; telephone (10); **appareil (photo) numérique** *m.* (*still*) digital camera (10); **qui est à l'appareil?** who's calling? (10)
apparemment *adv.* apparently
apparence *f.* appearance
apparenté *adj.* related; **mot** (*m.*) **apparenté** cognate (*word*)
apparition *f.* appearance
appartement (*fam.* **appart**) *m.* apartment (4)
appartenir (*like* **tenir**) **à** *irreg.* to belong to
appel *m.* call; **faire appel à** to appeal to; to require, call for
appeler (j'appelle) to call (10); to name; **comment s'appelle... ?** what's . . . name?; **comment vous appelez-vous? (comment t'appelles-tu?)** what's your name? (1); **je m'appelle...** my name is . . . (1); **s'appeler** to be named (13)

appétit *m.* appetite; **bon appétit** *interj.* enjoy your meal
appliquer to apply
apporter to bring, carry; to furnish (6)
apprécier to appreciate, value
apprendre (*like* **prendre**) *irreg.* to learn; to teach (6); **apprendre à** to learn (how) to
apprentissage (*m.*) **des langues** language learning
approcher to approach
approprié *adj.* appropriate
après *prep.* after (2); afterward (5); **après avoir (être)...** after having . . . ; **d'après** *prep.* according to
après-midi *m.* or *f.* afternoon; **cet après-midi** this afternoon (5); **de l'après-midi** in the afternoon (6); **tous les après-midi** every afternoon (10)
arabe *m.* Arabic (*language*)
arachide *f.* peanut(s)
arbre *m.* tree (5)
archéologique *adj.* archeological
archéologue *m., f.* archeologist
archi-comble full of people
architecte *m., f.* architect (14)
arène(s) *f.* (*pl.*) arena, bullring (12)
argent *m.* money (7); silver; **argent liquide** cash (14)
argot *m.* slang
arme *f.* weapon, arm
armée *f.* army; **armée de métier** professional army
armoire *f.* wardrobe; closet (4)
aromaticien(ne) *m., f.* perfume maker
arranger to arrange
arrêter (de) to stop, cease (12); **s'arrêter** to stop (*oneself*) (13)
arrière *adv.* back; **arrière-grand-parent** *m.* great-grandparent (5)
arrivant(e) *m., f.* newcomer
arrivée *f.* arrival (9)
arriver to arrive, come (3); to happen
arrondissement *m.* district, section (*of Paris*) (11)
arroser to water (*plants*)
art *m.* art; **œuvre** (*f.*) **d'art** work of art (12)
artichaut *m.* artichoke
artifice: feux (*m. pl.*) **d'artifice** fireworks
artisan(e) *m., f.* artisan, craftsperson (14)
artisanal *adj.* craft
artisanat *m.* handicrafts, arts and crafts
artiste *m., f.* artist (12)
artistique *adj.* artistic
ascenseur *m.* elevator
Asiatique *m., f.* person from Asia
Asie *f.* Asia
aspiré *adj.* aspirate
asseoir (*p.p.* **assis**) *irreg.* to seat; **s'asseoir** to sit down
asservi *adj.* enslaved
assez *adv.* somewhat (3); rather, quite; **assez de** *adv.* enough (6)
assiette *f.* plate (6)
assise *f.* foundation
assistance *f.* assistance, help; audience
assistant(e) *m., f.* assistant; **assistant(e) administratif/ive** administrative assistant
assisté *adj.* supported, assisted
assister à to attend, go to (*concert, etc.*) (15)
associer to associate
assortiment *m.* assortment
assurance *f.* assurance; insurance; **assurances-automobile** *pl.* car insurance
assurer to insure; to assure; to ensure
atelier *m.* workshop; (*art*) studio
athlète *m., f.* athlete
atmosphère *f.* atmosphere (16)
atours *m. pl.* finery, attire
atout *m.* asset
attacher to attach
attaquer to attack
atteindre (*like* **craindre**) *irreg.* to reach, attain
attendre to wait, wait for (5)
attention *f.* attention; **faire attention (à)** to pay attention (to); to be careful (of), watch out (for) (5)
attentivement *adv.* attentively
attirer to attract
attrait *m.* attraction, lure; charm
attraper to catch
attribuer to attribute
auberge *f.* inn; **auberge de jeunesse** youth hostel (9)
aucun(e) (ne... aucun[e]) *adj., pron.* none; no one, not one, not any; anyone; any
audace *f.* daring innovation
audacieux/euse *adj.* daring
auditeur/trice *m., f.* listener
auditoire *m.* audience
augmentation *f.* increase (14); **augmentation de salaire** salary raise (14)
augmenter to increase (16)
aujourd'hui *adv.* today (1); nowadays
auprès de *prep.* with, to
aurore *f.* dawn
aussi *adv.* also; so; as; **aussi... que** as . . . as (14); **moi aussi** me too (3)
aussitôt *conj.* immediately, at once; **aussitôt que** as soon as (14)
Australie *f.* Australia
autant (de) *adv.* as much, so much, as many, so many; **autant (de)... que** as much (many) . . . as (15); **autant que** as much as
auteur *m.* author; **auteur dramatique** playwright (12)
authentique *adj.* authentic, genuine
autobus (*fam.* **bus**) *m.* (*city*) bus (5)
autocar *m.* (*interurban*) bus (9)
automatique *adj.* automatic; **consigne** (*f.*) **automatique** coin locker (9); **guichet** (*m.*) **automatique** automatic teller machine (ATM) (14)
automne *m.* autumn, fall; **en automne** in the autumn (5)
automobile (*fam.* **auto**) *f., adj.* automobile, car
autonome autonomous
autoportrait *m.* self-portrait
autorisé permitted
autoritaire *adj.* authoritarian
autoroute *f.* highway, freeway (9)
autour de *prep.* around
autre *adj., pron.* other (4); another; *m., f.* the other; *pl.* the others, the rest; **autre chose** something else (7); **d'autres** other(s) (15); **entre autres** among other things; **l'autre / les autres** the other(s) (15); **un(e) autre** another (15)
autrefois *adv.* formerly, in the past (11)
autrement *adv.* otherwise; **autrement dit** in other words
Autriche *f.* Austria
auxiliaire *m., Gram.* auxiliary (verb)
avaleur/euse (*m., f.*) **de feu** fire swallower
avance *f.* advance; **à l'avance** beforehand; **en avance** early (6)
avancé *adj.* advanced
avant *adj.* before (*in time*); *prep.* before, in advance of; *m.* front; **avant de** + *inf.* (*prep.*) before; **avant-goût** *m.* foretaste; **avant-hier** *adv.* the day before yesterday (7); **avant tout** *prep.* above all
avantage *m.* advantage, benefit; **tirer avantage de** to take advantage of
avare *adj.* stingy, tightfisted
avec *prep.* with (2)
avenir *m.* future (14); **à l'avenir** from now on, in the future (14)
aventure *f.* adventure; **partir à l'aventure** to leave with no itinerary
aventurier/ière *m., f.* adventurer (adventuress)
averti *adj.* warned; informed
avertir to warn
aveugle *adj.* blind; **dégustation** (*f.*) **à l'aveugle** blind tasting
avion *m.* airplane (9); **billet** (*m.*) **d'avion aller-retour** round-trip plane ticket; **en avion** by plane
avis *m.* opinion; **à votre (ton) avis** in your opinion (11); **changer d'avis** to change one's mind
avocat(e) *m., f.* lawyer (14)
avoir (*p.p.* **eu**) *irreg.* to have (3); **avoir (vingt) ans** to be (twenty) years old (3); **avoir besoin de** to need (3); **avoir chaud** to be warm (hot) (3); **avoir confiance en** to have confidence in; **avoir de la chance** to be lucky (3); **avoir de la fièvre** to have a fever; **avoir droit à** to have a right to; **avoir du mal à** to have trouble (difficulty); **avoir envie de** to feel like; to want (3); **avoir faim** to be hungry (3); **avoir froid** to be (feel) cold (3); **avoir honte (de)** to be ashamed (of) (3); **avoir horreur de** to hate; **avoir l'air (de)** to seem, look (like) (3); **avoir le temps (de)** to have the time (to); **avoir lieu** to take place; **avoir mal (à)** to have pain; to hurt (13); **avoir peur (de)** to be afraid (of) (3); **avoir raison** to be right (3); **avoir rendez-vous avec** to have a meeting (date) with (3); **avoir soif** to be thirsty (3); **avoir sommeil** to be sleepy (3); **avoir tort** to be wrong (3); **il n'y a pas de quoi** you're welcome (7); **il y a** there is, there are (1); ago (8); **j'aurai droit à quoi** I'll be entitled to what
avouer to confess, admit
avril April (1)
Azur: Côte (*f.*) **d'Azur** French Riviera

babouche *f.* (Turkish) slipper
baccalauréat (*fam.* **bac**) *m.* baccalaureate (*French secondary school degree*)
badiner to banter, joke
bafouille *f., fam.* letter
bagages *m. pl.* luggage
bagarre *f.* fight, brawl
bagnole *f., fam.* car, jalopy
baguette (de pain) *f.* French bread, baguette (6)
baie *f.* bay
baigner: ça baigne it's chill, it's going great
se baigner to bathe (*oneself*) (13); to swim (13)
bain *m.* bath; swim; **maillot** (*m.*) **de bain** swimsuit (3); **salle** (*f.*) **de bains** bathroom (5)
baiser *m.* kiss
baisse *f.* lowering, reduction
baisser: faire baisser to lower

bal *m.* dance, ball
balade *f., fam.* walk, drive, outing
se balader *fam.* to go for a walk (drive, outing)
balancer: se balancer to sway
balayé *adj.* swept away
balcon *m.* balcony (5)
balle *f.* (*small*) ball; tennis ball
ballon *m.* (*soccer, basket*) ball; balloon; **ballon à air chaud** hot-air balloon
balnéaire *adj.* seaside
banal *adj.* commonplace
banane *f.* banana (6)
banc *m.* bench
bancaire *adj.* banking, bank; **carte** (*f.*) **bancaire** bank (ATM/credit) card (14); **compte** (*m.*) **bancaire** bank account
bande *f.* band; group; gang; (*cassette, video*) tape; **bande dessinée** comic strip, cartoon (15); *pl.* comics
banlieue *f.* suburbs (11); **en banlieue** in the suburbs
banlieusard *m., f.* suburbanite, commuter
banque *f.* bank (11)
baptiser to baptize; to name
bar *m.* bar; snack bar; pub
barde *f.* bard (*layer of bacon on a roast*)
barreau *m.* bar (*of a cage*)
barrer to bar, block; **se barrer** *fam.* to run off, clear out
barrière *f.* gate, fence; barrier
bas(se) *adj.* low; **à bas...** down with . . . ; **là-bas** *adv.* over there (10); **Pays-Bas** *m. pl.* the Netherlands, Holland
base *f.* base; basis, foundation; **base de données** database; **être à la base de** to be at the root of
base-ball *m.* baseball; **jouer au base-ball** to play baseball
baser to base; **se baser sur** to be based on
basilique *f.* basilica
basket-ball (*fam.* **basket**) *m.* basketball; **jouer au basket** to play basketball
bassin *m.* ornamental pond
bassiste *m., f.* bass guitarist; bass player
bataille *f.* battle
bateau *m.* boat (8); **bateau à voile** sailboat (8); **bateau de croisière** cruise ship; **bateau-mouche** *m. tourist boat on the Seine;* **en bateau** by boat, in a boat; **faire du bateau** to go boating (8)
bâtiment *m.* building (11)
bâtir to build (12)
battre (*p.p.* **battu**) *irreg.* to beat; to battle with; **se battre** to fight
bavard *adj.* talkative
bavardage *m.* chattering
bavarder to chat; to talk
bavaroise *f.* mousse (*dessert*)
bavette: bifteck (*m.*) **bavette** sirloin of beef
beau (bel, belle [beaux, belles]) *adj.* handsome; beautiful (3); **à la belle étoile** under the stars; **beau-frère** *m.* brother-in-law; stepbrother (5); **beau-père** *m.* father-in-law; stepfather (5); **belle-mère** *f.* mother-in-law; stepmother (5); **belle-sœur** *f.* sister-in-law; stepsister (5); **il fait beau** it's nice (weather) out (5)
beaucoup (de) *adv.* very much, a lot (1); much, many (6)
beauté *f.* beauty
bébé *m.* baby
bécane *f., fam.* bike
becquée *f.* beakful
beignet *m.* doughnut; fritter
belette *f.* weasel
belge *adj.* Belgian; **Belge** *m., f.* Belgian (*person*) (2)
Belgique *f.* Belgium (2, 8)
belle (see **beau**)
bénédiction *f.* blessing
bénéficier (de) to profit, benefit (from)
bénévolat *m.* volunteerism
bénévole *m., f., adj.* volunteer
béquille *f.* crutch
béret *m.* beret (3)
besoin *m.* need; **avoir besoin de** to need (3)
bête *f.* animal, beast
beur *m., f.* second-generation North African living in France
beurre *m.* butter (6)
beurré *adj.* buttered
bibliothèque (*fam.* **bibli**) *f.* library (2)
bicentenaire *m.* bicentennial
bicyclette *f.* bicycle (8); **faire de la bicyclette** to go bicycling (8)
bide: faire un bide *fam.* to flop; to bomb (as a theatre production)
bien *adv.* well (1); (*fam.*) good, quite; much; comfortable; **aimer bien** to like; **bien** (*m.*) **commun** common good (16); **bien sûr** *interj.* of course; **ça va bien** fine (things are going well) (1); **eh bien** *interj.* well (10); **je vais bien** I'm fine; **s'amuser bien** to have a good time; **s'entendre bien** to get along (well); **très bien** very well (good) (1); **vouloir bien** to be willing; to agree
bien-être *m.* well-being; welfare
bienfaisant *adj.* refreshing; beneficial
bientôt *adv.* soon (5); **à bientôt** *interj.* see you soon (1)
bienvenu(e) *adj., interj.* welcome
bière *f.* beer (6)
bifteck *m.* steak (6)
bijou *m.* jewel (14); piece of jewelry
bilingue *adj.* bilingual
billet *m.* bill (*currency*); ticket (9); **billet aller-retour** round-trip ticket; **billet d'avion (de train)** plane (train) ticket; **composter son billet** to stamp (punch) one's ticket
biologie *f.* biology (2)
biologique *adj.* (*fam.* **bio**) biological; organic
bip *m.* beep (*answering machine*)
biscuit (sec) *m.* cookie
bise *f., fam.* kiss, smack; **faire la bise** to kiss on both cheeks (*in greeting*); **(grosses) bises** love and kisses
bisou *m., fam.* kiss (*child's language*); **(gros) bisous** love and kisses
bistro *m.* bar, pub; neighborhood restaurant
bizarre *adj.* strange, odd; **il est bizarre que** + *subj.* it's strange (bizarre) that
blaff *m.* broth (in Martinique)
blague *f.* joke (15)
blanc(he) *adj.* white (3); **coup** (*m.*) **à blanc** blank shot
blancheur *f.* whiteness
blé *m.* wheat; *fam.* cash
blessé wounded
bleu *adj.* blue (3)
blog *m.* blog
blogueur/blogueuse *m., f.* blogger
blond(e) *m., f., adj.* blond (3)
bloqué *adj.* stuck, held up (*in traffic*); **être bloqué** to have a mental block
blouson *m.* windbreaker; jacket (3)
bobo *adj.* hipster
bœuf *m.* beef (6); **consommé** (*m.*) **de bœuf** beef consommé; **filet** (*m.*) **de bœuf** beef fillet; **rôti** (*m.*) **de bœuf** roast beef
bof *interj.* I dunno; not really; so-so
boire (*p.p.* **bu**) *irreg.* to drink (6); **boire un coup** to have a drink
bois *m.* forest, woods (11); wood
boisson *f.* drink, beverage (6); **boisson gazeuse** soft drink
boîte *f.* box; can; nightclub (15); **boîte (de conserve)** can (*of food*) (7); **boîte aux lettres** mailbox (10); **boîte de nuit** nightclub; **boîte vocale** voice mail (10)
bol *m.* wide cup; bowl (6)
bombe: faire la bombe *fam.* to celebrate, have a party
bon(ne) *adj.* good (4); right, correct; *f.* maid, chambermaid; **ah bon?** oh, really?; **bon anniversaire** *interj.* happy birthday; **bon appétit** *interj.* enjoy your meal; **bon marché** *adj., inv.* inexpensive; **bon voyage** *interj.* have a good trip; **bonne chance** *interj.* good luck; **bonne route** *interj.* have a good trip; **de bonne heure** early (6); **il est bon que** + *subj.* it's good that (16)
bonbon *m.* (*piece of*) candy
bonheur *m.* happiness
bonjour *interj.* hello, good day (1)
bonsoir *interj.* good evening (1)
bonté *f.* kindness
bord *m.* board; edge, bank, shore; **à bord** on board; **au bord de** on the banks (shore, edge) of
bordé *adj.* edged, lined
bordelais *adj.* Bordeaux-style
border to line, edge
borne *f.* terminal; pay point
borné *adj.* limited; restricted
Bosnie-Herzégovine *f.* Bosnia-Herzegovina
bosser *fam.* to work
bottes *f. pl.* boots (3)
boubou *m. long tunic worn by black North Africans*
bouche *f.* mouth (13)
boucher/ère *m., f.* butcher (14)
boucherie *f.* butcher shop (7); **boucherie-charcuterie** *f.* combination butcher and deli
boucler to buckle
bouddhisme *m.* Buddhism
bouffe *f.* (*fam.*) food, grub; **faire une petite bouffe** have a light meal
bouger (nous bougeons) to move, budge
bougie *f.* candle
bouillabaisse *f. fish chowder typical of southern France*
bouillir (*p.p.* **bouilli**) *irreg.* to boil; **faire bouillir** to bring to a boil
boulangerie *f.* bakery (7); **boulangerie-pâtisserie** *f.* bakery-pastry shop
boule *f.* ball
boulot *m., fam.* job; work
bouquin *m., fam.* book
bouquiniste *m., f.* secondhand bookseller (*especially along the Seine in Paris*)
bourgeois *adj.* bourgeois; middle-class
Bourgogne *f.* Burgundy
bourguignon(ne) *adj.* from Burgundy; **bœuf bourguignon** beef stew with red wine sauce

bourse (*f.*) **d'études** scholarship, study grant; **Bourse** *f.* stock exchange
bout *m.* end; **au bout de** to the end of; **jusqu'au bout** until the very end
bouteille *f.* bottle (6)
boutique *f.* shop, store
bouton *m.* button; push-button
branché *adj., fam.* trendy
brancher to connect (up); **se brancher (sur)** to link oneself (with); to go online (on the Internet)
bras *m. s., pl.* arm (13)
brasser to mix, stir
brasserie *f.* bar, brasserie
bref/ève *adj.* short, brief; *adv.* in short, in brief
Brésil *m.* Brazil (8)
Bretagne *f.* Brittany
breton(ne) *adj.* Breton; **Breton(ne)** *m., f.* Breton (*person*); **Far** (*m.*) **breton** traditional cake from Brittany
bribes *f. pl.* scraps, snippets
bricolage *m.* do-it-yourself work, puttering around (15)
bricoler to putter around, do odd jobs (15)
brièvement *adv.* briefly
brillant *adj.* brilliant; shining
briller to shine, gleam
brique *f.* brick
briser to break
bronchite *f.* bronchitis
bronzer to get a suntan (8)
brosse *f.* brush (13); **brosse à dents** toothbrush
brosser to brush; **se brosser les cheveux (les dents)** to brush one's hair (teeth) (13)
brousse *f.* (*African, Australian*) bush (country)
bru *f.* daughter-in-law (5)
bruit *m.* noise (5)
brûlant *adj.* burning; urgent
brûlé *adj.* burned, burnt; **crème** (*f.*) **brûlée** *custard topped with caramelized sugar*
brumeux/euse *adj.* foggy, misty
brun brown; **la sauce brune** gravy
brutal *adj.* violent, rough
Bruxelles Brussels
bûche *f.* log; **bûche de Noël** Yule log (*pastry*)
bûcheron(ne) *m., f.* woodcutter
budget *m.* budget (14); **budget militaire** military budget (16)
buée *f.* condensation; steam
buffet (*m.*) **de la gare** train station restaurant (9)
bureau *m.* desk (1); office (2), study (5); **bureau de change** money exchange (office) (14); **bureau de poste** post office (10); **bureau de tabac** (*government-licensed*) tobacconist (10)
bus *m.* (*city*) bus
but *m.* goal; objective; **ligne** (*f.*) **de but** goal, goal line (*soccer*)

ça *pron.* this, that; it (7); **ça cloche** things aren't going right; **ça m'est égal** it's all the same to me; **ça peut aller** all right, pretty well (1); **ça va?** how's it going? (1); **ça va** fine (things are going well) (1); **ça va bien (mal)** things are going well (badly) (1); **comme ci, comme ça** so-so (1)
cabine *f.* cabin; booth; **cabine téléphonique** telephone booth
cabinet *m.* office; **cabinet medical** doctor's office (13)
câble *m.* cable; cable TV (10); **télévision** (*f.*) **par câble** cable TV
câblé *adj.* wired; equipped for cable TV
cachemire *m.* cashmere
cacher to hide
cacheter (je cachette) to seal (*envelope*)
cadeau *m.* present, gift (10)
cadien(ne) *adj.* Cajun
cadre *m.* frame; setting, framework; middle (upper) manager (14)
café *m.* café (2); (cup of) coffee (2); coffee-flavored; **café au lait** coffee with milk; **café-tabac** *m.* bar- tobacconist (*government-licensed*) (11)
cafetière *f.* coffeepot, coffeemaker
cahier *m.* notebook (1); workbook
caisse *f.* cash register
calcul *m.* calculation; arithmetic; calculus; **faire des calculs** to do calculations
calculer to calculate, figure; **machine** (*f.*) **à calculer** adding machine
calendrier *m.* calendar
Californie *f.* California
californien(ne) *adj.* Californian
calme *m., adj.* calm (3)
calmer to calm (down)
calorique *adj.* caloric; **très (peu) calorique** high (low) in calories
camarade *m., f.* friend, companion; **camarade de chambre** roommate (3); **camarade de classe** classmate, schoolmate
Cameroun *m.* Cameroon
caméscope (numérique) *m.* (digital) camcorder, video camera (10)
camion *m.* truck (9)
camp (*m.*) **de travail forcé** forced laber camp
campagne *f.* country(side) (8); campaign; **à la campagne** in the country; **campagne électorale** election campaign; **pain** (*m.*) **de campagne** country-style bread, wheat bread (7); **pâté** (*m.*) **de campagne** terrine, (country-style) pâté (7)
camper to camp
campeur/euse *m., f.* camper
camping *m.* camping (8); **faire du camping** to go camping (8)
Canada *m.* Canada (2, 8)
canadien *adj.* Canadian; **Canadien(ne)** *m., f.* Canadian (*person*) (2)
canal (*pl.* **canaux**) *m.* channel; canal
canapé *m.* sofa, couch (4)
canard *m.* duck; *tr. fam.* newspaper; **confit** (*m.*) **de canard** duck conserve
canari *m.* canary
cancre *m.* dunce
candélabre *m.* candelabra
candidat(e) *m., f.* candidate; applicant
candidature *f.* candidacy; **poser sa candidature** to apply (14)
caniche *m.* poodle
canicule *f.* heat wave
canne (*f.*) **à sucre** sugarcane
cannelle *f.* cinnamon
canon *adj., fam.* sexy, gorgeous (*a woman*)
cap *m.* cape (*strip of land*)
capitale *f.* capital (*city*)
capter to pick up (a radio signal)
car *conj.* for, because
caractère *m.* character (*personality*)
caractériser to characterize; **se caractériser par** to be characterized (distinguished) by
caractéristiques *f.* characteristics
carafe *f.* carafe; pitcher (6)
Caraïbes *f. pl.* Caribbean (*islands*)
caravane *f.* caravan; (camping) trailer
carburateur *m.* carburetor
cardiaque *adj.* cardiac
cardinal: points (*m. pl.*) **cardinaux** compass points, directions
cargaison *f.* cargo
caricaturiste *m., f.* caricaturist, cartoonist
carnaval *m.* carnival
carnet *m.* booklet; **carnet d'adresses** address book; **carnet de chèques** checkbook (14)
carotte *f.* carrot (6)
carré *adj.* square (*geometry*)
carreau *m.* tile, window pane; **à carreaux** checkered, checked
carrefour *m.* intersection; crossroads (11)
carrière *f.* career
cartable *m.* schoolbag
carte *f.* card (3); menu (7); map (*of region, country*) (11); *pl.* (playing) cards; **carte bancaire** bank (ATM/credit) card (14); **carte d'anniversaire** birthday card; **carte de crédit** credit card (14); **carte de débit** debit card (14); **carte d'embarquement** boarding pass (9); **carte d'étudiant** student ID card; **carte d'identité** ID card (8); **carte postale** postcard (10); **carte routière** road map; **jouer aux cartes** to play cards (3)
carton *m.* box
cartonner *fam.* to score a success
cas *m.* case; **dans ce cas** in this case (situation); **en cas de** in case of; **en tout cas** in any case, at any rate; **selon le cas** as the case may be
casque *m.* helmet (8); headset
casquette *f.* cap; baseball cap (3)
casser to break; **se casser** *fam.* to leave (a place)
casserole *f.* saucepan
casse-dalle *m., fam.* sandwich
casse-tête *m.* puzzle, riddle game
cassette *f.* cassette tape (*video or audio*); **cassette vidéo** videotape; **lecteur** (*m.*) **de cassettes** cassette deck, cassette player
cata: cèst la cata! *fam.* It's a catastrophe!
catégorie *f.* category, class
catégorique *adj.* categorical, flat
cathédrale *f.* cathedral (12)
cauchemar *m.* nightmare
cause: à cause de because of
cave *f.* cellar
CD (les CD) *m.* CD (4); **lecteur** (*m.*) **de CD** compact disc player (4)
ce (c') (cet, cette, ces) *pron., adj.* this, that (7); **ce week-end** this weekend; **c'est-à-dire (que)** that is, I mean (10); **c'est moi.** It's me. (10); **c'est un(e)...** it's a (an) . . . ; **cet après-midi (ce matin, ce soir)** this afternoon (morning, evening) (5); **qu'est-ce que c'est?** what is it? (1); **qui est-ce?** who is it? (1)
cédérom (CD-ROM) *m.* CD-ROM
cédille *f.* cedilla **(ç)**
ceinture *f.* belt; **ceinture de sécurité** seat belt
cela (ça) *pron.* this, that
célèbre *adj.* famous
célébrer (je célèbre) to celebrate (6)
célébrité *f.* celebrity
céleri *m.* celery

célibataire *adj.* single (*person*) (5); *n. m., f.* single person (13)
cellulaire *m.* cellular phone
celui (ceux, celle, celles) *pron.* the one, the ones; this one, that one; these, those
cendres *f. pl.* ashes
cendrier *m.* ashtray
censé: être censé(e) + *inf.* to be supposed to (*do s.th.*)
cent *adj.* one hundred
centaine *f.* about one hundred
centrale *f.* power station; **centrale nucléaire** nuclear power plant (16)
centre *m.* center; **centre d'hébergement** shelter; **centre-ville** *m.* downtown (11)
cependant *conj.* however, nevertheless
céramique *f.* pottery, ceramics
cercle *m.* circle
céréales *f. pl.* cereal; grains
cérémonie *f.* ceremony (13)
cerise *f.* cherry
cerné de surrounded by
certain *adj.* sure; particular; certain (15); *pl., pron.* certain ones, some people; **il est certain que** + *indic.* it's certain that (16)
certificat *m.* certificate, diploma
ces (see **ce**)
cesser to stop, cease
c'est-à-dire *conj.* that is to say, I mean
cet (see **ce**)
chacun(e) *m., f., pron.* each (one), every one (15)
chagrin *m.* grief
chaîne *f.* television channel; network (10); chain
chair *f.* meat; flesh
chaise *f.* chair (1)
chaleur *f.* heat; warmth
chaleureux/euse *adj.* warm; friendly
chambre *f.* room; bedroom (4); hotel room; **camarade** (*m., f.*) **de chambre** roommate (3); **chambre de bonne** (4) garret; maid's room
chameau *m.* camel
champ *m.* field
champagne *m.* champagne, sparkling wine (*from Champagne*)
champignon *m.* mushroom (6)
champion(ne) *m., f.* champion
chance *f.* luck; possibility; opportunity; **avoir de la chance** to be lucky (3); **bonne chance** *interj.* good luck; **pas de chance** no luck; **quelle chance** what luck
chancelant unsteady, faltering
chandail *m.* sweater
change *m.* currency exchange; **bureau** (*m.*) **de change** money exchange (office) (14); **taux** (*m.*) **de change** exchange rate (14)
changement *m.* change
changer (nous changeons) to change; to exchange (*currency*) (14); **changer d'avis** to change one's mind; **changer de l'argent** to exchange currency
chanson *f.* song (15); **chanson de variété** popular song (15)
chant *m.* song
chanter to sing
chanteur/euse *m., f.* singer
chantilly *f.* whipped cream; **à la chantilly** with whipped cream
chapeau *m.* hat (3)
chapitre *m.* chapter
chaque *adj.* each, every (4)
charbon *m.* coal; charcoal
charcuterie *f.* deli; cold cuts; pork butcher's shop, delicatessen (7); **boucherie-charcuterie** *f.* combination butcher and deli
charge (*f.*); **charges comprises** utilities included; **pris/en/charge par** taken care of by
chargé (de) *adj.* in charge (of), responsible (for); heavy, loaded (with); busy
chargement *m.* loading; shipping; **gare** (*f.*) **de chargement** loading dock
charger (nous chargeons) to load; **charger de** to ask (*s.o. to do s.th.*); **se charger de** to take responsibility for, take care of
charlotte *f.* charlotte (*cake with whipped cream and fruit*)
charmant *adj.* charming (3)
charmer to charm, enchant
charmeur (*m.*) **de serpents** snake charmer
charolais *adj.* of (from) Charolais
charte *f.* charter, title
chasse *f.* hunt, hunting
chasser to hunt; to chase away
chat(te) *m., f.* cat (4)
châtain *adj.* brown, chestnut-colored (*hair*) (3)
château *m.* castle, chateau (11)
chatier to punish
chaud *adj.* warm; hot; **avoir chaud** to be warm (hot) (3); **il fait chaud** it's hot (5)
chauffeur/euse *m., f.* chauffeur; driver; **chauffeur/euse de taxi** taxi(cab) driver
chaussée *f.* pavement; **rez-de-chaussée** *m.* ground floor (5)
chaussettes *f. pl.* socks (3)
chaussures *f. pl.* shoes (3); **chaussures de ski (de montagne)** ski (hiking) boots (8)
chavirer to capsize
chef *m.* leader; head; chef, head cook; **chef d'entreprise** company head, top manager, boss (14)
chef-d'œuvre *m.* (*pl.* **chefs-d'œuvre**) masterpiece (12)
chemin *m.* way (*road*) (11); path; **chemin de fer** railroad
chemise *f.* shirt (3)
chemisier *m.* (*woman's*) shirt, blouse (3)
chèque *m.* check (14); **carnet** (*m.*) **de chèques** checkbook (14); **chèque de voyage** traveler's check; **compte-chèques** *m.* checking account (14); **déposer un chèque** to deposit a check; **encaisser (toucher) un chèque** to cash a check; **faire un chèque** to write a check (14)
cher/ère *adj.* expensive; dear (3)
chercher to look for (2); to pick up (*a passenger*); **chercher à** to try to (12)
chéri(e) *m., f.* darling
cheval (*pl.* **chevaux**) *m.* horse (8); **à cheval** on horseback; **faire du cheval** to go horseback riding (8); **queue** (*f.*) **de cheval** ponytail
cheveux *m. pl.* hair (3); **se brosser les cheveux** to brush one's hair (13)
chèvre *f.* (she-) goat
chez at the home (establishment) of (5); **chez moi** at my place
chic *adj., often inv.* chic, stylish (3)
chien(ne) *m., f.* dog (4)
chiffre *m.* number, digit; **chiffre d'affaires** turnover (*in business*); **chiffre record** record number
chimie *f.* chemistry (2)
chimique *adj.* chemical; **produit** (*m.*) **chimique** chemical
chimiste *m., f.* chemist
Chine *f.* China (2, 8)
chinois *adj.* Chinese; *m.* Chinese (*language*) (2); **Chinois(e)** *m., f.* Chinese (*person*) (2)
choc *m.* clash; shock; jolt
chocolat *m.* chocolate; hot chocolate (6); **éclair** (*m.*) **au chocolat** chocolate eclair; **mousse** (*f.*) **au chocolat** chocolate mousse; **pain** (*m.*) **au chocolat** chocolate croissant
chocolaterie *f.* chocolate shop
chocolatier/ière *m., f.* chocolate maker
choisir (de) to choose (to) (4)
choix *m.* choice
chômage *m.* unemployment (14); **taux** (*m.*) **de chômage** unemployment rate (14)
chômeur/euse *m., f.* unemployed person (14)
choquer to shock
chose *f.* thing; **autre chose** something else (7); **quelque chose** something (9); **quelque chose de** + *adj.* something + *adj.* (15)
chou *m.* cabbage; (*fam.*) darling; **chou-fleur** (*pl.* **choux-fleurs**) *m.* cauliflower
choucroute *f.* sauerkraut
chrétien(ne) *adj.* Christian
chronique *adj.* chronic
chronologique *adj.* chronological
ci: comme ci, comme ça so-so (1); **ci-dessous** *adv.* below; **ci-dessus** *adv.* above, previously
ciboulette *f.* chive(s)
cidre *m.* cider
ciel *m.* sky; **gratte-ciel** *m. inv.* skyscraper
cigare *m.* cigar
cils *m. pl.* eyelashes
cimetière *m.* cemetery
cinéaste *m., f.* filmmaker (12)
ciné-club *m.* film club
cinéma (*fam.* **ciné**) *m.* movies; movie theater (2)
cinglé(e) *m., f.* lunatic, crazy person
cinq *adj.* five (1)
cinquante *adj.* fifty (1); **les années** (*f. pl.*) **cinquante** the decade (era) of the fifties
cinquième *adj.* fifth (11)
circonflexe *m.* circumflex (*accent*) **(ê)**
circonstance *f.* circumstance
circuit *m.* organized tour
circulation *f.* traffic; circulation
circuler to circulate; to travel
cire *f.* wax
ciré *adj.* polished; waxed
cirque *m.* circus
cirrhose *f.* cirrhosis
citadin(e) *m., f.* city-dweller
citation *f.* quotation
cité *f.* area in a city; **cité universitaire** (*fam.* **cité-U**) university dormitory (2)
citer to cite, name; to quote
citoyen(ne) *m., f.* citizen (16)
citron *m.* lemon; **citron pressé** fresh lemon juice; **citron vert** lime (*fruit*)
cive *f.* chive
civil: état (*m.*) **civil** marital (civil) status
clair *adj.* light, bright; light-colored; clear; evident; **il est clair que** + *indic.* it's clear that (16)
clandestin *adj.* clandestine, secret
claquer *fam.* spend

clarinette *f.* clarinet
classe *f.* class; classroom; *adj., fam.* chic, stylish; **camarade** (*m., f.*) **de classe** classmate; **classe affaires (économique)** business (tourist) class (9); **première (deuxième [seconde]) classe** first (second) class (9); **salle** (*f.*) **de classe** classroom (1)
classement *m.* classification
classer to classify; to sort; to rate; **se classer** to come in; to rank
classique *adj.* classical; classic; **musique** (*f.*) **classique** classical music
clavier *m.* keyboard (10)
clé, clef *f.* key (5); **mot clé** *m.* key word
clic *m.* click
client(e) *m., f.* customer, client
clientèle *f.* clientele, customers
climat *m.* climate
climatisé *adj.* air-conditioned
cliquer (sur) to click (on) (10)
cloche *f.* bell
clocher *fam.* to be cockeyed; to go wrong; **ça cloche** things are going wrong
clos *m.* field
clou (*m.*) **de girofle** clove
club *m.* club (*social, athletic*); **ciné-club** *m.* film club
coca *m., fam.* cola drink
cocasse *adj.* comical, funny
cocher to check off (*list*)
coco: noix (*f.*) **de coco** coconut; **lait** (*m.*) **de coco** coconut milk
cocotier *m.* coconut tree
cocotte *f.* stewpot, casserole
code *m.* code; **code postal** postal (zip) code
cœur *m.* heart (13); **au cœur de** at the heart (source) of; **par cœur** by heart (12)
coexister to coexist
coffre *m.* trunk (*of car*) (9)
coffret *m.* box; lunch box
coiffeur/euse *m., f.* hairdresser; barber (14)
coiffure *f.* hair style; **salon** (*m.*) **de coiffure** beauty salon
coin *m.* corner (11)
colis *m.* package, parcel (10)
collant *m.* pantyhose
collectif/ive *adj.* collective
collectionner to collect
collège *m.* (*French*) *secondary school*
collègue *m., f.* colleague
colocataire (*fam.* **coloc**) *m., f.* housemate, roommate
colocation *f.* house or apartment sharing
colombage *m.* half-timbers
Colombie *f.* Colombia; **Colombie-Britannique** *f.* British Columbia
colonie *f.* colony
colonisateur/trice *m., f.* colonizer
colonisé *adj.* colonized
colonne *f.* column
combatif/ive *adj.* fighting, combative
combattre (*like* **battre**) *irreg.* to fight
combien (de)? *adv.* how much? (1), how many? (4); **c'est combien?** how much is it? (1) **depuis combien de temps... ?** (for) how long . . . ? (9); **pendant combien de temps... ?** (for) how long . . . ? (9)
combinaison *f.* combination
combiner to combine
comédie *f.* comedy
comédien(ne) *m., f.* stage actor; comedian (12)
comète *f.* comet
comique *m., f.* comedian, comic; *adj.* funny, comical, comic
commande *f.* order (*in business, restaurant*)
commandement *m.* command (*military leadership*)
commander to order (*in a restaurant*) (6)
comme *adv.* as, like, how; **comme ci, comme ça** so-so (1)
commencement *m.* beginning
commencer (nous commençons) (à) to begin (to) (2); **commencer par** to begin by (*doing s.th.*)
comment *adv.* how; **comment** what, how (1); **comment allez-vous? (comment vas-tu?)** how are you? (1); **comment ça va?** how are you?, how's it going? (1); **comment dit-on... en français?** how do you say . . . in French?; **comment est-il/elle?** what's he/she/it like?; **comment s'appelle-t-il/elle?** what's his/her name?; **comment vous appelez-vous? (comment t'appelles-tu?)** what's your name? (1)
commentaire *m.* remark, comment; commentary
commenter to comment on
commerçant(e) *m., f.* shopkeeper (14); *adj.* commercial, shopping
commerce *m.* business (2)
commercial *adj.* commercial, business; **directeur/trice** (*m., f.*) **commercial(e)** business manager (14)
commissariat *m.* police station (11)
commission *f.* commission; errand
commode *f.* chest of drawers (4); *adj.* convenient
commun *adj.* ordinary, common; shared; **bien** (*m.*) **commun** common good (16); **en commun** in common; **transports** (*m. pl.*) **en commun** public transportation
communauté *f.* community
commune *f.* district
communicatif/ive *adj.* communicative
communication *f.* communication; phone call
communiquer to communicate
compact: disque (*m.*) **compact** compact disc
compagnie *f.* company
compagnon/compagne *m., f.* companion
comparaison *f.* comparison
comparer to compare
compartiment *m.* compartment (9)
compatriote *m., f.* fellow countryman (-woman)
complément *m.* complement; **pronom** (*m.*) **complément d'objet (in)direct** *Gram.* (in) direct object pronoun
complémentaire *adj.* complementary
complet/ète *adj.* complete; whole
compléter (je complète) to complete, finish
compliqué *adj.* complicated
comportement *m.* behavior
composé *adj.* composed; **passé** (*m.*) **composé** *Gram.* compound past tense
composer to compose; to make up; **composer le numéro** to dial the (phone) number (10)
compositeur/trice *m., f.* composer (12)
composter to stamp (*date*); to punch (*ticket*)
compréhensif/ive *adj.* understanding
compréhension *f.* understanding
comprendre (*like* **prendre**) *irreg.* to understand; to comprise, include (6); **je ne comprends pas** I don't understand (1)
comprimé *m.* tablet, pill
compris *adj.* included (7); **tout compris** all inclusive
comptabilité *f.* accounting
comptable *m., f.* accountant (14); **expert(e)-comptable** *m., f.* certified public accountant
compte *m.* account; **à son compte** for oneself (14); **compte bancaire** bank account; **compte d'épargne** savings account (14); **travailler pour (à) son compte** to be self-employed (14)
compter to plan (to do something); to intend; to count (14); to have; to include; **compter sur** to count on, rely on (s.o. or s.th.)
concentrer to concentrate
concerner to concern; **en ce qui concerne** concerning
concevoir (*like* **recevoir**) *irreg.* to conceive, design
concierge *m., f.* caretaker, super, janitor; concierge
concilier to reconcile
conclu (*p.p. of* **conclure**) *adj.* settled, agreed upon
concours *m. s.* competition; competitive exam
conçu (*p.p. of* **concevoir**) *adj.* designed, devised, conceived
concurrence *f.* competition; trading
concurrencer to rival, compete with
concurrent(e) *m., f.* competitor
condamner to condemn
condition *f.* condition; situation; **à condition de** provided, providing
conditionnel *m., Gram.* conditional
conducteur/trice *m., f.* driver (9); engineer (*train*)
conduire (*p.p.* **conduit**) *irreg.* to drive (9); to take; to lead; **permis** (*m.*) **de conduire** driver's license
conduite *f.* behavior, conduct
confection *f.* making (*clothing*)
conférence *f.* lecture (12); conference
confiance *f.* confidence; **avoir confiance en** to have confidence in; to trust; **faire confiance à** to trust in
confié (à) *adj.* entrusted (to)
confirmer to confirm
confiserie *f.* candy store
confit (*m.*) **de canard** duck conserve
confiture *f.* jam
conflit *m.* conflict (16)
confondre to mix up, confuse
confondu *adj.* mixed, confused
conformiste *m., f., adj.* conformist (3)
confort *m.* comfort; amenities
confortable *adj.* comfortable
congé *m.* vacation, leave (*from work*)
Congo *m.* Congo (8); **République** (*f.*) **Démocratique du Congo** Democratic Republic of Congo (8)
congolais *adj.* Congolese; **Congolais(e)** *m., f.* Congolese (*person*)
congrès *m.* meeting, convention
conjugaison *f., Gram.* (verb) conjugation
conjuguer to conjugate
connaissance *f.* knowledge; acquaintance; **faire connaissance** to get acquainted; **faire la connaissance de** to meet (*for the first time*), make the acquaintance of (5)
connaisseur/euse *m., f.* connoisseur

connaître (*p.p.* **connu**) *irreg.* to know, be familiar with (11); **se connaître** to know one another; to meet
connecté logged on, connected (*to the Internet*)
connerie *f., tr. fam.* stupid mistake
connexion *f.* link, connection; **connexion ADSL** DSL connection/line (10)
connu *adj.* known; famous
conquérir (*p.p.* **conquis**) *irreg.* to conquer
consacrer to devote
se consacrer à to devote oneself to
conscience *f.* conscience; **prendre conscience de** to become aware of
conseil *m.* (piece of) advice; council; **donner des conseils à** to give advice to
conseiller (à, de) to advise; to suggest (12)
conseiller/ère *m., f.* adviser; **conseiller/ère d'orientation** guidance counselor
conservation *f.* conserving; preservation (16)
conservatoire *m.* conservatory
conserve *f.* preserve(s), canned food; *pl.* canned goods (7); **boîte** (*f.*) **de conserve** can of food (7)
conserver to conserve, preserve (16)
considération: prendre en considération to take into consideration
considérer (je considère) to consider (6)
consigne *f.* instruction(s); **consigne (automatique)** coin locker (9)
consommateur/trice *m., f.* consumer
consommation *f.* consumption; consumerism
consommé *m.* clear soup, consommé
consommer to consume (16)
conspirer à to conspire to
constamment *adv.* constantly (12)
constater to notice; to remark
constituer to constitute
constructeur *m.* maker; constructor
constructif/ive *adj.* constructive
construire (*like* **conduire**) *irreg.* to construct, build (9)
consulter to consult; **consulter l'annuaire** to look up a phone number (10)
contacter to contact
conte *m.* tale, story; **conte de fée** fairy tale
contempler to contemplate, meditate upon
contemporain *adj.* contemporary
contenir (*like* **tenir**) *irreg.* to contain
content *adj.* happy, pleased (3); **être content(e) de** (+ *inf.*) to be happy about (to); **être content(e) que** + *subj.* to be happy that
contenter to please
contenu *m.* content
contester to dispute; to answer
conteur/euse *m., f.* storyteller
continuer (à) to continue (to) (11)
contracter to get, contract (*a disease*)
contraire: vent (*m.*) **contraire** headwind
contrairement à contrary to, unlike
contrat *m.* contract
contravention *f.* traffic ticket
contre *prep.* against; **le pour et le contre** the pros and cons; **manifester contre** to demonstrate against (16)
contrôle *m.* control, overseeing; inspection
contrôler to inspect, monitor (14)
contrôleur/euse *m., f.* ticket collector; conductor
convaincant *adj.* convincing
convaincre (*p.p.* **convaincu**) *irreg.* to convince
convenable *adj.* proper; appropriate
convenir (*like* **venir**) *irreg.* to be suitable
converger (nous convergeons) (vers) to converge (on), lead (toward)
convertisseur *m.* converter
convoquer to summon, invite, convene
coordonner to coordinate
copain (copine) *m., f., fam.* friend, pal (7); boyfriend (girlfriend) (7)
copier to copy
copieux/euse *adj.* copious, abundant
coq *m.* rooster; **coq au vin** coq au vin (*chicken prepared with red wine*)
coquelicot *m.* poppy
coquillages *m. pl.* seashells
corbeau *m.* crow
corps *m. s.* body (13)
correctement *adv.* correctly
correspondance *f.* correspondence
correspondant(e) *m., f.* newspaper correspondent; *adj.* corresponding
correspondre to correspond
corriger (nous corrigeons) to correct
Corse *f.* Corsica
cortège *m.* procession
cortisone *f.* cortisone
cosmopolite *adj.* cosmopolitan
costume *m.* (*man's*) suit; costume (3)
costumé: soirée (*f.*) **costumée** costume party
costumier/ière *m., f.* costume designer
côte *f.* coast; chop (7); rib; rib steak; side; **côte d'agneau (de porc)** lamb (pork) chop; **Côte d'Azur** (French) Riviera; **Côte d'Ivoire** *f.* Cote d'Ivoire (2, 8)
côté *m.* side; **(d')à côté** (from) next door; **à côté (de)** *prep.* by, near; beside, next to (4); at one's side; **mettre de côté** to set aside
coton *m.* cotton
cou *m.* neck (13)
couchage: sac (*m.*) **de couchage** sleeping bag (8)
coucher to put to bed; **se coucher** to go to bed (13)
couchette *f.* berth (*train*) (9)
coucou *interj., fam.* peek-a-boo
coudre (*p.p.* **cousu**) *irreg.* to sew; **machine** (*f.*) **à coudre** sewing machine
coulé *adj.* cast
couleur *f.* color; **de quelle couleur est... ?** what color is . . . ?; **en couleur(s)** in color; colored
coulis *m.* purée
couloir *m.* hall(way) (4)
coup *m.* blow; **boire un coup** to have a drink; **coup à blanc** blank shot; **coup de foudre** flash of lightning (13); love at first sight (13); **coup de pouce** little push (in the right direction); **coup de téléphone** telephone call; **coup d'œil** glance, quick look; **tout à coup** *adv.* suddenly (11)
coupe *f.* trophy, cup; ice cream sundae; **Coupe d'Europe** European Cup (*soccer*); **Coupe du Monde** World Cup (*soccer*)
couper to cut (off, up); **couper la ligne** to cut off (*phone call*)
couple *m.* (*engaged, married*) couple
cour *f.* court (*legal, royal*)
courage *m.* courage; spirit; **bon courage** *interj.* cheer up, be brave
courageux/euse *adj.* courageous (3)
couramment *adv.* fluently (12)
courant *adj.* general, everyday; **être au courant de** to be up (to date) with
coureur/euse *m., f.* runner; **coureur/euse cycliste** bicycle racer
courir (*p.p.* **couru**) *irreg.* to run (13)
couronne *f.* crown; royalty
couronné *adj.* crowned
courriel *m., fam.* e-mail message (10)
courrier *m.* mail (10); **courrier électronique** e-mail (*in general*)
cours *m. s.* course (2); class; exchange rate (14); price; **au cours de** during; **cours d'eau** river, waterway; **cours du jour** today's exchange rate; **suivre un cours** to take a course
course *f.* race; errand; **faire les courses** to do errands; to shop (5)
court *adj.* short (3); *m.* (tennis) court; **à court terme** in the short term (run)
court-bouillon *m.* broth
couscous *m.* couscous (*North African cracked-wheat dish*)
couscoussier *m.* couscous pan (*with steamer*)
cousin(e) *m., f.* cousin (5)
coût *m.* cost; **coût de la vie** cost of living (14)
couteau *m.* knife (6)
coûter to cost
coutume *f.* custom, tradition
couture *f.* sewing; clothes design; ***haute couture** high fashion
couturier/ière *m., f.* clothes designer; dressmaker
couvert (de) *adj.* covered (with); *m.* table setting; **mettre le couvert** to set the table (10)
couverture *f.* coverage; cover
couvrir (*like* **ouvrir**) *irreg.* to cover (14)
covoiturage *m.* carpooling (16)
crabe *m.* crab (*seafood*)
craindre (*p.p.* **craint**) *irreg.* to fear
craquer to crack, snap
cravate *f.* tie (3)
crayon *m.* pencil (1)
créateur/trice *m., f.* creator
créativité *f.* creativity
crèche *f.* day-care center
crédit *m.* credit; **carte** (*f.*) **de crédit** credit card (14)
credo *m.* creed, system of beliefs
créer to create
crème *f.* cream (6); *m.* coffee with cream; **crème brulée** *custard topped with caramelized sugar;* **crème fraîche** clotted cream, crème fraîche; **crème glacée** *Q.* ice cream; **crème solaire** suntan lotion (8)
crêpe *f.* crepe, French pancake
crevé *adj., fam.* exhausted, wiped out
crevette *f.* shrimp
cri *m.* cry, shout
crier to cry out; to shout
crise *f.* crisis; **crise économique** recession; depression
critère *f.* criterion
critique *m., f.* critic
critiquer to criticize
croire (*p.p.* **cru**) **(à/en)** *irreg.* to believe (in) (10); **croire que** to believe that
croisière *f.* cruise; **bateau** (*m.*) **de croisière** cruise ship
croissant *m.* croissant (*roll*) (6); *adj.* growing
croisé: mers croisées *choppy seas, waves*

croix *f.* cross
croyance *f.* belief
cru *adj.* raw; *m.* vintage; vineyard or wine-producing region; **lait** (*m.*) **cru** unpasteurized milk
crustacé *m.* crustacea, shellfish
cuillère *f.* spoon (6); **cuillère à soupe** soup spoon, tablespoon (6); **petite cuillère** teaspoon
cuillerée *f.* spoonful (*measure*)
cuir *m.* leather; **en cuir** (*made of*) leather
cuire: faire cuire to cook (*food*)
cuisine *f.* cooking (6); food, cuisine; kitchen (5); **faire la cuisine** to cook (5); **nouvelle cuisine** light (low-fat) cuisine
cuisiner to cook
cuisinette *f.* kitchenette
cuisinier/ière *m., f.* cook, chef
cuisse *f.* leg; thigh
cuisson *f.* cooking (*process*)
cuit *adj.* cooked
culinaire *adj.* culinary, cooking
culotte *f.* breeches
cultivé *adj.* educated; cultured
cultiver to cultivate; to grow (*crops*)
culture *f.* education; culture
culturel(le) *adj.* cultural
cure *f.* course of treatment
curieux/euse *adj.* curious (3)
curiosité *f.* curiosity
curriculum (*m.*) **vitæ** résumé (14)
cybercafé *m.* Web (Internet) café
cybermarché *m.* Web (Internet) market
cyclable: piste (*f.*) **cyclable** bike path
cyclisme *m.* cycling (15)
cycliste *m., f.* cyclist, bicycle rider
cynique *adj.* cynical
cynisme *m.* cynicism

d'abord *adv.* first, first of all, at first (11)
d'accord *interj.* all right, O.K., agreed (2)
dalle: avoir la dalle to be hungry; **casse-dalle** *m.* sandwich
dame *f.* lady, woman; **messieurs dames** *colloq.* ladies and gentlemen
Danemark *m.* Denmark
dangereux/euse *adj.* dangerous
dans *prep.* within, in (2); **dans quatre jours** in four days (from now)
danse *f.* dance; dancing
danser to dance (2)
danseur/euse *m., f.* dancer
darne *f.* steak (*fish*)
date *f.* date (*time*); **quelle est la date (d'aujourd'hui)?** what's today's date? (1)
dater de to date from (12)
datte *f.* date (*fruit*)
d'autres *pron.* others (15)
davantage *adv.* more
de (d') *prep.* of, from, about (2); **de nouveau** again (11); **de rien** not at all; don't mention it; you're welcome (1); **de temps en temps** from time to time (2)
débarquement *m.* disembarkation, landing
débarquer to land
débat *m.* debate
débit: carte de débit debit card (14)
débouché *m.* opening, (job) prospect
déboucher to come out, lead to
debout *adj., inv., adv.* standing up
se débrouiller to manage (13)
début *m.* beginning; **au début (de)** in (at) the beginning (of)
débutant(e) *m., f.* beginner, novice
débuter to begin, start
décapotable *f.* convertible (*car*)
décembre December (1)
décevoir to disappoint
déchets *m. pl.* waste (material) (16); **déchets industriels** industrial waste; debris; **déchets nucléaires** nuclear waste
déchirer to rip; *fam.* to be the height of fashion
décidément *adv.* decidedly; definitely
décider (de) to decide (to) (12)
décision *f.* decision; **prendre une décision** to make a decision
déclencher to release, activate
déclin *m.* decline
déconseillé *adj.* not recommended
décor *m.* setting
décoratif/ive *adj.* decorative
décorer (de) to decorate (with)
découler to follow from; to ensue
découper to cut up
découragé *adj.* discouraged
décourager to discourage
découverte *f.* discovery
découvrir (*like* **ouvrir**) *irreg.* to discover (14)
décrire (*like* **écrire**) *irreg.* to describe (10)
décrocher *fam.* to get, receive
déçu *adj.* disappointed
dédié *adj.* consecrated, dedicated
défaite *f.* defeat
défaut *m.* defect, fault
défavoriser to penalize, put at a disadvantage
défendre to defend; to prohibit, disallow
défenseur *m.* defender, champion
défi *m.* challenge (16)
défiance *f.* mistrust
défilé *m.* fashion show
défiler to file past; to unwind
défini: article (*m.*) **défini** *Gram.* definite article
définir to define
définitif/ive *adj.* definitive, permanent
déforestation (*f.*) **tropicale** tropical rainforest deforestation (16)
dégager (nous dégageons) to release; to clear; to bring out
dégâts *m. pl.* damage, harm
dégénérer (je dégénère) to degenerate
dégouliner to drip
dégourdir to bring the circulation back to; to warm up
degré *m.* degree
déguiser to disguise
dégustation *f.* tasting
déguster to taste (*wine*)
dehors *adv.* outdoors; outside; **en dehors de** *prep.* outside
déjà *adv.* already; ever (9)
déjeuner to have lunch (6); *m.* lunch (6); **petit déjeuner** breakfast (6)
delà: au-delà de *prep.* beyond
délai *m.* wait, time period
délégué(e) *m., f.* delegate
délice *m.* delight
délicieux/euse *adj.* delicious
délinquance *f.* criminality
délire: en délire ecstatic; *adj., fam.* great, fantastic
demain *adv.* tomorrow (5)
demande (*f.*) **d'emploi** job application (14)
demander (de) to ask (for, to), request (2); **se demander** to wonder (13)
se démarquer (par) to stand out, distinguish oneself
déménagement *m.* move out (of a home)
déménager (nous déménageons) to move out (*change residence*) (4)
demeure *f.* residence
demeurer to remain
demi *adj.* half; **demi-frère** *m.* half brother; stepbrother (5); **demi-sœur** *f.* half sister; stepsister (5); **et demi(e)** half past (the hour) (6)
démocratie *f.* democracy
démocratique: République (*f.*) **Démocratique du Congo** Democratic Republic of Congo (8)
démodé *adj.* old-fashioned
démolir to demolish, destroy
démonstratif/ive *adj.* demonstrative
dénoncer (nous dénonçons) to denounce
dent *f.* tooth (13); **brosse** (*f.*) **à dents** toothbrush; **se brosser les dents** to brush one's teeth (13)
dentelle *f.* lace
dentiste *m., f.* dentist (14)
dépannage *m.* emergency repair
départ *m.* departure (9); **point** (*m.*) **de départ** starting point
se dépêcher to hurry (13); **dépêche-toi!** hurry up! (6)
dépendant *adj.* dependent
dépendre de to depend on
dépense *f.* expense; spending (14)
dépenser to spend (*money*) (10)
dépit: en dépit de *prep.* in spite of
déporté *adj.* deported
déposer to deposit (14); **déposer de l'argent (un chèque)** to deposit money (a check) (14); **déposer la monnaie** to deposit change (10)
dépot-vente *m.* resale store
dépravation *f.* depravity
dépression *f.* depression, breakdown
déprime *f., fam.* blues
déprimé *adj.* depressed
depuis *prep.* since, for (9); **depuis combien de temps... ?** (for) how long . . . ? (9); **depuis longtemps** for a long time; **depuis quand... ?** since when . . . ? (9)
député *m.* delegate, deputy
déranger (nous dérangeons) to disturb, bother
dernier/ière *adj.* last (4, 7); most recent; past; **la dernière fois** the last time; **l'an dernier (l'année dernière)** last year
dernièrement *adv.* recently
se dérouler to take place, happen
derrière *prep.* behind (4)
dès *prep.* from (*then on*); **dès que** *conj.* as soon as (14)
désaccord *m.* disagreement
désagréable *adj.* disagreeable, unpleasant (3)
désavantage *m.* disadvantage
descendre to go down (*street, river*) (5); to get off (5); to take down; **descendre à (sur)** to go down (*south*) to; **descendre de** to get down (from), get off
déséquilibre *m.* imbalance
désert *m.* desert; wilderness
déserter to desert; to run away
desertique *adj* desert; barren; arid

désespéré *adj.* desperate
désespoir *m.* despair, hopelessness
désigner to designate
désir *m.* desire
désirer to desire, want (15)
désolé *adj.* sorry (16); **(je suis) désolé(e)** I'm sorry
désordonné *adj.* disorganized
désordre *m.* disorder, confusion; **en désordre** disorderly; disheveled (4)
désormais *adv.* henceforth
dessert *m.* dessert (6)
dessin *m.* drawing
dessiné: bande (*f.*) **dessinée** comic strip, cartoon (15); *pl.* comics
dessiner to draw (10)
dessous: au-dessous de *prep.* below; **ci-dessous** *adv.* below
dessus: au-dessus de *prep.* above; **ci-dessus** *adv.* above, previously
destin *m.* destiny
destination *f.* destination; **à destination de** to, for (9); in the direction of; heading for
destinée *f.* destiny, future
détail *m.* detail; **en détail** in detail
détaillé *adj.* detailed
détecteur *m.* detector
se détendre to relax (13)
détente *f.* relaxation
déterminer to determine
détester to detest; to hate (2)
détour *m.* detour
détruire (*like* **conduire**) *irreg.* to destroy (9)
dette *f.* debt
deux *adj.* two (1); **tous (toutes) les deux** both (of them)
deuxième *adj.* second (11); **deuxième classe** *f.* second class; **deuxième étage** third floor (*in the U.S.*) (5)
devant *prep.* before, in front of (4)
développé *adj.* developed; industrialized
développement *m.* development (16); developing (*photo*); **développement durable** sustainable development; **pays** (*m.*) **en voie de développement** developing country
développer to develop (16); **se développer** to develop
devenir (*like* **venir**) *irreg.* to become (8)
deviner to guess (12)
devinette *f.* riddle, conundrum
dévoiler to reveal, disclose
devoir (*p.p.* **dû**) *irreg.* to owe; to have to, be obliged to (7); *m.* duty; *m. pl.* homework; **faire ses devoirs** to do one's homework (5); **je devrais** I should (15)
dévorant *adj.* all-consuming
d'habitude *adv.* habitually, usually (5)
diagnostic *m.* diagnosis; prognosis
diapositive *f.* (*photographic*) slide
dicter to dictate
dictionnaire *m.* dictionary (2)
diététique *adj.* dietetic
Dieu *m.* God; **croire en Dieu** to believe in God
différemment *adv.* differently
différend *m.* disagreement
différent *adj.* different (3)
difficile *adj.* difficult (3)
difficulté *f.* difficulty
diffuser to broadcast; to disseminate
digne *adj.* worthy
dignité *f.* dignity
diligemment *adv.* diligently
dimanche *m.* Sunday (1); **le dimanche** on Sundays (5)
diminuer to lessen, diminish, lower (16)
dinde *f.* turkey
dîner to dine, have dinner (6); *m.* dinner (6)
diplomate *m., f.* diplomat; *adj.* diplomatic, tactful
diplomatique *adj.* diplomatic (*of the diplomatic corps*)
diplôme *m.* diploma
diplômé(e) *m., f.* graduate; holder of a diploma
dire (*p.p.* **dit**) *irreg.* to say; to tell, relate (10); **c'est-à-dire que** that is to say, namely, I mean (10); **entendre dire que** to hear that; **que veut dire... ?** what does . . . mean?; **se dire** to say to one another; **vouloir dire** to mean
direct *adj.* direct; **en direct** live (*broadcasting*); **pronom** (*m.*) **(complément) d'objet direct** *Gram.* direct object pronoun
directeur/trice *m., f.* manager, head (14); **directeur/trice commercial(e)** business manager (14)
direction *f.* direction; steering (*auto*)
directives *f. pl.* rules of conduct, directives
diriger (nous dirigeons) to direct (14); to govern, control
discothèque (*fam.* **disco**) *f.* discothèque
discours *m. s.* discourse; speech
discret/ète *adj.* discreet
discuter (de) to discuss
disparaître (*like* **connaître**) *irreg.* to disappear
disparition *f.* disappearance; **en voie de disparition** endangered (*species*)
disponible *adj.* available
disposer to arrange
dispute *f.* quarrel
disputer to contest; to play; to fight (over); **se disputer** to argue (13)
disque *n.* record, recording; **disque compact** compact disc
dissertation *f.* essay, term paper
dissimuler to hide
dissiper to dissipate; to dispel
distance *f.* distance; **mettre à distance** to separate
distinguer to differentiate; **se distinguer** to distinguish oneself
distraction *f.* recreation; entertainment; distraction
se distraire (*p.p.* **distrait**) *irreg.* to have fun, amuse oneself
distribuer to distribute
distributeur *m.* distributor; **distributeur automatique** automatic teller machine (ATM)
divers *adj.* varied, diverse (1)
se diversifier to diversify
se divertir to amuse oneself, have a good time
divertissant *adj.* amusing
divisé (par) *adj.* divided (by)
divorcé *adj.* divorced (5)
divorcer (nous divorçons) to get a divorce, divorce
dix *adj.* ten (1); **dix-sept (-huit, -neuf)** *adj.* seventeen (eighteen, nineteen) (1)
dixième *adj.* tenth
dizaine *f.* about ten
djellaba *f.* djellaba (hooded Moroccan robe for men)
docteur *m.* doctor
doctorat *m.* doctorate
documentaire *m.* documentary (film) (10)
doigt *m.* finger (13)
domaine *m.* domain; specialty
domestique *m., f.* servant; *adj.* domestic; **animal** (*m.*) **domestique** pet
dominant: vent (*m.*) **dominant** prevailing wind
dominer to dominate
dommage! *interj.* too bad! (16); **il est dommage que** + *subj.* it's too bad that (16)
don *m.* gift
donc *conj.* then; therefore (4)
données: base (*f.*) **de données** database
donner to give (2); **donner des conseils** to give advice; **donner rendez-vous à** to make an appointment with; **donner sur** to overlook
dont whose, of whom, of which (14)
dorer: faire dorer to brown (*in cooking*); **se dorer au soleil** to sunbathe
dormir *irreg.* to sleep (8)
dortoir *m.* dormitory
dos *m. s., pl.* back (13); **sac** (*m.*) **à dos** backpack (3)
dossier *m.* document; file
douane *f.* customs (*at the border*)
doubler to double; to pass (*in a car*)
douche *f.* shower (*bath*) (4); **prendre une douche** to take a shower
se doucher to take a shower (13)
doudou *f., fam.* (*West Indies*) girlfriend
doué *adj.* gifted, talented
douleur *f.* pain, ache (13); grief
douloureux/euse *adj.* painful, unhappy
doute *m.* doubt; **sans doute** probably
douter to doubt (16); **douter de** to be suspicious of
doux (douce) *adj.* sweet; **à feu doux** over a low flame (*cooking*); **petits pois** (*m. pl.*) **doux** sweet peas
douzaine *f.* dozen; about twelve
douze *adj.* twelve (1)
douzième *adj.* twelfth
draguer *fam.* to come on to, flirt with
dragueur/euse *m., f.* flirt
dramatique: art (*m.*) **dramatique** theater, theater arts
drame *m.* drama
drap *m.* sheet (*bed*)
drapeau *m.* flag
dresser to set up
drogue *f.* drug(s)
droit *m.* law (2); right (*legal*); **droits civils** civil rights (16); **droit d'entrée** entrance fee
droit *adj.* right; straight; **Rive** (*f.*) **droite** Right Bank (*in Paris*) (11); **tout droit** *adv.* straight ahead (11)
droite *f.* right, right-hand; **à droite (de)** *prep.* on (to) the right (of) (4)
drôle *adj.* funny, odd (3)
duc *m.* duke
dur *adj.* hard
durable lasting, enduring; **développement** (*m.*) **durable** sustainable development
durant *prep.* during
durée *f.* duration, length
durer to last, continue; to endure; to last a long time
DVD *m.* DVD (1); **lecteur** (*m.*) **de DVD** DVD player (1)
dynamique *adj.* dynamic (3)

eau *f.* water (6); **cours** (*m.*) **d'eau** river, waterway; **eau minérale** mineral water (6)
ébène *f.* ebony
ébloui *adj.* dazzled
ébranlé *adj.* shaken, shattered
écart *m.* gap; difference
écarté *adj.* removed
échange *m.* exchange
échanger (nous échangeons) to exchange (10)
échapper (à) to get away (from); **s'echapper** to escape
s'échauffer to warm up
échec *m.* failure; *pl.* chess (3)
échelle *f.* scale; ladder
échouer to fail
éclair *m.* éclair (*pastry*) (7)
éclaircie *f.* clearing (*in weather*)
éclairer to light, illuminate
éclater to break out (*war*); **s'éclater** *fam.* to have a great time, have fun
école *f.* school (10); **école primaire (secondaire)** primary (secondary) school
écolier/ière *m., f.* pupil, schoolchild
écologie *f.* ecology
écologique (*fam.* **écolo**) *adj.* ecological
écologiste *m., f.* ecologist, environmentalist (16); *adj.* ecological
économe *adj.* thrifty, economical
économie *f.* economics (2); economy; *pl.* savings; **faire des économies** to save (up) money (14)
économique *adj.* economic; financial; economical; **classe** (*f.*) **économique** tourist class (9); **sur le plan économique** economically speaking
économiser to save (*money*) (14)
Écosse *f.* Scotland; **Nouvelle-Écosse** *f.* Nova Scotia
écoute *f.* listening; **à l'écoute** tuning in
écouter to listen to (2)
écran *m.* screen (1, 10); monitor (10); **écran solaire** sunblock (8); **le petit écran** television
écraser to crush
écrevisse *f.* crayfish (7)
écrire (*p.p.* **écrit**) **(à)** *irreg.* to write (to) (10)
écriture *f.* writing; handwriting
écrivain (femme écrivain) *m., f.* writer (12)
écumoire *f.* skimmer (*in cooking*)
édifice *m.* (public) building
éditeur/trice *m., f.* editor; publisher
édition *f.* publishing; edition; **maison** (*f.*) **d'édition** publisher, publishing house
éducatif/ive *adj.* educational
éducation *f.* upbringing; breeding; education
éduqué *adj.* educated; brought up
effacer to erase, wipe out; **s'effacer (nous nous effaçons)** to fade; to stay in the background
effectif/ive *adj.* effective
effectuer to carry out, make
effet *m.* effect; **en effet** as a matter of fact, indeed
efficace *adj.* efficient
effort *m.* effort, attempt; **faire des efforts pour** to try (make an effort) to
égal *adj.* equal (16); **cela (ça) m'est égal** I don't care, it's all the same to me
également *adv.* equally; likewise, also
égaler to equal
égalité *f.* equality
égard (*m.*): **à cet égard** in this respect
égaré *adj.* scattered, lost
église *f.* church (11)
égoïste *adj.* selfish (3)
égorger (nous égorgeons) to slit the throat of
Égypte *f.* Egypt
eh bien *interj.* well, well then (10)
élaborer to refine; to develop
s'élancer (nous nous élançons) to rush out
électeur/trice *m., f.* voter (16)
électoral *adj.* election, electoral
électricité *f.* electricity
électrique *adj.* electric
électronique: adresse (*f.*) **électronique** e-mail address; **courrier** (*m.*) **électronique** e-mail; **message** (*m.*) **électronique** e-mail message
élégant *adj.* elegant (3)
élève *m., f.* pupil, student
élevé *adj.* high; raised, built
éliminé *adj.* eliminated
élire (*like* **lire**) *irreg.* to elect (16)
elle *pron., f. s.* she; her; it; **elle-même** *pron., f. s.* herself (12); **elles** *pron., f. pl.* they; them
élu *adj.* elected
emancipé *adj.* emancipated
embarquement: carte (*f.*) **d'embarquement** boarding pass (9)
embarquer to embark, get on
embarrassé *adj.* embarrassed; ill-at-ease; bothered
embauche *f.* hiring; **entretien** (*m.*) **d'embauche** job interview
embaucher to hire (16)
embouteillage *m.* traffic jam
embrassade *f.* hugging and kissing, embrace
embrasser to kiss; to embrace; **je t'embrasse** love (*closing of letter*); **s'embrasser** to kiss; to embrace (13)
émérite *adj.* highly skilled; emeritus
émettre (*like* **mettre**) *irreg.* to broadcast
émeute *f.* riot
émigré(e) *m., f.* émigré, expatriate
émission *f.* program; broadcast (10); **émission de musique** music program (10); **émission de télé réalité** reality show (10)
emménager (nous emménageons) to move in (4)
emmener (j'emmène) to take (*s.o. somewhere*); to take along (12)
empêcher (de) to prevent (from) (12); to preclude
empereur *m.* emperor
emplacement *m.* location
emploi *m.* use; job, position (14); **demande** (*f.*) **d'emploi** job application (14); **marché** (*m.*) **de l'emploi** job market (14); **offre** (*f.*) **d'emploi** job offer
employé(e) *m., f.* employee (14); white-collar worker; (sales) clerk; **employé(e) de** s.o. employed by
employer (j'emploie) to use; to employ
employeur/euse *m., f.* employer
emporter to take (*s.th. somewhere*); to take out (*food*); to carry away
emprunt *m.* loan (14)
emprunter (à) to borrow (from) (11)
ému *adj.* moved
en *prep.* in (2); in, by (*train, plane, bus*) (9); to; like; in the form of; *pron.* of them; of it; some, any (11); **de temps en temps** from time to time (2); **en automne** in autumn (5); **en avance** early (6); **en dehors de** outside; **en effet** indeed; **en été** in summer (5); **en face de** across from (4); **en général** in general (2); **en hiver** in winter (5); **en profondeur** in depth; **en retard** late (6); **en train de** in the process of; **qu'en penses-tu?** what do you think of that? (11)
encadrement *m.* training, supervision; framework
encaisser to cash (*a check*)
enceinte *f.* enclosure; **dans l'enceinte de** within (the boundary of)
encens *m.* incense
encercler to circle, encircle
enchaîné *adj.* chained, fettered
enchanté *adj.* enchanted; pleased (to meet you)
enchère *f.* bid; **vente** (*f.*) **aux enchères** auction
enchérir to bid
encore *adv.* still (9); again; yet; even; more; **encore de** more; **encore un peu** a little more; **ne... pas encore** not yet (9); **ou encore** or else
encourager (nous encourageons) (à) to encourage (to)
encyclopédie *f.* encyclopedia
endormir (*like* **dormir**) *irreg.* to put to sleep; **s'endormir** to fall asleep (13)
endroit *m.* place, spot (8)
énergie *f.* energy; **énergie nucléaire (solaire)** nuclear (solar) energy (16)
énergique *adj.* energetic
énervant *adj.* aggravating, irritating
énervé *adj.* on edge, nervous
enfance *f.* childhood
enfant *m., f.* child (5); **petit-enfant** *m.* grandchild (5)
enfer *m.* hell
enfermer to lock up
enfin *adv.* finally, at last (11)
enflammer to kindle (*imagination*)
enfouir to bury
engagé *adj.* involved, politically active, politically committed
engagement *m.* (*political*) commitment
engager (nous engageons) to begin, start; **s'engager (dans)** to get involved (*in a public issue*) (16)
énigme *f.* riddle, enigma
enlever (j'enlève) to remove, take off
ennemi(e) *m., f.* enemy
ennui *m.* trouble; problem (9); worry; boredom
ennuyer (j'ennuie) to bother; to bore; **s'ennuyer** to be bored (13); **s'ennuyer à mourir** to be bored to death
ennuyeux/euse *adj.* boring; annoying
énoncé *m.* statement, utterance
énorme *adj.* enormous, huge
énormément *adv.* enormously, tremendously
enquête *f.* survey, poll
enregistrer to record; to check in
enrichissement *m.* enrichment
enseignant(e) *m., f.* teacher, instructor
enseignement *m.* teaching; education
enseigner (à) to teach (to) (12)
ensemble *adv.* together (8); *m.* ensemble; whole
ensoleillé *adj.* sunny
ensuite *adv.* then, next (11)
entendre to hear (5); **entendre dire que** to hear that; **entendre parler de** to hear about; **s'entendre (avec)** to get along (with) (13)

entente *f.* (mutual) understanding
enterré *adj.* buried
enthousiasme *m.* enthusiasm
enthousiaste *adj.* enthusiastic (3)
entier/ière *adj.* entire, whole, complete; **en entier** in its entirety
entourer (de) to surround (with)
entraînement *m.* practice, training
entraîner to bring about, lead to; **s'entraîner** to train, work out
entraîneur/euse *m., f.* trainer
entre *prep.* between, among (4)
entrecôte *f.* rib steak
entrée *f.* entrance, entry; admission; first course (*meal*) (7); **droit** (*m.*) **d'entrée** entrance fee
entreprendre to undertake
entrepreneur/euse *m., f.* entrepreneur
entreprise *f.* business, company (14); **chef** (*m.*) **d'entreprise** company head, top manager, boss (14)
entrer (dans) to enter (8)
entretien *m.* maintenance; conversation; **entretien (d'embauche)** job interview (14)
énumérer (j'énumère) to spell out, recite; to list, enumerate
envahir to invade
enveloppe *f.* envelope (10)
envers *prep.* toward
envie *f.* desire; **avoir envie de** to want; to feel like (3)
environ *adv.* about, approximately; *m. pl.* environs; **dans les environs** in the vicinity
environnement *m.* environment (16)
envoi *m.* sending
envoyer (j'envoie) (a) to send (to) (10)
éolienne *f.* windmill; windpump
épais *adj.* thick
s'épanouir to bloom
épargne: compte (*m.*) **d'épargne** savings account (14)
s'éparpiller to scatter
épaule *f.* shoulder
épice *f.* spice
épicé *adj.* spicy
épicerie *f.* grocery store (7)
épicier/ière *m., f.* grocer
épinards *m. pl.* spinach
époque *f.* period (*of history*) (12); **à l'époque (de)** at the time (of); **meubles** (*m. pl.*) **d'époque** antique furniture
épouser to marry
époux (épouse) *m., f.* husband; wife; **époux** *m. pl.* married couple
épreuve *f.* test; event (*sports*)
éprouver to feel; to experience
épuiser to use up, exhaust (16)
équilibre *m.* equilibrium, balance
équipage *m.* crew
équipe *f.* team (15); **sports** (*m. pl.*) **d'équipe** team sports; **travail** (*m.*) **d'équipe** teamwork
équipé *adj.* equipped
équipement *m.* equipment; gear
s'équiper to equip oneself
équitation *f.* horseback riding (8); **faire de l'équitation** to go horseback riding
erreur *f.* error; mistake
erroné *adj.* wrong, erroneous
escalade *f.* (mountain) climbing
escalader to climb, scale
escale: faire escale à to stop over at
escalier *m.* stairs, stairway (5)
escalope *f.* (*veal*) scallop
escargot *m.* snail; escargot (7)
escarpement *m.* steep slope
esclavage *m.* slavery
esclave *m., f.* slave
espace *m.* space; **espaces verts** open spaces, greenbelts
espadrilles *f. pl.* fabric sandals, espadrilles
Espagne *f.* Spain (2, 8)
espagnol *adj.* Spanish; *m.* Spanish (*language*) (2); **Espagnol(e)** *m., f.* Spaniard (*person*) (2)
espèces *f. pl.* species
espérer (j'espère) to hope (6)
espoir *m.* hope
esprit *m.* mind; spirit; wit
essai *m.* attempt, try; **mariage** (*m.*) **à l'essai** trial marriage
essaimer to spread, expand
essayer (j'essaie) (de) to try (to) (12)
essence *f.* gasoline, gas (9); **faire le plein (d'essence)** to fill the tank (9)
essentiel(le) *adj.* essential (3); **il est essentiel que** + *subj.* it's essential that (16)
essentiellement *adv.* largely, mainly
est *m.* east; **à l'est** to the east (9)
estampe *f.* engraving
esthétique *adj.* aesthetic
estimer to consider; to believe; to estimate (16)
et *conj.* and (2); **et demi(e)** half past (the hour) (6); **et puis** and (then), next (7); **et quart** quarter past (the hour); **et vous? (et toi?)** and you?; how about you? (1)
établir to establish, set up (16)
établissement *m.* establishment
étage *m.* floor (*of building*); **premier (deuxième) étage** second (third) floor (*in the U.S.*) (5)
étagère *f.* shelf (4)
étape *f.* stage; stopping place
état *m.* state (8); condition; **état civil** marital (civil) status; **États-Unis** *m. pl.* United States (of America) (2, 8); **homme (femme) d'état** statesman (-woman)
été *m.* summer; **en été** in summer (5); **job** (*m.*) **d'été** summer job
s'étendre to sprawl
étendue *f.* area, expanse
éternel(le) *adj.* eternal
éternité *f.* eternity
étincelle *f.* sparkle, sparkling
étiquette *f.* label
étoile *f.* star; **à la belle étoile** in the open air
étonné *adj.* surprised; astonished (16)
étouffer to suffocate
étrange *adj.* strange; **il est étrange que** + *subj.* it's strange that (16)
étranger/ère *adj.* foreign; *m., f.* stranger; foreigner; **à l'étranger** abroad, in a foreign country (9); **langue** (*f.*) **étrangère** foreign language
être (*p.p.* **été**) *irreg.* to be (2); **c'est (ce n'est pas)** it's (it isn't) (1); **c'est combien?** how much is it? (1); **comment est-il/elle?** what's he/she like?; **être en train de** to be in the process of, be in the middle of (15); **il est... heure(s)** it is . . . o'clock (6); **n'est-ce pas?** isn't it (so)?, isn't that right? (3); **nous sommes lundi (mardi...)** it's Monday (Tuesday . . .) (1); **peut-être** *adv.* perhaps, maybe; **quel jour sommes-nous (est-ce)?** what day is it? (1); **quelle heure est-il?** what time is it? (6); **qui est-ce?** who is it? (1)
étroit *adj.* narrow
étude *f.* study; *pl.* studies; **bourse** (*f.*) **d'études** scholarship, study grant; **faire des études** to study
étudiant(e) *m., f., adj.* student (1); **carte** (*f.*) **d'étudiant** student ID card
étudier to study (2)
euh... *interj.* uhmm . . . (10)
euphorisant *m.* producing a sense of euphoria
euro *m.* euro (*European currency*)
Europe *f.* Europe; **coupe** (*f.*) **d'Europe** European Cup (*soccer*)
européen(ne) *adj.* European; **Européen(ne)** *m., f.* European (*person*); **Union** (*f.*) **européenne (UE)** European Union (EU)
eux *pron., m. pl.* them; **eux-mêmes** *pron., m. pl.* themselves (12)
s'évader to escape
évaluer to appraise, evaluate
s'éveiller to wake up
événement *m.* event (12)
évidemment *adv.* evidently, obviously (12)
évident *adj.* obvious, clear; **il est évident que** + *indic.* it is clear that (16)
éviter to avoid
évoluer to evolve, advance, develop
évoquer to evoke, call to mind
exact *adj.* precise, true; **oui, c'est exact** yes, that's correct
exactement *adv.* exactly
exagérer (j'exagère) to exaggerate
examen (*fam.* **exam**) *m.* test, exam (2); examination; **passer un examen** to take an exam (4); **réussir à un examen** to pass a test
examiner to inspect, examine
exaspérant *adj.* exasperating
exaspéré *adj.* exasperated
excéder (j'excède) to exceed
excellent *adj.* excellent (3)
excentricité *f.* eccentricity
excentrique *adj.* eccentric (3)
excepté *prep.* except
exceptionnel(le) *adj.* exceptional
excès *m.* excess
excitant *adj.* exciting
excité *adj.* excited
exclamer to exclaim
exclu(e) *m., f.* excluded (*people*)
exclure (*p.p.* **exclu**) *irreg.* to exclude, rule out
exclusivement *adv.* exclusively
exclusivité *f.* exclusive rights, coverage
excursion *f.* excursion, outing; **faire une excursion** to go on an outing
s'excuser to apologize (13); **excusez-moi (excuse-moi)** excuse me, pardon me (1)
exemplaire *adj.* exemplary; *m.* copy
exemple *m.* example; **par exemple** for example (16)
exercer (nous exerçons) to exercise, exert (*control, influence*)
exercice *m.* exercise
exigeant *adj.* demanding; difficult
exigence *f.* demand
exiger (nous exigeons) to require; to demand (16)
exil *m.* exile
exilé *adj.* exiled
exister to exist
exode *m.* exodus

expatrié *adj.* expatriated
s'expatrier to leave one's country
expédition *f.* trip
expérience *f.* experience; experiment
expert(e) *m., f.* expert; **expert(e)-comptable** *m., f.* certified public accountant
explication *f.* explanation
expliquer to explain
exploité *adj.* exploited
exploiter to make use of, make the most of
explorateur/trice *m., f.* explorer
explorer to explore
exportation *f.* export(s)
s'exporter to be exported
exposé *m.* presentation, exposé; *adj.* displayed
exposer to expose, show; to display
exposition *f.* exhibition; show (12)
expression *f.* expression; term (1); **liberté** (*f.*) **d'expression** freedom of expression (16)
exprimer to express; **exprimer une opinion** to express an opinion (16); **s'exprimer** to express oneself
exquis *adj.* exquisite
extraire to extract
extrait *m.* excerpt; extract
extraordinaire *adj.* extraordinary (3)
extrasensoriel(le) *adj.* extra-sensory
extrêmement *adv.* extremely
extrémiste: idées (*f.*) **extrémistes** extremist ideas (16)

fabrication *f.* manufacture, making
fabriquer to manufacture, make
fabuleux/euse *adj.* fabulous
fac *f., fam.* **(faculté)** university department or school
façade *f.* façade, face (*of a building*)
face: en face (de) *prep.* opposite, facing, across from (4); **face à** facing; **face à face** face to face
fâché *adj.* angry (16)
fâcher to anger; **se fâcher** to get angry (13)
fâcheux/euse *adj.* unfortunate; troublesome; **il est fâcheux que** + *subj.* it is unfortunate that (16)
facile *adj.* easy (3)
facilité *f.* ease, easiness
faciliter to facilitate, make easier
façon *f.* way, manner, fashion; **de façon (logique)** in a (logical) way
facteur/trice *m., f.* factor; letter carrier (14)
faculté *f.* ability; (*fam.* **fac**) division (*academic*) (2); **faculté des lettres** School of Arts and Letters; **faculté des sciences** School of Science
faible *adj.* weak; small
failli: j'ai failli... I nearly . . .
faim *f.* hunger; **avoir faim** to be hungry (3)
faire (*p.p.* **fait**) *irreg.* to do; to make (5); to form; to be; **faire appel à** to appeal to; to require, call for; **faire attention (à)** to pay attention (to) (5); to watch out (for); **faire baisser** to lower; **faire beau (il fait beau)** to be good weather (it's nice out) (5); **faire bouillir** to boil; **faire chaud (il fait chaud)** to be warm, be hot (out) (it's warm, it's hot) (5); **faire confiance à** to trust; **faire connaissance** to get acquainted; **faire cuire** to cook; **faire de la bicyclette** to cycle, go (bi)cycling (8); **faire de la peinture (de la musique, de la poterie)** to paint (play music, do ceramics); **faire de la planche à voile** to go windsurfing; **faire de la plongée sous-marine** to go scuba diving (8); **faire de la politique** to go in for politics; **faire de la voile** to go sailing (5); **faire de l'aérobic** to do aerobics (5); **faire de l'alpinisme** to go mountain climbing (8); **faire de l'équitation** to go horseback riding (8); **faire des économies** to save (up) money (14); **faire des études** to study; **faire des glissades** *Q.* to go tobogganing; **faire des moulinets avec les bras** to whirl one's arms about; **faire des projets** to make plans; **faire des recherches** to do research; **faire dorer** to brown (*in cooking*); **faire du bateau** to go boating (8); **faire du bruit** to make noise; **faire du camping** to camp, go camping; **faire du cheval** to go horseback riding (8); **faire du covoiturage** to carpool, rideshare; **faire du jogging** to run, jog (5); **faire du magasinage** *Q.* to go shopping; **faire du patin à glace** to go ice-skating; **faire du patin à roues alignées** to do in-line skating; **faire du recyclage** to recycle; **faire du shopping** to go shopping; **faire du ski (alpin)** to ski (downhill) (5); **faire du ski de fond** to go cross-country skiing; **faire du ski nautique** to go waterskiing; **faire du snowboard** to go snowboarding; **faire du soleil (il fait du soleil)** to be sunny (it's sunny) (5); **faire du sport** to play, do sports (5); **faire du théâtre** to act; **faire du tourisme** to go sightseeing; **faire du vélo (de montagne)** to go cycling (mountain biking) (5); **faire du vent (il fait du vent)** to be windy (it's windy) (5); **faire escale à** to stop over at; **faire faire** to have done, make (*s.o.*) do (*s.th.*); **faire frais (il fait frais)** to be cool (out) (it's cool) (5); **faire froid (il fait froid)** to be cold (out) (it's cold) (5); **faire grève** to strike, go on strike (16); **faire la bise** to kiss on both cheeks (*in greeting*); **faire la connaissance de** to meet (*for the first time*) (5); **faire la cuisine** to cook (5); **faire la fête** to party; **faire la lessive** to do the laundry (5); **faire la queue** to stand in line (5); **faire la sieste** to take a nap; **faire la vaisselle** to wash (do) the dishes (5); **faire le lit** to make the bed; **faire le marché** to do the shopping, go to the market (5); **faire le ménage** to do the housework (5); **faire le plein** to fill it up (gas tank) (9); **faire le tour de** to go around; to tour; **faire les courses** to do errands (5); **faire les valises** to pack one's bags; **faire mauvais (il fait mauvais)** to be bad weather (out) (it's bad out) (5); **faire partie de** to belong to; **faire preuve de** to show; **faire ses devoirs** to do one's homework (5); **faire son possible** to do one's best; **faire un chèque** to write a check (14); **faire un pique-nique** to go on a picnic; **faire un safari** to go on a safari; **faire un temps pourri** *fam.* to be rotten weather; **faire un tour (en voiture)** to take a walk (ride) (5); **faire un voyage** to take a trip (5); **faire une erreur** to make a mistake; **faire une excursion** to go on an outing; **faire une promenade** to take a walk (5); **faire une randonnée (pédestre)** to go hiking (8); **faire une réservation** to make a reservation; **faire une visite** to pay a visit; **quel temps fait-il?** how's the weather? (5)
fait *m.* fact; *adj.* made; **tout à fait** *adv.* completely, entirely
falaise *f.* cliff
falloir (*p.p.* **fallu**) *irreg.* to be necessary (8); to be lacking; **il faut** + *inf.* it is necessary to, one must; one needs (8)
fameux/euse *adj.* famous
familial *adj.* family
famille *f.* family (5); **en famille** with one's family; **fonder une famille** to start a family
fanatique (*fam.* **fan**) *m., f.* fan; fanatic, zealot
fanatisme *m.* fanaticism
fantaisie: bijoux (*m. pl.*) **fantaisie** costume jewelry
fantaisiste *adj.* fanciful, whimsical
fantôme *m.* ghost
Far (*m.*) **breton** traditional cake from Brittany
farine *f.* flour
fascinant *adj.* fascinating
fasciné *adj.* fascinated
fatal *adj.* fatal; unlucky; fateful
fatigant *adj.* tiring
fatigué *adj.* tired (3)
fauché *adj., fam.* broke, without money
se faufiler to creep; to thread one's way; to sidle
faut (il) it is necessary to, one must; one needs (8)
faute *f.* fault, mistake
fauteuil *m.* armchair
faux (fausse) *adj.* false (4)
faveur: en faveur de in favor of
favorable: être favorable à to be in favor of (favorably disposed to)
favori(te) *adj.* favorite
favoriser to further, favor
fax *m.* fax (10)
fée *f.* fairy; **conte** (*m.*) **de fée** fairy tale
félicitations *f. pl.* congratulations
féminin *adj.* feminine; female
femme *f.* woman (2); wife (5); **femme d'affaires** businesswoman; **femme d'état** stateswoman; **femme écrivain** writer (12); **femme médecin** doctor, physician (14); **femme peintre** painter (12); **femme poète** poet (12); **femme politique** politician; **femme sculpteur** sculptor (12); **jeune femme** young woman (3)
fenêtre *f.* window (1)
fente *f.* slot
fer *m.* iron; **chemin** (*m.*) **de fer** railroad
ferme *f.* farm
fermer to close
fermeture *f.* closing
fermier/ière *m., f.* farmer
ferraille *f.* scrap iron, metal
ferroviaire *adj.* rail, railroad
fête *f.* holiday; celebration, party (7); saint's day, name day; *pl.* Christmas season; **faire la fête** to party; **fête des patrons** saint's day; **fête des Rois** Feast of the Magi, Epiphany; **jour** (*m.*) **de fête** holiday
fêter to celebrate; to observe a holiday
feu (*pl.* **feux**) *m.* fire; traffic light; **à feu doux** on low heat (*cooking*); **feux d'artifice** fireworks
feuille *f.* leaf
feuilleté *adj.* flaky (*pastry*)
feuilleton *m.* soap opera (10)

fève *f.* bean
février February (1)
fez *m.* fez (*feltcap*)
fiable *adj.* reliable
fiançailles *f. pl.* engagement (13)
fiancé(e) *m., f.* fiancé, fiancée
se fiancer (nous nous fiançons) to get engaged (13)
fibre *f.* fiber, filament
fiche *f.* index card; form (to fill out); deposit slip
fichier *m.* file (10)
fictif/ive *adj.* fictitious; imaginary
fier/ière *adj.* proud (3)
fierté *f.* pride
fièvre *f.* fever
figure *f.* figure, important person
figurer to appear
fil *m.*: **coup** (*m.*) **de fil** telephone call
filer to trail, follow
filet *m.* fillet (*fish, meat*) (7); **filet de porc (de bœuf)** pork (beef) fillet
filiale *f.* subsidiary; branch (*office*)
fille *f.* girl (3); daughter (5); **jeune fille** girl, young lady; **petite-fille** granddaughter (5)
film *m.* movie, film (2)
fils *m.* son (5); **petit-fils** grandson (5)
filtrage *m.* filtration, filtering
fin *f.* end; **à la fin de** at the end of; **en fin d'après-midi** in the late afternoon; **fin 1996** at the end of 1996; *adj.* fine, delicate; **extra-fin** *adj.* superfine; **mi-fin** *adj.* medium-cut (*vegetables*)
finalement *adv.* finally
finaliser to complete
finance *f.* finance; *pl.* finances
financier/ière *adj.* financial, monetary
finir (de) to finish (4); **finir par** to end (finish) by (*doing s.th.*) (4)
Finlande *f.* Finland
firme *f.* firm, company
fiscalité *f.* tax system, taxes
fixer to fasten; to make firm
flacon *m.* small bottle (*with stopper*)
flamand *m.* Flemish (*language*)
flâner to stroll (12)
flash (d'informations) *m.* newsbrief
flatté *adj.* flattered
fleur *f.* flower (4); **chou-fleur** *m.* cauliflower; **fleur de lys** fleur de lis, trefoil
fleurette *f.* floret
fleurir to flower; to flourish
fleuve *m.* (*large*) river (8)
Floride *f.* Florida
flûte *f.* flute
foie *m.* liver; **pâté** (*m.*) **de foie gras** goose liver pâté
foire *f.* fair, exhibition; marketplace
fois *f.* time, occasion; times (*arithmetic*); **à la fois** at the same time; **la première (dernière) fois** the first (last) time; **une fois** once (11); **une fois par semaine** once a week (5)
folklorique *adj.* traditional; folk (*music, etc.*)
foncé *adj.* dark
fonction *f.* function, use
fonctionnaire *m., f.* civil servant (14)
fonctionner to function, work
fond *m.* bottom; background; back; **ski** (*m.*) **de fond** cross-country skiing (8)
fondamental *adj.* fundamental, basic
fondateur/trice *m., f.* founder
fondation *f.* founding, inception
fonder to found; **fonder une famille** to start a family
fonds *m. pl.* fund
fondre to melt
fondue *f.* fondue (*Swiss melted cheese dish*)
fontaine *f.* fountain
fonte *f.* cast iron
football (*fam.* **foot**) *m.* soccer; **football américain** football; **match** (*m.*) **de foot** soccer game
footballeur/euse *m., f.* soccer player
footing *m.* jogging
force *f.* strength; **à force de** as a result of; **en force** in force; **force est de** + *inf.* one must
forcément *adv.* necessarily
forcer (nous forçons) to force, compel
forêt *f.* forest (8)
forgé: fer (*m.*) **forgé** wrought iron
formalité *f.* formality
formation *f.* education, training
forme *f.* form; shape; figure; **en (bonne, pleine) forme** physically fit; **en forme de** in the form of; **sous forme de** in the form of
formel(le) *adj.* formal
formellement *adv.* positively, categorically
former to form, shape; to train
formidable terrific, great
formule *f.* formula; plan
formuler to formulate, make up
fort *adj.* strong; heavy; *adv.* strongly; loudly; very (14); **parler fort** to speak loudly
fortifier to fortify
fou (fol, folle) *adj.* crazy, mad; **fou (folle)** *m., f.* insane (crazy) person
foudre *f.* lightning; **coup** (*m.*) **de foudre** flash of lightning (13); love at first sight (13)
foulard *m.* scarf
foule *f.* crowd (15)
fourchette *f.* fork (6)
fournir to furnish, supply
fournisseur (*m.*) **d'accès** service provider (*Internet*)
foyer *m.* hearth; home; student residence; **femme** (*f.*) **au foyer** homemaker
frais *m., pl.* expenses, costs (14); **frais de scolarité** school, university (tuition) fees
frais (fraîche) *adj.* cool; fresh (6); **crème fraîche** clotted cream, crème fraîche; **faire frais (il fait frais)** to be cool (out) (it's cool) (5); **produits** (*m.*) **frais** fresh products (6)
fraise *f.* strawberry (6)
framboise *f.* raspberry
franc(he) *adj.* frank; fruitful; honest
français *adj.* French; *m.* French (*language*); **Français(e)** *m., f.* Frenchman (-woman) (2)
France *f.* France (2, 8)
franchement *adv.* frankly (12)
franchir to cross
francophile *m., f.* Francophile (*person who admires France or the French*)
francophone *adj.* French-speaking
francophonie *f.* French-speaking world
frangin(e) *m., f. fam.* brother (sister)
frapper to strike
fraternité *f.* brotherhood, fraternity
fredonner to hum
freinage *m.* braking system (*auto*)
fréquemment *adv.* frequently, often
fréquent *adj.* frequent, common
fréquenter to go to often
frère *m.* brother (5); **beau-frère** brother-in-law (5); **demi-frère** half brother; stepbrother (5)
fric *m., fam.* money
fricassée *f.* (chicken) stew; fricassee
frigo *m., fam.* fridge, refrigerator
fringue *f., fam.* clothes
fripe *f. s.* secondhand clothing
frisé *adj.* curly
frites *f. pl.* French fries (6); **moules** (*f.*)**-frites** mussels with French fries; **steak** (*m.*)**-frites** steak with French fries
froid *adj.* cold; *m.* cold; **avoir froid** to be cold (3); **faire froid (il fait froid)** to be cold (out) (it's cold) (5)
fromage *m.* cheese (6)
front *m.* forehead
frontière *f.* border
frotter to rub
fruit *m.* fruit (6); **jus** (*m.*) **de fruit** fruit juice
fumer to smoke (2)
fumeur/euse *m., f.* smoker; **zone** (*f.*) **fumeurs (non-fumeurs)** smoking (nonsmoking) section
furax *adj., fam.* angry, furious
furieux/euse *adj.* furious (16)
fusée *f.* rocket
fût *m., fam.* pair of pants
futur *m., Gram.* future (*tense*); *adj.* future
futuriste *adj.* futuristic

gabarit *m.* size, stature
gagner to win; to earn (14); **gagner du temps** to save time
gai *adj.* cheerful
galère: C'était la galère! *fam.* It was hell!
galerie *f.* gallery; roof rack (*auto*)
galette *f.* pancake; tart, pie
gant *m.* glove (8)
garagiste *m., f.* mechanic, garage owner
garanti *adj.* guaranteed
garçon *m.* boy (3); café waiter
garder to keep, retain; **garder la ligne** to keep one's figure
gardien(ne) *m., f.* guard
gare *f.* station; train station (9); **buffet** (*m.*) **de la gare** train station restaurant (9); **gare de chargement** loading dock
garer to park; **se garer** to be parked
gars *m., fam.* guy; boy
gaspillage *m.* wasting, waste (16)
gaspiller to waste (16)
gastronome *m., f.* gourmet
gastronomie *f.* gastronomy, good food
gastronomique *adj.* gastronomic
gâteau *m.* cake (6)
gâter to spoil
gauche *adj.* left; *f.* left; **à gauche (de)** *prep.* on the (to the) left (of) (4); **Rive** (*f.*) **gauche** Left Bank (*in Paris*) (11); **se lever du pied gauche** to get up on the wrong side of the bed
gaz *m.* gas
gazeux/euse: boisson (*f.*) **gazeuse** soft drink (6)
gênant *adj.* bothersome, annoying
gendre *m.* son-in-law (5)
généalogique *adj.* genealogical; family
général *m., adj.* general; **en général** generally (2); **quartier** (*m.*) **général** headquarters
généraliste *m., f.* general practitioner (MD)
générer (je génère) to generate

généreux/euse *adj.* generous
génétique *adj.* genetic
Genève Geneva
génial *adj.* brilliant, inspired; *fam.* neat, delightful, cool
génie *m.* genius; engineering (2)
genou (*pl.* **genoux**) *m.* knee (13)
genre *m.* type, style, kind
gens *m. pl.* people; **jeunes gens** young men; young people
gentil(le) *adj.* nice, pleasant; kind (3)
gentillesse *f.* kindness, niceness
gentiment *adv.* nicely
géographe *m., f.* geographer
géographie (*fam.* **géo**) *f.* geography (2)
géographique *adj.* geographical
géologie *f.* geology (2)
géométrie *f.* geometry
Géorgie *f.* Georgia (*country*)
gerbe: donner la gerbe à (*qqn*) to make (*s.o.*) want to vomit
gérer (je gère) to manage (14)
geste *m.* gesture
gestion *f.* management
gigantesque *adj.* gigantic
gingembre *m.* ginger
girofle *m.* cloves
glace *f.* ice cream (6); ice; mirror; **patin** (*m.*) **à glace** ice-skating
glacé: crème (*f.*) **glacée** *Q.* ice cream
glissade: faire des glissades *Q.* to go tobogganing
se glisser to slip into
gloire *f.* glory
glorieux/euse *adj.* glorious
glorifier to glorify
golfe *m.* gulf
gomme *f.* eraser
gommier *m.* gum tree
gorge *f.* throat (13); gorge; **avoir mal à la gorge** to have a sore throat (13)
gosse *m., f. fam.* kid, child
gothique *adj.* Gothic (12)
gourmand(e) *adj.* gluttonous, greedy; *m., f.* glutton, gourmand
gousse (*m.*): **gousse d'ail** clove of garlic
goût *m.* taste; **avant-goût** *m.* foretaste
goûter *m.* afternoon snack (6); *v.* to taste; to eat (7)
goutte *f.* drop (*liquid*)
gouvernement *m.* government (16)
gouverner to rule; to govern
gouverneur *m.* governor
grâce *f.* grace; pardon; **jour** (*m.*) **d'action de grâce** Thanksgiving Day; **grâce à** thanks to
gramme *m.* gram
grammaire *f.* grammar
grand *adj.* great; large, tall; big (3); **arrière-grand-parent** *m.* great-grandparent; **grand magasin** *m.* department store; **grand-maman** *f.* grandma, granny; **grand-mère** *f.* grandmother (5); **grand-parent** (*pl.* **grands-parents**) *m.* grandparent (5); **grand-père** *m.* grandfather (5); **grande surface** *f.* mall; superstore; **grandes écoles** *f. pl. French government graduate schools*; **grandes vacances** *f. pl.* summer vacation (from school); **Train** (*m.*) **à grande vitesse (TGV)** (*French high-speed*) bullet train
grandeur *f.* size
grandir to grow; to grow up
gras(se) *adj.* fat; oily; rich; **en caractères gras** in boldface print; **pâté** (*m.*) **de foie gras** goose liver pâté
gratin *m.* gratin, cheese-topped dish
gratte-ciel *m., inv.* skyscraper
gratuit *adj.* free (*of charge*) (11)
grave *adj.* grave, serious; **accent** (*m.*) **grave** grave accent **(è)**
gravure *f.* printing, engraving
Grèce *f.* Greece (8)
grec(que) *adj.* Greek
greffe *f.* transplant
grenouille *f.* frog
grève *f.* strike, walkout (16); **faire grève** to strike (16)
griffe *f.* claw
grille *f.* grid
grillé *adj.* toasted; grilled; broiled
griller: faire griller to broil; to toast
grimpeur/euse *m., f.* climber
grippe *f.* flu, influenza
gris *adj.* gray (3)
gros(se) *adj.* large; fat; thick (4); **grosses bises (gros bisous)** *fam.* hugs and kisses (*closing of letter*)
grossir to gain weight
guéri *adj.* cured, healed (13)
guérison *f.* recovery
guerre *f.* war (16); **Première (Deuxième [Seconde]) Guerre mondiale** First (Second) World War
guetter to watch out for, be on the lookout for
guichet *m.* (ticket) window (9); counter, booth; **guichet automatique** automatic teller machine (ATM) (14)
guide *m., f.* guide; *m.* guidebook; instructions
Guinée *f.* Guinea
guirlande *f.* garland; Christmas lights
guitare *f.* guitar (4); **jouer de la guitare** to play the guitar
Guyane *f.* Guyana
gym (*ab.* **gymnastique**) *f.* fitness training
gymnase *m.* gymnasium (2)

habilement *adv.* skillfully
s'habiller to get dressed (13)
habit *m.* clothing, dress
habitacle *m.* passenger compartment
habitant(e) *m., f.* inhabitant; resident
habitation *f.* lodging, housing; **habitations à loyer modéré (H.L.M.)** *publicly subsidized apartment blocks* (*France*)
habiter to live (2)
habitude *f.* habit; **d'habitude** *adv.* usually, habitually (5)
habitué (à) *adj.* accustomed (to)
habituel(le) *adj.* usual
***hacher** to chop (up)
haïr to hate
Haïti *m.* Haiti (8)
***harceler** to harass, torment
***hardi** *adj.* bold, daring
***haricot** *m.* bean; **haricots** (*pl.*) **mange-tout** string beans; sugar peas; **haricots verts** green beans (6)
***harissa** *m., f.* hot chili sauce
***hasard** *m.* chance, luck; **jeux** (*m. pl.*) **de hasard** games of chance (15); **par hasard** by accident, by chance
***hasardeux/euse** *adj.* dangerous, hazardous
***hâte** *f.* haste; **à la hâte** hastily
***haut** *adj.* high; higher; tall; upper; *m.* top; height; **à voix haute** *adv.* in a loud voice, aloud; **de haut** high (*in measuring*); **du haut de** from the top of; **haute couture** *f.* high fashion; **là-haut** *adv.* up there
***hauteur** *f.* height
hébergement *m.* lodging, accommodations; shelter
héberger (nous hébergeons) to shelter
hectare *m.* hectare (slightly less than 2.5 acres)
hein? *interj.* eh?
hélas *interj.* alas
hépatite *f.* hepatitis
herbe *f.* herb
héritage *m.* legacy, inheritance
héritier *m.* heir
***héros** *m.* (*f.* **héroïne**) hero, heroine
hésiter (à) to hesitate (to)
heure *f.* hour; time; **à l'heure** on time (9); per hour; **à n'importe quelle heure** at any time; **à quelle heure... ?** (at) what time . . . ? (6); **à tout à l'heure** see you soon; **dans une heure** in one hour; **de bonne heure** early (6); **de l'heure** an hour, per hour; **demi-heure** *f.* half hour; **il est... heure(s)** it is . . . o'clock (6); **il est l'heure de** + *inf.* it's time to . . . ; **quelle heure est-il?** what time is it? (6); **tout à l'heure** in a while (5)
heureusement *adv.* fortunately, luckily
heureux/euse *adj.* happy; fortunate (3)
Hexagone *m.* (metropolitan) France
hic *m., fam.* snag, problem
hier *adv.* yesterday (7); **avant-hier** day before yesterday (7); **hier matin** yesterday morning; **hier soir** last night (7)
histoire *f.* history (2); story
historien(ne) *m., f.* historian
historique *adj.* historical (12)
hiver *m.* winter; **en hiver** in the winter (5)
H.L.M. (habitations à loyer modéré) *f. pl. publicly subsidized apartment blocks* (*France*)
hollandais *adj.* Dutch
***homard** *m.* lobster
hommage *m.* homage, respects; **en hommage à** in recognition of
homme *m.* man (2); **homme d'affaires** businessman; **homme politique** politician; **jeune homme** young man (3)
honnête *adj.* honest
honorer to honor
***honte** *f.* shame; **avoir honte (de)** to be ashamed (of) (3)
hop: et hop! *interj.* bingo!
hôpital *m.* hospital (11)
horaire *m.* schedule (12)
horodateur *m.* parking ticket machine
horreur *f.* horror; **avoir horreur de** to hate, detest; **j'ai horreur de...** I can't stand . . .
***hors de** *prep.* outside, beyond
***hors-d'œuvre** *m. inv.* appetizer (7)
hospitalier/ière *adj.* hospitable
hôtel *m.* hotel (11); **hôtel de ville** town hall, city hall
hôtellerie *f.* hotel business or management
hôtesse *f.* hostess; **hôtesse de l'air** flight attendant (9)
huile *f.* oil; **huile de tournesol** sunflower seed oil; **huile d'olive** olive oil (7); **sardines** (*f. pl.*) **à l'huile** sardines in oil (7)
***huit** *adj.* eight (1)
***huitième** *m.* one-eighth; *adj.* eighth (11)
huître *f.* oyster (7)

humain *adj.* human; *m.* human being; **corps** (*m.*) **humain** human body; **sciences** (*f. pl.*) **humaines** social sciences
humanitaire *adj.* humanitarian
humeur *f.* mood; temperament
humidité *f.* humidity, dampness
humour *m.* humor
hybride *adj.* hybrid; **voiture** (*f.*) **hybride** hybrid car (16)
s'hydrater to become hydrated
hymne *m.* hymn
hypocrisie *f.* hypocrisy
hypocrite *adj.* hypocritical (3)

ici *adv.* here (2)
idéal *m.* ideal; *adj.* ideal (3)
idéaliste *m., f.* idealist; *adj.* idealistic (3)
idée *f.* idea; **idées extrémistes** extremist ideas (16)
identifier to identify
identité *f.* identity; **carte** (*f.*) **d'identité** ID card (8)
idiome *m.* language
ignorer to not know; to have no experience of
il *pron., m. s.* he; it; there; **il faut** + *inf.* it is necessary to; one needs (8); **il n'y a pas de quoi** *interj.* you're welcome (7); **il y a** there is/are (1); ago; **il y a... que** for (*period of time*); it's been . . . since; **y a-t-il... ?** is/are there . . . ? (1)
île *f.* island (11)
illimité *adj.* unlimited
illuminer to light up
illustrer to illustrate
ils *pron., m. pl.* they
image *f.* picture, image
imaginer to imagine
imiter to imitate
immédiatement *adv.* immediately
immeuble *m.* apartment or office building (4)
immigré(e) *m., f.* immigrant
imparfait *m., Gram.* imperfect (*verb tense*)
impatience *f.* impatience; **avec impatience** impatiently
impératif *m., Gram.* imperative, command
impératrice *f.* empress
imperméable *m.* raincoat (3)
impersonnel(le) *adj.* impersonal
s'implanter to take hold
impliqué *adj.* implicated, involved
important *adj.* important (3); large, great; **il est important que** + *subj.* it's important that (16)
importer to import; to matter; **n'importe (où)** any(where)
imposer to impose
impossible *adj.* impossible; **il est impossible que** + *subj.* it's impossible that (16)
impôts *m. pl.* (*direct*) taxes (16)
impressionnant *adj.* impressive
impressionné *adj.* impressed
impressionnisme *m.* impressionism (*art*)
impressionniste *m., f., adj.* impressionist (*art*)
imprévisible *adj.* unpredictable
imprimante *f.* (*computer*) printer (10)
imprimer to print
improviste: à l'improviste unexpectedly, without warning
inacceptable *adj.* unacceptable
inaugurer to unveil
incarner to embody
incendie *f.* blaze, fire
incertitude *f.* uncertainty
inclure (*p.p.* **inclus**) *irreg.* to include
inconfortable *adj.* uncomfortable
inconnu *adj.* unknown
incontestablement *adv.* unquestionably
inconvénient *m.* disadvantage
incorporer to incorporate
incroyable *adj.* unbelievable, incredible
Inde *f.* India
indéfini *adj.* indefinite; **pronom** (*m.*) **indéfini** *Gram.* indefinite pronoun
indéniable *adj.* undeniable
indépendance *f.* independence; **fête** (*f.*) **de l'Indépendance** Independence Day
indépendant *adj.* independent; **travailleur/euse** (*m., f.*) **indépendant(e)** self-employed worker (14)
indicatif *m., Gram.* indicative
indication *f.* instruction(s)
indice *m.* indication, sign
indicible *adj.* inexpressible
indiquer to show, point out (15)
indirect *adj.* indirect; **pronom** (*m.*) **d'objet indirect** *Gram.* indirect object pronoun
indiscrèt *adj.* indiscreet
indispensable *adj.* indispensable; **il est indispensable que** + *subj.* it's indispensable that (16)
individu *m.* individual
individualisé *adj.* individualized
individualiste *adj.* individualistic, nonconformist (3)
industrialisé *adj.* industrialized
industrie *f.* industry
industriel(le) *adj.* industrial (16); *m.* manufacturer; **déchets** (*m. pl.*) **industriels** toxic waste (16)
inédit *adj.* original
inégalité *f.* inequality
inertie *f.* inertia
inexact *adj.* incorrect
inférer (j'infère) to infer
infernal *adj.* terrible
infini *adj.* infinite
infinitif *m., Gram.* infinitive
infirmier/ière *m., f.* (hospital) nurse
influencer (nous influençons) to influence
infographie *f.* computer graphics
informaticien(ne) *m., f.* computer scientist
information *f.* (*fam.* **info**) information; *pl.* (*fam.* **infos**) news (broadcast) (10); **flash** (*m.*) **d'informations** newsbrief
informatique *f., adj.* computer science (2)
informé *adj.* informed; **bien (mal) informé** well (badly) informed
informel(le) *adj.* informal
informer to inform
ingénieur *m.* engineer (14)
inhabituel(le) *adj.* unusual
initiateur/trice *m., f.* innovator, pioneer
initiation *f.* initiation, introduction
initiative: syndicat (*m.*) **d'initiative** (local) chamber of commerce; tourist information bureau (11)
initier (à) to introduce (*s.o.*) (to) (*activity, sport, cuisine, etc.*)
injure *f.* insult
injuste *adj.* unjust, unfair; **il est injuste que** + *subj.* it's unfair that (16)
innovant *adj.* innovative
inondation *f.* flood
inoubliable *adj.* unforgettable
inquiéter (j'inquiète) to trouble, concern, worry; to threaten
inquiétude *f.* worry
inscription *f.* inscription; matriculation; registration
inscrire (*like* **écrire**) *irreg.* to inscribe; **s'inscrire (à)** to join; to enroll; to register
insister to insist; **insister sur** to stress; to emphasize
insolite *adj.* unusual
inspirer to inspire; **s'inspirer de** to be inspired by
installation *f.* moving in; installation
installer to install; to set up; **s'installer** to settle down, settle in (13); to settle in (*to a new house*)
instant *m.* moment
instantané *adj.* instant
instituer to institute, set up
instituteur/trice *m., f.* elementary (primary) school teacher
instructeur/trice *m., f.* instructor
instrument *m.* instrument; **jouer d'un instrument** to play a musical instrument (3)
insuffisant *adj.* insufficient
insupportable *adj.* unbearable, insufferable
intègre *adj.* honest, upright
s'intégrer (je m'intègre) (à) to integrate oneself, get assimilated (into)
intégrisme *m.* fundamentalism (16)
intellectuel(le) *adj.* intellectual (3); *m., f.* intellectual (*person*)
intelligemment *adv.* intelligently
intempéries *f. pl.* bad weather
intention *f.* intention; meaning; **avoir l'intention de** to intend to
interdiction *f.* prohibition
interdire (*like* **dire, vous interdisez**) *irreg.* to forbid; to prohibit
interdit *adj.* forbidden; prohibited
intéressant *adj.* interesting (3)
intéresser to interest (14); **s'intéresser à** to be interested in
intérêt *m.* interest, concern
interlocuteur/trice *m., f.* speaker, interlocutor
internaute *m., f.* Internet user
Internet *m.* Internet (10); **sur Internet** on the Internet (10)
interprète *m., f.* singer, performer
interrogatif/ive *adj., Gram.* interrogative
interroger (sur) (nous interrogeons) to question, ask (about)
intervenir (*like* **venir**) *irreg.* to intervene
intervention *f.* intervention; speech; operation
interview *f.* interview (*journalism*)
interviewé(e) *m., f.* interviewee
interviewer to interview
intime *adj.* intimate; private; **journal** (*m.*) **intime** private diary
intimité *f.* intimacy
intouchable *adj.* untouchable
introduire to introduce
intrus(e) *m., f.* intruder
inutile *adj.* useless; **il est inutile que** + *subj.* it's useless that (16)
inventaire *m.* inventory
inventer to invent
inverser to reverse
investir to invest; **s'investir** to invest oneself
invité(e) *m., f.* guest, invitee
inviter to invite
iPod *m.* iPod (4)
ironie *f.* irony

irrégulier/ière *adj.* irregular
irrésistible *adj.* compelling
irrité *adj.* irritated, sore
islamiste *m., f.* Islamist, Muslim
isolé *adj.* isolated, alone
isolement *m.* isolation, loneliness
issu *adj.* stemming from
Italie *f.* Italy (2, 8)
italien *adj.* Italian; *m.* Italian (*language*) (2); **Italien(ne)** *m., f.* Italian (*person*) (2)
italique *m.* italic; **en italique** in italics
itinéraire *m.* itinerary; **tracer un itinéraire** to map out an itinerary
ivoire *m.* ivory; **Côte d'Ivoire** *f.* Cote d'Ivoire
ivoirien(ne) *adj.* of (from) the Ivory Coast Republic; **Ivoirien(ne)** *m., f.* native (inhabitant) of the Ivory Coast Republic

jamais *adv.* ever; **ne… jamais** *adv.* never (9)
jambe *f.* leg (13)
jambon *m.* ham (6)
janvier January (1)
Japon *m.* Japan (2, 8)
japonais *adj.* Japanese; *m.* Japanese (*language*) (2); **Japonais(e)** *m., f.* Japanese person (2)
jardin *m.* garden (5)
jardinage *m.* gardening (15); **faire du jardinage** to garden
jaune *adj.* yellow (3)
je (j') *pron., s.* I
jean(s) *m.* (*blue*) jeans (3)
jésuite *adj., m.* Jesuit
jeter (je jette) to throw, throw away; **ne jetez plus** don't throw away any more
jeu (*pl.* **jeux**) *m.* game; game show; **jeu de mots** pun, play on words (15); **jeu télévisé** game show (10); **jeux de *hasard** games of chance (15); **jeux de société** board games, group games (15); **jeux vidéo** video games
jeudi *m.* Thursday (1); **le jeudi** on Thursdays (5)
jeune *adj.* young (4); *m. pl.* young people, youth; **jeune femme** *f.* young woman (3); **jeune fille** *f.* girl, young lady; **jeune homme** *m.* young man (3); **jeunes gens** *m. pl.* young men; young people; **jeunes mariés** *m. pl.* newlyweds, newly married couple
jeunesse *f.* youth, young people; **auberge** (*f.*) **de jeunesse** youth hostel (9)
job *m.* job; odd job; **job d'été** summer job
Joconde: la Joconde *Mona Lisa*
jogging *m.* jogging; **faire du jogging** to run, jog (5)
joie *f.* joy
joindre (*p.p.* **joint**) *irreg.* to join; to reach; to attach; to add
joint *adj.* connected, reachable
joli *adj.* pretty (4)
jouer to play (3); **jouer à** to play (*a sport or game*) (3); to play at (*being*); **jouer de** to play (*a musical instrument*) (3); **jouer un rôle** to play a role
jouet *m.* toy
joueur/euse *m., f.* player
jour *m.* day (1); **au jour le jour** from day to day; **chaque jour** every day; **dans quatre jours** in four days (5); **de nos jours** these days, nowadays, currently; **du jour** today's (*menu, exchange rate*); **jour d'action de grâce** Thanksgiving Day; **par jour** per day, each day; **plat** (*m.*) **du jour** today's special (*restaurant*); **quel jour est-ce (aujourd'hui)?** what day is it today? (1); **quel jour sommes-nous?** what day is it? (1); **quinze jours** two weeks; **tous les jours** every day (5); **un jour** someday (14)
journal (*pl.* **journaux**) *m.* newspaper (2); **journal intime** private journal, diary; **journal télévisé** television news program (10)
journaliste *m., f.* reporter, journalist (2)
journée *f.* (*whole*) day (6)
joyau *m.* jewel
joyeux *adj.* joyful, merry
juger to judge
Juif/Juive *m., f.* Jewish person
juillet July (1)
juin June (1)
jupe *f.* skirt (3); **minijupe** *f.* miniskirt
jurer to swear
jus *m.* juice; **jus de fruit** fruit juice; **jus d'orange** orange juice (6)
jusqu'à (jusqu'en) *prep.* up to, as far as (11); until
juste *adj.* just; right, exact; *adv.* just, precisely; accurately; **il est juste que** + *subj.* it's fair (equitable) that (16)
justifier to justify

kabyle *m.* Kabylian (*language*)
kaki *adj. inv.* khaki
kasbah *m.* casbah (walled citadel of some Arab cities)
kawa *m., fam.* coffee
kif-kif: c'est kif-kif *fam.* (it's) all the same
kiffer *fam.* to like
kilo(gramme) (kg) *m.* kilogram (7)
kilomètre (km) *m.* kilometer
kiosque *m.* kiosk; newsstand (10)
KO *adj. inv.* exhausted

la (l') *art., f. s.* the; *pron., f. s.* it, her
là *adv.* there; **là-bas** *adv.* over there (10); **oh, là, là** *interj.* good heavens, my goodness
laboratoire (*fam.* **labo**) *m.* laboratory; **laboratoire de langues** language lab (2)
lac *m.* lake (8); **au bord du lac** on the lakeshore
lâcher to let go
laisser to let; to leave (*behind*) (7); **laisser** + *inf.* to let, allow
lait *m.* milk (6); **café** (*m.*) **au lait** coffee with hot milk
laitier/ière *adj.* dairy, milk
laitue *f.* lettuce (6)
lampe *f.* lamp (4); flashlight; **lampe torche** flashlight
lancer (nous lançons) to launch; to start up; **se lancer dans** to take on, embark on
langage *m.* language (system of symbols)
langue *f.* language; tongue; **apprentissage** (*m.*) **des langues** language learning; **laboratoire** (*m.*) **de langues** language lab (2); **langue étrangère** foreign language; **langue maternelle** native language; **langues vivantes** modern languages
lapin *m.* rabbit
large *adj.* wide; extensive; **au large de Dakar** off (of) Dakar
larme *f.* tear (drop)
las(se) weary (16)
latin: Quartier (*m.*) **latin** Latin Quarter (*in Paris*)
lauréat(e) *m., f.* (award) winner
laurier *m.* laurel, bay; **feuille** (*f.*) **de laurier** bay leaf
lavabo *m.* bathroom sink (4)
lavande *f.* lavender
lave-vaisselle *m.* (*automatic*) dishwasher
laver to wash; **se laver** to wash (*oneself*) (13); **se laver les mains** to wash one's hands
laveuse *f.* washing machine
le (l') *art., m. s.* the; *pron., m. s.* it, him
leçon *f.* lesson
lecteur/trice *m., f.* reader; *m.* disk drive; **lecteur de DVD** DVD player (1)
lecture *f.* reading (15)
légalisation *f.* legalization (16)
légendaire *adj.* legendary
légende *f.* legend
léger/ère *adj.* light; lightweight; slight; mild
légume *m.* vegetable (6)
lendemain *m.* day after
lent *adj.* slow
lequel (laquelle, lesquels, lesquelles) *pron.* which one, who, whom, which (15)
les *art., pl., m., f.* the; *pron., pl., m., f.* them
lessive *f.* laundry; **faire la lessive** to do the laundry (5)
lettre *f.* letter (10); *pl.* literature; humanities; **arts** (*m.*) **et lettres** humanities; **boîte** (*f.*) **aux lettres** mailbox (10); **faculté** (*f.*) **des lettres** School of Arts and Letters; **mettre une lettre à la poste** to mail a letter (10); **poster une lettre** to mail a letter
leur *adj., m., f.* their; *pron., m., f.* to them; **le/la/les leur(s)** *pron.* theirs
lever (je lève) to raise, lift; **levez la main** raise your hand; **se lever** to get up; to get out of bed (13)
levier *m.* lever
lèvres *f. pl.* lips; **rouge** (*m.*) **à lèvres** lipstick (13)
lézard *m.* lizard
liaison *f.* liaison; love affair
Liban *m.* Lebanon (2, 8)
libanais *adj.* Lebanese; **Libanais(e)** *m., f.* Lebanese person (2)
libéral *adj.* liberal; **professions** (*f. pl.*) **libérales** professions (*private practice*)
libérer (je libère) to free
liberté *f.* freedom; **liberté d'expression** freedom of expression (16)
librairie *f.* bookstore (2)
libre *adj.* free; available; vacant; **plongée** (*f.*) **libre** snorkeling (8); **temps** (*m.*) **libre** leisure time (15); **union** (*f.*) **libre** cohabitation, common-law marriage
libre-service *m. inv.* self-service
Libye *f.* Libya
licence *f.* French university degree (*U.S. bachelor's degree*)
lien *m.* tie, bond, link
lier to link
lieu *m.* place (2); **au lieu de** *prep.* instead of, in the place of; **avoir lieu** to take place
ligne *f.* line; bus line; figure; **couper la ligne** to cut off (*phone call*); **en ligne** online; **garder la ligne** to keep one's figure; **ligne de but** goal, goal line; **ligne fixe** (telephone) landline
lilas *m. inv.* lilac
limite *f.* limit, deadline; **limite de vitesse** speed limit
limiter to limit
limonade *f.* lemonade; soft drink

linge *m.* laundry
linguiste *m., f.* linguist
linguistique *f.* linguistics (2)
liqueur *f.* liquor; liqueur
liquide *m., adj.* liquid; cash; **argent** (*m.*) **liquide** cash (14)
lire (*p.p.* **lu**) *irreg.* to read (10)
liseuse *f.* e-reader (10)
lisible *adj.* legible
liste *f.* list
lit *m.* bed (4); **faire son lit** to make one's bed; **wagon-lit** *m.* sleeping car
litre *m.* liter
littéraire *adj.* literary
littérature *f.* literature (2)
livraison *f.* delivery
livre *m.* book (1); **livre numérique** e-book (10); **livre papier** print book (10)
locataire *m., f.* renter
location *f.* rental; rent (4)
logement *m.* lodging(s), place of residence (4)
loger to reside, live
logiciel *m.* software (program) (10); **logiciel de navigation** browser
logique *m.* logic; *adj.* logical
loi *f.* law
loin *adv.* far; **loin de** *prep.* far from (4)
loisir *m.* leisure; *pl.* leisure activities (15)
Londres London
long(ue) *adj.* long (3); **le long de** (all) along; **tout au long de** throughout
longtemps *adv.* (for) a long time; **il y a longtemps** a long time ago
lors de at the time of
lorsque *conj.* when
loterie *f.* lottery
loto *m.* lottery
louer to rent (4); to reserve; **à louer** for rent
Louisiane *f.* Louisiana
loup *m.* wolf
lourd *adj.* heavy
loyer *m.* rent (*payment*)
ludique *adj.* playful
lui *pron., m., f.* he; it; to him; to her; to it; **lui-même** *pron., m. s.* himself (12)
lumière *f.* light; **Siècle** (*m.*) **des lumières** Age of Enlightenment
lumineux: voyant lumineux *m.* indicator light
lundi *m.* Monday (1); **le lundi** on Mondays (5)
lune *f.* moon
lunettes *f. pl.* (eye)glasses (8); **lunettes de ski** ski goggles (8); **lunettes de soleil** sunglasses (8)
lutter to fight
luxe *m.* luxury
luxueux/euse *adj.* luxurious
lycée *m.* lycée (*French secondary school*)
lycéen(ne) *m., f.* secondary school student
lyonnais *adj.* of (from) Lyon
lyrique *adj.* lyrical
lys: fleur (*f.*) **de lys** fleur de lis, trefoil

ma *adj., f. s.* my; **pour ma part** in my opinion, as for me (16)
mâcher to chew
machine *f.* machine; **machine à café** coffee-maker; **machine à calculer** calculator; **machine à coudre** sewing machine
madame (Mme) (*pl.* **mesdames**) *f.* Madam, Mrs. (ma'am) (1)
mademoiselle (Mlle) (*pl.* **mesdemoiselles**) *f.* Miss (1)
magasin *m.* store, shop (3); **grand magasin** department store; **magasin d'alimentation** food store
magasinage *m., Q.* shopping; **faire du magasinage** to go shopping
magazine *m.* (*illustrated*) magazine (4)
Maghreb *m.* Maghreb, North Africa
maghrébin *adj.* from the Maghreb; North African
magique *adj.* magic, magical
magnifique *adj.* magnificent (12)
mai May (1)
maillot *m.* jersey, T-shirt; **maillot de bain** swimsuit (3); **maillot jaune** yellow jersey (*worn by current leader in the Tour de France*)
main *f.* hand (13); **sac** (*m.*) **à main** handbag, purse (3); **se laver les mains** to wash one's hands; **se serrer la main** to shake hands
maintenant *adv.* now (2); **à partir de maintenant** from now on (14)
maintenir to maintain
maintien *m.* keeping, upholding
maire *m.* mayor
mairie *f.* town (city) hall (11)
mais *conj.* but (2); **mais non** (but) of course not; **mais si** of course (*affirmative answer to negative question*)
maison *f.* house, home (4); company, firm; **à la maison** at home; **Maison-Blanche** *f.* White House; **maison d'édition** publishing company; **repas** (*m.*) **fait maison** home-made meal
maître (maîtresse) *m., f.* master (mistress)
maîtriser to master, have a command of (14)
majestueux/euse adj. majestic, stately
majeur *adj.* major
majoritairement *adv.* mostly, in the majority
majorité *f.* majority
mal *adv.* badly (1); *m.* evil; pain (*pl.* **maux**); **aller mal** to feel bad (ill); **avoir du mal à** to have trouble (difficulty); **avoir mal (à)** to hurt, have a pain; **avoir mal à la tête (au ventre)** to have a headache (stomachache) (13); **ça va mal** bad(ly) (things are going badly) (1); **(le) plus mal** worse (worst); **pas mal** not bad(ly) (1); **pas mal de** a lot of
malade *m., f.* sick person; patient; *adj.* sick (13)
maladie *f.* illness, disease; **assurances** (*f. pl.*) **maladie** health insurance
malaise *m.* uneasiness
malchance *f.* bad luck, misfortune
mâle *adj.* male
malgré *prep.* in spite of
malheur *m.* unhappiness
malheureusement *adv.* unfortunately; sadly
malheureux/euse *adj.* unhappy; miserable
maltraité *adj.* mistreated
maman *f., fam.* mom, mommy
mamie *f., fam.* grandma
mamours: se faire des mamours (*m. pl., fam.*) to bill and coo, neck, sweet-talk
mandat *m.* mandate, term in office
mange-tout: ***haricots** (*m. pl.*) **mange-tout** string beans; sugar peas
manger (nous mangeons) to eat (2); *n. m.* food; **salle** (*f.*) **à manger** dining room (5)
mangeur/euse *m., f.* eater
mangue *f.* mango
maniable *adj.* easy to handle, manageable
manier to wield; to handle
manière *f.* manner, way; **bonnes manières** good manners
manifestation (*fam.* **manif**) *f.* (*political*) demonstration; **manifestation sportive** sporting event (15)
manifester (pour, contre) to demonstrate (for, against) (16)
manne *f.* manna, godsend
mannequin *m.* fashion model
manque *m.* lack, shortage
manquer to lack; **manquer à** to be missed by
manteau *m.* coat, overcoat (3)
se maquiller to put on makeup (13)
marais *m.* marsh, swamp
marbre *m.* marble
marchand(e) *m., f.* merchant, shopkeeper; **marchand(e) de vin** wine merchant (14)
marchander to bargain
marche *f.* walking (15); step (*stair*)
marché *m.* market; deal, transaction; **bon marché** *adj. inv.* cheap, inexpensive; **faire le marché** to do the shopping, go to the market (5); **marché aux puces** flea market; **marché de l'emploi** job market (14); **marché en plein air** outdoor market
marcher to walk (13); to work (*machine, object*)
mardi *m.* Tuesday (1); **le mardi** on Tuesdays (5)
mari *m.* husband (5)
mariage *m.* marriage; wedding (13); **mariage à l'essai** trial marriage
marié *adj.* married (5); **nouveaux mariés** *m. pl.* newlyweds, newly married couple (13)
se marier (avec) to get married (to) (13)
marin *adj.* maritime, of the sea; **plongée** (*f.*) **sous-marine** scuba diving (8); **sous-marin** (*m.*) submarine
marmite *f.* soup pot
Maroc *m.* Morocco (2, 8)
marocain *adj.* Moroccan; **Marocain(e)** *m., f.* Moroccan (*person*) (2)
marque *f.* trade name, brand, make
marquer to mark; to indicate
marrant *adj., fam.* funny, hilarious
marre: avoir marre de *fam.* to be fed up with
se marrer to have a good time
marron *adj. inv.* brown (3); *m.* chestnut; **dinde** (*f.*) **aux marrons** turkey with chestnuts
mars March (1)
martiniquais *adj.* Martinican; **Martiniquais(e)** *m., f.* Martinican (*person*)
masculin *adj.* masculine
masque *m.* mask
masqué *adj.* masked
master *m.* masters degree (*in France*)
mât *m.* pole, climbing pole
match *m.* game (15); **match de foot(ball) (de rugby)** soccer game (rugby match)
matérialiste *adj.* materialistic
matériau (*pl.* **matériaux**) *m.* material; building material
matériel *m.* material(s); **matériel(le)** *adj.* material
maternel(le) *adj.* maternal; **(école)** (*f.*) **maternelle** nursery school, preschool; **langue** (*f.*) **maternelle** native language
maternité *f.* maternity, childbearing
mathématiques (*fam.* **maths**) *f. pl.* mathematics (2)

matière *f.* academic subject (2); material; **en matière de** in the matter of, as far as . . . is concerned
matin *m.* morning; **ce matin** this morning (5); **du matin** in the morning (6); **petit matin** early morning; **tous les matins** every morning (10)
matinal *adj.* morning
matinée *f.* morning (*duration*) (7)
mauvais *adj.* bad (4); **il fait mauvais** it's bad (weather) out (5); **le/la plus mauvais(e)** the worst; **plus mauvais(e)** worse
me (m') *pron., s.* me, to me, for me
mec *m., fam.* guy
mécanicien(ne) *m., f.* mechanic
mécanisme *m.* mechanism
médaille *f.* medal
médecin (femme médecin) *m., f.* doctor, physician (14); **médecin généraliste** general practitioner
médias *m. pl.* media (16)
médicament *m.* medication; drug
médiéval *adj.* medieval (12)
médina *f.* medina (old part of city in Morocco)
méditer to meditate
mégalithique *adj.* megalithic
meilleur *adj.* better (14); **le/la/les meilleur(e)(s)** the best
mél *m.* e-mail (10)
mélange *m.* mixture
mélanger (nous mélangeons) to mix
mêlée *f.* scrum (*rugby*)
se mêler to mingle
membre *m.* member
même *adj.* same (8); itself; very same; *adv.* even (8); **de même** *adv.* likewise; **en même temps** at the same time; **le/la/les même(s)** the same one(s) (15); **moi-même** *pron.* myself (12); **quand même** anyway, even so
mémoire *m.* memory; *pl.* memoirs
ménage *m.* housekeeping; household; **faire le ménage** to do the housework (5); **scène** (*f.*) **de ménage** domestic squabble
ménager/ère *adj.* household; **tâches** (*f. pl.*) **ménagères** household tasks
mener (je mène) (à) to lead (to)
mensuel(le) *adj.* monthly
menthe *f.* mint (*leaves*)
mentionner to mention
menton *m.* chin
menu *m.* menu; fixed-price menu (7)
mer *f.* sea, ocean (8); **au bord de la mer** at the seashore
merci *interj.* thank you (1); **merci beaucoup** thank you very much (1)
mercredi *m.* Wednesday (1); **le mercredi** on Wednesdays (5)
mère *f.* mother (5); **belle-mère** mother-in-law; stepmother (5); **grand-mère** grandmother (5)
méridien *m.* meridian
mérite *m.* merit, worth
mériter to deserve, be worth
merveille *f.* marvel; **à merveille** *adv.* marvelously
merveilleux/euse *adj.* wonderful
mes *adj., m., f., pl.* my
mesdames *f., pl.* ladies
message (*m.*) **électronique** e-mail message
messager/ère *m., f.* messenger
messe *f.* (*Catholic*) Mass
messieurs dames ladies and gentlemen
mesure *f.* measure; **dans une moindre mesure** to a lesser extent; **prendre des mesures** to take measures; **sur mesure** custom-made
météo *f., fam.* weather forecast (5)
méthode *f.* method
métier *m.* trade, profession (14); **armée** (*f.*) **de métier** professional army
métissage *m.* mixing of races
mètre *m.* meter
métro *m.* subway (*train, system*) (9); **station** (*f.*) **de métro** metro station (11)
métropole *m.* metropolis
métropolitain *adj.* metropolitan; from (of) mainland France
mets *m. s.* food, dish
metteur/euse (*m., f.*) **en scène** producer; film or theater director
mettre (*p.p.* **mis**) *irreg.* to place, put (10); to put on (10); to turn on; to take (*time*); to admit, grant; **mettre à mort** to put to death; **mettre en valeur** to emphasize; **mettre la table (le couvert)** to set the table (10); **mettre ses vêtements** to get dressed; **mettre une lettre à la poste** to mail a letter (10); **se mettre à** to begin to (*do s.th.*) (13)
meuble *m.* piece of furniture (5); **meubles d'époque** antique furniture
meublé *adj.* furnished
meuf *f., fam.* chick, woman, girl
meule *f., fam.* moped
meurs, meurt (see **mourir**)
mexicain *adj.* Mexican; **Mexicain(e)** *m., f.* Mexican (*person*) (2)
Mexico Mexico City
Mexique *m.* Mexico (2, 8)
mi-: (à la) mi-juin (in) mid-June
micro-ordinateur (*fam.* **micro**) *m.* desktop computer (10)
midi noon; Midi *m. south-central region of France*; **après-midi** *m.* or *f.* afternoon; **de l'après-midi** in the afternoon (6); **il est midi** it's noon (6)
miel *m.* honey
mien(ne)(s) (le/la/les) *pron., m., f.,* mine
mieux *adv.* better (15); **aimer mieux** to prefer (2); **il vaut mieux que** + *subj.* it's better that (16); **mieux (le mieux)** better (the best) (15); **tant mieux** so much the better (15)
mièvrerie *f.* sentimentality, soppiness, mush
mijoter to simmer
milieu *m.* environment; milieu, setting; middle; **au milieu de** in the middle of
militaire *adj.* military; **budget** (*m.*) **militaire** military budget (16)
militairement *adv.* militarily
militer pour (contre) to militate, argue for (against)
mille *adj.* thousand (7)
millénaire *m.* one thousand; millennium; *adj.* millennial
milliard *m.* billion (7)
milliardaire *m., f.* billionaire
millier *m.* (around) a thousand
million *m.* million (7)
mince *adj.* thin; slender
minceur *f.* leanness, slenderness
mine *f.* appearance, demeanor; mine; **vous n'avez pas bonne mine** you don't look well
minéral: eau (*f.*) **minérale** mineral water (6)
minier/ière *adj.* mining
minijupe *f.* miniskirt
ministre *m.* minister; **premier ministre** prime minister
minuit midnight; **il est minuit** it's midnight (6)
minute *f.* minute; **dans dix minutes** in ten minutes
miraculeux/euse *adj.* miraculous
miroir *m.* mirror (4)
mise *f.* placement; **mise à distance** separating; **mise en circulation** putting into circulation; **mise en place** placement
misère *f.* misery, poverty
missionnaire *m., f.* missionary
mixeur *m.* mixer
mixité *f.* diversity
mixte *adj.* mixed
mobile *m.* cell phone (10)
mobiliser to mobilize
mobilité *f.* mobility
mobylette *f.* moped
mode *f.* fashion, style; *m.* form, mode; *adj.* fashionable; **à la mode** in style; **créateur/trice** (*m., f.*) **de mode** fashion designer
modèle *m.* model; pattern
modéré *adj.* moderate; **habitations** (*f. pl.*) **à loyer modéré (H.L.M.)** *publicly subsidized apartment blocks* (*France*)
modernité *f.* modernity
modeste *adj.* modest, humble (3)
modifié *adj.* modified
moi *pron. s.* I, me; **c'est moi.** it's me (10); **chez moi** at my place; **excusez-moi** excuse me; **moi aussi** me too (3); **moi-même** *pron.* myself (12); **moi non plus** me neither (3); **selon moi** in my view
moindre *adj.* less, lesser; **dans une moindre mesure** to a lesser extent; **le/la/les moindre(s)** the least
moine *m.* monk
moins *adv.* less; minus; **au moins** at least; **le moins** the least; **moins de...** fewer than (*with numbers*); **moins le quart** quarter to (the hour) (6); **moins... que** less . . . than (14); **plus ou moins** more or less
mois *m.* month (1); **par mois** per month
moitié *f.* half
môme *m.,f., fam.* kid
moment *m.* moment; **au dernier moment** at the last moment; **au moment de partir** upon leaving; **en ce moment** now, currently; **pour le moment** for the moment
momie *f.* mummy
mon *adj., m. s.* my
monde *m.* world (8); people; society; **Coupe** (*f.*) **du Monde** World Cup (*soccer*); **Tiers-Monde** *m.* Third World; **tour** (*m.*) **du monde** trip around the world; **tout le monde** everybody, everyone (7)
mondial *adj.* world; worldwide; **Première (Deuxième [Seconde]) Guerre** (*f.*) **mondiale** First (Second) World War
mondialement *adv.* throughout the world
mondialisation *f.* globalization (16)
monétaire *adj.* monetary
moniteur *m.* monitor; screen (10)
monnaie *f.* coins, change (10); currency (*units*); **déposer la monnaie** to deposit change (10)
monsieur (M.) (*pl.* **messieurs**) *m.* Mister; gentleman; sir (1); **croque-monsieur** *m.* *grilled ham and cheese sandwich*

montagne *f.* mountain (8); **à la montagne** in the mountains; **chaussures** (*f.*) **de montagne** hiking boots (8); **faire du vélo de montagne** to go mountain biking
montant *m.* sum, amount (14); total
monter (dans) to set up, organize; to put on; to carry up; to go up; to climb (into) (8); **en montant à bord** embarking, getting on board
montre *f.* watch; wristwatch
montrer to show (3)
monumental *adj.* huge
moquer: se moquer de to make fun of (14)
moqueur/euse *adj.* mocking
moral *m.* morale, spirits
morale *f.* moral philosophy
moralement in one's morale; morally
moralité *f.* morals, morality
morceau *m.* piece (7); **morceau de gâteau** piece of cake
mordre to bite; **être mordu de** to be crazy about, smitten with
morosité *f.* gloominess, moroseness
morphinique *adj.* containing morphine
mort *f.* death; *adj.* dead; **mettre à mort** to put to death; **mort de fatigue** dead-tired; **nature** (*f.*) **morte** still life
mosaïque *f.* mosaic
mosquée *f.* mosque
mot *m.* word (1); **jeu** (*m.*) **de mots** pun, play on words (15); **mot apparenté** related word, cognate; **mot clé** key word
moteur (*m.*) **de recherche** search engine
motivation *f.* motive; **lettre** (*f.*) **de motivation** cover letter, letter in support of one's application
motivé *adj.* motivated
motocyclette (*fam.* **moto**) *f.* motorcycle (9)
mouche *f.* fly, housefly; **bateau-mouche** (*pl.* **bateaux-mouches**) *m. tourist boat on the Seine*
moudre to grind
moule *f.* mussel (*seafood*)
moulinet: faire des moulinets avec les bras to whirl one's arms about
mourant *adj.* dying
mourir (*p.p.* **mort**) *irreg.* to die (8); **s'ennuyer à mourir** to be bored to death
mousse (*f.*) **au chocolat** chocolate mousse
mousser to bubble; to sparkle
moustique *m.* mosquito
mouton *m.* sheep
mouvement *m.* movement
moyen *m.* mean(s); way; **moyen de transport** means of transportation (9); **un bon (meilleur) moyen** a good (better) way
moyen(ne) *adj.* average; all right (*in response to* **comment vas-tu?**) **cadre** (*m.*) **moyen** middle manager; **des classes** (*f.*) **moyennes** middle classes; **de taille moyenne** of medium height (3); **Moyen Âge** *m. s.* Middle Ages (12)
moyennant *prep.* in return for (which)
moyenne *f.* average; **en moyenne** on (an) average
mp3 *m.* mp3 player (10)
muet(te) *adj.* mute
multinationale *f.* multinational (corporation)
multiplier to multiply
mur *m.* wall (4)
muraille *f.* wall
musée *m.* museum (11)
musical (*pl.* **musicaux**) *adj.* musical
Musicien(ne) *m., f.* musician (12)
musique *f.* music (2); **musique classique** classical music
Musulman(e) *m., f.* Muslim
mutation *f.* change, alteration
myrtille *f.* huckleberry; blueberry
mystère *m.* mystery

nacre *f.* mother-of-pearl; *m.* pearly (*color*)
nager (nous nageons) to swim (8)
naïf/ive *adj.* naive (3); simple
naissance *f.* birth
naissant *adj.* emerging
naître (*p.p.* **né**) *irreg.* to be born (8)
nana *f., fam.* babe (pretty girl)
nappe *f.* tablecloth (6)
narrateur/trice *m., f.* narrator
natal *adj.* native
natation *f.* swimming
nation *f.* nation; **Organisation des Nations Unies (ONU)** United Nations (UN)
nationaliste *m., f.* nationalist; *adj.* nationalistic, nationalist
nationalité *f.* nationality (2)
nature *f.* nature (16); **nature morte** still life
naturel(le) *adj.* natural; **ressources** (*f. pl.*) **naturelles** natural resources (16); **sciences** (*f. pl.*) **naturelles** natural sciences (2)
nautique *adj.* nautical; **ski** (*m.*) **nautique** water-skiing (8)
navarin *m.* stew; lamb stew
navet *m., fam.* bad film, flop
navigateur *m.* browser (10)
navigation: logiciel (*m.*) **de navigation** browser (*Internet*)
naviguer to navigate, to browse (10)
navire *m.* ship
n'dolé *m.* hearty soup of Cameroon
ne (n') *adv.* no; not; **ne... aucun(e)** none, not one; **ne... jamais** never, not ever (9); **ne... ni... ni** neither . . . nor; **ne... pas** no; not; **ne... pas du tout** not at all (9); **ne... pas encore** not yet (9); **ne... personne** no one, nobody (9); **ne... plus** no more, no longer (9); **ne... que** only (9); **ne... rien** nothing (9); **n'est-ce pas?** isn't it (so)?, isn't that right? (3)
néanmoins *adv.* nevertheless
nécessaire *adj.* necessary; **il est nécessaire que** + *subj.* it's necessary that (16)
nécessité *f.* need
nécessiter to require, necessitate
né(e) (see **naître**)
néfaste *adj.* harmful
négatif/ive *adj.* negative
négativement *adv.* negatively
négociateur/trice *m., f.* negotiator
négocier to negotiate
nègre (négresse) *m., f.* Negro (Negress)
négrier/ière: traite (*f.*) **négrière** slave trade
négritude *f.* Negritude (*1930s Black consciousness movement*)
neige *f.* snow; **surf** (*m.*) **des neiges** snowboarding
neiger (il neigeait) to snow; **il neige** it's snowing (5)
nénuphar *m.* water lily
nerveux/euse *adj.* nervous (3)
net(te) *adj.* clear; net (*price*)
nettoyer (je nettoie) to clean
neuf *adj.* nine (1)
neuf (neuve) *adj.* new, brand-new; **quoi de neuf?** what's new?; **remettre à neuf** to restore; **Terre-Neuve** *f.* Newfoundland
neutre *adj.* neutral
neuvième *adj.* ninth (11)
neveu *m.* nephew (5)
nez *m.* nose (13)
ni *conj.* neither; nor; **ne... ni... ni** neither . . . nor
niçois(e) *adj.* of/from Nice
nièce *f.* niece (5)
niveau *m.* level; **niveau de vie** standard of living (16)
noces: repas (*m.*) **de noces** wedding meal/party; **voyage** (*m.*) **de noces** honeymoon trip
Noël *m.* Christmas; **bûche** (*f.*) **de Noël** Yule log (*pastry*); **père** (*m.*) **Noël** Santa Claus; **réveillon** (*m.*) **de Noël** *midnight Christmas dinner*
noir *adj.* black (3)
noisette *f.* hazel nut
noix *f.* nut; **noix de coco** coconut
nom *m.* noun; name; **au nom de** in the name of
nombre *m.* number (1); quantity; **nombres** (*pl.*) **ordinaux** ordinal numbers
nombreux/euse *adj.* numerous; **famille** (*f.*) **nombreuse** large family
nommer to name; to appoint
non *interj.* no; not (1); **moi non plus** me neither (3); **non plus** neither, not . . . either
nord *m.* north; **Amérique** (*f.*) **du Nord** North America; **au nord** to the north (9); **Nord-américain(e)** *m., f.* North American (*person*); **nord-est** *m.* northeast; **nord-ouest** *m.* northwest
normal *adj.* normal; **il est normal que** + *subj.* it's normal that (16)
normalement *adv.* usually
normand *adj.* Norman; **à la normande** in the Norman style
Normandie *f.* Normandy
Norvège *f.* Norway
nos *adj., m., f., pl.* our
notamment *adv.* notably; especially
note *f.* note; grade (*academic*); **bonnes (mauvaises) notes** good (bad) grades; **prendre des notes** to take notes
noter to notice; to note, write down
notre *adj., m., f., s.* our
nôtre(s): le/la/les nôtre(s) *pron., m., f.* ours; our own
nourrir to nourish
nourrissant *adj.* nourishing
nourriture *f.* food (6)
nous *pron., pl.* we; us; **nous-mêmes** *pron., pl.* ourselves (12); **nous sommes lundi (mardi...)** it's Monday (Tuesday . . .) (1); **quel jour sommes-nous?** what day is it? (1)
nouveau (nouvel, nouvelle [nouveaux, nouvelles]) *adj.* new (3); **à nouveau** once more; **de nouveau** again (11); **nouveaux mariés** *m. pl.* newlyweds, newly married couple (13); **la nouvelle cuisine** *lighter, low-fat cooking style*; **La Nouvelle-Orléans** New Orleans; **Nouveau-Brunswick** *m.* New Brunswick; **Nouveau-Mexique** *m.* New Mexico; **Nouvel An** *m.* New Year's; **Nouvelle-Écosse** *f.* Nova Scotia
nouveauté *f.* novelty

nouvelle *f.* piece of news; short story; *pl.* news, current events; **bonne (mauvaise) nouvelle** good (bad) news
novembre November (1)
nu *adj.* naked
nuage *m.* cloud
nuageux/euse *adj.* cloudy; **le temps est nuageux** it's cloudy (5)
nucléaire *adj.* nuclear; **armes** (*f. pl.*) **nucléaires** nuclear weapons; **centrale** (*f.*) **nucléaire** nuclear power plant; **déchets** (*m. pl.*) **nucléaires** nuclear waste (16); **énergie** (*f.*) **nucléaire** nuclear power (16)
nuit *f.* night (7); **boîte** (*f.*) **de nuit** nightclub, club; **de nuit** at night
nul(le) *adj.*, null; worthless; *fam.* no good
numérique digital; **appareil** (*m.*) **(photo) numérique** digital camera (10); **livre** (*m.*) **numérique** e-book (10); **télévision** (*f.*) **numérique terrestre (la TNT)** high-definition television (10)
numéro *m.* number (10); **composer le numéro** to dial the number (10); **numéro de téléphone** telephone number (10)
numéroter to number
nuque *f.* nape, back of the neck
nymphéa *m.* white water lily

obéir to obey
objectif *m.* goal, objective
objet *m.* object; objective; **pronom** (*m.*) **complément d'objet direct (indirect)** *Gram.* direct (indirect) object pronoun
obligatoire *adj.* obligatory; mandatory; **service** (*m.*) **(militaire) obligatoire** mandatory military service
obligatoirement *adv.* necessarily, obligatorily
obligé *adj.* obliged, required; **être obligé de** to be obliged to
observateur/trice *m., f.* observer
observer to observe
obsolète *adj.* obsolete, outdated
obtenir (*like* **tenir**) *irreg.* to obtain, get (8)
obtention *f.* obtaining; achieving
occasion *f.* opportunity; occasion; bargain
occident *m.* the west
occidental *adj.* (*pl.* **occidentaux**) western, occidental; **Afrique** (*f.*) **occidentale** western Africa; **Virginie-Occidentale** *f.* West Virginia
occupé *adj.* occupied; busy
occuper to occupy; **s'occuper de** to look after, take care of
océan *m.* ocean, sea; **océan Atlantique** Atlantic Ocean
Océanie *f.* Oceania, the South Sea Islands
ocre *adj.* ochre (yellow-earth color)
octobre October (1)
odeur *f.* odor, smell
odorat *m.* sense of smell
œil (*pl.* **yeux**) *m.* eye (13); **coup** (*m.*) **d'œil** glance, quick look
œnologue *m., f.* oenologist, wine expert
œuf *m.* egg (6)
œuvre *f.* work; artistic work; **chef-d'œuvre** (*pl.* **chefs-d'œuvre**) *m.* masterpiece (12); ***hors-d'œuvre** *m. inv.* appetizer (7); **œuvre d'art** work of art (12)
officiel(le) *adj.* official
offre *f.* offer; **offre d'emploi** job offer
offrir (*like* **ouvrir**) *irreg.* to offer (14)
oie *f.* goose; **la Mère l'Oie** Mother Goose
oignon *m.* onion (7); **soupe** (*f.*) **à l'oignon** (French) onion soup
oiseau *m.* bird
olive *f.* olive; **huile** (*f.*) **d'olive** olive oil (7)
olivier *m.* olive tree
ombre *f.* shadow; shade
ombrelle *f.* parasol
omelette *f.* omelet
on *pron. s.* one, they, we
oncle *m.* uncle (5)
onze *adj.* eleven (1)
onzième *adj.* eleventh (11)
opéra *m.* opera (15)
opérateur *m.* operator **opérateur de téléphonie mobile** cell phone service provider
opinion *f.* opinion; **exprimer une opinion** to express an opinion (16); **opinion publique** public opinion (16)
opposé *m.* the opposite
opter pour to opt for, choose
optimiste *m., f.* optimist; *adj.* optimistic (3)
or *m.* gold
orage *m.* storm
orageux/euse *adj.* stormy; **le temps est orageux** it's stormy (5)
orange *adj. inv.* orange (3); *m.* orange (*color*); *f.* orange (*fruit*) (6); **jus** (*m.*) **d'orange** orange juice (6)
orchestre *m.* orchestra; band
ordinaire *adj.* ordinary, regular (3)
ordinal *adj.* ordinal; **nombres** (*m. pl.*) **ordinaux** ordinal numbers
ordinateur (*fam.* **ordi**) *m.* computer (1); **micro-ordinateur** *m.* desktop computer; **ordinateur de bureau (de table)** desktop computer (10); **ordinateur portable** (*fam.* **portable** *m.*) laptop computer (10)
ordonner to order (*s.o. to do s.th.*)
ordre *m.* order; command; **dans le bon ordre** in the right order; **dans l'ordre chronologique** in chronological order; **en ordre** orderly, neat (4)
oreille *f.* ear (13)
organique *adj.* organic
organiser to organize
organisme *m.* organization, institution; organism
oriental (*pl.* **orientaux**) *adj.* Oriental
orientation *f.* orientation; direction; **conseiller/ère** (*m., f.*) **d'orientation** guidance counselor
s'orienter to orient oneself, get one's bearings
oriflamme *f.* banner, standard (*flag*)
originaire (*adj.*) **de** native to
original (*pl.* **originaux**) *adj.* original; eccentric
originalité *f.* originality, imagination
origine *f.* origin; **d'origine algérienne** of Algerian origin (background); **pays** (*m.*) **d'origine** native country, nationality
ornement *m.* ornament; embellishment, adornment
orteil *m.* toe
os *m.* bone
ou *conj.* or; either (2); **ou bien** or else
où *adv.* where (4); *pron.* where, in which, when (14); **où est… ?** where is . . . ?
ouah ouah! bow-wow!, woof!
oublier (de) to forget (to) (8)
ouest *m.* west; **à l'ouest** to the west (9); **Afrique** (*f.*) **de l'ouest** West Africa; **nord-ouest** *m.* northwest; **ouest-africain** *adj.* West African; **sud-ouest** *m.* southwest
ouf *interj.* phew, whew
oui *interj.* yes (1); **oui, mais…** yes, but . . . (10)
ouïe *f.* sense of hearing
ouragan *m.* hurricane
outil *m.* tool
ouvert *adj.* open; frank
ouverture *f.* opening
ouvrier/ière *m., f.* (*manual*) worker, laborer (14)
ouvrir (*p.p.* **ouvert**) *irreg.* to open (14)

pacifiste *adj.* pacifistic
pacsé *adj.* legally joined by a PACS
page (*f.*) **d'accueil** homepage
pager *m.* pager
pain *m.* bread (6); **baguette** (*f.*) **de pain** (French) bread, baguette; **pain au chocolat** chocolate croissant; **pain de campagne** country-style bread, wheat bread (7)
pair: au pair au pair (*child care by foreign student*)
paix *f.* peace
palais *m.* palace (12)
palier *m.* (stair) landing; **voisin(e)** (*m., f.*) **de palier** neighbor living on the same landing
palmarès *m.* record of achievement
palmeraie *f.* palm grove
palmier *m.* palm tree
pamplemousse *m.* grapefruit
Paname *m. fam.* Paris
pané *adj.* fried in breadcrumbs
panier *m.* basket
panne *f.* (*mechanical*) breakdown; **en panne de débouchés** faced with an absence of job openings
panneau *m.* billboard, sign
panoramique *adj.* with a panoramic view
pantalon *m.* (pair of) pants (3)
pantoufle *f.* slipper (13)
papa *m., fam.* dad, daddy
papier *m.* paper; **livre** (*m.*) **papier** print book (10)
papy *m., fam.* grandpa
Pâques *f. pl.* Easter
paquet *m.* package
par *prep.* by, through, with (4, 12); **commencer (finir) par** to begin (end up) by; **par avion** air-mail; **par cœur** by heart (12); **par exemple** for example (16); **par *hasard** by chance; **par jour (semaine,** *etc.***)** per day (week, etc.); **par ordre chronologique** in chronological order; **par rapport à** in comparison with, in relation to; **par terre** on the ground (4); **une fois par semaine** once a week (5)
paradis *m.* paradise
paradoxalement *adv.* paradoxically
paradoxe *m.* paradox
paragraphe *m.* paragraph
paraître (*like* **connaître**) *irreg.* to appear (16)
paralysé *adj.* paralyzed; strike-bound
parapluie *m.* umbrella (8)
parasol *m.* beach umbrella; parasol
parc *m.* park (11); **parc d'attraction** theme park
parce que *conj.* because (4)
parcourir (*like* **courir**) *irreg.* to cover, travel; to skim
parcours *m. s.* distance, journey, course
pardon *interj.* pardon (me) (1)
pareil(le) *adj.* the same, similar

parent(e) *m., f.* parent; relative (5); **arrière-grand-parent** *m.* great-grandparent (5); **grand-parent** grandparent (5); **parent(e) proche** close relative
parenthèse *f.* parenthesis; **entre parenthèses** in parentheses
paresseux/euse *adj.* lazy (3)
parfait *adj.* perfect
parfaitement *adv.* perfectly (14)
parfois *adv.* sometimes (9)
parfum *m.* perfume; flavor
parfumé *adj.* fragrant; flavorful
pari *m.* bet, wager; **pari perdu** lost bet
parier to bet, wager
parisien(ne) *adj.* Parisian (3); **Parisien(ne)** *m., f.* Parisian (*person*)
parking *m.* parking lot
parlement *m.* parliament
parler (à, de) to speak (to, of) (2); to talk (2); *m.* speech
parmi *prep.* among
parole *f.* word; *pl.* lyrics
parquet *m.* wooden (parquet) floor
part *f.* share, portion; **à part** besides; separately; **c'est de la part de X** X is calling; **de ma part** for me, on my behalf; **pour ma part** in my opinion, as for me (16); **quelque part** somewhere
partager (nous partageons) to share
partenaire *m., f.* partner
partenariat *m.* partnership
parti *m.* (*political*) party (16)
participant(e) *m., f.* participant
participe *m., Gram.* participle
participer à to participate in
particulier/ière *adj.* particular, special; **en particulier** in particular
partie *f.* part; **faire partie de** to be part of
partir (*like* **dormir**) **(à, pour, de)** *irreg.* to leave (for, from) (8); **à partir de** *prep.* starting from; **à partir de maintenant** from now on (14); **partir à l'aventure** to leave with no itinerary; **partir en vacances** to leave on vacation
partisan(e) *m., f.* supporter, advocate
partitif/ive *adj., Gram.* partitive
partout *adv.* everywhere (11)
parvenir (*like* **venir**) **à** *irreg.* to succeed in
pas (ne… pas) not; **ne… pas du tout** not at all (9); **ne… pas encore** not yet (9); **n'est-ce pas?** isn't it (so)?, isn't that right? (3); **pas à pas** step-by-step; **pas du tout** not at all; **pas mal** not bad(ly) (1)
passage *m.* passage; passing; **lieu** (*m.*) **de passage** crossing point, passageway
passager/ère *m., f.* passenger (9)
passant(e) *m., f.* passerby
passé *m.* past; *adj.* past, gone, last (7); **l'année** (*f.*) **passée** last year; **participe** (*m.*) **passé** *Gram.* past participle; **passé composé** *Gram.* compound past tense; **passé simple** *Gram.* past tense (*literary*)
passeport *m.* passport (8)
passer to pass, spend (*time*) (6); to put through to (*by phone*); to show, play (*a film, record*); **passer (par)** to pass (by, through) (8); **passer sur** to go over; **passer les vacances** to spend one's vacation; **passer un examen** to take an exam (4); **qu'est-ce qui se passe?** what's happening?, what's going on? (15); **se passer** to happen, take place (15); to go
passe-temps *m. inv.* pastime, hobby (15)
passionné(e) *m., f.* enthusiast; *adj.* enthusiastic; passionate
se passionner pour to be excited about
pasteur *m.* (*Protestant*) minister
pastilla *f.* pastilla (*Moroccan pastry and meat dish*)
patate *f., fam.* potato
pâté *m.* liver paste, pâté; **pâté de campagne** (country-style) pâté (7); **pâté de foie gras** goose liver pâté
paternel(le) *adj.* paternal
pâtes *f. pl.* pasta, noodles (7)
patience *f.* patience; **avoir de la patience** to be patient; **perdre patience** to lose patience
patient *m., f.* (*hospital*) patient; *adj.* patient (3)
patienter to wait (patiently)
patin *m.* skate, ice skate; **faire du patin à glace** to go ice-skating; **faire du patin à roues alignées** to do in-line skating
patiner to skate
pâtisserie *f.* pastry; pastry shop (7); **boulangerie-pâtisserie** *f.* bakery-pastry shop
pâtissier/ière *m., f.* pastry shop owner; pastry chef
patrie *f.* native land
patrimoine *m.* legacy; heritage (12)
patron(ne) *m., f.* boss, employer; **fête** (*f.*) **des patrons** saint's day
pause *f.* pause, break
pauvre *adj.* poor; unfortunate (3)
pauvreté *f.* poverty
pavillon *m.* house, lodge
payé *adj.* paid, paying
payer (je paie) to pay, pay for (10)
pays *m.* country, nation (2); **pays en voie de développement** developing nation; **Pays-Bas** *m. pl.* Netherlands, Holland; **pays d'origine** native country
paysage *m.* landscape; scenery
paysan(ne) *m., f.* peasant, farmworker
peau *f.* skin
pêche *f.* peach; fishing (15); **aller à la pêche** to go fishing (8); **avoir la pêche** *fam.* to feel great, like a million bucks
pêcheur/euse *m., f.* fisherman (woman)
pécule *m., fam.* savings
pédagogique *adj.* pedagogical, teaching
pédaler to pedal
pédestre *adj.* pedestrian; **randonnée** (*f.*) **pédestre** hike; hiking
peigne *m.* comb (13)
se peigner to comb one's hair (13)
peindre (*like* **craindre**) *irreg.* to paint (12)
peintre (femme peintre) *m., f.* painter (12)
peinture *f.* painting (12); paint(s); **faire de la peinture** to paint
peler to peel
peloton: en peloton *m.* in a pack (*of people*)
pendant *prep.* for, during (9); **pendant combien de temps… ?** (for) how long . . . ? (9); **pendant les vacances** during vacation; **pendant que** *conj.* while
pénible *adj.* painful; hard, difficult
péniche *f.* barge
Pennsylvanie *f.* Pennsylvania
pensée *f.* thought; idea
penser to think (10); to reflect; to expect, intend; **je ne pense pas** I don't think so; **penser** + *inf.* to plan on (*doing s.th.*); **penser à** to think of, think about (11); **penser de** to think of, have an opinion about (11); **qu'en penses-tu?** what do you think about it? (11); **que pensez-vous de… ?** what do you think of . . . ? (11)
penseur/euse *m., f.* thinker
pensif/ive *adj.* pensive, thoughtful
perception (*f.*) **extrasensorielle** extrasensory perception (ESP)
perché *adj.* perched, sitting (on)
perdre to lose; to waste (5); **perdre patience** to lose patience; **se perdre** to get lost (13)
père *m.* father (5); **beau-père** father-in-law; stepfather (5); **grand-père** grandfather (5)
perfectionner to perfect
performant *adj.* competitive; highly capable
péril *m.* danger; **mettre en péril** to endanger
période *f.* period (*of time*)
péripétie *f.* adventure; event, episode
perle *f.* pearl
permanence: en permanence *adv.* permanently
permettre (*like* **mettre**) **(de)** *irreg.* to permit, allow (to), let (12)
permis *m.* permit, license; **permis de conduire** driver's license; **permis de travail** work permit
perruque *f.* wig
persévérant *adj.* persevering, dogged (3)
persil *m.* parsley
personnage *m.* (*fictional*) character; personality, celebrity
personnalisé *adj.* personalized
personnalité *f.* personality
personne *f.* person (3); **ne… personne** nobody, no one (9)
personnel(le) *adj.* personal
personnellement *adv.* personally (16)
perspective *f.* view; perspective
persuader to persuade, convince
perte *f.* loss
peser to weigh
pessimiste *adj.* pessimistic (3)
pétanque *f.* bocce ball, lawn bowling (*southern France*) (15)
pétiller to fizz
petit *adj.* little; short (3); very young; *m. pl.* young ones; little ones; **petit(e) ami(e)** *m., f.* boyfriend, girlfriend; **petit déjeuner** *m.* breakfast (6); **petit écran** *m.* television; **petit matin** *m.* early morning; **petit-enfant** *m.* grandchild (5); **petit-fils** *m.* grandson (5); **petite cuillère** *f.* teaspoon; **petite-fille** *f.* granddaughter (5); **petites annonces** *f. pl.* classified ads (10); **petits pois** *m. pl.* peas; **un petit peu** a little (bit)
pétrole *m.* oil, petroleum
peu *adv.* little; few; not very; hardly (3); **à peu près** *adv.* nearly; **encore un peu** a little more; **il est peu probable que** + *subj.* it's doubtful that (16); **peu à peu** little by little; **peu calorique** low in calories; **peu de** few (6); **un peu** a little (3); **un peu (de)** a little (of) (6)
peuple *m.* nation; people (*of a country*)
peuplé (de) *adj.* filled (with), full (of); populated
peur *f.* fear; **avoir peur (de)** to be afraid (of) (3)
peut-être *adv.* perhaps, maybe (5)
pharaon *m.* Pharaoh
phare *m.* beacon
pharmacie *f.* pharmacy, drugstore (11)
pharmacien(ne) *m., f.* pharmacist (14)

phénomène *m.* phenomenon
philanthrope *m., f.* philanthropist
philosophe *m., f.* philosopher
philosophie (*fam.* **philo**) *f.* philosophy (2)
philosophique *adj.* philosophical
photocopieur *m.* photocopy machine (10)
photographe *m., f.* photographer
photo(graphie) *f.* picture, photograph; **appareil (photo) numérique** *m.* digital camera (10); **prendre des photos** to take photos
photographique *adj.* photographic
phrase *f.* sentence
physique *f.* physics (2); *adj.* physical
piano *m.* piano; **jouer du piano** to play the piano
pianoter to tap away on
piaule *f., fam.* digs, place (*residence*)
pièce *f.* piece; room (*of a house*) (5); coin; **monter une pièce** to put on a play; **pièce de collection** collector's item; **pièce de monnaie** coin; **pièce de théâtre** (*theatrical*) play (12)
pied *m.* foot (13); **à pied** on foot (9); **se lever du pied gauche** to get up on the wrong side of the bed
piège *f.* trap, trick
pierre *f.* stone
pieu *m., fam.* bed
pile *f.* battery; stack; support
pilote *m., f.* pilot (9); driver
piment *m.* chili, pepper
pinard *m., fam.* wine
pincée *f.* pinch, dash (*cooking*)
pique-nique *m.* picnic (15); **faire un pique-nique** to go on a picnic
pique-niquer to have a picnic
piqûre *f.* injection, shot (13)
pire *adj.* worse (14); **le/la/les pire(s)** the worst
pirogue *f.* dugout canoe
pis *adv.* worse; **le pis** the worst; **tant pis** too bad (15)
piscine *f.* swimming pool (11)
piste *f.* path, trail; course; slope; lead (14); **piste cyclable** bicycle path
pitchoune *f., fam.* girl
pittoresque *adj.* picturesque
place *f.* place; position; (public) square (11); seat (12); **à votre (ta) place** in your place, if I were you (15); **mise** (*f.*) **en place** placement
placer (nous plaçons) to place, put
plafond *m.* ceiling
plage *f.* beach (8); **serviette** (*f.*) **de plage** beach towel (8)
plaidoyer *m.* defense, plea
se plaindre (de) (*like* **craindre**) *irreg.* to complain (about)
plaine *f.* plain
plaire (*p.p.* **plu**) **à** *irreg.* to please; **en français, s'il vous plaît** in French, please; **s'il te (vous) plaît** *interj.* please (1)
plaisir *m.* pleasure
plan *m.* plan; diagram; map (*of a city*) (11); **sur le plan économique** economically speaking
planche *f.* board; **faire de la planche à voile** to windsurf; **planche à voile** windsurfer (8)
plancher *m.* floor
planète *f.* planet
planifier to plan
plante *f.* plant
planter to plant
planteur *m.* planter, plantation owner
plaque *f.* package (*of frozen food*); **plaque tournante** linchpin; hub
plaquer to tackle (*U.S. football*)
plat *m.* dish (*type of food*); course (*meal*) (7); *adj.* flat; **plat de résistance** main course, dish; **plat du jour** today's special (*restaurant*); **plat principal** main course, main dish (7)
plein (de) *adj.* full (of); complete; **activités** (*f. pl.*) **de plein air** outdoor activities (15); **faire le plein** to fill it up (*gas tank*) (9); **marché** (*m.*) **en plein air** outdoor market; **plein de** a lot of
plénitude *f.* plenitude; richness
pleurer to cry, weep
pleuvoir (*p.p.* **plu**) *irreg.* to rain (7); **il pleut** it's raining (5)
plier to fold
plombier *m.* plumber (14)
plongée *f.* diving; **faire de la plongée libre** to go snorkeling (8); **faire de la plongée sous-marine** to go scuba diving (8)
plonger (nous plongeons) to dive, plunge
pluie *f.* rain
plumard *m., fam.* bed
plumer to pluck
plupart: la plupart (de) most (of), the majority (of) (12)
pluriel *m., Gram.* plural
plus (de) *adv.* more; plus; **de plus en plus** more and more; **en plus** in addition; **le plus** + *adv.* most; **le/la/les plus** + *adj.* most; **moi non plus** me neither; **ne... plus** no longer, no more (9); **plus... que** more . . . than (14); **plus tard** later
plusieurs (de) *adj., pron.* several (of) (6)
plutôt *adv.* instead; rather
poche *f.* pocket (10)
poème *m.* poem (12)
poésie *f.* poetry (12)
poète (femme poète) *m., f.* poet (12)
poétique *adj.* poetic, poetry
poids *m.* weight
poignée (*f.*) **de main** handshake
point *m.* point; spot; **être sur le point de** + *inf.* to be on the verge of; **point cardinal** compass point; **point de départ** starting point; **point de rencontre** meeting point; **point de vue** point of view; **point fort** strong point; *adv.* **ne... point** not at all
pointe *f.* point, tip; *pl.* headlands
pointillisme *m.* pointillism (*style of painting*)
pointu *adj.* pointed, sharp
pointure *f.* (shoe) size
poire *f.* pear (6)
pois *m. pl.* peas; dots; **à pois** polka-dotted; **petits pois** peas
poisson *m.* fish (6)
poissonnerie *f.* fish market (7)
poivrade: sauce (*f.*) **poivrade** *vinaigrette dressing with pepper*
poivre *m.* pepper (6); **steak** (*m.*) **au poivre** pepper steak
poivrer to pepper
poivron *m.* bell pepper
poli *adj.* polite (12); polished
police *f.* police; **agent** (*m.*) **de police** police officer (14); **poste** (*m.*) **de police** police station (11)
policier/ière *adj.* pertaining to the police; *m.* police officer; **roman** (*m.*) **policier** detective novel
poliomyélite *f.* polio(myelitis)
politicien(ne) *m., f.* politician
politique *f.* politics; policy (16); *adj.* political; **faire de la politique** to go in for politics; **homme (femme) politique** *m., f.* politician (16)
Polononais(e) *m., f.* Polish person
polonais *adj.* Polish
polyvalent *adj.* multipurpose; versatile
polluant *adj.* polluting
polluer to pollute (16)
Polynésie (*f.*) **française** French Polynesia
pomme *f.* apple (6); **jus** (*m.*) **de pomme** apple juice; **pomme de terre** potato (6); **tarte** (*f.*) **aux pommes** apple tart
pompe *f., fam.* shoe
pompier *m.* fire fighter
ponctuation *f.* punctuation
ponctuel *adj.* punctual
pont *m.* bridge
populaire *adj.* popular; common; of the people
popularité *f.* popularity
porc *m.* pork (6); **côte** (*f.*) **de porc** pork chop
portable *m.* laptop computer (1, 10); **téléphone portable** cell phone (10)
porte *f.* door (1); stop, exit (*metro*); gate
porter to wear; to carry (3); **prêt-à-porter** *m.* ready-to-wear (*clothing*)
porto *m.* port (*wine*)
portugais *adj.* Portuguese
Portugal *m.* Portugal (8)
poser to put (down); to state, pose; to ask; **poser sa candidature** to apply; to run (*for office*) (14); **poser une question** to ask a question (11)
positif/ive *adj.* positive
positionnement *m.* positioning
posséder (je possède) to possess (10)
possesseur/euse *m., f.* owner
possessif/ive *adj.* possessive
possession *f.* possession; **prendre possession de** to take possession of
possibilité *f.* possibility
possible *adj.* possible; **aussi souvent que possible** as often as possible; **faire son possible** to do one's best; **il est possible que** + *subj.* it's possible that (16)
postal *adj.* postal, post; **carte** (*f.*) **postale** postcard (10); **code** (*m.*) **postal** postal code, zip code
poste *m.* position; employment; *f.* mail (10); **bureau** (*m.*) **de poste** post office (10); **La Poste** post office; postal service (10); **poste** (*m.*) **de police** police station (11)
poster to mail (10)
postuler to apply (*for a job*)
potasser *fam.* to study
pote *m., fam.* buddy
poterie *f.* pottery
poubelle *f.* garbage can
pouce *m.* thumb; inch; **coup** (*m.*) **de pouce** little push (in the right direction)
poudre: en poudre *f.* powdered
poule *f.* hen
poulet *m.* chicken (6)
poupée *f.* doll

pour *prep.* for, in order to (2); **le pour et le contre** the pros and cons; **manifester pour** to demonstrate for (16); **pour ma part** in my opinion, as for me (16); **pour que** + *subj.* in order to
pourboire *m.* tip, gratuity (7)
pourcentage *m.* percentage
pourquoi *adv., conj.* why (4)
pourri: faire un temps pourri *fam.* to be rotten weather
poursuivre (*like* **suivre**) *irreg.* to pursue (12)
pourtant *adv.* yet, nevertheless
pousser to push; to grow; to move (*s.o. to do s.th.*)
poutine *f.* poutine (Quebec dish of French fries with cheese and gravy)
pouvoir (*p.p.* **pu**) *irreg.* to be able to, can (7); *m.* power, strength; **ça peut aller** all right, pretty well (1); **il se peut que** + *subj.* it's possible that (16); **je pourrais** I could (7); **pouvoir** (*m.*) **d'achat** purchasing power (16)
pratique *adj.* practical; *f.* practice; use; **travaux** (*m. pl.*) **pratiques** hands-on learning
pratiquer to play, perform (*sport, activity*)
préalablement *adv.* beforehand
préavis: sans donner de préavis without notice
précaire fragile, precarious
précédent *adj.* preceding
précéder (je précède) to precede
précieusement *adv.* preciously
précipiter to rush, hurry
précieux/euse *adj.* precious
précis *adj.* precise, accurate (3)
préciser to clarify, specify
précision *f.* precision; piece of information
précoce *adj.* precocious
prédiction *f.* prediction, forecast
prédilection *f.* partiality, predilection
prédire (*like* **dire, vous prédisez**) *irreg.* to predict, foretell
préférable *adj.* preferable, more advisable; **il est préférable que** + *subj.* it's preferable that (16)
préféré *adj.* favorite, preferred (5)
préférence *f.* preference; **de préférence** preferably
préférer (je préfère) to prefer, like better (6)
préfrit *adj.* pre-fried
préjugé *m.* prejudice
prélèvement (*m.*) **automatique** automatic payment/withdrawal (14)
premier/ière *adj.* first (4); *f.* opening night, premiere; **le premier janvier** the first of January; **premier étage** *m.* second floor (*in the U.S.*) (5); **premier ministre** *m.* prime minister; **première classe** *f.* first class (9)
prendre (*p.p.* **pris**) *irreg.* to take (6); to have (to eat, to drink) (6); to order (6); **prendre au sérieux** to take seriously; **prendre conscience de** to realize, become aware of; **prendre des notes** to take notes; **prendre des vacances** to take vacation; **prendre du temps** to take a long time (6); **prendre l'avion** to take a plane; **prendre possession de** to take possession of; **prendre rendez-vous** to make an appointment (date); **prendre son temps** to take one's time (6); **prendre un repas** to have a meal (6); **prendre un verre** *fam.* to have a drink (*with s.o.*) (6); **prendre une douche** to take a shower; **prendre une photo** to take a photo; **se prendre pour** to believe oneself to be
prénom *m.* first name, Christian name
préoccupé *adj.* worried, preoccupied (16)
préoccuper to concern; **se préoccuper de** to concern, preoccupy oneself with; to worry about
préparatifs *m. pl.* preparations
préparer to prepare (5); **préparer un examen** to study for an exam; **se préparer (à)** to prepare oneself, get ready (for) (13)
près (de) *adv.* near, close to (4); **à peu près** nearly; **tout près** very near
présence *f.* presence; attendance
présent *m.* present (*time*); *adj.* present; **à présent** now, at the present time
présentement *adv.* presently, currently
présenter to present; to introduce; to put on (*a performance*); **je vous (te) présente...** I want you to meet . . . ; **se présenter** to run for office; to introduce oneself
préserver to preserve
président(e) *m., f.* president
présidentiel(le) *adj.* presidential
présider to preside
presque *adv.* almost, nearly
presse *f.* press (*media*)
pressé *adj.* in a hurry, rushed; **citron** (*m.*) **pressé** fresh lemon juice
prestigieux/ieuse *adj.* prestigious
prêt *adj.* ready (3); **prêt-à-porter** *m.* ready-to-wear clothing
prétendre to claim (to be); **prétendre à** to lay claim to
prétentieux/euse *adj.* pretentious
prêter (à) to lend (to) (11)
prétexte *m.* pretext, excuse
preuve *f.* proof; **faire preuve de** to show
prévision *f.* prediction
prévoir (*like* **voir**) *irreg.* to foresee, anticipate
prévu *adj.* expected, anticipated; **comme prévu** as planned
prier to pray; to beg, entreat; to ask (*s.o.*); **je vous (t')en prie** please; you're welcome (7)
primaire *adj.* primary; **école** (*f.*) **primaire** primary school
principal *adj.* principal, main, most important; **plat** (*m.*) **principal** main course (7)
principe *m.* principle
printanier/ière *adj.* spring(like); with vegetables (*in cooking*)
printemps *m.* spring; **au printemps** in the spring (5)
priorité *f.* priority
pris (see **prendre**)
prise *f.* taking
prisme *m.* prism
prisonnier/ière *m., f.* prisoner
privé *adj.* private
privilégié *adj.* privileged
privilégier to favor
prix *m.* price (7); prize
probabilité *f.* probability
probable *adj.* probable; **il est peu probable que** + *subj.* it's doubtful that (16); **il est probable que** + *indic.* it's probable that (16)
problématique *f.* problem, issue
problème *m.* problem (16)
procédé *m.* process, method
procéder (je procède) to proceed
processus *m.* process
prochain *adj.* next; coming; **à la prochaine** until next time; **la rentrée prochaine** beginning of next academic year; **la semaine prochaine** next week (5)
prochainement *adv.* soon, shortly
proche (de) *adj., adv.* near, close; *m. pl.* close relatives; **futur** (*m.*) **proche** *Gram.* immediate (near) future
producteur/trice *m., f.* producer
produire (*like* **conduire**) *irreg.* to produce (9)
produit *m.* product (6); **produit chimique** chemical; **produits frais** fresh products (6)
professeur (*fam.* **prof**) *m.* professor, instructor (*male or female*) (1); **professeur des écoles** *m., f.* primary school teacher (14)
professionnel(le) *adj.* professional
profil *m.* profile; outline; cross section
profiter de to take advantage of, profit from; **profitez-en donc** take advantage of it
profiterole *f.* profiterole (*small cream puff*)
profond *adj.* deep
profondément *adv.* deeply, profoundly
profondeur: en profondeur in depth
programme *m.* program; agenda
programmer to program; to plan
progrès *m. s.* progress
progresser to advance, make progress
projection *f.* projection, showing
projet *m.* project; *pl.* plans (5); **projets d'avenir** future plans
prolifération *f.* proliferation (16)
promenade *f.* walk; ride; **faire une promenade** to take a walk (5)
promener (je promène) to take out walking, take for a walk; **se promener** to go for a walk (drive, ride), take a walk (13)
promesse *f.* promise
promettre (*like* **mettre**) **(de)** *irreg.* to promise (to)
promotion *f.* promotion; sale, store special; **en promotion** on special
promouvoir (*p.p.* **promu**) *irreg.* to promote
pronom *m., Gram.* pronoun; **pronom accentué (indéfini, interrogatif, personnel, relatif)** *Gram.* disjunctive, stressed (indefinite, interrogative, personal, relative) pronoun; **pronom complément d'objet direct (indirect)** *Gram.* direct (indirect) object pronoun
pronominal *adj., Gram.* pronominal; **verbe** (*m.*) **pronominal** *Gram.* pronominal (reflexive) verb
prononcé *adj.* pronounced
prononcer to pronounce
prononciation *f.* pronunciation
propagation *f.* spread
propos *m.* talk; utterance; **à propos** by the way; **à propos de** about
proposer to propose; to offer (14)
proposition *f.* proposal; offer
propre *adj.* own; clean; **propre à** characteristic of
propriétaire (*fam.* **proprio**) *m., f.* owner; landlord
propriété *f.* property
prospectus *m.* handbill, leaflet
protéger (je protège, nous protégeons) to protect (16)
prouver to prove
provenir (*like* **venir**) *irreg.* to come (descend) from

province *f.* province; **ville** (*f.*) **de province** country town
provincial *adj.* small-town; *n. m.* small-town person
provision *f.* supply; *pl.* groceries
provoquer to provoke
proximité *f.* proximity, closeness; **à proximité de** near
prudent *adj.* careful; cautious
prune *f.* plum
psychiatre *m., f.* psychiatrist
psychologie (*fam.* **psycho**) *f.* psychology (2)
psychologique *adj.* psychological
psychologue *m., f.* psychologist
public (publique) *adj.* public (11); *m.* public; audience; **opinion** (*f.*) **publique** public opinion (16); **télévision** (*f.*) **publique** government-owned television (10)
publicité (*fam.* **pub**) *f.* commercial, advertisement; advertising (10)
publier to publish
puce *f.* flea; **marché** (*m.*) **aux puces** flea market; **excité comme une puce** as excited as a flea (at a cat show)
puériculteur/trice *m., f.* daycare teacher, nursery nurse
puis *adv.* then, next (11); besides (7); **et puis** and then; and besides (7)
puissance *f.* power, strength
puissant *adj.* powerful; **tout-puissant** *adj.* all-powerful
puit *m.* well
pull-over (*fam.* **pull**) *m.* sweater (3)
pulpeux/euse *adj.* fleshy
pur *adj.* pure
purée *f.* purée (*e.g., mashed potatoes*)
pureté *f.* purity
puzzle *m.* puzzle
pyjama *m. s.* pajamas

quai *m.* quay; platform (*train station*) (9)
qualificatif/ive *adj.* qualifying
qualité *f.* quality; characteristic
quand *adv., conj.* when (4); **depuis quand** since when (9); **quand même** even so; anyway (16)
quant à *adv.* as for; regarding
quantité *f.* quantity
quarantaine *f.* quarantine
quarante *adj.* forty (1)
quart *m.* quarter; fourth; quarter of an hour; **et quart** quarter past (the hour) (6); **moins le quart** quarter to (the hour) (6); **un quart de vin** a quarter liter carafe of wine
quartier *m.* quarter, neighborhood (2); **quartier général** headquarters; **Quartier latin** Latin Quarter (district) (*in Paris*)
quasi-totalité *f.* nearly all
quatorze *adj.* fourteen (1)
quatorzième *adj.* fourteenth
quatre *adj.* four (1)
quatre-vingts *adj.* eighty
quatrième *adj.* fourth
que (qu') what (4); that, which; whom (14); **ne... que** *adv.* only (9); **parce que** because (4); **que pensez-vous de... ?** what do you think about . . . ? (11); **que veut dire... ?** what does . . . mean?; **qu'en penses-tu?** what do you think of that? (11); **qu'est-ce que** what (*object*) (4); **qu'est-ce que c'est?** what is it? (1); **qu'est-ce qui** what (*subject*) (15); **qu-est-ce qui se passe?** what's happening?, what's going on? (15)
Québec *m.* Quebec (*province*); (2, 8); **Québec** Quebec (*city*)
québécois *m.* Quebecois (*language*); *adj.* from (of) Quebec; **Québécois(e)** *m., f.* Quebecois (*person*)
quel(le)(s) *interr. adj.* what, which (7); what a; **à quelle heure... ?** (at) what time . . . ? (6); **quel âge avez-vous?** how old are you?; **quel jour sommes-nous (est-ce)?** what day is it? (1); **quel temps fait-il?** how's the weather? (5); **quelle est la date?** what is the date? (1); **quelle heure est-il?** what time is it? (6)
quelque(s) *adj.* some, any; a few (15); **quelque chose** *pron.* something (9); **quelque chose de** + *adj.* something + *adj.* (15); **quelque part** *adv.* somewhere
quelquefois *adv.* sometimes (2)
quelques-uns/unes *pron., pl.* some, a few (15)
quelqu'un *pron., neu.* someone, somebody (9)
question *f.* question; **poser une question (à)** to ask a question (11)
quête *f.* quest, search
queue *f.* line (*of people*); **faire la queue** to stand in line (5); **queue de cheval** ponytail
qui *pron.* who, whom (4); who, that, which (14); **qu'est-ce qui** what (*subject*); **qui est à l'appareil?** who's calling? (10); **qui est-ce?** who is it? (1); **qui est-ce que** whom (*object*) (15); **qui est-ce qui** who (*subject*)
quiche *f.* quiche (*egg custard pie*); **quiche lorraine** *egg custard pie with bacon*
quinze *adj.* fifteen (1); **quinze jours** two weeks
quinzième *adj.* fifteenth
quitter to leave (*s.o. or someplace*) (8); **se quitter** to separate, leave one another
quoi (à quoi, de quoi) *pron.* which; what; **à quoi sert-il?** what is it for?; **il n'y a pas de quoi** you're welcome (7); **j'aurai droit à quoi** I'll be entitled to what; **n'importe quoi** anything; no matter what
quotidien(ne) *adj.* daily, everyday (13); *n. m.* daily life; **dépenses** (*f. pl.*) **du quotidien** everyday living expenses

raccrocher to hang up (the telephone)
racine *f.* root
racisme *m.* racism
raconter to tell, relate (a story) (10); **qu'est-ce que tu racontes / vous racontez?** what are you talking about? (15)
rage: faire rage to rage; to be fierce
ragoût *m.* meat stew, ragout
raï *m.* raï (type of Moroccan music)
raide *adj.* stiff; straight (*hair*) (3)
raideur *f.* stiffness
raisin *m.* grape
raison *f.* reason; **avoir raison** to be right (3)
raisonnable *adj.* reasonable; rational (3)
raisonnement *m.* (logical) argument, reasoning
raisonneur/euse *adj.* argumentative; reasoning
râler *fam.* to complain
ralliement *m.* rallying
rallonger (nous rallongeons) to prolong, lengthen
rame *f.* oar; paddle
ramener (je ramène) to bring back
ramer to row
randonnée *f.* hike; **faire une randonnée (pédestre)** to go hiking (8)
rang *m.* rank, ranking; row
ranger to put away, tidy up
rapatriement *m.* repatriation
raper to grate
rapide *adj.* rapid, fast; **restauration** (*f.*) **rapide** fast food
rapidement *adv.* quickly
rappeler (je rappelle) to remind; **se rappeler** to recall, remember (13)
rapport *m.* relation; **rapports familiaux** family relationships; **par rapport à** in comparison with, in relation to
rapporter to bring back; to return; to report
rapprocher to relate; **se rapprocher (de)** to draw nearer (to)
rarement *adv.* rarely (2)
raser to raze, demolish; **se raser** to shave (oneself) (13)
rasoir *m.* razor (13)
rassembler to put back together, reassemble; to gather together, assemble
rassurant *adj.* reassuring
rassurer to reassure
rater to miss, not find
rationnellement *adv.* reasonably, rationally
rattraper to recapture
ravi *adj.* delighted
ravissant *adj.* charming, delightful; beautiful
rayé *adj.* striped
rayon (*m.*) **de soleil** ray of light
réactionnaire *adj.* reactionary, very conservative
réagir to react
réaliser to carry out, fulfill; to create (14)
réaliste *adj.* realistic (3)
réalité *f.* reality; **en réalité** actually
rebondir to bounce (back)
récemment *adv.* recently, lately (12)
recensement *m.* census
récent *adj.* recent, new, late
réception *f.* hotel (lobby) desk; receiving, receipt
recette *f.* recipe
recevoir (*p.p.* **reçu**) *irreg.* to receive (10)
rechange: ampoule (*f.*) **de rechange** spare lightbulb
rechargement *m.* recharging; refilling
réchauffement (*m.*) **de la planète** global warming (16)
recherche *f.* (*piece of*) research; search; **à la recherche de** in search of; **faire des recherches** to do research; **moteur** (*m.*) **de recherche** search engine
rechercher to research; to seek out; to strive for; **recherché** *adj.* sought after
réclamer to call for, demand
récolte *f.* harvest
récolter to harvest
recommandation *f.* recommendation
recommander to recommend
recommencer (nous recommençons) to start again
réconcilier to reconcile; **se réconcilier** to make up (*with somebody*)
reconnaître (*like* **connaître**) *irreg.* to recognize (16)
reconnu *adj.* known, recognized
recours: avoir recours à to have recourse, turn to
recruter to recruit (14)
reçu *m.* receipt (14); (see **recevoir**)

recueil *m.* collection (12)
reculer to move backward; to recoil; to delay
récupérer (je récupère) to recover, get back
recyclage *m.* recycling (16)
recycler to recycle (16)
rédacteur/trice *m., f.* writer; editor (14)
rédaction *f.* writing, preparing (*documents*)
rédiger (nous rédigeons) to write, write up, compose
redoutable *adj.* formidable, fearsome
réduction *f.* reduction; discount
réduire (*like* **conduire**) *irreg.* to reduce (9)
réduit *adj.* reduced; discounted
rééducation *f.* rehabilitation
réel(le) *adj.* real, actual
référence *f.* reference
réfléchir (à) to reflect (upon); to think (about) (4)
reflet *m.* reflection
refléter (je reflète) to reflect, mirror
réflexion *f.* reflection, thought
réforme *f.* reform (16)
réformer to reform
reformuler to reformulate
refrain *m.* chorus, refrain
refus *m.* refusal
refuser (de) to refuse (to) (12)
se régaler to feast on, treat oneself
regard: porter un regard (sur) to have a viewpoint (about)
regarder to look at, watch (2); **se regarder** to look at oneself, look at each other (13)
régime *m.* diet; régime (7)
régional (*pl.* **régionaux**) *adj.* local, of the district
règle *f.* rule
règlement *m.* rules, regulations
régler (je règle) to regulate, adjust; to settle
règne *m.* reign
regretter to regret, be sorry (16)
regrouper to regroup
régulier/ière *adj.* regular
régulièrement *adv.* regularly
reine *f.* queen (12)
rejoindre (*like* **craindre**) *irreg.* to (re)join
réjouissance *f.* rejoicing
relatif/ive *adj.* relative; **pronom** (*m.*) **relatif** *Gram.* relative pronoun
relation *f.* relation; relationship; **en relation avec** in contact with
relativement *adv.* relatively
relevé *m.* bank statment
se relaxer to relax
relier to tie, link
religieux/euse *adj.* religious
reliure *f.* bookbinding
remarquable *adj.* remarkable, outstanding
remarquer to notice
remède *m.* remedy; treatment
remercier (de) to thank (for); **(je ne sais pas) comment vous (te) remercier** I don't know how to thank you
remerciements *m. pl.* thanks
remettre (*like* **mettre**) *irreg.* to hand in; to replace; to deliver; **remettre à neuf** to restore
rempart *m.* wall (of a city)
remplacer (nous remplaçons) to replace
rempli *adj.* filled, full
remplir to fill (in, out, up)
remporter to win
rémunéré *adj.* compensated, paid
Renaissance *f.* Renaissance (12)
rencard *m.* date; appointment
rencontre *f.* meeting, encounter (13); **point** (*m.*) **de rencontre** meeting point
rencontrer to meet, encounter; **se rencontrer** to meet; to get together (13)
rendez-vous *m.* meeting, appointment; date (13); meeting place; **avoir rendez-vous avec** to have a meeting (date) with (3); **donner rendez-vous à** to make an appointment with
rendre to give (back), return; to hand in (5); to render, make; **rendre visite à** to visit (*s.o.*) (5); **se rendre à** to go to
renoncer to reject; to give up (*s.th.*)
renouveler (je renouvelle) to renew
rénover to renew
renseignement *m.* (*piece of*) information
se renseigner sur to make inquiries about
rentrée *f.* going back to school; **rentrée prochaine** beginning of next academic year
rentrer to return, go home (8)
réparation *f.* repair
réparer to repair
réparti *adj.* spread out
repartir (*like* **partir**) *irreg.* to leave (again)
répartition *f.* dividing up; distribution
repas *m.* meal (6); **repas fait maison** homemade meal
repeindre (*like* **craindre**) *irreg.* to repaint
repérer (je repère) to spot, locate, find
répertoire *m.* directory (*Internet*)
répéter (je répète) to repeat; **répétez (répète)** repeat (1)
réplique *f.* replica
répondeur (téléphonique) *m.* answering machine
répondre (à) to answer, respond (5)
réponse *f.* answer, response
reportage *m.* reporting; commentary
repos *m.* rest
reposant *adj.* restful
reposer to put down, set down; **se reposer** to rest (13)
reprendre (*like* **prendre**) *irreg.* to take (up) again; to have more (*food*)
représentant(e) *m., f.* representative
représentatif/ive *adj.* representative
représenter to represent
reprise: à plusieurs reprises several times
reprocher to reproach (*s.o. for s.th.*)
reproduire (*like* **conduire**) *irreg.* to reproduce, copy
république *f.* republic; **République Démocratique du Congo** Democratic Republic of Congo (2, 8)
répudié *adj.* repudiated, renounced
réputé *adj.* famous
réseau *m.* network
réservation *f.* reservation; **faire une réservation** to make a reservation
réservé (à) *adj.* reserved (for)
réserver to reserve; to keep in store
résidence *f.* residence; apartment building; **résidence universitaire** dormitory building
résider to reside
résistance: plat (*m.*) **de résistance** main dish, course
résister à to resist
résolument *adv.* resolutely, steadfastly
résonner to resonate, reverberate, resound
résoudre (*p.p.* **résolu**) *irreg.* to solve, resolve
respecter to respect, have regard for
respectueux/euse *adj.* respectful
respirer to breathe
responsabilité *f.* responsibility
responsable *m., f.* supervisor; staff member; *adj.* responsible
ressemblance *f.* resemblance
ressembler à to resemble; **se ressembler** to look alike, be similar
ressentir (*like* **dormir**) *irreg.* to feel
ressource *f.* resource; **ressources naturelles** natural resources (16)
restaurant (*fam.* **resto**) *m.* restaurant (2); **restaurant universitaire** (*fam.* **resto-U**) university cafeteria (2)
restaurateur/trice *m., f.* restaurant owner
restauration *f.* restoration; restaurant business; **restauration rapide** fast food
reste *m.* rest, remainder
rester to stay, remain (5); to be remaining; **il nous reste encore...** we still have . . .
restituer to return, restore
restreint *adj.* limited, restrained
résultat *m.* result
résulter de to stem from, result from
résumé *m.* summary, résumé
rétablir to reestablish
retard *m.* delay; **en retard** late (6)
retirer to withdraw (14); to derive, gain
retour *m.* return; **au retour** upon returning; **billet** (*m.*) **aller-retour** round-trip ticket
retourner to return; to go back (8)
retraite *f.* retirement; pension (16)
retraité(e) *m., f.* retiree, retired person
retransmission *f.* broadcast; rebroadcast (10); **retransmission sportive** sports broadcast (10)
retrouver to find (again); to regain; **se retrouver** to meet (again)
réunion *f.* meeting; reunion
réunir to collect, gather together; **se réunir** to get together; to hold a meeting
réussir (à) to succeed (at), be successful (in); to pass (*a test*) (4)
réussite *f.* success, accomplishment
revanche *f.* revenge
rêve *m.* dream; **un emploi** (*m.*) **de rêve** a "dream" job
réveil *m.* alarm clock (4)
réveiller to wake, awaken (*s.o.*); **se réveiller** to awaken, wake up (13)
Réveillon *m.* Christmas Eve (New Year's Eve) dinner
révéler to reveal
revendication *f.* demand; claim
revenir (*like* **venir**) *irreg.* to return; to come back (*someplace*) (8)
revenus *m. pl.* personal income
rêver (de, à) to dream; to dream (about, of) (2)
réviser to review, revise
révision *f.* review; revising
revivre (*like* **vivre**) *irreg.* to relive
revoir (*like* **voir**) *irreg.* to see again (10); **au revoir** good-bye (1)
révolte *f.* rebellion, revolt
révolutionnaire *adj.* revolutionary
révolutionner to revolutionize
revue *f.* magazine; review; journal (10)
rez-de-chaussée *m.* ground floor, first floor (5)
rhume *m.* (head) cold
riad (*see* **ryad**)
riche *adj.* rich (3)
richesse *f.* wealth; blessing

rideau (*pl.* **rideaux**) *m.* curtain (4)
ridicule *adj.* ridiculous
rien (ne… rien) *pron.* nothing (9); **de rien** *interj.* not at all, don't mention it; you're welcome (1)
rigoler *fam.* to amuse, entertain; to be kidding
rire (*p.p.* **ri**) *irreg.* to laugh (15); *m.* laughter
risette *f., fam.* smile
risque *m.* risk
risquer to risk
rissoler to brown (*cooking*)
rivage *m.* shore, beach coast
rivaliser avec to rival, compete with
rive *f.* (river)bank; **Rive gauche (droite)** the Left (Right) Bank (*in Paris*) (11)
rivière *f.* river, tributary
riz *m.* rice
robe *f.* dress (3)
robinet *m.* faucet, tap
rocheux/euse *adj.* rocky
roi *m.* king (12); **fête** (*f.*) **des Rois** Feast of the Magi, Epiphany
rôle *m.* part, character, role; **à tour de rôle** in turn, by turns; **jouer le rôle de** to play the part of
romain *adj.* Roman (12)
roman *m.* novel (10); **roman de science-fiction** science fiction novel; **roman policier** detective novel
romancier/ière *m., f.* novelist
romantique *m., f., adj.* romantic
romantisme *m.* romanticism
rompre (avec) (*p.p.* **rompu**) *irreg.* to break (with)
rond *adj.* round; *m.* (smoke) ring
rondelle *f.* round slices
rose *adj.* pink (3); *f.* rose
rôti *m.* roast (7)
roue *f.* wheel; **faire du patin à roues alignées** to do in-line skating
rouge *adj.* red (3); **rouge** (*m.*) **à lèvres** lipstick (13)
roulé *adj.* rolled (up)
rouler to travel (*in a car, on a bike*) (9); to roll (along)
route *f.* road, highway (8); **en route** on the way, en route
routier/ière *adj.* (pertaining to the) road; **carte** (*f.*) **routière** road map; **sécurité** (*f.*) **routière** highway safety
routinier/ière *adj.* routine, following a routine
roux (rousse) *m., f.* redhead; *adj.* redheaded; red (*hair*) (3)
royaume *m.* kingdom
rubrique *f.* headline; section
rue *f.* street (4)
ruelle *f.* alley; narrow street; lane
ruine *f.* ruin; decay; collapse
ruiné *adj.* ruined
russe *adj.* Russian; *m.* Russian (*language*); **Russe** *m., f.* Russian (*person*) (2)
Russie *f.* Russia (2, 8)
ryad *m.* Moroccan villa
rythme *m.* rhythm (16)

sa *adj., f. s.* his; her; its; one's
sable *m.* sand
sac *m.* sack; bag; handbag; **sac à dos** backpack (3); **sac à main** handbag (3); **sac de couchage** sleeping bag (8)
sachet *m.* packet
sacré *adj.* sacred; *fam.* darn
sacrifier to sacrifice
safran *m.* saffron
saharien(ne) *adj.* saharan
sage *m.* wise man; *adj.* good, well-behaved
saignant *adj.* rare (*meat*)
Saint-Sylvestre *f.* New Year's Eve
saison *f.* season
saisonnier/ière *adj.* seasonal
salade *f.* salad; lettuce (6)
salaire *m.* salary (14); **augmentation** (*f.*) **de salaire** salary raise (14)
salarié(e) *m., f.* salaried employee; **travailleur/euse** (*m., f.*) **salarié(e)** salaried worker (14)
saler to salt
salle *f.* room; auditorium; **salle à manger** dining room (5); **salle de bains** bathroom (5); **salle de classe** classroom (1, 5); **salle de sports** gymnasium
salon *m.* salon; living room; **salon de coiffure** hairdresser, beauty salon
saltimbanque *m., f.* acrobat; traveling performer
saluer to greet; **se saluer** to greet each other
salut *m.* health; *interj.* hi; bye (1)
salutation *f.* greeting
samedi *m.* Saturday (1); **le samedi** on Saturdays (5)
sandales *f. pl.* sandals (3)
sans *prep.* without; **sans-abri (sans-domicile)** *m., f. inv.* homeless (*person, people*) (16); **sans doute** probably (16)
santé *f.* health (13); **à votre (ta) santé** *interj.* cheers, to your health
sardines (*f. pl.*) **(à l'huile)** sardines (in oil) (7)
satellite: télévision (*f.*) **satellite** satellite television (10)
satisfaisant *adj.* satisfying
satisfait *adj.* satisfied; pleased
sauce *f.* sauce; gravy; salad dressing
saucisse *f.* sausage (7)
saucisson *m.* (hard) salami
sauf *prep.* except
saumon *m.* salmon (7); **darne** (*f.*) **de saumon** salmon steak
sauté *adj.* pan-fried, sautéed
sauter to jump
sauve-qui-peut *m., inv.* stampede
sauver to save, rescue (16)
savane *f.* savanna
saveur *f.* flavor
savoir (*p.p.* **su**) *irreg.* to know (how, a fact) (11)
savon *m.* soap
scandaleux/euse *adj.* scandalous
scanner *m.* scanner (10)
scénario *m.* screenplay, script
scène *f.* stage; scenery; scene; **scène de ménage** domestic squabble
science *f.* science; **faculté** (*f.*) **des sciences** School of Science; **science-fiction** science fiction; **sciences humaines** humanities; **sciences naturelles** natural sciences (2)
scientifique *m., f.* scientist; *adj.* scientific
scolaire *adj.* pertaining to schools, school, academic; **frais** (*m. pl.*) **scolaires** tuition, fees; **zone** (*f.*) **scolaire** school zone
scolarité: frais (*m. pl.*) **de scolarité** tuition, fees
scotché (à) *adj., fam.* glued (to)
scrupuleusement *adj.* scrupulously
sculpté *adj.* sculpted
sculpteur (femme sculpteur) *m., f.* sculptor (12)
se (s') *pron.* oneself; himself; herself; itself; themselves; to oneself, etc.; each other
sec (sèche) *adj.* dry; **biscuit** (*m.*) **sec** cookie, wafer
séché *adj.* dried
second *adj.* second; **seconde classe** second class; **Seconde Guerre** (*f.*) **mondiale** Second World War
secondaire *adj.* secondary; **école** (*f.*) **secondaire** secondary school
secours *m. s.* help, assistance, aid; *pl.* rescue services; **trousse** (*f.*) **de secours** first-aid kit
secrétaire *m., f.* secretary (14)
section *f.* section; division
sécurité *f.* safety; sense of security; **ceinture** (*f.*) **de sécurité** seat belt; **sécurité routière** highway safety; **sécurité sociale** Social Security
séducteur/trice *m., f.* charmer; seducer/seductress
séduire (*like* **conduire**) *irreg.* to charm, win over; to seduce
sein: au sein de within
seize *adj.* sixteen (1)
seizième *adj.* sixteenth
séjour *m.* living room (5); stay, sojourn
sel *m.* salt (6)
sélectionner to select
selon *prep.* according to (8); **selon moi** according to me, in my opinion
semaine *f.* week (1); **la semaine prochaine (passée)** next (last) week (5); **toutes les semaines** every week (10); **une fois par semaine** once a week (5)
semblable (à) *adj.* like, similar (to)
sembler to seem; to appear; **il semble que** + *subj.* it seems that (16)
semestre *m.* semester
semoule *f.* semolina
sénateur *m.* senator
Sénégal *m.* Senegal (2, 8)
sénégalais *adj.* Senegalese; **Sénégalais(e)** *m., f.* Senegalese person (2)
senior *m., f.* senior citizen
sens *m.* meaning; sense; way, direction; **bon sens** common sense; **dans ce sens** to that end (effect)
sensibiliser (à) to make (*s.o.*) sensitive (to)
sensoriel(le) *adj.* sensory; **perception** (*f.*) **extrasensorielle** extra-sensory perception
sentiment *m.* feeling
sentir (*like* **dormir**) *irreg.* to feel, sense; to smell (8); **se sentir** to feel; **sentir bon (mauvais)** to smell good (bad)
séparé *adj.* separated
sept *adj.* seven (1)
septembre September (1)
septième *adj.* seventh
sera (see **être**)
sereine *adj.* clear; serene
série *f.* series (10); **série télévisée** serial drama (10)
sérieusement *adv.* seriously
sérieux/euse *adj.* serious (3); **prendre au sérieux** to take seriously
serpent *m.* snake
serré *adj.* tight, snug
serrer to hug, embrace; **se serrer la main** to shake hands

serveur/euse *m., f.* bartender; waiter, waitress (7)
service *m.* favor; service; military service; serve (*tennis*); **station-service** *f.* gas station (9)
serviette *f.* napkin (6); towel; briefcase; **serviette de plage** beach towel (8)
servir (*like* **dormir**) *irreg.* to serve (8); **à quoi sert-il?** what is it for?; **servir à** to be of use in, be used for
ses *adj. m., f. pl.* his; her; its; one's
seuil *m.* threshold; doorstep
seul *adj.* alone; single
seulement *adv.* only (9)
sexisme *m.* sexism (16)
short *m.* (*pair of*) shorts (3)
si *adv.* so (very); so much; yes (*response to negative question*) (9); **si (s')** *conj.* if; whether (4); **même si** even if; **s'il vous (te) plaît** please (1)
sida (SIDA) *m.* AIDS
siècle *m.* century (12); **Siècle des lumières** Age of Enlightenment
siège *m.* seat (9); place; headquarters
sien: le/la/les sien(ne)(s) *pron., m., f.* his/hers
sieste *f.* nap; **faire la sieste** to take a nap
signe *m.* sign, gesture
signer to sign
signifier to mean
significatif/ive *adj.* significant
silencieux/euse *adj.* silent
simplement *adv.* simply
simplicité *f.* simplicity
sincère *adj.* sincere (3)
sincérité *f.* sincerity
se singulariser to distinguish oneself
singularité *f.* peculiarity
singulier/ière *adj.* singular; *m., Gram.* singular (*form*)
sinon *prep.* if not; otherwise
site *m.* site (10)
situer to situate, find; **se situer** to be situated; to be located
six *adj.* six (1)
sixième *adj.* sixth
ski *m.* skiing; ski (8); **chaussures** (*f. pl.*) **de ski** ski boots (8); **faire du ski** to ski (5); **lunettes** (*f. pl.*) **de ski** ski goggles (8); **ski alpin** downhill skiing (8); **ski de fond** cross-country skiing (8); **ski nautique** water-skiing (8); **station** (*f.*) **de ski** ski resort
skier to ski (2)
skieur/euse *m., f.* skier
smartphone *m.* smartphone (1)
SMS *m.* text message (10)
SNCF (Société nationale des chemins de fer français) *f. French national train system*
snob *adj. inv.* snobbish (3)
snowboard: faire du snowboard to go snowboarding
sociabilité *f.* sociability
sociable *adj.* sociable (3)
social *adj.* social; **logement** (*m.*) **social** housing project; **sécurité** (*f.*) **sociale** Social Security; **siège** (*m.*) **social** head office, headquarters
société *f.* society; organization; company (14); **jeux** (*m. pl.*) **de société** board games, group games (15)
sociologie (*fam.* **socio**) *f.* sociology (2)
sœur *f.* sister (5); **belle-sœur** sister-in-law (5); **demi-sœur** half sister; stepsister
soi (soi-même) *pron., neu.* oneself (12); **chez soi** at one's own place, home
soie *f.* silk
soif *f.* thirst; **avoir soif** to be thirsty (3)
soigner to take care of; to treat (14)
soigneusement *adv.* carefully
soin *m.* care; **avec soin** carefully
soir *m.* evening; **ce soir** tonight, this evening (5); **ce soir-là** that evening; **demain soir** tomorrow evening; **du soir** in the evening, at night (6); **hier soir** last night; **le lundi (le vendredi) soir** on Monday (Friday) evenings (5); **tous les soirs** every evening (10)
soirée *f.* party (3); evening (7)
sois gentil! *interj.* be nice! (6)
soit: quel(le)(s) que soit (soient)... whatever may be . . .
soixante *adj.* sixty (1)
sol: sous-sol *m.* basement, cellar (5)
solaire *adj.* solar; **crème** (*f.*) **solaire** suntan lotion (8); **écran** (*m.*) **solaire** sunblock (8); **énergie** (*f.*) **solaire** solar energy (16)
soldat *m.* soldier
solde *f.* (*soldier's*) pay, wages; **en solde** *m.* on sale
sole *f.* sole (*fish*) (7)
soleil *m.* sun; **faire du soleil (il fait du soleil)** to be sunny (out) (it's sunny) (5); **le roi Soleil** the Sun King (Louis XIV); **lunettes** (*f. pl.*) **de soleil** sunglasses (8)
solidaire *adj.* showing solidarity, loyal
solidarité *f.* solidarity; interdependence
solide *adj.* solid, sturdy
solitaire *adj.* solitary; single; alone (3)
solitude *f.* loneliness; solitude (16)
sombre *adj.* dark; gloomy
sommeil *m.* sleep; **avoir sommeil** to be sleepy (3); **le plein sommeil** deep in sleep
sommet *m.* summit, top
somnambule *m. f.* sleepwalker
somptueux/euse *adj.* sumptuous
son *adj., m. s.* his; her; its; one's; *n. m.* sound
sonate *f.* sonata
sondage *m.* opinion poll, survey (16)
songer à to think of (about)
sonner to ring (*telephone*)
sonnette *f.* bell; doorbell
sonore *adj.* sound
sophistiqué *adj.* sophisticated
sorte *f.* sort, kind; manner
sortie *f.* exit; going out; evening out
sortir (*like* **dormir**) *irreg.* to leave; to take out; to go out (8)
sot(te) *adj.* stupid, foolish
souci *m.* care, worry
se soucier de to worry about
soucoupe (*f.*) **volante** flying saucer
soudain *adv.* suddenly (11)
souffle *m.* breath of air; puff of wind
souffrance *f.* suffering
souffrir (*like* **ouvrir**) *irreg.* to suffer (14)
souhait *m.* wish, desire
souhaiter to wish, desire (16)
souk *m. North African market*
soulagement *m.* relief
soulager (nous soulageons) to relieve
soulever (je soulève) to excite; to bring up
souligner to underline, emphasize
soumission *f.* subservience, submissiveness
soupe *f.* soup; **cuillère** (*f.*) **à soupe** tablespoon, soup spoon (6)
sourcil *m.* eyebrow
sourd *adj.* deaf
souriant *adj.* smiling
sourire (*like* **rire**) *irreg.* to smile; *m.* smile
souris *f.* mouse (1)
sournois *adj.* sly, shifty
sous *prep.* under, beneath (4); in (*rain, sun*); **sous (la) forme de** in the form of
sous-marin *adj.* underwater; *m.* submarine; **plongée** (*f.*) **sous-marine** scuba diving (8)
sous-sol *m.* basement, cellar (5)
soutenir (*like* **tenir**) *irreg.* to support (16); to assert
soutien *m.* support
souvenir *m.* memory, recollection; souvenir
se souvenir (*like* **venir**) **de** *irreg.* to remember (13)
souvent *adv.* often (2)
spécial (*pl.* **spéciaux**) *adj.* special
spécialisé *adj.* specialized
spécialiste (en) *m., f.* specialist (in)
spécialité *f.* specialty (*in cooking*)
spectacle *m.* show; performance (15)
spectaculaire *adj.* spectacular
spectateur/trice *m., f.* viewer, spectator
spirituel(le) *adj.* spiritual; witty
splendeur *f.* splendor
spontané *adj.* spontaneous
sport *m.* sport(s) (2); **faire du sport** to do (participate in) sports (5); **magasin** (*m.*) **de sports** sporting goods store; **salle** (*f.*) **de sport** gymnasium
sportif/ive *adj.* athletic; sports-minded (3); **manifestation** (*f.*) **sportive** sporting event (15); *m., f.* athlete; **retransmission** (*f.*) **sportive** sports broadcast (10)
squelette *m.* skeleton
stable *adj.* stable; **emploi** (*m.*) **stable** steady job
stade *m.* stadium
stage *m.* training course; practicum, internship (14)
standardiste *m., f.* switchboard operator
station *f.* resort (*vacation*); station; **station de métro** subway station (11); **station de ski** ski resort; **station-service** *f.* gas station, garage (9)
stationnement *m.* parking
statut *m.* status
steak *m.* (beef) steak; **steak au poivre** pepper steak; **steak frites** steak with French fries
stéréotypé *adj.* stereotyped
steward *m.* flight attendant, steward (9)
stimuler to stimulate
stipuler to stipulate
stratégie *f.* strategy
stricte *adj.* strict
studette *f.* small studio (apartment) with shared bathroom (4)
studieux/ieuse *adj.* studious
studio *m.* studio (apartment) (4)
stupide *adj.* stupid; foolish; **il est stupide que** + *subj.* it's idiotic that (16)
style *m.* style; **style de vie** lifestyle
styliste *m., f.* fashion designer
stylo *m.* pen (1)
subir to undergo, be subjected to
subjonctif *m., Gram.* subjunctive (*mood*)
substantif *m., Gram.* noun, substantive
substituer to substitute
subtil *adj.* subtle
subventionner to support, back (*financially*)

se succéder (ils se succèdent) to follow one another
succès *m.* success; **à succès** successful
successeur *m.* successor
succession *f.* series, succession
sucre *m.* sugar (6); **canne** (*f.*) **à sucre** sugarcane
sucré *adj.* sweetened
sud *m.* south; **Amérique** (*f.*) **du Sud** South America; **au sud** to the south (9); **sud-est (-ouest)** southeast (-west)
Suède *f.* Sweden
suffire (*p.p.* **suffi**) to be enough
suggérer (je suggère) to suggest
se suicider to commit suicide
Suisse *f.* Switzerland (2, 8); **suisse** *adj.* Swiss; **Suisse** *m., f.* Swiss person (2)
suite: et ainsi de suite and so on; **tout de suite** immediately (5)
suivant *adj.* following
suivi (de) *adj.* followed (by)
suivre (*p.p.* **suivi**) *irreg.* to follow; to take (*a class, a course*) (12)
sujet *m.* subject; topic
super *adj. inv., fam.* super, fantastic
superbe *adj.* magnificent, superb
supérieur *adj.* superior; upper
supermarché *m.* supermarket
supplément *m.* supplement, addition; supplementary charge
supplémentaire *adj.* supplementary, additional
supportable *adj.* bearable, tolerable
supporter to bear, tolerate; **supporter** *m.* fan (sports)
supposer to suppose
supprimer to abolish, suppress
sur *prep.* on, on top (of) (4); over; out of; about; **donner sur** to overlook
sûr *adj.* sure, certain (16); safe; **bien sûr** of course; **il est sûr que** + *indic.* it is certain that (16)
surchargé *adj.* overloaded
surdoué *adj.* gifted
sûrement *adv.* definitely, certainly
surf (*m.*) **des neiges** snowboarding
surface *f.* surface; **grande surface** shopping mall, superstore
surfer to surf; **surfer sur le Web** to surf the web (10)
surgelé *adj.* frozen
surnom *m.* name, family name
surnommer to nickname
surpopulation *f.* overpopulation (16)
surprenant *adj.* surprising
surpris *adj.* surprised (16)
surtout *adv.* especially; above all (10)
survenir (*like* **venir**) *irreg.* to happen
survêtement *m.* track suit, sweat suit
survivre (*like* **vivre**) *irreg.* to survive
survol *m.* browsing (*Internet*)
survoler to fly over
susceptible (de) *adj.* capable of, likely to
suspect(e) *m., f.* suspect
symbole *m.* symbol
symboliser to symbolize
symétrique *adj.* symmetrical
sympathique (*fam., inv.* **sympa**) *adj.* nice, friendly (3)
symphonie *f.* symphony
syndicat (*m.*) **d'initiative** (local) chamber of commerce, tourist information bureau (11)
synonyme *m.* synonym; *adj.* synonymous
système *m.* system

ta *adj., f. s., fam.* your
tabac *m.* tobacco; **bureau** (*m.*) **de tabac** (*licensed*) tobacco store; **café-tabac** *m.* bar-tobacconist (11)
table *f.* table (1); **à table** at (to) the table
tableau *m.* (chalk)board (1); painting (12); chart
tablette *f.* bar (*of chocolate*); a tablet computer, an iPad (1)
tâche *f.* task; **tâches ménagères** household tasks
taille *f.* waist; build; size; **de taille moyenne** of medium height (3)
tailleur *m.* (*woman's*) suit (3)
tailleuse *f.* tailoress
tajine *m.* tajine (a Moroccan stew)
talonnade *f.* heel; back-heel (*rugby, soccer*)
tambour *m.* drum
tandis que *conj.* while, whereas
tannage *m.* tanning (process)
tant *adj.* so much; so many; **tant de** so many, so much; **tant mieux** so much the better (15); **tant pis** too bad (15)
tante *f.* aunt (5)
taper to type; to be scorching; **se taper la cloche** to have a good meal
tapis *m.* rug (4)
tapisserie *f.* tapestry
tarbouche *m.* brimless hat worn by Muslim men
tard *adv.* late; **il est tard** it's late; **plus tard** later
tarif *m.* tariff; fare, price
tarifaire *adj.* tariff
tarte *f.* tart; pie (6); **tarte aux pommes** apple tart; **tarte tatin** upside-down apple tart
tartine *f. bread and butter sandwich*
tas: des tas de lots of, piles of
tasse *f.* cup (6)
tatouage *m.* tattoo
tatoueur *m.* tatooer
taux *m.* rate; **taux de change** exchange rate (14); **taux de chômage** unemployment rate (14)
taxe *f.* indirect tax
taxi *m.* taxi; **chauffeur/euse** (*m., f.*) **de taxi** cab driver
tchao *interj.* good-bye
tchatcher to talk
te (t') *pron., s., fam.* you; to you, for you; **s'il te plaît** *interj.* please (1)
technicien(ne) *m., f.* technician
technique *f.* technique; *adj.* technical
techno *adj.* synthesized (music)
technologie *f.* technology
tee-shirt (*pl.* **tee-shirts**) *m.* T-shirt (3)
tel(le) *adj.* such; **tel père, tel fils** like father, like son; **tel que** such as
télécarte *f.* telephone calling card
télécharger (nous téléchargeons) to download (10)
télécommande *f.* remote control (10)
télécopieur *m.* fax machine
téléphone *m.* telephone (4); **numéro** (*m.*) **de téléphone** telephone number (10); **téléphone fixe** landline (12); **téléphone portable** cell phone (10)
téléphoner (à) to phone, telephone (3); **se téléphoner** to call one another
téléphonique: répondeur (*m.*) **téléphonique** (telephone) answering machine
téléspectateur/trice *m., f.* television viewer
télévisé *adj.* televised; **jeu** (*m.*) **télévisé** game show (10); **journal** (*m.*) **télévisé** television news program (10)
téléviseur (*fam.* **télé**) *m.* television set (10)
télévision (*fam.* **télé**) *f.* television (1); **télévision numérique terrestre (TNT)** high-definition television (10); **télévision par câble (le câble)** cable television (10); **télévision publique** government-owned television; **télévision satellite** satellite television (10)
tellement *adv.* so; so much (11)
témoin *m.* witness; **être témoin de** to witness
tempérament *m.* temperament, personality
température *f.* temperature
tempête *f.* storm
temporaire *adj.* temporary
temporel(le) *adj.* temporal, pertaining to time
temps *m.* time; weather (5); *Gram.* tense; **avoir le temps de** to have time to; **de temps en temps** from time to time (2); **depuis combien de temps... ?** since when . . . ?, (for) how long . . . ? (9); **en même temps** at the same time; **en temps de pluie** in rainy weather; **faire un temps pourri** to be rotten weather; **gagner du temps** to save time; **il est temps de** it's time to; **le temps est nuageux** it's cloudy (5); **le temps est orageux** it's stormy (5); **passer du temps** to spend time; **pendant combien de temps... ?** (for) how long . . . ? (9); **perdre du temps** to waste time; **prendre le temps (de)** to take the time (to); **quel temps fait-il?** how's the weather? (5); **temps libre** leisure time (15); **tout le temps** always, the whole time
tendance *f.* tendency; trend; **avoir tendance à** to have a tendency to
tendinite *f.* tendonitis
tendre *adj.* tender, sensitive; soft
tenir (*p.p.* **tenu**) *irreg.* to hold; to keep; **tenir à** to be keen about (16); **tenir au courant** to keep up to date; **tenir un journal** to keep a diary
tennis *m.* tennis; *pl.* tennis shoes (3); **court** (*m.*) **de tennis** tennis court; **jouer au tennis** to play tennis
tentant *adj.* tempting
tentation *f.* temptation
tente *f.* tent (8)
tenter (de) to try, attempt (to)
terme *m.* term; expression; **à court (long) terme** in the short (long) run
terminer (qqch) to finish (*s.th.*); to end (*s.th.*); **se terminer** to end
terrain *m.* field; ground; **terrain** (*m.*) **de camping** campground; **tout-terrain** *adj.* all-terrain (*vehicle*)
terrasse *f.* terrace, patio (5)
terre *f.* land; earth; **Terre** the planet Earth; **Terre Neuve** *f.* Newfoundland; **par terre** on the ground (4); **pomme** (*f.*) **de terre** potato (6)
terrine *f.* (*type of*) pâté, terrine
territoire *m.* territory
terrorisme *m.* terrorism (16)
tes *adj., m., f. pl., fam.* your

tête *f.* head (13); **avoir mal à la tête** to have a headache (13); **casse-tête** *m.* puzzle; **tête-à-tête** tête-à-tête, intimate conversation
texte *m.* text; passage; **traitement** (*m.*) **de texte** word processing (10)
texto *m.* text message (10)
textoter to text (*fam.*)
TGV (Train à grande vitesse) *m.* (*French high-speed*) bullet train
thé *m.* tea (6)
théâtre *m.* theater (12); **faire du théâtre** to act, do theater; **pièce** (*f.*) **de théâtre** (*theatrical*) play (12)
théorie *f.* theory
thermes *m. pl.* thermal baths
thon *m.* tuna
tiède *adj.* lukewarm, tepid
tiens *interj.* well, well (*expresses surprise*); you don't say; **ah, tiens...** oh, there's . . .
tiers *m.* one-third; *adj.* third; **Tiers-Monde** *m.* Third World
tigre *m.* tiger
timbre *m.* stamp; postage stamp (10)
timide *adj.* shy; timid
tiré (de) *adj.* drawn, adapted (from)
tirer to pull, draw (out); **tirer avantage de** to take advantage of
tissu *m.* cloth, fabric
titre *m.* title; degree
TNT (télévision numérique terrestre) *f.* high-definition television (10)
toi *pron., s., fam.* you; **et toi?** and you?, how about you? (1); **toi-même** *pron.* yourself (12)
toilettes *f. pl.* bathroom, toilet (4); **faire sa toilette** to wash up
toit *m.* roof
tolérance *f.* tolerance
tolérer to tolerate, stand for
tomate *f.* tomato (6)
tombe *f.* tomb, grave
tomber to fall (8); **tomber amoureux/euse (de)** to fall in love (with) (13)
ton *adj., m. s., fam.* your; **à ton avis** in your opinion (11)
tondeuse *f.* lawn mower
tondre to mow (*lawn*)
tonton *m., fam.* uncle
torche: lampe (*f.*) **torche** flashlight
tort *m.* wrong; **avoir tort** to be wrong (3)
se tortiller to twist, wriggle
tortueux/euse *adj.* twisting
tôt *adv.* early; **il est tôt** it's early
totalement *adv.* totally, completely
totalité *f.* totality, entire amount
touche *f.* key (*keyboard*); stroke
toucher (à) to touch (14); to concern; to cash (*a check*) (14)
toujours *adv.* always (2); still
tour *f.* tower (11); *m.* walk, ride; turn; tour; trick; **à tour de rôle** in turn, by turns; **faire le tour de** to go around, take a tour of; **faire un tour (en voiture)** to take a walk (ride) (5)
tourisme *m.* tourism; **faire du tourisme** to go sightseeing
touriste *m., f.* tourist
touristique *adj.* tourist
tourmenté *adj.* uneasy; tortured
tournant: plaque (*f.*) **tournante** linchpin; hub
tourné (*adj.*) **vers** facing
tourner (à) to turn (11); to film (a movie)
tournesol *m.* sunflower; **huile** (*f.*) **de tournesol** sunflower seed oil
tournoi *m.* tournament
tousser to cough
tout(e) (*pl.* **tous, toutes**) *adj., pron.* all; every (10); everything (9); each; any; **tout** *adv.* wholly, entirely, quite, very, all; **à tout à l'heure** see you soon; **avant tout** *prep.* above all; **en tout** altogether, in all; **en tout cas** in any case, at any rate; **haricots** (*m. pl.*) **mange-tout** green beans; sugar peas; **je n'aime pas du tout...** I don't like . . . at all; **ne... pas du tout** not at all (9); **pas du tout** not at all; **tous ensemble** all together; **tous les après-midi** every afternoon (10); **tous (toutes) les deux** both (of them); **tous les jours** every day (5, 10); **tous les matins** every morning (10); **tous les soirs** every evening (10); **tout à coup** suddenly (11); **tout à fait** completely, entirely; **tout à l'heure** in a while (5); **tout au long de** throughout; **tout de suite** immediately (5); **tout droit** *adv.* straight ahead (11); **tout le monde** everybody, everyone (7); **tout le temps** always, the whole time; **tout va bien** everything is going well; **tout-puissant** *adj.* all-powerful; **tout-terrain** *adj.* all-terrain (*vehicle*); **toute la matinée (la journée, la soirée, la nuit)** all morning (day, evening, night) (7); **toutes les deux heures** every two hours; **toutes les semaines** every week (10)
toutefois *adv.* however
tracasserie *f.* harassment, hassle
tracer (nous traçons) to draw; to trace out; **tracer un itinéraire** to map out an itinerary
tracteur *m.* tractor
traditionnel(le) *adj.* traditional
traduction *f.* translation
traduire (*like* **conduire**) *irreg.* to translate (9)
trafic *m.* traffic
train *m.* train (9); **billet** (*m.*) **de train** train ticket; **en train** by train; **être en train de** to be in the process of (15); **prendre le train** to take the train; **Train à grande vitesse (TGV)** (*French high-speed*) bullet train; **train-train** (*m.*) **quotidien** daily grind, routine
trait *m.* feature, trait
traite *f.* trade; **traite négrière** slave trade
traité *adj.* treated, dealt with
traitement *m.* treatment; **traitement de texte** word processing (10)
traiter to treat; **traiter de** to deal with
traiteur *m.* caterer, deli owner; delicatessen
trajet *m.* trip; distance
tranche *f.* slice (7); block, slab
trancher to slice, cut up
tranquille *adj.* quiet, calm
tranquillité *f.* tranquility; calm
transformer to transform, change; **se transformer** to change
translucide *adj.* translucent
transmettre (*like* **mettre**) *irreg.* to transmit, convey
transport(s) *m.* transportation; **moyen** (*m.*) **de transport** means of transportation (9); **transports en commun** public transportation
transporter to carry, transport
trapéziste *m., f.* trapeze artist
travail (*pl.* **travaux**) *m.* work (2); project; job; employment; **langue** (*f.*) **de travail** working language; **travail d'équipe** teamwork; **travaux** (*pl.*) **pratiques** hands-on (practical) work
travaillé *adj.* finely worked; intricate; polished
travailler to work (2); **travailler à (pour) son compte** to be self-employed (14)
travailleur/euse *m., f.* worker (14); *adj.* hardworking (3); **travailleur/euse indépendant(e)** self-employed worker (14); **travailleur/euse salarié(e)** salaried worker (14)
travers: à travers *prep.* through
traversée *f.* crossing
traverser to cross (9)
treize *adj.* thirteen (1)
treizième *adj.* thirteenth
tréma *m.* dieresis, umlaut **(ë)**
tremplin *m.* diving board; springboard
trentaine *f.* about thirty
trente *adj.* thirty (1)
très *adv.* very; most; very much; **très bien** *interj.* very well (good) (1); **très bien, merci** *interj.* very well, thank you; **très (peu) calorique** high (low) in calories
trésor *m.* treasure
trésorier/ière *m., f.* treasurer
tricolore *m.* French flag (*blue, white, red*)
trimestre *m.* trimester; quarter (*academic*)
triomphe *m.* triumph, success
triompher to triumph
tripes *f. pl.* tripe
triste *adj.* sad (3)
trois *adj.* three (1)
troisième *adj.* third
tromper to deceive; **se tromper (de)** to make a mistake; to be wrong (13)
trompette *f.* trumpet
trop (de) *adv.* too; too much (of); too many (of) (6)
trophée *m.* trophy
troquet *m., fam.* bar
trottoir *m.* sidewalk
troubler to trouble, disturb
troupeau *m.* herd
trousse *f.* case; kit; **trousse de secours** first-aid kit
trouver to find (2); to deem; to like; **se trouver** to be located (situated, found) (13)
truffe *f.* truffle
truite *f.* trout
tu *pron., s., fam.* you
tube *m., fam.* hit (song)
tuer to kill
Tunisie *f.* Tunisia (2, 8)
tunisien *adj.* Tunisian; **Tunisien(ne)** *m., f.* Tunisian (*person*) (2)
turc (turque) *adj.* Turkish
Tweet *m.* tweet
type *m.* type, kind; *fam.* guy, fellow
typique *adj.* typical

un(e) (*pl.* **des**) *art.*, a, an; *adj., pron.* one (1); **un(e) autre** another (15); **un jour** someday (14); **un peu** a little (3); **un peu (de)** a little (of) (6); **une fois** once (11); **une fois par semaine** once a week (5)
unanime *adj.* unanimous
uni *adj.* united; plain, solid (*color*); **États-Unis** *m. pl.* United States; **Organisation** (*f.*) **des Nations Unies (ONU)** United Nations (UN)

uniformisateur *adj.* making s.th. uniform, all the same
uniformiser to make uniform
union *f.* union; marriage; **Union européenne (UE)** European Union (EU); **union libre** living together, common-law marriage
unique *adj.* only, sole; single; singular
uniquement *adv.* only
s'unir to unite
unité *f.* unity; unit; department
univers *m. s.* universe
universel(le) *adj.* universal
universitaire *adj.* (*of or belonging to the*) university; **cité** (*f.*) **universitaire** (*fam.* **cité-U**) university dormitory; **résidence** (*f.*) **universitaire** dormitory; **restaurant** (*m.*) **universitaire** (*fam.* **resto-U**) university cafeteria (2)
université *f.* university (2)
urbain *adj.* urban, city
urgent *adj.* urgent; **il est urgent que** + *subj.* it's urgent that (16)
usage *m.* use; custom
ustensile *f.* kitchenware, cookware
utile *adj.* useful; **il est utile que** + *subj.* it's useful that (16)
utilisateur/trice *m., f.* user
utilisation *f.* use
utiliser to use, utilize
utilité *f.* use; utility, usefulness

vacances *f. pl.* vacation (5); **grandes vacances** summer vacation; **partir (aller) en vacances** to leave on vacation; **passer les vacances** to spend one's vacation; **pendant les vacances** during vacation
vacancier/ère *m., f.* vacationer
vache *f.* cow
vachement *adv., fam.* very, tremendously
vague *f.* (*ocean*) wave; **nouvelle vague** new wave (*trend*)
vaincre (*p.p.* **vaincu**) *irreg.* to win; to triumph
vaisselle *f. s.* dishes; **faire la vaisselle** to wash (do) the dishes (5)
valable *adj.* valid
valeur *f.* value; worth
valise (*fam.* **valoche**) *f.* suitcase (8); **faire sa valise** to pack one's bag
vallée *f.* valley
valoir (*p.p.* **valu**) *irreg.* to be worth (16); **il vaut mieux que** + *subj.* it is better that (16)
valorisé *adj.* valued
valoriser to value
vanille *f.* vanilla
vaniteux/euse *adj.* vain
variante *f.* variation
varier to vary; to change
variété *f.* variety, type; **chanson** (*f.*) **de variété** popular song (15); **spectacle** (*m.*) **de variétés** variety show; floor show (in a restaurant) (15)
Varsovie *f.* Warsaw
vaste *adj.* vast; wide, broad
va-t'en! *interj. fam.* get going!, go away! (13)
vaut (see **valoir**)
veau *m.* veal (7); calf; **escalope** (*f.*) **de veau** veal scaloppini
vedette *f.* star, celebrity (*male or female*)
végétarien(ne) *m., f., adj.* vegetarian
véhicule *m.* vehicle
veille *f.* the day (evening) before; eve
Veinard! *interj. fam.* Lucky you!
vélo *m., fam.* bike; **à/en vélo** by bike; **faire du vélo** to go cycling (5)
velours *m.* velvet
vendanges *m. pl.* grape harvest
vendeur/euse *m., f.* salesperson
vendre to sell (5); **à vendre** for sale
vendredi *m.* Friday (1); **le vendredi** on Fridays (5); **le vendredi soir** on Friday evenings (5)
se venger (nous nous vengeons) to avenge oneself; to take revenge
venir (*p.p.* **venu**) *irreg.* to come (8); **venir de** + *inf.* to have just (*done s.th.*) (8)
vent *m.* wind; **faire du vent (il fait du vent, il y a du vent)** to be windy (it's windy) (5); **vent alizé** trade wind
vente *f.* sale; sales; **vente aux enchères** auction
venter to be windy; **il vente** it's windy (5)
ventre *m.* abdomen, belly; stomach (13)
verbe *m.* verb; language
vérifier to verify
véritable *adj.* true; real
vérité *f.* truth
verlan *m.* *French form of slang that reverses syllables* **(l'envers→verlan)**
verre *m.* glass (6); **prendre un verre** *fam.* to have a drink (*with s.o.*) (6); **un verre de** a glass of
verrouillable *adj.* lockable
vers *prep.* around, about (*with time expressions*); toward, to; about; **tourné** (*adj.*) **vers** facing
verser to pour
version *f.* version; **en version originale** original version, not dubbed (*movie*)
vert *adj.* green (3); (*politically*) "green"; **citron** (*m.*) **vert** lime (*fruit*); **espace** (*m.*) **vert** open space, greenbelt; ***haricots** (*m. pl.*) **verts** green beans (6); **poivron** (*m.*) **vert** green (bell) pepper; **tourisme** (*m.*) **vert** ecotourism
veste *f.* sports coat, blazer (3); **veste de montagne** hiking (ski) jacket
veston *m.* suit jacket (3)
vêtement *m.* garment; *pl.* clothes, clothing
viande *f.* meat (6)
vibrer to vibrate
victime *f.* victim (*male or female*)
victoire *f.* victory
vide *adj.* empty; **vide-grenier** *m.* garage sale
vidéo *f., fam.* video(cassette); *adj. inv.* video; **caméra** (*f.*) **vidéo** video camera; **cassette** (*f.*) **vidéo** videocassette; **jeux** (*m. pl.*) **vidéo** video games
vidéothèque *f.* video store
vie *f.* life (2); **coût** (*m.*) **de la vie** cost of living (14); **niveau** (*m.*) **de vie** standard of living (16)
Vietnam *m.* Vietnam (2, 8)
vietnamien *adj.* Vietnamese; **Vietnamien(ne)** *m., f.* Vietnamese person (2)
vieux (vieil, vieille) *adj.* old (4); **mon vieux (ma vieille)** old friend, buddy
vif (vive) *adj.* lively; bright
vigne *f.* vine; vineyard
vignoble *m.* vineyard
villa *f.* bungalow; single-family house; villa
villageois *adj.* village style
ville *f.* city (1); **centre-ville** *m.* downtown (11); **en ville** in town, downtown
vin *m.* wine (6); **coq** (*m.*) **au vin** coq au vin (*chicken prepared with red wine*); **marchand(e)** (*m., f.*) **de vin** wine merchant (14)
vingt *adj.* twenty (1); **vingt et un (vingt-deux...)** *adj.* twenty-one (twenty-two . . .) (1)
vingtaine *f.* about twenty
vingtième *adj.* twentieth
violet(te) *adj.* purple, violet (3); *m.* violet (*color*)
violon *m.* violin
violoncelle *m.* cello
virelangue *m.* tongue twister
virement *m.* transfer (money) (14)
Virginie *f.* Virginia; **Virginie-Occidentale** West Virginia
visa *m.* visa (8); signature
visage *m.* face (13)
vis-à-vis (de) *adv.* opposite, facing; toward
viser à to aim to; to set out to
visibilité *f.* visibility
visionnaire *m., f.* visionary
visionner to watch, view
visite *f.* visit (2); **faire une visite** to pay a visit; **rendre visite à** to visit (*s.o.*) (11)
visiter to visit (*a place*) (2); **je peux la visiter** I may visit it
visiteur/euse *m., f.* visitor
vitæ: curriculum (*m.*) **vitæ** résumé (14)
vite *adv.* quickly, fast, rapidly; **il faut faire vite** we have to move fast; **venez vite** come quickly
vitesse *f.* speed; **limite** (*f.*) **de vitesse** speed limit; **Train** (*m.*) **à grande vitesse (TGV)** (*French high-speed train*) bullet train
vitres *f. pl.* windows
vitrine *f.* display window, store window
vivant *adj.* living; **langues** (*f. pl.*) **vivantes** modern languages
vive... *interj.* long live . . .
vivre (*p.p.* **vécu**) *irreg.* to live (12); **facile (difficile) à vivre** easy (hard) to live with; **vive...** *interj.* long live (hurrah for) . . .
vocabulaire *m.* vocabulary
vocal: boîte (*f.*) **vocale** voice mail (10)
vœu (*pl.* **vœux**) *m.* wish
voici *prep.* here is/are (2)
voie *f.* way, road; course; lane; railroad track; **pays** (*m.*) **en voie de développement** developing nation
voilà *prep.* there is/are (2)
voile *m.* veil; *f.* sail; **bateau** (*m.*) **à voile** sailboat (8); **faire de la voile** to go sailing (5); **planche** (*f.*) **à voile** windsurfer
voilier *m.* sailboat
voir (*p.p.* **vu**) *irreg.* to see (10)
voire *adv.* indeed
voisin(e) *m., f.* neighbor; **voisin(e) de palier** neighbor living on the same landing
voiture *f.* car, automobile (4); train car; **faire un tour en voiture** to take a ride (5); **voiture hybride** hybrid car (16)
voiture-restaurant *f.* dining car (*train*)
voix *f.* voice; **à voix haute** *adv.* in a loud voice; aloud
vol *m.* flight (9)
volaille *f.* poultry
volant: objet (*m.*) **volant non identifié (O.V.N.I.)** unidentified flying object (UFO); **soucoupe** (*f.*) **volante** flying saucer
volcan *m.* volcano

voler to fly; to steal; **qui vole un œuf vole un bœuf** once a thief always a thief
volley-ball (*fam.* **volley**) *m.* volleyball; **jouer au volley** to play volleyball
volontaire *m., f., adj.* volunteer
volontiers *adv.* gladly
volonté *f.* will, willingness
volupté *f.* voluptuous pleasure
vos *adj., m., f. pl.* your
voter to vote
votre *adj., m., f.* your; **à votre avis** in your opinion (11)
vôtre(s): le/la/les vôtre(s) *pron., m., f.* yours; *pl.* your close friends, relatives
vouloir (*p.p.* **voulu**) *irreg.* to wish, want (7); **je voudrais** I would like (6); **que veut dire... ?** what does . . . mean?; **vouloir bien** to be willing; to agree (7); **vouloir dire** to mean (7)
vous *pron.* you; yourself; to you; **chez vous** where you live, your place; **et vous?** and you?, how about you? (1); **s'il vous plaît** please (1); **vous-même** *pron.* yourself (12)
voyage *m.* trip; **agence** (*f.*) **de voyages** travel agency; **bon voyage** *interj.* have a good trip; **chèque** (*m.*) **de voyage** traveler's check; **faire un voyage** to take a trip (5); **partir (s'en aller) en voyage** to leave on a trip; **projets** (*m. pl.*) **de voyage** travel plans
voyager (nous voyageons) to travel (8)
voyageur/euse *m., f.* traveler
voyant(e) *m., f.* fortune-teller, medium; **voyant** (*m.*) **lumineux** indicator light
voyelle *f.* vowel
voyons,... let's see, . . . (10)
vrai *adj.* true, real (4); **il est vrai que** + *indic.* it's true that (16)
vue *f.* view; panorama; sight; **en vue de** with a view toward; **point** (*m.*) **de vue** point of view

wagon *m.* train car (9); **wagon-lit** *m.* sleeping car; **wagon-restaurant** *m.* dining car
Wallonie *f.* Wallonia (*French-speaking Belgium*)
W.-C. *f. pl.* restroom, toilet (4)
Web *m.* (World Wide) Web (10)
week-end *m.* weekend; **ce week-end** this weekend (5); **le week-end** on weekends (5)
Wi-Fi *m.* Wi-Fi (wireless) connection (10)

xénophobie *f.* xenophobia

y *pron.* there (11); **il n'y a pas de...** there isn't (aren't) . . .; **il y a** there is (are) (1); ago (8); **qu'est-ce qu'il y a dans... ?** what's in . . . ?; **y a-t-il... ?** is (are) there . . . ?
yeux (*pl.* of **œil**) *m.* eyes (13)

zèbre *m.* zebra
zéro *m.* zero
zone *f.* zone, area
zoologique *adj.* zoological; **jardin** (*m.*) **zoologique** (*fam.* **zoo**) zoological gardens, zoo
zouk *m.* zouk music (of Guadeloupe, Martinique, Haiti)

Lexique anglais-français

This English-French end vocabulary contains the words in the active vocabulary lists of all chapters. See the introduction to the *Lexique français-anglais* for a list of abbreviations used.

abdomen ventre *m.* (13)
able: to be able pouvoir *irreg.* (7)
abolish abolir (16)
about (*with time expressions*) vers (6)
abroad à l'étranger (9)
accept accepter (de) (12)
accident accident *m.* (16)
accomplish réussir (4)
according to selon (8)
account compte *m.* (14); **checking account** compte-chèques *m.* (14); **savings account** compte d'épargne (14)
accountant comptable *m., f.* (14)
acquaintance: to make the acquaintance (of) faire la connaissance (de) (5)
across from en face de (4)
act *v.* agir (4)
activities (leisure) loisirs *m. pl.* (15); **outdoor activities** activités (*f.*) de plein air (15)
actor acteur/trice *m., f.* (12)
address adresse *f.* (10)
adore adorer (2)
ads (classified) petites annonces *f. pl.* (10)
advertisement, advertising publicité *f.* (10)
advise conseiller (à, de) (15)
aerobics aérobic *f.* (5); **to do aerobics** faire de l'aérobic (5)
afraid: to be afraid of avoir peur de (3)
after après (2, 5)
afternoon après-midi *m.* (5); **afternoon snack** goûter *m.* (6); **this afternoon** cet après-midi (5)
afterward après (5)
again de nouveau (11)
age âge *n. m.*; **Middle Ages** le Moyen Âge (12)
ago il y a (8)
agree vouloir (*irreg.*) bien (7)
agreeable agréable (3)
agreed d'accord (2)
ahead: straight ahead tout droit (11)
airplane avion *m.* (9)
airport aéroport *m.* (9)
alarm clock réveil *m.* (4)
Algeria Algérie *f.* (2, 8)
Algerian (*person*) Algérien(ne) *m., f.* (2)
all *adj.*, tout, toute, tous, toutes (9); *pron.* tout(e); **all right** ça peut aller (1); moyen (1); **not at all** ne... pas du tout (9)
allow (to) permettre (de) (12)
almost presque (6)
already déjà (9)
also aussi
always toujours (2)
American (*person*) Américain(e) *m., f.* (2)
amount montant *m.* (14)
amusing amusant(e) (3)
and et (2); **and you?** et vous? (et toi?) (1)
angry fâché(e) (16); **to get angry** se fâcher (13)
another un(e) autre (15)
answer *v.* répondre à (5)
antique *adj.* ancien(ne) (4)
any en *pron.* (11)
anyway quand même (16)
apartment appartement *m.* (4); **apartment building** immeuble *m.* (4); **studio apartment** studio *m.* (4)
apologize s'excuser (13)
apparatus appareil *m.* (10)
appear avoir l'air (3); paraitre *irreg.* (16)
appetizer *hors-d'œuvre *m. inv.* (7)
apple pomme *f.* (7)
application (job) demande (*f.*) d'emploi (14)
apply (*for a job*) poser sa candidature (14)
appointment: to have an appointment avoir (*irreg.*) rendez-vous (3)
April avril (1)
architect architecte *m., f.* (14)
arena arènes *f. pl.* (12)
argue se disputer (13)
arm bras *m. s., pl.* (13)
around (*with time expressions*) vers (6)
arrival arrivée *f.* (9)
arrive arriver (3)
art art (*m.*); **work of art** œuvre (*f.*) d'art (12)
artisan artisan(e) *m., f.* (14)
artist artiste *m., f.* (14)
as . . . as aussi... que (14); **as far as** jusqu'à (11); **as for me** pour ma part (16); **as much (many) . . . as** autant (de)... que (15); **as soon as** dès que (14), aussitôt que (14)
ashamed: to be ashamed avoir (*irreg.*) honte (3)
ask (for) demander (2); **to ask a question** poser une question (12)
asleep: to fall asleep s'endormir *irreg.* (13)
at à (2)
athletic sportif/ive (3)
atmosphere atmosphère *f.* (16)
attend assister à (15)
attendant (flight) hôtesse (*f.*) de l'air (9), steward *m.* (9)
attention: to pay attention (to) faire (*irreg.*) attention (à) (5)
August août (1)
aunt tante *f.* (5)
automatic teller (ATM) guichet (*m.*) automatique (14)
automobile voiture *f.* (4)
autumn automne *m.* (5); **in autumn** en automne (5)
awaken se réveiller (13)

back dos *m. s., pl.* (13)
backpack sac (*m.*) à dos (3)
bad mauvais(e) *adj.* (4); **bad(ly)** mal *adv.*; **it's bad (out)** il fait mauvais (5); **not bad(ly)** pas mal (1); **things are going badly** ça va mal (1); **to feel bad (ill)** aller (*irreg.*) mal (5); **too bad!** dommage! *interj.* (16)
badly *adv.* mal (1)
bag: sleeping bag sac (*m.*) de couchage (8)
baguette baguette (*f.*) (de pain) (6)
bakery boulangerie *f.* (7)
balcony balcon *m.* (5)
ball: bocce ball pétanque *f.* (15)
bank banque *f.* (11); **bank (ATM/credit) card** carte (*f.*) bancaire (14); **bank statment** *m.* relevé (14) **the Left Bank** (*in Paris*) Rive (*f.*) gauche (11); **the Right Bank** (*in Paris*) Rive (*f.*) droite (11)
bar-tobacconist café-tabac *m.* (11)
basement sous-sol *m.* (5)
bathe se baigner (13)
bathroom salle (*f.*) de bains (5); **bathroom sink** lavabo *m.* (4)
be être (*irreg.*) (2); **here is/are** voici (2); **how are you?** comment allez-vous? (comment vas-tu?) (1); **it's a . . .** c'est un (une)... (1); **there is/are** il y a; voilà; **to be in the middle (the process) of** être en train de (15)
beach plage *f.* (8); **beach towel** serviette (*f.*) de plage (8)
beans: green beans *haricots (*m. pl.*) verts (6)
beautiful beau, bel, belle (beaux, belles) (3)
because parce que (4)
become devenir *irreg.* (8)
bed lit *m.* (4); **to go to bed** se coucher (13)
bedroom chambre *f.* (4)
beef bœuf *m.* (6)
beer bière *f.* (6)
begin commencer (2); **to begin to** (*do s.th.*) se mettre (*irreg.*) à (+ *inf.*) (13)
behind derrière (4)
Belgian (*person*) Belge *m., f.* (2)
Belgium Belgique *f.* (2, 8)
believe croire *irreg.* (10); estimer (16); **to believe in (that)** croire à/en (que)
beret béret *m.* (3)
berth couchette *f.* (9)
beside à côté de (4)
best le mieux *adv.* (15); le/la/les meilleur(e)(s) *adj.*
better meilleur(e) *adj.*; mieux *adv.* (15); **it is better that** il vaut mieux que + *subj.* (16); **so much the better** tant mieux (15)
between entre (4)
bicycle bicyclette *f.* (8), vélo *m.*; **by bike** à vélo (9); **to go bicycling** faire (*irreg.*) de la bicyclette, du vélo (5)
big grand(e) (3)
bill (*in a restaurant*) addition *f.* (7); (*currency*) billet *m.*
biology biologie *f.* (2)
black noir(e) (3)
blackboard tableau (noir) *m.* (1)
blazer veste *f.* (3)
blond(e) blond(e) (3)
blouse chemisier *m.* (3)
blue bleu(e) (3)
board games jeux (*m. pl.*) de société (15)
boarding pass carte (*f.*) d'embarquement (9)
boat bateau *m.* (8); **sailboat** bateau à voile (8)
boating: to go boating faire du bateau (8)
bocce ball pétanque *f.* (15)
body corps *m.* (13)
book livre *m.* (1); **e-book** livre (*m.*) numérique (10); **print book** livre (*m.*) papier (10)
bookstore librairie *f.* (2)
boots bottes *f. pl.* (3); **hiking boots** chaussures (*f. pl.*) de montagne (8); **ski boots** chaussures (*f. pl.*) de ski (8)
bore: to be bored s'ennuyer (13)

born: to be born naître *irreg.* (8)
borrow (from) emprunter (à) (11)
boss chef (*m.*) d'entreprise (14)
bottle bouteille *n. f.* (6)
boulevard boulevard *m.* (11)
bowling (lawn) pétanque *f.* (15)
boy garçon *m.* (3)
boyfriend copain *m.* (7)
brave courageux/euse (3)
Brazil Brésil *m.* (8)
bread pain *m.* (6); **country-style wheat bread** pain de campagne (7)
breakfast petit déjeuner *m.* (6)
bring apporter (6); **to bring** (*s.o. somewhere*) amener
broadcast émission *n. f.* (10); **sports broadcast** retransmission (*f.*) sportive (10); **to broadcast** émettre (*irreg.*)
brother frère *m.* (5); **brother-in-law** beau-frère *m.* (5)
brown (*hair*) châtain(e) (3); marron *inv.* (3)
browse naviguer (10)
browser navigateur *m.* (10)
brush (one's hair, teeth) se brosser (les cheveux, les dents) (13); brosse *f.* (13)
budget budget *m.* (14)
build bâtir (6)
building bâtiment *m.* (1); immeuble (*office, apartment*) *m.* (4)
bus (*city*) autobus *m.* (5); (*interurban*) autocar *m.* (9)
business commerce *m.* (2); **business class** classe (*f.*) affaires (9); **business manager** directeur/trice commercial(e) (14)
but mais (2)
butcher boucher/ère *m., f.* (14); **butcher shop** boucherie *f.* (7); **pork butcher's shop** charcuterie *f.* (7)
butter beurre *m.* (6)
buy *v.* acheter (8)
by à (2); en (2); par (12); **by (train, plane, bus)** en (9); **by bike** à velo (9)

cable TV câble *m.* (10)
café café *m.* (2)
cafeteria (university) restaurant (*m.*) universitaire (resto-U) (2)
cake gâteau *m.* (6)
call *v.* appeler (10); **who's calling?** qui est à l'appareil? (10)
calm calme (3)
camcorder (digital) caméscope *m.* (10)
camera (digital) appareil (*m.*) (photo) numérique (10); **digital video camera** caméscope *m.* (10)
camping camping *m.* (8); **to go camping** faire (*irreg.*) du camping
can (*to be able*) pouvoir *irreg.* (7)
can (of food) boîte (*f.*) (de conserve) (7)
Canada Canada *m.* (2, 8)
Canadian (*person*) Canadien(ne) *m., f.* (2)
cancel annuler (11)
canned goods conserves *f. pl.* (7)
cap casquette *f.* (3)
car voiture *f.* (4); **train car** wagon *m.* (9)
carpooling covoiturage *m.* (16)
carafe carafe *f.* (6)
card carte *f.* (3); **bank (ATM/credit) card** carte bancaire (14); **credit card** carte de crédit (14); **debit card** carte de débit (14); **to play cards** jouer aux cartes (3)
careful: to be careful faire (*irreg.*) attention (à) (5)
Caribbean Islands Antilles *f. pl.* (1)
carrier (letter) facteur/trice *m., f.* (14)
carrot carotte *f.* (6)
carry apporter (7); porter (3)
cartoon bande (*f.*) dessinée (15)
case: in that case alors (4)
cash argent (*m.*) liquide (14); **to cash** (*a check*) toucher (14), encaisser
castle château *m.* (11)
cathedral cathédrale *f.* (12)
celebrate fêter, célébrer (6)
celebration fête *f.* (7)
cell phone mobile *m.* (10); téléphone portable *m.* (10)
century siècle *m.* (12)
ceremony cérémonie *f.* (13)
certain certain(e) (16); sûr(e) (16)
chair chaise *f.* (1)
chalkboard tableau (noir) *m.* (1)
challenge défi *n. m.* (16)
chance: games of chance jeux (*m. pl.*) de hasard (15)
change monnaie *n. f.* (10); *v.* changer (14)
channel (*television*) chaîne *f.* (10)
chateau château *m.* (11)
check (*in a restaurant*) addition *f.* (7); (*bank*) chèque *m.* (14); **to cash a check** toucher un chèque (14), encaisser un chèque; **to write a check** faire (*irreg.*) un chèque (14)
check *v.* contrôler
cheese fromage *m.* (6)
chemistry chimie *f.* (2)
chess échecs *m. pl.* (3)
chest (of drawers) commode *f.* (4)
chestnut (*hair color*) châtain (3)
chicken poulet *m.* (6)
child enfant *m., f.* (5)
China Chine *f.* (2, 8)
Chinese (*person*) Chinois(e) *m., f.* (2); (*language*) chinois *m.* (2)
chocolate chocolat *m.* (6)
choose choisir (4)
chop (*meat*) côte *n. f.* (7)
church (*Catholic*) église *f.* (11)
citizen citoyen(ne) *m., f.* (16)
city ville *f.* (2)
civil civil(e); **civil rights** droits (*m. pl.*) civils (16); **civil servant** fonctionnaire *m., f.* (14)
class (business) classe (*f.*) affaires (9); **first class** première classe (9); **second class** deuxième classe (9); **tourist class** classe économique (9)
classical classique
classified ads petites annonces *f. pl.* (10)
classroom salle (*f.*) de classe (1)
clear *adj.* clair(e) (16)
clerk (sales) employé(e) (14)
click (on) cliquer (sur) (10)
climb *v.* monter (8)
clock (alarm) réveil *m.* (4)
close to près de (4)
closet armoire *f.* (4)
cloudy: it's cloudy le temps est nuageux (5)
clubbing: to go clubbing aller en boîte (15)
coat manteau *m.* (3); **sports coat** veste *f.* (3)
coffee (cup of) un café *m.* (2)
coin locker consigne *f.* (automatique) (9)
coins monnaie *f.* (10)
cold froid *m.*; **it's cold** il fait froid (5); **to be cold** avoir (*irreg.*) froid (3)
collection collection *f.* (15); recueil *m.* (12)
comb peigne *n. m.* (13); **to comb one's hair** se peigner (13)
come venir *irreg.* (8); **to come back to** (*someplace*) revenir *irreg.* (8)
command: to have a command of maîtriser (14)
commercial publicité *n. f.* (10)
common good bien (*m.*) commun (16)
compact disc (CD) player lecteur (*m.*) de CD (4)
company entreprise *f.* (14); société *f.* (14); **company head** chef (*m.*) d'entreprise (14)
compartment (*train*) compartiment *m.* (9)
composer compositeur/trice *m. f.* (12)
computer ordinateur *m.* (1); **computer science** informatique *f.* (2); **desktop computer** ordinateur (*m.*) de bureau (de table) (10), micro-ordinateur (micro) *m.* (10); **laptop computer** ordinateur (*m.*) portable (portable *m.*) (1, 10)
concern *v.* toucher (14)
conflict conflit *n. m.* (16)
conformist conformiste (3)
Congo (Democratic Republic of) République (*f.*) Démocratique du Congo (2, 8)
conservation conservation *f.* (16)
conserve conserver (16)
consider estimer (16)
constantly constamment (12)
construct construire *irreg.* (9)
consume consommer (16)
continue continuer (11)
cooking cuisine *f.* (6); **to cook** faire (*irreg.*) la cuisine (5)
cool *adj.* frais (fraîche); **it's cool** il fait frais (5)
corner coin *m.* (11)
cost of living coût (*m.*) de la vie (14)
costs frais *m. pl.* (14)
Cote d'Ivoire Côte d'Ivoire *f.* (2, 8)
country (*nation*) pays *m.* (2); **country(side)** campagne *f.* (8)
couple (*engaged, married*) couple *m.* (13)
courageous courageux/euse (3)
course (*academic*) cours *m.* (2); **course** (*meal*) plat *m.* (7); **first course** entrée *f.* (7); **main course** plat (*m.*) principal (7)
cousin cousin(e) *m., f.* (5)
cover *v.* couvrir *irreg.* (14)
craftsperson artisan(e) *m., f.* (14)
crayfish écrevisse *f.* (7)
cream crème *f.* (6); **ice cream** glace *f.* (6)
credit card carte (*f.*) de crédit (14)
croissant croissant *m.* (6)
cross *v.* traverser (9); **cross-country skiing** ski (*m.*) de fond (8)
crowd foule *n. f.* (15)
cup tasse *f.* (6); **cup of coffee** un café *m.* (2); **wide cup** bol *m.* (6)
cured guéri(e) (13)
current events actualité *f.* (14)
curtain rideau *m.* (4)
cycling cyclisme *m.* (15); vélo *m.*; **to go cycling** faire (*irreg.*) du vélo (5)

daily quotidien(ne) (13)
dance *v.* danser (2)
date (from) *v.* dater (de) (12); **to have a date** avoir (*irreg.*) rendez-vous (3); **what is the date?** quelle est la date? (1)
daughter fille *f.* (5); **daughter-in-law** bru *f.* (5)

day jour *m.* (1); **all day** toute la journée (7); **every day** tous les jours (5); **the day before yesterday** avant-hier (7); **what day is it?** quel jour sommes-nous? (1); **whole day** journée *f.* (7)
dear cher/ère (3)
debit card carte de débit (14)
decade: the decade of (the fifties) les années (cinquante) *f. pl.* (8)
December décembre (1)
decide décider (de) (12)
delay retard *n. m.* (6)
delicatessen charcuterie *f.* (7)
demand *v.* exiger (16)
demonstrate (for/against) manifester (pour/contre) (16)
dentist dentiste *m., f.* (14)
departure départ *m.* (9)
deposit (change) *v.* déposer (14); déposer (la monnaie) (10)
describe décrire *irreg.* (10)
desire *v.* désirer (15); souhaiter (16)
desk bureau *m.* (1)
desktop computer micro (-ordinateur) *m.* (10), ordinateur de bureau (de table) (10)
dessert dessert *m.* (6)
destroy détruire *irreg.* (9)
detest détester (2)
develop développer (16)
development développement *m.* (16)
dial (the number) composer (le numéro) (10)
dice dés *m. pl.* (4)
dictionary dictionnaire *m.* (2)
die *v.* mourir *irreg.* (8)
diet régime *n. m.* (7)
different différent(e) (3)
difficult difficile (3)
digital camera appareil (*m.*) numérique (10)
dine dîner (6)
dining room salle (*f.*) à manger (5)
dinner dîner *m.* (6); **to have dinner** dîner (6)
direct *v.* diriger (14)
directory (online) annuaire (*m.*) éléctronique (10)
disagreeable désagréable (3)
discover découvrir *irreg.* (14)
dishes vaisselle *f. s.*; **to wash (do) the dishes** faire (*irreg.*) la vaisselle (5)
district quartier *m.* (2); arrondissement *m.* (11)
division (*academic*) faculté *f.* (2)
divorced divorcé(e) (5)
do faire *irreg.* (5); **do-it-yourself work** bricolage *m.* (15)
doctor médecin *m.*, femme médecin *f.* (14); **doctor's office** cabinet (*m.*) medical (13)
documentary documentaire *n. m.* (10)
dog chien(ne) *m., f.* (4)
door porte *f.* (1)
dormitory cité (*f.*) universitaire (cité-U) (2)
doubt *v.* douter (16); **without a doubt** sans doute (16)
downhill skiing ski (*m.*) alpin (8)
download *v.* télécharger (10)
downtown centre-ville *m.* (11)
draw dessiner (10)
drawers (chest of) commode *f.* (4)
dream (of) *v.* rêver (de) (2)
dress robe *f.* (3); **to get dressed** s'habiller (13)
drink (soft) boisson (*f.*) (gazeuse) (6); **to drink** boire *irreg.* (6)
drive *v.* conduire *irreg.* (9)
driver conducteur/trice *m., f.* (9)
drugstore pharmacie *f.* (11)
DSL connection/line connexion (*f.*) ADSL (10)
during pendant (9)
DVD player lecteur (*m.*) de DVD (1)
dynamic dynamique (3)

each (one) chacun(e) *pron.* (15); chaque *adj.* (4)
ear oreille *f.* (13)
early de bonne heure (6); tôt (6); en avance (6)
earn gagner (14)
east est *m.* (9); **to the east** à l'est (9)
easy facile (3)
eat manger (2); **eat a meal** prendre un repas (6)
e-book livre (*m.*) numérique (10)
eccentric excentrique (3)
eclair éclair (*pastry*) *m.* (7)
economics économie *f.* (2)
editor rédacteur/trice *m., f.* (14)
egg œuf *m.* (6)
eight *huit (1)
eighteen dix-huit (1)
eighth le/la *huitième (11)
elect élire *irreg.* (16)
eleven onze (1)
eleventh le/la onzième (11)
else (s.th.) autre chose (7)
e-mail message mél *m.* (10); courriel *m.* (10)
employee employé(e) *m., f.* (14); **s.o. employed (by)** employé(e) (de) (14)
encounter rencontre *n. f.* (13); **to encounter** rencontrer (13)
end by (*doing s.th.*) finir par (12)
energy énergie *f.* (16); **nuclear/solar energy** énergie (*f.*) nucléaire/solaire (16)
engage: to get engaged se fiancer (13)
engagement fiançailles *f. pl.* (13)
engineer ingénieur *m.* (14)
engineering génie *m.* (2)
England Angleterre *f.* (2, 8)
English (*person*) Anglais(e) *m., f.* (2); (*language*) anglais *m.* (2)
enough (of) assez de (6)
enter entrer (8)
enthusiastic enthousiaste (3)
envelope enveloppe *f.* (10)
environment environnement *m.* (16)
environmentalist écologiste *m., f.* (16)
equal égal(e) (16)
era: the era of (the fifties) les années (cinquante) *f. pl.* (8)
e-reader liseuse *f.* (10)
errands courses *f. pl.*; **to do errands** faire (*irreg.*) les courses (5)
especially surtout (10)
essential essentiel(le) (16)
establish établir (16)
establishment: at the establishment of chez (5)
estimate *v.* estimer (16)
even so quand même (16)
evening soir *m.* (6); **all evening** toute la soirée (7); **entire evening** soirée *f.* (7); **good evening** bonsoir (1); **in the evening** du soir (6); **Monday/Friday evenings** le lundi/le vendredi soir (5); **this evening** ce soir (5)
event événement *m.* (12); **sporting event** manifestation (*f.*) sportive (15)
ever: have you ever . . . ? avez-vous (as-tu) déjà… ? (9)
every tout, toute, tous, toutes (10); **every day (afternoon, morning, evening)** tous les jours (après-midi, matins, soirs) (5); **every week** toutes les semaines (10)
everybody tout le monde (7)
everyday quotidien(ne) *adj.* (13)
everyone tout le monde (9)
everything tout (9)
everywhere partout (11)
evidently évidemment (12)
exam examen *m.* (2); **to take an exam** passer un examen (4); **to pass (an exam)** réussir à (4)
example: for example par exemple (16)
exchange *v.* échanger (10); **exchange rate** cours (*m.*) (14), taux (*m.*) de change (14); **money exchange (office)** bureau (*m.*) de change (14)
excuse (oneself) s'excuser (13); **excuse me** excusez-moi (1)
exhaust *v.* épuiser (16)
exhibit exposition *n. f.* (12)
expense dépense *f.* (14); **expenses** frais *m. pl.* (14)
expensive cher/ère (3)
express an opinion exprimer une opinion (16)
expression: freedom of expression liberté (*f.*) d'expression (13)
extremist ideas idées (*f.*) extrémistes
eye œil *m.* (13) (*pl.* yeux) (3)

face visage *n. m.* (13)
fair *adj.* juste (16)
fall automne *n. m.* (5); **in fall** en automne (5)
fall *v.* tomber (8); **to fall in love (with)** tomber amoureux/euse (de) (13)
false faux (fausse) (4)
familiar: to be familiar with connaître *irreg.* (11)
family famille *f.* (5)
far from loin de (4)
farmer agriculteur/trice *m., f.* (14)
fat *adj.* gros(se) (4)
father père *m.* (5); **father-in-law** beau-père *m.* (5); **stepfather** beau-père *m.* (5)
favorite préféré(e) (5)
fax fax *m.* (10)
February février (1)
feel sentir *irreg.* (8); **to feel bad** aller (*irreg.*) mal (5); **to feel like** avoir (*irreg.*) envie de (3)
few: a few *adj.* quelques; quelques-uns/unes *pron.* (9)
fifteen quinze (1)
fifth le/la cinquième *m., f.* (11)
fifty cinquante (1)
file fichier *m.* (10)
fill it up faire (*irreg.*) le plein (9)
fillet (*beef, fish, etc.*) filet *m.* (7)
film film *m.* (2)
filmmaker cinéaste *m., f.* (12)
finally enfin (11)
find *v.* trouver (2)
fine bien (15); ça va bien (1)
finger doigt *m.* (13)
finish finir (de + *inf.*) (4); **to finish by** (*doing s.th.*) finir par (+ *inf.*) (4)
first d'abord *adv.* (11); premier/ière *adj.* (4); **first of all (at first)** d'abord (11)
fish poisson *m.* (6); **fish store** poissonnerie *f.* (7); **fishing** pêche *f.* (15); **to go fishing** aller (*irreg.*) à la pêche (8)
five cinq (1)
fixed-price menu menu *m.* (7)
flash of lightning coup (*m.*) de foudre (13)

flight vol *m.* (9); **flight attendant** hôtesse (*f.*) de l'air (9); steward *m.* (9)
floor: ground floor rez-de-chaussée *m.* (5); **second floor** (*in the U.S.*) premier étage *m.* (5); **third floor** (*in the U.S.*) deuxième étage *m.* (5)
flower fleur *f.* (4)
fluently couramment (12)
follow suivre *irreg.* (12)
food nourriture *f.* (6)
foot pied *m.* (13); **on foot** à pied (9)
for pour (2); (*time*) depuis (9), pendant (9); (*flight*) à destination de (9); **for example** par exemple (16); **for oneself** à son compte (14)
foreign étranger/ère (2); **in a foreign country** à l'étranger (9); **foreign language** langue (*f.*) étrangère (2)
forest bois *m.* (11); forêt *f.* (8)
forget (to) oublier (de) (8)
fork fourchette *f.* (6)
former ancien(ne) (4)
formerly autrefois (11)
fortunate heureux/euse (3)
forty quarante (1)
found: to be found se trouver (13)
four quatre (1)
fourteen quatorze (1)
fourth le/la quatrième (11); **one-fourth** quart *m.* (6)
France France *f.* (2, 8)
free gratuit(e) (11); **free time** temps (*m.*) libre (15)
freedom (of expression) liberté (*f.*) (d'expression) (16)
French (*person*) Français(e) *m., f.* (2); (*language*) français *m.*; **French fries** frites *f. pl.* (6); **in French, please** en français, s'il vous plaît (1)
fresh frais (fraîche) (5)
Friday vendredi *m.* (1)
friend ami(e) *m., f.* (2); copain/copine (7)
friendship amitié *f.* (13)
fries frites *f. pl.* (6)
from de (2); **from time to time** de temps en temps (2); **from now on** à l'avenir (14), à partir de maintenant (14)
front: in front of devant (4)
fruit fruit *m.* (6); **fruit juice** jus (*m.*) de fruit (6)
fun *adj.* amusant(e) (3); **to have fun** s'amuser (à) (13)
fundamentalism intégrisme *m.* (16)
funny drôle (3)
furious furieux/euse (16)
furniture (piece of) meuble *m.* (5)
future avenir *m.* (14); **in the future** à l'avenir (14)

game (*sport*) match (15); **games of chance** jeux (*m. pl.*) de *hasard (15); **group, social games** jeux (*m. pl.*) de société (15)
garden jardin *n. m.* (5)
gardening jardinage *m.* (15)
garlic ail *m.* (15)
garret chambre (*f.*) de bonne (4)
gas station station-service *f.* (9)
gasoline essence *f.* (9)
generally en général (2)
geography géographie *f.* (2)
geology géologie *f.* (2)
German (*person*) Allemand(e) *m., f.* (2); (*language*) allemand *m.* (2)
Germany Allemagne *f.* (2, 8)
get obtenir *irreg.* (8); **get going!** va-t'en! (13); **to get along (with)** s'entendre (avec) (13); **to get off, down from** descendre (de) (5); **to get up** se lever (13)
gift cadeau *m.* (10)
girl fille *f.* (3)
girlfriend copine *f.* (7)
give donner (2); **to give back** rendre (5)
glass verre *m.* (6); **(eye)glasses** lunettes *f. pl.* (8)
global warming réchauffement (*m.*) de la planète (16)
globalization mondialisation *f.* (16)
glove gant *m.* (8)
go: to go aller *irreg.* (5); **go away!/get going!** allez-vous-en! (va-t'en!) (13); **how's it going?** ça va? (1); **things are going well** ça va (1); **to be going** (*to do s.th.*) aller + *inf.* (5); **to go back** retourner (8); **to go clubbing** aller en boîte (15); **to go down** (*a street, a river*) descendre (5); **to go fishing** aller à la pêche (8); **to go home** rentrer (8); **to go off, go away** (*to work*) s'en aller *irreg.* (13); **to go out** sortir *irreg.* (de) (8); **to go up** monter (8); **what's going on?** qu'est-ce qui se passe? (15)
goggles: ski goggles lunettes (*f. pl.*) de ski (8)
good bien *adv.* (15); bon(ne) *adj.* (4); **common good** bien (*m.*) commun (16); **good-bye** au revoir (1); **good day** bonjour (1); **good evening** bonsoir (1); **that's good** tant mieux (15)
Gothic gothique (12)
government gouvernement *m.* (16)
grandchild petit-enfant *m.* (5)
granddaughter petite-fille *f.* (5)
grandfather grand-père *m.* (5)
grandmother grand-mère *f.* (5)
grandparent grand-parent *m.* (5)
grandson petit-fils *m.* (5)
gray gris(e) (3)
great-grandparent arrière-grand-parent *m.* (5)
Greece Grèce *f.* (8)
green vert(e) (3); **green beans** *haricots (*m. pl.*) verts (6)
grocery store épicerie *f.* (7)
ground: on the ground par terre (4); **ground floor** rez-de-chaussée *m.* (5)
group games jeux (*m. pl.*) de société (15)
guess *v.* deviner (12)
guitar guitare *f.* (4)
gymnasium gymnase *m.* (2)

habitually d'habitude (5)
hair cheveux *m. pl.* (3)
hairdresser coiffeur/euse *m., f.* (14)
Haiti Haïti *m.* (8)
half demi(e) (6); **half brother** demi-frère *m.* (5); **half past (the hour)** et demi(e) (6); **half sister** demi-sœur *f.* (5)
hall couloir *m.* (4); **lecture hall** amphithéâtre *m.* (2); **town hall** mairie *f.* (11)
ham jambon *m.* (6)
hand main *f.* (13); **to hand in** rendre (5)
handbag sac (*m.*) à main (3)
handsome beau, bel, belle (beaux, belles) (3)
happen se passer (15); **what's happening?** qu'est-ce qui se passe? (15)
happy heureux/euse (3)
hardly peu (3)
hardworking travailleur/euse (3)
hat chapeau *m.* (3)
have avoir *irreg.* (3); **to have** (*to eat; to order*) prendre *irreg.* (6); **to have a drink** (with *s.o.*) prendre un verre (6); **to have breakfast** prendre le petit déjeuner (6); **to have to** devoir *irreg.* (7)
head tête *f.* (13); directeur/trice *m., f.* (14); **company head** chef (*m.*) d'entreprise (14)
healed guéri(e) (13)
health santé *f.* (13)
hear entendre (5)
heart cœur *m.* (13); **by heart** par cœur (12)
height: medium height de taille moyenne (3)
hello bonjour (1); (*telephone*) allô (10)
helmet casque *m.* (8)
help *v.* aider (14)
here ici (1); **here is/are** voici (2)
heritage patrimoine *m.* (12)
hi salut (1)
high-definition television TNT *f.*; télévision (*f.*) numérique terrestre
highway autoroute *f.* (9)
hike randonnée *n. f.* (8); **hiking boots** chaussures (*f. pl.*) de montagne (8); **to go hiking** faire (*irreg.*) une randonnée (pédestre) (8)
hire embaucher (16)
historical historique *f.* (13)
history histoire *f.* (2)
hobby passe-temps *m.* (15)
holiday fête *f.* (1)
home maison *f.* (4); **at the home of** chez (5); **to go home** rentrer (8)
homeless sans-abri *m., f. inv.* (16)
homework devoirs *m. pl.*; **to do homework** faire (*irreg.*) ses devoirs (5)
hope *v.* espérer (6)
horse cheval *m.* (8); **to go horseback riding** faire (*irreg.*) du cheval (8)
hospital hôpital *m.* (9)
hostel: youth hostel auberge (*f.*) de jeunesse (9)
hot chaud; **it's hot** il fait chaud (5); **to be hot** avoir (*irreg.*) chaud (3)
hotel hôtel *m.* (9)
hour heure *f.* (6); **quarter before the hour** moins le quart (6)
house maison *f.* (4)
housework: to do the housework faire (*irreg.*) le ménage (5)
how comment (1); **how are you?** comment allez-vous? (comment vas-tu?) (1); **how much is it?** c'est combien? (1); **how many?** combien (de)? (4); **how much?** combien (de)? (1); **how's it going?** ça va? (1)
hungry: to be hungry avoir (*irreg.*) faim (4)
hurry *v.* se dépêcher (13); **hurry up!** dépêche-toi! (6)
hurt *v.* avoir (*irreg.*) mal (à) (13)
husband mari *m.* (5)
hybrid voiture (*f.*) hybride (16)

ice cream glace *f.* (6)
ID card carte (*f.*) d'identité (8)
idealistic idéaliste (3)
if si; **if I were you** à ta (votre) place (15)
immediately tout de suite (5)
impatient impatient(e) (3)
important important(e) (3)
impossible: it is impossible that il est impossible que + *subj.* (16)

in à (2); en (2); dans; **in four days (from now)** dans quatre jours (5); **in order to** pour (4); **in the afternoon** de l'après-midi (6)
include comprendre *irreg.* (6)
increase augmentation *n. f.* (14)
indispensable indispensable (16)
individualistic individualiste (3)
industrial industriel(le) (16)
inflation inflation *f.* (16)
information: tourist information bureau syndicat (*m.*) d'initiative (11)
injection piqûre *f.* (13)
inspect contrôler (16)
instructor professeur *m., f.* (1)
intellectual intellectuel(le) (3)
intelligent intelligent(e) (3)
interest *v.* intéresser (14)
interesting intéressant(e) (3)
Internet Internet (10); **on the Internet** sur Internet (10)
internship stage *m.* (14)
intersection carrefour *m.* (11)
interview (job) entretien *m.* (14)
involve: to get involved (in) (*a public issue, cause*) s'engager (dans) (16)
iPad tablette *f.* (1)
iPod iPod *m.* (4)
island île *f.* (11)
isn't it so? n'est-ce pas? (3)
it's a/an . . . c'est un(e)… (1)
it's me. c'est moi. (10)
Italian (*person*) Italien(ne) *m., f.* (2); (*language*) italien *m.* (2)
Italy Italie *f.* (2, 8)
Ivory Coast See Cote d'Ivoire

jacket (ski) anorak *m.* (8); **suit jacket** veston *m.* (3)
January janvier (1)
Japan Japon *m.* (2, 8)
Japanese (*person*) Japonais(e) *m., f.* (2); (*language*) japonais *m.* (2)
jeans jean *m.* (3)
jewel bijou *m.* (14)
job market marché (*m.*) de l'emploi (14)
jog faire (*irreg.*) du jogging (5)
joke blague *n. f.* (15)
juice (orange) jus (*m.*) (d'orange) (6)
July juillet (1)
June juin (1)
just: to have just done s.th. venir (*irreg.*) de + *inf.* (8)

keen: to be keen about tenir à (16)
key clé, clef *f.* (5)
keyboard clavier *m.* (10)
kilo kilo(gramme) *m.* (7)
kiosk kiosque *m.* (10)
kiss *v.* s'embrasser (13)
kitchen cuisine *f.* (5)
knee genou *m.* (*pl.* genoux) (13)
knife couteau *m.* (6)
know connaître *irreg.* (11); **to know (how)** savoir *irreg.* (11)

lake lac *m.* (8)
lamp lampe *f.* (4)
language (foreign) langue (*f.*) (étrangère) (2)
laptop computer portable *m.* (1, 10)
large gros(se) (4)
last dernier/ière (4, 7); passé(e) (7); **last night** hier soir (7)
late en retard (6)
laugh *v.* rire *irreg.* (15)
laundry: to do the laundry faire (*irreg.*) la lessive (5)
law droit *m.* (2)
lawn bowling pétanque *f.* (15)
lawyer avocat(e) *m., f.* (14)
lazy paresseux/euse (3)
lead (clue) *n.* piste *f.* (14)
learn apprendre *irreg.* (à) (6)
leave (for, from) partir *irreg.* (à, de) (8); **to leave** (*behind*) laisser (7); **to leave** (*go out*) sortir *irreg.* (8); **to leave** (*s.o. or someplace*) quitter (8)
Lebanon *m.* Liban (2, 8)
Lebanese (*person*) Libanais(e) *m., f.* (2)
lecture conférence *f.* (12); **lecture hall** amphithéâtre *m.* (2)
left: on the left à gauche (4); **the Left Bank** (*in Paris*) Rive (*f.*) gauche (11)
leg jambe *f.* (13)
legacy patrimoine *m.* (12)
legalization légalisation *f.* (16)
leisure activities loisirs *m. pl.* (15)
lend (to) prêter (à) (11)
less . . . than moins… que (14)
let's see, . . . voyons,… (10)
letter lettre *f.* (10); **letter carrier** facteur/trice *m., f.* (14)
lettuce laitue *f.* (6), salade *f.* (6)
library bibliothèque *f.* (2)
life vie *f.* (2)
lightning: flash of lightning coup (*m.*) de foudre (13)
like aimer (2); **I would like** (*to do s.th.*) je voudrais (+ *inf.*) (6); **to like better** aimer mieux (2)
likeable sympa(thique) (13)
likely probable (16)
line: to stand in line faire (*irreg.*) la queue (5)
linguistics linguistique *f.* (2)
lipstick rouge (*m.*) à lèvres (13)
listen écouter (2)
literature littérature *f.* (2)
little: a little (of) un peu (de) (3)
live habiter (2); vivre *irreg.* (12)
living: cost of living coût (*m.*) de la vie (14); **living room** séjour *m.* (5); **standard of living** niveau (*m.*) de vie (16)
loaf (of bread) baguette (*f.*) (de pain) (6)
loan emprunt *m.* (14)
locate: to be located se trouver (13)
locker (coin) consigne (*f.*) automatique (9)
lodging logement *m.* (4)
loneliness solitude *f.* (16)
long long(ue) (3)
longer: no longer ne… plus (9)
look (at) regarder (8); **to look (like)** avoir (*irreg.*) l'air (de) (3); **to look at oneself, look at each other** se regarder (13); **to look for** chercher (2); **to look up** (*a phone number*) consulter l'annuaire (10)
lose perdre (5); **to get lost** se perdre (13)
lot: a lot (of) beaucoup (de) (1, 6)
lotion, suntan crème (*f.*) solaire (8)
love *v.* adorer (2); aimer (2); amour *n. m.* (13); **love at first sight** coup (*m.*) de foudre (13); **lover; loving** amoureux/euse (13); **to fall in love (with)** tomber amoureux/euse (de) (13)
lucky: to be lucky avoir (*irreg.*) de la chance (8)
lunch déjeuner *m.* (6); **to have lunch** déjeuner (6)
ma'am Madame (Mme) (1)
magazine (*illustrated*) magazine *m.* (4); (*journal*) revue *f.* (10)
magnificent magnifique (12)
maid's room chambre (*f.*) de bonne (4)
mail *v.* poster (10); **mail (a letter)** *v.* mettre (une lettre) à la poste (10); *n.* courrier *m.*; poste *f.*
mailbox boîte (*f.*) aux lettres (10)
main dish plat (*m.*) principal (7)
majority: the majority of la plupart de (12)
make faire *irreg.* (5); **make fun of** se moquer de (14); **to make (happen)** réaliser (14)
makeup: to put on makeup se maquiller (13)
man homme *m.* (2); **young man** jeune homme *m.* (13)
manage gérer (14)
manager directeur/trice *m., f.* (14); **middle/senior manager** cadre *m.* (14); **top manager** chef (*m.*) d'entreprise (14)
many: how many? combien (de)? (4)
map plan (*city*) *m.* (11); carte (*of a region, country*) *f.* (11)
March mars (1)
market marché *m.*; **to go to the market** faire (*irreg.*) le marché (5); **job market** marché (*m.*) de l'emploi (14)
marriage mariage *m.* (13)
married marié(e) (5); **to get married** se marier (avec) (13)
Martinique Martinique *f.* (1)
master *v.* maîtriser (14)
masterpiece chef-d'œuvre *m.* (*pl.* chefs-d'œuvre) (12)
mathematics (math) mathématiques (maths) *f. pl.* (2)
May mai (1)
maybe peut-être (5)
me: as for me pour ma part (16); **it's me.** c'est moi. (10); **me neither** moi non plus (3); **me too** moi aussi (3)
meal repas *m.* (6)
mean *v.* vouloir (*irreg.*) dire (7); **I mean . . .** c'est-à-dire… (10)
meat viande *f.* (6)
media médias *m. pl.* (16)
medieval médiéval(e) (12)
medium: of medium height de taille moyenne (3)
meet se rencontrer (13); **to meet (for the first time)** faire (*irreg.*) la connaissance (de) (5)
meeting rencontre *f.* (13); **to have a meeting** avoir (*irreg.*) rendez-vous (3)
mention: don't mention it de rien (1)
menu carte *f.* (7); **fixed-price menu** menu *m.* (7)
merchant (wine) marchand(e) (de vin) (14)
messy en désordre (4)
metro station station (*f.*) de métro (11)
Mexican (*person*) Mexicain(e) *m., f.* (2)
Mexico Mexique *m.* (2, 8)
middle: Middle Ages Moyen Âge *m. s.* (12); **to be in the middle of** être (*irreg.*) en train de (15)
midnight: it is midnight il est minuit (6)
military budget budget (*m.*) militaire (16)
milk lait *m.* (6)
mirror miroir *m.* (4)
Miss Mademoiselle (Mlle) (1)
mixture mélange *m.* (7)
Monday lundi *m.* (1); **it's Monday** nous sommes lundi

money argent *m.* (7); **money exchange (office)** bureau (*m.*) de change (14)
monitor (computer) écran *m.* (10); moniteur *m.* (10); *v.* contrôler (14)
month mois *m.* (1)
monument monument *m.* (11)
more . . . than plus... que (14); **no more** ne... plus (9)
morning matin *m.* (5); **all morning** matinée toute la matinée (7); **entire morning** matinée *f.* (7); **in the morning** du matin (6); **this morning** ce matin (5)
Moroccan (*person*) Marocain(e) *m., f.* (2)
Morocco Maroc *m.* (2, 8)
most (of) la plupart (de) (12)
mother mère *f.* (5)
mother-in-law belle-mère *f.* (5)
motorcycle motocyclette, moto *f.* (9)
mountain montagne *f.* (8); **to go mountain climbing** faire (*irreg.*) de l'alpinisme (8)
mouse souris *f.* (1, 10)
mouth bouche *f.* (13)
move in emménager (4)
move out déménager (4)
movie film *m.* (2); **movie theater; movies** cinéma *m.* (2)
mp3 player mp3 *m.* (10)
Mr. Monsieur (M.) (1)
Mrs. Madame (Mme) (1)
much bien *adv.*; **as much/many . . . as** autant (de)... que (15); **how much?** combien (de)? (1); **so much the better** tant mieux (15); **too much** trop de (6); **very much** beaucoup (1)
municipal municipal(e) (11)
museum musée *m.* (11)
mushroom champignon *m.* (6)
music musique *f.* (2)
musician musicien(ne) *m., f.* (12)
must: one must (not) il (ne) faut (pas) + *inf.* (8)
myself moi-même (12)

naive naïf/ïve (3)
name(d): my name is . . . je m'appelle... (10); **to be named** s'appeler (13); **what's your name?** comment vous appelez-vous? (comment t'appelles-tu?) (10)
napkin serviette *f.* (6)
natural naturel(le); **natural resources** ressources (*f. pl.*) naturelles (16)
nature nature *f.* (16)
navigate naviguer (10)
necessary: it is necessary that il est nécessaire que + *subj.* (16); **it is necessary to** il faut + *inf.* (8); **to be necessary** falloir *irreg.* (8)
neck cou *m.* (13)
necktie cravate *f.* (3)
need *v.* avoir (*irreg.*) besoin de (3); **one needs** il faut (8); il est nécessaire de (16)
neighbor voisin(e) *m., f.* (4)
neighborhood quartier *m.* (2)
nephew neveu *m.* (5)
nervous nerveux/euse (3)
network (*television*) chaîne *f.* (10)
never ne... jamais (9)
new nouveau, nouvel, nouvelle (nouveaux, nouvelles) (3)
newlyweds nouveaux mariés *m. pl.* (13)
news (*TV program*) informations *f. pl.* (10)
newspaper (news [on television]) journal *m.* (*pl.* journaux) (2)
newsstand kiosque *m.* (10)
next ensuite, puis *adv.* (11); prochain(e) *adj.*; **next to** à côté de (4); **next week** la semaine prochaine (5)
nice beau (*weather*) (5); gentil(le) (3); agréable (3); sympathique (sympa *inv.*) (3); **be nice!** soyez gentil! (6); **it's nice (out)** il fait beau (5)
niece nièce *f.* (5)
night nuit *f.* (7); **all night** toute la nuit (7); **at night** du soir (6); **last night** hier soir (7)
nine neuf (1)
nineteen dix-neuf (1)
ninth le/la neuvième (11)
no non (1); **no longer, no more** ne... plus (9); **no one, nobody** ne... personne (9)
noise bruit *m.* (5)
noon midi (6)
normal normal(e) (16)
north nord *m.* (9); **to the north** au nord (9)
nose nez *m.* (13)
not (at all) ne... pas (du tout) (9); **not bad(ly)** pas mal (1); **not very** peu (3); **not yet** ne... pas encore (9)
notebook cahier *m.* (1)
nothing ne... rien (9)
novel roman *m.* (10)
November novembre (1)
now maintenant (2); **from now on** à l'avenir (14), à partir de maintenant (14)
nuclear: nuclear energy énergie (*f.*) nucléaire (16); **nuclear power plant** centrale (*f.*) nucléaire (16)
number (telephone) numéro *m.* (de téléphone) (10); **to dial the number** composer le numéro (10)

obliged: to be obliged to devoir *irreg.* (7)
obtain obtenir *irreg.* (8)
ocean mer *f.* (8)
o'clock: it is . . . o'clock il est... heures (6)
October octobre (1)
odd drôle (3)
of de (2); **of which** dont (14)
offer *v.* offrir *irreg.* (14)
office bureau *m.* (2); **doctor's office** cabinet (*m.*) medical (13)
officer (police) agent (*m.*) de police (14)
often souvent (2)
oil (olive) huile *f.* (d'olive) (7)
okay d'accord (2)
old ancien(ne) (4); vieux, vieil, vieille (4)
on (top of) sur (4); **on the ground** par terre (4); **on** (*bicycle, horseback, foot*) à (9)
once une fois (11); **all at once** tout d'un coup (11); **once a week** une fois par semaine (5)
one un(e) (1)
onion oignon *m.* (7)
only ne . . . que (9); seulement (9)
open *v.* ouvrir *irreg.* (14)
opera opéra *m.* (15)
opinion: in my opinion pour ma part (16); à mon avis (11); **in your opinion** à votre (ton) avis (11); **public opinion** opinion (*f.*) publique (16); **to express an opinion** exprimer une opinion (16); **to have an opinion about** penser de (11)
optimistic optimiste (13)
or ou (2)
orange orange *inv.* (3); (*fruit*) orange *f.* (6); **orange juice** jus (*m.*) d'orange (6)
order: in order/orderly en ordre (4); **in order to** pour (2); **to order** commander (6), prendre *irreg.* (*in a restaurant*) (6)
other autre (4); **others** d'autres (15); **the other(s)** l'/les autre(s) (15)
outdoors de plein air; **outdoor activities** activités (*f.*) de plein air (15)
over there là-bas (10)
overpopulation surpopulation *f.* (16)
owe devoir *irreg.* (7)
oyster huître *f.* (7)

package colis *m.* (10)
pain douleur *f.* (13); **to have pain** avoir (*irreg.*) mal (à) (3)
paint *v.* peindre *irreg.* (12)
painter artiste peintre *m., f.* (14); peintre *m.*, femme peintre *f.* (12)
painting peinture *f.* (12); tableau *m.* (12)
palace palais *m.* (12)
pants pantalon *m. s.* (3)
pardon (me) pardon (1)
Parisian *adj.* parisien(ne) (3)
park parc *n. m.* (11)
party soirée *f.* (3); fête *f.* (7); **political party** parti *m.* (16)
pass (*time*) passer (6); **boarding pass** carte (*f.*) d'embarquement (9); **to pass** (*a test*) réussir à (4); **to pass by** passer par (8)
passenger passager/ère *m., f.* (9)
passport passeport *m.* (8)
past passé *n. m.* (8)
pasta pâtes *f. pl.* (7)
pastry, pastry shop pâtisserie *f.* (7)
pâté (country-style) pâté *m.* (de campagne) (7)
patient *adj.* patient(e) (3)
patrimony patrimoine *m.* (12)
pay *v.* payer (10); **to pay attention (to)** faire (*irreg.*) attention (à) (5)
payment: automatic payment/withdrawal prélevement automatique (14)
pear poire *f.* (6)
pen stylo *m.* (1)
pencil crayon *m.* (1)
pension retraite *f.* (16)
pepper poivre *m.* (6)
perfectly parfaitement (14)
performance spectacle *m.* (15)
period (*of history*) époque *f.* (12)
permit (to) *v.* permettre *irreg.* (de) (12)
person personne *f.* (3)
personally personnellement (16)
pessimistic pessimiste (3)
pharmacist pharmacien(ne) *m., f.* (14)
pharmacy pharmacie *f.* (11)
philosophy philosophie *f.* (2)
phone See **telephone.**
photocopy machine photocopieur *m.* (10)
physics physique *f.* (2)
picnic pique-nique *m.* (15)
pie tarte *f.* (6)
piece morceau *m.* (7); **piece of furniture** meuble *m.* (5)
pilot pilote *n. m., f.* (9)
pink rose (3)
place endroit *n. m.* (8); lieu *n. m.* (2); **place of residence** logement *m.* (4); **to place (put)** mettre *irreg.* (10)
plans projets *m. pl.* (5)
plate assiette *f.* (6)
platform (*train station*) quai *m.* (9)
play (*theater*) pièce (*f.*) de théâtre (12); *v.* jouer (3); **to play** (*a musical instrument*) jouer de (3); **to play** (*a sport or game*) jouer à (3); faire de (5)

player (DVD) lecteur *m.* (de DVD) (4, 10)
pleasant gentil(le) (3); agréable (3)
please *interj.* s'il vous (te) plaît (1)
plumber plombier *m.* (14)
pocket poche *f.* (10)
poem poème *m.* (12)
poet poète *m.*, femme poète *f.* (12)
poetry poésie *f.* (12)
point out indiquer (15)
police officer agent (*m.*) de police (14); **police station** commissariat *m.* (11), poste (*m.*) de police (11)
policy politique *f.* (16)
polite poli(e) (12)
politely poliment (12)
political party parti *m.* (16)
politician homme politique *m.*, femme politique *f.* (16)
politics politique *f.* (16)
pollute polluer (16)
pollution pollution *f.* (16)
pool (swimming) piscine *f.* (11)
poor pauvre (3)
popular song chanson (*f.*) de variété (15)
pork porc *m.* (6); **pork butcher's shop (delicatessen)** charcuterie *f.* (7)
Portugal Portugal *m.* (8)
possess *v.* posséder (10)
possible possible; **it is possible that** il est possible que + *subj.* (16), il se peut que + *subj.* (16)
post office bureau (*m.*) de poste (10); La Poste (10)
postcard carte (*f.*) postale (10)
poster affiche *f.* (4)
potato pomme (*f.*) de terre (6)
power: purchasing power pouvoir (*m.*) d'achat (16)
prefer aimer mieux (2); préférer (6)
preferable préférable (16)
preferred préféré(e) (5)
preoccupied préoccupé(e) (16)
prepare préparer (5)
pretty joli(e) (4)
prevent (from) empêcher (de) (12)
price prix *m.* (7); **fixed-price menu** menu *m.* (7)
primary school teacher professeur (*m.,f.*) des écoles (14)
print book livre (*m.*) papier (10)
printer (computer) imprimante *f.* (10)
problem ennui *m.* (9); problème *m.* (16)
process: to be in the process of être (*irreg.*) en train de (15)
produce *v.* produire *irreg.* (9)
product produit *m.* (6); **fresh products** les produits frais (6)
professor professeur *m., f.* (1)
program (*TV, radio*) émission *f.* (10); **music program (on TV)** émission de musique (10)
proliferation prolifération *f.* (16)
propose *v.* proposer (14)
protect protéger (16)
protection protection *f.* (16)
proud fier/ère (3)
psychology psychologie *f.* (2)
public public (publique) (11); **public opinion** opinion (*f.*) publique (16)
pun jeu (*m.*) de mots (15)
purchasing: purchasing power pouvoir (*m.*) d'achat (16)
pursue poursuivre *irreg.* (12)
put (on) mettre *irreg.* (8)
putter (around) bricoler (15); **puttering (around)** bricolage *m.* (15)

quarter (*one-fourth*) quart *m.* (6); **quarter** (*district*) quartier *m.* (2); **quarter past (the hour)** et quart (6); **quarter to (the hour)** moins le quart (6)
Quebec (*province*) Québec *m.* (2, 8); (*city*) Québec *m.*
queen reine *f.* (12)
question: to ask a question poser une question (à) (11)
quiet tranquille *adj.* (4)

radio radio *f.* (2)
rain *v.* pleuvoir *irreg.* (7); **it's raining** il pleut (5)
raincoat imperméable *m.* (3)
raise *v.* augmenter (16); *n.* augmentation (*f.*) de salaire (14)
rarely rarement (2)
rate (of exchange) cours *m.* (14), taux (*m.*) de change (14); **(of unemployment)** taux de chômage (14)
razor rasoir *m.* (13)
read lire *irreg.* (10)
reading lecture *f.* (15)
ready prêt(e) (3); **to get ready** se préparer (13)
realistic réaliste (3)
really vraiment (12)
reasonable raisonnable (3)
receipt reçu *m.* (14)
receive recevoir *irreg.* (10)
recognize reconnaître *irreg.* (16)
recruit *v.* recruter (14)
recycle recycler (16)
recycling recyclage *m.* (16)
red rouge (3); **red** (*hair*) roux (rousse) (3)
redheaded roux (rousse) (3)
reform réforme *f.* (16)
refuse (to) refuser (de) (12)
regret *v.* regretter (16)
relate (*tell*) raconter (1)
relax se détendre (13)
relieved soulagé(e) (16)
remain rester (5)
remember se rappeler (13); se souvenir *irreg.* (de) (13)
remote control télécommande *f.* (10)
Renaissance Renaissance *f.* (12)
rent *v.* louer (4); location *f.* (3)
repeat répéter (1)
reporter journaliste *m., f.* (2)
require exiger (16)
rescue *v.* sauver (16)
residence: university residence complex cité (*f.*) universitaire (cité-U) (2)
resource: natural resources ressources (*f. pl.*) naturelles (16)
rest *v.* se reposer (13)
restaurant restaurant *m.* (2)
résumé curriculum (*m.*) vitæ (C.V.) (14)
return (give back) rendre (5); (*go home*) rentrer (8); (*go back*) retourner (8); (*come back to someplace*) revenir *irreg.* (8)
review revue *n. f.* (10)
rhythm rythme *m.* (16)
ride: to take a ride faire (*irreg.*) un tour (en voiture) (5)
right *n.* droit *m.* (16); **civil rights** droits civils (16); **on (to) the right** à droite (4); **the Right Bank** (*in Paris*) Rive (*f.*) droite (11); **to be right** avoir (*irreg.*) raison (3)
river fleuve *m.* (8)
road route *f.* (8)
roast rôti *m.* (7)
roll *v.* rouler (9)
Roman romain(e) (12)
room pièce *f.* (5); (*bedroom*) chambre *f.* (4, 5)
roommate camarade (*m., f.*) de chambre (4)
rug tapis *m.* (4)
run courir *irreg.* (13); faire (*irreg.*) du jogging (5)
Russia Russie *f.* (2, 8)
Russian (*person*) Russe *m., f.* (2)

sad triste (3)
sailboat bateau (*m.*) à voile (8)
sailing voile *f.*; **to go sailing** faire (*irreg.*) de la voile (5)
salad salade *f.* (6)
salami saucisson *m.* (7)
salaried worker travailleur/euse (*m., f.*) salarié(e) (14)
salary salaire *m.* (14)
salmon saumon *m.* (7)
salt sel *m.* (6)
same même; **the same one(s)** le/la/les même(s) (15)
sandals sandales *f. pl.* (3)
sardines (in oil) sardines *f. pl.* (à l'huile) (7)
satellite TV télévision (*f.*) satellite (10)
Saturday samedi *m.* (1)
sausage saucisse *f.* (7)
save (*rescue*) sauver (16); **savings account** compte (*m.*) d'épargne (14); **to save (up) money** faire (*irreg.*) des économies (14)
say dire *irreg.* (10)
scanner scanner *m.* (10)
schedule horaire *m.* (12)
school école *f.* (10); **primary school teacher** professeur des écoles *m., f.* (14)
screen écran *m.* (1, 10)
scuba diving plongée (*f.*) sous-marine (8); **to go scuba driving** faire (*irreg.*) de la plongée sous-marine (8)
sculptor sculpteur *m.*, femme sculpteur *f.* (14)
sculpture sculpture *f.* (14)
sea mer *f.* (8)
season saison *f.* (5)
seat siège *m.* (9); (*theater*) place *f.* (12)
second deuxième *m., f.* (11); **second class** (*in a train*) deuxième classe (9); **second floor** (*in the U.S.*) premier étage *m.* (5)
secretary secrétaire *m., f.* (14)
section (*of Paris*) arrondissement *m.* (11)
see voir *irreg.* (10); **let's see, . . .** voyons… (10); **see you soon** à bientôt (5); **to see again** revoir *irreg.* (10)
seems: it seems that il semble que + *subj.* (16); **to seem** avoir (*irreg.*) l'air de (3)
self-employed: self-employed worker travailleur/euse (*m., f.*) indépendant(e) (14); **to be self-employed** travailler à son compte (14)
sell vendre (5)
send envoyer (10)
Senegal Sénégal *m.* (2, 8)
Senegalese (*person*) Sénégalais(e) *m., f.* (2)
sense *v.* sentir *irreg.* (8)
September septembre (1)
series série *f.* (10); **drama series** (*on TV*) série télévisée (10)
serious sérieux/euse (3)

serve servir *irreg.* (8)
set the table mettre le couvert (10)
settle (down, in) s'installer (13)
seven sept (1)
seventeen dix-sept (1)
several plusieurs (6)
sexism sexisme *m.* (16)
shave *v.* se raser (13)
shelf étagère *f.* (4)
shirt chemise *f.* (3)
shoes chaussures *f. pl.* (3); **tennis shoes** tennis *m. pl.* (3)
shop (*store*) magasin *m.* (3); **butcher shop** boucherie *f.* (7); **pastry shop** pâtisserie *f.* (7)
shopkeeper commerçant(e) *m., f.* (14)
shopping: to do the shopping faire (*irreg.*) le marché (5)
short court(e) (*hair*) (3); petit(e) (*person*) (3)
shorts short *m. s.* (3)
shot (injection) piqûre *f.* (13)
show spectacle *n. m.* (15); **TV show** émission *f.* (10); **game show** jeu (*m.*) télévisé (10); **reality show** émission (*f.*) de télé réalité (10); **variety/floor show** spectacle de variétés (15); **to show** indiquer (15); montrer (3)
shower douche *f.* (4); **to take a shower** prendre une douche, se doucher (13)
sick malade (13)
since depuis (9); **since when** depuis quand (9)
sincere sincère (3)
sing chanter
single (*person*) *adj.* célibataire (5); *n. m., f.* celibataire (13)
sir Monsieur (M.) (1)
sister sœur *f.* (5); **sister-in-law** belle-sœur *f.* (5)
site site *m.* (10)
situate: to be situated se trouver (11)
six six (1)
sixteen seize (1)
sixty soixante (1)
ski ski *n. m.* (8); **ski boots** chaussures (*f. pl.*) de ski (8); **ski goggles** lunettes (*f. pl.*) de ski (8); **ski jacket** anorak *m.* (8); **to ski** faire (*irreg.*) du ski (5), skier (2)
skiing ski *m.*; **cross-country skiing** ski de fond (8); **downhill skiing** ski alpin (8); **to go skiing** faire (*irreg.*) du ski (5); **waters-kiing** ski nautique (8)
skirt jupe *f.* (3)
sleep *v.* dormir *irreg.* (8)
sleeping bag sac (*m.*) de couchage (8)
sleepy: to be sleepy avoir (*irreg.*) sommeil (3)
slice tranche *f.* (7)
slipper pantoufle *f.* (13)
small petit(e) (3)
smartphone smartphone *m.* (1)
smell *v.* sentir *irreg.* (8)
smoke *v.* fumer (2)
smoker fumeur/euse *m., f.*
snack: afternoon snack goûter *m.* (6)
snobbish *adj.* snob (3)
snorkeling plongée (*f.*) libre (8)
snow neige *n. f.*; **to snow** neiger; **it's snowing** il neige (5)
so alors (4); *adv.* tellement (11); **so much the better** tant mieux (15); **so-so** comme ci, comme ça (1)
soap opera feuilleton *m.* (10)
sociable sociable (3)
sociology sociologie *f.* (2)
socks chaussettes *f. pl.* (3)
sofa canapé *m.* (4)
software program logiciel *m.* (10)
solar energy énergie (*f.*) solaire (16)
sole (*fish*) sole *f.* (7)
solitude solitude *f.* (16)
some en *pron.* (11); quelques-uns/unes *pron.* (15); quelques *adj.* (15)
someday un jour (14)
someone quelqu'un (de) (15)
something quelque chose (de) (9); **something else** autre chose (7)
sometimes parfois (9); quelquefois (2)
somewhat assez (3)
son fils *m.* (5); **son-in-law** gendre *m.* (5)
song chanson *f.* (15); **popular song** chanson de variété (15)
soon bientôt (5); **as soon as** aussitôt que (14); dès que (14); **see you soon** à bientôt (1)
sorry désolé(e) (16); **to be sorry** regretter (16)
source source *f.* (16)
south sud *m.* (9); **to the south** au sud (9)
Spain Espagne *f.* (2, 8)
Spaniard Espagnol(e) *m., f.* (2); (*language*) espagnol *m.* (2)
speak parler (2)
spend (*money*) dépenser (10); (*time*) passer (6)
spoon (soup) cuillère *f.* (à soupe) (6)
sport(s) sport *m.* (2); **sporting event** manifestation (*f.*) sportive (15); **sports coat** veste *f.* (3); **sports-minded** sportif/ive (3); **to do sports** faire (*irreg.*) du sport (5)
spring printemps *m.* (5); **in spring** au printemps (5)
square (*in city*) place *f.* (11)
stairway escalier *m.* (5)
stamp timbre *m.* (10)
stand: to stand in line faire (*irreg.*) la queue (5)
standard: standard of living niveau (*m.*) de vie (16)
state état *m.* (8); **United States** États-Unis *m. pl.* (8)
station (subway) station (*f.*) de métro (11); **police station** commissariat *m.* (11); poste (*m.*) de police (11); **service station** station-service *f.* (9); **train station** gare *f.* (9)
stay *v.* rester (5)
steak bifteck *m.* (6)
stepbrother demi-frère *m.* (5)
stepfather beau-père *m.* (5)
stepmother belle-mère *f.* (5)
stepsister demi-sœur *f.* (5)
steward, stewardess steward *m.* (9), hôtesse (*f.*) de l'air (9)
still encore (9)
stomach ventre *m.* (13)
stop *v.* arrêter (de) (12); s'arrêter (13)
store magasin *m.* (3); **fish store** poissonnerie *f.* (7); **grocery store** épicerie *f.* (7)
stormy: it's stormy le temps est orageux (5)
straight (*hair*) raide (3); **straight ahead** tout droit (11)
strange étrange (16)
strawberry fraise *f.* (6)
street rue *f.* (4)
strike *n.* grève *f.* (16); **to strike** faire (*irreg.*) grève (16)
stroll *v.* flâner (12)
student étudiant(e) *m., f.* (1)
studio (apartment) studio *m.* (4)
study étudier (2)
stylish chic *inv.* (3)
suburbs banlieue *f.* (11)
subway métro *m.* (9); **subway station** station (*f.*) de métro (11)
succeed réussir (à) (4)
success réussite *f.*
suddenly soudain (11); tout à coup (11)
suffer souffrir *irreg.* (14)
sugar sucre *m.* (6)
suit (*man's*) costume *m.* (3); (*woman's*) tailleur *m.* (3); **suit jacket** veston *m.* (3)
suitcase valise *f.* (8)
sum montant *m.* (14)
summer été *m.* (5); **in summer** en été (5)
sun soleil *m.*; **it's sunny** il fait du soleil (5)
sunblock écran (*m.*) solaire (8)
Sunday dimanche *m.* (1)
sunglasses lunettes (*f. pl.*) de soleil (8)
suntan: to get a suntan bronzer (8)
suntan lotion crème (*f.*) solaire (8)
support *v.* soutenir *irreg.* (16)
sure sûr(e) (16)
surf the web surfer sur le Web (10)
surprised étonné(e) (16); surpris(e) (16)
survey sondage *n. m.* (16)
sweater pull-over *m.* (3)
sweetheart amoureux/euse *m., f.* (13)
swim *v.* nager (8); se baigner (13)
swimming pool piscine *f.* (11)
swimsuit maillot (*m.*) de bain (3)
Swiss (*person*) Suisse *m., f.* (2)
Switzerland Suisse *f.* (2, 8)

table table *f.* (1); **set the table** mettre le couvert (10)
tablet (computer) tablette *f.* (1)
take prendre *irreg.* (6); **to take** (*a course*) suivre *irreg.* (12); **to take** (*s.o. somewhere*) emmener (12); **to take a ride** faire (*irreg.*) un tour (5); **to take a shower** se doucher (13); **to take a trip** faire (*irreg.*) un voyage (5); **to take a walk** faire (*irreg.*) un tour (5) faire (*irreg.*) une promenade (5); se promener (13); **to take an exam** passer un examen (4); **to take place** se passer (15); **to take one's time** prendre son temps (6); **to take (a long) time** prendre du temps (6)
tall grand(e) (3)
talk: what are you talking about? qu'est-ce que tu racontes / vous racontez? (15)
taste *v.* goûter (7)
taxes impôts *m. pl.* (16)
tea thé *m.* (6)
teach enseigner (à) (12); apprendre (à) (6)
teacher professeur *m., f.* (1); **primary school teacher** professeur des écoles *m., f.* (14)
team équipe *f.* (15)
telephone téléphone *n. m.* (4); (*receiver*) appareil *n. m.* (10); **cell phone** mobile *m.* (10), téléphone (*m.*) portable (4, 10); **telephone number** numéro (*m.*) de téléphone (10); **to telephone** téléphoner (à) (3)
television télévision *f.* (1); **cable television** câble *m.* (10); **television channel/network** chaîne *f.* (10); **high-definition television** TNT (télévision numérique terrestre) *f.* (10); **satellite television** télévision satellite (10); **television news program** journal (*m.*) télévisé (10) (See also **broadcast, program, series, show.**)
tell dire *irreg.* (10); raconter (10)
teller: automatic teller machine (ATM) guichet (*m.*) automatique (14)
ten dix (1)

tennis shoes tennis *m. pl.* (3)
tent tente *f.* (8)
terrace terrasse *f.* (5)
terrorism terrorisme *m.* (16)
test examen *m.* (2); **to pass a test** réussir à un examen (4); **to take a test** passer un examen (4)
text message SMS *m.* (10); texto *m.* (10)
thank you (very much) merci (beaucoup) (1); **to thank** remercier
that cela (ça) *pron.;* que *conj.* (4, 14); qui *rel. pron.* (4, 14); ce, cet, cette, ces *demonstrative adj.* (7); **that is** c'est-à-dire (10)
theater théâtre *m.* (12); (*movie*) cinéma *m.* (2)
then (and) (et) alors (4); ensuite; puis (11)
there là *adv.*; y *pron.* (11); **is/are there . . . ?** il y a… ? (1); **over there** là-bas (10); **there is/are** voilà (2); il y a (1)
therefore alors (4); donc (4)
thick gros(se) (4)
think (about) réfléchir (à) (4); **to think (of, about)** penser (à) (10); **to think (have an opinion) about** penser de (11); **what do you think about . . . ?** que pensez-vous (penses-tu) de… ? (11); **what do you think of that?** qu'en pensez-vous (penses-tu)? (11)
third floor (*in the U.S.*) deuxième étage *m.* (5)
thirsty: to be thirsty avoir (*irreg.*) soif (3)
thirteen treize (1)
thirty trente (1)
this cela (ça) *pron.*; ce, cet, cette, ces *adj.* (7)
three trois (1)
throat gorge *f.* (13)
through par (12)
Thursday jeudi *m.* (1)
ticket billet *m.* (6); **ticket window** guichet *m.* (9)
tidy en ordre (4)
tie (*necktie*) cravate *f.* (3)
time fois *f.* (5); heure *f.* (9); temps *m.* (5); **at what time . . . ?** à quelle heure… ? (6); **free time** temps libre (15); **from time to time** de temps en temps (2); **not on time** en retard (6); **on time** à l'heure (9); **the time is . . . o'clock** il est… heures (6); **to pass, spend time** passer du temps (6); **what time is it?** quelle heure est-il? (6)
tip pourboire *n. m.* (7)
tired fatigué(e) (3)
to à (3); (*flight*) à destination de (9)
tobacconist (bar) café-tabac *m.* (11)
tobacco store bureau (*m.*) de tabac (10)
today aujourd'hui (1)
together ensemble (8)
tomato tomate *f.* (6)
tomorrow demain (5)
too: me too moi aussi (3); **too bad!** dommage! *interj.* (16); **too much of, too many of** trop de (6)
tooth dent *f.* (13)
top: on top of sur (4)
touch *v.* toucher (14)
tourist class classe (*f.*) économique (9); **tourist information bureau** syndicat (*m.*) d'initiative (11)
towel: beach towel serviette (*f.*) de plage (8)
tower tour *f.* (11)
town hall mairie *f.* (11)
trade métier *n. m.* (14)
train train *m.* (9); **train car** wagon *m.* (9); **train station** gare *f.* (9)
transfer (money) virement *m.* (14)
translate traduire *irreg.* (9)
transportation: means of transportation moyen (*m.*) de transport (9)
travel *v.* voyager (8); (*in a car, on a bike*) rouler (9)
treat *v.* soigner (14)
tree arbre *m.* (5)
trip: to take a trip faire (*irreg.*) un voyage (5)
trouble ennui *m.* (9)
truck camion *m.* (9)
true vrai(e) (4); **it's true that . . .** il est vrai que… (16)
trunk coffre *m.* (9)
try (to) essayer (de) (14); chercher (à) (12)
T-shirt tee-shirt *m.* (3)
Tuesday mardi *m.* (1)
Tunisia Tunisie *f.* (2, 8)
Tunisian (*person*) Tunisien(ne) *m., f.* (2)
turn *v.* tourner (11)
TV télévision *f.* (5)
twelve douze (1)
twenty vingt (1): **twenty-one** vingt et un (1); **twenty-two** vingt-deux (1)
two deux (1)

ugly laid(e) (4)
uhmm . . . euh… *interj.* (10)
umbrella parapluie *m.* (8)
uncle oncle *m.* (5)
under sous (4)
understand comprendre *irreg.* (6); **I don't understand** je ne comprends pas (1)
unemployment chômage *m.* (14); **unemployed person** chômeur/euse (14); **unemployment rate** taux (*m.*) de chômage (14)
unfair: it is unfair that il est injuste que + *subj.* (16)
unfortunate pauvre (3); **it is unfortunate that** il est fâcheux que + *subj.* (16)
United States États-Unis *m. pl.* (2, 8)
university université *f.* (2); **university cafeteria** restaurant (*m.*) universitaire (resto-U) (2); **university dormitory** cité (*f.*) universitaire (cité-U) (2)
unjust injuste (16)
unlikely peu probable (16)
until jusqu'à (11)
up to jusqu'à (11)
urgent urgent(e) (16)
useful utile (16)
useless inutile (16)
use up épuiser (16)
usually d'habitude (5)

vacation vacances *f. pl.* (5)
variety show spectacle (*m.*) de varietés (15)
veal veau *m.* (7)
vegetable légume *m.* (6)
very très (1); fort *adv.* (14); **not very** peu (3); **very much** beaucoup (1); **very well, good** très bien (1)
Vietnam Vietnam *m.* (2, 8)
violet violet(te) (3)
visa visa *m.* (8)
visit visite *n. f.* (2); **to visit** (*a place*) visiter (2); **to visit** (*s.o.*) rendre visite à (11)
voice mail boîte (*f.*) vocale (10)
voter électeur/trice *m., f.* (16)

wait (for) attendre (5)
waiter, waitress serveur/euse *m., f.* (7)
wake up se réveiller (13)
walk *v.* marcher (13); **to take a walk** se promener (15); faire (*irreg.*) un tour (5); faire (*irreg.*) une promenade (5); **walking** marche *f.* (15)
wall mur *m.* (4)
want avoir (*irreg.*) envie de (3); désirer (15); vouloir *irreg.* (7)
war guerre *f.* (16)
wardrobe armoire *f.* (4)
warm: to be warm avoir (*irreg.*) chaud (3)
wash (*oneself*) se laver (13)
waste gaspillage *n. m.* (16); (*material*) déchet *n. m.* (16); **to waste** perdre (5); gaspiller (16)
watch *v.* regarder (2); **to watch out (for)** faire (*irreg.*) attention (à) (5)
water (mineral) eau (*f.*) (minérale) (6)
waterskiing ski (*m.*) nautique (8)
way (*road*) chemin *m.* (11)
wear porter (3)
weather temps *m.* (5); **how's the weather?** quel temps fait-il? (5); **it's bad (nice) weather** il fait mauvais (beau) (5); **weather forecast** météo *f.* (5)
Web Web *m.* (10)
Wednesday mercredi *m.* (1)
weary las(se) (16)
week semaine *f.* (1); **every week** toutes les semaines (10); **next week** la semaine prochaine (5); **once a week** une fois par semaine (5)
weekend: on weekends le week-end (6); **this weekend** ce week-end (5)
welcome: you're welcome de rien (1); il n'y a pas de quoi (7); je vous en prie (7)
well bien *adv.* (1); *interj.* eh bien,… (10); **pretty well** ça peut aller (1); **things are going well** ça va bien (1); **very well** très bien (1)
west ouest *m.* (9); **to the west** à l'ouest (9)
what que (4); qu'est-ce que (1); qu'est-ce qui (15); quel(le) (7); **what?** comment? (1); **what is it?** qu'est-ce que c'est? (4)
when quand (4); lorsque; où *relative pron.* (4); **since when** depuis quand (9)
where où (4)
which lequel, laquelle, lesquels, lesquelles (15); que, qui *relative pron.* (4); quel, quelle, quels, quelles *interr. adj.* (7); **of which** dont (14)
while: in a while tout à l'heure (5)
white blanc(he) (3); **white-collar worker** employé(e) *m., f.* (14)
who qui (4); qui est-ce qui (14); **who is it?** qui est-ce? (1); **who's calling?** qui est à l'appareil? (10)
whom qui (4); qui est-ce que; que (14); **of whom** dont (14)
whose dont (14)
why pourquoi (4)
wife femme *f.* (5)
Wi-Fi (wireless) connection Wi-Fi *m.* (10)
willing: to be willing vouloir (*irreg.*) bien (7)
win *v.* gagner (14)
wind vent *m.*; **it's windy** il fait du vent, il y a du vent (5)
windbreaker blouson *m.* (3)
window fenêtre *f.* (1); **(ticket) window** guichet *m.* (9)
windsurfing planche (*f.*) à voile (8); **to go windsurfing** faire (*irreg.*) de la planche à voile
wine vin *m.* (6); **wine merchant** marchand(e) (*m., f.*) de vin (14)
winter hiver *m.* (5); **in winter** en hiver (5)
wish *v.* souhaiter (16)

with avec (2); par (12)
withdraw retirer (14)
withdrawal: automatic withdrawal/payment prélèvement automatique (14)
without: without a doubt sans doute (16)
woman femme *f.* (2); **young woman** jeune femme *f.* (3)
wonder se demander (13)
wood(s) bois *m.* (11); forêt *f.* (8)
word mot *m.* (1); **word processing** traitement (*m.*) de texte (10)
work travail *n. m.* (2); **do-it-yourself work** bricolage *m.* (15); **work (of art)** œuvre *f.* (d'art) (12); **to work** travailler (2); (*machine or object*) marcher
worker travailleur/euse *m., f.* (14); (*manual*) ouvrier/ière *m., f.* (14); **salaried worker** travailleur/euse *m., f.* salarié(e) (14); **self-employed worker** travailleur/euse (*m., f.*) indépendant(e) (14); **white-collar worker** employé(e) *m., f.* (14)
world monde *m.* (8); **World Wide Web** Web *m.* (10)
worse pire (14)
worth: to be worth valoir *irreg.* (16)
write (to) écrire *irreg.* (à) (10)
writer écrivain *m.*, femme écrivain *f.* (12)
wrong: to be wrong avoir (*irreg.*) tort (3); se tromper (13)
year an *m.* (1); **entire year** année *f.*; **to be (vingt) years old** avoir (*irreg.*) (twenty) ans (3)
yellow jaune (3)
yes oui (1); si (*response to negative question*) (9); **yes, but . . .** oui, mais... (10)
yesterday hier (8); **the day before yesterday** avant-hier (8)
yet: not yet ne... pas encore (9)
you: and you et vous (et toi) (1)
young *adj.* jeune (4); **young lady** jeune fille *f.* (3); **young man** jeune homme *m.* (3)
youth: youth hostel auberge (*f.*) de jeunesse (9)

Credits

Image Researcher: Judy Mason
Interior Designer: Preston Thomas
Cover Designer: Preston Thomas

Photo Credits

Design Elements
Headphones: © Istockphoto.com/cherkas; Keyboard keys: © Istockphoto.com/malerapaso; Communication icon (couple): © Ariel Skelley/Blend Images/Corbis: Banners for Lea, Hassan, Juliette, and Hector: © McGraw-Hill Education.

Chapter 1

Opener (both): © McGraw-Hill Education; **p. 7** (top): © McGraw-Hill Education; **p. 7** (bottom): © Paul Edmondson/Corbis; **p. 12:** © Hemis/Alamy; **p. 16:** Masterfile RF; **p. 18:** © McGraw-Hill Education; **p. 19:** © Paul Edmondson/Corbis; **p. 28:** © McGraw-Hill Education.

Chapter 2

Opener (top): © McGraw-Hill Education; Opener (bottom): Universal Images Group/DeAgostini/Alamy; **p. 31** (both): © McGraw-Hill Education; **p. 41:** © Owen Franken; **p. 44:** © Tom Craig/Alamy; **p. 46–47:** © McGraw-Hill Education; **p. 48:** © Comstock Images/Getty Images RF; **p. 48** (inset): © McGraw-Hill Education; **p. 51:** © Owen Franken; **p. 57:** © McGraw-Hill Education.

Chapter 3

Opener (top): © McGraw-Hill Education; Opener (bottom): © Hendrik Ballhausen/picture-alliance/dpa/AP Images; **p. 61** (both): © McGraw-Hill Education; **p. 70**: © Corbis/PunchStock RF; **p. 73:** © Owen Franken; **p. 74–76:** © McGraw-Hill Education; **p. 79:** © McGraw-Hill Education; **p. 83:** Courtesy of Les Petites, Paris. © Owen Franken; **p. 85** (top): © Joel Saget/AFP/Getty Images; **p. 85** (bottom): © Owen Franken; **p. 87:** © McGraw-Hill Education.

Chapter 4

Opener (top): © McGraw-Hill Education; Opener (bottom): © Mike McQueen/Corbis; **p. 91** (both): © McGraw-Hill Education; **p. 95:** © Journal-Courier/Steve Warmowski/The Image Works; **p. 96:** © Owen Franken; **p. 98:** © McGraw-Hill Education; **p. 102–103:** © McGraw-Hill Education; **p. 104:** © Magwitch/Alamy; **p. 106:** Courtesy of booking.com/© Owen Franken; **p. 110:** PhotoAlto/Alix Minde/Getty Images RF; **p. 112:** © Andy Brilliant; **p. 113:** *Chambre d'Arles*, 1888, Oil on canvas, 56.5 x 74.0 cm. Gogh, Vincent van. Musée d'Orsay Paris. Photo: Alfredo Dagli Orti/The Art Archive/Corbis; **p. 114:** © McGraw-Hill Education; **p. 116** (top): © McGraw-Hill Education; **p. 116** (bottom): Courtesy of FeuFollet/Photo by Blake Bumpus; **p. 117** (top): © McGraw-Hill Education; **p. 117** (bottom): © Corbis.

Chapter 5

Opener (top): © McGraw-Hill Education; Opener (bottom): © Camera Lucida/Alamy; **p. 119** (top): © McGraw-Hill Education; **p. 119** (bottom): © Allison Michael Orenstein/Getty Images; **p. 121:** © Owen Franken; **p. 131:** © Oote Boe/Alamy; **p. 132:** © McGraw-Hill Education; **p. 133:** © Allison Michael Orenstein/Getty Images; **p. 134:** © William Ryall RF; **p. 136:** © Sami Sarkis France/Alamy; **p. 140:** © Robert Harding Picture Library Ltd/Alamy; **p. 141:** © The Gallery Collection/Corbis; **p. 143:** © McGraw-Hill Education.

Chapter 6

Opener (top): © McGraw-Hill Education; Opener (bottom): © Alex Segre/Alamy Images; **p. 147** (top): © McGraw-Hill Education; **p. 147** (bottom): © MBI/Alamy RF; **p. 152:** © McGraw-Hill Education; **p. 154:** © Imageshop/Alamy RF; **p. 156:** © George Jurasek/Getty Images RF; **p. 160:** © McGraw-Hill Education; **p. 161:** © MBI/Alamy RF; **p. 167:** © Steve Cole/Getty Images RF; **p. 170** (top): © Maggie Janik Photography; **p. 170** (bottom): © Tracy Hebden; **p. 171–172:** © McGraw-Hill Education.

Chapter 7

Opener (top): © McGraw-Hill Education; Opener (bottom): © Dennis Macdonald/Getty Images; **p. 175** (top): © McGraw-Hill Education; **p. 175** (bottom): © Dave Stamboulis/Getty Images RF; **p. 179** (top): © William Ryall RF; **p. 179** (bottom left): © Walter Pietsch/Alamy; **p. 179** (bottom right): © Foodcollection; **p. 181:**© Ingram Publishing/Superstock RF; **p. 182:** © Jon Hicks/Corbis; **p.184:** © Brett Stevens/cultura/Corbis; **p. 186:** © McGraw-Hill Education; **p. 187:** © Dave Stamboulis/Getty Images RF; **p. 189:** © Owen Franken/Corbis; **p. 191:** © McGraw-Hill Education; **p. 193:** © Mark Harris/Getty Images RF; **p. 194:** © PhotoEdit; **p. 195** (top): © Comstock/Jupiter Images RF; **p. 195** (top middle): Markus Guhl/Getty Images RF; **p. 195** (bottom middle): © FoodCollection RF; **p. 195** (bottom): © Hemera Technologies/JupiterImages RF; **p. 196:** © J.Riou/photocuisine/Corbis; **p. 197:** © Michael Mahovlich/Getty Images RF; **p. 198:** © McGraw-Hill Education.

Chapter 8

Opener (top): © McGraw-Hill Education; Opener (bottom): © imagebroker/Alamy RF; **p. 201** (top): © Dennie Cody/Getty Images; **p. 201** (bottom): © Jon Arnold/Agency Jon Arnold Images/age fotostock; **p. 203**: © Tom Stewart/Corbis; **p. 206** (top): Courtesy of IBM Archives; **p. 206** (middle): © Roger-Viollet, Paris/The Image Works; **p. 206** (bottom): © Bettmann/Corbis; **p. 208** (top): © Pixtal/age footstock; **p. 208** (bottom): © Purestock/Getty Images; **p. 211** (bottom): © Marco Albonico/age fotostock; **p. 212** (both): © McGraw-Hill Education; **p. 214:** © Owen Franken; **p. 216:** © Dennie Cody/Getty Images; **p. 217:** © Jon Arnold/Agency Jon Arnold Images/age fotostock; **p. 218:** © D. Hurst/Alamy RF; **p. 220:** © Author's Image/PunchStock RF; **p. 222:** © McGraw-Hill Education; **p. 223:** © Corbis/Royalty-Free; **p. 226** (top): © Corbis/Royalty-Free; **p. 226** (bottom): © Jean du Boisberranger/Hemis/Corbis; **p. 228:** © McGraw-Hill Education; **p. 230** (top): © McGraw-Hill Education; **p. 230** (bottom): © Sophie Bassouls/Sygma/Corbis; **p. 231** (top): © McGraw-Hill Education; **p. 231** (bottom): © SEYLLOU/AFP/Getty Images.

Chapter 9

Opener (top): © McGraw-Hill Education; Opener (bottom): © Bryan F. Peterson/Corbis; **p. 233:** © McGraw-Hill Education; **p. 239:** © Owen Franken/Corbis; **p. 241:** © McGraw-Hill Education; © Owen Franken; **p. 243:** © Owen Franken; **p. 244:** © McGraw-Hill Education; **p. 253:** © Robert Gray/Alamy; **p. 254** (top): © incamerastock/Alamy; **p. 254** (bottom): © Horacio Villalobos/epa/Corbis; **p. 256:** © Gero Breloer/epa/Corbis.

Chapter 10

Opener (top): © McGraw-Hill Education; Opener (bottom): © Jacques Brinon/AP Images; **p. 259** (top): © McGraw-Hill Education; **p. 259** (bottom): © Owen Franken; **p. 266** (left): © Fabrice Lerouge/Getty Images; **p. 266** (inset): © McGraw-Hill Education; **p. 268:** © Owen Franken; **p. 270:** © claude thibault/Alamy; **p. 273:** © Owen Franken; **p. 274:** © McGraw-Hill Education; **p. 275:** © Owen Franken; **p. 277:** © Mark Dierker/McGraw-Hill RF; **p. 278:** © Glenn Paulina/TRANSTOCK/Corbis; **p. 280:** © OJO Images/Getty Images RF; **p. 281:** © Owen Franken; **p. 282:** © David Hanover/Stone/Getty Images; **p. 285:** © McGraw-Hill Education.

Chapter 11

Opener (top): © McGraw-Hill Education; Opener (bottom): © Jean-Pierre Lescourret/Corbis; **p. 289** (top): © McGraw-Hill Education; **p. 289** (bottom): © René Mattes/Hemis/Corbis; **p. 294:** © Loïc Venance/AFP/Getty Images; **p. 297:** © Owen Franken/ Corbis; **p. 298:** © Benoit Roland/The Image Works; **p. 299:** © Russell Kord/Alamy; **p. 301:** © Owen Franken; **p. 302:** © McGraw-Hill Education; **p. 303:** © René Mattes/Hemis/Corbis; **p. 304:** © Art Media/Heritage-Images/The Image Works; **p. 305:** © Jacques Guillard/Scope; **p. 306:** © Giraudon/Art Resource; **p. 307:** © Greg Balfour Evans/Alamy; **p. 311:** © Doug Armand/Getty Images; **p. 314:** © Juniors Bildarchiv GmbH/Alamy; **p. 316:** © McGraw-Hill Education.

Chapter 12

Opener (top): © McGraw-Hill Education; Opener (bottom): © Gala/SuperStock; **p. 319** (top): © McGraw-Hill Education; **p. 319** (bottom): © Christine Osborne/Corbis; **p. 320** (top): © Franz-Marc Frei/Corbis; **p. 320** (bottom): © Jahan/Explorer/Science Source; **p. 321** (left): © Owen Franken; **p. 321** (right): © Vanni Archive/Corbis; **p. 322** (top): © Images de Paris/Alamy; **p. 322** (bottom left): © Keren Su/Corbis; **p. 322** (bottom right): © Steve Vidler/SuperStock; **p. 325:** Gogh, Vincent van (1853–1890) *Self-Portrait*. 1889. Oil on canvas, 65 x 54.5 cm. Location: Musée d'Orsay, Paris, France. Photo: Erich Lessing/Art Resource; **p. 326:** © Erich Lessing/Art Resource, NY; **p. 327:** © Tate Gallery, London/Art Resource, NY; **p. 334:** © McGraw-Hill Education; **p. 335:** © Christine Osborne/Corbis; **p. 336** (top): © Comstock Images/Getty Images; **p. 336** (bottom): © McGraw-Hill Education; **p. 339:** © Paul Seheult/Eye Ubiquitous/Corbis; **p. 341:** © Ingram Publishing RF; **p. 342:** © Corbis/Royalty Free; **p. 343:** © Gauguin, Paul (1848–1903) *Women of Tahiti or On the Beach.* 1891. Oil on canvas, 69.0 x 91.5 cm. Photo: Hervé Lewandowski. Location: Musée d'Orsay, Paris, France. Réunion des Musées Nationaux/Art Resource, NY; **p. 346:** © Globe Photos; **p. 347:** Chagall, Marc (1887–1985) © ARS, NY *The Song of Songs, IV,* 1958. Oil on canvas, 50 x 61 cm. Musée National message biblique Marc Chagall, Nice, France. Gerard Blot/Réunion des Musées Nationaux/Art Resource, NY; **p. 348:**

© McGraw-Hill Education; **p. 350** (top): © Photononstop/SuperStock; **p. 350** (bottom): © Hulton-Deutsch/Corbis; **p. 351** (top): © Demetrio Carrasco/Getty Images; **p. 351** (bottom): © Magritte, René (1898-1967) © ARS, NY. *Le Maître d'école*, 1954. Oil on canvas, 81 x 60 cm. Location: Private Collection. Herscovici/Art Resource, NY.

Chapter 13

Opener (top): © McGraw-Hill Education; Opener (bottom): © blickwinkel/Alamy Images; **p. 353** (top): © McGraw-Hill Education; **p. 353** (bottom): © Animals/Animals; **p. 356:** © Owen Franken; **p. 358:** © Owen Franken; **p. 360:** © Owen Franken; **p. 361:** © Fototeca Storica Nazionale/Getty Images RF; **p. 364:** © McGraw-Hill Education; **p. 365:** © Animals/Animals; **p. 368** (top): © Nik Wheeler; **p. 368** (bottom): © McGraw-Hill Education; **p. 372:** © Comstock/PunchStock RF; **p. 374:** © McGraw-Hill Education.

Chapter 14

Opener (top): © McGraw-Hill Education; Opener (bottom): © Christophe Boisvieux/Corbis; **p. 377** (bottom): © Directphoto.org/Alamy RF; **p. 377** (top): © McGraw-Hill Education; **p. 382:** © Owen Franken; **p. 383:** © Christopher Bissell/Getty Images; **p. 384** (top): © McGraw-Hill Education; **p. 386** (top): © Owen Franken; **p. 386** (bottom): Courtesy of Dell; **p. 389:** © Bruce Paton/Panos Pictures; **p. 390** (bottom): © McGraw-Hill Education; **p. 391:** © Directphoto.org/Alamy RF; **p. 392** (left): © Comstock Images/Getty Images; **p. 392** (right): © McGraw-Hill Education; **p. 395:** © DAJ/Getty Images RF; **p. 397:** © Jean-Pierre Lescourret/Corbis; **p. 399:** © William Ryall 2010; **p. 401:** © Purestock/Superstock RF; **p. 403** (top): © Farrell Grehan/Photo Researchers; **p. 403** (bottom): © Hiroko Masuike/AP Images; **p. 404:** © Alfred/SIPA/AP Images; **p. 405:** McGraw-Hill Education.

Chapter 15

Opener (top): © McGraw-Hill Education; Opener (bottom): © Gail Mooney/Corbis; **p. 409** (top): © Paul Seheult/Eye Ubiquitous/Corbis; **p. 409** (bottom): © Morgan David de Lossy/Corbis; **p. 411:** © Owen Franken; **p. 413:** © Purestock/SuperStock RF; **p. 420:** © McGraw-Hill Education; **p. 421:** © Owen Franken; **p. 422:** © Paul Seheult/Eye Ubiquitous/Corbis; **p. 423:** © Morgan David de Lossy/Corbis; **p. 424:** © Owen Franken; **p. 427:** © Patrick Ward/Alamy; **p. 430:** © Nik Wheeler/Alamy; **p. 432:** © MARCEL MOCHET/AFP/Getty Images; **p. 434:** © McGraw-Hill Education.

Chapter 16

Opener (top): © McGraw-Hill Education; Opener (bottom): © Roger Ressmeyer/Corbis; **p. 437** (top): © McGraw-Hill Education; **p. 437** (bottom): © Owen Franken/Corbis; **p. 442:** © Richard Wareham Fotografie/Alamy; **p. 443:** © Facelly/Sipa Press; **p. 448** (both): © McGraw-Hill Education; **p. 452:** © McGraw-Hill Education; **p. 453:** © Owen Franken/Corbis; **p. 454:** © Antoine Antoniol/Getty Images; **p. 460:** © William Ryall RF; **p. 462:** © Donald Stampfli/AP Images; **p. 464:** © McGraw-Hill Education; **p. 466** (top): © Jack Fields/Corbis; **p. 466** (bottom): © Dan Christensen; **p. 467** (top): © David Giral/Alamy; **p. 467** (bottom): © Pimental Jean/Kipa Collection/Corbis.

Text Credits

Pages 111: From "Avantages et pièges de la colocation" by Sebastien Thomas, *Quo*. Used by permission of Hachette Filipacchi Associés, Levallois-Perret Cx, France; **170:** Adapted from "Blaff de poissons," http://www.antilles-martinique.com/recettes.html; **314:** «Le chat abandonné» by Paul Degray in *Poésies et jeux de langage CP/CE1*, Christian Lamblin, © Éditions Retz 2003; **346:** "Déjeuner du matin" in *Paroles* by Jacques Prévert, © Éditions GALLIMARD; **372:** "Pour toi mon amour" in *Paroles* by Jacques Prévert, © Éditions GALLIMARD; **432:** Adapted from "Traversée de l'Atlantique à la rame en solitaire" by Nicolas Gonidec, www.antourtan.org. Used by permission; **462:** From *La Réclusion solitaire* by Tahar Ben Jelloun, © by Éditions Denoël, 1976.

Realia Credits

Pages 16: Holidays in Suisse, États-Unis, France: *Air Canada Magazine*; **26:** Ad from the Internet site www.letudiant.fr. Used by permission; **35–36:** Flags © Liber Kartor, Sweden; **55:** Text, logo, and photo used courtesy of Programme spécial de français, École des langues vivantes, Université Laval, Québec; **71:** Magazines Canada 1998: Writer/Art Director, Dennis Bruce; Art, Jerzy Kolacz; **82:** © Yayo/Cartoonists & Writers Syndicate, www.nytsyn.com/cartoons; **124:** *Dernières Nouvelles d'Alsace*; **159:** © *L'Express* 1998; **177:** Restaurant La Guirlande de Julie, Paris, France; **233, 245:** BlaBlaCar website screenshot used by permission; **236:** Text: SNCF; **283:** Book cover *Comment être le meilleur sur Meetic* used by permission of Éditions First; **292:** © MICHELIN Paris Hotel & Restaurants—Permission No. 06-US-006; **380:** Jean-Pierre Adelbert; **426:** Data from Ministère de la Culture et de la Communication *in Francoscopie 1999* by Gérard Mermet (Paris: Larousse); **439:** Parigramme.

Index

Part 2: Topics

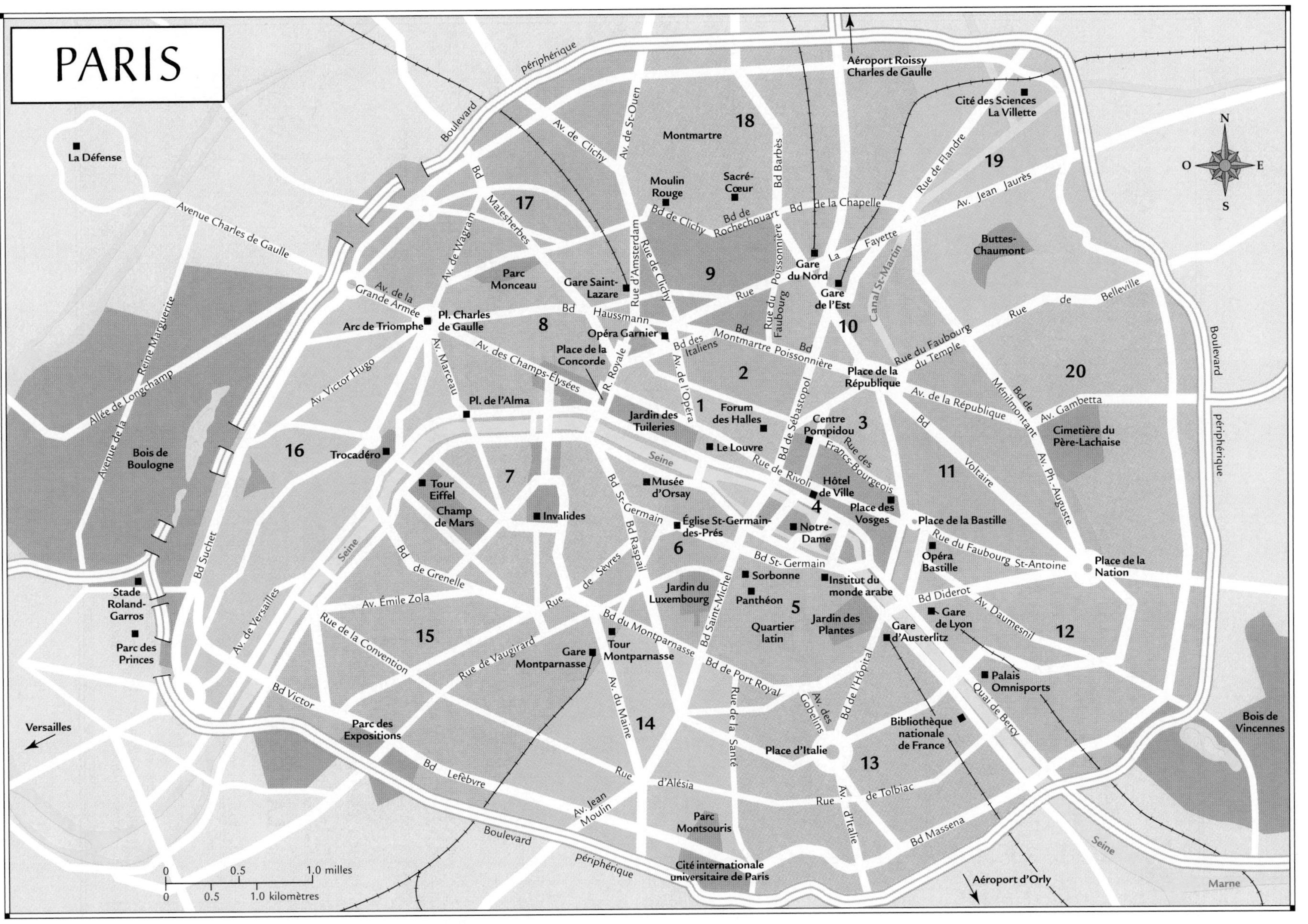
PARIS
La Défense
Avenue Charles de Gaulle
Allée de Longchamp
Avenue de la Reine Marguerite
Bois de Boulogne
Stade Roland-Garros
Parc des Princes
Bd Suchet
Versailles
Boulevard périphérique
Av. de Clichy
Av. de St-Ouen
Montmartre
18
Moulin Rouge
Sacré-Cœur
Bd Barbès
Bd de Clichy
Bd de Rochechouart
Bd de la Chapelle
Aéroport Roissy Charles de Gaulle
Cité des Sciences La Villette
Rue de Flandre
19
Av. Jean Jaurès
Buttes-Chaumont
N
O
E
S
17
Bd Malesherbes
Av. de Wagram
Parc Monceau
Gare Saint-Lazare
Rue d'Amsterdam
Rue de Clichy
9
Rue La Fayette
Gare du Nord
Gare de l'Est
Canal St-Martin
Rue de Belleville
Av. de la Grande Armée
Arc de Triomphe
Pl. Charles de Gaulle
8
Bd Haussmann
Opéra Garnier
Rue du Faubourg Poissonnière
10
Bd Montmartre Poissonnière
Bd des Italiens
Place de la Concorde
R. Royale
Av. de l'Opéra
2
Place de la République
Rue du Faubourg du Temple
20
Bd de Ménilmontant
Av. Gambetta
Av. Victor Hugo
Av. Marceau
Av. des Champs-Élysées
Pl. de l'Alma
1
Forum des Halles
Jardin des Tuileries
Av. de la République
Cimetière du Père-Lachaise
16
Trocadéro
Le Louvre
Centre Pompidou
3
Bd de Sébastopol
Rue des Francs-Bourgeois
Bd Voltaire
11
Av. Ph.-Auguste
Seine
Rue de Rivoli
Hôtel de Ville
Tour Eiffel
7
Musée d'Orsay
4
Place des Vosges
Place de la Bastille
Champ de Mars
Invalides
Bd St-Germain
Église St-Germain-des-Prés
Notre-Dame
Rue du Faubourg St-Antoine
Opéra Bastille
Place de la Nation
6
Bd Raspail
Bd de Grenelle
Rue de Sèvres
Bd St-Germain
Sorbonne
Institut du monde arabe
Jardin du Luxembourg
Panthéon
5
Bd Diderot
Av. Daumesnil
Gare de Lyon
12
Av. Émile Zola
Av. de Versailles
Rue de la Convention
15
Rue de Vaugirard
Gare Montparnasse
Tour Montparnasse
Bd du Montparnasse
Bd Saint-Michel
Quartier latin
Jardin des Plantes
Gare d'Austerlitz
Bd de Port Royal
Bd de l'Hôpital
Palais Omnisports
Quai de Bercy
Bd Victor
Parc des Expositions
Av. du Maine
14
Rue de la Santé
Av. des Gobelins
Bibliothèque nationale de France
Bois de Vincennes
Place d'Italie
13
Bd Lefebvre
Rue d'Alésia
Av. Jean Moulin
Rue de Tolbiac
Av. d'Italie
Parc Montsouris
Bd Massena
Seine
Cité internationale universitaire de Paris
Aéroport d'Orly
Marne
0
0.5
1.0 milles
0
0.5
1.0 kilomètres

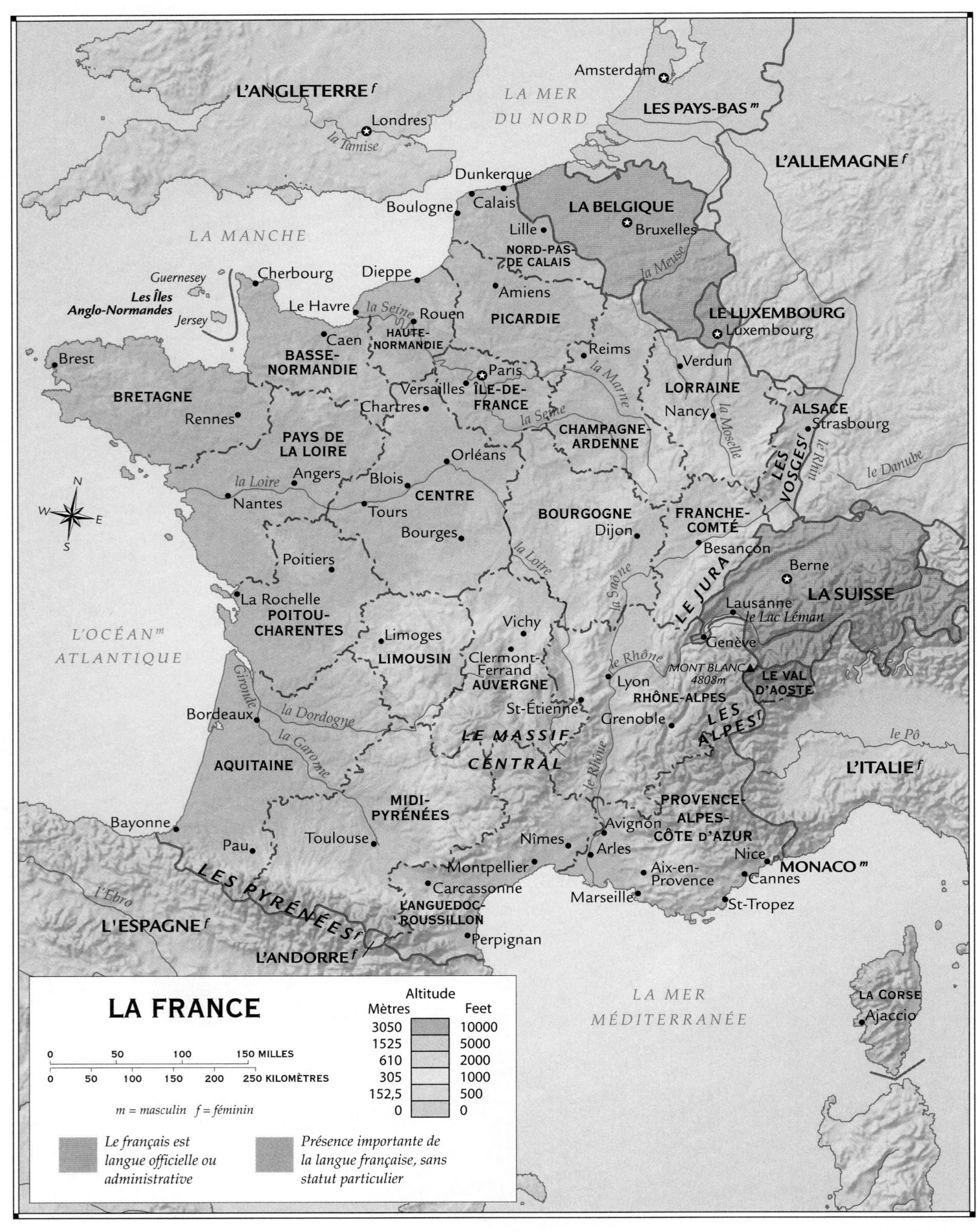

LA FRANCE
L'ANGLETERRE f
Londres
la Tamise
LA MER DU NORD
Amsterdam
LES PAYS-BAS m
L'ALLEMAGNE f
Dunkerque
Calais
Boulogne
LA BELGIQUE
Bruxelles
Lille
LA MANCHE
NORD-PAS-DE CALAIS
Amiens
PICARDIE
la Meuse
LE LUXEMBOURG
Luxembourg
Guernesey
Les Îles Anglo-Normandes
Jersey
Cherbourg
Dieppe
Le Havre
la Seine
Rouen
HAUTE-NORMANDIE
Caen
BASSE-NORMANDIE
Brest
BRETAGNE
Rennes
Reims
Verdun
la Marne
Paris
Versailles
ÎLE-DE-FRANCE
LORRAINE
Nancy
la Moselle
ALSACE
Strasbourg
LES VOSGES f
le Rhin
Chartres
la Seine
CHAMPAGNE-ARDENNE
PAYS DE LA LOIRE
Orléans
le Danube
Angers
Blois
la Loire
Nantes
CENTRE
Tours
Bourges
BOURGOGNE
Dijon
FRANCHE-COMTÉ
Besançon
Poitiers
la Loire
la Saône
Berne
LE JURA
LA SUISSE
Lausanne
le Lac Léman
La Rochelle
POITOU-CHARENTES
L'OCÉAN m ATLANTIQUE
Limoges
LIMOUSIN
Vichy
Clermont-Ferrand
AUVERGNE
Genève
le Rhône
MONT BLANC 4808m
LE VAL D'AOSTE
Lyon
RHÔNE-ALPES
Gironde
Bordeaux
la Dordogne
St-Étienne
Grenoble
LES ALPES f
la Garonne
LE MASSIF CENTRAL
le Pô
AQUITAINE
le Rhône
L'ITALIE f
MIDI-PYRÉNÉES
PROVENCE-ALPES-CÔTE D'AZUR
Bayonne
Pau
Toulouse
Nîmes
Avignon
Arles
Nice
MONACO m
Montpellier
Aix-en-Provence
Cannes
LES PYRÉNÉES f
l'Ebro
Carcassonne
Marseille
St-Tropez
L'ESPAGNE f
LANGUEDOC-ROUSSILLON
Perpignan
L'ANDORRE f
LA MER MÉDITERRANÉE
LA CORSE
Ajaccio
N
S
E
W
0 50 100 150 MILLES
0 50 100 150 200 250 KILOMÈTRES
m = masculin f = féminin
Altitude
Mètres Feet
3050 10000
1525 5000
610 2000
305 1000
152,5 500
0 0
Le français est langue officielle ou administrative
Présence importante de la langue française, sans statut particulier

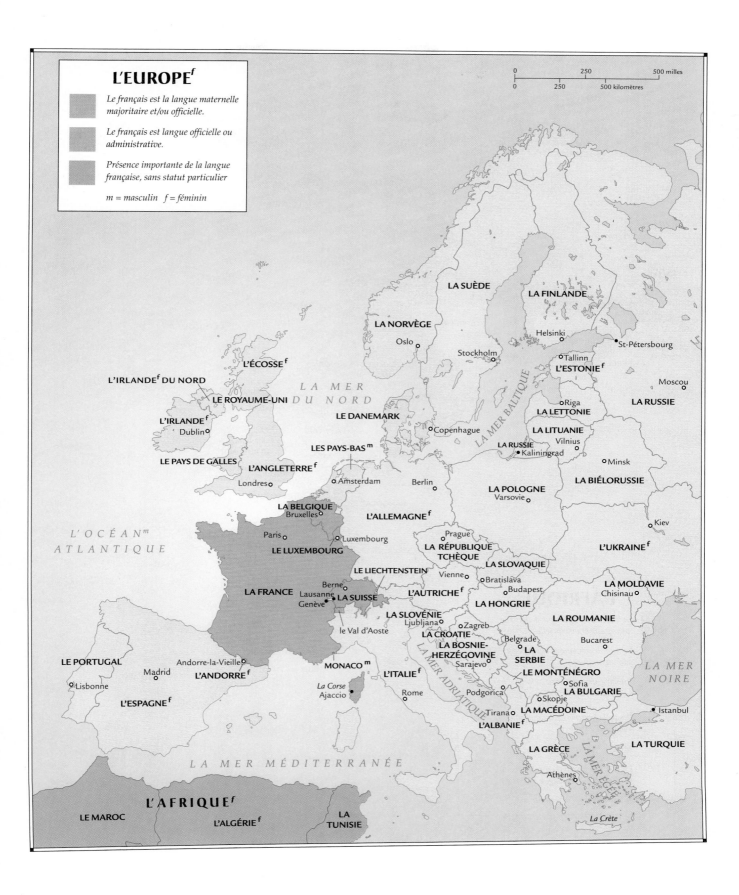
L'EUROPE f
Le français est la langue maternelle majoritaire et/ou officielle.
Le français est langue officielle ou administrative.
Présence importante de la langue française, sans statut particulier
m = masculin f = féminin
0 250 500 milles
0 250 500 kilomètres
LA SUÈDE
LA FINLANDE
LA NORVÈGE
Oslo
Helsinki
St-Pétersbourg
Stockholm
Tallinn
L'ESTONIE f
L'ÉCOSSE f
L'IRLANDE f DU NORD
LA MER DU NORD
LE ROYAUME-UNI
LA MER BALTIQUE
Moscou
Riga
LA RUSSIE
LA LETTONIE
L'IRLANDE f
LE DANEMARK
Dublin
Copenhague
LA LITUANIE
LA RUSSIE
Vilnius
Kaliningrad
LES PAYS-BAS m
LE PAYS DE GALLES
Minsk
L'ANGLETERRE f
Londres
Amsterdam
Berlin
LA BIÉLORUSSIE
LA POLOGNE
Varsovie
LA BELGIQUE
Bruxelles
L'ALLEMAGNE f
Kiev
L'OCÉAN m ATLANTIQUE
Paris
Luxembourg
Prague
LA RÉPUBLIQUE TCHÈQUE
L'UKRAINE f
LE LUXEMBOURG
LA SLOVAQUIE
LE LIECHTENSTEIN
Vienne
Bratislava
LA MOLDAVIE
Berne
Budapest
LA FRANCE
Lausanne
LA SUISSE
L'AUTRICHE f
Chisinau
Genève
LA HONGRIE
LA SLOVÉNIE
LA ROUMANIE
Ljubljana
Zagreb
le Val d'Aoste
LA CROATIE
Belgrade
Bucarest
LA BOSNIE-HERZÉGOVINE
LA SERBIE
LE PORTUGAL
Andorre-la-Vieille
Sarajevo
LA MER NOIRE
MONACO m
Madrid
L'ANDORRE f
L'ITALIE f
LE MONTÉNÉGRO
Lisbonne
Sofia
La Corse
LA BULGARIE
Ajaccio
Rome
Podgorica
Skopje
L'ESPAGNE f
LA MER ADRIATIQUE
Tirana
LA MACÉDOINE
Istanbul
L'ALBANIE f
LA GRÈCE
LA TURQUIE
LA MER MÉDITERRANÉE
LA MER EGÉE
Athènes
L'AFRIQUE f
LE MAROC
L'ALGÉRIE f
LA TUNISIE
La Crète

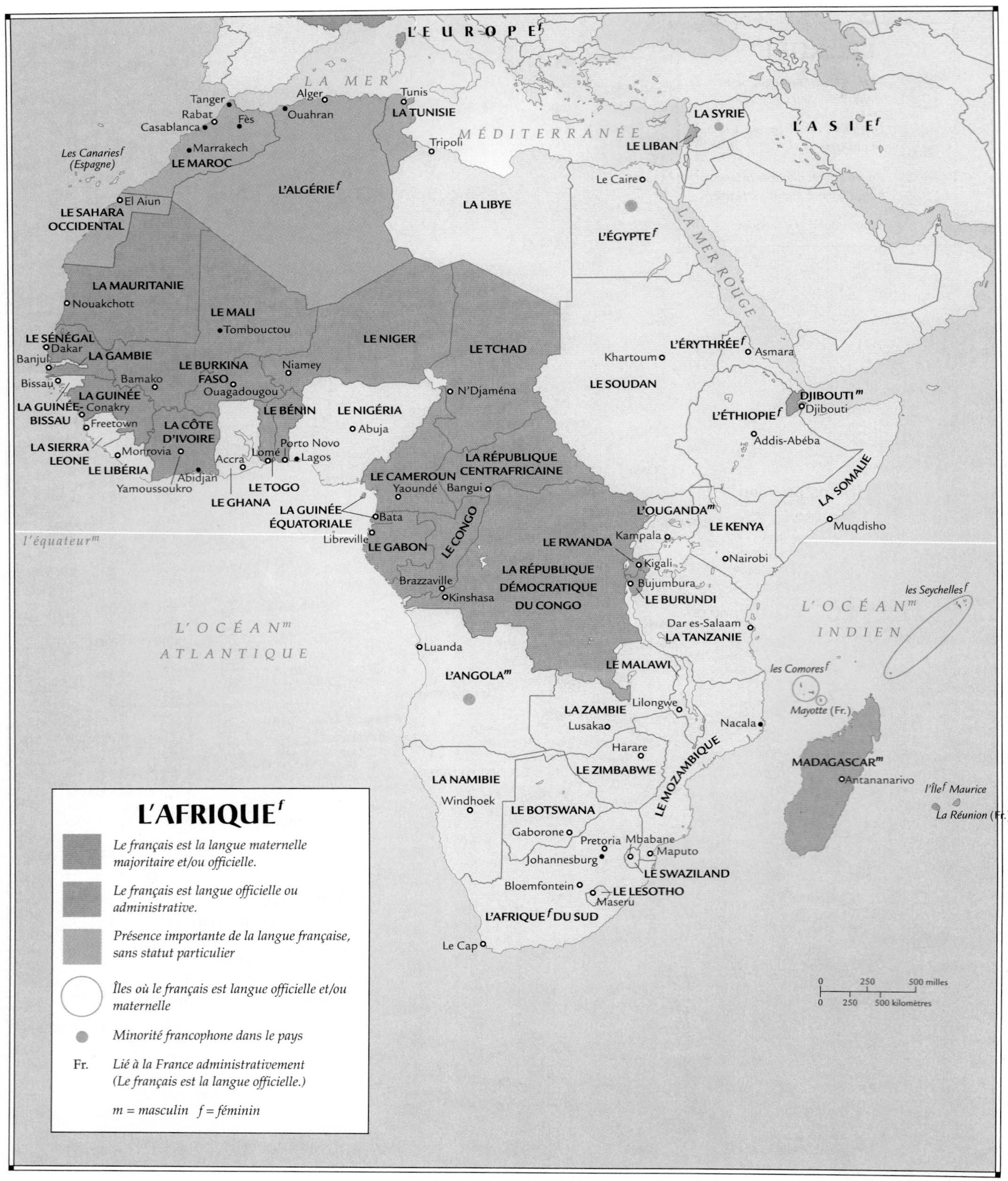
L'AFRIQUE[f]
Le français est la langue maternelle majoritaire et/ou officielle.
Le français est langue officielle ou administrative.
Présence importante de la langue française, sans statut particulier
Îles où le français est langue officielle et/ou maternelle
Minorité francophone dans le pays
Fr. Lié à la France administrativement (Le français est la langue officielle.)
m = masculin f = féminin
L'EUROPE[f]
L'ASIE[f]
LA MER MÉDITERRANÉE
LA MER ROUGE
L'OCÉAN[m] ATLANTIQUE
L'OCÉAN[m] INDIEN
l'équateur[m]
LE MAROC
L'ALGÉRIE[f]
LA TUNISIE
LA LIBYE
L'ÉGYPTE[f]
LA SYRIE
LE LIBAN
LE SAHARA OCCIDENTAL
LA MAURITANIE
LE MALI
LE NIGER
LE TCHAD
LE SOUDAN
L'ÉRYTHRÉE[f]
DJIBOUTI[m]
L'ÉTHIOPIE[f]
LA SOMALIE
LE SÉNÉGAL
LA GAMBIE
LA GUINÉE-BISSAU
LA GUINÉE
LA SIERRA LEONE
LE LIBÉRIA
LA CÔTE D'IVOIRE
LE BURKINA FASO
LE GHANA
LE TOGO
LE BÉNIN
LE NIGÉRIA
LE CAMEROUN
LA RÉPUBLIQUE CENTRAFRICAINE
LA GUINÉE ÉQUATORIALE
LE GABON
LE CONGO
LA RÉPUBLIQUE DÉMOCRATIQUE DU CONGO
L'OUGANDA[m]
LE KENYA
LE RWANDA
LE BURUNDI
LA TANZANIE
L'ANGOLA[m]
LA ZAMBIE
LE MALAWI
LE MOZAMBIQUE
LE ZIMBABWE
LA NAMIBIE
LE BOTSWANA
LE SWAZILAND
LE LESOTHO
L'AFRIQUE[f] DU SUD
MADAGASCAR[m]
Les Canaries[f] (Espagne)
les Comores[f]
Mayotte (Fr.)
les Seychelles[f]
l'Île[f] Maurice
La Réunion (Fr.)
Tanger
Rabat
Casablanca
Fès
Marrakech
Alger
Ouahran
Tunis
Tripoli
Le Caire
El Aiun
Nouakchott
Tombouctou
Dakar
Banjul
Bissau
Bamako
Conakry
Freetown
Monrovia
Yamoussoukro
Abidjan
Accra
Lomé
Porto Novo
Lagos
Ouagadougou
Niamey
Abuja
N'Djaména
Yaoundé
Bangui
Bata
Libreville
Brazzaville
Kinshasa
Luanda
Khartoum
Asmara
Djibouti
Addis-Abéba
Muqdisho
Kampala
Nairobi
Kigali
Bujumbura
Dar es-Salaam
Lilongwe
Lusaka
Harare
Nacala
Antananarivo
Windhoek
Gaborone
Pretoria
Johannesburg
Mbabane
Maputo
Bloemfontein
Maseru
Le Cap
0 250 500 milles
0 250 500 kilomètres

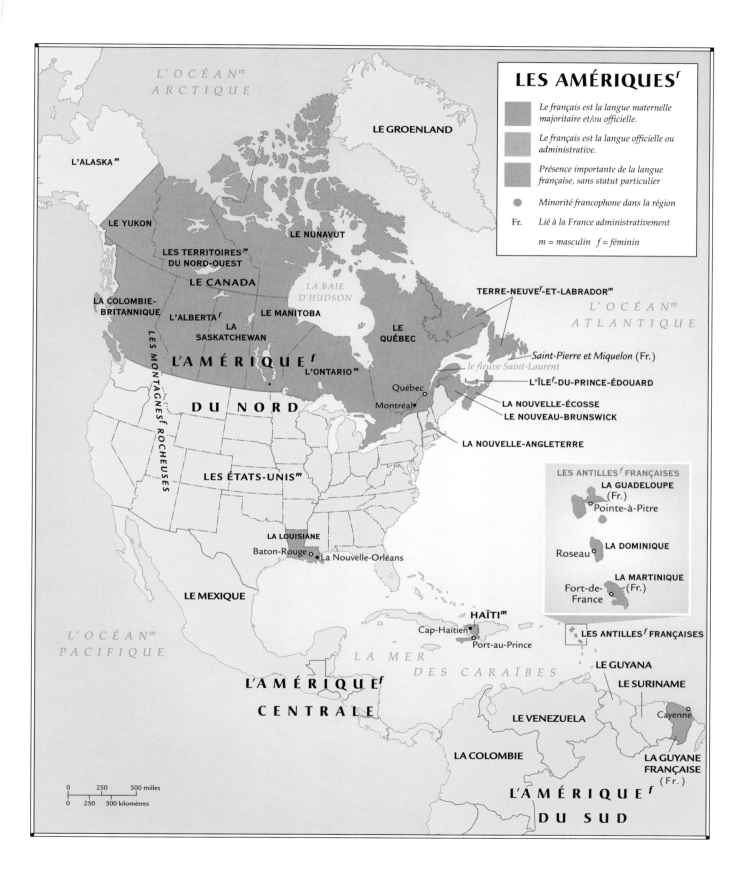
LES AMÉRIQUES[f]
Le français est la langue maternelle majoritaire et/ou officielle.
Le français est la langue officielle ou administrative.
Présence importante de la langue française, sans statut particulier
Minorité francophone dans la région
Fr. Lié à la France administrativement
m = masculin f = féminin
L'OCÉAN[m] ARCTIQUE
LE GROENLAND
L'ALASKA[m]
LE YUKON
LE NUNAVUT
LES TERRITOIRES[m] DU NORD-OUEST
LE CANADA
LA BAIE D'HUDSON
LA COLOMBIE-BRITANNIQUE
L'ALBERTA[f]
LA SASKATCHEWAN
LE MANITOBA
LE QUÉBEC
TERRE-NEUVE[f]-ET-LABRADOR[m]
L'OCÉAN[m] ATLANTIQUE
Saint-Pierre et Miquelon (Fr.)
le fleuve Saint-Laurent
L'AMÉRIQUE[f] DU NORD
L'ONTARIO[m]
LES MONTAGNES[f] ROCHEUSES
Québec
Montréal
L'ÎLE[f]-DU-PRINCE-ÉDOUARD
LA NOUVELLE-ÉCOSSE
LE NOUVEAU-BRUNSWICK
LA NOUVELLE-ANGLETERRE
LES ÉTATS-UNIS[m]
LES ANTILLES[f] FRANÇAISES
LA GUADELOUPE (Fr.)
Pointe-à-Pitre
LA DOMINIQUE
Roseau
LA MARTINIQUE (Fr.)
Fort-de-France
LA LOUISIANE
Baton-Rouge
La Nouvelle-Orléans
LE MEXIQUE
HAÏTI[m]
Cap-Haïtien
Port-au-Prince
LES ANTILLES[f] FRANÇAISES
L'OCÉAN[m] PACIFIQUE
LA MER DES CARAÏBES
LE GUYANA
LE SURINAME
L'AMÉRIQUE[f] CENTRALE
LE VENEZUELA
Cayenne
LA COLOMBIE
LA GUYANE FRANÇAISE (Fr.)
L'AMÉRIQUE[f] DU SUD
0 250 500 milles
0 250 500 kilomètres

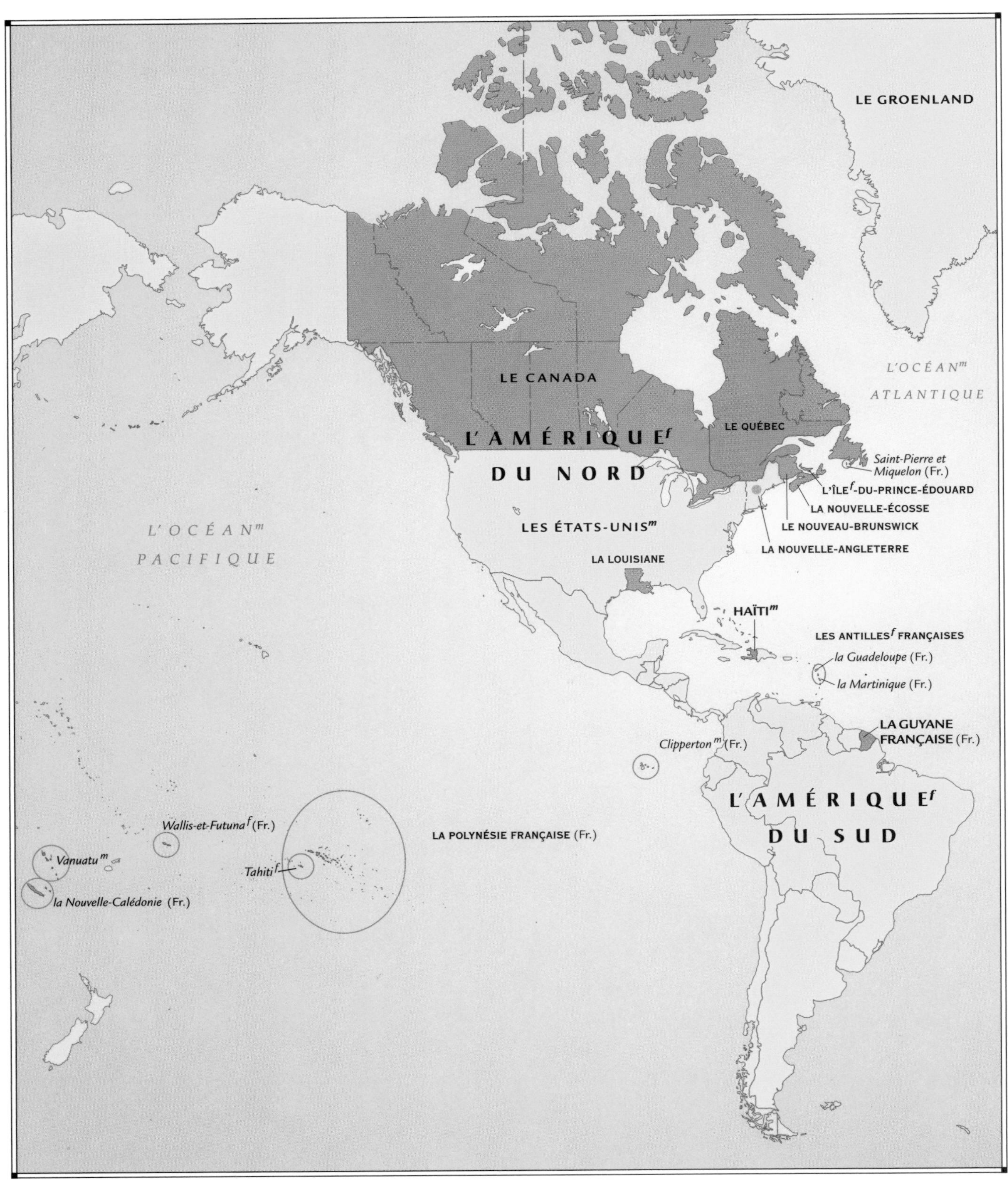
LE GROENLAND
L'OCÉANm
ATLANTIQUE
LE CANADA
LE QUÉBEC
L'AMÉRIQUEf
DU NORD
Saint-Pierre et
Miquelon (Fr.)
L'ÎLEf-DU-PRINCE-ÉDOUARD
LA NOUVELLE-ÉCOSSE
LE NOUVEAU-BRUNSWICK
LA NOUVELLE-ANGLETERRE
L'OCÉANm
PACIFIQUE
LES ÉTATS-UNISm
LA LOUISIANE
HAÏTIm
LES ANTILLESf FRANÇAISES
la Guadeloupe (Fr.)
la Martinique (Fr.)
LA GUYANE
FRANÇAISE (Fr.)
Clippertonm (Fr.)
L'AMÉRIQUEf
DU SUD
Wallis-et-Futunaf (Fr.)
LA POLYNÉSIE FRANÇAISE (Fr.)
Vanuatum
Tahitif
la Nouvelle-Calédonie (Fr.)